FAMILY
HEALTH GUIDE
AND
MEDICAL
ENCYCLOPEDIA

Reader's Digest

FAMILY HEALTH GUIDE

and

MEDICAL ENCYCLO-PEDIA

Based on the medical writings of
BENJAMIN F. MILLER, M.D.

The Reader's Digest Association, Inc.
Pleasantville, New York   Montreal

Family Health Guide and Medical Encyclopedia (Revised Edition)

Editor: James A. Maxwell
Art Director: Paul Jensen
Senior Editor: Walter Fox
Associate Editor: Inge N. Dobelis
Assistant Artist: Elizabeth Barth
Research Editor: Peter Ferrara
Editorial Assistant: Brenda Nicholls

Acknowledgments

The editors of Reader's Digest are deeply grateful to the physicians, dentists, and health organizations that assisted in the preparation of this work.

Chief Consultant
EZRA LAMDIN, M.D.
Former Director, Division of Scientific Affairs, American Heart Association

Stewart Cooper, M.D.
Royal Victoria Hospital and McGill University, Montreal
Edward Alfred Davies, M.D.
Director of Pediatrics, Lenox Hill Hospital, New York, New York
Hilliard Dubrow, M.D., F.A.C.S.
Associate Professor of Obstetrics and Gynecology, Cornell Medical College, New York, New York
Henry J. Heimlich, M.D.
Director of Surgery, The Jewish Hospital, Cincinnati, Ohio
Leonard Jackson, M.D.
Grace Dart Hospital, Montreal
Harold I. Kaplan, M.D.
Professor of Psychiatry, New York Medical College, New York, New York
Harold F. Klein, D.M.D.
Louisville, Kentucky
Henry Rosenberg, M.D.
University of Pennsylvania School of Medicine, Philadelphia, Pennsylvania

American Cancer Society, Inc.
American Diabetes Association, Inc.
American Heart Association, Inc.
American Leprosy Missions, Inc.
American Lung Association
American Social Health Association
Arthritis Foundation
Asthma and Allergy Foundation of America
Center for Disease Control (U.S. Public Health Service)
Cooley's Anemia Foundation, Inc.
Dairy Council of Metropolitan New York
Epilepsy Foundation of America
Kidney Foundation of New York
Muscular Dystrophy Association, Inc.
National Center for Health Statistics (Division of Vital Statistics)
National Council on Alcohol
National Institute for Occupational Safety and Health (NIOSH)
National Multiple Sclerosis Society
The Nutrition Foundation, Inc.
Parkinson's Disease Foundation
Planned Parenthood Federation of America, Inc.
The Sickle Cell Disease Foundation of Greater New York
United Cerebral Palsy Association
The Visiting Nurse Service of New York

Contents

Part 1

FAMILY HEALTH GUIDE

A Guide to Good Health

When you buy an automobile, a refrigerator, or any other piece of intricate equipment, you undoubtedly receive and follow instructions telling you how to maintain your purchase. This chapter also deals with maintenance—maintenance of that most precious, complex, and varied mechanism, the human body. The effects of fresh air, cleanliness, sleep, posture, exercise, smoking, and alcohol are among the topics covered here. The food you eat also belongs in this category, but because the subject is so large, all of Chapter 2 is devoted to it.

CLEANLINESS

As you read this section, keep in mind that every human being is unique. Most doctors agree that what is best for one patient may not necessarily be ideal for all. And what is customary for one may seem strange to another. For example, the average American takes more baths than his European counterpart. This is not because Americans are inherently cleaner than other peoples, but because most United States citizens have more efficient, modern plumbing and an ample water supply. Also, they live in a culture that equates cleanliness with virtue. While daily bathing is a fine idea in hot weather, two or three baths a week are enough for a person who is not physically active. Your personal situation and your personal preference should, of course, determine your bathing habits.

THE AIR YOU BREATHE

"Fresh air" is a frequently misunderstood term. Unless a room is completely sealed up, enough air comes in around doors and windows to provide oxygen for breathing. Whether more air should be circulated through the room will depend upon one's own comfort and desires.

A few generations ago, air in itself was considered dangerous. Doctors blamed drafts for any number of illnesses, a belief still held by many people. Night air, which was supposed to carry disease-laden vapors—called miasmas—was viewed as especially hazardous. As a result, many

of our ancestors accustomed themselves to wearing several layers of underclothing in all seasons and to sleeping with their windows tightly closed. Babies were wrapped up like mummies.

With discoveries such as the fact that malaria was caused by mosquitoes and not by night air, the pendulum began to swing in the opposite direction. Practically every family now had its fresh-air fiend who went around flinging windows wide open, to the discomfort of everyone else. Determined to give their children all the benefits of the newly discovered "fresh air," ultramodern parents would force the tots to stay outdoors regardless of the temperature. A not too active child would often suffer frostbitten fingers and toes. In winter, bedrooms of both young and old were like refrigerators.

There is no evidence to prove that one practice is significantly more healthful than another. Each person needs to find the condition to which his body responds best.

Room Temperature

There is, of course, a problem when it comes to getting along with people whose standard of comfort differs from your own. The average person seems to do well with a room temperature that ranges between 68° and 74°F. As an energy conservation measure, it has been suggested that thermostats be set at 68°F. If you like to be warmer or colder than your associates, try to take care of this by the clothing you wear. Happily, the recent fashion trend of several layers of clothing and the emphasis upon casual, easy to

The air we breathe

Air, the mixture of gases called the atmosphere, extends as a thin blanket over the surface of the earth. Oxygen makes up about a fifth of the atmosphere and it is essential for the respiration of all living things—a man dies if deprived of oxygen for more than a few minutes. In industrial and heavy traffic areas, the air may become polluted and contain substances which can be harmful if breathed in.

Exosphere, the outermost layer of the atmosphere, contains hardly any gas molecules and stretches away from the earth into the near vacuum of space

Ionosphere, extending from 50 to 300 miles above the ground, contains electrically charged gas atoms which can act as a "mirror" for radio waves bouncing off the bottom of the layer. Temperature gradually rises with altitude, reaching 1832°F (1000°C) at the top of the ionosphere

Stratosphere is a 40-mile thick layer of thin air ending 50 miles above the ground. At its center is a band of air at about freezing point containing ozone, which acts as a filter to block most of the ultraviolet rays from the sun

Troposphere, the layer of air 10 miles thick above the ground, holds all the clouds and weather. In this layer, air pressure falls from about 14½ lb. per sq. in. at sea level to only 1½ lb. per sq. in. 10 miles up, where the temperature is −67°F (−55°C). Men need breathing apparatus at altitudes over 25,000 ft (about 5 miles up)

care for garments make it a simple matter to choose a wardrobe for style as well as comfort. Garments should be loose enough not to restrict the body and to permit the absorption or evaporation of perspiration.

Heating Appliances

Most of us enjoy the benefits of central heating. But extremely cold weather or simply the pleasure of looking at an open fire causes many people to employ additional sources of heat. Under certain circumstances, this can be dangerous.

Coal, wood, or gas burned in fireplaces or stoves produces fumes containing carbon monoxide, a colorless, odorless but highly poisonous gas. When such heating methods are used, make certain that air is entering the room. If the doors and windows fit so snugly that you do not feel any air coming in when you place your hand near the sills, be sure to open a window slightly. Always be careful to protect a gas flame from drafts that might blow it out and cause unburned gas to pour into the room. This has been the source of many serious accidents. While their operation may be more costly, electric heaters and stoves provide clean heat and do not produce fumes.

Air Conditioning

Air conditioning has become so common that few of us could avoid it even if we wanted to. Certainly it is a great aid to comfort. Your air conditioner should have a thermostat so that the temperature of each room can be adjusted to individual comfort and health requirements. But it is important that the body be allowed to make an adjustment to varying climatic conditions, a necessity for maintaining a healthy, sturdy constitution. For instance, going from an air-conditioned apartment to an air-conditioned car to an air-conditioned office and then back home again at the end of the day deprives the system of this opportunity. Walking and other open-air exercises in all seasons put your body through this adjustment cycle.

On the other hand, air conditioning can be a real lifesaver. Hot, humid weather places added strain on the circulatory system. Persons suffering from some types of heart disease may find this added strain intolerable. Under such circumstances, living in an air-conditioned environment during the summer months may be prescribed by your physician.

Composition of air

Nitrogen	78.1 percent
Oxygen	20.9 percent
Argon	0.93 percent
Carbon dioxide and other gases	0.07 percent

Pure dry air contains about 78 percent nitrogen—a colorless, odorless gas which takes no part in respiration—and about 21 percent oxygen. The remaining 1 percent is mainly argon, with traces of other inert gases such as helium, neon, krypton, and xenon. There is also at least 0.03 percent of carbon dioxide, although the concentration of this gas may be higher in some places. But the air most people have to breathe is not completely pure: it contains water vapor, dust, pollen, and germs. Near towns, cities, and highways, it may also contain poisonous gases such as nitrogen dioxide and sulfur dioxide, as well as lead compounds and other pollutants. Most of these substances get into the air from the burning of coal, oil, and gasoline, and if the air does not rise because it is colder than the air above it, the concentration of these pollutants presents a hazard, especially to people with disorders of the heart and lungs. The human body has defense mechanisms against many of them but, if they fail, inhaling dust and poisonous gases may aggravate or cause lung disorders, pollen can give rise to allergies such as hay fever, and germs which penetrate the body's defenses can enter the lungs and cause disease.

Humidity and Comfort

Humidity—the moisture content of the air—is also a factor influencing health. Again, this is a matter of individual preference. Some people feel well in cold-weather climates where the indoor air is extremely dry. For other people this dry atmosphere causes irritation of the nose and throat. For the latter group, room or heating-system humidifiers that put moisture into the air may be of enormous help.

Some people welcome summer when the air is warm and moist. Others are so oppressed by excessive humidity that they need a fan or an air conditioner. Because perspiration evaporates more readily in dry air, thus cooling the body, most people mind the heat less when it is not combined with dampness.

A number of room dehumidifiers have come on the market recently. Consult a reliable consumer-rating service before buying one.

HOBBIES

Hobbies not only provide relaxation, they also help maintain the zest for living that doctors have come to realize is immensely important to your health.

Ideally, each of us should have indoor and outdoor hobbies that provide genuine satisfaction. A hobby need not be expensive. Indeed, some of them—such as gardening, furniture refinishing, sewing, or embroidering—can more than pay for themselves. You don't have to stick with a particular hobby forever; many people change their hobbies every year or so.

Adult education is becoming more and more popular as a part-time activity. The motives for enrollment range from completing degree requirements to acquiring new knowledge or skill for its own sake, to developing a hobby. Newspapers and magazines are full of advertisements and notices for adult education courses in colleges and universities everywhere. Your local public school board may also offer adult courses at night. The Adult Education Association of the U.S.A., 810 18th Street NW, Washington, D.C. 20006, will tell you about the opportunities in your area.

Just be certain that the activity is something you want to do, that it provides enjoyment and relaxation, and is, in the end, worth doing. A mere time-filler soon becomes boring.

Finally, do not wait until you are retired before beginning to cultivate a hobby or interests. How you develop your activities as a young person and continue them into middle age will largely determine how enjoyably you will spend your later years.

REST AND SLEEP

The amount of sleep necessary for good health varies tremendously from person to person. Eight hours each night appear to be average, but the real test is how you feel. If you are truly rested in the morning and have sufficient energy to carry on the day's activities, your sleeping pattern is providing all you need. If not, chronic fatigue may accumulate and contribute to what can become a serious illness.

Some men and women find that they can get along on fewer than eight hours of sleep a night as they grow older. But if you are concerned that you are really not getting enough sleep, discuss it with your doctor. It is altogether possible that you are getting less sleep because you need less. (Inability to sleep is discussed under INSOMNIA in the encyclopedia section; see also SLEEP.)

As important as the need for a good night's sleep is the need for rest during the day. Business

13

Stages of sleep

There are four main stages of sleep; the first two correspond to light or paradoxical sleep, and stages three and four occur during deep or orthodox sleep. Regular swings from light to deep sleep occur during the night. These different sleep stages are probably brought about by chemical processes in the brain, which first suppress the activity of the brain center controlling wakefulness, and then induce sleep. Each type of sleep shows changes in the pattern of brain waves, which can be recorded by an electroencephalograph (EEG) machine. In orthodox sleep, for example, the brain produces large, slow waves. At this point muscles are relaxed, breathing is even, and temperature and blood pressure are low. During paradoxical sleep brain activity speeds up. There are rapid eye movements, which give this type of sleep its other name—REM sleep. At the same time body muscles move, although neck muscles are slack. Pulse and blood pressure become irregular, and dreaming occurs during REM sleep. As the hours pass, the periods of REM sleep increase, and dreams become longer and more bizarre.

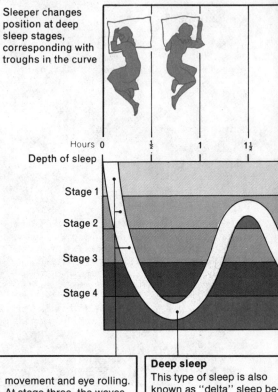

Sleeper changes position at deep sleep stages, corresponding with troughs in the curve

Falling asleep

When the eyes are shut before sleep, brain waves registered by the EEG trace show the pattern of relaxation (below left). These waves become small and irregular as the sleeper drifts into a state of drowsiness, or stage one sleep (center). The descent into stage two sleep is marked by body movement and eye rolling. At stage three, the waves become slower (below right). Stage four sleep, the deepest kind, produces a craggy outline.

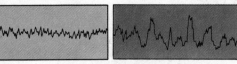

Deep sleep

This type of sleep is also known as "delta" sleep because of the large, slow waves recorded by the EEG (below right). During deep sleep the muscles are relaxed, breathing is even, and body temperature and blood pressure are down. At this time the sleeper is most likely to change position, as

men, professional people, executives, and many others who not only work hard but are also under heavy stress could live more comfortably and probably longer if they managed to get some rest during the day. Even a brief period of relaxation would be healthful. A simple measure such as having lunch in a quiet restaurant instead of a noisy one can provide this change of pace. When the weather is pleasant it would be beneficial to bring lunch from home, take a leisurely stroll, and eat in a park.

Franklin D. Roosevelt and Winston Churchill amazed their colleagues by being able to take five-minute naps during the day, almost at will. These short periods of total relaxation renewed their energy, as charging does a battery's.

Many people find it refreshing to rest at home for half an hour when they return from work instead of rushing directly to the dinner table. Most men and women are more tired than hungry at the end of a day. Delaying the evening meal to allow time for unwinding will greatly lessen the possibility of irritability that is simply the result of tension. It will make the dinner hour a more pleasant time for the family to be together and share the day's experiences.

The relaxation that comes from engaging in pleasant recreation at least once a week is necessary to most people. And more and more, it is being recognized that a yearly vacation helps to safeguard good health and improve the on-the-job performance.

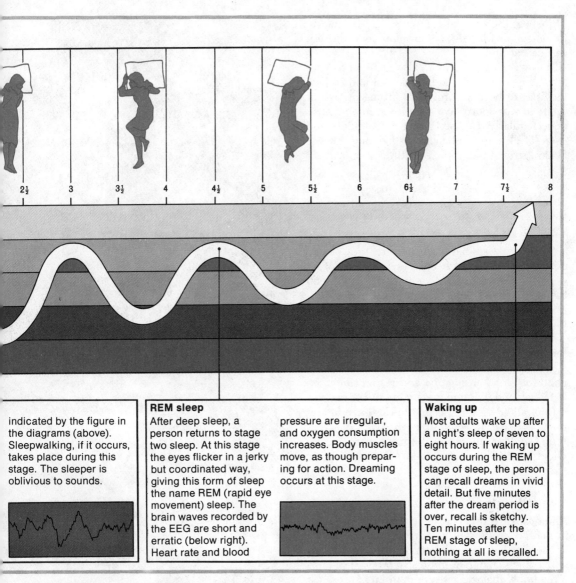

| | 2½ | 3 | 3½ | 4 | 4½ | 5 | 5½ | 6 | 6½ | 7 | 7½ | 8 |

indicated by the figure in the diagrams (above). Sleepwalking, if it occurs, takes place during this stage. The sleeper is oblivious to sounds.

REM sleep
After deep sleep, a person returns to stage two sleep. At this stage the eyes flicker in a jerky but coordinated way, giving this form of sleep the name REM (rapid eye movement) sleep. The brain waves recorded by the EEG are short and erratic (below right). Heart rate and blood pressure are irregular, and oxygen consumption increases. Body muscles move, as though preparing for action. Dreaming occurs at this stage.

Waking up
Most adults wake up after a night's sleep of seven to eight hours. If waking up occurs during the REM stage of sleep, the person can recall dreams in vivid detail. But five minutes after the dream period is over, recall is sketchy. Ten minutes after the REM stage of sleep, nothing at all is recalled.

EXERCISE AND SPORTS

In the matter of exercise, perhaps more than in any other subject taken up in this chapter, the factors of individual likes and dislikes and bodily reactions are tremendously important. If you are thinking of trying something new, such as handball or tennis, talk it over with your doctor, particularly if you are entering the middle or later years of life. Some people can safely engage in very strenuous sports and exercises, even until they are very old. Others need to start limiting such activity relatively early in life. On the basis of this knowledge about your own medical condition and the history of illness and longevity in your ancestors, your doctor can advise you. (See Chapter 9 for the importance of periodic medical checkups.)

Choice of Sports and Athletics

The fun and competition of an athletic game stimulate interest so that you enjoy your exercise. But many young people, especially young men, become proficient in sports that cannot be carried into later life. Some of these, such as boxing, carry the continual threat of body injury. Highly competitive sports, such as football, baseball, basketball, and soccer, do not serve a useful purpose in the individual health program in later life. Either they are too strenuous, or they require more participants than can be conveniently assembled by a busy adult with a job and family.

Moreover, the stress of competition, particularly to someone with a risk of coronary heart disease, can be harmful.

It is wise for the athletically inclined to take advantage of their local high school and college facilities to become proficient in one or two of the following sports. We have listed some that, if done regularly, can be carried into middle and even late life to the benefit of body and muscle health, strength and good posture:

Swimming	Hiking
Golf	Badminton
Tennis	Squash
Dancing	Horseback Riding
Canoeing	

These are desirable sports because they can be done alone or require only one or two other persons, need not be competitive, and lend themselves to weekend relaxation. Married couples can enjoy them together, later participating in them with their children.

"Ballroom" dancing—including square and folk dancing—is excellent exercise for persons of all ages. It gives the muscles a workout and is good for blood circulation and respiration.

Hiking and swimming are good sports for persons of all ages. Many communities have indoor pools, so that it is possible to swim the year round. Indoor, all-weather tennis courts are also widely available. None of these sports needs to be overly expensive.

The Exercise Routine

Americans are always ready to try the newest fad in matters relating to health. Almost as popular as the diet fads (see Chapter 2) are some recent odd notions about exercise. Rigorous programs often imply that exercise is a punishment for past excesses, that once the offending bulge has been smoothed or the desired size reached, the effort should cease.

Exercising (like eating sensibly) should never be a crash program, but rather a lifetime involvement. Nor should it be a kind of penance, something you feel you *must* do. Therefore, you should find the regimen that can be a source of enjoyment to you. If you enjoy listening to music, exercise along with your favorite performers. If you don't like working out in a gym by yourself, join a group, or form one of your own by getting together with a few friends who also prefer companionship. Regular exercise not only promotes muscle tone, it eases tensions that build up daily. A workout is the simplest way to combat lower-

Daily exercise

The best kinds of routine exercises are activities such as walking, cycling, and swimming. Many people get enough exercise in their ordinary daily routine, but some prefer to do a "daily dozen"— an organized program of exercises designed to tone up individual groups of muscles. These should be chosen with care and, especially in someone past middle age, only after seeking a

Knee raising

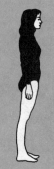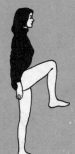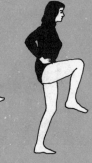

1 Stand straight-backed, with your feet together and your hands at your sides.

2 Raise your right knee as high as possible; repeat with the left leg. Raise each leg 5-10 times.

3 For variation, try the same exercise with your hands on your hips.

Leg raising sideways

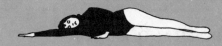

1 Lie on your side, with your legs straight and the lower arm stretched under your head and along the floor.

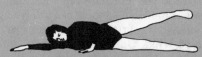

2 Raise your leg about 18 inches and lower it slowly. Repeat 5-10 times; then repeat the exercise with other leg.

doctor's advice. For example, if you are not used to regular physical activity, bending down to touch your toes with your legs straight can cause more back trouble than it cures. The exercises described here can be done by men or women. If you want to try them, begin with easy exercises and do each one only a few times. Do not avoid the early exercises because they are easy. They are designed not to tax your strength: their purpose is to strengthen the muscles gradually so that you can work up to the more demanding exercises and perform them without unnecessary strain. Special exercises for women after pregnancy are given on pp. 176 and 177.

Bending sideways

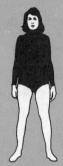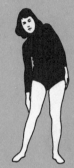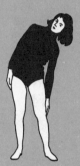

1 Stand upright with your feet slightly apart and your hands at your sides.

2 Bend sideways from the waist, pushing your hand as far down your leg as you can.

3 Repeat on the other side; do not bend forward. Bend 5-10 times to each side.

Arm circling

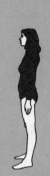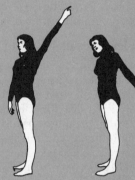

1 Stand upright with your feet apart and your hands at your sides.

2 Swing your left arm forward in a large circle 5-10 times; repeat with your right arm.

3 Repeat, but circling your arms backward. Do 5-10 circles with each arm.

Head and shoulders raising

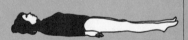

1 Lie on your back, with your legs straight and toes pointed, arms at your sides.

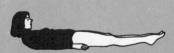

2 Raise your head and shoulders off the floor and lower them again. Repeat 6-12 times.

Leg raising in front

1 Lie on your back, with your legs and arms straight, and hands flat on the floor.

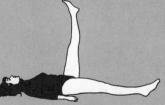

2 Raise your left leg until it is upright and lower it slowly 4-8 times; then repeat with right leg.

Press-ups

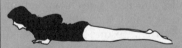

1 Lie face downward, with legs straight and toes pointed, and hands under your shoulders.

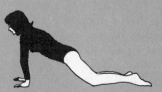

2 Push your body off the floor, but not your knees and shins. Repeat 5-10 times.

back syndrome and sagging abdomen, two of the most common afflictions resulting from our sedentary way of life.

Daily exercise, plus a sensible diet, is the answer to the question, "What do I do about my growing waistline?", which is asked by most men over 35. Such a program will also counteract middle-aged spread, the combination of fat and poor muscle tone around thighs and buttocks that afflicts many women in their forties and fifties.

Your local Y.M./Y.W.C.A. or Y.M./Y.W.H.A. will be able to provide you with a variety of exercises that are simple, effective, and approved by medical authorities. Or follow the simple exercise program illustrated in this chapter.

The Pleasures of Walking

If you do not care for sports or games and cannot bear to commit yourself to even five minutes of daily exercise, all is not lost. A brisk, regular walk will do a great deal for your muscle tone, circulation, and general health. Instead of driving all the way to work, you might park a mile or so from your office and take your walk at the beginning and end of your workday. If you must use the parking facilities at your place of work, park in the area of the lot that is farthest away from the entrance to the building. In short, create your own opportunities to walk. This is only a modest amount of exercise, but it will give you a chance to relax a little before and after the pressures of the day.

YOUR POSTURE

Good posture is an expression of good health rather than a major factor in producing it. As a rule, a healthy person will automatically find a position that is comfortable and attractive.

Certain posture rules are worth putting into practice every day. At work, at school, or at home, your chair should feel comfortable and should give sufficient support so that your back rests against the chair's back. The chair should be strong and solid enough to take your weight comfortably and should not sag or rock when you sit in it. The choice of a well-designed chair is especially important if you sit for extended periods at your work—for example, as a typist or other office worker. Sit squarely, with both feet placed on the floor a short distance in front of your chair. Avoid such bad habits as wrapping one leg around the leg of the chair.

If you travel a great deal by car, you will find it helpful to pull the driver's seat as far forward

Avoiding back trouble

One of the penalties that mankind pays for having adopted an upright posture during the course of evolution, instead of going on all fours, is that human beings are prone to back trouble. The bones of the human spinal column are separated by disks of cartilage, which allow the spine to bend in any direction. But the more the spine bends, the greater is the strain put on the disks. If the spine is bent and, at the same time, compressed—as when someone stoops to lift a heavy weight—the disks may be squeezed and deformed so that they stick out. Protrusion of a disk causes trouble only if it presses on the spinal cord or on a nerve running from the cord. Back trouble can be prevented as long as the spine is kept as upright as possible in all lifting movements, since this avoids pressure on the disks and reduces the risk of protrusion.

Spine straight   Spine curved   Spine strained with disks pinched

Vertebrae and disks Between all but the uppermost pair of vertebrae, disks act as shock absorbers and allow bending of the spine. Each disk consists of a wide rim of cartilage with a pulpy center. Bending of the spine can nip the disk; extreme pressure can cause it to spread outwards, touch a nerve, and cause pain in an area of the body served by that nerve.

Reaching to the floor

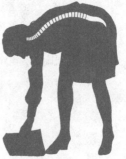

Wrong Legs straight, spine flexed

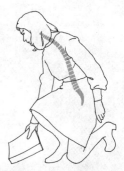

Right Knees bent, back hollow, minimum flexing

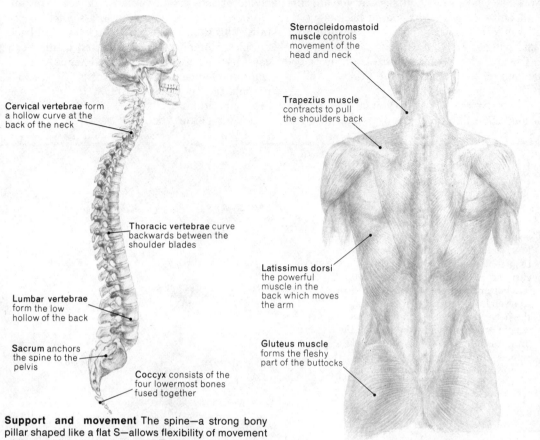

Sternocleidomastoid muscle controls movement of the head and neck

Cervical vertebrae form a hollow curve at the back of the neck

Trapezius muscle contracts to pull the shoulders back

Thoracic vertebrae curve backwards between the shoulder blades

Latissimus dorsi the powerful muscle in the back which moves the arm

Lumbar vertebrae form the low hollow of the back

Sacrum anchors the spine to the pelvis

Gluteus muscle forms the fleshy part of the buttocks

Coccyx consists of the four lowermost bones fused together

Support and movement The spine—a strong bony pillar shaped like a flat S—allows flexibility of movement while providing general support. There are 24 vertebrae in the main part of the spine; all are basically similar in structure, but they differ in size. The vertebrae, and the disks between them, are thickest where they have to bear the greatest weight, in the low, lumbar region.

Muscles of the back and spine Pairs of muscles arranged in a V-shape, upright or reversed, join the spine to control movement. The trapezius, for example, controls bracing of the shoulders.

Bending to the oven

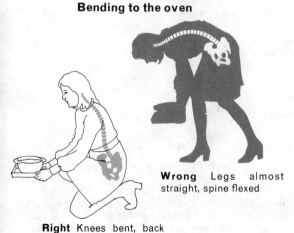

Wrong Legs almost straight, spine flexed

Right Knees bent, back retains its natural shape

Kneeling on the floor

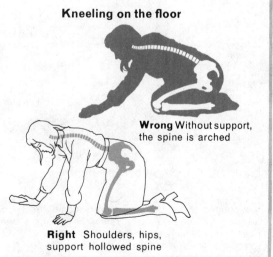

Wrong Without support, the spine is arched

Right Shoulders, hips, support hollowed spine

as possible when driving. In this way you are able to sit quite straight, with ample back support, and can press down on the accelerator rather than having to stretch the leg at an angle to reach it. This upright driving posture is the least demanding on the muscles of the back as well as on those of the leg.

If your work requires that you be on your feet for long hours at a time, it is important that you find a relaxed, attractive stance that feels restful. Do not try to stand as erect as a soldier on parade. This stance will strain the knees and back muscles. Slumping in a too-relaxed manner can cause backache as well as other ailments. An easy, comfortable manner, with buttocks "tucked in," permits the abdomen and chest to be in their proper positions.

If your posture does not satisfy you, try to

Lifting and carrying

Lifting not only involves muscles in the arms but also uses the back muscles, which contract and compress the joints in the spine. If these joints are already compressed by extreme bending at the hips, damage can result and cause pain by pressure on the spinal nerves. When carrying a weight, even a large handbag, it is better to support it above the hips; the weight is then transferred, through the pelvis, equally to both legs. If the weight is carried below the level of the hips, it is borne on one leg only, and the spine is curved sideways; again, backache can result from continually straining to keep the body upright.

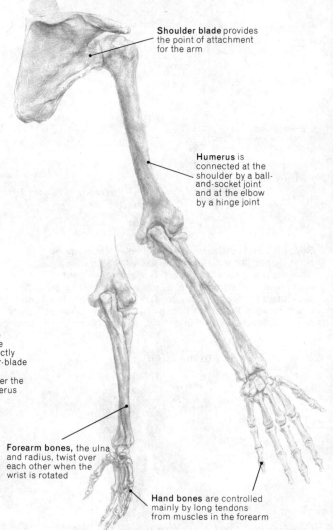

Shoulder blade provides the point of attachment for the arm

Humerus is connected at the shoulder by a ball-and-socket joint and at the elbow by a hinge joint

Forearm bones, the ulna and radius, twist over each other when the wrist is rotated

Hand bones are controlled mainly by long tendons from muscles in the forearm

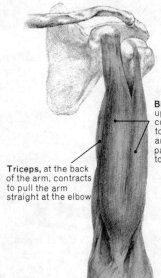

Biceps has two upper ends, one connected directly to the shoulder-blade and the other passing to it over the top of the humerus

Triceps, at the back of the arm, contracts to pull the arm straight at the elbow

Muscles in the upper arm Contraction of the biceps and brachialis muscles raises the forearm. The triceps, which continues over the elbow, straightens the arm and allows the forearm to be moved across the body.

Rotation of the wrist The lower end of the radius bone in the arm rotates round the ulna, carrying with it the carpal bones of the wrist. Movement is limited by a triangular ligament joining the forearm bones. Overstretching the ligaments causes a sprained wrist.

improve it with exercise. If, after several months, you are still troubled by problems with your posture, see your doctor for a checkup and get his advice.

Posture During and After Pregnancy

Because of the pull on the muscles of the back and the abdomen during pregnancy, many women lose their good posture and figure during pregnancy and never regain them. Prenatal exercises are designed to help a woman maintain good posture and keep fit while she is pregnant. In addition, if there is undue strain on her abdominal and back muscles, her doctor may prescribe a maternity corset.

After the baby is born, the mother should carry through the series of exercises presented in Chapter 14. These will help bring back the strength of

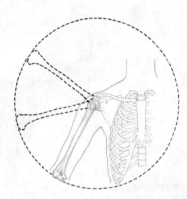

A circle of movement A ball-and-socket joint allows the head of the humerus to rotate in the shoulder blade so that the arm can be held in any position.

Lifting from the floor

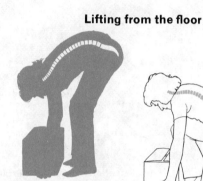

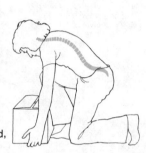

Wrong Arms outstretched, spine bent almost double

Right Arms, knees, and hips bent reduce spine curvature

Carrying on the hip

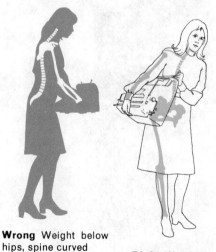

Wrong Weight below hips, spine curved

Right Weight on hips transferred to both legs

Carrying on the arm

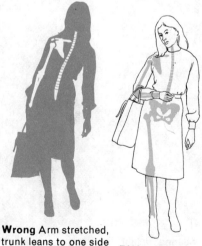

Wrong Arm stretched, trunk leans to one side

Right Weight above hips, trunk upright

Standing and pushing

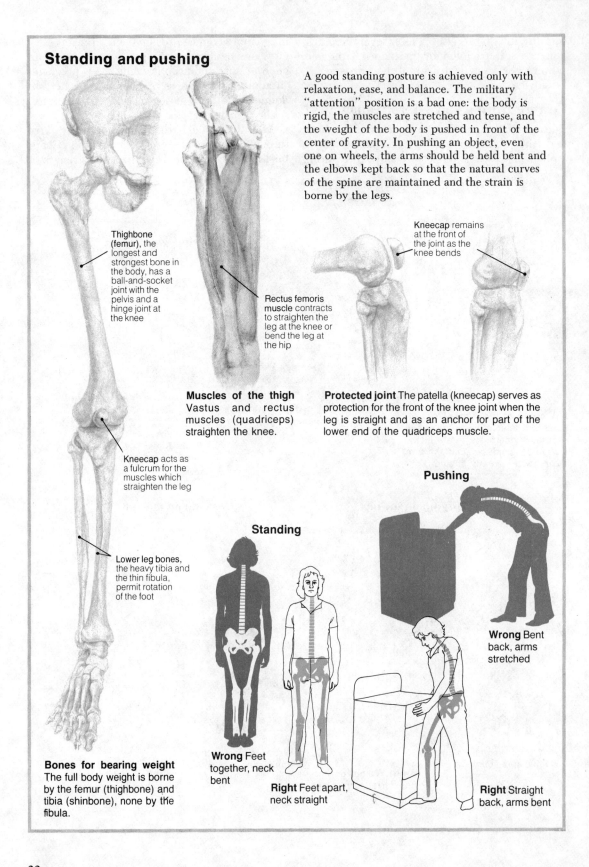

A good standing posture is achieved only with relaxation, ease, and balance. The military "attention" position is a bad one: the body is rigid, the muscles are stretched and tense, and the weight of the body is pushed in front of the center of gravity. In pushing an object, even one on wheels, the arms should be held bent and the elbows kept back so that the natural curves of the spine are maintained and the strain is borne by the legs.

Thighbone (femur), the longest and strongest bone in the body, has a ball-and-socket joint with the pelvis and a hinge joint at the knee

Rectus femoris muscle contracts to straighten the leg at the knee or bend the leg at the hip

Kneecap remains at the front of the joint as the knee bends

Muscles of the thigh Vastus and rectus muscles (quadriceps) straighten the knee.

Protected joint The patella (kneecap) serves as protection for the front of the knee joint when the leg is straight and as an anchor for part of the lower end of the quadriceps muscle.

Kneecap acts as a fulcrum for the muscles which straighten the leg

Pushing

Standing

Lower leg bones, the heavy tibia and the thin fibula, permit rotation of the foot

Wrong Bent back, arms stretched

Bones for bearing weight The full body weight is borne by the femur (thighbone) and tibia (shinbone), none by the fibula.

Wrong Feet together, neck bent

Right Feet apart, neck straight

Right Straight back, arms bent

22

the abdominal muscles. Many women have borne half a dozen children and have retained youthful, trim figures.

Posture for Children

Problems of posture in children are discussed in Chapter 16.

DRINKING AND SMOKING

Before we take up these subjects individually, we wish to remind you that we are discussing them as they relate to general body care. Smoking and drinking were once considered matters of morals and one's own conscience. If you believe this, you should consult your spiritual adviser. We are limiting ourselves here to telling you what medical science has discovered to date about the effect of certain substances upon your body.

Alcohol

Although generally considered a stimulant, alcohol is actually a depressant. It *seems* to lessen fatigue and make you energetic; it takes the brakes off certain processes. Even a small amount of alcohol lessens the inhibitions that normally govern our behavior. This makes us feel relieved and free.

Alcohol can be harmful in certain diseases. People who consider a drink of whiskey as the initial step in all first-aid treatment can, therefore, do a great deal of damage. For example, alcohol is definitely harmful in cases of heatstroke and snakebite. If you or anyone in your family is ill, be sure to discuss the matter of alcohol with your doctor before giving it to the patient.

Alcohol for the Normal, Healthy Individual

There is no firm evidence that moderate drinking will cause disease, injure the health, or shorten the life of the normal adult. What do we mean by moderate drinking? There are no specific limits, because the amount that different people can tolerate varies considerably. Most doctors would describe the moderate drinker as one who takes one or two drinks a day—a couple of highballs each containing two ounces of whiskey, or a quart of beer during the course of several hours. To the moderate drinker alcoholic beverages are taken for relaxation, never as a constant necessity. The moderate drinker does not become intoxicated. Yet even under these relaxed, pleasurable circumstances there may be some impairment of judgment or coordination. There are people who ought not to drive a car after sipping even a small glass of sherry.

Excessive Drinking

By excessive drinking we mean drinking to the point where it interferes with one's job, one's family life, and one's relationship to society. Some degree of intoxication is the inevitable result of drinking alcohol. That is its pharmacological action. And most people are able to determine for themselves just how much is enough. However, alcohol affects judgment just when discretion is most needed—when one has already had a few drinks. Charts showing the relationship between the number of drinks, the time between them, and the person's weight are available from the National Council on Alcoholism to help you determine what the limit on your drinking should be. If there is no affiliate in your community, write to the Council at 733 Third Avenue, New York, N.Y. 10017.

Intoxication can be simply unpleasant in a social gathering. Excessive drinkers are almost inevitably bores; with their judgment and perception gone awry, they have not much sense of what they are saying or how often they may have already said it. But this phenomenon is minor compared to the danger that exists when an intoxicated person has to assume responsibilities he is incapable of fulfilling, such as driving a car.

Excessive drinkers create other problems for themselves. They often fail to eat properly and otherwise neglect the rules of good health, thereby suffering a number of illnesses as an indirect consequence of their drinking. Recently it has been shown that cancer of the mouth can be associated with heavy drinking. (See ALCOHOLISM in the encyclopedia section.)

The Chronic Alcoholic

There are some people to whom drinking too much comes easily. They depend on alcohol as a drug. It is now thought that there may be a genetic predisposition to alcoholism. The individual who has evidence of alcoholism in his or her family would do well to be cautious about drinking. Once alcoholism has become established it is extremely difficult to overcome without help. It leads to permanent damage throughout the body and especially to the liver. The brain is affected as well. One should be on guard if he begins to use alcohol for any purpose but the social pleasures with which it is most commonly associated.

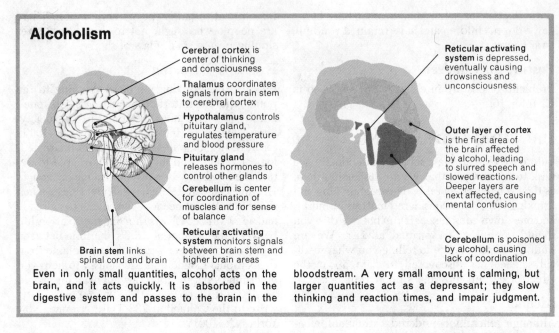

Alcoholism

Cerebral cortex is center of thinking and consciousness

Thalamus coordinates signals from brain stem to cerebral cortex

Hypothalamus controls pituitary gland, regulates temperature and blood pressure

Pituitary gland releases hormones to control other glands

Cerebellum is center for coordination of muscles and for sense of balance

Reticular activating system monitors signals between brain stem and higher brain areas

Brain stem links spinal cord and brain

Reticular activating system is depressed, eventually causing drowsiness and unconsciousness

Outer layer of cortex is the first area of the brain affected by alcohol, leading to slurred speech and slowed reactions. Deeper layers are next affected, causing mental confusion

Cerebellum is poisoned by alcohol, causing lack of coordination

Even in only small quantities, alcohol acts on the brain, and it acts quickly. It is absorbed in the digestive system and passes to the brain in the bloodstream. A very small amount is calming, but larger quantities act as a depressant; they slow thinking and reaction times, and impair judgment.

Chronic Alcoholism—a disease. Every responsible medical organization has defined alcoholism as a disease. If you have a question relating to the use of alcohol by yourself or someone close to you, remember that it is a serious *medical* problem. Avoiding action may result in many social problems and, possibly, further sickness, even death. A physician will treat this problem sympathetically, but professionally. Alcoholism cannot be "handled" solely by a loving family, an attentive spouse, or helpful neighbors. It is a disease. The afflicted person needs experienced care.

You may wish to consult Alcoholics Anonymous (AA) or an affiliate of the National Council on Alcoholism in your community. These organizations can direct you to treatment facilities in your area and send you other helpful information about available assistance.

TOBACCO

We now know enough about the relation between smoking and several serious diseases to say, "Tobacco is bad for you." The advice of many physicians to patients is simply: If you don't smoke, don't start. If you do smoke, stop. If you can't stop, then at least cut down. (The dangers and diseases associated with smoking are discussed in the entry on SMOKING in the encyclopedia section.)

It would be simple to order everyone to stop smoking—but not very realistic. Although it is the single biggest environmental cause of cancer in men and women, smoking is a habit that is extremely difficult to break.

How to Stop Smoking

There are about 40 million *ex*-smokers in the United States, some of whom once smoked as many as four packs of cigarettes a day and now do not smoke at all. Here are some suggestions as to how to rid yourself of this harmful habit:

1. Write down your reasons for wanting to stop smoking and make a list of your reasons for continuing to smoke.
2. Change to a low-tar/low-nicotine brand.
3. Select a date to quit. Give yourself plenty of time—five or six weeks if you feel you need it.
4. Chart your smoking habits for two weeks. The simplest way is to wrap a piece of paper around your pack of cigarettes and mark it whenever you take a cigarette. Make a special note of the cigarettes that are most important to you (those immediately after meals, for example), the ones that are least important (perhaps those smoked while driving to work), and the one that tastes especially good to you (the first of the day, for instance).
5. Each night repeat at least 10 times one of your reasons for not smoking.
6. Eliminate at least one cigarette from your routine—the one you found you desired least (or most).
7. Quit on the day you selected—and keep very busy. Go to movies; take long walks; exercise.

Give yourself plenty of substitutes for smoking: water, gum, raisins, carrots, celery. Start a new activity if you need to, such as needlepoint, whittling—something to involve your attention and your hands.

Do not be discouraged. If you don't make it the first time, try again. Many ex-smokers quit many times before finally succeeding.

It is possible that you will gain weight when you stop smoking. Don't worry about it. When your body has adjusted to its new, healthful way of life you will be able to get down to the proper size and shape.

The American Cancer Society has some very helpful materials on the benefits of giving up smoking. They will even provide you with instructions on conducting a smoke-withdrawal program in your community. (Many people find it helpful to be part of a group.) If there is no branch in your area, write to American Cancer Society, 777 Third Avenue, New York, N.Y. 10017.

COFFEE AND TEA

Both coffee and tea contain caffeine, a stimulating compound. In moderate amounts these beverages are not harmful. The use of more than three or four cups of coffee or tea per day may, however, lead to restlessness, overactivity, nervousness, insomnia, and excessive urination. Each person needs to find the correct amount for his particular system and life-style. Some people can drink coffee or tea shortly before going to bed without affecting their sleep; others find that the caffeine in these beverages keeps them awake for hours.

Coffee and tea should not be given to children. Even when so much water is added that there is practically no caffeine present in a cup of these beverages, they should not be substituted for nutritious drinks such as milk and fruit juices, which growing children and adolescents need even more than adults. (The caffeine in cocoa is negligible.)

COLA DRINKS

The average cola drink contains the same amount of caffeine as a cup of coffee. If you use these drinks, set a daily quota for yourself that will keep you from suffering any of the symptoms caused by too much caffeine. With children exercise the same restraint with these drinks as you do with coffee and tea.

HOW MUCH WATER SHOULD YOU DRINK?

The amount of water you drink each day is usually correctly adjusted by your sense of thirst. The body loses about a quart of water daily in the form of perspiration on the skin and as water vapor expired into the air from the lungs. This loss of water plus the quart or more contained in the daily urine must be supplied chiefly by:

1. Water in solid foods. For example, vegetables and fruits are high in water content.
2. Water in fluids such as milk, soups, and beverages.
3. Water taken as such. This will balance any difference between the above intake and the output.

In hot weather, or when you work in a hot area, your body requires more water to compensate for the loss through sweating. Heavy perspiration may result in the loss of many quarts of water a day. After strenuous physical activity, it is important to replace this water.

MEDICINES, DRUGS, AND NARCOTICS

Since the 1950's a revolution has taken place in the field of medicine. As a result, the public can now be protected against or cured of many ailments that, in the past, had been disabling or fatal, or had required tedious weeks for recovery. But there have been bad side effects accompanying a number of the new cures. A new category of illnesses has arisen, caused by the administration of medicines and drugs.

More than ever before, it is of vital importance that you use only those medicines your doctor recommends for you and use them exactly as he directs. Your doctor is aware of the dangerous side effects of many medicines. The practices of using an old medication to treat apparently similar symptoms occurring months or years later, or of taking a medicine prescribed for a friend who had the same complaint are worse than foolish. They are extremely dangerous.

Pregnant women should be particularly careful to avoid all medicines except those ordered by their own physician. A seemingly innocent preparation may harm the woman or the fetus. No more shocking example of this can be given than that which occurred when thalidomide was introduced. Created as a sedative and sleep inducer, it was sold without prescription in several foreign countries. Its hideous side effects soon became apparent. Infants whose mothers had used the drug were born with deformed or rudimentary arms, sometimes little more than flippers. Thousands of such deformed babies were born in Germany, England, France, Belgium, Australia, and Canada. Women and children in the United States were spared this nightmare only through the caution exercised by Dr. Frances O. Kelsey, a medical officer of the U.S. Food and Drug Administration. Because she believed it had not been properly tested, she refused to license thalidomide for sale in this country, and brought about the withdrawal of the drug for experimental use.

From the 1950's to the early 1970's, many doctors prescribed DES, or diethylstilbestrol, for pregnant women in danger of having a miscarriage. Studies now show that the daughter of a woman who took DES may have a predisposition to vaginal cancer, or may have trouble carrying a child. A woman who knows or suspects that she was exposed to DES should tell her gynecologist who will probably suggest more frequent checkups.

Such seemingly harmless standbys of the family medicine cabinet as aspirin and bicarbonate of soda should not be taken indiscriminately either. Aspirin, for example, has been known to cause bleeding in peptic ulcers. Excessively high doses of certain vitamins, especially A and D, have been known to be harmful. This is not to say that one should be fearful of all medicines. We only want to emphasize the warning that they should not be taken without your doctor's advice. Pain, indigestion, and other symptoms are indications that something is wrong within the body—that the system is out of balance. If any symptom is severe or persists, consult your doctor to find what the trouble is and correct it. Do not obscure symptoms by self-medication. Let your doctor prescribe for you.

Sleeping pills should be taken only upon a doctor's prescription. In many states they cannot be obtained without one. This is a wise provision, for they can be extremely hazardous to health.

Amphetamines to pep you up or stifle the appetite can also be very harmful. Most doctors no longer prescribe them.

Painkillers such as codeine (related to morphine and opium) are habit-forming. Only a physician knows when more powerful narcotics such as morphine and codeine should be administered to relieve intolerable pain. Otherwise, even the most high-minded individual runs a very grave risk of becoming addicted, with resulting deterioration of body and mind. (See also the entry on DRUG ADDICTION in the encyclopedia section.)

If you feel a desire to use these drugs, or if you do use them or have used them in the past, you should discuss the matter very frankly with your doctor. He will pass no moral judgment on you, but will advise you how to prevent or to overcome the habit before it is too late.

"ONLY ONE TO A CUSTOMER"

Your body is the one machine that is unconditionally guaranteed to last a lifetime. How long and how good a lifetime this will be depends on you—on whether you neglect or abuse your body out of carelessness or ignorance, or treat it with the respect that such a wonderful and complicated organism deserves.

Eating Wisely and Controlling Your Weight

CHAPTER 2

It's an old saw but a true one: You are—more or less—what you eat. Medical science finds more and more evidence of a basic relationship between the kinds of food people consistently eat and the state of their health. Overweight and underweight are the most obvious results of a faulty diet. But food is also implicated in the cause of other, less obvious problems. Heart disease and diabetes are prime examples; anemia is less life-threatening but affects more people than do the other two disorders. This chapter deals with the basic facts about nutrition. By knowing them, you will find it is easy to choose the foods that not only satisfy appetite and taste, but also provide the essentials for good health.

BALANCED NUTRITION

The quality of your diet helps to determine from day to day whether you have a high level of energy, whether your hair and skin are healthy, and whether your teeth and bones are strong. Even though you may never have experienced prolonged hunger, the foods you habitually choose may provide such a poorly balanced diet that you are in a state of chronic and dangerous undernourishment.

The elements of good nutrition are easy to find in the foods we eat every day; the problem is to obtain them in sufficient quantities and in the right combinations. While we all know the advertised value of apples in keeping the doctor away, no reasonable person expects to live on apples alone—or on whole wheat, or hamburgers, or packaged "high protein" breakfast substitutes. Instead, the sensible person tries to attain a balance and is aware of the necessity of combining foods from the four main food categories: the milk group, the meat group, vegetables and fruits, and breads and cereals.

The milk group consists of milk and everything made from it, such as cheese, ice cream, and yogurt. The meat group also includes fish, poultry, and eggs, as well as dried beans, peas, and nuts as alternates. Fruits comprise citrus fruits, apples, peaches, and berries among others. Vege-

The four basic food groups

Milk Group: whole, skim, evaporated, instant, non-fat, dry, or buttermilk
Daily requirements: Adults: 2 cups
Children: 3-4 cups
Alternatives: 1 oz American cheese = ¾ cup milk
½ cup cottage cheese = ⅓ cup milk

Meat Group: beef, veal, lamb, pork, fish, eggs, dry beans, dry peas, and nuts
Daily requirements: 2 or more servings (1 serving = 2-3 oz cooked lean meat, fish, or poultry).
Alternatives: 2 eggs (unless there are cholesterol restrictions), or one cup cooked dried beans, or 4 tbsp peanut butter.

Vegetable-Fruit Group: spinach, carrots, broccoli, sweet potatoes, cabbage, turnip greens, kale, oranges, grapefruit, apricots.
Daily requirements: 4 or more servings (1 serving = ½ cup vegetables or fruits). Include a dark, leafy green or deep yellow vegetable for vitamin A every other day and 2 or 3 daily servings of other vegetables including potatoes.

Bread-Cereal Group: whole grain, dark and rye breads; rice, noodles, or cornmeal.
Daily requirements: 4 or more servings (1 serving = 1 slice of bread, or 1 oz cereal, or ⅓ to ½ cup cooked cereal, noodles, rice, etc.).

tables include such foods as yellow squash, carrots, turnips, and green spinach. Breads and cereals, ideally made from whole grains, include noodles and rice. The chart on page 27 shows the quantities from each food group that will insure a generally well-balanced diet.

What is Food Made of?

Foods are composed of the same chemicals that make up our bodies. But when we talk about diet, we classify foods according to the kinds of nutrients they provide that are essential to our

Nutrients in common foods

The table below gives the percentages of the U.S. Recommended Daily Allowances for eight essential nutrients yielded by measured amounts of various foods. For one week keep a list of what you eat each day. Compare the size of your portions with those in the table, and work out the total

Percentage of U.S. Recommended Daily Allowance

—equals less than 2 percent

	Amount	Weight in grams	Calories	Protein	Vitamin A	Vitamin C	Thiamine (B₁)	Riboflavin (B₂)	Niacin (B₃)	Calcium	Iron
MILK GROUP											
Butter or fortified margarine	1 tbsp	14	100	—	10	—	—	—	—	—	—
Cheese, Amer., Swiss, pasteurized	1 oz	28	105	15	6	—	—	7	—	22	2
Cheese, cottage, regular, creamed	1 cup	245	260	70	8	—	4	35	—	25	4
Ice cream, regular, all flavors	1 cup	133	260	15	10	2	4	15	—	20	—
Milk, skim	1 cup	245	90	20	—	4	6	25	—	30	—
Milk, whole	1 cup	244	160	20	6	4	4	25	—	30	—
Yogurt, plain, low fat	1 cup	245	120	20	4	4	6	25	—	30	—
MEAT GROUP											
Bacon, crisp (20 strips per lb)	2 strips	15	90	10	—	—	6	2	4	—	2
Beans, Gt. Northern, dried, cooked	1 cup	180	210	30	—	—	15	8	6	8	25
Beef, ground, regular, broiled	3 oz	85	270	50	—	—	4	10	25	—	15
Beef rump, roasted, lean only	3 oz	85	180	60	—	—	4	10	20	—	15
Chicken, broiled, no skin	3 oz	85	120	45	2	—	2	10	40	—	8
Cod, broiled with butter	3 oz	85	140	60	4	—	4	6	15	2	4
Egg, raw, boiled or poached	1 large	50	80	15	10	—	2	8	—	2	6
Flounder, baked with butter	3 oz	85	170	60	—	4	4	4	10	2	6
Frankfurter, heated, (8 per lb)	1 frank	56	170	15	—	—	6	6	6	—	4
Ham, cured, baked, lean only	3 oz	85	160	50	—	—	35	10	20	—	15
Lamb, leg, roast, lean only	3 oz	85	160	60	—	—	10	15	25	2	10
Lentils, dry, cooked	1 cup	200	210	35	—	—	10	8	6	4	25
Liver, beef, fried	3 oz	85	200	50	910	40	15	210	70	—	40
Peanuts, roasted, salted	1 cup	144	840	80	—	—	30	10	120	10	15
Peanut butter	1 tbsp	16	90	8	—	—	2	2	10	—	2
Peas, split, dry, cooked	1 cup	200	230	35	2	—	20	10	8	2	20
Pork loin, roasted, lean only	3 oz	85	220	60	—	—	60	15	30	2	20
Pork sausage, link	2 links	27	130	10	—	—	15	6	4	—	4
Salmon, pink, canned, with bones	3 oz	85	100	30	—	—	2	8	30	15	4
Sardines, canned in oil, drained	3 oz	85	170	45	4	—	2	10	25	35	15
Shrimp, fresh, fried	3 oz	85	190	40	—	—	2	4	10	6	10
Soybeans, dry, cooked	1 cup	180	230	45	2	—	25	10	6	15	25
Sunflower seeds, dry, hulled	1 cup	145	810	80	2	—	190	20	40	15	60
Tuna, canned in water, drained	3 oz	85	110	50	—	—	—	6	60	—	8
Veal cutlet, braised or broiled	3 oz	85	180	50	—	—	4	10	25	—	15
VEGETABLE-FRUIT GROUP											
Apple, raw, with skin	1 med	150	80	—	2	10	2	2	—	—	2
Apricots, canned in syrup	1 cup	258	220	2	90	15	4	2	4	2	4
Asparagus, cooked	4 spears	60	10	2	10	25	6	6	4	2	2
Avocado	1/2 med	180	200	4	8	35	10	20	10	2	4
Banana (8-3/4 in. long)	1 fruit	175	100	2	4	20	4	4	4	—	4
Beans, baby lima, frozen, cooked	1 cup	180	210	20	8	35	10	6	10	6	25
Beans, green, fresh, cooked	1 cup	125	30	4	15	25	6	6	4	6	4
Beans, yellow or wax, fresh, cooked	1 cup	125	30	2	6	25	6	6	4	6	4
Beet greens, cooked, drained	1 cup	145	25	4	150	35	6	15	2	15	15
Beets, canned, whole, drained	1 cup	160	60	2	—	8	2	2	—	2	6

bodies' growth and health. These nutrients comprise *proteins, carbohydrates, fats, minerals,* and *vitamins.*

Proteins. These are the basic substance of our bodies, the stuff out of which every cell is built.

When eaten in foods, proteins also provide energy. Foods vary in the amount and quality of the protein they contain. Top-quality protein, with the essential amino acids, is of animal origin: meat, fish, eggs, milk. But dried beans, peas, and nuts rank almost as high. Breads, cereals, and some

daily percentage of the U.S. RDA for each nutrient supplied by your fare. Most people do not need 100 percent of each of these nutrients, but if your

score is markedly low in any area, you should consider modifying your diet. See also page 42.

	Amount	Weight in grams	Calories	Protein	Vitamin A	Vitamin C	Thiamine (B₁)	Riboflavin (B₂)	Niacin (B₃)	Calcium	Iron
Broccoli, cooked	1 stalk	180	45	8	90	270	10	20	6	15	8
Brussels sprouts, cooked	1 cup	155	60	10	15	230	8	15	6	4	10
Cabbage, cooked, drained	1 cup	145	30	2	4	80	4	4	2	6	2
Cabbage, raw, finely shredded	1 cup	90	22	2	2	70	2	2	2	4	2
Cantaloupe, ripe	1/2 med	477	80	2	180	150	8	4	8	4	6
Carrots, cooked, sliced	1 cup	155	50	2	330	15	6	4	4	6	4
Cauliflower, buds, cooked	1 cup	125	30	4	2	120	8	6	4	2	4
Cherries, raw, sweet, pitted	1 cup	145	100	2	4	25	4	6	4	4	4
Collards, cooked, drained	1 cup	190	60	10	300	240	15	20	10	35	8
Corn, ear 5 in. long	1 ear	140	70	4	6	10	6	4	6	—	2
Dandelion greens, cooked, drained	1 cup	105	35	4	250	30	10	10	—	15	10
Eggplant, diced, cooked	1 cup	200	40	4	—	10	6	4	4	2	6
Grapefruit, raw, white	1/2 med	241	45	—	—	70	4	2	—	2	2
Grapefruit juice, canned, unsweetened	1 cup	247	100	2	—	140	4	2	2	2	6
Grapes, raw, with skin	1 cup	153	70	2	2	6	4	2	2	2	2
Lettuce, iceberg, chopped or shredded	1 cup	55	8	—	4	4	2	2	—	2	2
Mushrooms, canned, solids and liquid	1 cup	244	40	8	—	6	2	35	25	2	6
Onions, mature, cooked, drained	1 cup	210	60	4	2	25	4	4	2	4	4
Orange juice, from frozen concentrate	1 cup	249	120	2	10	200	15	2	4	2	2
Orange, raw, 2-5/8 in. diam	1 fruit	180	60	2	6	110	8	2	2	6	2
Peach, raw, yellow flesh, 2-1/2 in. diam	1 fruit	115	40	—	25	10	2	2	4	—	2
Pear, raw, with skin	1 med	180	100	2	—	10	2	4	—	2	2
Peas, green, canned, drained	1 cup	170	150	10	25	25	10	6	6	4	20
Peppers, sweet, green, cooked, sliced	1 cup	135	25	2	10	220	6	6	4	2	4
Pineapple, canned, chunks and syrup	1 cup	255	190	2	2	30	15	2	2	2	4
Potato, sweet, baked in skin	1 med	146	160	4	180	40	6	4	4	4	6
Potato, white, baked, with skin	1 med	202	150	6	—	50	10	4	15	2	6
Raisins, seedless, pressed down	1 cup	165	480	6	—	4	10	8	4	10	30
Spinach, cooked, drained	1 cup	180	40	8	290	80	8	15	4	15	20
Squash, winter varieties, mashed	1 cup	205	130	6	170	45	6	15	6	6	8
Strawberries, raw	1 cup	149	60	2	2	150	2	6	4	4	8
Tomato, raw, ripe, with skin, 7 oz	1 fruit	200	40	4	35	70	8	4	6	2	4
Tomatoes, canned, solids and liquid	1 cup	241	50	4	45	70	8	4	8	2	6
Turnip greens, cooked, drained	1 cup	145	30	4	180	170	15	20	4	25	8
Turnips, cooked, diced, drained	1 cup	155	35	2	—	60	4	4	2	6	4
BREAD-CEREAL GROUP											
Bread, French, enriched, 5 × 2-1/2 × 1 in.	1 slice	35	100	4	—	—	10	4	6	2	10
Bread, whole wheat, firm crumb	1 slice	25	60	4	—	—	4	2	4	2	4
Cereal flakes, average 59 varieties	1 oz	28	110	4	20	20	25	25	20	—	20
Corn grits, degermed, enriched	1 cup	245	130	4	240	—	6	4	4	—	4
Macaroni, spaghetti, enriched, cooked	1 cup	130	190	10	—	—	15	8	8	2	8
Noodles, egg, enriched	1 cup	160	200	10	2	—	15	8	10	2	8
Oatmeal, regular or quick cooking	1 cup	240	130	8	—	—	15	2	—	2	8
Rice, white, unenriched, cooked	1 cup	205	220	6	—	—	2	2	4	2	2

Percentage of U.S. Recommended Daily Allowance

vegetables also provide protein, but in smaller quantities.

Carbohydrates. More commonly known as starches and sugars, carbohydrates provide the body with energy and heat. Digestive juices convert these foods into glucose, the form of sugar found in the blood. Glucose is used by the body's cells as the fuel for all cellular activity. Carbohydrates also supply needed bulk or roughage in the form of cellulose, the fibrous material present in many vegetables.

Fats. Fats are a superconcentrated source of energy, giving more than twice as much as either carbohydrates or proteins. Many foods that contain fat also supply vitamins A, D, and E. Common sources of fats are butter, salad dressing and cooking oils, most cheeses, nuts, milk, fatty meats, and eggs.

Minerals. Minerals required by the body include calcium, iodine, and iron. Calcium is supplied by milk and milk products and is also present in certain vegetables such as turnips and mustard greens, cabbage, and watercress. Iodine is found in produce grown near the seacoast and in iodized salt. The chief source of iron is liver, but it is also available in enriched and whole-grain cereals, lean meats, shellfish, dried beans and peas, green vegetables, dried fruits, and egg yolk. Other essential minerals include magnesium,

phosphorus, sodium, and potassium—all of which are found in a variety of foods. Special sources for these are given on page 42.

Vitamins. Vitamins can be obtained from an assortment of common foods. There are a dozen vitamins that are essential to good health. A well-balanced diet should ideally supply all necessary vitamins, although many people take a daily multivitamin capsule as a supplement. (For further information about nutrients, see the entries CALCIUM; CARBOHYDRATE; FAT; IODINE; PROTEIN; VITAMIN in the encyclopedia section.)

CALORIES AND CHOLESTEROL

We hear a great deal about calories in food, especially in regard to diets that are designed to add or reduce weight. Calories are not nutrients but simply units of measurement that determine the energy value of food. (One calorie, where used as a dietary unit, is the amount of heat needed to raise the temperature of one kilogram of water one degree centigrade.) High-calorie foods are usually rich in fat or contain large amounts of carbohydrates or protein that have the same number of calories per gram.

Your body requires a certain number of calories in order to function efficiently. If your diet provides too few calories, your body will begin to consume its stored proteins and fats in order to supply the energy it needs. If you eat more calo-

Calories needed each day

The required daily intake of calories from food depends largely on such factors as age, sex, and physical activity (activity decreases in later life, and women are generally less active than men). The greater the activity, the greater the number of calories required to supply the energy expended. An elderly housewife may require only 1800 calories, whereas a middle-aged woman needs 2000; a girl student should have 2100 calories a day, but a man student of the same age needs as many as 2800; and a man who works in an office probably needs only 2700 calories each day, whereas a coal miner or a forestry worker doing heavy manual work needs 3100. An adolescent boy needs about 500 calories a day less than an equally active man, a pregnant woman needs an extra 300 calories, and a mother breast-feeding her baby needs 500 extra.

	Age	Calories per day	Range
Children	1-3	1300	900-1800
	4-6	1700	1300-2300
	7-10	2400	1650-3300
Males	11-14	2700	2000-3700
	15-18	2800	2100-3900
	19-22	2900	2500-3300
	23-50	2700	2300-3100
	51-75	2400	2000-2800
	76+	2050	1650-2450
Females	11-14	2200	1500-3000
	15-18	2100	1200-3000
	19-22	2100	1700-2500
	23-50	2000	1600-2400
	51-75	1800	1400-2200
	76+	1600	1200-2000
Pregnant		+300	
Lactating		+500	

During childhood there is little difference between the calorie requirement of boys and girls. After puberty, boys need a higher intake, and the difference continues throughout life.

ries than your system can use, however, your body will store the excess food as fat.

The amount of calories you need is determined by your body size and the kinds of daily activities in which you participate. A six-foot-tall, cross-country skier obviously needs more calories than a five-foot-tall chess player. Men generally need more calories than women. Active children and growing teenagers must have them in abundance. But a 65-year-old man usually needs fewer calories than he consumed when he was 45 years old.

If you feel that you are too heavy, or not heavy enough, you can adjust your caloric intake to compensate for the discrepancy. Check your weight against the weight chart shown on page 34; if there is a marked difference between your actual weight and the desirable weight given for a person of your height, age, and build, you should consider going on a diet.

Overweight Can Be Dangerous

By definition, an obese person weighs 30 percent or more over his ideal weight. Even if you are not that severely overweight, you should be alert to the potential problems too much poundage may cause. The obese person may suffer from one or more of the following nine disabilities: (1) an overworked heart and circulatory system; (2) shortness of breath; (3) a tendency to high blood pressure; (4) early symptoms of diabetes if he or she unknowingly has this disease; (5) poor adjustment to hot weather and changes of temperature;

(6) increased strain on joints and ligaments, often leading to chronic back and joint pains; (7) reduced capacity for physical activities; (8) greater susceptibility to infectious diseases; and (9) personality problems. In fact, medical evidence shows that overweight shortens the life span.

If you are overweight—and a medical checkup indicates no physiological cause—then you can assume that your excess weight is a result of an imbalance between the amount and kinds of food you eat and the amount of energy you expend in physical activity.

The Cholesterol Problem

Cholesterol, a fatty substance in the blood vessels, is either manufactured naturally by the body or is obtained from animal and other fats (called "saturated fats") in food. In excessive amounts, cholesterol can cause health problems. Americans, who generally eat a diet heavy in cholesterol-rich foods, have an alarmingly high rate of heart disease, which is the leading cause of death in the United States. The close relationship between cholesterol and heart disease, while it has not yet been absolutely proven, is accepted by almost all medical authorities. They believe that hardening of the arteries (arteriosclerosis) is probably linked to excess blood cholesterol, which forms deposits on the insides of blood vessels. As the deposits increase, the passageways of the circulatory system gradually narrow, until the flow of blood is obstructed. When the choles-

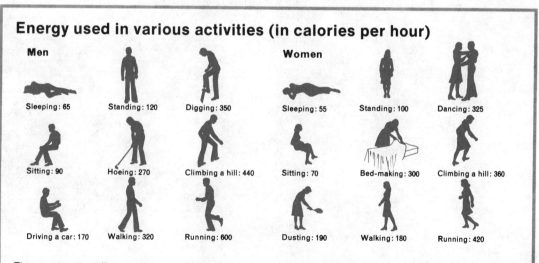

Energy used in various activities (in calories per hour)

Men

Sleeping: 65 Standing: 120 Digging: 350

Sitting: 90 Hoeing: 270 Climbing a hill: 440

Driving a car: 170 Walking: 320 Running: 600

Women

Sleeping: 55 Standing: 100 Dancing: 325

Sitting: 70 Bed-making: 300 Climbing a hill: 360

Dusting: 190 Walking: 180 Running: 420

The greater the effort, the more calories are consumed. Women do not use as much energy as men because they generally weigh less and usually have more body fat to retain heat; the difference in energy used applies to all activities—even sleeping, sitting, or standing still.

Calories in common foods

Carbohydrates, obtained from starchy food such as bread and potatoes, provide most of our energy. In Western countries they supply between 40 and 50 percent of the calories needed each day. Fats provide about 35–40 percent, and the remainder is supplied by proteins, from food such as meat, fish, and cheese, which build new body tissues. Fats are the most concentrated source of calories and can supply twice as much energy as can a similar weight of carbohydrates or proteins. As long as the correct balance of carbohydrates, fats, and proteins is maintained, the most important aspect of plan-

ning a daily intake of food is to ensure that it contains the right number of calories to meet your individual calorie requirement. This is determined by your age, sex, build, and occupation (see p. 30). Vitamins and minerals are also essential components in a well-balanced diet, and details of these are given on pp. 28–30 and 42, and in Part III. The calorie count of other important foods is given in the chart on pp. 28–29. The standard measures used in this calorie chart are: 1 cup = 8 fluid ounces, 1 fluid ounce = 2 tablespoons, and 3 teaspoons = 1 tablespoon.

Food	Portion	Calories
Applesauce, unsweetened	1 cup	100
Apricots, raw, with skin	3 med	60
Bagel, 3-in. diam	1 bagel	165
Beans, red kidney, canned	1 cup	230
Beef, dried, chipped, creamed	1 cup	380
Beef rib roast, lean and fat	3 oz	370
Beer	12 oz	150
Blueberries, raw	1 cup	90
Bluefish, broiled with butter	3 oz	140
Bologna	1 oz	80
Bread, rye, 18 slices per lb	1 slice	60
Bread, white, 18 slices per lb	1 slice	70
Brownie, with nuts	1 brownie	100
Cake, devil's food layer, av	1/16 of cake	290
Cake, pound, plain loaf	1 slice	150
Carrot, raw, 5-1/2 × 1 in.	1 carrot	20
Catsup	1 tbsp	16
Celery, wide stalk 8 in. long	1 stalk	8
Cheese, Cheddar, natural	1 oz	110
Cheese, cream	1 oz	110
Chicken, fried	1 drumstick	90
Chocolate candy, milk, plain	1 oz	150
Clams, raw	4–5 clams	60
Cod, broiled with butter	3 oz	140
Coffee, plain	1 cup	2
Cola beverage	1 cup	90
Coleslaw with mayonnaise	1 cup	170
Cookies, chocolate chip, av	1 cookie	50
Crackers, graham, 2-1/2 in. square	2 crackers	60
Crackers, saltine, packet	4 crackers	50
Cream, heavy, unwhipped	1 tbsp	60
Cream, imitation, powdered	1 tsp	10
Cream, imitation, whipped	1 tbsp	10
Cucumber, raw, sliced	1 cup	16
Custard, milk, baked	1 cup	310
Dates, pitted, chopped	1 cup	490
Doughnuts, cake type, med	1 cake	160
Figs, canned, with syrup	1 cup	220
French dressing	1 tbsp	70
Gelatin dessert, plain	1 cup	140
Ginger ale	1 cup	70
Haddock, fried	3 oz	140
Honey	1 tbsp	60
Jelly, jam, preserves	1 tbsp	60
Lamb chop, loin, lean and fat	3-1/2 oz	360

Food	Portion	Calories
Liquors, 80–90 proof	1 oz	70
Liverwurst (braunschweiger)	1 oz	90
Macaroni and cheese, homemade	1 cup	430
Mayonnaise	1 tbsp	100
Milk, canned, evaporated	1 cup	350
Milk, skim, dry, reconstituted	1 cup	80
Molasses, blackstrap	1 tbsp	45
Muffin, bran, 2-5/8-in. diam	1 muffin	100
Muffin, corn, 2-3/8-in. diam	1 muffin	130
Mushrooms, raw, sliced	1 cup	70
Oil, salad	1 tbsp	120
Oysters, raw, shelled	1 cup	160
Pancake, plain, 4-in. diam	1 cake	60
Pickle, dill, 3-3/4-in. long	1 pickle	8
Pie, apple, 2 crust, 9-in. diam	1/6 of pie	400
Pie, pecan, 9-in. diam	1/6 of pie	580
Pie, pumpkin, 9-in. diam	1/6 of pie	320
Pineapple, raw, diced	1 cup	80
Plum, raw, with skin	1 med	30
Popcorn, popped, plain	1 cup	25
Pork, butt, lean and fat	3 oz	300
Pork, spareribs, braised	3 oz	370
Potatoes, French-fried, frozen	10 pieces	110
Pudding, made with mix, milk	1 cup	320
Pudding, bread, with raisins	1 cup	500
Pudding, rice, with raisins	1 cup	390
Quinine water, sweetened	1 cup	70
Raspberries, red, raw	1 cup	70
Salami, dry, hard type	1 oz	130
Sauerkraut, with liquid	1 cup	40
Sherbet	1 cup	260
Soup, cream of mushroom	1 cup	220
Soup, onion	1 cup	70
Soybeans, sprouted seeds, raw	1 cup	50
Sugar, brown, packed	1 cup	820
Sugar, white, granulated	1 cup	770
Syrup, blend, chiefly corn	1 tbsp	60
Tea, plain	1 cup	4
Tomato juice, canned	1 cup	45
Tongue, beef, braised	3 oz	210
Turkey, light meat, no skin	3 oz	150
Watermelon, wedge 4 × 8 in.	1 piece	110
Welsh rarebit	1 cup	420
Wine, dessert	1 oz	40
Wine, table	1 oz	25

terol buildup occurs in an artery carrying blood to the heart, the end result is often a heart attack.

Your blood cholesterol level can be determined by a blood test. If it is too high, your doctor will prescribe a low-cholesterol diet. Because the diet of most Americans is far too rich in cholesterol-bearing foods, many nutritionists recommend that *all* of us restrict our intake of certain kinds of food. The principal dietary villains are fatty meats and shellfish, egg yolk, and any food containing the fatty components of milk—whole milk, butter, cream, whole-milk cheeses. Also implicated in cholesterol formation are the saturated fats: hydrogenated, solid vegetable shortening or margarine made from hydrogenated oils, and coconut oil.

A low-cholesterol diet emphasizes lean meats, poultry and fish, all skim-milk products, and foods prepared with "polyunsaturated" fats—oil made from corn, safflower seed, cottonseed, sesame seed, or sunflower seed.

Fortunately, those persons who follow a low-cholesterol diet accomplish more than just lowering the quantity of saturated fats they consume. Rich foods such as chocolate are eliminated because they contain these fats. Such sweet foods as cakes and ice cream are avoided because of their egg content. Therefore, the caloric total of a low-cholesterol diet is usually lower than that of an ordinary diet. This may result in a loss of excess weight and a lowering of the blood-sugar level that is important in reducing the risk of diabetes. A low-cholesterol diet may also lead to a decrease in hypertension, the high blood pressure many people have—often without knowing it—that is a major factor in causing strokes.

Fattening Foods

If you are concerned about excess weight and know that it is not caused by any functional disorder of your body, you can easily set up a regime of regular exercise combined with dieting that should result in a slow but steady weight loss. Before you plan your diet, you should know what types of food are high in calories and fattening, so that you can avoid them as much as possible.

Generally, all foods that are rich in fat are fattening. These include the following:
Butter, margarine, cream
Certain cheeses
Oils, salad dressings, mayonnaise
Foods fried in deep fat
Ice cream
Nuts

Chocolate
Fatty meats
Foods that are heavy in starch or sugar are equally fattening. The chief ones are:
Potatoes
Bread, crackers
Cookies, cakes, pastries, candy
Rice
Noodles, macaroni
Figs, dates, and other dried fruits
Canned fruits in sugar syrup
Carbonated drinks
Alcoholic drinks

On the opposite side of the caloric scale, there are many nourishing foods that will add minimal numbers of calories to your diet:
Eggs
Lean meats
Skim milk and all skim-milk products—cottage cheese, skim-milk yogurt
Fresh fruits
Vegetables

Remember that the way food is prepared may add calories to your diet. A boiled egg has about 77 calories; fried, it has 110. A half-cup of boiled potatoes equals 55 calories; a half-cup of potatoes when French fried has about 150 calories.

Although eggs are rich in cholesterol, or saturated fat, the usual low-calorie diet lays heavy stress on eggs because they are an excellent and inexpensive source of protein. Egg yolk contains saturated fat, however, and is generally omitted from or restricted in low-cholesterol diets; but egg *white* can be eaten without ill effects.

If you intend to go on a reducing diet but are concerned about cholesterol, you should check with your doctor first. This is especially recommended to young people or women of child-bearing age, because these two groups most need the kind of protein found in eggs and fatty meats. Your doctor will test your blood-cholesterol level and, if it is too high, will suggest modifications in your low-calorie diet.

Weight and Exercise

There are 150 calories in a glass of beer. If your body does not need the energy these calories provide, and if you don't want the beer to end up as fatty tissue, you will have to run for 15 minutes, swim for 22 minutes, or walk for 28 minutes in order to burn up the extra calories.

Exercise is vital in taking off excess weight. A daily exercise program may not cause the pounds to melt away overnight, but it will diminish body fat, improve muscle tone, improve the efficiency

Desirable weights for men and women

Weight depends as much on build as on height. The desirable weight—the weight medical records show is associated with good health—can vary up to 22 pounds, depending on the build of the person. The tables below show desirable weights for men and women of ages 25 and over, in indoor clothing. For women between 18 and 25, subtract 1 pound for every year below 25.

Men

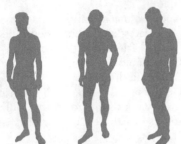

| Height | | Weight (in pounds) | | |
ft	in	Small build	Medium build	Large build
5	1	112–120	118–129	126–141
5	2	115–123	121–133	129–144
5	3	118–126	124–136	132–148
5	4	121–129	127–139	135–152
5	5	124–133	130–143	138–156
5	6	128–137	134–147	142–161
5	7	132–141	138–152	147–166
5	8	136–145	142–156	151–170
5	9	140–150	146–160	155–174
5	10	144–154	150–165	159–179
5	11	148–158	154–170	164–184
6	0	152–162	158–175	168–189
6	1	156–167	162–180	173–194
6	2	160–171	167–185	178–199
6	3	164–175	172–190	182–204

Women

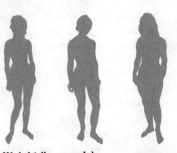

| Height | | Weight (in pounds) | | |
ft	in	Small build	Medium build	Large build
4	8	92–98	96–107	104–119
4	9	94–101	98–110	106–122
4	10	96–104	101–113	109–125
4	11	99–107	104–116	112–128
5	0	102–110	107–119	115–131
5	1	105–113	110–122	118–134
5	2	108–116	113–126	121–138
5	3	111–119	116–130	125–142
5	4	114–123	120–135	129–146
5	5	118–127	124–139	133–150
5	6	122–131	128–143	137–154
5	7	126–135	132–147	141–158
5	8	130–140	136–151	145–163
5	9	134–144	140–155	149–168
5	10	138–148	144–159	153–173

with which your body burns carbohydrates (see METABOLISM in the encyclopedia section), and lower your pulse rate and blood pressure.

You should be aware of your body's limitations, however. If you are not accustomed to strenuous exercise, a mile-long jog can be dangerous as well as exhausting. Instead, it would be wise to plan a program of mild exercise daily: sports, if you have always engaged in them; walking; or even a short exercise routine in your bedroom. But no matter which regimen of exercise you choose, do it as regularly and habitually as brushing your teeth. You will discover in a few weeks how easy it is to do, and how much better you feel for having done it.

EATING PATTERNS: HOW TO CHANGE THEM

Many people do not eat more or less than they need to maintain their ideal weight. When they

exercise, they eat more; when they eat a heavy meal at noon, they feel no need to eat a heavy dinner. Their appetites are regulated by their physical requirements and are in balance.

With other people, though, eating habits are not in balance with their bodies' needs. The compulsive cake-snacker, the teenager who lives on hamburgers and milk shakes, the habitual second-helping eater are all the victims of habit—and habit can be changed.

Emotional factors play an important part in overeating and undereating. People who feel lonely and unwanted often eat a great deal because it is one of their few pleasures. Women with small children frequently overeat simply out of boredom or to calm their anxiety. Worry and tension, or the desire for attention and sympathy, can cause undereating, too. Deep psychological problems, often signaled by disastrous eating habits, call for the help of a specialist. But for most people the will to change and the knowledge of how to do so are sufficient reasons to alter their diet and reduce or gain weight.

Losing Weight. If you decide to reduce, here are a few simple hints to start with: Try not to snack between meals, but if you do, eat low-calorie fruits or raw vegetables. Remove temptation—if the candy you usually eat is not in the house, you won't eat any. Learn to recognize the high-calorie foods and go easy on them at mealtime. Avoid alcoholic beverages and soft drinks containing large amounts of sugar. Introduce new, low-calorie foods into your diet slowly, and if you really don't like them, drop them. Try eating cereal and fruit with no sugar added; you will be astonished at how quickly you can lose the taste for superimposed sweetness. Try black coffee or plain unsweetened tea for a change. Remember that it's not a tragedy if you leave the table feeling slightly hungry. In fact, it is proof that you are doing something right!

Except when you are eating, don't think about food. If you feel hungry, take a walk or clean the garage. If you feel *really* hungry, have a glass of water (0 calories), or two stalks of celery (under 20 calories), or a cup of tomato juice (under 45 calories). Teach your body to accept nonsweet, nonstarch, nonfat foods; and after a while your system will respond by learning to like them.

Three Squares a Day? If you are accustomed to three meals daily, don't change your eating pattern—but *do* pay special attention to breakfast. A good, high-protein breakfast will eliminate that mid-morning slump and reduce your hunger for lunch. In fact, nutritionists now say that the first meal of the day is the most important. Make sure that it includes fruit or juice, skim milk in some

---

A diet to lose weight by

These sample menus for three days will cut your intake of calories to 1,200 per day and still provide all necessary nutrients.

1st Day (1,200 calories)

Breakfast
Grapefruit (1/2 med)
Wheat flakes (1 oz)
Skim milk (1 1/2 cups)
Coffee (black), if desired

Lunch
Chef's salad:
  Julienne chicken (1 oz)
  Cheddar cheese (1/2 oz)
  Hard-boiled egg (1/2 egg)
  Tomato (1 large)
  Cucumber (6 slices)
  Endive (1/2 oz)
  Lettuce (1/8 head)
  French dressing (2 tbsp)
Rye wafers (4 wafers)
Skim milk (1 cup)

Dinner
Beef pot roast (3 oz)
Mashed potatoes (1/3 cup)
Green peas (1/2 cup)
Whole wheat bread (1 slice)
Margarine (1/2 tsp)
Fruit cup
  Orange (1/2 small)
  Apple (1/2 small)
  Banana (1/2 med)

Snack between meals
Banana (1/2 med)

2nd Day (1,200 calories)

Breakfast
Orange juice (1/2 cup)
Soft-boiled egg (1 egg)
Whole wheat toast (1 slice)
Margarine (1 tsp)
Skim milk (1 cup)
Coffee (black), if desired

Lunch
Sandwich:
  Enriched bread (2 slices)
  Boiled ham (1 1/2 oz)
  Mayonnaise (2 tsp)
  Mustard
  Lettuce (1 large leaf)
Celery (1 small stalk)
Radishes (4 radishes)
Dill pickle (1/2 large)
Skim milk (1 cup)

Dinner
Roast lamb (3 oz)
Rice, converted (1/2 cup)
Spinach (3/4 cup)
Lemon (1/4 med)
Salad:
  Peaches, canned (1/2 peach)
  Cottage cheese (2 tbsp)
  Lettuce (1 large leaf)

Snack between meals
Apple (1 med)

3rd Day (1,200 calories)

Breakfast
Tomato juice (1/2 cup)
French toast
  Bread (1 slice)
  Egg (1/2 beaten)
  Milk
Margarine (1 tsp)
Jelly (1 1/2 tsp)
Skim milk (1 cup)
Coffee (black), if desired

Lunch
Tuna fish salad
  Tuna fish (2 oz)
  Hard-boiled egg (1/2 egg)
  Celery (1 small stalk)
  Lemon juice (1 tsp)
  Dressing (1 1/2 tsp)
  Lettuce (1 large leaf)
Whole wheat bread (2 slices)
Margarine (1 tsp)
Carrot sticks (1/2 carrot)
Skim milk (1 cup)

Dinner
Beef liver (2 oz)
Green snap beans (2/3 cup)
Shredded cabbage with vinegar dressing (2/3 cup)
Roll, enriched (1 small)
Margarine (1/2 tsp)
Grapes (1 small bunch)

Snack between meals
Orange (1 med)

form (yogurt, for instance), meat or an egg (omit the egg if you are on a low-cholesterol diet), and whole-grain cereal or bread.

As for your other meals, make sure they are adequate but not huge. Don't overeat at any meal, because you will only increase your body's expectation for even more at the next round. Many people find they are happier with four or

five small meals each day, rather than three large ones. You might experiment with a light lunch and dinner, plus a nourishing snack in the mid-afternoon and another in the evening.

A Word of Caution Before Dieting

If you are considerably overweight or have symptoms that indicate a physiological problem,

Calorie-rated menus

Age, sex, occupation, and mode of living (active or sedentary) determine your caloric needs. Sample diets, ranging from 2,000 to 3,500 calories per day are shown here. For perfect balance, any diet should contain 64 percent (about 10 ounces)

of carbohydrates, 21 percent (about 3¼ ounces) of fat, 14 percent (about 2½ ounces) of proteins, and 1 percent (about a seventh of an ounce) of vitamins and minerals. The meals set out here are only examples; unless otherwise stated, the

2,000 calories per day

Number of calories required by a moderately active woman and a man over 65. Slimming diet for a man doing light work or a very active woman.

Breakfast		425
Grapefruit	½ med	45
Oatmeal	1 cup	130
with whole milk	½ glass	80
with sugar	2 tsp	30
Egg (scrambled)	1 med	110
Tea/coffee (with milk)	1 cup	15
with sugar	1 tsp	15

Lunch		625
Sardines (packed in oil)	3 oz	175
Lettuce (iceberg)	½ head	30
Tomato	1 med	40
Mayonnaise	1 tbsp	100
Bread (rye)	2 slices	120
Milk (whole)	1 glass	160

Dinner		705
Pork chop (thick-cut)	1 med	260
Applesauce	½ cup	115
Peas	½ cup	60
with butter	1 pat	50
Greens (mustard)	1 cup	35
Melon (cantaloupe)	½ melon (5″ diam.)	60
with ice cream	3 oz	95
Tea/coffee (with milk)	1 cup	15
with sugar	1 tsp	15

Snack		250
Pear	1 med	100
Chocolate chip cookies	3 med	150

2,500 calories per day

Calories required by a man in a sedentary occupation, such as an office worker, and by an active woman.

Breakfast		645
Grapefruit juice	1 cup	100
Cereal (corn flakes)	1 cup	100
with whole milk	½ glass	80
with sugar	1 tbsp	40
Toast (enriched white)	2 slices	140
with butter	1 pat	50
Bacon	2 strips	90
Tea/coffee (with milk)	1 cup	15
with sugar	2 tsp	30

Lunch		630
Egg salad sandwich:		
eggs	2 med	160
mayonnaise	1 tbsp	100
bread (enriched white)	2 slices	140
Milk (whole)	1 glass	160
Apple	1 med	70

Dinner		1035
Beef, steak (broiled)	3 oz	375
Spinach (cooked)	1 cup	40
Potato	1 med	90
with butter	1 pat	50
Lettuce (iceberg)	½ head	30
with vinegar	1 tbsp	00
with oil	1 tbsp	125
Vanilla pudding (starch base)	1 cup	280
Tea/coffee (with milk)	1 cup	15
with sugar	2 tsp	30

Snack		185
Oatmeal cookie	1 med	120
Orange	1 med	65

see your doctor before attempting to diet. He will determine whether a disease is associated with your weight problem and will help you to devise a diet designed specifically for your needs.

Weight-Reducing Drugs. Never take them without a doctor's prescription. They can be dangerous, addicting, or simply a waste of money.

Your Water Intake. The body needs adequate water and other fluids. Decreasing the amount of water you drink or sweating it off in a sauna may cause a quick loss of weight, but it is an illusory loss. You will regain the weight as soon as you replace the water that you have eliminated. Insufficiency of liquids will play havoc with your heart, circulatory system, and kidneys.

portions are those given in the caloric chart on p. 32. Roast veal or pork (410 calories per 4 ounces) can be substituted for other meats if adjustments are made so that the total caloric intake is not exceeded. If early morning coffee is drunk, each

cup (with milk) adds 15 calories to the intake; and every teaspoon of sugar adds another 15 calories. The caloric values of made-up dishes, such as soups, stews, pies, and puddings, are governed by their contents.

3,000 calories per day
Calories required by a man, up to 65 years of age, in a moderately active occupation and by an extremely active woman.

Breakfast		610
Orange juice	1 cup	110
Eggs (poached)	2 med	160
Bacon	2 strips	90
Toast (rye)	2 slices	120
with butter	2 pats	100
Tea/coffee (with milk)	1 cup	15
with sugar	1 tsp	15

Lunch		660
Cheeseburger:		
beef (ground)	3 oz	245
cheese (American)	1 oz	105
hamburger roll (enriched)	1 roll	140
Pickle	1 med	10
Milk (whole)	1 glass	160

Dinner		1430
Chicken breast (broiled)	1 med (6 oz)	310
Broccoli	2 cups	80
with butter	1 pat	50
Sweet potato	1 med	155
with butter	1 pat	50
Avocado salad:		
avocado	½ med	185
vinegar	1 tbsp	00
oil (corn)	1 tbsp	125
lemon juice (fresh)	1 tsp	10
Bread (rye)	1 slice	60
with butter	1 pat	50
Milk (whole)	1 glass	160
Fruit cocktail	1 cup	195

Snack		300
Pound Cake	1 slice (½" thick)	140
Milk (whole)	1 glass	160

3,500 calories per day
Calories for an extremely active man, such as one doing heavy manual work, up to 60 years old. No woman requires such a calorie intake.

Breakfast		775
Orange juice	1 cup	110
Oatmeal	1 cup	130
with whole milk	½ glass	80
with honey	2 tsp	40
Eggs (soft-boiled)	2 med	160
Bacon	2 strips	90
Toast (whole wheat)	1 slice	60
with butter	1 pat	50
Tea/coffee (with milk)	1 cup	15
with sugar	2 tsp	30

Lunch		1110
Tuna	6 oz	340
Bread (rye)	2 slices	120
Tomatoes	2 med	80
Dressing (Thousand Island)	2 tbsp	160
Doughnuts	2 plain	250
Milk (whole)	1 glass	160

Dinner		1295
Tomato juice	1 cup	45
Liver (beef)	6 oz	390
with onions (fried)	1 cup	60
Carrots (cooked)	2 cups	90
with butter	1 pat	50
Spinach (cooked)	1 cup	40
Potato	1 med	90
with butter	1 pat	50
Lettuce (iceberg)	½ head	30
with dressing (French)	1 tbsp	65
Milk (whole)	1 glass	160
Strawberries	1 cup	55
with cream (light)	2 tbsp	90
Tea/coffee	1 cup	05
with cream (light)	1 tbsp	45
with sugar	2 tsp	30

Snack		325
Apple	1 med	70
Banana	1 med	100
Cherries	1 cup	105
Chocolate chip cookie	1 med	50

Fad Diets. Such diets, discussed in greater detail later in this chapter, are often dangerous. A diet that is extremely restrictive, consisting, for example, of nothing but grapefruit, or steak, or lettuce and cottage cheese, may result in loss of weight. Such a diet may also ruin your health. So consult your doctor before embarking on any such programs.

Do You Need to Gain Weight?

Fat people are always overweight, but thin people are not necessarily underweight. How can you tell if your weight is normal for you? Compare your actual weight with the figures given in the weight table on page 34. If you are 10 or 15 pounds below the desirable weight listed for your height and build, and if your body is bony, with only a thin covering of muscle tissue on your back, buttocks, and thighs, you are very likely underweight.

Let your doctor decide whether your extreme thinness is due to ill health or to your failure to eat enough of the right kinds of food. If he thinks that your diet is inadequate, he will be able to guide you to the calorie-rich foods suitable for your needs.

Concentrate on high-calorie foods such as cream soups, chowders, mayonnaise, cereals with milk or cream, and cream-rich desserts. But be sure to check first with your doctor about the cholesterol problem because you will probably be eating large quantities of whole-milk food and eggs.

Peas, potatoes, and lima beans provide more carbohydrates than the leafy vegetables you may have been eating, but don't give up salads. They help with digestion; and because of all the starches and sugars in your new regimen, you will need to maintain some bulk in your diet. Try not to eat sweets; they only increase the possibility of tooth decay and give you few nutrients beyond the sugar they contain. Snacks such as fruit, peanut butter, and eggnog furnish protein, minerals, and vitamins as well as calories.

Be sure to watch your weight. If you find that you are developing a sweet tooth and adding pounds rapidly, slow down—and check with your doctor. He may wish to modify your diet.

Special Diets

For Children. Infants have their own special needs, and their diets are determined by those needs. The question of when milk should be supplemented with cereals, vegetables, meat, and solid foods will be determined by the baby's

How the body deals with food

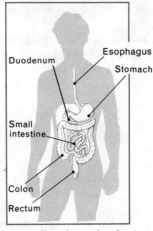

Duodenum
Esophagus
Stomach
Stomach
Small intestine
Colon
Rectum

It usually takes a day for food to pass all the way from the mouth and through the alimentary canal to the rectum; and it may be several days before the last of the waste products from that meal have been disposed of. Contraction and relaxation of the muscles in the walls of the stomach and the intestines propel the food on its way. All food consists of four basic components: carbohydrates, fats, proteins, and water. Each, except water, is broken down into simpler substances by enzymes in the various digestive juices: carbohydrates into sugars, fats into glycerol and fatty acids, and proteins into their constituent amino acids. These simpler substances are carried in the bloodstream and the lymph system to be stored until they are required or are used in bodily processes. Most of the water is also removed from food in the intestine and passed into the circulation.

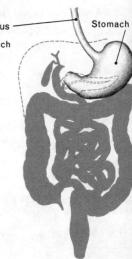

Chewed food passes through the esophagus into the stomach where, as chyme, it is stored for three to four hours.

Mouth and gullet During chewing and swallowing, enzymes in saliva begin the breakdown of starch to sugars

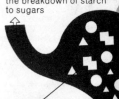

Gastric juices from glands in the stomach begin the digestion of proteins

▲ **Protein** Mainly in meat, fish, and eggs
■ **Carbohydrate** in sugar and starchy foods
● **Fat** in meat, dairy products, margarine, and cooking oil

Stomach Chewed food mixes with saliva and passes to the stomach. Gastric juices from glands in the stomach begin the digestion of proteins.

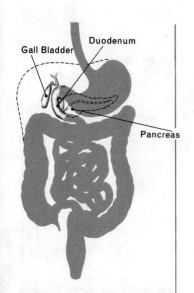

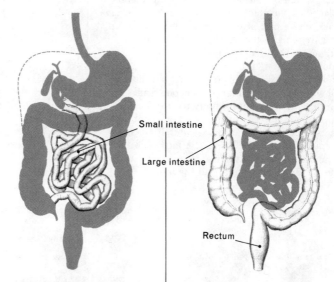

From the stomach, food passes into the duodenum, the first 10-12 inches of the small intestine, where it is partially or completely digested by the action of pancreatic juices.

From the duodenum, food enters the small intestine, a 22-foot coiled tube. Proteins and fats are broken down, and digestion of all the food eaten is completed.

Within five hours of leaving the stomach, food enters the 4½-foot colon, or large intestine. It is some hours before the indigestible residue reaches the rectum.

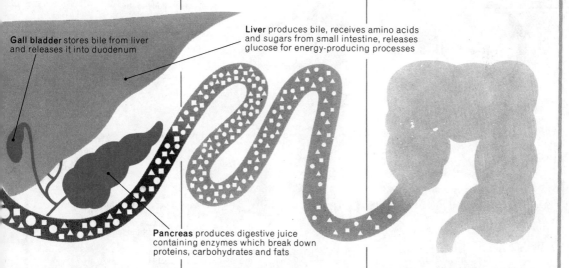

Gall bladder stores bile from liver and releases it into duodenum

Liver produces bile, receives amino acids and sugars from small intestine, releases glucose for energy-producing processes

Pancreas produces digestive juice containing enzymes which break down proteins, carbohydrates and fats

Duodenum Here bile from the liver emulsifies fats. Enzymes in the pancreatic juice begin to digest fats, continue the digestion of proteins and complete the breakdown of carbohydrates into sugars.

Small intestine At this stage the food is in liquid form and most of the nutrients are passed into the body via the hair-like tentacles (villi) that line the inner walls of the small intestine.

Colon While the indigestible food residues – in liquid form – are in the colon, water is extracted and passed into a network of blood vessels, leaving a residue of semi-solid waste matter as feces.

How the body handles fluids

More than 60 percent of the body is composed of water, which is continually being changed and replaced by the consumption of liquids, either as drinks or as a part of solid foods. The amount in the body remains the same, controlled by the workings of the kidneys, and the surplus is disposed of through the bladder, lungs, intestines, and skin. The kidneys act as a filter as well as an absorption unit. If someone drinks more than the amount his body requires, he urinates more to lose the excess; if he is hot and sweats a lot, he becomes thirsty and drinks more to replace the fluid he has lost. A fairly constant amount of water is lost in the feces and as water vapor in air breathed out from the lungs.

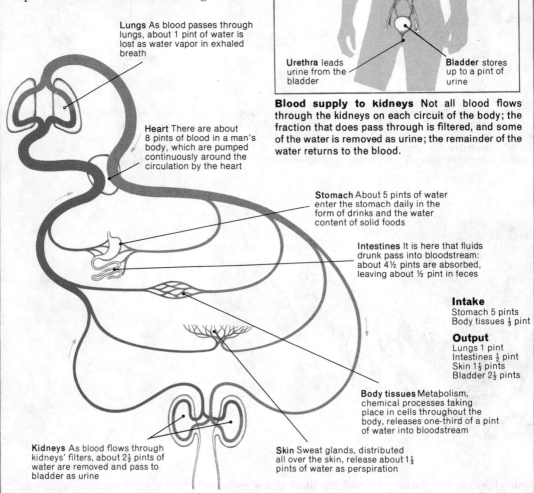

Heart pumps blood to and from the kidneys

Kidneys filter impurities and water from the blood

Ureters carry urine to the bladder

Urethra leads urine from the bladder

Bladder stores up to a pint of urine

Blood supply to kidneys Not all blood flows through the kidneys on each circuit of the body; the fraction that does pass through is filtered, and some of the water is removed as urine; the remainder of the water returns to the blood.

Lungs As blood passes through lungs, about 1 pint of water is lost as water vapor in exhaled breath

Heart There are about 8 pints of blood in a man's body, which are pumped continuously around the circulation by the heart

Stomach About 5 pints of water enter the stomach daily in the form of drinks and the water content of solid foods

Intestines It is here that fluids drunk pass into bloodstream: about 4½ pints are absorbed, leaving about ½ pint in feces

Intake
Stomach 5 pints
Body tissues ⅓ pint

Output
Lungs 1 pint
Intestines ½ pint
Skin 1⅓ pints
Bladder 2½ pints

Body tissues Metabolism, chemical processes taking place in cells throughout the body, releases one-third of a pint of water into bloodstream

Kidneys As blood flows through kidneys' filters, about 2½ pints of water are removed and pass to bladder as urine

Skin Sweat glands, distributed all over the skin, release about 1⅓ pints of water as perspiration

Daily intake and output A person in a temperate climate needs to take in about 5 pints of water each day. A further half pint is generated by chemical processes in the body tissues. All this water passes into the bloodstream, from which it is lost in four ways, so that a fluid balance is maintained. Most is lost in urine, some as sweat, some as vapor in the breath, and a little in the feces.

growth and digestive abilities. (For a discussion of infants' diets, see Chapter 14.)

From the time the doctor says that your child can eat everything, his diet will be much the same as that of the normal adult, except that the child needs more milk and the extra energy that high-calorie foods provide. But do not encourage your child to eat sweets. Too much sugar may take away a child's desire to eat regular meals and ruin his teeth. Bread and cheese are far more nourishing than a chocolate bar.

For Adolescents. During their rapid growth in adolescence, boys and girls need extra milk, proteins, and vitamins. It is essential that they eat a balanced diet, supplemented by additional food and milk between meals to fuel their growing bodies. Good dietary habits are especially important at this age. (See also Chapter 17.)

For Pregnant Women. The pregnant woman must supply her own body with good nourishment and at the same time eat foods that will build her baby's bones and tissues. It is essential that pregnant women pay particular attention to their diet, under the supervision of a doctor. (See also Chapter 13.)

For Older People. Retired and aged persons tend to burn fewer calories and to need fewer fats and carbohydrates than younger people. At the same time their bodies may require additional minerals and vitamins—particularly vitamin D, which helps keep bones strong, and the controversial vitamin E, which some experts believe is capable of retarding the aging process. As one advances in age, a cholesterol-restricted diet becomes more important.

Low-Salt or Low-Sodium Diets. A diet excessively high in salt often results in *edema,* the retention of fluid in the body tissues. For people who have hypertension (high blood pressure), fluid retention can be dangerous, and they are often put on a low-salt diet. The salt used in cooking and table salt itself are both eliminated, while salted foods such as bacon, bread, and cheese are severely restricted. Salt-free diets are prescribed for pregnant women who gain too much weight, and for certain cases of obesity.

Vegetarian Diets. There are three kinds: the least restrictive, which bars meat but permits all other types of food including fish; the more restrictive, which bars meat and fish but allows inclusion of such animal products as milk, cheese, and eggs; and the most rigorous form, which confines the diet exclusively to plants and plant products. For the last type of vegetarian diet, maintaining an adequate protein intake may be difficult unless the dieter is a trained nutritionist. With careful planning and a great deal of knowledge, however, it is possible to devise a diet with sufficient protein from wheat germ, brewer's yeast, soybeans, nuts, whole grains, fruits, vegetables, and vegetable oils. But such a diet cannot be recommended without the advice of a nutritionist. A protein-rich vegetarian diet should contain milk products, eggs, and fish, which is as rich in protein as meat.

Given the current high cost of meat and its equally high cholesterol content, a modified vegetarian diet might well appeal to overweight, cost-conscious dieters.

Some Recent Diet Fads

The Low-Carbohydrate, High-Fat Diet. Introduced for weight reducing, this diet eliminates carbohydrate-rich foods, but encourages fat intake. In addition to increasing cholesterol consumption and raising the risks of arteriosclerosis, this diet may also be responsible for inducing other ailments as, for example, gout. Some dieters report an initial loss of weight, but others complain of fatigue and irritability. Nutritionists generally believe the diet is essentially useless and potentially harmful.

The High-Protein Diet. Another weight-reducing regimen, this one emphasizes the eating of meat, milk, and vegetable protein, and the lowering or elimination of sugar and starch as well as animal fats. If you are interested, consult your doctor; he may be concerned about the low-carbohydrate levels in high-protein diets.

The Macrobiotic Diet. This diet, which has attained considerable notoriety, is an extreme vegetarian regimen. If followed faithfully, it may produce serious nutritional deficiencies, scurvy, and actual starvation. Most nutritionists advise against it.

CAN A DIET CURE WHAT AILS YOU?

We often hear about diets that will prevent acid or alkaline stomach; cure constipation, skin disease, cancer, and tooth decay; increase virility; or guarantee long life. Some special diets are useful and necessary—for example, diabetic diets, low-salt diets for hypertension, or low-cholesterol diets to reduce the risk of arteriosclerosis. Constipation and acne can often be relieved by eating or not eating certain foods. But by and large, it is necessary to determine first whether your symptoms are the result of some nutritional lack, or whether they are organically caused. Your doctor should be consulted before you make a drastic change in what you eat.

While a weight-reducing diet may not cure your particular ailments, the experience of many successful dieters has shown that a proper diet will make you feel better and enjoy a fuller life.

Nutrients: Recommended Daily Dietary Allowances

The amounts of nutrients listed below are considered adequate for maintaining good nutrition by the Food and Nutrition Board of the National Academy of Sciences. The chart shows the nutritional needs of men and women at various stages of life.

Age	Protein (grams)	Vitamin A (retinol equiv.)	Vitamin D (μg of cholecalciferol)	Vitamin E (mg alpha-tocopherol equiv.)	Vitamin C (mg)	Thiamine (mg)	Riboflavin (mg)	Niacin (mg)	Vitamin B6 (mg)	Folic Acid (μg)	Vitamin B12 (μg)	Calcium (mg)	Phosphorous (mg)	Magnesium (mg)	Iron (mg)	Zinc (mg)	Iodine (μg)
Infants																	
To 6 mos	kg x 2.2	420	10	3	35	0.3	0.4	6	0.3	30	0.5	360	240	50	10	3	40
To 1 yr	kg x 2.0	400	10	4	35	0.5	0.6	8	0.6	45	1.5	540	360	70	15	5	50
Children																	
1-3	23	400	10	5	45	0.7	0.8	9	0.9	100	2.0	800	800	150	15	10	70
4-6	30	500	10	6	45	0.9	1.0	11	1.3	200	2.5	800	800	200	10	10	90
7-10	34	700	10	7	45	1.2	1.4	16	1.6	300	3.0	800	800	250	10	10	120
Males																	
11-14	45	1000	10	8	50	1.4	1.6	18	1.8	400	3.0	1200	1200	350	18	15	150
15-18	56	1000	10	10	60	1.4	1.7	18	2.0	400	3.0	1200	1200	400	10	15	150
19-22	56	1000	7.5	10	60	1.5	1.7	19	2.2	400	3.0	800	800	350	10	15	150
23-50	56	1000	5	10	60	1.4	1.6	18	2.2	400	3.0	800	800	350	10	15	150
51 +	56	1000	5	10	60	1.2	1.4	16	2.2	400	3.0	800	800	350	10	15	150
Females																	
11-14	46	800	10	8	50	1.1	1.3	15	1.8	400	3.0	1200	1200	300	18	15	150
15-18	46	800	10	8	60	1.1	1.3	14	2.0	400	3.0	1200	1200	300	18	15	150
19-22	44	800	7.5	8	60	1.1	1.3	14	2.0	400	3.0	800	800	300	18	15	150
23-50	44	800	5	8	60	1.0	1.2	13	2.0	400	3.0	800	800	300	18	15	150
51 +	44	800	5	8	60	1.0	1.2	13	2.0	400	3.0	800	800	300	10	15	150
Pregnant	+ 30	+ 200	+ 5	+ 2	+ 20	+ 0.4	+ 0.3	+ 2	+ 0.6	+ 400	+ 1.0	+ 400	+ 400	+ 150	*	+ 5	+ 25
Lactating	+ 20	+ 400	+ 5	+ 3	+ 40	+ 0.5	+ 0.5	+ 5	+ 0.5	+ 100	+ 1.0	+ 400	+ 400	+ 150	*	+ 10	+ 50

*The increased requirement during pregnancy and lactation cannot be met by the iron content of habitual American diets nor by the existing iron stores of many women; therefore the use of 30-60 milligrams of supplemental iron is recommended.

More about minerals

Magnesium. Deficiencies in magnesium are rare in the United States. Good sources of the mineral are seafood, beef liver, whole grains, milk, molasses, dark green leafy vegetables, dried fruits, avocados, nuts, and sesame seeds.

Potassium. Recommended dietary requirements have not yet been established for potassium, but most experts believe that between 1875 and 5625 milligrams a day are sufficient for most adults. The average diet supplies enough for most people. Sources of potassium are lean meats, fish, pan-fried or baked potatoes, lima beans, soybeans, broccoli, brussels sprouts, raw cabbage, green leafy vegetables, winter squash, prune juice, orange juice, papayas, avocados, bananas, dates, sunflower seeds, peanuts, milk products, and whole grains.

Sodium. Although recommended dietary allowances for sodium are not definitely established, many experts believe 1100–3300 milligrams a day are adequate. The average individual probably consumes 5 to 20 times as much as he or she needs. High sources of sodium are table salt (¼ teaspoon supplies 500 mg), baking powder, baking soda, seafood, poultry, meats, oatmeal, farina, cottage cheese, peanut butter, beets, carrots, celery, mushrooms (canned or cooked), and processed meats, vegetables and soups.

CHAPTER 3

The Parts of Your Body: How They Function, the Care They Need

What is good health? One answer might be: the absence of disease. But a better definition would be: the most efficient working and interaction of the many parts of the body. Our pattern of living and our emotional state affect almost all parts of our body. Preventive medicine, which is largely up to us, is simply knowing how to take the best possible care of ourselves so that the body can operate in good health.

This chapter basically describes most of the individual parts of the body and gives commonsense advice on how to care for them. It does not attempt to discuss every possible illness involving every part. The teeth and gums, for instance, and the endocrine glands are discussed in Chapters 4 and 5 respectively, and Chapter 8 is devoted to the mind and emotions. Although the parts of the body are dealt with separately, remember that they function together. Caring for any part is helping to care for the whole.

THE INTERNAL PARTS

The following internal parts and organs are discussed in this section. External parts are discussed later in the chapter.

Brain	Stomach, intestines
Nervous System	Rectum
Heart	Liver
Lungs	Gallbladder
Blood	Kidneys
Bones, joints, ligaments	Urinary bladder
Muscles, tendons	Appendix

This section is written to counteract such misinformation as "a chronic pain in the back means you have kidney trouble," or "you should take pills to stimulate your liver." It will answer such questions as whether you should do something to protect your heart and lungs and whether certain foods are good for your brain.

Brain

The human brain is surely an awe-inspiring phenomenon. Fortunately, this intricate three-pound structure—the controlling organ of our bodies—is well defended against injuries. The bony shield of the skull, wrapped in the resilient scalp and lined within by a tough membrane called *dura mater* (or "hard mother" in Latin), protects the brain admirably against blows and falls. As a further protective device, the brain is surrounded by fluid that helps absorb traumatic shocks. Superb as these defenses are, man himself, with his modern automobiles and passion for speed and for certain violent sports can deal dangerous blows to the brain.

Protecting the Brain. To protect our brains against severe trauma, we need to know the hazards of such sports as football, baseball (when batting), and diving, and how to avoid injuries to the skull. Concern for safety does not make you "chicken"; prudence marks you as a sensible person. Motorcyclists and equestrians should always wear hard hats. Automobile drivers should refrain from reckless driving and unsafe automobiles. He or she should always use seat belts while riding in a car—preferably the harness type—to provide the best protection for the head and upper torso.

Excessive use of alcohol not only interferes with safe driving, it is an internal threat to the tissues of the brain. Young people should be thoroughly indoctrinated on the fiercely destructive potential of such drugs as LSD and "speed." Amphetamines and the psychedelic and opiate drugs can alter one's perception so that driving is

43

unsafe for anyone under their influence. Worse, many of these drugs themselves are known to cause brain damage and to bring on psychotic states. (For further information about alcoholism, see Chapter 1; for drug abuse, see Chapter 17.)

Workers should alert themselves to any physical as well as chemical hazards that can endanger the brain or nervous system on the job. (Some of these hazards are discussed in Chapter 7).

If you are the victim of an accident and suffer a serious blow to the head, watch for such symptoms as vomiting, dizziness, or impaired vision. The classical bump on the head can become dangerous if collected fluid presses on the lining of the brain. (See the entry HEMATOMA in the encyclopedia section.)

Keeping the Brain in Good Working Order. You can help your brain to stay healthy and work at top efficiency by providing it with sufficient sleep. The amount of sleep necessary differs with individuals, but generally children require about

The nervous system—the master of the body

The central nervous system consists of the brain, the spinal cord, and the body's nerve network. This complex system is based on one kind of cell—the neuron. The brain, the mass of tissue inside the head, has the greatest number of these cells, most of which are in its outer part, the cerebrum. Below the cerebrum is the cerebellum and the brain stem, which is linked to the spinal cord.

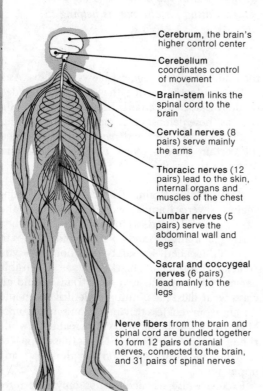

Cerebrum, the brain's higher control center

Cerebellum coordinates control of movement

Brain-stem links the spinal cord to the brain

Cervical nerves (8 pairs) serve mainly the arms

Thoracic nerves (12 pairs) lead to the skin, internal organs and muscles of the chest

Lumbar nerves (5 pairs) serve the abdominal wall and legs

Sacral and coccygeal nerves (6 pairs) lead mainly to the legs

Nerve fibers from the brain and spinal cord are bundled together to form 12 pairs of cranial nerves, connected to the brain, and 31 pairs of spinal nerves

Nerve pathways to the brain

The spinal cord is a column of nervous tissue extending two-thirds of the way down the backbone. The nerves attached to it spread throughout the body and carry impulses to and from the brain.

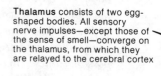

Thalamus consists of two egg-shaped bodies. All sensory nerve impulses—except those of the sense of smell—converge on the thalamus, from which they are relayed to the cerebral cortex

Hypothalamus below the thalamus, contains centers for the regulation of body temperature and blood pressure. It also regulates the drives of hunger, thirst, and sex, and may be the source of emotional reactions, such as fear and anger

Pituitary gland is a tiny rounded organ attached to the base of the brain by a slender stalk. It is the master endocrine gland of the body; its secretions activate other glands. For example, pituitary hormones stimulate the ovaries in women and so control the menstrual cycle

Olfactory bulbs lie beneath the front of the cerebral hemispheres, directly above the nasal cavity. The bulbs receive smell impulses from the olfactory nerves, and relay them to the brain

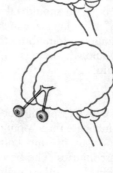

Optic nerve contains nerve fibers from the retina in the eye. It transmits information destined for the visual center at the back of the brain

Brain stem, a bundle of nerve tissue at the base of the brain, consists of the midbrain, the pons, and the medulla oblongata, which have centers controlling the heart, the lungs, and the digestive system

12 hours and adults need between six and eight hours to feel refreshed. When body and mind tell you they are tired, don't interfere by overstimulating your brain with too much caffeine from coffee or tea or by the use of "pep pills" (amphetamines), which can produce dangerous mental disorders. Similarly, most sleeping pills that promise a good night's sleep are essentially useless. If anxiety or discomfort are interfering with your sleep, discuss the problem with your doctor before resorting to pills.

Do you need special "brain foods" and tonics to keep your brain in good working order? *No!* The well-balanced diets described in Chapter 2 will provide the brain with all the vitamins and nourishment it requires. Fish is not any better for the brain than any other protein food.

Dangers to the Brain. Some of aging's harmful effects on the brain can be prevented or diminished by following suggestions given in the discussion of high blood pressure (Chapter 2), of

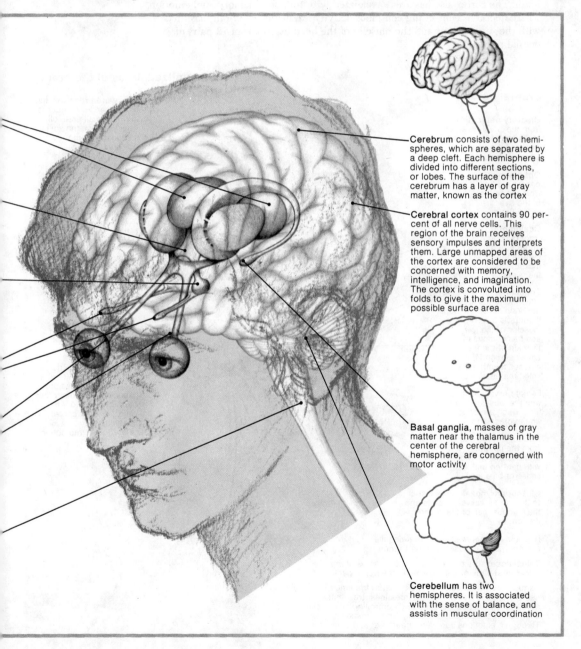

Cerebrum consists of two hemispheres, which are separated by a deep cleft. Each hemisphere is divided into different sections, or lobes. The surface of the cerebrum has a layer of gray matter, known as the cortex

Cerebral cortex contains 90 percent of all nerve cells. This region of the brain receives sensory impulses and interprets them. Large unmapped areas of the cortex are considered to be concerned with memory, intelligence, and imagination. The cortex is convoluted into folds to give it the maximum possible surface area

Basal ganglia, masses of gray matter near the thalamus in the center of the cerebral hemisphere, are concerned with motor activity

Cerebellum has two hemispheres. It is associated with the sense of balance, and assists in muscular coordination

45

hardening of the arteries (Chapter 22), and of other conditions that weaken the arteries of the brain.

Remember that the brain reacts quickly to diseases in other parts of the body. Dizziness, fainting, impaired memory, and other symptoms can be owing to conditions in and around the brain, such as sinus trouble or a tumor. These symptoms also can be the result of poisons because damaged kidneys are not removing toxic materials from the blood. Headaches have a variety of causes and should be brought to a doctor's

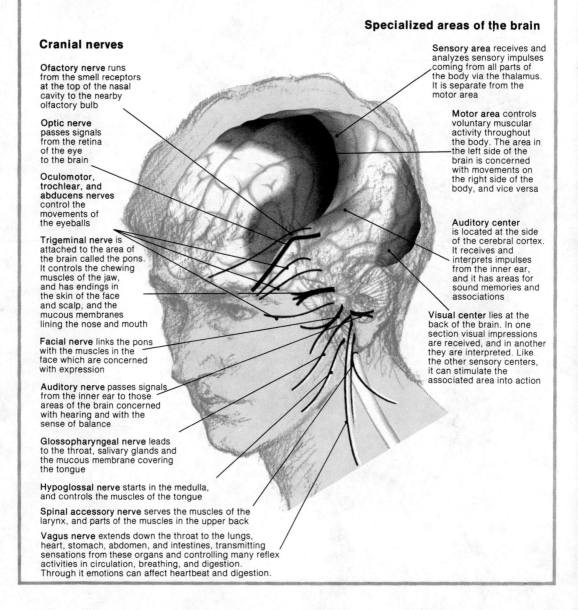

The brain—the center of decision and control

Areas for dealing with sense impressions and coordinating muscular movement are found in the cortex, the outer layer of the two cerebral hemispheres of the brain. The cortex also has areas associated with thought, memory, and emotion, where decisions controlling conscious activity are made. The brain has links with the sense organs and the muscles of the head by means of 12 pairs of cranial nerves.

Cranial nerves

Ofactory nerve runs from the smell receptors at the top of the nasal cavity to the nearby olfactory bulb

Optic nerve passes signals from the retina of the eye to the brain

Oculomotor, trochlear, and abducens nerves control the movements of the eyeballs

Trigeminal nerve is attached to the area of the brain called the pons. It controls the chewing muscles of the jaw, and has endings in the skin of the face and scalp, and the mucous membranes lining the nose and mouth

Facial nerve links the pons with the muscles in the face which are concerned with expression

Auditory nerve passes signals from the inner ear to those areas of the brain concerned with hearing and with the sense of balance

Glossopharyngeal nerve leads to the throat, salivary glands and the mucous membrane covering the tongue

Hypoglossal nerve starts in the medulla, and controls the muscles of the tongue

Spinal accessory nerve serves the muscles of the larynx, and parts of the muscles in the upper back

Vagus nerve extends down the throat to the lungs, heart, stomach, abdomen, and intestines, transmitting sensations from these organs and controlling many reflex activities in circulation, breathing, and digestion. Through it emotions can affect heartbeat and digestion.

Specialized areas of the brain

Sensory area receives and analyzes sensory impulses coming from all parts of the body via the thalamus. It is separate from the motor area

Motor area controls voluntary muscular activity throughout the body. The area in the left side of the brain is concerned with movements on the right side of the body, and vice versa

Auditory center is located at the side of the cerebral cortex. It receives and interprets impulses from the inner ear, and it has areas for sound memories and associations

Visual center lies at the back of the brain. In one section visual impressions are received, and in another they are interpreted. Like the other sensory centers, it can stimulate the associated area into action

46

How the brain prepares the body for conflict

The two divisions of the autonomic nervous system regulate the heart and blood vessels, lungs, stomach, and some sexual organs and endocrine glands. The sympathetic nerves increase their activity; the parasympathetic nerves decrease it. When a person is confronted with situations of emotional stress, involving fear or anger, the brain sends messages along the sympathetic nerves to change the activity of the organs to prepare the body for emergency action.

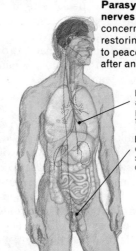

Parasympathetic nerves are concerned with restoring the body to peaceful activity after an emergency

Heart slows down and the blood pressure falls after the danger is over

Bladder can be contracted and its sphincter may open, causing urination

Sympathetic nerves. Through the sympathetic nerves, the brain mobilizes the body for action to meet possible danger

Iris changes size. When someone is frightened or angry, the brain stimulates the sympathetic nerves to this part of the eye, causing the pupils to open wide

Salivary glands produce less saliva, so that the mouth goes dry

Lungs and windpipe are affected under stress; breathing becomes faster, so that the body gets more oxygen

Heart pumps faster during times of fear and anger. Normally you are unaware of the beating of the heart, but its increased activity in times of excitement raises the blood pressure, pumping more blood to supply energy for muscles

Adrenal glands at the top of the kidneys secrete the hormone adrenaline, which prepares the body to fight or run away

Liver releases glucose under emotional stress, providing extra energy for muscles

Stomach and intestines have their blood diverted to the heart, central nervous system, and muscles, so that they can operate under stress. The wavelike movements of the intestinal walls stop, and the various sphincters close

Sphincter at the end of the rectum closes in times of stress, so that defecation is prevented

attention if they are unusually severe or persistent or fail to respond to aspirin. Convulsions are also signals that require special attention—*immediate* attention if they are accompanied by a high fever. (See also HEADACHE; CONVULSIONS in the encyclopedia section.) In other words, *any* unusual brain symptoms call for a complete medical checkup by your doctor.

Nervous System

If we compare the brain to a telephone switchboard, we can think of the rest of the nervous system as trunk and branch lines that directly connect all our sensations and activities with that center. The nerve network instantaneously carries millions of messages from the outside world and from within our own bodies to various parts of the brain, and conversely, all the nerve impulses from the brain to the different parts of our body. The decision, for instance, to move the big toe will race at a speed of 225 miles per hour from the head to the foot of a six-foot man in one-fiftieth of a second. In addition to the 51 billion nerve units in the brain, there are billions of receptors throughout the body for receiving and transmitting sensations of vision, hearing, pressure, heat, cold, taste, and many others. Even pain has its purpose, for it is the nervous system's way of alerting us to trouble within our bodies. (For a fuller discussion, see the entries NERVE; NERVOUS SYSTEM in the encyclopedia section.)

Many complaints loosely labeled "nervous disorders" are not organic (or physical) problems of the nervous system at all. They are the expression of some emotional stress we may be undergoing, and are more properly considered psychological symptoms. (For emotional troubles, which are best treated by a psychologist, psychiatrist, or psychoanalyst, see the discussion in Chapter 8.)

Sharp pains in the legs or face, however, may

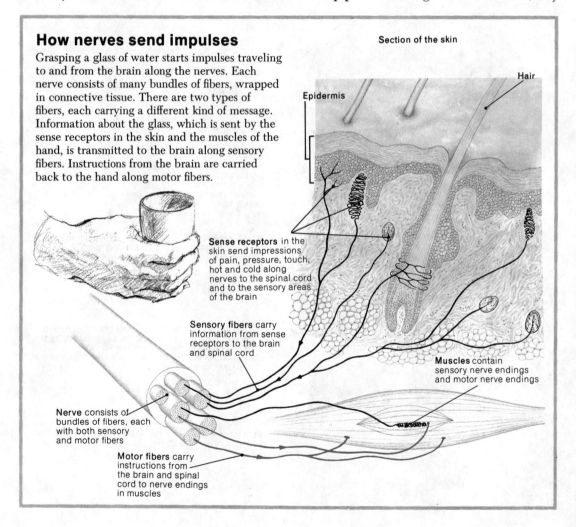

How nerves send impulses

Grasping a glass of water starts impulses traveling to and from the brain along the nerves. Each nerve consists of many bundles of fibers, wrapped in connective tissue. There are two types of fibers, each carrying a different kind of message. Information about the glass, which is sent by the sense receptors in the skin and the muscles of the hand, is transmitted to the brain along sensory fibers. Instructions from the brain are carried back to the hand along motor fibers.

Section of the skin

Hair

Epidermis

Sense receptors in the skin send impressions of pain, pressure, touch, hot and cold along nerves to the spinal cord and to the sensory areas of the brain

Sensory fibers carry information from sense receptors to the brain and spinal cord

Muscles contain sensory nerve endings and motor nerve endings

Nerve consists of bundles of fibers, each with both sensory and motor fibers

Motor fibers carry instructions from the brain and spinal cord to nerve endings in muscles

indicate problems with the nerves themselves. Some common ailments such as NEURITIS and NEURALGIA are discussed in Chapter 23 as well as in the encyclopedia section.

There is little you need do to protect your nervous system other than to keep healthy, active, and alert.

The Heart

The heart, lungs, and some 100,000 miles of blood-filled vessels together make up the circulatory system by which oxygen and other vital elements are carried to nourish the live cells in all parts of the body. The heart is the muscular pump that keeps it all going—a pear-shaped organ not much bigger than your fist. This organ, composed of four chambers with valves in them, is located a little to the left of center in the chest. The heart's function, like its position, is central to life.

The heart is by no means a delicate organ. Surgeons can sew up wounds in the heart, repair or replace its valves, and correct some malformations. Protected by the resilient ribs, the heart is rarely damaged by a blow. A healthy heart responds with ease to extraordinary demands made upon it.

Heart Diseases. Why, then, is heart disease America's number-one killer, accounting for more deaths than even cancer or accidents? The answer is found in the life-style of our Western technological societies, where cholesterol-rich diets, lack of exercise, and the stresses of competition act together to undermine the health of the heart. Women, once considered low risks for heart attacks, are entering the statistics in greater numbers as their lives become less sheltered.

Despite the sophisticated surgical and medical techniques now available, heart diseases are not so much cured as mitigated by treatment. For the heart—perhaps more than for any other organ—prevention of problems is the best cure. If you observe the following precautions and live a life free from the more hazardous habits, you probably need not worry much about your heart.

Remember that the heart is a muscle, and like any muscle it must receive an adequate supply of oxygen in order to function well. Therefore, anything that tends to impede the availability of oxygen to the heart or to obstruct the coronary arteries may starve the heart muscle for oxygen and do damage to the area of the heart those arteries serve. (See HEART DISEASE in the encyclopedia section.)

The heart's pacemaker

Without an internal control, the rate of heartbeats, about 72 per minute, would be insufficient to meet the demands made by the extensive range of the body's activities. But the heart has a pacemaker that raises the pulse rate as the demand arises. The firing of two masses of nerve tissue—the sinoatrial (SA) node and the atrioventricular (AV) node—sets up impulses that pass from the upper chamber of the heart to the lower chamber through conductive tissue known as the Bundle of His. The SA node fires the faster and sets the pace at which the heart pumps.

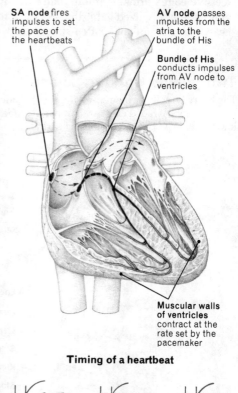

SA node fires impulses to set the pace of the heartbeats

AV node passes impulses from the atria to the bundle of His

Bundle of His conducts impulses from AV node to ventricles

Muscular walls of ventricles contract at the rate set by the pacemaker

Timing of a heartbeat

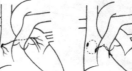

Heartbeat starts in the SA node and its impulses spread in one-tenth of a second across the two atria, causing them to contract

There is a delay of one-tenth of a second before the impulses are picked up by the AV node and passed on to the Bundle of His

In another tenth of a second, impulses from the AV node spread through the bundle of His, making the ventricles contract

Dangers to the Heart. High among our risky habits is smoking. Even an occasional cigarette puts a strain on the heart, and heavy smokers run a proven risk of heart disease. Smoking speeds up the heartbeat, raises blood pressure, and produces changes in the blood that may harm its oxygen-carrying capacity. Though not inhaling the smoke is certainly better than inhaling it, even pipe and cigar smoking carry a risk of cancer; so the best precaution is not to begin smoking at all. The next best course is to quit smoking as soon as possible. For help in giving up cigarettes, contact your local branch of the American Cancer Society or the American Heart Association.

Excessive coffee drinking (more than five cups a day) is another civilized habit that bodes ill for the heart. As a stimulant, coffee speeds up the rate of heartbeat, but there is also the possibility that a substance found in the coffee bean tends to increase the saturated fats in the blood. (For more information about smoking and coffee drinking, see Chapter 1.)

Drug abuse also affects the heart in dangerous and damaging ways. For example, sniffing glue for a "high" introduces a chemical into the bloodstream that reduces the rate of the heartbeat; collapse and sudden death have been known to occur as a result of this practice.

People who are overweight are continuously and unnecessarily taxing their hearts and substantially increasing their chances of developing heart disease. Increased blood pressure and blood-fat abnormalities often accompany weight problems, not to mention the anxieties and emotional problems that afflict overweight people.

Two pumps working as one

The heart is really two pumps lying side by side, and each has an upper and a lower chamber. Blood enters the upper chambers, and is pumped out of the lower ones. The two halves of the heart are separated by a wall of muscle.

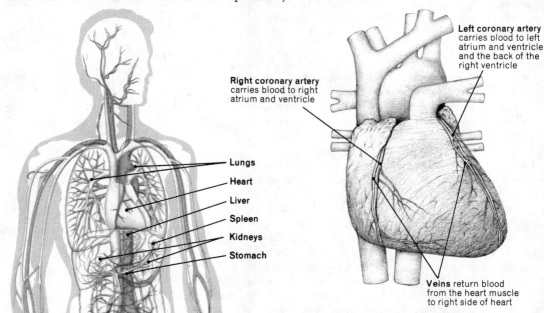

Left coronary artery carries blood to left atrium and ventricle and the back of the right ventricle

Right coronary artery carries blood to right atrium and ventricle

Lungs
Heart
Liver
Spleen
Kidneys
Stomach

Veins return blood from the heart muscle to right side of heart

What the heart does The heart lies in front of the lungs in the chest cavity, slightly to the left of the body, and protected by the surrounding rib cage. Without a continuous supply of blood, the body cannot function. To maintain this supply, the heart has to work nonstop, receiving deoxygenated blood on the right side and pumping it into the lungs to be oxygenated; oxygenated blood returns to the left side of the heart, which pumps it around the circulation.

The heart's own blood supply The heart is a muscle and needs its own supply of blood to keep it beating. This flows through a network of coronary arteries branching from the aorta. As a person grows older, blood may settle and clot in the hardened arteries, restricting the flow. Blockage of a coronary artery starves part of the heart muscle of blood and causes a form of heart attack, called coronary thrombosis. Blockage of a main artery may result in death.

The cause of obesity is not in the genes, but in eating habits developed in childhood, and these can be changed. (For information about a proper diet, see Chapter 2.)

Protecting Your Heart. Exercise is beneficial to the heart because it relaxes you and reduces the effect of the stresses and tensions endemic in modern life. Stress alone may not kill us, but financial worry, job pressure, and the continuous demands of family problems all increase our blood pressure. (See the entry HYPERTENSION in the encyclopedia section.) There is some evidence to suggest that overly ambitious and competitive people run a higher risk of heart disease than do easygoing types. Headaches, fatigue, and a noticeable decrease in sexual activity are early warnings of stress that should be controlled be-

fore they put their heavy hand on your heart.

Are some people more susceptible to heart disease than others? Statistics say yes. If other members of your family have died of heart attacks at an early age, or if they have a tendency to high blood pressure, gout, or diabetes, you should make your doctor aware of the facts. Your regular checkup should include an electrocardiogram (EKG), a painless test for measuring certain activities of the heart. Though not an all-inclusive diagnostic tool, periodic EKG's are useful in measuring some changes your heart may have undergone.

Every pain in the chest does not signal a heart attack. In rare cases a heart attack may occur without any pain. But anyone who experiences a brief, squeezing pain in the chest or down the left arm while exerting himself or after eating a

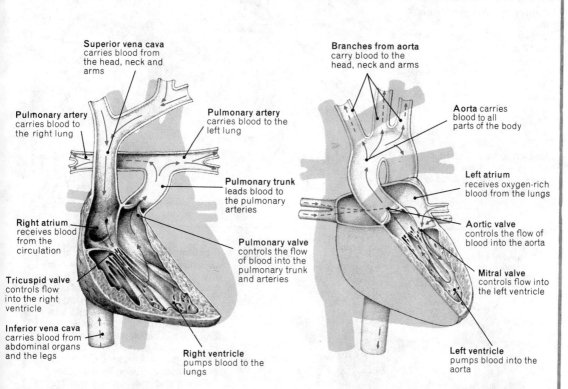

Superior vena cava carries blood from the head, neck and arms

Branches from aorta carry blood to the head, neck and arms

Pulmonary artery carries blood to the right lung

Pulmonary artery carries blood to the left lung

Aorta carries blood to all parts of the body

Pulmonary trunk leads blood to the pulmonary arteries

Left atrium receives oxygen-rich blood from the lungs

Right atrium receives blood from the circulation

Pulmonary valve controls the flow of blood into the pulmonary trunk and arteries

Aortic valve controls the flow of blood into the aorta

Mitral valve controls flow into the left ventricle

Tricuspid valve controls flow into the right ventricle

Inferior vena cava carries blood from abdominal organs and the legs

Right ventricle pumps blood to the lungs

Left ventricle pumps blood into the aorta

Incoming blood Deoxygenated blood flows into the right upper chamber (atrium), which is separated from the lower chamber (ventricle) by a one-way valve. When pressure in the atrium is greater than that in the ventricle, the leaves of the valve are pushed downward and blood flows through until the two pressures are equal. Contraction of the muscle surrounding the ventricle pumps the blood through the pulmonary valve along the pulmonary artery and to the lungs.

Outgoing blood Oxygenated blood flows from the lungs through pulmonary veins into the upper chamber on the left side of the heart. The greater pressure in the left atrium forces the blood through a one-way valve into the left ventricle below it. Muscle surrounding the ventricle contracts and pumps the blood through a valve into the aorta, to be circulated throughout the body and ultimately returned as deoxygenated blood to the right side of the heart.

How the lungs work

Breathing is controlled by changes in the volume of the chest cavity, brought about mainly by muscular movements of the diaphragm. Expansion and contraction of the lungs to fill the cavity result in lower and higher air pressures within them, which are equalized with the atmospheric pressure as air is forced into and out of the lungs.

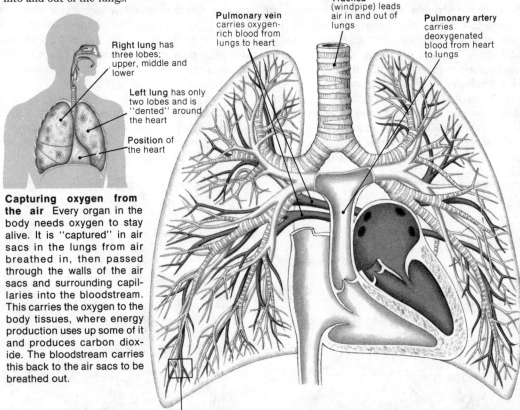

Right lung has three lobes; upper, middle and lower

Left lung has only two lobes and is "dented" around the heart

Position of the heart

Pulmonary vein carries oxygen-rich blood from lungs to heart

Trachea (windpipe) leads air in and out of lungs

Pulmonary artery carries deoxygenated blood from heart to lungs

Capturing oxygen from the air Every organ in the body needs oxygen to stay alive. It is "captured" in air sacs in the lungs from air breathed in, then passed through the walls of the air sacs and surrounding capillaries into the bloodstream. This carries the oxygen to the body tissues, where energy production uses up some of it and produces carbon dioxide. The bloodstream carries this back to the air sacs to be breathed out.

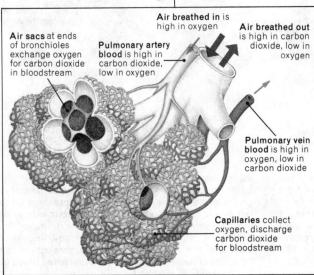

Air sacs at ends of bronchioles exchange oxygen for carbon dioxide in bloodstream

Pulmonary artery blood is high in carbon dioxide, low in oxygen

Air breathed in is high in oxygen

Air breathed out is high in carbon dioxide, low in oxygen

Pulmonary vein blood is high in oxygen, low in carbon dioxide

Capillaries collect oxygen, discharge carbon dioxide for bloodstream

Exchange of gases Respiratory passages in each lung terminate in minute air sacs called alveoli. These are in contact with a network of capillary blood vessels surrounding them. The different oxygen and carbon dioxide concentrations in the blood in the capillaries and in the air in the alveoli cause the two to exchange gases. Carbon dioxide, at a higher concentration in the blood, leaves it and enters the lungs. Oxygen, which initially has a higher concentration in the lungs, leaves them and enters the blood. In the blood, oxygen combines with the red coloring matter, hemoglobin, which transports it, pumped by the heart, to all the organs and tissues in the body.

heavy meal, should report it to his doctor. (See the entry ANGINA PECTORIS in the encyclopedia section.)

If any member of your family has a serious heart ailment, you should enroll in classes given by the American Red Cross in cardiac resuscitation, i.e., what to do if someone's heart stops beating. Many lives have been saved by quick administration of mouth-to-mouth resuscitation combined with heart massage. (These techniques are described in the FIRST AID section.)

The great enemies of your heart are the following illnesses: coronary heart disease, diabetes, hardening of the arteries, hypertension, hyperthyroidism, nephritis (or Bright's disease), rheumatic fever, and syphilis. (Refer to these entries in the encyclopedia section so that you will be alerted to their dangers and know what medical science has learned about their prevention and treatment.)

Lungs

The breath of life is the business of our two lungs. They supply the body with oxygen. The blood picks up in the lungs' capillaries the oxygen that the tissues must have and carries it in its red cells throughout the body. Carbon dioxide, which the tissues give off as a waste product, is carried back to the lungs and expelled. Like the heart, the lungs are completely encased by the ribs of the chest cavity, or thorax.

Protecting our lungs is harder in today's industrial world than it was in the past because the carbons and chemicals of the urban air enter our lungs and bloodstream. These pollutants are a major factor in the increase of respiratory diseases. Still, commonsense precautions will go a long way toward protecting the lungs.

Smoking is not only self-pollution; evidence exists that cigarettes also affect the air others breathe. Smoking is known to increase your chances of getting lung and throat cancer, emphysema, and heart disease. Even the milder forms of smoking—such as a pipe, whose smoke you do not inhale—bear the risk of tongue or mouth cancer. (See the entry SMOKING in the encyclopedia section, and the discussion of lung cancer in Chapter 22.)

If you work in any occupation where dust, gases, and smoke are inhaled, learn the medical risks involved with your job. Some industrial materials such as silica and asbestos cause irreversible damage to the lungs by the time any symptoms appear. (For further information about industrial disease, see Chapter 7.)

Lung infections that accompany a cold are usually thrown off easily. The cough, irritating as it is, is the lungs' way of ridding themselves of obstructive mucus, or sputum, and this serves a useful purpose. If a cough hangs on when you are otherwise well, however, or if you are suddenly short of breath, check with your doctor to determine the cause. (See the entry ASTHMA in the encyclopedia section.) A serious cold, if untreated, can develop into bronchitis, pneumonia, or influenza, which are particularly dangerous to the elderly. Pleurisy, an infection involving the pleura, the outer lining of the lung, can produce sharp pain when you inhale. (See also the entries on these diseases in the encyclopedia section.) For information on what to do in case of choking, consult the FIRST AID section.

Blood

Blood is the elixir of life. Its red color comes from the trillions of red cells in the blood that carry oxygen to the organs and tissues and remove the carbon dioxide from them. The white blood cells protect the body from infections by devouring dangerous bacteria. Tiny bodies called platelets help the blood to coagulate—that is, to form blood clots so that serious bleeding will not result from a cut or wound. All these cells speed about the body suspended in plasma, a clear liquid that conveys important enzymes, proteins, and hormones to all parts of the body and helps remove waste materials. The blood also serves as a thermostat, keeping temperature equal throughout the body.

The blood types, which are important where transfusions of whole blood (but not of plasma) are concerned, are not arranged according to race. The blood of a black or Chinese person may match that of a Scandinavian, for instance, while that of his own brother may not match. (See the entry BLOOD TYPE in the encyclopedia section.)

The lack of the Rh (rhesus) factor in the blood can cause incompatibility in case of a transfusion. About 15 percent of all people do not have this factor in their blood; they are called "Rh negatives" and should have transfusions of whole blood taken only from other Rh negatives. The baby of an Rh-negative mother and an Rh-positive father may (in about 4 percent of such cases) suffer from a blood disorder that was often fatal in the past but is now counteracted by transfusions of blood from an Rh-negative person. (For a fuller discussion, see the entry RH FACTOR in the encyclopedia section.)

Your blood does not need to be "purified," so

The blood flow around the body

The supply of blood, which is necessary for every organ and tissue to remain alive, is maintained by a continuous circulation through arteries, capillaries, and veins.

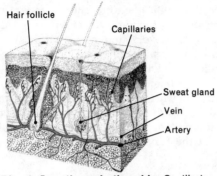

Hair follicle

Capillaries

Sweat gland

Vein

Artery

Blood flow through the skin Capillaries carry blood for the hair follicles and sweat glands. No blood vessels extend to the outer layers of skin, which consist of dead cells.

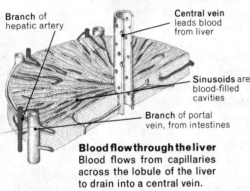

Branch of hepatic artery

Central vein leads blood from liver

Sinusoids are blood-filled cavities

Branch of portal vein, from intestines

Blood flow through the liver Blood flows from capillaries across the lobule of the liver to drain into a central vein.

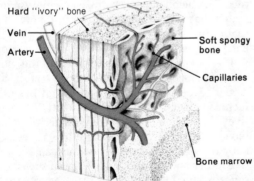

Hard "ivory" bone

Vein

Artery

Soft spongy bone

Capillaries

Bone marrow

Blood flow through the bones About 5 million red cells for the blood are made every second in the bone marrow and penetrate the thin walls of capillaries in the bones.

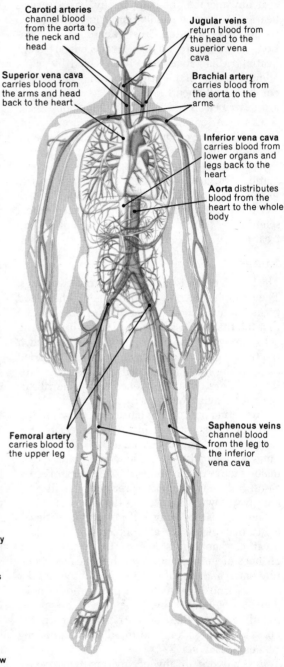

Carotid arteries channel blood from the aorta to the neck and head

Superior vena cava carries blood from the arms and head back to the heart

Jugular veins return blood from the head to the superior vena cava

Brachial artery carries blood from the aorta to the arms.

Inferior vena cava carries blood from lower organs and legs back to the heart

Aorta distributes blood from the heart to the whole body

Femoral artery carries blood to the upper leg

Saphenous veins channel blood from the leg to the inferior vena cava

From artery to vein The general flow of blood is from an artery, through arterioles to a set of capillaries, then through venules—which group to form veins—back to the heart. Exchanges of gases, food, and waste materials between the blood and body tissues take place through the walls of the capillaries.

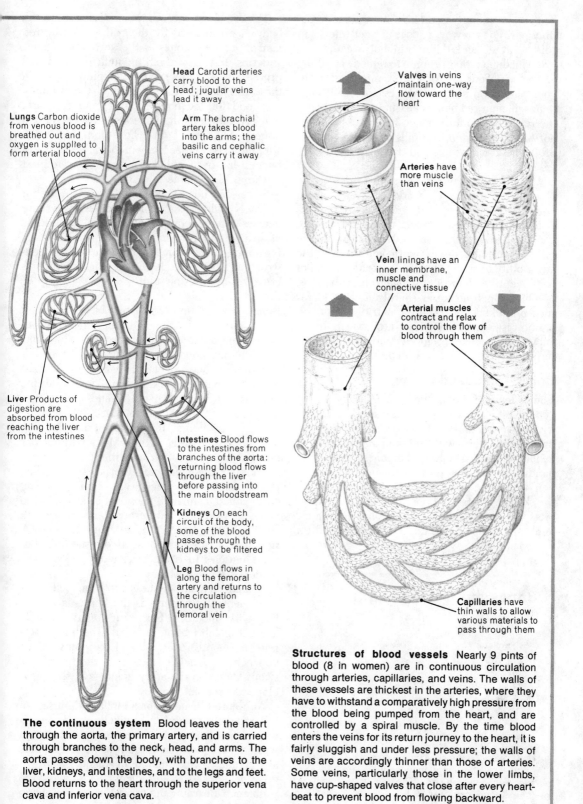

Head Carotid arteries carry blood to the head; jugular veins lead it away

Arm The brachial artery takes blood into the arms; the basilic and cephalic veins carry it away

Lungs Carbon dioxide from venous blood is breathed out and oxygen is supplied to form arterial blood

Liver Products of digestion are absorbed from blood reaching the liver from the intestines

Intestines Blood flows to the intestines from branches of the aorta: returning blood flows through the liver before passing into the main bloodstream

Kidneys On each circuit of the body, some of the blood passes through the kidneys to be filtered

Leg Blood flows in along the femoral artery and returns to the circulation through the femoral vein

Valves in veins maintain one-way flow toward the heart

Arteries have more muscle than veins

Vein linings have an inner membrane, muscle and connective tissue

Arterial muscles contract and relax to control the flow of blood through them

Capillaries have thin walls to allow various materials to pass through them

The continuous system Blood leaves the heart through the aorta, the primary artery, and is carried through branches to the neck, head, and arms. The aorta passes down the body, with branches to the liver, kidneys, and intestines, and to the legs and feet. Blood returns to the heart through the superior vena cava and inferior vena cava.

Structures of blood vessels Nearly 9 pints of blood (8 in women) are in continuous circulation through arteries, capillaries, and veins. The walls of these vessels are thickest in the arteries, where they have to withstand a comparatively high pressure from the blood being pumped from the heart, and are controlled by a spiral muscle. By the time blood enters the veins for its return journey to the heart, it is fairly sluggish and under less pressure; the walls of veins are accordingly thinner than those of arteries. Some veins, particularly those in the lower limbs, have cup-shaped valves that close after every heartbeat to prevent blood from flowing backward.

don't waste money on tonics that could not possibly purify it anyway. It does not get thicker in cold weather and thinner in hot weather, so avoid medicines that promise to remedy anything of the sort. Your doctor can examine a drop of your blood and find out whether or not it contains sufficient red blood cells and whether or not the red cells contain enough hemoglobin. So do not waste money on iron pills or tonics that you probably do not need—and that may upset your digestion.

All that a healthy person needs to do for the blood is to maintain an adequate diet, avoid poisonous substances, and guard against infections of the bloodstream. If you are a woman about 40 years of age who is taking contraceptive pills, you should discuss with your doctor the advisability of switching to a less chancy form of contraceptive; the risk of stroke from embolisms, or blood clots, increases sharply at age 40 for such pill-takers. (See also the entries EMBOLISM; BLOOD DISEASE; BLOOD POISONING; ANEMIA in the encyclopedia section; for a more detailed description of the blood, see BLOOD.)

Bones, Joints, and Ligaments

The skeleton of the upright human, composed of 206 bones in the adult, provides support, mobility, and protection for the vital organs. The spinal column, along with the skull and rib cage, is called the *axial* skeleton. The bones of the arms, hands, legs, and feet, plus the shoulder and pelvic bones, make up the *appendicular* skeleton. Just as the skull protects the brain, so the rib cage protects the lungs and heart. But the intricately jointed bones of hands and feet are devised for movement.

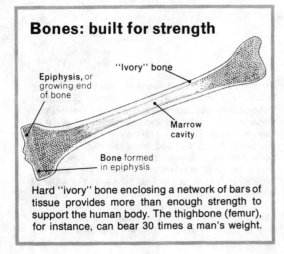

Bones: built for strength

Epiphysis, or growing end of bone

"Ivory" bone

Marrow cavity

Bone formed in epiphysis

Hard "ivory" bone enclosing a network of bars of tissue provides more than enough strength to support the human body. The thighbone (femur), for instance, can bear 30 times a man's weight.

The red blood cells, suppliers of oxygen to the body, are produced by the trillions in the red marrow of such bones as the vertebrae, femur, and ribs. If you are getting sufficient iron and proteins in your diet, you are helping to nourish these red blood cells. Vitamins of the B family are good for the bone marrow, and the hard, outer structure of the bones requires calcium, a mineral found in both whole and skim milk. Vitamin D is also necessary in the manufacture of bone; it has been added as a supplement to most of the milk available in stores.

Generally, bone is as strong as cast iron, but infinitely lighter and more flexible. Its rigidity enables us to bear our own weight, plus the stress of lifting and carrying. But the mechanically ingenious joints—some of ball-and-socket construction, others like levers or hinges—make us creatures of amazing agility.

Bone Connections. Ligaments, bands of tough tissue, connect the bones to one another when they come together to form a joint. The joints provide the smooth, gliding surfaces at the ends of bones so that movements can be carried out easily and painlessly. Nature provides a flexible material called cartilage for the ends of the bones involved in our bodily movements. This material decreases friction so that fingers, arms, and legs can move thousands of times daily without our being conscious of their activities.

To bind the bones together and strengthen joints, nature uses a special type of tough binding cords called ligaments. These are attached to the bones so well that only exceptional strains will tear the elastic ligament away from the bone. A similar type of tough connective tissue that connects muscles to bones is called a tendon, but tendons do not stretch.

A final element in the smooth and effective movement of our joints is the bursa—a sac, or bag, with smooth surfaces that contains a small amount of lubricating material. The bursas permit the smooth functioning of the joints. When you get housemaid's knee, it is the bursa that swells. (See also the entry BURSITIS in the encyclopedia section.)

An injured ligament or an inflamed bursa can be extremely painful. A strained joint is one in which the ligament has been severely stretched without being torn; in a sprain, some of the fibers are actually torn. Injured ligaments require a great deal of rest to help them heal, so avoid the problem by learning the correct use of your body in lifting and in strenuous sports. You can protect

The scaffolding of the body

The body owes its shape and support to the skeleton—a scaffolding consisting of hundreds of jointed bones. Contraction of muscles anchored to the bones brings about all bodily movements, such as grasping, carrying, bending, walking, and running.

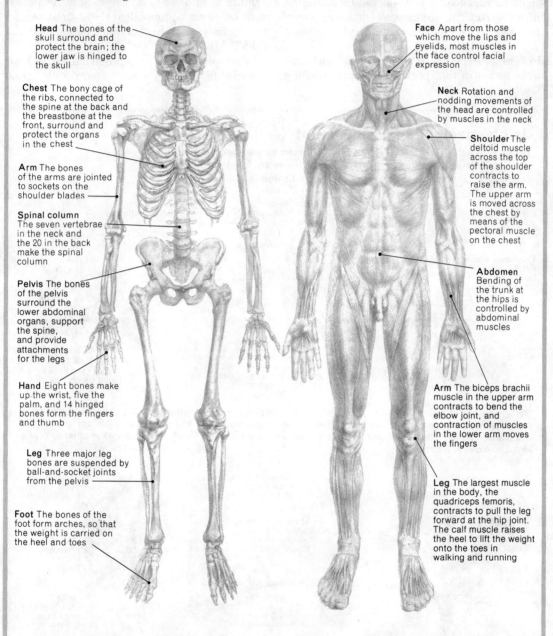

Head The bones of the skull surround and protect the brain; the lower jaw is hinged to the skull

Chest The bony cage of the ribs, connected to the spine at the back and the breastbone at the front, surround and protect the organs in the chest

Arm The bones of the arms are jointed to sockets on the shoulder blades

Spinal column The seven vertebrae in the neck and the 20 in the back make the spinal column

Pelvis The bones of the pelvis surround the lower abdominal organs, support the spine, and provide attachments for the legs

Hand Eight bones make up the wrist, five the palm, and 14 hinged bones form the fingers and thumb

Leg Three major leg bones are suspended by ball-and-socket joints from the pelvis

Foot The bones of the foot form arches, so that the weight is carried on the heel and toes

Face Apart from those which move the lips and eyelids, most muscles in the face control facial expression

Neck Rotation and nodding movements of the head are controlled by muscles in the neck

Shoulder The deltoid muscle across the top of the shoulder contracts to raise the arm. The upper arm is moved across the chest by means of the pectoral muscle on the chest

Abdomen Bending of the trunk at the hips is controlled by abdominal muscles

Arm The biceps brachii muscle in the upper arm contracts to bend the elbow joint, and contraction of muscles in the lower arm moves the fingers

Leg The largest muscle in the body, the quadriceps femoris, contracts to pull the leg forward at the hip joint. The calf muscle raises the heel to lift the weight onto the toes in walking and running

Bones More than 206 bones support the adult body and provide protection for organs such as the brain, heart, and lungs. They also store minerals necessary for the body, and make blood cells.

Muscles These provide about 42 percent of a man's weight and 36 percent of a woman's. All movement requires muscular contraction, which pulls one bone or set of bones toward another.

your joints from strain by practicing good posture and by keeping your weight down. Overweight people are constantly overloading the joints of the knees, feet, and spine. Unusual pain or inflammation or swelling in the joints can indicate a number of possible ailments and should be checked by your doctor. (See also the entries ARTHRITIS; BONE; BONE DISEASE; JOINT; LIGAMENT; SPRAIN in the encyclopedia section.)

How to Protect the Bones. A good diet and safety measures that prevent accidents provide the best protection you can give your bones and ligaments. Accidents do happen, however, and if the victim is suffering great pain or you notice a deformity of any injured part, it is possible that the bone is fractured. *Do not move a person if a fracture of the back or neck is suspected.* If the fracture is in a limb, however, and the person must be moved, immobilize the injured section with splints. (For further information, see the FIRST AID section.)

When properly set by a physician, bones have remarkable healing powers. As people grow

Joints: designed for movement

Rotating, hinging, and sliding movements between various bones are made possible by joints. The rubbing surfaces of the bones are lined with smooth cartilage, and the bones are held in position by ligaments.

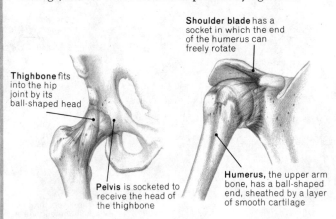

Shoulder blade has a socket in which the end of the humerus can freely rotate

Forearm bones, the ulna and radius, form a sliding joint with the bones of the wrist

Wrist is made up of eight small bones bound together by ligaments

Thighbone fits into the hip joint by its ball-shaped head

Pelvis is socketed to receive the head of the thighbone

Humerus, the upper arm bone, has a ball-shaped end, sheathed by a layer of smooth cartilage

Finger bones each have a hinged joint with bones of the wrist

Ball-and-socket swivel In this type of joint, the rounded end of one bone fits into a cupped depression in another to allow movement in any plane. The shoulder (right) and hip are examples: the arms and legs can move in a circle.

Sliding joint Jointed surfaces in the wrist and ankle are almost flat and slide over one another to give a range of movements.

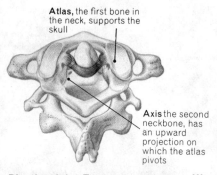

Atlas, the first bone in the neck, supports the skull

Humerus, the upper arm bone, hinges in a hollow at the end of the ulna

Lower arm bones, the radius and ulna complete the hinge joint at the elbow

Thighbone hinges against two semi-circles of cartilage in the knee joint

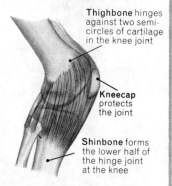

Kneecap protects the joint

Axis the second neckbone, has an upward projection on which the atlas pivots

Shinbone forms the lower half of the hinge joint at the knee

Pivoting joint The head can rotate from side to side or nod back and forth by means of the pivot joint in the neck.

Hinged joints In the elbow (left), knee (right) and fingers, the jointed ends of the bones glide face-to-face. They are connected by strong ligaments that prevent any sideways movement, and bending is in one plane only, with the joint bending like a hinge.

older, however, the bones become more brittle and heal less easily. For this reason, physicians fear certain fractures in the elderly more than in young people. A family with an older member should be especially cautious about icy steps, floor clutter, or anything else that could cause a fall. (For information about precautions against accidents in the home, see Chapter 21.)

Backache is so common that it could almost be considered one of the penalties we pay for walking upright. We are not personally responsible for our state of evolution, but when we put undue strain on out-of-condition muscles—such as by digging up the garden after spending a sedentary winter—we are tempting fate. Persistent backache should be treated with rest and a doctor's attention. You can help a strained back by sleeping on a hard bed and sitting in straight chairs only. (See also the entries BACKACHE; VERTEBRAL DISK in the encyclopedia section.)

Muscles and Tendons

Carrying out the enormous variety of the body's movements is the job of the muscles. Even when we stand perfectly still, muscles are at work supporting our weight and maintaining our balance. While we sleep the muscles of our internal organs continue their motions.

Those quick-acting muscles under our direct, conscious control are known as voluntary muscles. Under the microscope they appear as parallel bundles of long, striped fibers. Each fiber is about the thickness of a hair, yet it can support 1,000 times its own weight. Because this type of muscle tissue is usually attached to the bone, it is also called skeletal muscle. Many of the muscles, like the bones themselves, do double duty: they protect the nerves, blood vessels, and vital organs from blows, as well as move and support the various parts of the body.

There is another group of muscles in the body over which we have little or no conscious control: the involuntary muscles. They propel food along the intestine, control our breathing, direct the dilation and contraction of the eye's pupil, and perform many other automatic functions. The fibers of these smooth muscles are smaller and more delicate than those of the skeletal muscles, and their actions are controlled by a different part of the brain than that which governs the voluntary muscles.

Watch a child learning to write or a tennis player practicing his serve, and you realize how much of our pleasure and competence in life come from the conscious mastery of our volun-

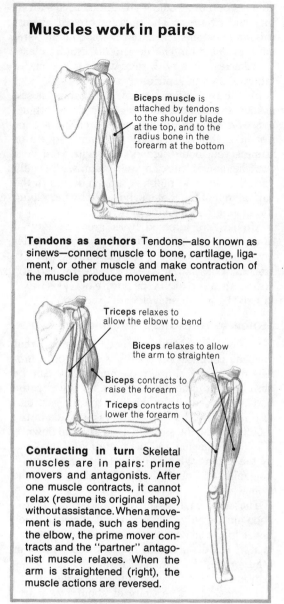

Muscles work in pairs

Biceps muscle is attached by tendons to the shoulder blade at the top, and to the radius bone in the forearm at the bottom

Tendons as anchors Tendons—also known as sinews—connect muscle to bone, cartilage, ligament, or other muscle and make contraction of the muscle produce movement.

Triceps relaxes to allow the elbow to bend

Biceps relaxes to allow the arm to straighten

Biceps contracts to raise the forearm

Triceps contracts to lower the forearm

Contracting in turn Skeletal muscles are in pairs: prime movers and antagonists. After one muscle contracts, it cannot relax (resume its original shape) without assistance. When a movement is made, such as bending the elbow, the prime mover contracts and the "partner" antagonist muscle relaxes. When the arm is straightened (right), the muscle actions are reversed.

tary muscles. Healthy muscles are important to our sense of well-being, our grace, coordination, and energy. But only properly exercised muscles stay in good condition; the reduced muscle tone that goes with a sedentary life can lead to poor circulation and a sense of physical depression. If muscles are not used at all because of prolonged bedrest or other immobilization, they become weak and atrophied. (For information on keeping muscles in good condition through exercise and sports, see Chapter 1.)

Almost everyone has experienced a charley horse. This results from too violent use of a muscle or group of muscles—for instance, in shoveling the first snow. The muscles protest against this unaccustomed activity by becoming sore, stiff, and painful. The discomfort usually clears up in a few days with rest, warm baths, and a tablet or two of aspirin.

Muscle twitchings result from various causes, usually minor ones such as temporary fatigue, overwork of a group of muscles, nervousness, or insomnia. If muscle twitches become frequent or painful, you should discuss them with your doctor. The same is true of muscle cramps, especially ones that occur at night. A sudden cramp in the calf or arch of the foot can be eased by massaging the muscle and walking slowly.

Muscles are affected by a great variety of disorders. (For more information about muscles and muscular disorders, see the entries MUSCLE; MUSCLE CONTRACTION; MUSCULAR DYSTROPHY; MYALGIA; MYASTHENIA GRAVIS; PARALYSIS; PARKINSONISM in the encyclopedia section.)

Stomach, Intestines, and Rectum

The fuel of the body is food. Digestion, that amazing chemical process by which food is broken down into simpler elements that can be absorbed into the bloodstream for use by the body, is carried out by the digestive, or gastrointestinal, tract. The first action takes place in the mouth, where the process of food breakdown is begun by chewing and the secretion of enzymes by the salivary glands. Food then passes down a long muscular tube called the esophagus into the stomach.

The stomach rests in the upper part of the abdominal cavity. Discomforts that occur much lower in the abdomen are not really "stomachaches," but disturbances felt in the intestines or other organs. The stomach is rather like a wineskin in shape and, when fully distended after a large meal, has a capacity of about $2\frac{1}{2}$ quarts.

The strong, muscular action of the stomach churns up the food and mixes it with digestive enzymes and acids that help break down food into forms that the body can absorb. Additional juices from the pancreas, liver, and gallbladder are mixed in when the food enters the duodenum, at the entry to the small intestine.

The small intestine is longer but narrower than the large intestine. It is in the small intestine that the useful proteins, carbohydrates, and fats, now converted to simpler substances, are absorbed through the intestinal walls into the bloodstream and lymphatic system. At the end of the small intestine about all that is left of the food is waste solids, which then pass through the large intestine and are eliminated.

Digestive Complaints. Hardly anyone has gotten through childhood, much less middle age, without discomfort of some kind in the digestive system. Even people who brag of having an "iron stomach" have trouble with their digestion at some time. The stomach is not made of iron, but it will function well if we treat it with respect. Hasty, inadequate meals, too many fatty foods, or tensions at the dinner table can lead to intestinal rebellion. Be careful about taking alcohol, coffee, or aspirin on an empty stomach; these often irritate the stomach lining and may create a preulcerous condition.

Indigestion and what is loosely called "heartburn" (an irritation of the lower esophagus) are not caused by an "acid stomach." Acid is a natural and necessary part of the stomach's digestive function; therefore, most "aids to digestion" and "stomach sweeteners" will do nothing to help and may do harm. However, if heartburn is fairly constant, see your doctor. The condition is sometimes a symptom of an ulcer.

Aids to Digestion. You can help the process of digestion by eating foods such as whole grains, green vegetables, and fruits that provide the "roughage" necessary for well-functioning bowels. Every individual has his own rate of elimination; for some it is an everyday affair, but for others who are equally healthy it may be twice a day or every other day. Fussing about the regularity of bowel movements is totally unnecessary and, in fact, may actually make constipation worse rather than cure it, especially in children. Likewise, enemas taken to "clean out the colon" can be both physically and psychologically harmful.

If constipation does occur, do not get into the habit of taking laxatives; their constant use may aggravate the condition by desensitizing the lining of the intestines. If you are occasionally constipated, it is safe to take mild laxatives such as one or two tablespoonfuls of milk of magnesia. (See the discussion of constipation in Chapter 24.) Acute constipation is often troublesome for the elderly, for women after childbirth, and for people with hemorrhoids, and should be treated by a doctor. In rare cases, an obstruction in the intestine may be responsible.

It must be remembered that indigestion is not a disease, but a condition or group of symptoms that can be caused by any number of actual diseases. Even a skilled physician often finds it a long and difficult task to determine the cause—and hence the treatment—of indigestion.

If a mildly upset stomach troubles you occasionally, you can try some of the following remedies at home: a level teaspoonful of bicarbonate of soda in a pleasant-tasting drink; a liquid antacid; or a pharmacist's preparation of rhubarb and soda. Constant and repetitive use of bicarbonate of soda, however, or of commercial antacid preparations that contain it, has a bad effect on people on salt-restricted diets. Furthermore, such dosing may obscure the real cause of the discomfort.

Be sure to see a doctor if you suffer persistently or repeatedly from any of the following symptoms: nausea, vomiting, excessive belching, fullness or burning sensation in the abdomen, cramps, indigestion, constipation, diarrhea. And also see your physician if you pass stools that are blood-streaked or unusually foul-smelling, or if your bowel habits change markedly for a prolonged period of time. (See also the entries COLON; INDIGESTION; INTESTINE; STOMACH in the encyclopedia section.)

Liver

If you place your left hand over the lowermost ribs on the right side of your chest, it will cover the liver, the largest internal organ in your body. The liver has about 500 known functions and perhaps more that are unknown. Products of digestion that are absorbed into the bloodstream from the stomach and intestines travel straight to the liver for further processing. The liver completes the transformation of sugars into glycogens for storage, breaks down proteins and synthesizes new ones, and stores vitamins. The liver also helps detoxify harmful substances in the blood. Bile, a greenish, bitter fluid that is extremely important to the digestion of fats, is produced by the liver.

A diet rich in proteins and carbohydrates is essential to the healthy functioning of the liver. In fact, in many countries malnutrition is one of the chief causes of liver ailments. In the United States alcoholism is the disease that most commonly threatens the liver. Heavy drinkers (who often do not eat properly) introduce so much alcohol into the bloodstream that the liver's tissues are hardened, a condition called cirrhosis of the liver.

If infection or some form of poisoning causes damage to the liver, a condition known as jaundice can develop. This results in a yellowing of the skin and the whites of the eyes owing to an excess of a substance found in bile. Jaundice is considered to be more of a sign than a disease; its presence may be the first indication that there is trouble with the liver. You should report the condition to your doctor immediately.

One infection that causes a jaundiced, or yellow, look is infectious hepatitis, one of the most common of all liver diseases. The virus is passed from person to person mainly through stools and urine, although dogs can also transmit hepatitis and travelers can contract it from contaminated water and food. A contaminated blood transfusion or an improperly sterilized hypodermic needle may also spread the disease, but the latter problem is being eliminated by the more widespread use of disposable needles.

If you think you have been directly exposed to a person with hepatitis, your doctor may recommend a shot of gamma globulin to boost your defenses against infection. If someone in your family should contract the disease, he need not be isolated, but scrupulous care should be taken about disposal of excreta and contaminated objects. Make sure the patient does not sneeze or cough directly on other people.

Liver problems often announce themselves by fever, vomiting, and a sudden change in the color of the stool. Either very black or oddly pale stools or unusually dark urine should be reported immediately to your doctor. (See also the entries HEPATITIS; JAUNDICE; LIVER in the encyclopedia section.)

Gallbladder

The gallbladder, a kind of pocket in the channel through which the bile flows from the liver into the intestine, acts as a storage place for the bile.

There is nothing you need to do about the everyday care of your gallbladder except to keep your weight normal. Obesity probably increases the tendency toward gallbladder disease. Women who have had several children are more likely to suffer from gallstones, in general, after their fortieth birthday. About twice as many women as men have this problem. Some people have gallstones and never know it, because the stones never move into a position to block a duct or cause irritation.

But if inflammation occurs, your doctor has ways of stimulating the flow of bile and of decreasing the infection in the gallbladder. In extreme cases, it is possible to remove the gallbladder entirely, for the body can function without it. Recently, tests in using drugs to dissolve gallstones have been successful, but the treatment is still in the experimental stage. (For a fuller discussion, see the entries GALLBLADDER; GALLSTONE in the encyclopedia section.)

Kidneys

The twin kidneys, together with the urinary bladder and the tubes leading to and from it, form the urinary tract. The kidneys, about the size of Idaho potatoes, are set on either side of the backbone, just above the hips. These remarkable organs filter about 15 gallons of blood per hour, eliminating from it waste products and excess water, as well as extra sodium (salt), potas-

sium, urea, and other substances. These rejects from the blood are deposited in the urinary bladder as urine. When a person drinks a large amount of fluid, the kidneys excrete the excess, but in hot weather, when extra fluid is lost by perspiration, the kidneys excrete relatively less. The kidneys also play a role in regulating blood pressure and producing red blood cells.

Despite ads for patent medicines, kidneys do not need to be "flushed" or "stimulated." To help your kidneys regulate the body's supply of fluids, simply drink the amount of liquids your thirst dictates. Less than a pint a day is too little. Go easy on coffee because its caffeine acts as a diu-

The kidney: system of a million filters

The kidneys have two functions: to remove waste products from the blood and to regulate the salt and liquid content of the body. Filtering is done through 1¼ million microscopic tubules in each kidney. About 2 pints of blood pass through the kidneys each minute; only a small fraction is purified, and it takes about 50 minutes for the whole of the body's blood volume to be cleansed. Excess water and the dissolved waste products are released and form urine, which is stored in the bladder.

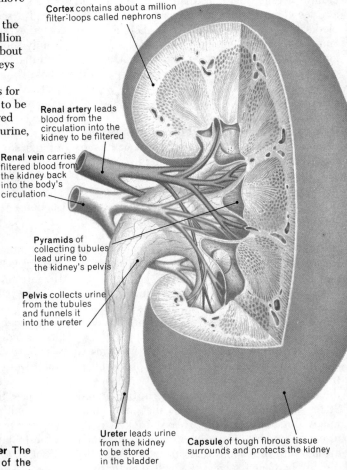

Cortex contains about a million filter-loops called nephrons

Renal artery leads blood from the circulation into the kidney to be filtered

Renal vein carries filtered blood from the kidney back into the body's circulation

Pyramids of collecting tubules lead urine to the kidney's pelvis

Pelvis collects urine from the tubules and funnels it into the ureter

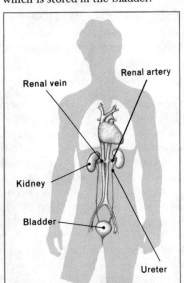

Renal artery

Renal vein

Kidney

Bladder

Ureter

Ureter leads urine from the kidney to be stored in the bladder

Capsule of tough fibrous tissue surrounds and protects the kidney

Position of the kidneys and bladder The kidneys lie high up towards the back of the abdomen, one on each side of the spinal column. A tube called the ureter connects each kidney with the bladder, where urine collects to be passed through the urethra.

retic, a substance that stimulates the kidneys to excrete more liquids than they ordinarily would. Controlling your coffee intake will help the kidneys to function more naturally. Remember that a urine test should be part of your regular checkup.

Like the gallbladder and urinary bladder, kidneys can develop hard stones that may cause blockage or pain. Do not take home remedies to dissolve them. One of the causes may be an untreated infection of the urinary tract that spreads upward, but people who are confined to bed or have infections elsewhere in the body also tend to develop stones. A stone trying to pass

down the urinary tract can cause extreme pain and obviously needs immediate attention. (See the entries KIDNEY; KIDNEY STONE in the encyclopedia section.)

The kidneys' location in the body makes them vulnerable to damage from accidents. Very high blood pressure, heart failure, and infections such as those caused by streptococci can also harm them. Great strides have been made in recent years, however, in helping people with kidney failure to lead almost normal lives. Surgically, kidney transplants have had considerable success, especially when the new kidney comes from someone in the immediate family. This transplant is possible for the donor because we can all live perfectly well with only one healthy kidney.

A substitute for surgery is dialysis, an expensive method by which a patient's blood supply is periodically filtered by a machine that removes the toxic waste products normally excreted by the kidneys. Dialysis is usually done in a hospital, although in some areas of the country a machine can be rented for use at home. The current development of cheaper, smaller machines may permit more patients to "wash their blood" at home. There is even hope that portable dialysis machines will soon be available. (For further information, see KIDNEY DISEASE; NEPHRITIS in the encyclopedia section.)

Urinary Bladder

Through two tubes called ureters, the urinary bladder receives waste products, including urea, from the kidneys. After a sufficient quantity has collected, it is eliminated by urination through the tube called the urethra.

Between the ages of two and five, the average child's urinary bladder doubles in size. At the same time, the natural process of maturation helps him gradually to gain control over the voluntary sphincter muscles that control urination. It is not unusual, however, for lack of control to persist beyond the fifth year, particularly in boys. Time and parental patience are the best cure, for additional anxiety only adds to a child's bedwetting difficulties. (See ENURESIS in the encyclopedia section.)

Infections and inflammations are fairly common in the urinary system, especially in the bladder. They are more common in women than in men. (See the entry CYSTITIS in the encyclopedia section.)

In older men, it is not unusual for an enlarged prostate gland to cause blockage of the urinary tract at some point. Incontinence, or the inability

Artery, a branch of the renal artery, carries incoming blood into the outer layer, or cortex, of the kidney

Arteriole is a small artery that takes blood to a single nephron

Glomerulus is a knot of capillary blood vessels from which water and chemicals pass into the tubule

Blood flow through the kidneys Blood enters the kidneys through the renal artery and then flows through fine capillaries into the tubules. Water and dissolved chemicals pass from the blood through the walls of capillary blood vessels into the cup-shaped Bowman's capsule and the looped kidney tubule. Farther along the tubule, chemicals needed by the body pass back into the capillaries. The filtered blood then joins the other blood in capillary veins.

to control urination, is common in elderly people, but it can occur as the result of an infection as well. Any pain, burning sensation, or difficulty in urinating requires the attention of a doctor.

Appendix

Near the juncture of the small intestine and the large intestine is a little, wormlike appendage called the vermiform appendix. This apparently useless structure, whose function may have disappeared during the course of evolution, can be a source of serious or even fatal illness. No age group is immune to it, but it seems to occur more frequently to children and young people than it does to mature men and women.

If your appendix is inflamed, the pain may not always be in the lower right portion of the abdomen; it may be felt in the area around the navel as well. Usually, the area of the appendix is tender when pressed. There may be fever and vomiting. If you suspect appendicitis, do not apply a hot water bottle or take medicines, especially laxatives, because you run the risk of rupturing the infected appendix. Call your doctor or go to the nearest emergency ward of a hospital as quickly as possible. (See also the entry APPENDIX in the encyclopedia section.)

THE EXTERNAL PARTS

This section discusses the following external organs of the body, which are more subject to injury and localized infection than are the internal ones:

Genitals (male)	Throat and tonsils
Genitals (female)	Larynx, trachea, and neck
Eyes	Feet
Ears	Skin
Nose	Hair and scalp
Lip, mouth, and tongue	Fingernails

Male Genitals

For a description of the male reproductive system, see the entry GENITALS in the encyclopedia section.

Is Circumcision Necessary? The foreskin (prepuce) of a boy covers the tip (glans) of the penis. In a newborn male, it is normally attached to the glans, and should not be drawn back, even for cleaning. Later the adhesions disappear.

Circumcision is a quick operation that removes the foreskin. If performed during the first weeks of a baby's life, the procedure is relatively simple and has no psychological effect on the child.

In most cases, there is no medical reason for circumcision. The presence of the foreskin in later life does not necessarily attract infection if good hygiene is maintained. But the operation is advisable if the foreskin covers the entire end of the penis so as to obstruct the passage of urine, or if it is so tight that irritation results. Circumcision can be performed later in life if it becomes medically necessary, but for a developing child or youth, the experience of the operation can be psychologically damaging. (For further discussion, see Chapter 14 and the encyclopedia entry CIRCUMCISION.)

Cleansing the Genitals. The genitals should be kept clean and free from infection. Uncircumcised males should pull back the foreskin and wash off any secretions with soap and water as frequently as required to keep the penis clean. The genitals should be protected from blows and other injuries during strenuous sports such as football. In hot weather, perspiration may cause sore spots from chafing, especially on the inner thigh. To avoid this, wash often and dust with pure talcum powder. (For further information about male genitals, see the entries GONORRHEA; SYPHILIS; VENEREAL DISEASE in the encyclopedia section.)

Female Genitals

The term "female genitals" usually refers to the external organs, or vulva, comprising the labia, the hymen, and the clitoris. (See the entry VULVA in the encyclopedia section.) For information on pregnancy and childbirth, see Chapter 13; infertility and sterility are discussed in Chapter 12 and in the entry STERILITY in the encyclopedia section; menstruation and the menopause are covered in Chapter 19.

Hygiene. Feminine hygiene does not require the taking of douches because nature has provided for the cleansing of the internal passages. Altogether too many women have been persuaded to take frequent douches of antiseptic solutions because of advertising claims that imply no woman can be dainty or clean without such cleansing. Actually, antiseptic douches may cause irritation if they destroy the vaginal bacteria, a natural and important part of the body's defenses. Similarly, vaginal deodorants serve no useful purpose at all and can cause irritation.

Should external or internal pads be used during the menstrual period? This depends entirely on individual choice; either method is safe.

Infections. Any unusual itching, soreness, or milky discharge may indicate an infection in the vaginal area. This is fairly common (especially following the use of antibiotics), and most such irritations can be promptly analyzed and treated by your doctor. (For more information, see the entries LEUKORRHEA; VAGINITIS; VENEREAL DISEASE in the encyclopedia section.)

Eyes

The eye is like a camera. The front part consists of the cornea—the transparent area in the center—surrounded by the sclera, as the white of the eye is called. Behind the cornea is the colored part, or iris, in the middle of which is the pupil, which, like a shutter, grows larger or smaller to control the amount of light let into the "camera." The clear, transparent lens, located slightly in back of the iris, focuses the image on the retina, which is about three-quarters of an inch behind the lens. The optic nerve carries the image from the retina to the brain. The eye also contains muscles to help do this work and different types of fluid to keep the parts in good working condi-

The structure of the eyeball

The eyeball is a nearly perfect sphere approximately an inch in diameter. It is set in a protective bony socket lined with fatty tissue, and it is controlled by three pairs of strong muscles. The main parts of its structure are three concentric layers: the sclera, the choroid, and the retina.

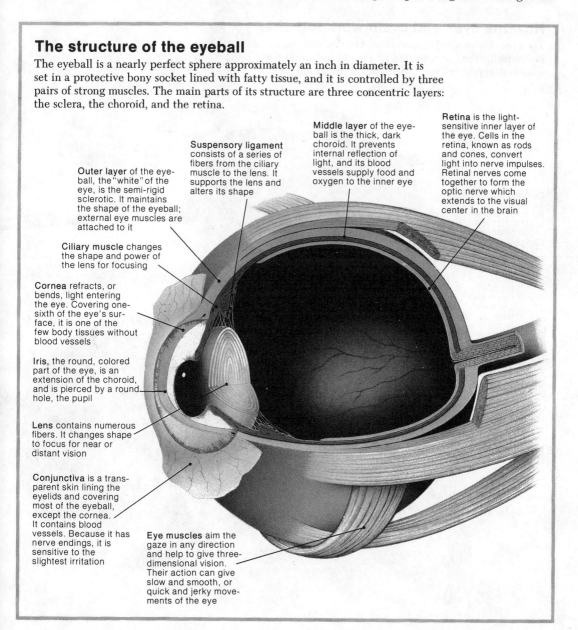

Outer layer of the eyeball, the "white" of the eye, is the semi-rigid sclerotic. It maintains the shape of the eyeball; external eye muscles are attached to it

Suspensory ligament consists of a series of fibers from the ciliary muscle to the lens. It supports the lens and alters its shape

Middle layer of the eyeball is the thick, dark choroid. It prevents internal reflection of light, and its blood vessels supply food and oxygen to the inner eye

Retina is the light-sensitive inner layer of the eye. Cells in the retina, known as rods and cones, convert light into nerve impulses. Retinal nerves come together to form the optic nerve which extends to the visual center in the brain

Ciliary muscle changes the shape and power of the lens for focusing

Cornea refracts, or bends, light entering the eye. Covering one-sixth of the eye's surface, it is one of the few body tissues without blood vessels

Iris, the round, colored part of the eye, is an extension of the choroid, and is pierced by a round hole, the pupil

Lens contains numerous fibers. It changes shape to focus for near or distant vision

Conjunctiva is a transparent skin lining the eyelids and covering most of the eyeball, except the cornea. It contains blood vessels. Because it has nerve endings, it is sensitive to the slightest irritation

Eye muscles aim the gaze in any direction and help to give three-dimensional vision. Their action can give slow and smooth, or quick and jerky movements of the eye

tion. (See also the entry EYE in the encyclopedia section.)

Most people consider blindness an affliction to be avoided at all costs. Yet an amazing number of individuals live with a partial loss or distortion of sight without being aware of it; they simply assume that the world is as they see it. If you have to hold this book close to your nose to make out the print, or are holding it at arm's length, the chances are that you should have your eyes examined. Even people who know they need their vision corrected put off an examination, perhaps because they don't like the idea of wearing glasses. Serious eye conditions have been neglected in this way, sometimes with tragic consequences. Yet the reward of a periodic eye checkup is often a brighter and clearer world.

Young children should have a vision test well before they start school, preferably by age three or four. There are ways of testing the eyesight of children who do not yet know their letters, so don't put off an eye examination simply because

How the eyes and brain work together

The eyes receive visual impressions, but the brain makes sense of them. Light rays entering the eye strike the retina and trigger off nerve impulses to the brain, which interprets, or "sees", them as a series of pictures.

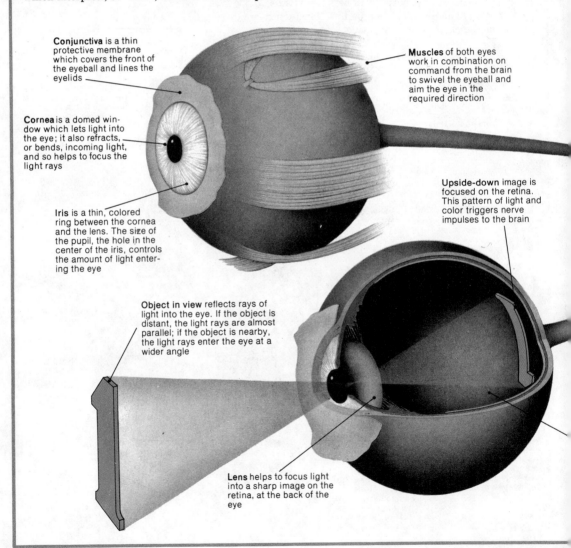

Conjunctiva is a thin protective membrane which covers the front of the eyeball and lines the eyelids

Cornea is a domed window which lets light into the eye; it also refracts, or bends, incoming light, and so helps to focus the light rays

Iris is a thin, colored ring between the cornea and the lens. The size of the pupil, the hole in the center of the iris, controls the amount of light entering the eye

Muscles of both eyes work in combination on command from the brain to swivel the eyeball and aim the eye in the required direction

Upside-down image is focused on the retina. This pattern of light and color triggers nerve impulses to the brain

Object in view reflects rays of light into the eye. If the object is distant, the light rays are almost parallel; if the object is nearby, the light rays enter the eye at a wider angle

Lens helps to focus light into a sharp image on the retina, at the back of the eye

your three-year-old has not yet mastered the alphabet. Usually a test can be done during the child's regular pediatric checkup. If an obvious eye problem is noticed—such as a turned or crossed eye, sties, inability to see in dim light, constant rubbing of the eye—the child should have immediate attention. The younger the child, the easier it is to reverse certain eye conditions. (For further information, see the entries AMBLYOPIA; GLAUCOMA; COLOR BLINDNESS; NIGHT BLINDNESS in the encyclopedia section.)

Remember that any sudden change in your vision needs looking into because it could be the symptom of an illness. But aside from the important periodic eye examination, what else can you do to protect your eyes?

Protect Against Injuries. The eyes are amazingly well protected by the bony forehead and cheekbones, and by the quick reflexes of the eyelids. Still, you cannot be too careful about guarding your eyes against accidents at home or at work.

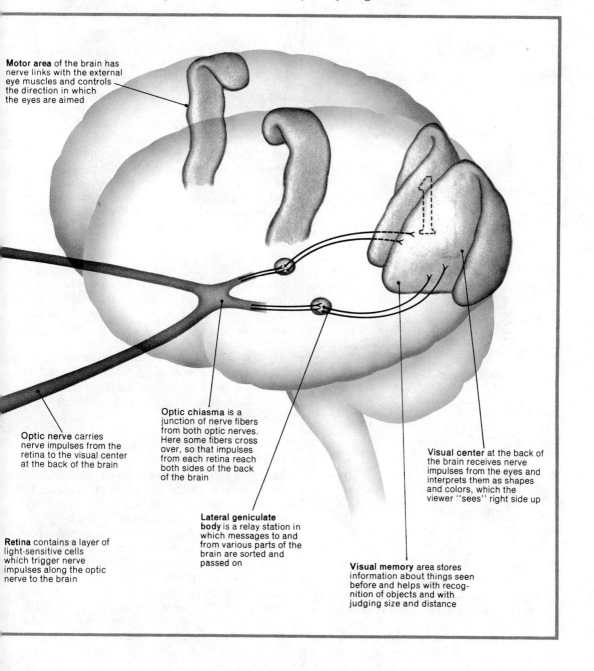

Motor area of the brain has nerve links with the external eye muscles and controls the direction in which the eyes are aimed

Optic nerve carries nerve impulses from the retina to the visual center at the back of the brain

Optic chiasma is a junction of nerve fibers from both optic nerves. Here some fibers cross over, so that impulses from each retina reach both sides of the back of the brain

Visual center at the back of the brain receives nerve impulses from the eyes and interprets them as shapes and colors, which the viewer "sees" right side up

Lateral geniculate body is a relay station in which messages to and from various parts of the brain are sorted and passed on

Retina contains a layer of light-sensitive cells which trigger nerve impulses along the optic nerve to the brain

Visual memory area stores information about things seen before and helps with recognition of objects and with judging size and distance

Eye movements

Two sets of muscles on each eye control eye movements. The contraction of two or more of them gives sideways, up-and-down, and rotating movements. Weakness in one or more muscles can cause strabismus, commonly known as cross-eye or wall-eye.

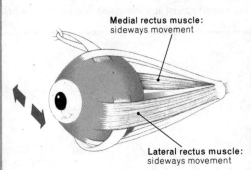

Medial rectus muscle:
sideways movement

Lateral rectus muscle:
sideways movement

Sideways movement The medial rectus and the lateral rectus muscles can move the eyeball only from side to side.

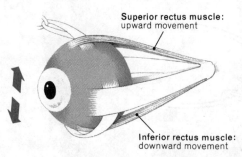

Superior rectus muscle:
upward movement

Inferior rectus muscle:
downward movement

Up-and-down movement Contractions mainly of the rectus muscles are used to make the eye move up and down.

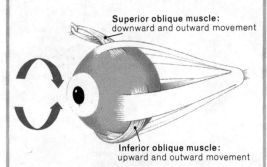

Superior oblique muscle:
downward and outward movement

Inferior oblique muscle:
upward and outward movement

Rotating movement Oblique muscles acting with one or more of the rectus muscles cause the eyes to roll.

Some of the chemicals most damaging to eyes are right under your kitchen sink. Be sure to read all the small-print precautions on cleaning and woodworking fluids, and never throw out the label; it may contain information important to the doctor in an emergency. If such fluids do get into your eye, immediately run as much water into the eye as you can. Speed in irrigating the eye after injury is extremely important to prevent damage. If there is redness and pain, keep up the irrigating process for at least half an hour. An injured eye should always be checked by a doctor.

Guard Against Infections. Many infections affect the eye, the most common of which is conjunctivitis, or pink eye, which is often contracted at public swimming places. Conjunctivitis is extremely contagious; so it is important that the sufferer does not share washcloths and towels with other people and that he wash his hands after touching his face. The symptoms of conjunctivitis—redness, sticky discharge—are similar to those of other types of eye infection, so do not attempt to treat the condition at home. A doctor can make a proper diagnosis and prescribe appropriate medication that will clear up the condition.

Women should avoid any eye cosmetics that claim to dye the lashes for longer than a day. Such eye makeup may be harmful. Mascara is usually harmless, however, unless you experience an adverse reaction to it; but all eye cosmetics should be washed off at night.

Prevent Eyestrain. Eyestrain is probably the most common eye complaint. Usually caused by overtiredness (from lack of sleep) or by glare (as from water or snow), such stress reddens the eyes and makes them smart.

Can drops help eyestrain? *No.* Popularly advertized preparations for "tired eyes" do nothing that your own natural tearing (which is slightly antiseptic) and a night's rest won't do better. You can take care of the symptoms of eyestrain by resting the eyes, or by putting a few drops of cold water (*not* boric acid solution) in the eye.

The best cure for eyestrain is to end the conditions that are causing it. Improper lighting, especially when reading or doing other close work, is a frequent cause of eyestrain, but it does not cause permanent damage to the eyes. Be sure that your light bulbs are strong enough (75 to 100 watts) to furnish proper lighting. Hold your book or paper about 16 to 18 inches away from your

How the eye focuses

Focusing involves bending light rays to make them converge on the retina. The cornea does some of this work, but fine adjustments are made by the lens, which changes shape. This pliability is controlled by the ciliary muscles. As a person gets older, the lens becomes less flexible, and some focusing power is lost.

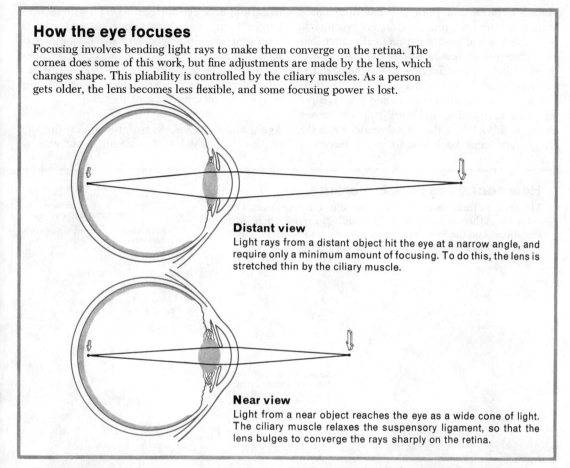

Distant view
Light rays from a distant object hit the eye at a narrow angle, and require only a minimum amount of focusing. To do this, the lens is stretched thin by the ciliary muscle.

Near view
Light from a near object reaches the eye as a wide cone of light. The ciliary muscle relaxes the suspensory ligament, so that the lens bulges to converge the rays sharply on the retina.

eyes and a little lower than eye level. Reading when you are lying on your back in bed or propped up on an elbow will strain your eyes, and so will reading for a long time in a moving train or car. Rest your eyes from time to time by looking off into the distance.

If you are in the bright sun, sunglasses will protect your eyes from glare. In selecting a pair of sunglasses, make sure they noticeably reduce the brilliance of bright sunlight. If you already wear ordinary glasses for reading and/or distance viewing, have a pair of sunglasses ground to your prescription rather than clip a pair of possibly inferior sun screens over your carefully made regular lenses. Remember, sunglasses *never* make it safe for you to look directly at the sun—even during an eclipse!

Movies and television can cause eyestrain if viewed for long periods. Looking at a flickery motion picture, sitting too far on the side of a theater, or watching television in too dark a room can tire your eyes. Children's television habits should be controlled so that they give their

eyes (and minds) a rest after about an hour of watching. Neither you nor they should sit too close to the television set; six feet is a minimum distance.

Eyeglasses. A most important source of eyestrain is in the eyes themselves. A large number of people are nearsighted, farsighted, or astigmatic—conditions usually caused by irregularities in the shape of the eyeball. Fortunately, these conditions are readily corrected by wearing the proper eyeglasses. Ideally, an ophthalmologist (eye specialist) should conduct the eye examination and make out your prescription for glasses. If an ophthalmologist is not available, a good optometrist can perform the same service. Do not buy "over-the-counter" glasses simply because they seem to fit your immediate needs and are less expensive; the cost to your eyes may be incalculable.

Athletes and people who find regular glasses inconvenient or object to them for cosmetic reasons now have an alternative—contact lenses.

Made of translucent plastic, these tiny lenses, ground to your own prescription, are worn right over the cornea, and are practically invisible. The closeness of the lenses to the eyes makes them actually more effective than regular glasses for some types of vision disorders.

Wearers of contact lenses should take scrupulous care in washing and sterilizing the lenses, and must follow their doctor's directions exactly. Great care must be taken to avoid infection, irritation, and eye fatigue. Wear the lenses no longer than your doctor suggests and consult with him as soon as you feel any discomfort or pain. It is necessary to return for a checkup every six months to a year. Contact lenses are not advised for people with corneal scratches and scarring or inflammation of the eyes.

Aging and the Eyes. As we grow older, the lens of the eye, which automatically contracts or

---

How sound reaches the brain

The ear is in three parts: the outer, middle, and inner ears. The outer ear gathers sound waves; the middle ear passes them on as vibrations; and the inner ear converts them into nerve impulses which the brain interprets and "hears" as a series of sounds.

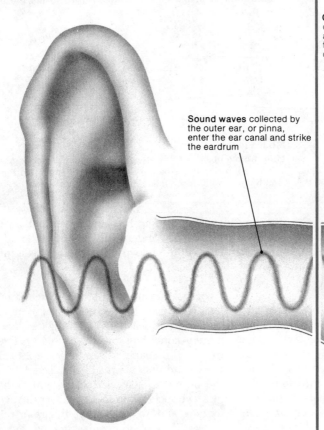

Sound waves collected by the outer ear, or pinna, enter the ear canal and strike the eardrum

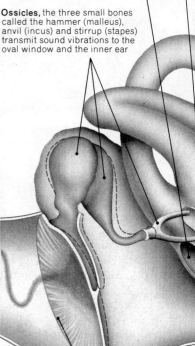

Oval window, pulsated by vibrations of the stirrup, presses on fluid in the coiled tubes of the cochlea

Round window expands outwards under internal pressure of the fluid in the cochlea

Ossicles, the three small bones called the hammer (malleus), anvil (incus) and stirrup (stapes) transmit sound vibrations to the oval window and the inner ear

Eardrum vibrates in step with the sound waves, and passes the vibrations on to three small interconnected bones in the middle ear

Outer ear
The outer ear consists of an external flap of cartilage called the pinna and the ear canal, which funnels sound waves on to the eardrum. The ear canal is about an inch long and is slightly arched in the middle. The entrance to the ear canal is guarded by a layer of wax, also known as cerumen, secreted by small glands in the wall of the canal. Hairs and wax trap any tiny particles of dust and dirt, preventing them from drifting along the canal towards the eardrum.

Middle ear
Vibrations of the eardrum are passed on by the three tiny bones of the middle ear—the hammer, anvil, and stirrup—to the oval window of the inner ear; these bones are also called the ossicles. The Eustachian tube leads to the back of the throat, where it is closed by a valve.

relaxes to adjust our focus, becomes less elastic. At age 45 the lens is only about half as elastic as it was at age 30. After 45, most people need reading glasses. The condition—known as presbyopia—is progressive; that is, it tends to get worse as age increases, so that the glasses may have to be changed every one to three years.

Glaucoma, one of the most widespread causes of blindness, particularly affects people over age 35. If you have glaucoma, or even a tendency toward it (your doctor can tell you), you should be aware that the use of antihistamines and certain sleeping pills or tranquilizers can be dangerous; many of these preparations contain ingredients that increase the pressure in the eyeball.

Ears

The ear is made up of three parts: the outer ear, the middle ear, and the inner ear. The part you see—the lobe and the ear canal—makes up the

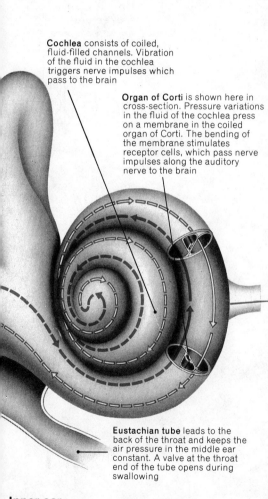

Cochlea consists of coiled, fluid-filled channels. Vibration of the fluid in the cochlea triggers nerve impulses which pass to the brain

Organ of Corti is shown here in cross-section. Pressure variations in the fluid of the cochlea press on a membrane in the coiled organ of Corti. The bending of the membrane stimulates receptor cells, which pass nerve impulses along the auditory nerve to the brain

Eustachian tube leads to the back of the throat and keeps the air pressure in the middle ear constant. A valve at the throat end of the tube opens during swallowing

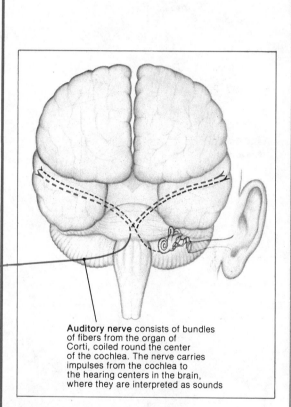

Auditory nerve consists of bundles of fibers from the organ of Corti, coiled round the center of the cochlea. The nerve carries impulses from the cochlea to the hearing centers in the brain, where they are interpreted as sounds

Inner ear

The inner ear consists of the cochlea and the auditory nerve. The cochlea contains three parallel channels of fluid, which are vibrated by the stirrup. Waves travel from the oval window along one channel around the coils of the cochlea, and return along another channel to the round window. Pressure changes in the fluid trigger impulses to the brain.

Brain

From the cochlea, impulses travel along the auditory nerve to the brain, which interprets them as sounds. The nerve leads to various parts of the hearing center: high notes end deep in the center, low notes are heard at the surface. Along the auditory pathway are junctions at which the brain stops unwanted sounds, and prevents very loud sounds from possibly damaging the ear.

How the ear balances the body

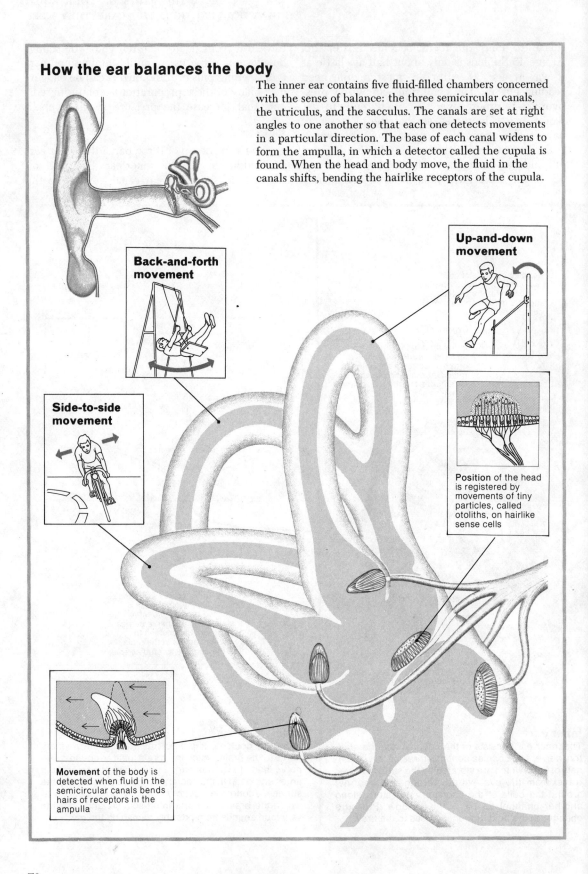

The inner ear contains five fluid-filled chambers concerned with the sense of balance: the three semicircular canals, the utriculus, and the sacculus. The canals are set at right angles to one another so that each one detects movements in a particular direction. The base of each canal widens to form the ampulla, in which a detector called the cupula is found. When the head and body move, the fluid in the canals shifts, bending the hairlike receptors of the cupula.

Up-and-down movement

Back-and-forth movement

Side-to-side movement

Position of the head is registered by movements of tiny particles, called otoliths, on hairlike sense cells

Movement of the body is detected when fluid in the semicircular canals bends hairs of receptors in the ampulla

outer ear. The canal leads to the eardrum and the *middle ear* in which lie the three tiny bones of hearing, called the hammer, anvil, and stirrup because of their resemblance to those objects. The middle ear is connected to the upper rear part of the throat by the Eustachian tube, and to the mastoid cells inside the temporal bone in the skull just behind the outer ear. The *inner ear* contains the semicircular canals, or labyrinth, which are essential to our sense of balance, and the cochlea, in which nerves analyze the sounds transmitted through the outer and middle ears and carry them to the brain. (For a fuller description, see the entries EAR; MOTION SICKNESS in the encyclopedia section.)

Infections of the Ear. Middle-ear infections do not usually come from outside, but from the nose and throat via the Eustachian tube. That is why inflamed tonsils and adenoids, a severe cold, sore throat, or sinusitis are usually accompanied by a sense of pressure or pain in the ears.

If the middle ear becomes seriously infected, hearing may be threatened. Children are especially susceptible to middle-ear infections. Since the development of antibiotics, however, middle-ear infections can usually be controlled and mastoiditis prevented.

Infections of the outer ear involving the lining of the auditory canal are common. They may be caused by fungi or by germs, resulting in boils on the canal. Eczema frequently affects this area. If these exterior infections are ignored, they may travel inward and involve the eardrum and the middle ear.

Infections that injure the hearing can also be caused by foreign objects, such as beads or pencil erasers, which very young children sometimes push into the ear canal. Adults can cause similar trouble by cleaning their ears with hairpins, matchsticks, or other long, pointed objects. Follow this rule for cleaning the ear canal: what you cannot remove with your little finger (which has been thoroughly cleaned with soap and water) should be attended to by a doctor or a nurse at an ear clinic.

Anyone with an infection in the nose, sinuses, or throat should not go swimming, lest the infection spread to the ear. If you have a perforated eardrum, get your doctor's permission before swimming. (See also the entries EARACHE; EARDRUM in the encyclopedia section.)

Deafness. Infections are not the only cause of deafness. The changes of old age may gradually bring on deafness, which in many cases can be somewhat relieved by a doctor. Old people who can hear some sounds perfectly well but others not at all are suffering from a selective deafness in certain frequencies.

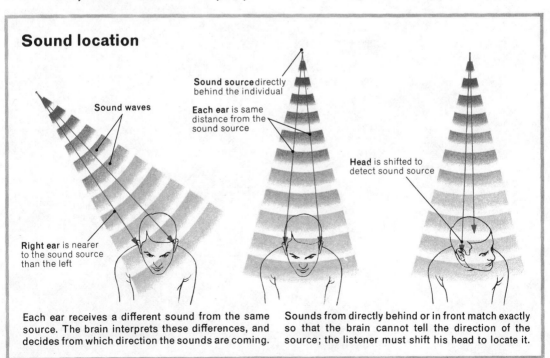

Sound location

Sound waves

Sound source directly behind the individual

Each ear is same distance from the sound source

Head is shifted to detect sound source

Right ear is nearer to the sound source than the left

Each ear receives a different sound from the same source. The brain interprets these differences, and decides from which direction the sounds are coming.

Sounds from directly behind or in front match exactly so that the brain cannot tell the direction of the source; the listener must shift his head to locate it.

A few types of deafness cannot be helped much by hearing aids, but many more can. Electronic transistors permit the creation of extremely effective, small hearing instruments. But make sure that a doctor, not a salesman, helps you choose the right kind of hearing aid. See if you can try the hearing aid at home for a while before committing yourself to a purchase; only you can tell how helpful the instrument is for hearing all kinds of sounds.

The general noise level of our world has risen so much in modern times as to be considered a disease factor in itself. Most adults who have been in the army, live in cities, or have subjected themselves to the intense decibles of rock music, suffer some hearing impairment, whether they know it or not. Protect yourself from loud noises by covering your ears or turning down the volume on the radio or record player. If noise is unavoidable, such as on the job, wear earmuffs.

The most important thing you can do to prevent deafness is to have the hearing of all members of the family tested regularly. See a doctor the minute you or your child feels any ear pain, has a discharge from the ear, complains of any unusual buzzing, ringing, or pressure in the ears,

The nose and the sense of smell

At the roof of the nose are two patches of receptors that make up the sense of smell. They consist of thousands of sensory hairs, embedded in a layer of mucus. Molecules of substances are drawn in through the nose, and circulate over these hairs. Some molecules dissolve in the mucus, causing olfactory hairs to send signals to the olfactory bulbs and the brain.

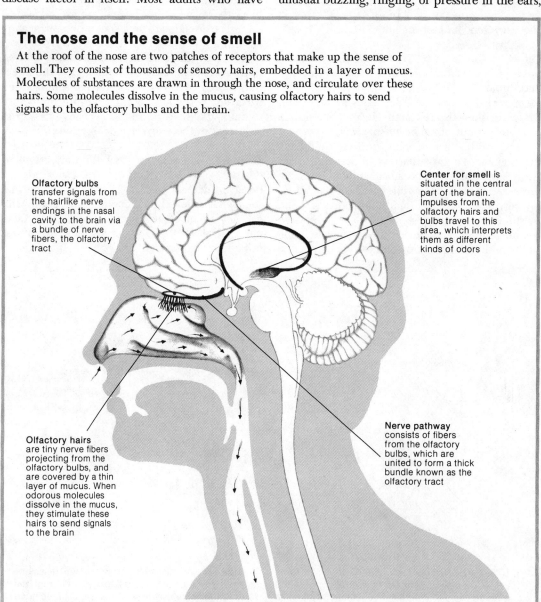

Olfactory bulbs transfer signals from the hairlike nerve endings in the nasal cavity to the brain via a bundle of nerve fibers, the olfactory tract

Center for smell is situated in the central part of the brain. Impulses from the olfactory hairs and bulbs travel to this area, which interprets them as different kinds of odors

Olfactory hairs are tiny nerve fibers projecting from the olfactory bulbs, and are covered by a thin layer of mucus. When odorous molecules dissolve in the mucus, they stimulate these hairs to send signals to the brain

Nerve pathway consists of fibers from the olfactory bulbs, which are united to form a thick bundle known as the olfactory tract

The threshold of smell

The ability to smell a particular substance depends on the concentration of it present in the air. The minimum amount that can be detected is known as the threshold of smell. The table shows the thresholds for six substances in a large room of 35,000 cubic feet. These thresholds vary according to circumstances; a rise in temperature raises the thresholds at which perfumes can be detected, and moist air intensifies all smells.

Amount of substance present in a large room of 35,000 cubic feet in volume (approximately 70 ft by 50 ft by 10 ft high):

Source of smell	Active principle	Minimum concentration (mg/1000 cu meters)
Vanilla	Vanillin	0·0002
Feces	Skatole	0·0004
Rotten cabbage	Mercaptan	0·04
Rancid butter	Butyric acid	1·0
Musk ox	Musk	7·0
Coal tar	Phenol	1200·0

or experiences any loss of hearing. (See also the entries DEAFNESS; HEARING in the encyclopedia section.)

Nose

The nose with its bones, cartilage, nerves, mucous membranes, and glands that secrete a watery fluid, is the organ of smell. Even more important, it is the means by which we take air into our bodies. We can—and some people do—breathe through the mouth, but the nose is a far better ventilator. It filters out dust, provides moisture, and acts as an air conditioner by warming the air we take in. (See also the entry NOSE in the encyclopedia section.)

Infections of the Nose. The most prevalent disease of the nose is also the most widespread disease in the world—the common cold. (For a discussion of this ailment, see the entry COMMON COLD in the encyclopedia section; other conditions causing congestion of the nose are discussed in the entries ADENOID; ALLERGY; HAY FEVER; RHINITIS; SINUSITIS.)

Ozena is a severe form of chronic infection of the nose and is characterized by an unpleasant odor. A persistent, foul-smelling discharge in children is usually caused by a foreign object, such as a bean or a small stone, that has become lodged deep in the nasal passage. Always have a doctor remove such an object.

Nosebleed. Nosebleeds are common, especially in children, and are usually harmless. But a nosebleed in an elderly person may be more serious. (See the entry NOSEBLEED in the encyclopedia section; for instructions on how to stop a nosebleed, consult the FIRST AID section.)

Caring for the Nose. Your nose needs little regular care. The dryness of many houses and apartments in winter tends to dry out the protective membranes of the nose. This irritation can be avoided by adding moisture to the atmosphere of your home with humidifiers or pans of water placed over heating grates or on radiators.

Do *not* use nose drops, sprays, or "sniffers" unless your doctor tells you to. They cure nothing and may cause irritation or injury. Do not pick your nose or pull out the hairs; unsightly nose hairs are best controlled by trimming carefully with a small scissors with blunted points.

For information on how to relieve nasal congestion in an infant, see the section on colds in Chapter 16.

Lips, Mouth, and Tongue

Most diseases and sores of the lips, tongue, and mouth are either very minor or very serious. The slight cracks from dried-out lips heal readily, and the irritating lumpy spots in the mouth called cankers disappear quickly. But other whitish spots, lumps, or sores may indicate early stages of cancer, or they may be signs of syphilis or some other serious disease. You can usually tell the mild from the serious conditions by the rapidity with which they heal. Any canker or fever sore or a lump that does not heal readily should be seen by a doctor. Pipe smokers should take special care to check out any irritation of the lips or the mouth, since pipe smoking can cause cancer.

Trench mouth (Vincent's angina) is a common infection characterized by sores and ulcers on the lining of the cheeks, the gums, and the back of the throat, but similar symptoms may be caused by other conditions. (See the entries VINCENT'S ANGINA; STOMATITIS in the encyclopedia section.)

Most lipsticks are harmless unless you happen to have an allergic reaction to them. Cracked, chapped, or sunburned lips will usually get better if you apply a soothing ointment such as petroleum jelly or cold cream.

The four basic tastes

There are four basic tastes—sweet, sour, salt, and bitter—and every taste sensation is made up of a combination of these aided by the sense of smell. The receptors of taste, the taste buds, are grouped on the surface of the tongue.

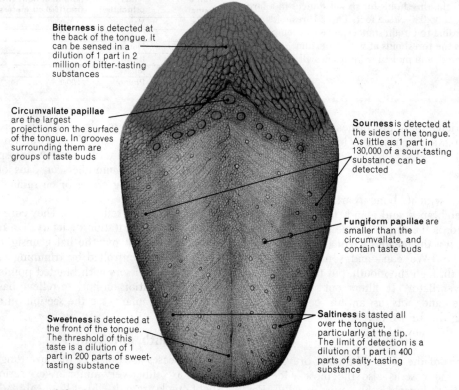

Bitterness is detected at the back of the tongue. It can be sensed in a dilution of 1 part in 2 million of bitter-tasting substances

Circumvallate papillae are the largest projections on the surface of the tongue. In grooves surrounding them are groups of taste buds

Sourness is detected at the sides of the tongue. As little as 1 part in 130,000 of a sour-tasting substance can be detected

Fungiform papillae are smaller than the circumvallate, and contain taste buds

Sweetness is detected at the front of the tongue. The threshold of this taste is a dilution of 1 part in 200 parts of sweet-tasting substance

Saltiness is tasted all over the tongue, particularly at the tip. The limit of detection is a dilution of 1 part in 400 parts of salty-tasting substance

Taste areas of the tongue

This muscular organ is covered with small humps, called papillae, which are surrounded by trenches. In the lining of some of these trenches are the openings of the taste buds. Each flask-shaped taste bud contains hairlike cells which project through its opening, and fibers which are attached to one of two major nerves leading to the brain. The tongue is sensitive to heat, cold, and touch, but only certain parts can detect specific tastes. This is due to the way in which the taste buds are distributed. For example, the bitterness of coffee can be tasted only at the back of the tongue, where the receptors are sensitive to this taste.

Your mouth does not need mouthwashes that claim to cure bad breath. Repeated use of antiseptic mouthwashes may damage the protective bacteria of the mouth; and chronic bad breath usually has a medical reason, such as infected teeth or gums. (See also the entry HALITOSIS in the encyclopedia section.)

Throat and Tonsils

For descriptions of the THROAT and the TONSILS, see those entries in the encyclopedia section.

Like your nose and mouth, your throat does not need sprays, gargles, or lozenges to keep it healthy. Avoid them because their regular use may cause irritation.

Sore throats are almost as common as colds, because a certain amount of inflammation in the throat usually results from the cold itself. A sore throat may also be caused by excessive smoking. If cutting down on your smoking and gargling every two or three hours with a third of a glassful of warm water containing two crushed aspirin tablets does not bring relief in a few days, visit your doctor or a hospital clinic. Serious conditions may begin with a sore throat.

Cancer of the lip, mouth, throat, and tongue are definitely connected with smoking, especially heavy smoking. Smokers should be alert to sores in these areas and should have any stubborn irritation checked at once by a doctor.

Taste messages to the brain

The sense of taste starts working when food is moistened in the mouth and shaped into a round bolus which can be swallowed. Food in solution stimulates the taste buds. Those at the front and the middle of the tongue send messages to the brain along the lingual nerve; those at the back of the tongue use the glossopharyngeal nerve. The brain sorts out these signals and identifies them as different tastes. Smell also aids the sense of taste. Food aromas pass into the nasal cavity and excite the olfactory sense.

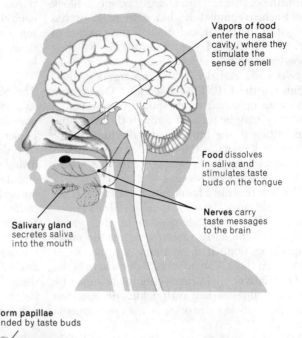

Vapors of food enter the nasal cavity, where they stimulate the sense of smell

Food dissolves in saliva and stimulates taste buds on the tongue

Nerves carry taste messages to the brain

Salivary gland secretes saliva into the mouth

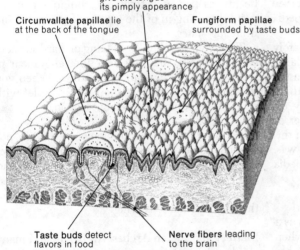

Filiform papillae give the tongue its pimply appearance

Circumvallate papillae lie at the back of the tongue

Fungiform papillae surrounded by taste buds

Taste buds detect flavors in food

Nerve fibers leading to the brain

The surface of the tongue

On the surface of the tongue are three different types of pimplelike projections called papillae. At the front are the most plentiful, the filiform; these give the tongue its furred appearance. Concentrated in the center of the tongue are the large fungiform papillae. At the back are eight or 10 papillae, known as the circumvallate, which are moundlike projections. Food particles dissolved in saliva flow into grooves around the papillae, which contain clusters of taste buds.

An acutely sore throat accompanied by a fever in either an adult or a child may mean trouble. It is an early symptom of the following diseases, which are discussed in the encyclopedia section: DIPHTHERIA, SCARLET FEVER, STREP THROAT, and TONSILLITIS. (See also the entry SORE THROAT in the encyclopedia section.)

Larynx, Trachea, and Neck

The larynx, which projects itself on the outside of the body as the Adam's apple, is part of the breathing apparatus. Its main function, however, is to act as a voice box in producing sounds.

Hoarseness is a sign that something may be wrong with your larynx. Naturally, if you have been shouting and cheering at a football game the day before, the reason is obvious. But if hoarseness or a change in your voice comes on without apparent cause and lasts longer than a few days, it may indicate a tumor, tuberculosis, or some other potentially serious condition of the larynx. Immediate attention is essential. See your doctor or the throat specialist he recommends without delay.

The trachea is the windpipe through which air enters and leaves the lungs. It is connected with the throat by way of the larynx. Although the trachea is protected by a lid (the epiglottis), food particles sometimes get into it; most of us have, on occasion, swallowed something the "wrong way." People, children particularly, have choked to death because an object, large enough to block the trachea completely, has entered it or has lodged in the throat and shut off the passage of air. This is one of the situations in which a knowledge of first aid can mean the difference between life and death. (For emergency treatment, see the FIRST AID section.) One reason why nose or throat drops should be avoided is that they may be inhaled through the windpipe and irritate it, the bronchi, and the lungs.

The neck contains the thyroid gland, which is discussed more fully in the entry THYROID GLAND in the encyclopedia section.

You are probably familiar with a fairly common condition of the neck, usually called swollen glands. This is an enlargement of the lymph nodes. (See the entry LYMPH NODE in the encyclopedia section.) If these glands are painful, it means that there is an infection somewhere in the head. Relatively painless swollen glands may be caused by illnesses such as Hodgkin's disease. (See the entry HODGKIN'S DISEASE in the encyclopedia section.)

Make it a rule to see a doctor immediately whenever a swelling occurs in any of the glands of the throat. Let him know if you notice unusual lumps of any kind. They may not mean anything serious, but the cause must be satisfactorily established. A stiff neck accompanied by fever or nausea may be a symptom of polio, although this disease is much less common than it once was. (See the entry STIFF NECK in the encyclopedia section.)

Feet

The feet are intricately designed to act both as a lever (when we move) and as a pedestal (when we stand). The anatomy of the human foot has changed hardly at all from the time of our most primitive ancestors; what has changed is the way we use our feet. We walk and run less. Moreover, we subject the bones and muscles of the feet to the strains of high heels and poorly fitting shoes. No wonder that so many middle-aged and elderly people suffer from foot problems.

Our feet perspire freely, and when they are enclosed for long periods in nonporous footwear—such as vinyl boots or shoes—the perspiration cannot evaporate. Peeling or cracking of the sole along the creases is a result of this overly humid condition. It is important to wash your feet daily, wear clean socks or stockings, and give your feet some time in the air. Cut toenails every one to two weeks. If hot weather tends to make your feet and ankles swell, wear comfortable, porous shoes, and prop your feet up for a rest each day. If the swelling is marked or persistent, see your doctor, because this condition is sometimes a symptom of disease in another part of the body.

The Shoes You Wear. Heels much higher than two inches tend to tilt the body forward, demanding a compensatory curving of the spine. Backache, foot pain, and foot deformities can be traced to prolonged use of high heels. But ill-fitting shoes, which cramp the toes or restrict the circulation, are perhaps worse. If your foot is normal, choose a flexible shoe with rounded, rather than pointed, toes and a straight inner border. A good-fitting shoe is about three-quarters to one inch longer than the foot by outside measurement, and it should fit well around the ankle and instep. A loose shoe, in which your foot slides forward enough to compress the toes, can be just as bad as a tight one. Bunions and the painful turning-in of the big toes can result from ill-fitting shoes.

Too much standing or walking on hard surfaces can cause footache, and poor foot alignment in standing or walking can cause strain. When you stand or walk, your feet should be parallel with each other, toeing neither out nor in.

Foot Troubles. If you think your feet are not normal, do not buy any kind of "remedial" shoes or get arch supports without consulting a doctor. You may be "correcting" the wrong thing; your troubles may be caused by something other than the shoes you are wearing.

Flatfeet and Fallen Arches. All babies and many children have the appearance of flatfeet because their developing arches are hidden in pads of fat. Even in adults, flatfeet need be no problem, as long as the feet are strong. If you are overweight, however, you are putting an unnecessary strain on the arches and muscles of your feet. Don't decide with the help of a shoe salesman that either flatfeet or fallen arches are your trouble; only a doctor can diagnose such conditions properly. (See also the entries FALLEN ARCH; FLATFOOT in the encyclopedia section.)

Corns and Calluses. A callus is a thickening or overgrowth of the skin in areas subjected to intermittent pressure. A corn is one type of callus that most often afflicts the toes of a person whose shoes pinch. These growths can be painful and

Feet

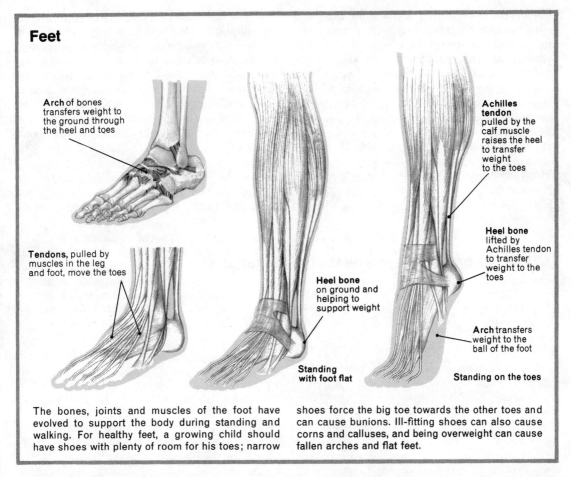

Arch of bones transfers weight to the ground through the heel and toes

Tendons, pulled by muscles in the leg and foot, move the toes

Achilles tendon pulled by the calf muscle raises the heel to transfer weight to the toes

Heel bone lifted by Achilles tendon to transfer weight to the toes

Heel bone on ground and helping to support weight

Arch transfers weight to the ball of the foot

Standing with foot flat

Standing on the toes

The bones, joints and muscles of the foot have evolved to support the body during standing and walking. For healthy feet, a growing child should have shoes with plenty of room for his toes; narrow shoes force the big toe towards the other toes and can cause bunions. Ill-fitting shoes can also cause corns and calluses, and being overweight can cause fallen arches and flat feet.

unsightly, and the best way to avoid or cure them is to purchase and wear better-fitting shoes. (See also the entries CORN; CALLUS in the encyclopedia section.)

Ingrown Toenails. This painful condition often occurs when shoes are so tight that they cause pressure on the sides and top of the toe, and the edge of the nail begins to cut into surrounding skin and tissue. A chronic inflammation can result. Cutting the toenail straight across, with the edges a bit longer than the middle, will help prevent it. (See also INGROWN TOENAIL in the encyclopedia section.)

Bunions. A bunion is a deformity of the big toe, almost always caused by wearing shoes that force it to turn in toward the other toes. It is frequently associated with flat or weak feet. In mild cases, the pain can be relieved by heat, and the condition will correct itself after properly fitting shoes have been worn for some time. In more severe cases, a physician should be consulted; a surgical operation may be necessary to correct the condition. (See also the entry BUNION in the encyclopedia section.)

Athlete's Foot (Dermatophytosis). This condition occurs when sweaty, damp feet become infected with a fungus. Usually there is itching and cracking between the toes, peeling, and sometimes raw blisters. It is a very annoying condition that can best be prevented by keeping the feet washed and by dusting a little talcum powder between the toes to absorb dampness. Cotton socks absorb perspiration better than wool or synthetics. Do not go barefoot in public bathing places or locker rooms where the fungus most often thrives. In summer, when the irritation is most likely to worsen, wear well-ventilated sandals or light, porous shoes. (For treatment of ATHLETE'S FOOT, see the entry in the encyclopedia section.)

Skin

As the largest organ of the body, the skin's most obvious function is to serve as a covering that protects the body against germs, cold, heat, and injury. Beyond that, our skin helps regulate the body's temperature by the evaporation of perspiration and by contracting or relaxing the superficial blood vessels to conserve or release heat.

A major organ of sense, the skin is laced with an elaborate network of nerve endings, but in varying concentrations. In some areas—such as the fingertips—the skin is extremely sensitive, while in others—such as the buttocks—it is not. Vitamin D is synthesized by the skin through the action of sunlight. When destroyed or injured in any part, the skin has extraordinary capacity for quick regeneration.

The skin reveals a great deal about how we feel physically and emotionally. The onset of sickness may make a person pale; embarrassment causes some of us to blush; a food allergy may announce itself by a rash. The skin is indeed our "birthday suit," reflecting the changes of adolescence and middle age. It is important to know, then, what types of care will help it and what will not. (For more information see the entry SKIN in the encyclopedia section.)

Care of the Skin. Normal skin needs chiefly to be kept clean with soap and water. Always use a clean washcloth, rinse thoroughly, and dry well.

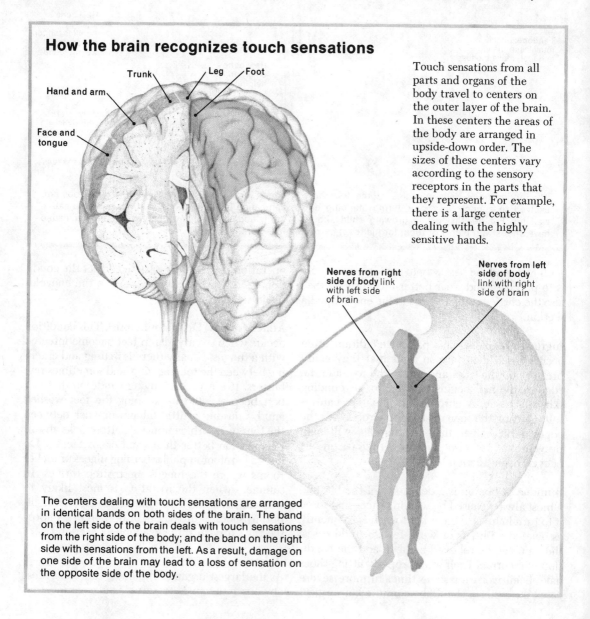

How the brain recognizes touch sensations

Trunk
Leg
Foot
Hand and arm
Face and tongue

Touch sensations from all parts and organs of the body travel to centers on the outer layer of the brain. In these centers the areas of the body are arranged in upside-down order. The sizes of these centers vary according to the sensory receptors in the parts that they represent. For example, there is a large center dealing with the highly sensitive hands.

Nerves from right side of body link with left side of brain

Nerves from left side of body link with right side of brain

The centers dealing with touch sensations are arranged in identical bands on both sides of the brain. The band on the left side of the brain deals with touch sensations from the right side of the body; and the band on the right side with sensations from the left. As a result, damage on one side of the brain may lead to a loss of sensation on the opposite side of the body.

There is no need for germicidal or antiseptic soaps to protect your skin against bacteria; they can be irritating, and healthy skin is not bothered by most germs that land on it. The best way to protect your skin against infection is to take care of cuts and abrasions properly. (See also the FIRST AID section.)

Shaving (for Men). Every man is absolutely sure that his method of shaving is the best ever devised. Whatever the method, an occasional cut or infection can result from shaving. The ordinary small cut will stop bleeding if you merely dab cold water on it with pieces of clean tissue. Then stick on a piece of dry tissue. Usually by the time the shave is finished, you can remove the tissue gently with cold water, and the bleeding has been effectively stanched.

In case of infection, shave around the infected area. Discontinue using a shaving brush if that is your method. Use a new blade each time, and shave the noninfected portions of the face first. If the infection covers a fairly large area, your doctor may want you to continue shaving daily, even over the infection, so that the medicine he prescribes can penetrate better into the infected hair follicles. Follow his advice.

Excess Hair in Women. Whether or not women wish to shave their legs or underarms is a matter of individual choice. Contrary to some old wives' tales, shaving does not cause hair to grow back coarser or thicker.

Excess hair on the face, which can be inherited or caused by a hormonal change in the body, may cause embarrassment for some women. The simplest method of eliminating it is to shave it off. Do not pluck or shave hair growing from a mole; trim it with scissors instead. Don't try to rub off facial hairs with a pumice stone, since this can irritate the skin. Wax treatments, more painful than shaving, last only until the hair grows back again. Chemical depilatories can be dangerous, especially if they get in your eyes. Remember that none of these methods will remove hair permanently.

The only permanent method is electrolysis, involving the insertion of a tiny needle into the hair follicle. It can be dangerous, unless done by an expert. (See also the entry ELECTROLYSIS in the encyclopedia section.)

Wrinkles. Wrinkles are part of the natural process of aging, and, for the most part, should be accepted gracefully. The millions of dollars women spend annually on cosmetics to avoid facial wrinkles are simply wasted.

Dermatologists place some of the blame for wrinkles on sunshine. This means you should be careful about the amount of sunshine you expose yourself to. If you prize a deep tan, be aware that constant tanning does have a drying and sagging effect on the skin. In most cases, you tan now and pay, in appearance, later.

Another cause of wrinkles, especially on the hands, is too much soap and water. The average housewife rinses her hands frequently and is likely to wash dishes several times a day. With that much washing away of the body's natural oils, it is wise to wear rubber gloves for household chores requiring water and to rub on a good hand lotion from time to time. This will also help protect the skin from eczema, an itchy, sometimes swelling irritation that, while not contagious, can be extremely hard to get rid of. A common cause of eczema is long exposure to detergents and other household chemicals.

The only way to eliminate facial wrinkles once they appear is by cosmetic surgery. Commonly called a "face-lift," the operation is expensive, and the effects last only a few years. Recently, operations for removing large bags under the eyes have also been done successfully.

Do not waste your money on lotions and creams that promise relief from wrinkles. Those containing skin food cannot do what they claim because, like any other organ, the skin is fed by the body's circulatory system. Lotions that contain hormones may be dangerous, and wearing a wrinkle mask to bed will do little good. Some cosmetic treatments provide a look of temporary improvement, either by stimulating circulation or by an astringent action that tightens the facial skin, but no permanent change is effected.

In general, the skin is better off without heavy applications of makeup, but most of the cosmetics on the market today will not hurt your skin unless you are allergic to them. Because pancake makeup, covering lotions, and powder may clog the pores, wash them off or remove them with cleansing cream every night.

Good diet, good health, exercise, and sleep will do more to keep the skin looking young than anything you can buy in a bottle. What else will help? A more cheerful and realistic attitude about aging.

Pigmentation and Sunburn. Skin color is determined by the inherited amount of a dark pigment, called melanin, in the skin. The purpose of melanin seems to be to protect the skin from harmful rays of the sun. Individuals with red hair and fair skin have less melanin than darker people, and because light individuals cannot produce enough to protect themselves, are more likely to suffer burning from exposure to the sun. If you tan easily, it is because the sun stimulates your skin to produce more of the pigmenting substance. A complete lack of this pigment, rare among humans, causes albinism, a condition characterized by pink irises, a pink-white skin, and white hair. Albino people must be extremely careful to avoid sunburn.

Freckles are caused by an excess of pigment in some patches of the skin. Don't bother with freckle removers; they do no good. The opposite condition, white spots called vitiligo, is owing to a lack of pigment in scattered patches.

Some women have found that contraceptive pills cause dark patches on the skin, especially around the hairline. If this happens, consult your doctor about discontinuing use of the pill.

A suntan does not benefit the skin. In fact, years of heavy tanning can age the skin, causing a leathery, wrinkled look or, in some cases, skin cancer. Nor do you get more vitamin D by tanning; your body needs only a minimal exposure to sunlight to make this vitamin. No matter how easily you think you tan, be careful to build up your exposure to the sun slowly to avoid serious sunburn. (For further information, see Chapter 7.)

Sunscreen lotions filter out some—but not all—of the sun's burning rays. Lotions that contain paraminobenzoic acid, or red veterinary petroleum, have been proven effective; they should be reapplied after swimming. Baby oil, olive oil, and mineral oil help prevent drying but have no special screening properties.

Only experience can teach you what your own tolerance is for the sun. Avoid making sunbathing a painful experience! (For treatment of severe SUNBURN, see that entry in the encyclopedia section; see also SUNSTROKE; HEAT PROSTRATION.)

Perspiration and Body Odor. The odor of perspiration is caused by the action of bacteria on organic elements in our perspiration. Though antibacterial or deodorant soaps control bacteria, they may be harmful. Probably the best way to combat perspiration odor is to wash frequently with regular soap and to use an antiperspirant that suppresses the production of perspiration in certain areas of the body, especially the armpits. Most of these preparations contain aluminum or

zinc salts and are safe—unless you happen to be allergic or sensitive to these chemicals. Do not use antiperspirants or any other preparation in an aerosol spray can; they can be dangerous to skin and lungs. Chlorophyll preparations do not reduce perspiration. You can check perspiration in the armpits and the hands or the feet with an antiperspirant, but the sweating apparatus must be free to work for most of the body.

Excessive perspiration may be caused by poor health; night sweats, for example, are characteristic of certain diseases. Emotional stress may also cause undue sweating. Truly offensive body odor, called bromidrosis, is relatively rare. (See the entry BROMIDROSIS in the encyclopedia section.)

Dry Skin, Oily Skin. Everyone's skin is different, partly because the sebaceous glands in our skin produce greater or lesser amounts of fats. It is possible to have dry skin on the hands and oily facial skin at the same time. Adolescence, a certain stage within the menstrual cycle, middle and old age, and even the weather all have an effect on the skin.

If your skin is too dry, avoid too much washing with soap and water; use a cleansing cream or oil, or a soap substitute. Try applying a lubricating cream at night that contains lanolin (never use pure lanolin) or cholesterol.

Oily skin, on the other hand, needs plenty of soap and water. But creams, greasy lotions, and heavy makeup—all of which can block the pores—should be avoided.

Rashes. Rashes have any number of causes: some occur as a symptom of certain diseases, such as German measles or, in babies, roseola infantum. Others seem to be reactions to emotional distress. Or the sudden onset of a rash may signal an allergic reaction to some plant or food. (See the entry ALLERGY in the encyclopedia section.)

Aside from applying a soothing lotion such as calamine to ease itching, you should not attempt to diagnose or treat a rash yourself; let your doctor determine its real cause. (Some common rashes of infants, such as DIAPER RASH and PRICKLY HEAT, are discussed in the encyclopedia section and in Chapter 14.)

Frostbite. Exposure to extreme cold can cause frostbite, a freezing of the tissues that may result in permanent damage. Fingers, toes, and the nose are particularly vulnerable to frostbite. Remember that wind aggravates the effect of low temperatures. Skiers and others who are outside for long periods in the cold are vulnerable to frost-bite in temperatures of between 8° and 15° F above zero. For warmth, clothes should be put on in layers, with the outer layer being windproof. Warm wool face masks can be worn to protect the face from cold and wind.

Freezing can occur without your being aware of it, but thawing out is a painful process that needs great care if the tissues are to survive unharmed. Under no circumstances should snow be rubbed on the frostbitten part, nor should you massage that part with your hands. (For information on how to treat FROSTBITE, see the entry in the encyclopedia section.)

Acne. As boys and girls approach maturity, their glandular activity increases, including that of the sebaceous glands of the skin. The increase in sebum production, combined with obstruction of the pores by dead cells which for some reason are not being cast off, sets the stage for acne. In general, boys suffer more than do girls from acne, but girls have it too, especially at the time of menstruation.

Although acne is not primarily caused by unclean skin or poor diet, some skin doctors (dermatologists) feel that cleanliness is essential for improvement of the condition, and recommend frequent, vigorous washing with regular soap and water to keep oils and bacteria on the surface of the skin to a minimum. And many teenagers have found that cutting down on such foods as sweets, nuts, chocolate, and fried foods has a good effect. Also, in the opinion of some doctors, foods that contain iodides, such as iodized salt, saltwater fish, spinach, and artichokes, may exacerbate the condition.

In serious cases of acne, preparations that cause inflammation and peeling of the skin have been used with good results. Those known to be somewhat helpful include benzoyl peroxide, sulfur, resorcinol, and salicylic acid. Sometimes an abrasive soap helps, but only if you do not have sensitive skin. Any preparation you use, however, should be approved by your doctor.

Blackheads are not specks of dirt, but are caused when the fatty material in a clogged pore comes into contact with the air. Squeezing them is a temptation to be avoided; it can lead to enlarged pores that may persist long after maturity has driven acne away. To remove them, use a blackhead extractor after softening the clogged pores with warm-water compresses.

Good care by a family physician or dermatologist will help avoid the permanent scarring or pocking that are the real cosmetic dangers of acne. If serious acne occurs in an adult, it may be the symptom of a larger hormonal disorder and should receive prompt medical attention.

Infections of the Skin. Although most germs do not affect the skin, it is exposed and can be infected by various microorganisms. Bacteria can cause boils or impetigo; viruses can induce fever blisters; parasites may be responsible for scabies; and fungi cause diseases such as athlete's foot.

Boils and Carbuncles. These skin eruptions are caused by pus-forming bacteria often present on the skin. The germs are unable to do any damage unless the skin's resistance has been lowered by such things as irritating friction, cuts, poor health, bad nutrition, or diabetes. A carbuncle is more serious than a boil because it is larger and goes deeper. Do not try to open a boil or carbuncle yourself, especially if it is on the face. Such self-medication can expose you to the danger of blood poisoning.

Boils and carbuncles respond readily to treatment by a physician, who may incise and open them, and/or use penicillin or other antibiotics. In addition, he will discover and eliminate their cause. Also see a doctor if you suffer from a carbuncle, or have a number of boils or experience them repeatedly. (For home treatment of an occasional, small boil, see the entry BOIL in the encyclopedia section.)

Impetigo. This infection is also caused by bacteria. It spreads quickly on the body, and is highly contagious, especially in infants and young children. It is characterized by yellowish crusts, often on the face, that look as though they had been applied to the skin. A doctor can easily cure impetigo before other infections set in. (See the entry IMPETIGO in the encyclopedia section.)

Fever Sores (Herpes Simplex). There are two similar varieties of this infection, each caused by a virus. The blisters usually occur with a fever or cold, and appear around the mouth and nose or in the genital area. Though they usually clear up in a week to 10 days, the virus itself is very hard to eliminate from the body and may cause recurrent attacks. Such factors as illness, emotional stress, or sunburn may cause the sores to reappear. A little petroleum jelly or zinc oxide ointment may be soothing. Recurrent fever sores should be seen by a doctor. (See also the entry FEVER SORE in the encyclopedia section.)

Shingles (Herpes Zoster). In this painful disorder a virus that infects part of a nerve causes an eruption that appears on the skin. There are some potentially dangerous complications from shingles in the eyes and nerves that should be treated immediately by a doctor. (See the entry SHINGLES in the encyclopedia section.)

Other Skin Infections. Remember that an infected cut or wound can also cause trouble. If the tissues surrounding a healing cut become red, swollen, or tender, or if redness starts to spread out from the area of the cut, the infection should be seen by a doctor. (For a description of other types of skin infections, see the encyclopedia entries for FOLLICULITIS; ERYSIPELAS; ITCHING.)

Birthmarks and Moles. Pigmented moles and the vascular areas, such as strawberry marks, are types of birthmarks. From time to time, they

How the skin heals

The skin is one of the body's chief barriers against infection, and any injury to it, such as a deep cut, sets in motion a swift and complex process of healing and self-repair.

The moment the skin is cut, the capillary blood vessels which are broken by the injury constrict to stem the flow of blood and to prevent germs from entering the bloodstream. Immediately afterward they open again to release substances from the blood that cause clotting.

One of these substances, the blood protein fibrin, knits the edges of the wound together with very fine

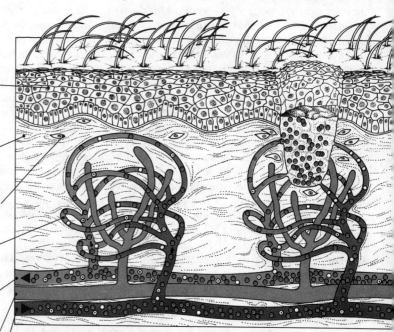

○ Neutrophils
◉ Monocytes
● Red blood cells

Section of unbroken skin
Internal parts of the body are protected by a barrier of skin

Skin with a cut
Any injury damages the barrier and exposes the body to infection

Epidermis is the tough outer covering of the skin. The flat, dead cells of the horny layer are shed constantly and replaced by others from deeper layers. It is made up of rapidly dividing cells

Dermis underlies the epidermis, and makes up the greater part of the total skin thickness. This layer of tissue contains cells which generate connective tissue

Fibroblasts are cells found in the dermis; they also migrate up to the wound from deeper skin layers. They divide to create new tissue after the cells of the dermis have been damaged

Capillaries are networks of tiny blood vessels branching off the small arteries in the dermis. The blood in them brings oxygen and nutrients to the skin, and carries away waste products

Veins collect blood from the capillaries in the skin and carry it back to the heart. Venous blood contains carbon dioxide and other waste products

Lymph vessels drain away tissue fluids such as blood plasma

Arteries carry oxygen-rich blood from the heart to the capillaries in the skin

Blood contains substances which, normally inactive, form clots if the skin is injured. Chief of these are the proteins prothrombin and fibrinogen. The cut fills with white blood cells which, with connective tissue cells, help to plug the opening of the wound

Platelets, small blood cells, help to block out blood vessels. They break up and release a chemical that initiates a chain of events to form fine threads of fibrin, which bridge the gap caused by the wound

should be checked by your doctor. Never attempt to remove either kind by yourself. If they are unsightly, they can be covered with a cosmetic preparation, or in many cases removed by surgery. Your doctor may feel it is best to remove any moles located on the palms, soles, or genitals. Any mole that starts to grow or bleed should be attended to immediately by a doctor. (See also the entries BIRTHMARK; MOLE in the encyclopedia section.)

Keloids and Xanthomas. Both of these growths are nonmalignant tumors. Keloids form in scars and should not be cut out, because they usually reappear in the new scar tissue. A doctor can remove them with radium or dry ice, although treatment is not always successful. Deposits of fat in the skin cause harmless yellow tumors (xanthomas) that can be removed by a physician if they are unsightly. (See also the entries KELOID; XANTHOMA in the encyclopedia section.)

threads. These eventually bridge the gap and harden into a scab, beneath which repair work can begin.

Six hours after the injury, white blood cells begin to break down and remove bacteria, debris, and other foreign matter from the wound. In the inner layer of the skin, the cells called fibroblasts move into the wound and create new tissue.

In the outer layer, the epidermal cells reproduce themselves to form a new surface. When this new layer is almost completed, the scab is sloughed off, leaving little sign of the cut.

One day later
First signs appear that the gap in the skin is being repaired

Two days later
Creation of new tissue continues under a protective scab

One week later
New tissue replacing the damaged skin may be completely formed

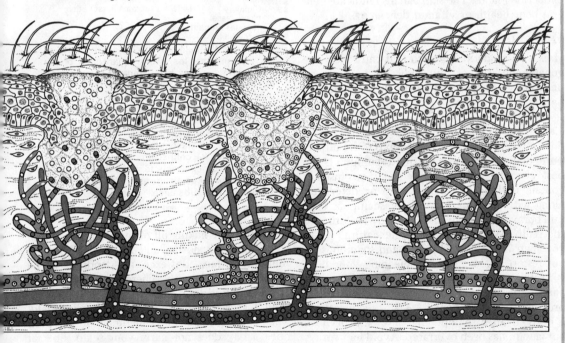

Neutrophils, the most common of the white blood cells, swarm into the wound from the surrounding blood vessels. They break down foreign particles and debris. Epidermal cells begin to multiply

Scab consists of hardened fibrin, which forms over the wound, and debris from injured tissue. Beneath this the epidermal cells unite to form a continuous layer. More white blood cells, known as monocytes, absorb the neutrophils and any remaining foreign matter

New epidermis is seen when the scab comes away. In the site of the wound are a few remaining white blood cells. At first, the tissue has more cells than the original, uninjured skin

Warts. A virus causes warts. Do not attempt to remove them yourself, for the only satisfactory methods of getting rid of them should be performed by a physician. Doctors often advise simply leaving them alone, because warts usually disappear by themselves in time.

Cancer. Skin cancer is often less serious than cancer in any other part of the body, because it can be diagnosed and removed early—provided no time is lost on dangerous home treatment. Basal cell carcinoma is a skin tumor that seldom spreads to other parts of the body, but it can spread locally. Any developing growth on the scalp or any other part of the skin should therefore be seen promptly by a doctor. (For a fuller discussion of CANCER, see Chapter 21; see also the entry CARCINOMA in the encyclopedia section.)

Never Neglect a Skin Disease. It is important to remember that in addition to the diseases mentioned above, a skin condition can indicate the presence of a deep-seated disease of the lungs, liver, heart, and many other organs, including the endocrine glands. The skin can also indicate general poor health or vitamin deficiency.

Hair and Scalp

Hair is an epidermal growth that can reflect the general condition of your body. For example, an underactive thyroid gland can cause dry, coarse hair.

Care of the Hair. Keep your hair clean. Wash it once a week, more often if it tends to be oily. A pure, plain toilet soap or a good shampoo is the best cleansing agent. Good shampoos usually contain nothing more than soap or detergent, along with some perfume. Poor shampoos contain borax or an alkali that is usually irritating to the scalp. Washing removes the natural oil in your hair along with the dirt, and shampoos do not restore these oils while cleaning your hair.

Protein conditioners, advertised to give the hair more "body," simply coat the hairs, but provide no lasting benefit. A little mineral oil rubbed in after shampooing may ease dryness, but lanolin has been overrated. Avoid hair sprays that come in aerosol cans; the materials in such containers can be dangerous to the eyes, skin, and lungs.

Keeping your hair clean and brushed is the best thing you can do for its health and looks. Remember to wash your brush and comb at least as often as you do your hair.

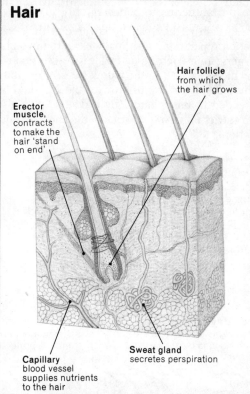

Hair

Hair follicle from which the hair grows

Erector muscle, contracts to make the hair 'stand on end'

Capillary blood vessel supplies nutrients to the hair

Sweat gland secretes perspiration

Apart from the palms of the hands, the soles of the feet and the lips, every square inch of the body surface grows hair. Some of these are so fine that they can hardly be seen, and the only noticeably hairy areas on both men and women are the scalp, armpits and pubic areas. Men also grow hair on their faces, and their body hair is generally thicker and more conspicuous than a woman's. Each hair grows from a bulb-like follicle, and is connected to a tiny erector muscle, which contracts to make the hair stand on end. Sebaceous glands astride the hair sheath secrete an oily substance.

Dandruff. The flaking off of the scalp's dead skin cells is perfectly normal and occurs on all parts of the body surface. But excessive dandruff can be annoying and unsightly. There is no proof that it is caused by a germ of any kind; nor does dandruff increase your chances of becoming bald. The best treatment is to shampoo often—even once a day does not harm your scalp. Special dandruff shampoos containing one or more of the following ingredients are sometimes helpful: sulfur, selenium sulfide, salicylic acid, and tar. Or you may want your doctor or a dermatologist to prescribe a shampoo tailored specifically for you. (See also the entry DANDRUFF in the encyclopedia section.)

Head Lice. These wingless little parasites often spread from person to person in crowded places such as schools. Lice leave tiny white eggs (nits) attached to the hairs, but the nits can be removed by using a very fine-toothed steel comb and by careful picking with your fingers. There are medicated shampoos your doctor may recommend that can be used to wash the hair. In severe cases, the doctor may recommend a very short haircut. These lice are different from the kind that settle in pubic hairs. (See the entry LOUSE in the encyclopedia section.)

Hair Bleaches and Dyes. Hair can be bleached by ordinary hydrogen peroxide to which a drop of ammonia has been added. Sodium perborate bleaches can be harmful, and all bleaching tends to alter the texture of the hair. Later, new hairs grow in with their original color.

Hair can also be dyed or tinted. If you wish to have your hair dyed, be sure to have a small lock tested first to find out whether the dye will irritate your scalp or cause a general illness. Always repeat the test process each time you have your hair redyed, because you can develop a sensitivity to the tint from repeated use.

Permanent Waves. How safe are permanents? The process depends on the action of chemicals that make the hair more pliable so that it takes the shape of the curler, and a second type of chemical that makes hair hold its new shape. Many people are allergic or sensitive to these chemicals. Always have a test curl made first, to be certain you will not suffer a reaction that may be severe. Great care should be taken to keep the waving lotions away from the eyes and any cuts or sores, and to remove them promptly if they do touch sensitive areas.

Home permanents contain much the same ingredients as those used in beauty parlors. You or the friend who gives you the permanent should make a test curl first, and you should be careful to keep the lotion away from your eyes and face—and from children. Follow the directions carefully. The American Medical Association, while recognizing these dangers, feels that home permanent kits are safe for normal use.

Baldness. The common (patterned) type of baldness is inherited. The gene that determines baldness is sex-linked, and the problem afflicts far more men than women. Unfortunately, there is no "wonder" preparation that will restore lost hair if your genes have determined that you will be bald. Once an area is bald, the hair follicles and the blood vessels and nerves that supply it cannot be restored.

Still, those miraculous tales of bald people who grew back a whole head of hair may be perfectly true. This can happen only if the original cause of baldness was a disease or temporary emotional shock that for some reason caused the hair to fall out—not if it is a baldness of the inherited type. When the condition is remedied, the still living hair follicles resume growing hairs.

Bald patches can sometimes result from local infection, rubbing—as from a tight hatband—or as a reaction to the chemical and radiation treatments that cancer patients undergo.

In some women, too, the hair may become thin. This is natural in the elderly, but it may result as well from a shortage of thyroid hormone.

If baldness is particularly distressing to you, do not waste money on "hair restorers," but spend it on a good toupee or wig, which, if carefully made to match your hair and skillfully fitted, are hard to distinguish from the real thing. Hair transplants, though painful and expensive, can offer an even more natural looking restoration. (See also the entries ALOPECIA; HAIR in the encyclopedia section.)

Fingernails

These horny outgrowths of skin cells reflect your general health, but the white spots that sometimes appear do not indicate sickness. Your fingernails need little care. In fact, most infections around the nails are usually caused by too much manicuring of the cuticle. Do not snip off cuticle tissue, but you may push it back gently, especially when it is soft, as after a bath. Do not use sharply pointed instruments for this or for cleaning under your nails. Dryness of the skin of the hands encourages hangnails, but a plain oil or hand cream will help correct this tendency. Any nail polish you fancy is safe to use, provided it does not cause irritation owing to an allergy or sensitivity.

Nails are often subject to bruises and injury. The deep red-to-black spot that may occur under a bruised nail is simply blood; and although it may take a long time to be reabsorbed by the body, the spot will eventually disappear. If a damaged nail comes off, or appears likely to come off before new nail tissue has formed underneath, protect the tender skin by wearing a small bandage. (See also NAIL in the encyclopedia section.)

4

CHAPTER

Care of the Teeth and Gums

Dentistry has made enormous strides in recent years. New, more efficient instruments, new techniques, new understanding of dental problems have made possible retention of teeth that once would have been extracted, more effective treatment of various diseases of the gums and teeth, painless procedures in nearly all fields of dentistry—to name but a few of the advances made. In this chapter we discuss some of these changes, describe the causes of many of the common diseases of the teeth and gums, and tell you what you can do to enjoy improved oral health.

MAJOR DENTAL PROBLEMS

Tooth decay—which your dentist calls dental caries—is the single most common disease in the United States. It is the chief cause of toothaches, cavities, and pulp abscesses. (See the entry DENTAL CARIES in the encyclopedia section.)

Pyorrhea—destruction of the bone tissue around the teeth—is another major dental disease. Untreated, it may cause bleeding of the gums, and the teeth may become so loose that they cannot be saved. It is, in fact, the primary reason for most extractions. Detected in its early stages, however, pyorrhea can be successfully treated, generally by a specialist called a periodontist. (For a fuller discussion, see the entry PYORRHEA in the encyclopedia section.)

Other dental troubles are the result of accidents, impacted teeth, and poor alignment of teeth. If the teeth are not correctly aligned, the bite does not work properly and chewing may be difficult or inadequate. The correction of this condition is known as orthodontics and specialists in this work are called orthodontists.

DENTISTRY

At one time, teeth were extracted as soon as they started to ache, or even before. Dentists now try to save every tooth they can. Although modern dentures are remarkable—natural in appearance and comfortable to wear—they cost time, trouble, and a considerable amount of money. More-

over, they seldom do as good a job of chewing as the natural teeth, and proper chewing has much to do with good digestion.

A major part of modern dentistry is reconstruction work—preparing and capping the teeth with porcelain or plastic that matches their natural color. The caps are joined permanently to the natural teeth and are rarely removed. Reconstruction work may involve only a few teeth or the entire mouth. It is undertaken for a variety of reasons—cosmetic, orthodontic, the repairing of teeth that have been broken, or the replacement of teeth that have been extracted. In this last case, the teeth on either side of the space left by the extraction are capped, and an artificial tooth, linked to the caps on either side, is placed between them.

Anesthetics

Years ago, dentists used anesthetics and analgesics only when extracting teeth. Today, most dentists use them with both children and adults for almost all uncomfortable procedures. The dentist may use a local anesthetic, injected around the nerves of the teeth and gums, which are first desensitized by the application of a topical anesthetic. He may use nitrous oxide gas, which the patient inhales. Nitrous oxide leaves the patient conscious and aware of the drilling, but sensation is so dulled that he or she experiences no discomfort. In the case of a patient who is particularly apprehensive or sensitive, the dentist may recommend a tranquilizer or a sedative, such as phenobarbital, to be taken a short while before the dental work is to be done.

The Dentist's Tools

Modern dental instruments, which enable the dentist to work quickly and gently, also keep discomfort at a minimum. Ultrasonic instruments are used for cleaning the teeth. Contemporary dental drills combine air turbines with a water spray, thus reducing heat and friction and the pain they create for a patient when a tooth is being drilled.

Choosing Your Dentist

Remember that however well qualified a dentist may be, personality is an extremely important factor. A dentist whom the patient finds sympathetic and understanding can relieve much of the fear and tension many of us associate with a visit to the dental office. And remember, too, that dentistry, like medicine, has become increasingly specialized as knowledge has increased. We have already mentioned the fields of orthodontics and periodontics. In addition, some dentists specialize in oral surgery (extractions and the repair of broken facial bones) and others in endodontics (saving teeth that have become abscessed). A pedodontist specializes in the care of children's teeth. Your family dentist (or your local dental school or dental association) will refer you to the appropriate dental specialist if his services are needed.

Replacing the Teeth

Contemporary dentistry has opened up some exciting possibilities for saving teeth that would previously have been unsalvageable, and for replacing teeth that have been lost. None of these techniques is everyday dental practice, but all of them are much more than experiments. One involves regeneration: If disease has destroyed the tissues and bone around a tooth, proper treatment can sometimes induce them to grow back, or regenerate. A second involves reimplantation. Under certain circumstances, a tooth that has been knocked out of place can be reinserted into its socket, reinforced, and encouraged to grow back into the jaw. Finally, a new technique, called implantation, can, under certain circumstances, be used to replace lost teeth. In this procedure, a special metal frame is placed on or in the jawbone and removable or permanent bridgework is attached to it. The specialists who perform this new type of dentistry are called implantologists.

YOUR TEETH

Nature provides all of us with two sets of teeth: the 20 deciduous (first, baby, or milk) teeth and the 32 permanent (second) teeth. It is a serious mistake to assume that the first teeth are less important than the second. If the first become badly decayed and have to be extracted, the permanent teeth may not come in properly, because every baby tooth reserves a space for the permanent tooth that will replace it. If the baby tooth is extracted before the permanent tooth has begun to appear, a space-maintaining device should be placed in the child's mouth by the dentist who removes the tooth.

Baby Teeth

The illustration on page 90 is a guide to the approximate ages at which the different teeth erupt. Notice the word "approximate;" ages vary with individual children, and your child's teeth may erupt earlier (or later) than the chart suggests. If, however, the teeth do not appear at about the times noted here, consult your dentist or physician, so that the reason can be discovered and the problem, if there is one, corrected.

Proper nourishment is essential to the development of both the first and second teeth. Cleanliness and dental care are equally important. So take your child to the dentist—either your family dentist or, if you prefer, a pedodontist—soon after the first 20 teeth have appeared (at two and a half to three years of age). The chances are that no treatment will be needed then. Therefore your child's first and crucial experience with the dentist will be a pleasant one.

Give your child a small, soft-bristle toothbrush of his or her own, to be used—with toothpaste—at the same time you are brushing your teeth. Children are great imitators, and imitation is a splended way for them to learn, especially if they are praised even when their efforts appear clumsy.

Impacted Teeth

An impacted tooth is one that is formed but does not come through the gums, or pushes only partway through. The last teeth to erupt—the third molars, or wisdom teeth—are the ones most likely to become impacted. If any tooth fails to come through, causing pain and swelling, consult your dentist. The surgery that may be necessary can usually be performed in the dentist's office, but if it is complicated, he may prefer to have it done in a hospital.

Teeth

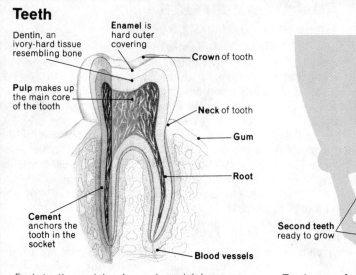

Dentin, an ivory-hard tissue resembling bone

Enamel is hard outer covering

Crown of tooth

Pulp makes up the main core of the tooth

Neck of tooth

Gum

Root

Cement anchors the tooth in the socket

Blood vessels

First teeth in position

Roots

Second teeth ready to grow

Each tooth consists of a root, containing nerves and blood vessels leading to the pulpy central part of the tooth; the root is bedded into the socket by bone-like cement. A layer of hard dentin surrounds the pulp, and the outermost layer consists of enamel, the hardest of all.

Teeth grow from the upper and lower jaws, the maxilla and mandible. This illustration shows the teeth of a child aged 3–5 years.

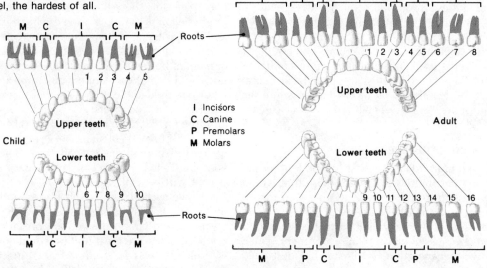

Roots

M C I C M

1 2 3 4 5

Upper teeth

Child

Lower teeth

6 7 8 9 10

Roots

M C I C M

I Incisors
C Canine
P Premolars
M Molars

M P C I C P M

1 2 3 4 5 6 7 8

Upper teeth

Adult

Lower teeth

9 10 11 12 13 14 15 16

M P C I C P M

A child's first set contains 20 teeth: eight incisors, four canines, and eight molars. These baby teeth are also known as milk, or deciduous, teeth.

Permanent teeth begin to appear at about the age of six. By age 21 there should be 32 teeth: eight incisors, four canines, eight premolars, and twelve molars. Some people never cut their rearmost molars (wisdom teeth).

Approximate ages at which teeth appear

1 central incisor: 7½ mos.
2 lateral incisor: 9 mos.
3 cuspid: 18 mos.
4 first molar: 14 mos.
5 second molar: 24 mos.
6 central incisor: 6 mos.
7 lateral incisor: 7 mos.
8 cuspid: 18 mos.
9 first molar: 15 mos.
10 second molar: 20 mos.

1 central incisor: 7-8 yrs.
2 lateral incisor: 8-9 yrs.
3 cuspid: 11-12 yrs.
4 first bicuspid: 10-11 yrs.
5 second bicuspid: 10-12 yrs.
6 first molar: 6-7 yrs.
7 second molar: 12-13 yrs.
8 third molar: 17-21 yrs.

9 central incisor: 6-7 yrs.
10 lateral incisor: 7-8 yrs.
11 cuspid: 9-10 yrs.
12 first bicuspid: 10-12 yrs.
13 second bicuspid: 11-12 yrs.
14 first molar: 6-7 yrs.
15 second molar: 11-13 yrs.
16 third molar: 17-21 yrs.

Faulty Alignment of Teeth

Some people have teeth that are irregular or that overlap or protrude unattractively. Sometimes the upper and lower teeth do not meet (occlude) properly. This may be because the first teeth failed to fall out when they should have, or because decay or accident caused them to be lost too soon—good reasons for taking your child to the dentist early. Another cause of a faulty bite is insufficient chewing; this usually happens when the diet is overloaded with soft foods. Like muscles, teeth need exercise to remain in good condition. (See the entries MALOCCLUSION and ORTHODONTICS in the encyclopedia section.)

Dental Caries

It is important to realize that dental caries is a disease, not a mysterious rotting of the teeth that must be accepted fatalistically. To understand how it develops, you should know something about the structure of the teeth.

Each tooth has a crown—the part that lies above the surface—and a root—the part that lies within the jaw. The root is covered with a thin, bonelike layer called cementum; the crown is covered with a coating of enamel, which is thickest on the grinding surface, where it wears down from use. Beneath the enamel lies the hard bone-like dentin, which covers the pulp chamber; and running from the chamber to the root is the root canal, which contains blood vessels and nerve fibers.

Dental caries almost always starts on the crown, in the enamel, with a pinhead-sized collection of bacteria and food. It is generally believed that most of these bacteria thrive best on starchy and sugary foods, which they convert into lactic acid. Although the tooth enamel is the strongest material in the body, able to withstand enormous biting pressures, it is extremely vulnerable to lactic acid, which quickly and permanently dissolves it. By creating minute pits and furrows on the surface of the tooth, the acid opens up new territory for the bacteria, which soon reach the softer, richer dentin, where they grow faster and spread rapidly. Finally they proceed into the root canal, attacking the nerves and causing great pain. (See the entry TOOTHACHE in the encyclopedia section.)

Infected pulp and decaying teeth make excellent breeding places for bacteria. They can cause localized abscesses, and may even enter the bloodstream to spread their poison to various parts of the body.

Filling Teeth

Enamel that has been destroyed by acid will not grow back again; neither will the dentin of a tooth destroyed by bacteria. For the dentist to save the tooth, he must remove the diseased portion and fill the cavity.

When the decay has extended into the pulp and root canal, the tooth may begin to ache. The nerve dies, and the infection spreads around the ends of the roots in the jawbone. The dentist tries to save most of the tooth by cleaning out the decay and the residue of the pulp and nerve. He sterilizes the root canal with an irrigational solution and antiseptics, then fills it and the cavity to seal them. If the infection continues or recurs, it may be necessary to perform an apicoectomy—a minor surgical procedure involving removal of the infected end of the root.

Why Do YOU Get So Many Cavities?

Some people seem to inherit so-called soft teeth, which decay more readily than teeth with a harder enamel. Others seem to be immune to dental caries, for reasons which are not yet known. Sometimes—again for unknown reasons—people have an immunity to caries during certain periods of their lives, usually from about 25 to 45 years of age.

Fluoridation

Extensive research has established that fluoride is an aid in reducing the amount of tooth decay, or preventing it entirely. Your dentist may apply it directly to your youngster's teeth. Many toothpastes now contain it. Fluoride tablets are sometimes recommended for young children who do not receive fluoride in any other form. But it is most effective when absorbed by the body through drinking water, and for this reason the drinking water in many communities is now fluoridated. In such communities, no added fluoride in toothpaste is needed although it may give added protection. Possible side effects of artificial fluoridation of water, however, is still a subject of debate in some scientific and lay circles. (For further discussion, see FLUORIDATION in the encyclopedia section.)

Can Anything Else Be Done to Prevent Dental Caries?

A great deal. Scientists are studying ways of attacking the bacteria that dissolve the enamel by producing acid. In addition, we ourselves can do some things to render them harmless. The first has to do with diet. Decay bacteria demand carbohydrates (sugar and starches) for food; it is these carbohydrates that are converted to lactic acid. Sweet carbonated beverages contain concentrated sugars. Pastries, pies, cookies, and ice cream also contain considerable sugar. The worst enemies of the teeth are all-day suckers, chewy candies, and sweetened chewing gum. A sweet tooth can ruin all the teeth!

Restrict Candy. Yet most children love sweets, and we do not like to remove them entirely from their diet. A sensible compromise is to restrict candy to a special, infrequent treat—but *not* just before bedtime, because children, as well as many adults, do not remove all candy and cake from their teeth when they brush. In addition, it is a good idea, after eating candy, to eat other foods, such as apples and raw carrots, that cleanse the teeth instead of sticking to them.

Dental Floss. The second important thing you can do to reduce tooth decay and to keep your teeth and gums healthy is to use unwaxed dental floss daily. This helps remove the thin, transparent film called plaque that builds up on the teeth and serves as the collecting point at which the bacteria begin the decay process. Flossing greatly reduces the plaque and thus reduces the incidence of decay.

Teeth Grinding (Bruxism)

Some people, both adults and children, grind their teeth during sleep or at other times, either because of a malocclusion or as a result of nervous tension. This habit, which is known as bruxism, can wear away the enamel. An alert dentist can usually recognize the symptoms of the problem, and may recommend reshaping the cusps of the teeth or the use of a plastic nightguard to be kept in the mouth during sleep to protect the tooth surfaces from the constant abrasion.

KEEPING YOUR TEETH CLEAN

Brush Your Teeth. The purpose of brushing the teeth is to help prevent decay by removing food particles from the surfaces of the teeth. The surfaces that need to be brushed most carefully are those between the teeth and in the crevices of the bicuspids and molars. Proper brushing also massages the gums and cleans the crevices where teeth and gums meet. The best times to brush your teeth—or to rinse your

mouth thoroughly with tap water or salt water, if it is not convenient for you to use a toothbrush—are after meals and before going to bed.

Have Two Good Toothbrushes. Two toothbrushes are necessary to make sure that each of them gets a chance to dry out thoroughly. This helps the bristles to remain in good condition longer. Rinse the brush in cold water after using it; any food particles that remain on it will provide an excellent breeding place for bacteria. Do not let your toothbrush touch the brushes others have been using.

Use a Safe Dentifrice. As yet, there is no perfect toothpaste or powder. Those containing harsh abrasives or strong antiseptics should be avoided. Rely on the recommendation of your dentist or of such nonprofit organizations as the United States Public Health Service or the Council on Dental Therapeutics of the American Dental Association. (For a fuller discussion, see DENTIFRICES in the encyclopedia section.)

Brush Properly. Proper brushing is an important step in dental health. Most dentists believe that a soft brush with rounded end bristles is the best kind to use, since such bristles actually work under the crevices between teeth and gums, and provide excellent cleaning action without damaging the gums. The brush should be held at an angle of about 45 degrees, with the bristles directed to the area where the gum meets the crown of the teeth. The brush should be moved in a short, vibrating action, with the teeth cleansed in groups of three or four at a time.

The Electric Toothbrush and Similar Devices. Some dentists believe electric toothbrushes massage the gums more thoroughly than hand brushes. Another electric dental device, manufactured under various trade names, emits a tiny stream of water under high pressure that flushes out food particles. Before you spend your money for either of these instruments, get your dentist's advice.

CARE OF ARTIFICIAL TEETH

Dentures should be removed and cleaned and the mouth rinsed after every meal, if possible. Do not use hot water, as it may warp or crack the dentures. Putting them in a glass of water overnight helps to keep them clean. Dentures should be checked regularly by your dentist to make certain that they have not warped and that a change in your mouth or gums has not altered or impaired their fit.

HALITOSIS (BAD BREATH)

Certain foods cause bad breath, and the condition almost always accompanies pyorrhea. It can also be caused by teeth and gums that are not clean or in good condition. In addition, halitosis may have medical causes, such as inflamed tonsils, infections in or behind the nose, disorders of the stomach or intestine, and uremia, among others. It is difficult to tell whether one has halitosis, but there is no need to worry about it or spend time and money on remedies. Your dentist or physician will tell you —and help you to find its cause and cure.

PERIODIC DENTAL CHECKUPS

How often should you see your dentist? As often as necessary. Let him decide. If dental decay is on the rampage, or you are fighting off a threatened case of pyorrhea, you may need to have a dental appointment every month. Under other circumstances, a visit once a year may be sufficient. Unless your dentist reminds you periodically, it would probably be advisable for you to make an appointment *now*—because the chances are you are overdue for a visit.

5 CHAPTER

Your Endocrine Glands and Their Hormones

Glands are organs that secrete and release substances essential for the proper functioning of the body. There are two types of glands: exocrine and endocrine. The exocrines have ducts that carry their secretions to particular parts of the body. The salivary glands that provide the mouth with saliva and the mammary glands that produce milk belong to this group, as do the glands that produce bile in the liver and digestive juices in the stomach.

Endocrine glands, the subject of this chapter, have no ducts and release their substances, called hormones, directly into the bloodstream. The endocrines and their hormones help to regulate such vital processes as growth, development, and reproduction as well as control the balance of salt and water in the body and the level of sugar in the blood.

THE FAMILY OF ENDOCRINE GLANDS

The endocrine glands form a complex, interdependent system. Removal or underfunctioning of one gland may seriously affect the functioning of others. Similarly, an increase in the functioning of one will change that of the others. This is one reason why it is extremely dangerous to dose oneself with hormones, glandular tissue, or glandular extract.

The Pituitary Gland

About the size of a pea, this gland lies in a small hollow well within the skull, at about the level of the top of the nose. It is connected to the part of the brain called the hypothalamus, and this link gives the brain direct control over the pituitary's hormone production. The most important function of the pituitary is to stimulate, regulate, and coordinate the functions of certain of the other endocrines. For this reason it is called the master gland. (See PITUITARY GLAND in the encyclopedia section.)

Diseases of the pituitary gland fortunately are relatively rare. Too little pituitary secretion causes certain types of dwarfism, while too much stimulates the body to grow to gigantic proportions. Pituitary tumors may press on the optic nerves, resulting in headaches and loss of vision. Another rare disease of the pituitary is diabetes insipidus, which causes excessive thirst and excessive secretion of urine. (See the entry DIABETES in the encyclopedia section.)

In some instances malfunction of the pituitary can be successfully treated with such medications as cortisone derivative and thyroid and sex-hormone extracts.

The Thyroid Gland

The thyroid gland is in front of the throat, below the Adam's apple and just above the breastbone. It is U-shaped, each end of the U flaring back into a lobe that is about the size of the big toe. The thyroid's hormonal production stimulates or affects almost every important body process, including the body's use of oxygen. Too much or too little of the hormone, called thyroxine, can cause serious health problems. (See THYROID GLAND in the encyclopedia section.)

Hypothyroidism. This is the name given a complete or partial deficiency of thyroid hormone. The specific reasons for the deficiency can range from a thyroid missing at birth to a lack of iodine needed for the manufacture of thyroxine.

A total lack of the hormone in a newborn infant because the thyroid is either missing or grossly underactive results in cretinism, a rare form of mental retardation and physical underdevelopment. Early diagnosis is vitally important, so that treatment with thyroid hormone may prevent severe retardation. A partial lack of thyroid hormone in later childhood—called juvenile myxedema—will also cause physical underdevelopment if treatment is not begun with thyroid hormone, extract, or synthetic substitutes. In a fully developed adult, severe hypo-

thyroidism—or myxedema—causes weight gain, puffy skin, excessive fatigue, dry hair and hair loss, and other serious effects. All these symptoms may be reversed by regular treatment.

Simple Goiter. The thyroid gland needs iodine for the manufacture of thyroxine, its major hormone product. Simple goiter is a symptom of a form of hypothyroidism in which insufficient iodine is available in the system for the proper

Control centers of body processes

Various functions and rhythms of the body are controlled by hormones, chemical messengers produced by the endocrine glands and discharged into the bloodstream. These glands include the pituitary, thyroid, parathyroids, adrenals, islets of Langerhans, and the sex glands or gonads. Some interaction takes place among all the endocrine glands, but only the hormones from the pituitary are able to control production of hormones in other glands. Most glands produce several types of hormones—the pituitary, for example, produces at least nine—and each type reaches its own target area in the body, no matter how far from the gland producing it.

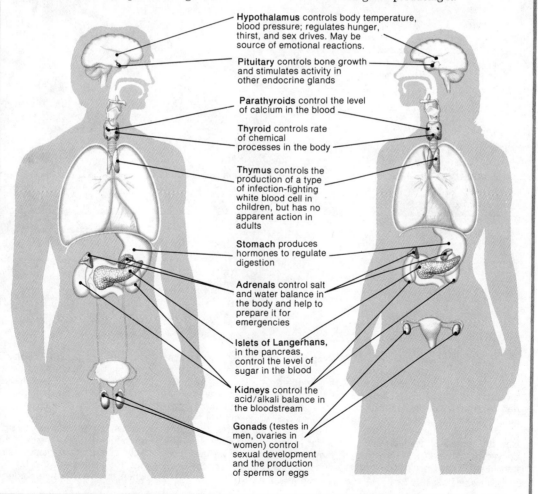

Hypothalamus controls body temperature, blood pressure; regulates hunger, thirst, and sex drives. May be source of emotional reactions.

Pituitary controls bone growth and stimulates activity in other endocrine glands

Parathyroids control the level of calcium in the blood

Thyroid controls rate of chemical processes in the body

Thymus controls the production of a type of infection-fighting white blood cell in children, but has no apparent action in adults

Stomach produces hormones to regulate digestion

Adrenals control salt and water balance in the body and help to prepare it for emergencies

Islets of Langerhans, in the pancreas, control the level of sugar in the blood

Kidneys control the acid/alkali balance in the bloodstream

Gonads (testes in men, ovaries in women) control sexual development and the production of sperms or eggs

Control of growth and development

The front lobe of the pituitary gland produces several hormones, of which seven have been identified. Three directly control body growth, milk production, and skin pigment; the other four stimulate the thyroid gland, adrenals, and gonads to secrete their own hormones to control body chemistry, prepare the body for stress, and control sexual development. None acts independently of the others.

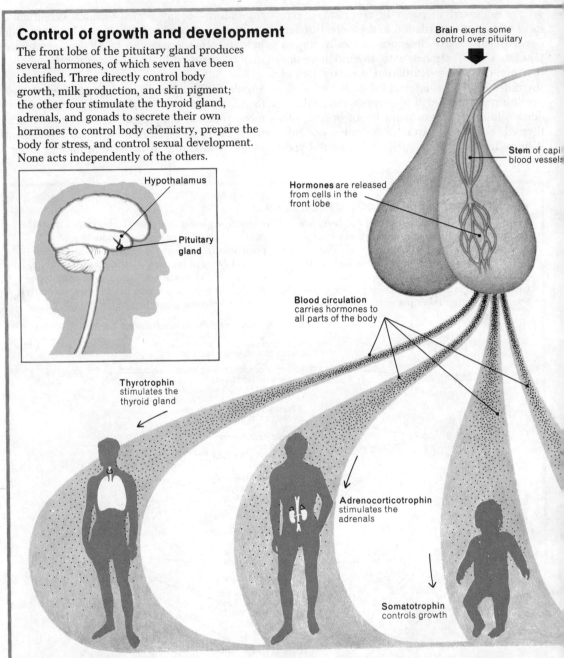

Brain exerts some control over pituitary

Stem of capi blood vessels

Hormones are released from cells in the front lobe

Hypothalamus

Pituitary gland

Blood circulation carries hormones to all parts of the body

Thyrotrophin stimulates the thyroid gland

Adrenocorticotrophin stimulates the adrenals

Somatotrophin controls growth

Controlling body chemistry
Under stimulation by a pituitary hormone, the thyroid gland secretes thyroxine hormones. These are carried to all body tissues, where they control chemical processes taking place in them. They speed up or slow down the rate at which food is converted into energy. A necessary constituent of the thyroid hormone is iodine, supplied in various foods.

Preparing the body for stress
Hormones from the adrenal glands are triggered off by one from the pituitary to regulate the way in which the body uses the products of digestion, as well as to control the balance of sodium, potassium, and water in the body. Some male and female sex hormones are also produced by the outer part, or cortex, of the adrenal glands.

Controlling growth The size of the growing body is affected by somatotrophin, a hormone secreted by the front lobe of the pituitary gland. This hormone acts directly to regulate the growth of nearly all bones and tissues, unlike other hormones from the pituitary which regulate the activity of individual glands. Its production ceases in the late teens when the body reaches adult size

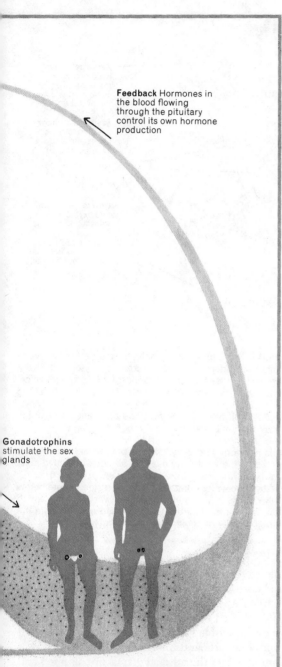

Feedback Hormones in the blood flowing through the pituitary control its own hormone production

Gonadotrophins stimulate the sex glands

Controlling sexual development
Hormones from the pituitary gland stimulate the testes in men and the ovaries in women to secrete sex hormones, which cause development of secondary sex characteristics in adolescence. In boys, they cause the growth of facial hair and deepening of the voice; in girls, they cause development of the breasts and the start of menstruation.

functioning of the gland. In its effort to produce more thyroxine the gland becomes enlarged; this swelling is known as goiter, and it may interfere with breathing or swallowing. A very small amount of iodine in the diet—e.g., that consumed in iodized table salt at meals—is usually sufficient to prevent simple goiter. Anyone with even a small goiter should consult a doctor, who can readily treat the condition. (See the entry GOITER in the encyclopedia section.)

Hyperthyroidism. A more serious type of neck goiter develops when the thyroid manufactures too much hormone. People with hyperthyroidism are nervous and irritable and suffer from insomnia. Heat makes them very uncomfortable. The excess secretion also produces heart palpitations that people frequently mistake for a true cardiac attack. Another symptom is loss of weight—in spite of the increased hunger that usually accompanies the malady. When severe, hyperthyroidism often causes the eyes to protrude, or bulge—a condition called exophthalmic goiter. (See EXOPHTHALMOS in the encyclopedia section.)

For many years the only treatment for hyperthyroidism was surgery, in which up to 90 percent of the gland was removed. Today combinations of drugs can help control excessively active thyroid hormone production or, where necessary, radioactive iodine can be used to lessen activity of the gland or make it completely inactive.

The Parathyroid Glands

There are four parathyroid glands, a pair on, or embedded in, each side of the thyroid gland in the neck. Each parathyroid is the size of a small pea. These glands help to regulate the level of calcium in the bloodstream which, in turn, helps to control the way the muscles receive nerve impulses from the brain.

In parathyroid deficiency, the calcium regulation is disturbed, and the muscles become subject to spasms, a condition known as tetany. The administration of parathyroid hormone—certain synthetically manufactured compounds—or a potent vitamin D preparation will keep the calcium level normal and stop the spasms. Taking calcium is also extremely helpful in such cases. (For a fuller discussion, see the entry TETANY in the encyclopedia section.)

The Adrenal Glands

These two glands fit like small cups, one on the top of each kidney. Each adrenal gland consists of two major parts: the cortex, or outer portion,

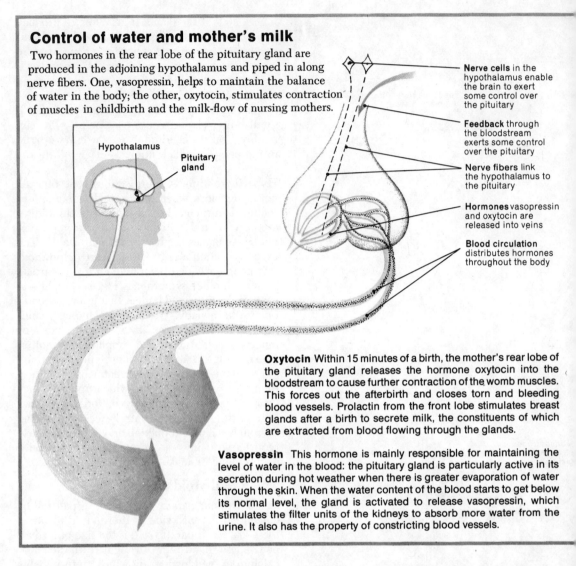

Control of water and mother's milk

Two hormones in the rear lobe of the pituitary gland are produced in the adjoining hypothalamus and piped in along nerve fibers. One, vasopressin, helps to maintain the balance of water in the body; the other, oxytocin, stimulates contraction of muscles in childbirth and the milk-flow of nursing mothers.

Hypothalamus

Pituitary gland

Nerve cells in the hypothalamus enable the brain to exert some control over the pituitary

Feedback through the bloodstream exerts some control over the pituitary

Nerve fibers link the hypothalamus to the pituitary

Hormones vasopressin and oxytocin are released into veins

Blood circulation distributes hormones throughout the body

Oxytocin Within 15 minutes of a birth, the mother's rear lobe of the pituitary gland releases the hormone oxytocin into the bloodstream to cause further contraction of the womb muscles. This forces out the afterbirth and closes torn and bleeding blood vessels. Prolactin from the front lobe stimulates breast glands after a birth to secrete milk, the constituents of which are extracted from blood flowing through the glands.

Vasopressin This hormone is mainly responsible for maintaining the level of water in the blood: the pituitary gland is particularly active in its secretion during hot weather when there is greater evaporation of water through the skin. When the water content of the blood starts to get below its normal level, the gland is activated to release vasopressin, which stimulates the filter units of the kidneys to absorb more water from the urine. It also has the property of constricting blood vessels.

and the medulla, or central section. The cortex, essential to life, secretes more than 30 hormones and regulates many of our metabolic processes.

The two main functions of the hormones of the adrenal cortex are: (1) the control of the proper salt and water content of the body; and (2) the regulation of carbohydrate, fat, and protein metabolism. In addition, the cortex secretes sex hormones, mainly androgens, similar to those produced by the testicles.

Atrophy or underfunctioning of the adrenal cortex produces Addison's disease, which results in loss of salt and water in the body. Symptoms include low blood pressure, weight loss, and general weakness. (See also ADDISON'S DISEASE in the encyclopedia section.) The pituitary hormone ACTH (adrenocorticotrophic hormone) stimu-lates secretion of certain hormones by the adrenal cortex, and can be used therapeutically if the adrenal gland is not completely atrophied. The ACTH used to treat humans is derived from the pituitaries of hogs and cattle. A synthetic adrenal hormone preparation can replenish the body's supply when the adrenal glands are diseased and underproductive. Administration of these hormones may bring about favorable results in the treatment of many other diseases, including rheumatic fever, arthritis, and asthma.

The overproduction of adrenal hormones results in Cushing's syndrome, which causes retention of salt and water, obesity of the face and trunk, and high blood pressure. (For a fuller discussion of CUSHING'S SYNDROME, see that entry in the encyclopedia section.)

Milk for the baby After puberty, estrogen and progesterone hormones from the ovaries cause development of the female breasts. In pregnancy, these hormones promote further growth, but there is a fall in their production when the placenta is released. Prolactin hormones from the pituitary gland take over three to four days after the birth and stimulate secretion of milk from the breast glands.

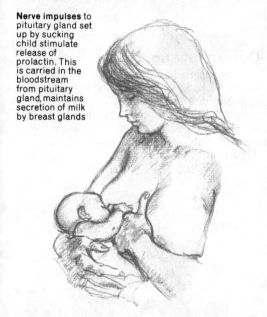

Nerve impulses to pituitary gland set up by sucking child stimulate release of prolactin. This is carried in the bloodstream from pituitary gland, maintains secretion of milk by breast glands

Supply and demand A sucking child sets up two different nerve impulses. One stimulates secretion of milk from the breast glands through the nipple: the other stimulates the pituitary gland to release prolactin to maintain secretion by glands within the breast.

The medulla of the adrenal gland produces the hormone called adrenaline, or epinephrine. The output of this hormone is immediately stepped up when one becomes angry, fearful, or excited. This state produces chemical changes that prepare the body for action.

The Islets of Langerhans in the Pancreas

Many years ago, a scientist named Paul Langerhans studied small clusters of cells that formed what he called "islands" scattered throughout the pancreas, the flat organ situated below and behind the stomach. The main part of the pancreas produces juices that play a major part in the digestion of proteins and fats, while the islets, or islands, of Langerhans, control the body's use of sugar through their secretion of two hormones, insulin and glucagon. Together, these hormones regulate the level of glucose (blood sugar) in the blood. Insulin enables the body to use, or burn, sugar and starch after they have been converted into glucose by the digestive juices. The body uses this glucose to provide heat and energy and to help in the utilization of other foods. Any sugar the normal body does not immediately need is stored in the liver as glycogen (stored carbohydrate) or converted into fat. Glucagon has the opposite action of insulin: it raises the blood sugar level and lowers the amount of glycogen in the liver.

Causes and Symptoms of Diabetes. When the islets of Langerhans fail to produce enough insulin to utilize the glucose in the body, the blood sugar level rises and glucose appears in the urine. This glandular disorder is known as diabetes mellitus, or simply, diabetes. Everyone should be alert for the following symptoms of diabetes:

1. Excessive hunger, thirst, and urination; in children, bed-wetting may be a sign.
2. Loss of weight, especially when normal consumption of food is maintained or increased.
3. Weakness, listlessness, and fatigue.
4. Decreased resistance to infection, often manifested in frequent boils or carbuncles, or (especially in elderly people) in gangrenous conditions, particularly in the feet.
5. Itching of the genitals. In females especially, the itching may be associated with a fungus infection of the genital region.

Before insulin was introduced, the only treatment for diabetics was severe limitation of sugars and starches in the diet. Dietary control is still in wide use today, and for mild, borderline diabetes in adults—usually those cases beginning after age 40—it can be the major element for controlling diabetes. But a restricted diet alone is wholly inadequate in advanced cases.

Today even the most serious types of diabetes can be controlled with insulin. The doctor will instruct the patient and family members in insulin injection techniques and will teach them how to make a simple test for sugar in the urine. But even with insulin injections, the diabetic must learn to regulate his diet. Deviation from the prescribed regimen can produce dangerous conditions such as insulin reaction and diabetic coma.

What to Do for Insulin Reaction (Hypoglycemia). If too much insulin is taken or too little food eaten to use that insulin, the blood sugar becomes dangerously low, and the urine contains no sugar instead of the small amount normally present. The skin turns pale, cold, and moist. Breathing is shallow. Dizziness, palpitations, and tremors may also occur. Severe reactions resemble symptoms of drunkenness, or the diabetic may become unconscious. A mild insulin reaction can be countered by eating a candy bar or two lumps of sugar or by drinking orange juice with two lumps of sugar dissolved in it. Tubes of concentrated glucose can also be squeezed between the lips of a patient who is conscious but not alert.

Diabetics should carry candy bars, sugar lumps, or glucose tubes at all times. Severe reactions should be treated by a doctor, but for emergencies diabetics and their families should always keep a supply of the hormone glucagon on hand. The doctor will instruct the patient and members of his family in its administration, which is by injection.

Control of calcium

Calcium, necessary for healthy bones and teeth, is taken into the body in food and extracted by the digestive system. The parathyroid glands in the neck monitor the level of calcium in the bloodstream and release a hormone that controls the exchange of calcium between bones and other tissues.

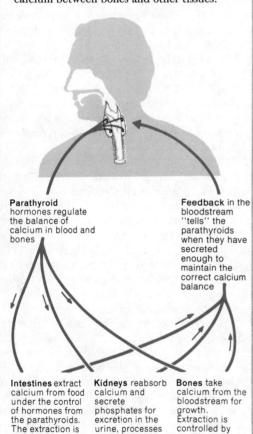

Parathyroid hormones regulate the balance of calcium in blood and bones

Feedback in the bloodstream "tells" the parathyroids when they have secreted enough to maintain the correct calcium balance

Intestines extract calcium from food under the control of hormones from the parathyroids. The extraction is greatest in a growing child, for building bones

Kidneys reabsorb calcium and secrete phosphates for excretion in the urine, processes controlled by the parathyroid hormones

Bones take calcium from the bloodstream for growth. Extraction is controlled by parathyroid hormones to maintain the required calcium level in the bloodstream

Control of sugar

Sugar, in the form of glucose, is required for generation of energy in the body. In addition to that in the blood, there is a reserve supply in the liver in the form of glycogen. Hormones released by the islets of Langerhans in the pancreas maintain the correct level of glucose in the blood.

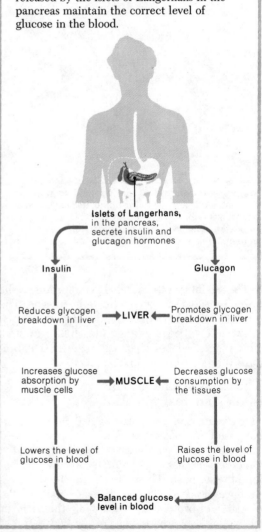

Islets of Langerhans, in the pancreas, secrete insulin and glucagon hormones

Insulin

Glucagon

Reduces glycogen breakdown in liver → **LIVER** ← Promotes glycogen breakdown in liver

Increases glucose absorption by muscle cells → **MUSCLE** ← Decreases glucose consumption by the tissues

Lowers the level of glucose in blood

Raises the level of glucose in blood

Balanced glucose level in blood

What to Do for Diabetic Coma (Hyperglycemia). This is the reverse of insulin reaction. Unable to use carbohydrates because of insulin lack, the body of a diabetic patient builds up excess ketone bodies, such as acetones. Diabetic coma (or diabetic acidosis) is usually caused by overeating, failure to take insulin, vomiting and diarrhea from any cause, and infections. The onset of diabetic acidosis is gradual, and the actual coma is fairly rare; but when it occurs, it is serious. The skin becomes flushed and dry, and the breath has a fruity odor from acetone. Breathing is deep and labored. Large amounts of sugar are present in the urine.

Call the doctor at once when you suspect diabetic coma. Keep the patient quiet and warm until help arrives. If symptoms seem severe and the doctor cannot be reached promptly, get the diabetic to a hospital, informing the doctor's answering service of your decision. Accurate information on the patient's insulin program and deviation from it or from his diet will help an emergency-room doctor begin countermeasures.

A diabetic should *always* carry an identification card. Symptoms of hyperglycemia can be mistaken for drunkenness or some other problem. Such a card has often saved a diabetic's life.

Care of the Feet for Diabetics. A great deal of emphasis is placed on foot care for the diabetic because there is danger of gangrene—a condition in which tissues actually die—if the feet are neglected. This is because diabetes often results in poor circulation especially in the feet and legs. Diabetics, particularly those over 45, should be meticulous about carrying out the following foot-care measures:

1. Wash the feet daily with soap and water, then dry thoroughly.
2. With an upward motion, massage feet and legs to the knee daily with lanolin.
3. Raise yourself on your toes 20 times, twice a day.
4. Have your toenails cut carefully by someone other than yourself, preferably a podiatrist, who must be told that you are diabetic. A podiatrist should deal with any ingrown toenails, but if you have to treat them yourself, use the method described under INGROWN TOENAIL in the encyclopedia section.
5. Wear shoes that are comfortable and wide enough not to rub against the feet.
6. Stockings or socks should be washed daily and should be free of imperfections that may irritate the skin.

For further information on any aspect of diabetes, write to the American Diabetes Association, Inc., 600 Fifth Avenue, New York, New York 10020.

The Sex Glands—or Gonads

The sex glands, or gonads, are the testes in men and the ovaries in women. The gonads are stimulated by the pituitary gland, which controls their activity by means of gonadotrophic hormones.

These hormones stimulate the testes to make sperm cells and the ovaries to produce egg cells. In addition, the gonads secrete hormones that affect the growth and well-being of the entire body.

The Male Sex Glands. The testes, or testicles, are a pair of oval glands, each about the size of a small plum. They are suspended in the pouchlike scrotum, and are connected to the body by the spermatic cords. Sperm passes from the testes through the spermatic cords to the prostate gland and the urethra and out through the penis. Each testicle consists of a set of tubules that produce sperm and a group of cells that manufacture hormones.

Starting at puberty, the cells secrete testosterone—the chief male sex hormone. Testosterone is responsible for the development of the male secondary sex characteristics during adolescence—the growth of the penis and the testicles, the deepening of the voice, the growth of pubic and facial hair, and the development of the characteristic male muscle and bone pattern. At the end of adolescence, the hormone speeds the fusing of the growing ends of bones with the main shafts, so that the growth of the bones has to stop.

The Female Sex Glands. The ovaries in women correspond to the testes in men. They are a pair of oval white bodies, about 1½ inches long, lying one on each side of the uterus and connected to it by the Fallopian tubes. The function of the ovaries is to produce egg cells, or ova, during a woman's reproductive years.

At birth the ovaries contain several hundred thousand Graafian follicles. Each follicle is a small, hollow ball about pinhead size in which an egg (ovum) may develop. At puberty the influence of a hormone from the pituitary gland begins to ripen the follicles. Normally, one follicle and egg mature each month, and an ovum is released into one of the Fallopian tubes. It is believed that the ovaries take turns in supplying eggs.

The hormones produced by the ovaries are the estrogens and progesterone. Estrogens are responsible for the general growth of the breasts at puberty, and for the development of the other secondary female sex characteristics, i.e., enlargement of the uterus and of the vagina, the distribution of body hair, and the typically feminine narrow shoulders and broad hips. The hormone progesterone chiefly builds up the lining of the uterus to make it ready to receive a fertilized egg cell.

Menstruation and Ovulation

Menstruation is the periodic discharge from the body of the extra blood and tissue that have been built up in preparation for pregnancy and have not been used. Although menstrual cycles vary, the time from one menstrual period to the next is usually about 28 days.

Doctors customarily count the first day of menstruation as Day 1 in the cycle. During the first 14 days of the cycle, the Graafian follicle and

Effects of some hormones

Gland or tissue	Hormones	Normal amount	Too little leads to	Too much leads to
Pituitary	Somatotrophin (growth hormone)	Controls bone growth	Underdevelopment (dwarfism)	Overdevelopment (gigantism; acromegaly)
	Thyrotrophin	Stimulates thyroid gland	Decreased thyroid activity (cretinism)	Increased thyroid activity
	Adrenocortico-trophin	Stimulates adrenal glands		Cushing's syndrome
	Follicle stimulating hormone	Stimulates ripening of ova in women and production of sperms in men	Underdevelopment of ovaries or testes	Premature sexual development
	Luteinizing hormone (in women) Interstitial-cell-stimulating hormone (in men)	Stimulates corpus luteum which prepares the uterus in early pregnancy Regulates production of testosterone	Indirectly causes miscarriage	
	Prolactin	Stimulates production of milk in mammary glands	Too little milk produced	Too much milk produced
	Vasopressin	Controls resorption of water by kidneys	Too much and too dilute urine	
	Oxytocin	Contracts muscles of womb in childbirth		
Thyroid	Thyroxine	Controls rate of metabolism and growth	Cretinism, myxedema	Increased thyroid activity
Parathyroids	Parathyroid hormone	Controls exchange of calcium and phosphate between blood, bones, intestines, and kidneys	Tetany and muscular spasms	Muscular weakness; deposits of calcium salts in the body
Thymus	Not known	Controls production of lymphocytes in young people		
Adrenals	Corticosterones	Control salt and water content of blood	Excessive excretion of salt and water; weakness; low blood pressure	Cushing's syndrome
	Adrenaline	Prepares body for emergency action		Raised blood pressure, sweating
Islets of Langerhans	Insulin	Controls conversion of glucose from the blood to glycogen in the liver	Diabetes mellitus	Low blood sugar
	Glucagon	Converts liver glycogen into glucose		

the egg within it grow until the follicle is several times its original pinhead size. While it is growing, the follicle makes the estrogen hormones.

On about Day 14, stimulated by the pituitary gland, the follicle bursts and the egg enters the Fallopian tube on its way down to the uterus. If any sperm cells are present in the tube at this time, fertilization may take place. The fertilized egg continues its 6½-day journey down the tube and implants itself in the wall of the uterus. Meanwhile, the ruptured follicle from which the

egg was discharged is transformed into a yellowish, solid ball called the corpus luteum (Latin for "yellow body"). This body produces another hormone, progesterone. (See the entries on MENSTRUATION and OVULATION in the encyclopedia section.) During the last 14 days of the cycle, the hormones produced by the corpus luteum stimulate the development of the tissues and blood supply in the uterus.

The fertilized egg secretes its own hormone. This hormone helps the corpus luteum to persist

Gland or tissue	Hormones	Normal amount	Too little leads to	Too much leads to
Stomach and intestines	Gastrin	Stimulates secretion of gastric juice		
	Secretin	Stimulates secretion of pancreatic juice		
	Cholecystokinin	Stimulates release of bile from gallbladder		
	Enterogastrone	Inhibits secretion of acid by glands in stomach		
Ovaries	Estrogens	Stimulate development of female organs and secondary sexual characteristics	Absent or reduced sexual development; failure of periods to start	Premature sexual development
	Progesterone	Prepares lining of uterus for implantation of embryo; development of placenta; suppression of ovulation in pregnancy; development of mammary glands	Possible miscarriage	
	Relaxin	Softening and widening of pubic symphysis during childbirth		
Testes	Testosterone	Stimulates development of male organs and secondary sexual characteristics	Absent or reduced sexual development	Premature sexual development
Placenta	Progesterone	Suppresses ovulation during pregnancy; causes development of mammary glands		
Embryo	"Organizers"	Stimulate the correct sequence of development in the womb		
Kidney	Renin	Raises blood pressure to work kidney's filters		
	Erythropoietin	Regulates production of red blood cells by bone marrow		
Nerve endings	Adrenaline or acetylcholine	Transmit nerve impulses between nerve cells		

and continue making estrogen and progesterone. In other words, the process is like a chain reaction, with one hormone prodding the other two hormones to keep going.

If pregnancy does not occur, the corpus luteum degenerates and its secretions halt. With the stopping of the hormones, the rich blood supply built up in the lining of the uterus sloughs off and leaves the body during menstruation.

Scientists have learned how to make synthetic hormones in the laboratory, so that the process of ovulation can be controlled at will. The contraceptive pill prevents pregnancy by halting ovulation. (This and other birth-control methods are discussed in Chapter 12, "Family Planning.")

A pregnant woman has an additional powerful producer of sex hormones. This temporary hormone-generator is the placenta, the disk of tissue inside the uterus that acts principally as a bridge between the blood circulations of the mother and the developing baby. The hormones from the placenta include progesterone, estrogen, and gonadotrophin, which stimulates the woman's ovaries into continued hormone production after the normal commands from her pituitary gland have been switched off. Some of the gonadotrophin is filtered from the blood by the kidneys, and released in the urine. It is the presence of this hormone in a woman's urine that makes possible one of the most reliable chemical tests for early pregnancy.

HORMONES FROM OTHER TISSUES

Various activities of the body are controlled by hormones produced by organs or tissues other than the endocrine glands. For instance, hormones play a vital role in the processes of digestion. Small glands in the lining of the stomach react to the presence of protein-rich foods by secreting the hormone gastrin, which stimulates the flow of gastric juices. Other glands in the walls of the intestine release secretin, a hormone which helps to control the production of bile by the liver. The same hormone probably stimulates the pancreas to release its digestive juices into the intestine.

Bile is stored in the gallbladder. When food containing fats leaves the stomach and enters the duodenum (the first part of the small intestine), its walls release another hormone, called cholecystokinin. This is carried in the bloodstream to the gallbladder, where it causes the walls of the organ to contract and squirt bile into the duodenum. Bile is needed for the digestion of fats, and the hormone is the messenger that "tells" the gallbladder to make the necessary bile available.

CHAPTER 6

Germs and How to Fight Them

Medically speaking, a germ is a microorganism too small to be seen by the unaided eye; usually the term refers to an organism likely to cause disease. But germs also perform many useful functions—such as helping man to make bread, cheese, beer, or wine. Without these beneficial microorganisms, nothing would decay in the soil, which then would become infertile.

Germs are also known as microbes. Because of their tiny size, germs were not detected until the 17th century, and it was not until 1862 that the French chemist Louis Pasteur discovered their importance. He found that they play a vital role in the decomposition or fermentation of food, and that heat could kill germs—the pasteurization process for purifying milk. This led to the modern antiseptic method for preventing the spread of disease.

This chapter defines the six types of germs and tells what diseases they cause. It describes how the body fights them and what doctors do to help in this fight. The ways germs can enter your body and the precautions you should take to prevent them from taking hold are also discussed.

TYPES OF GERMS

There are six types of germs or microorganisms that cause communicable diseases: *bacteria, protozoa, viruses, rickettsiae, parasitic worms,* and *fungi.* Knowing something about them will make it easier for you to maintain good health. (Further information on these germs and the diseases they cause can be found in the encyclopedia section.)

Bacteria

Bacteria are single-celled microorganisms; most of them are more beneficial than harmful to human life. Some bacteria draw nitrogen from the atmosphere and fix it in the soil for use by growing plants. Others decompose all living matter after it dies, returning its components to the earth in a natural recycling process.

But there are other kinds of bacteria that produce disease in living bodies. All can be killed with heat. Chemical disinfectants such as alcohol, mercury compounds, phenol, and carbolic acid can also kill these germs, but these chemicals are poisonous and must be used with caution.

Among the many bacteria-caused diseases are pneumonia, typhoid fever, tetanus (lockjaw), botulism, syphilis, and diphtheria. Many such diseases—but not all—can now be controlled or stopped by sulfa drugs and antibiotics. However, two diseases—tetanus and botulism—have resisted both of these medical tools.

Protozoa

Protozoa are one-celled animals that may be 50 times larger than bacteria but still cannot be seen without a microscope. One of the most common of these germs is the ameba type, some of which cause amoebic dysentery. The disease is spread by contamination of food or water with the eliminations of a human carrier, either directly or by flies and other insects. Another amebic type of protozoa causes inflammation of the mucous membranes in the mouth and is suspected of causing pyorrhea, a disease of the gums.

One class of protozoa causes African sleeping sickness, a disease spread by the tsetse fly. Protozoan parasites produce malaria, which is transmitted from human to human by the anopheles mosquito.

Viruses

Viruses are the smallest disease-producing organisms. They are so tiny that they cannot be seen through an ordinary microscope but require an electron microscope to show their shape and structure. Viruses are more primitive than other microorganisms in that they lack certain elements in their structure that would allow them to grow by themselves. Instead, a virus must invade a cell and change that cell's chemical organization to suit the virus' needs. This altered cell can cause disease at once, but often the virus-dominated cell remains dormant until some circumstance lowers the resistance of the host body, permitting the cell to become active.

Drugs that are effective against other types of germs cannot overcome viruses. Instead, immunizing techniques that cause the body to produce antibodies are used against them. In some instances, a person who has recovered from a mild case of a virus-caused disease will develop an immunity.

Viruses are extremely potent; very small numbers can start a disease. They cause a great many illnesses, including poliomyelitis, yellow fever, influenza, infectious hepatitis, rabies, smallpox, chicken pox, measles, and mumps. The common cold is also caused by viruses.

Rickettsiae

Rickettsiae are submicroscopic organisms that are smaller than bacteria but larger than viruses. They resemble true bacteria in structure, but they also are like viruses in that they require a living cell in which to grow and reproduce. Rickettsiae are carried from one person to another by means of a transmitting insect. The organisms are spread by the bites or feces of ticks, fleas, lice, and by mites that may inhabit the bodies of both animals and man. The rickettsiae enter the victim's bloodstream through a break in the skin.

Some rickettsiae are peculiar to insects of a specific area and cause regional diseases such as Rocky Mountain spotted fever, which is spread by a tick. Others are responsible for such wide-ranging diseases as typhus.

Parasitic Worms

Some of these parasites can be readily seen by the unaided eye, while others are so small they can only be identified with a microscope. The smallest are the size of a pinhead; the largest, a tapeworm, can grow to a length of 26 feet.

Parasitic worms enter the human body by a variety of means. Some hookworm larvae penetrate the bare skin of a foot and work their way to the intestines, where they settle and suck blood. Other worm larvae use intermediate hosts. Trichina roundworm larvae get into pig tissue and, if the hog flesh is not thoroughly cooked, are transmitted to man. They cause trichinosis, a disease in which the parasites eventually infest the victim's muscles.

Many parasitic worms such as the flukes (one of two types of flatworms) are more prevalent in the tropics than they are in North America. The tapeworm (the second type of flatworm) is found in North America and is taken into the body by the eating of beef, pork, or fish containing this parasite. Among the roundworms common in the southern United States are the pinworm, the intestinal roundworm, and the hookworm.

Parasitic worms cause a wide variety of illnesses ranging from serious swelling or gastric discomfort to jaundice or anemia—and sometimes result in blindness or death.

Fungi

Fungi are plants which lack chlorophyll (the green pigment in leafy plants) and feed on live and/or dead organic matter. They come in many sizes, ranging from huge mushrooms, or toadstools, to microscopic spores. There are about 10,000 species of fungi, but only an estimated 35 to 40 types of fungi spores can cause disease in man.

Most common fungi-related illnesses are those involving the skin. These include diseases known by such generic nicknames as athlete's foot, jockstrap itch, ringworm, and jungle rot. Other fungi germs can cause internal illnesses involving a variety of body organs and ranging from mild infections to deadly reactions. Fungi are responsible for diseases such as actinomycosis and moniliasis. Fortunately, most of the more serious disorders caused by fungi are relatively rare in the United States.

HOW THE BODY FIGHTS GERMS

However, the body is not helpless against germs. It has filters, such as the tiny hairs in the nose, to keep them out, and secretions, such as the tears, to kill them or wash them away. If germs do get into the blood, leukocytes (white blood cells) attack and devour them. When an infection develops, the number of these white cells increases

How the body fights infection

Infectious diseases are caused by viruses, bacteria, fungi, worms, and other parasites, which enter the body through the skin, nose, mouth, or other openings of the body. The body has various barriers against such invasions.

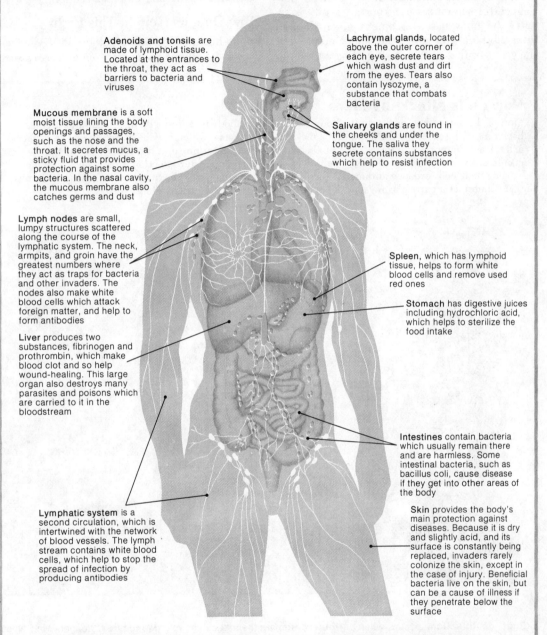

Adenoids and tonsils are made of lymphoid tissue. Located at the entrances to the throat, they act as barriers to bacteria and viruses

Lachrymal glands, located above the outer corner of each eye, secrete tears which wash dust and dirt from the eyes. Tears also contain lysozyme, a substance that combats bacteria

Mucous membrane is a soft moist tissue lining the body openings and passages, such as the nose and the throat. It secretes mucus, a sticky fluid that provides protection against some bacteria. In the nasal cavity, the mucous membrane also catches germs and dust

Salivary glands are found in the cheeks and under the tongue. The saliva they secrete contains substances which help to resist infection

Lymph nodes are small, lumpy structures scattered along the course of the lymphatic system. The neck, armpits, and groin have the greatest numbers where they act as traps for bacteria and other invaders. The nodes also make white blood cells which attack foreign matter, and help to form antibodies

Spleen, which has lymphoid tissue, helps to form white blood cells and remove used red ones

Stomach has digestive juices including hydrochloric acid, which helps to sterilize the food intake

Liver produces two substances, fibrinogen and prothrombin, which make blood clot and so help wound-healing. This large organ also destroys many parasites and poisons which are carried to it in the bloodstream

Intestines contain bacteria which usually remain there and are harmless. Some intestinal bacteria, such as bacillus coli, cause disease if they get into other areas of the body

Lymphatic system is a second circulation, which is intertwined with the network of blood vessels. The lymph stream contains white blood cells, which help to stop the spread of infection by producing antibodies

Skin provides the body's main protection against diseases. Because it is dry and slightly acid, and its surface is constantly being replaced, invaders rarely colonize the skin, except in the case of injury. Beneficial bacteria live on the skin, but can be a cause of illness if they penetrate below the surface

The skin is the first line of defense. Any wound through which germs might enter is soon closed by a blood clot, which also makes tissue repair possible. Secretions produced in the body openings and cavities also provide protection. Mucus from the membranes lining the nose and throat resists infection.

Tears wash germs from the eyes; saliva in the mouth and acid in the stomach destroy invaders. Because these barriers can fail to protect the body, another line of defense exists in the bloodstream and the lymphatic system, where white blood cells and antibodies combat invaders.

rapidly. Fever raises the body's temperature to inhibit or destroy germs.

The body has other resources as well. It manufactures substances that counteract the germs and render their poisons (toxins) harmless. These germ fighters are called antibodies, and the poison-control substances are known as antitoxins. After the body has overcome a given disease, these substances remain in the blood and prevent the germs of that disease from getting a foothold again. Physicians refer to this condition as an *acquired* immunity. People who are immune to a disease without ever having had it are said to have a *natural* immunity. Many immunities are partial or temporary. (See ANTIBODY; ANTITOXIN; IMMUNITY in the encyclopedia section.)

How Doctors Help in This Fight

Public-health measures together with vaccinations have all but eliminated some diseases such

How cells attack invaders

Most of the germs that penetrate the body are bacteria or viruses. These disrupt bodily functions and release poisons called toxins. Their effects are counteracted by the body's defensive cells.

Some body cells produce antibodies, substances that counteract a particular invader. Each antibody is tailor-made to combat a particular antigen—which may be a protein on the surface of a bacterium, or a toxin produced by the infection. After infection is past, the antibodies may remain in the bloodstream, giving immunity against similar invasions.

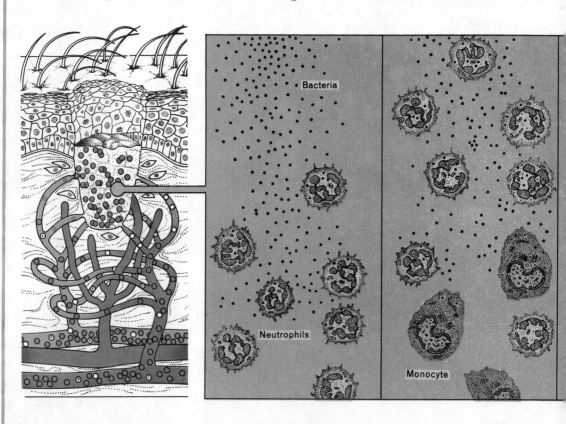

Start of infection occurs when germs enter the body through a cut. White blood cells engulf them, but if the germs are not destroyed by these cells, they may enter the blood and lymph streams and multiply, causing generalized "blood poisoning."

Neutrophils are the first defensive white cells to arrive at the site of an infection. Formed in the bone marrow and the spleen, they begin to engulf the bacteria, although their effectiveness against these infective invaders is short-lived.

Monocytes, longer-living types of white blood cells, move in after the neutrophils. These new arrivals turn into macrophages, cells that remove pathogens and disintegrating neutrophils. The macrophages also play a part in antibody formation.

as smallpox and polio. But no layman should make any assumptions about whether or not such protection is needed. A doctor's counsel and—when recommended—vaccination are always best.

Immunization. Immunization is a simple process. The doctor introduces a killed or weakened form of the germ, or a related strain of a similar but harmless disease, into the blood. For example, if the Sabin polio immunization is employed, the doctor or a nurse simply gives the patient a series of doses of a vaccine containing the attenuated, or weakened, virus. The patient's blood then creates antibodies to protect the individual from the assault of the disease germs. The introduction of material that has been modified or rendered harmless causes the body to create a resistance to certain germs; this is the principle on which all innoculation for immunization is based.

Body cells attack disease-causing bacteria, or pathogens, in various ways. Some antibodies break up bacteria before destroying them. Others prevent their growth by causing them to clump together; the clumped bacteria are then mopped up by white blood cells. Certain antibodies are antitoxins, which neutralize bacterial poisons.

Like bacteria, viruses stimulate the body cells to produce antibodies. In some diseases, such as smallpox, one infection produces long-term immunity. But in other cases, such as colds and influenza, the antibodies are effective only for a short time.

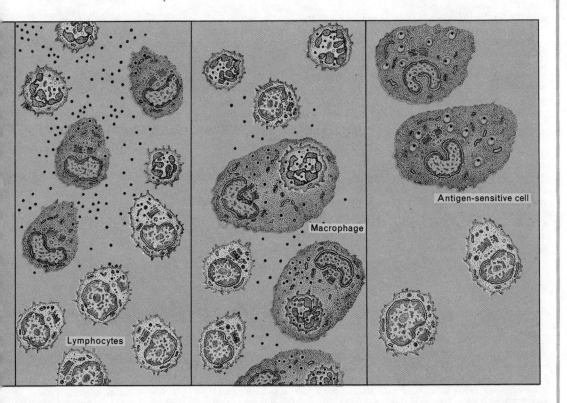

Antigen-sensitive cell

Macrophage

Lymphocytes

Lymphocytes, a third type of white blood cell, also enter infected areas. When these small cells come in contact with bacteria, they develop into larger cells. These new lymphocytes create plasma cells, which control antibody production.

Bacteria are eventually engulfed by macrophages and lymphocytes, and are also attacked and destroyed by antibodies. These substances are produced by plasma cells in the lymphatic system, through which they travel to infected areas.

End of infection occurs with the destruction of bacteria and the removal of debris. The bacterial antigens stimulate sensitive white cells to produce antibodies, which provide immunity against later attacks by the same invader.

Immunity acquired this way is *active* because it is the individual's body that makes the protective substances. The polio immunization, which has helped to nearly wipe out that disease, is an active immunity process. *Passive* immunity results from an injection by the doctor of antibodies created in another person or animal. For instance, the immune globulin used in antirabies treatment is a passive immunity substance.

Diseases to Be Immunized Against. Everyone should have a schedule of immunization recommended by a doctor following Public Health Service (PHS) guidelines. The PHS currently recommends immunization against poliomyelitis (infantile paralysis), diphtheria, whooping cough, tetanus, measles, rubella (German measles), and mumps. It is especially important to protect, i.e., immunize, young children and those who come into close contact with them against such diseases.

Measles, for example, is a very serious affliction that can lead to other diseases such as pneumonia and damage to the nervous system. Protective vaccination can be given to children at age 12 months or at any time thereafter.

Immunity: natural defense and medical technique

The body's ability to resist and overcome disease depends on immunity, a natural defensive mechanism that is due to the presence in the blood and lymph streams of substances called antibodies. These attack disease-causing invaders, and there is an antibody for each disease.

Someone who is immune to a particular disease has the correct antibody already in his system. If it is lacking, the body cells produce the necessary antibody when invaders attack. Once formed, a specific antibody can provide lifelong resistance against a particular invader.

Antigens, the foreign substances that invade the body, stimulate the production of antibodies. Some are manufactured by various white cells, such as plasma cells and lymphocytes. Other antibodies are derived from the protein gamma globulin present in the bloodstream.

Immunity to particular diseases can be deliberately built up before exposure to infection by using immunization. One method involves giving injections of dead or weakened strains of bacteria or viruses, called vaccines. These preparations are strong enough to help the body produce antibodies, but are too weak to cause a dangerous infection.

Another method is to give an injection of blood serum containing ready-made antibodies, either from another human being or from an animal.

Immunity

Natural immunity
The immunity with which a person is born is natural immunity. Human beings are naturally immune to many diseases that afflict animals—for instance, human beings cannot catch swine fever. Certain groups of people have greater immunity to some diseases than to others. For example, some primitive peoples are less immune to tuberculosis than are Americans.

Active immunity

Acquired through disease
Active immunity results when someone produces his own antibodies against a disease, usually after he has recovered from an illness. The body can produce many antibodies, some of which—such as those against measles—remain effective for years

Acquired through vaccine
Active immunity may be produced by using a vaccine, which consists of dead or weakened strains of disease-causing bacteria or viruses. When the vaccine is injected, it stimulates the body to produce antibodies, which combat any infection. It may cause mild symptoms of the disease

Passive immunity

Acquired from the mother
Immunity may be passed on to a child from his mother. It is acquired in the womb from the mother's bloodstream, or through the colostrum, the watery fluid that flows from the mother's breasts for two or three days after the child's birth

Acquired from another victim
Antibodies or antitoxins can be taken from the blood of someone who has had a disease, and given to another who is suffering from it. Alternatively, antibody formation can be stimulated in the blood of an animal, such as a horse. This kind of immunity is always short-lived

Rubella threatens the life of the unborn child. Vaccination is recommended for children between the age of 12 months and puberty because they are most likely to spread the disease to a pregnant woman. Nonpregnant adult women of childbearing age should take a blood test to determine their immunity against rubella. If they are not immune, they should have the vaccination, provided they take measures not to become pregnant for at least two months after receiving the vaccine.

The success of immunization in controlling or practically eliminating disease has made many people complacent about preventive measures. For instance, poliomyelitis, a terrible disease and once widespread, was dramatically defeated by the Salk and Sabin vaccines. This led many people to assume that polio was no longer a threat to anyone. But that is far from true. There may be less chance of contracting it and other diseases because of broad immunization programs; but most doctors, backed by the PHS and the American Academy of Pediatrics, strongly advise an innoculation program for every family member.

Certain diseases such as tetanus (lockjaw) are ever present, ready to strike the unprotected. Tetanus, once contracted by a person not immunized, presents a very dangerous opponent to the patient and the doctor. Thoughtful people will seek immunity not only for this kind of common threat but, under special circumstances or in particular areas, for rarer diseases such as yellow fever, tularemia, and Rocky Mountain spotted fever.

Immunization will usually protect you from developing certain diseases even if it is administered after the germs have gained a foothold in your body. For example, rabies can be conquered by immunization after exposure—that is, injections given between the time the germs start to grow in your body and the time they cause the symptoms to appear. Treatment should be immediate if there is reason to suspect that the germs have entered your body and are causing an infection.

Other injections will help your body to win its battle against some diseases even after the illness is well under way. In diphtheria, for example, the antitoxin can be injected to neutralize the toxic effect of the germs.

Other Protections. Chemical substances, such as the sulfa-based medicines, can be used to destroy germs which have invaded the body. Some chemicals such as chloroquine, which attacks malaria germs, can be used as a preventive before invasion takes place. Antibiotics fight germs in different but effective ways. Penicillin destroys bacteria cell walls as these germs divide in order to multiply. Other antibiotics inhibit or prevent bacterial growth so that the germs can be overcome by the body's natural defenses.

HOW GERMS GET INTO YOUR BODY

Your skin is an excellent coat of armor that keeps most germs out of the body. But cuts or other breaks in this covering, and openings such as the nose and mouth, provide opportunities for germs to enter. When you breathe and ingest food and liquid, germs frequently hitch a ride on these life-sustaining elements to find their way to places inside where they can comfortably settle and multiply.

Although some germs can directly penetrate the skin, most enter when the body's armor is cut, pierced, or otherwise rendered vulnerable by injury.

Nose, Throat, and Lungs

Many bacteria and viruses are spread and taken into the body through the nose and throat. Large numbers of germs thrive in moisture, and spitting, coughing, and sneezing keeps them circulating from person to person. When you sneeze, you may expel a spray of liquid drops extending several feet.

Other germs can ride aboard tiny bits of dust, dirt, cigarette smoke, or other foreign matter into the mouth, throat, and lungs, and weaken the body's defenses. For example, the particles in cigarette smoke have a definite, harmful effect on lung tissue and make that tissue more susceptable to assault by inhaled germs.

Among the many illnesses caused by germs inhaled with air are the common cold, pneumonia, scarlet fever, diphtheria, influenza, and meningitis. Colds or flu, serious enough in themselves, weaken the body's resistance and offer other germs such as streptococci and pneumococci a greater chance to get a foothold in your body and cause more dangerous diseases. A persistent cough, especially one that lasts more than several weeks, may indicate the development of a serious condition, and a doctor should be consulted.

Infection from Food and Water

Solid foods and liquids provide perfect vehicles for germs to use to get past the body's natural

How the body fights colds

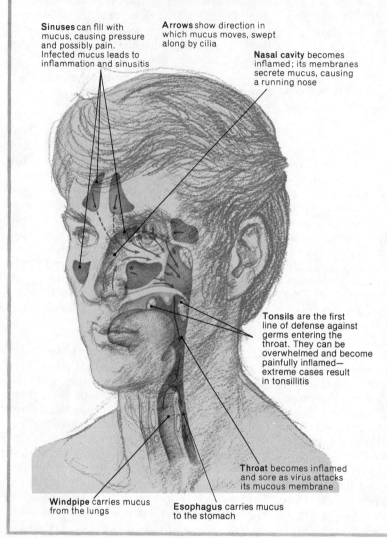

Sinuses can fill with mucus, causing pressure and possibly pain. Infected mucus leads to inflammation and sinusitis

Arrows show direction in which mucus moves, swept along by cilia

Nasal cavity becomes inflamed; its membranes secrete mucus, causing a running nose

Tonsils are the first line of defense against germs entering the throat. They can be overwhelmed and become painfully inflamed—extreme cases result in tonsillitis

Throat becomes inflamed and sore as virus attacks its mucous membrane

Windpipe carries mucus from the lungs

Esophagus carries mucus to the stomach

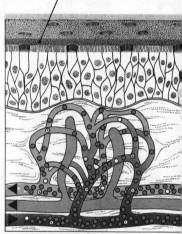

- ○ Neutrophils
- ⊙ Lymphocytes
- ● Red cells

Normal state of the membrane

Cilia, hair-like projections embedded in the mucus

Viruses, breathed in on airborne droplets from an infected person's sneeze, infiltrate the cells of the mucous membrane, which responds by secreting extra mucus.

armor. Many foods in their natural and uncooked states carry germs and the toxins they create. Even foods and liquids which have been thoroughly cleaned and boiled can be contaminated through improper and unsanitary handling by a germ carrier.

For example, amoebic dysentery is sometimes present in a public water system because the germs which cause it resist the chemicals used for purification. Typhoid fever, now relatively uncommon, is typical of the infections that can enter the body through the mouth. It is frequently transmitted in food, milk, or water that has been contaminated by feces.

Habits of cleanliness should be practiced by everyone, especially by those who handle and prepare food. Washing hands after going to the toilet and before eating should be as automatic as breathing.

Liquids. Water from the faucet in most cities is safe to drink. But if you live in the country or spend your vacation there, be careful about the drinking water. To be on the safe side, boil it for 10 minutes before drinking it.

Milk is a perfect culture medium for germs and thus requires especially careful preparation, preservation, and handling. *All* milk should be pasteurized. Raw (unpasteurized) milk—even from cattle certified as healthy—should be

A common cold is an infectious disease of the upper parts of the respiratory system—the nose and the throat. It can be caused by any one of a hundred or more viruses, and others are still being discovered.

Unlike bacteria, viruses multiply only within body cells. They also show preferences for certain types of tissue—for example, cold viruses infect only the membranes lining the nose and throat. Once inside these tissues, the viruses take control of the activities of the tissue cells, and begin to multiply rapidly. They kill the host cell, which

bursts and releases viruses that infect other cells. The virus stimulates the formation of antibodies, which may protect the patient against subsequent attacks by the same virus.

The symptoms of a cold appear 18-48 hours after infection. The nose begins to run, because the mucous membrane produces an excessive secretion of mucus to prevent the spread of the virus. This excess may fill the sinus cavities, causing a mild headache. The victim feels "low" and his joints may ache.

Onset of the cold　　**Peak of the cold**　　**End of the cold**

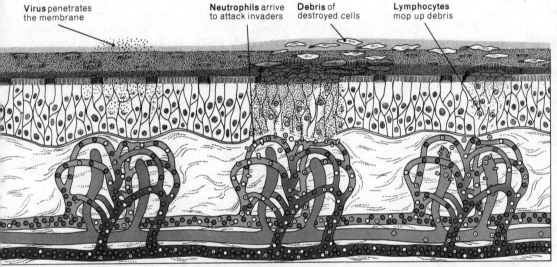

Virus penetrates the membrane

Neutrophils arrive to attack invaders

Debris of destroyed cells

Lymphocytes mop up debris

Cilia are tiny hairlike outgrowths from the cells of the mucous membranes which line the nose and windpipe. Their beating motion sweeps out mucus containing foreign matter.

White blood cells, such as neutrophils, rush to the site of the infection to attack the virus. As a result, antibodies are produced to neutralize the virus.

Infection ends after three or four days. Damaged membrane is shed on the fifth day, and new tissue is formed during the next two weeks. White cells are shed in the mucus.

scalded in a double boiler at 150° F for half an hour before being drunk. It should be stored under refrigeration to inhibit germ growth. And it should be kept in sterilized containers and away from sources of contamination.

Meats and Fish. Meats also carry disease. Pork may contain trichinae parasites and should be cooked thoroughly; pinkness of the flesh means the meat is underdone. Brucellosis (undulant fever) is a serious disease and can be acquired from pork, beef, and unpasteurized milk. Raw fish, beef, and pork may contain tapeworms. Thorough cooking of all meats and fish is the best protection.

Canned Foods. Improperly canned food is extremely dangerous. This is also true of home-preserved food whose containers have lost their airtightness. Such food can contain bacteria that cause food poisoning. One of the worst kinds, botulism, results from the toxin of a germ and produces a fatal paralysis. It is usually caused by home-canned food that was improperly processed. If you home-can food, use only the proven methods recommended by the U.S. Department of Agriculture and published in "Home and Garden Bulletin No. 8." You can get this publication by writing to the Superintendent of Documents, U.S. Government Printing Office, Washington, D.C. 20402.

Do not even taste canned food suspected of spoilage. Food from a bulging, punctured, or split container, or food that has an odd look or smell, can be deadly.

Baked Goods. Active germs may be lurking in bakery goods, especially those with custard fillings such as éclairs. Buy only fresh-baked goods from a clean, reliable bakery, and keep them refrigerated.

Refrigerating Food. One of the most frequent food infection problems results from poor refrigeration or none at all, thus allowing bacteria to grow. Every precaution should be taken to keep food that is susceptible to spoilage under proper refrigeration in order to prevent the growth of dangerous bacteria. In particular, moist salads and prepared dishes bought from trays in a store should be treated with caution. Many are made with milk or eggs, and unless fresh and well-refrigerated, they can harbor germ cultures.

Wounds and Scratches

All cuts, wounds, and scratches are potential entrances for germs. The damaged area should be washed with soap and water, then treated as explained in the FIRST AID section.

One of the most serious dangers from wounds and deep scratches is the germ causing tetanus (lockjaw). It is usually found in the soil—especially wherever there are horses, cows, and manure—and is also present in the dust of city streets. A deep puncture wound by a nail is serious; it is not the rust but the germs on the nail that cause infection.

The best preventive for tetanus is toxoid immunization. For children aged two months to six years, three doses at four to six weeks' intervals are recommended, with an additional dose at one year of age and another upon entering school. Thereafter, one dose every 10 years is advised. School-age children and adults who need immunization should get two doses at four to six weeks' intervals, a third dose at six to 12 months, and one every 10 years thereafter.

An injured person without toxoid immunization needs tetanus antitoxin (TAT). For those sensitive to this horse serum, tetanus immune globulin (TIG), made from human serum, can be substituted by the attending physician.

Animal Bites

Any animal bite that breaks the skin should be washed with soap and water, then covered with a sterile dressing. Do *not* use alcohol or other antiseptics. Always consult a doctor. (See also the FIRST AID section.)

Rabies is a virus disease that affects the brain and nervous system. It comes from a virus in the saliva of infected, warm-blooded wild and domestic animals such as dogs, cats, squirrels, and bats. If possible, the biting animal should be caught for examination by public health officials. Persons bitten by an infected animal or one suspected of rabies must receive treatment with either a combination of serum and vaccine, or of vaccine alone in some cases. Otherwise, rabies is fatal. If the bite of an infected animal is on the victim's head or neck, prompt treatment is vital because the virus can reach the brain rapidly.

All warm-blooded animals are potential rabies carriers, and any pet acting strangely should be examined by a veterinarian. Such pets should also be vaccinated against rabies if they roam free. Contact of any kind with a wild animal that behaves oddly—that is, approaches a human or does not run away—should be avoided. (See also the entry RABIES in the encyclopedia section.)

Insect Bites

Bites of insects are a source of infection because they often carry germs in their mouths or in their excrement. An insect bite breaks the body's skin armor, permitting germs to enter through the opening.

Germs that cause endemic typhus fever in Mexico and the southern United States are carried by fleas living on rats and other rodents. When the flea bites a human, the germs are transmitted. Similarly, Rocky Mountain spotted fever is transmitted by the bites of ticks.

Malaria and yellow fever are carried by certain mosquitoes. If you visit areas where malaria is prevalent, protect yourself against mosquitoes with a repellant and use mosquito netting over the bed. Although there is no immunization against malaria, your doctor can recommend effective prophylactic measures you should take in case you visit malaria-infested areas. (For further information about prevention of and treatment for insect bites, see Chapter 7.)

Physical Contact

The human reproductive process and customs related to it can result in contact with harmful germs. The urinogenital openings of the body are natural entrances for germs causing venereal diseases, which are spread by sexual contact. The germs causing two major venereal diseases,

114

Infectious diseases: causes and treatments

Disease	Germ	Transmission	Treatment	Prevention
Actinomycosis	Fungus		Antibiotics; sulfonamides	
Amebic dysentery	Protozoan (amoeba)	Food; water	Drugs	Hygiene
Anthrax	Bacteria (bacillus)	Contact (with animals)	Antibiotics	
Bilharziasis	Metazoan (trematode)	Water	Drugs	Avoid polluted water
Botulism	Bacteria (bacillus)	Food	Antiserum	Wholesome food
Brucellosis	Bacteria (brucella)	Milk; cattle	Antibiotics	Pasteurization of milk
Bubonic plague	Bacteria (pasteurella)	Rat flea bite	Antibiotics; sulfonamides	Hygiene; immunization
Chagas' disease	Protozoan (trypanosome)	Bug bite	Drugs	Hygiene
Chicken pox	Virus	Contact		Avoid contact
Cholera	Bacteria (vibrio)	Food; water	Saline drip; antibiotics	Immunization; hygiene
Diphtheria	Bacteria (bacillus)	Contact	Antitoxin; antibiotics	Immunization
Elephantiasis	Metazoan (filaria)	Mosquito bite	Drugs; surgery	Insecticides
Erysipelas	Bacteria (streptococcus)	Contact	Antibiotics	Hygiene
Gas gangrene	Bacteria (bacillus)	Contact	Antitoxin; antibiotics; surgery	Cleanse wounds
Gonorrhoea	Bacteria (diplococcus)	Contact	Antibiotics	
Influenza	Virus	Airborne droplets		Immunization
Leishmaniasis	Protozoan (flagellate)	Sand fly bite	Drugs	Hygiene
Leprosy	Bacteria (bacillus)	Prolonged contact	Drugs	
Malaria	Protozoan (plasmodium)	Mosquito bite	Drugs	Drugs
Measles	Virus	Contact		Immunization
Meningitis (bacterial)	Bacteria (diplococcus)	Contact	Antibiotics; sulfonamides	
Mononucleosis	Virus	Contact	Rest	
Mumps	Virus	Contact		Immunization
Pneumonia (lobar)	Bacteria (diplococcus)	Airborne droplets	Antibiotics; sulfonamides	
Poliomyelitis	Virus	Contact; droplets		Immunization
Psittacosis	Virus	Contact (with birds)	Antibiotics	Hygiene
Rabies	Virus	Animal bites	Early immunization	
Ringworm	Fungus	Contact	Antibiotics	Hygiene
Rubella (German measles)	Virus	Contact		Immunization
Shingles	Virus	Contact		
Sleeping sickness	Protozoan (trypanosome)	Tsetse fly bite	Drugs	
Smallpox	Virus	Contact		Immunization
Streptococcal infections	Bacteria (streptococcus)	Contact; droplets	Antibiotics	
Syphilis	Bacteria (spirochete)	Contact	Antibiotics	
Tetanus	Bacteria (bacillus)	Contact	Antitoxin; intensive care	Immunization
Thrush (moniliasis)	Fungus	Contact	Antibiotics	Hygiene
Tuberculosis	Bacteria (bacillus)	Airborne droplets; milk	Antibiotics	Immunization
Typhoid	Bacteria (bacillus)	Food; water	Antibiotics	Hygiene; immunization
Typhus	Rickettsia	Louse or flea bite	Antibiotics	Hygiene; immunization
Whooping cough	Bacteria	Contact; droplets	Antibiotics	Immunization
Yaws	Bacteria (spirochete)	Contact	Antibiotics	
Yellow fever	Virus	Mosquito bite		Immunization

Germs enter the body through the nose, throat, lungs, intestinal tract, or skin, and they may soon bring about a feverish reaction throughout the body. There are few effective drugs for treating virus infections, but antibiotics are available for most diseases caused by bacteria and rickettsiae. Protozoa and metazoa, which include worms, are disease-causing parasites that can be wiped out by drugs. Immunization is the best method of preventing diseases, such as diphtheria, whooping cough, poliomyelitis, and measles, which are caused by bacteria or viruses.

syphilis and gonorrhea, thrive in a warm, moist environment and are transmitted from one human to another by contact of mucous membrane surfaces. (See the entries CHANCROID; GONORRHEA; LYMPHOGRANULOMA VENEREUM; VENEREAL DISEASE in the encyclopedia section.)

TAKE REASONABLE PRECAUTIONS

Although germs are everywhere, there is no need to be intimidated by them. Like many other dangers to life and health, this threat can easily be minimized if you simply exercise common sense. For example, do not drink from glasses or use towels that have been used by others. Minimize your contacts with infected persons. When you are in an area where dangerous germs are known to exist in great numbers, follow recommended anti-infection procedures that have proved to be effective. Insect repellents, clothing and shoes that protect you from wounds, and the avoidance of food and water suspected of transmitting disease can all play major roles in keeping you healthy.

Soap and water can destroy or wash away many germs. Disinfectants are useful in inhibiting germs, but they can lull you into a false sense of security. Antiseptics such as a strong bleach will kill germs, but being poisonous, they can be dangerous if improperly handled. In general, soap and water, fresh air, and sunshine are the best everyday aids in killing germs.

Finally, if you know you have been exposed to dangerous germs and suspect infection, consult your physician at once. If you take reasonable precautions to keep germs away, you will find that you can get along very well in spite of them.

Keeping Healthy at Work and Play

CHAPTER 7

The mounting effects of our advanced technology on the environment have created serious health problems and dangers for all of us at work and at play. This chapter defines the health hazards that industrial workers, farmers, and business and professional people encounter in their work, and describes the proper safety measures necessary to guard against them. Here, too, are helpful health rules you should follow to make your vacation a healthy as well as a happy one. For instance, you will find a list of medical supplies you should take along on holidays, tips to prevent sunburn, ways to treat cases of plant poisoning and insect bites—and much more.

YOUR HEALTH AND SAFETY ON THE JOB

In recent years we have become increasingly aware of the close relationship between environment and health, and of the health problems our advanced technology has brought with it. The air has been polluted by noxious fumes; waterways have been ruined by industrial wastes; our food has been contaminated by these pollutants and by various additives and chemicals. In addition, working men and women are often exposed to serious health and safety hazards by their job environments. According to the National Safety Council, 13,000 Americans die yearly of job-related accidents, and a much greater number—estimated officially at 100,000 persons—die as a result of occupational diseases.

Industrial workers are not the only ones whose jobs can endanger their health and lives. Farm workers, too, face job-related health problems. And many business and professional workers develop a number of illnesses caused in large part by the emotional stress associated with their work.

Increasing recognition of these work-related problems by government, labor unions, employers, and the medical profession has brought about greater efforts to reduce environmentally produced health hazards. But in a highly industrialized society such as ours it is unlikely that such hazards can ever be entirely eliminated, or that

it will be possible to identify and deal with all of them before they have done some damage. Occupational diseases, for example, generally take years to develop. Indeed, the prime distinction between health and safety hazards is that safety hazards usually do immediate harm in one dramatic episode, while health hazards work more slowly and insidiously and produce recognizable damage only after a protracted period of time.

Fortunately, there are many things that you can do to protect yourself from the health and safety hazards associated with your work. Learning what these risks are is one way of arming yourself against them. This chapter describes some of the hazards and suggests ways to deal with them. (Health hazards involved in housework are reviewed in Chapter 21.)

General Health and Safety Rules at Work

You should go to work feeling rested and relaxed. Fatigue not only lowers your resistance to disease, but it also causes accidents. Excessive drinking is unwise at any time and is especially unwise on the evening before a working day. A worker should never drink so much that he suffers from a hangover at work.

Regular periods of rest are essential to good health. You should have one or two days off each week and should consider an annual vacation a necessity, not a luxury.

Find out the safety rules on your job and follow them closely. Make sure you know where the first aid station is located. Be sure your work area is adequately lighted. Poor lighting can cause accidents, eye fatigue, dizziness, and headaches. Company lavatories should be clean and adequately equipped; they should be inspected regularly by health officials.

At your place of work watch out for defective electrical wiring and for wet or slippery floors. The first should be corrected; the second guarded against. Practical jokers are a safety hazard, too, as are workers who do not know how to handle dangerous equipment. If a fellow worker has proved to be a danger to himself or his colleagues, you should take up the matter with someone in authority.

The Occupational Safety and Health Act of 1970 established workplace standards with which every employer must comply. If you believe that your job endangers your health or safety, try to get help either from the company management or from your union in correcting the condition. But if the condition is not corrected, then call or write the nearest area office of the Occupational Safety and Health Administration, U.S. Department of Labor. If it develops that the hazard is not covered by the Occupational Safety and Health Act, get in touch with the National Institute for Occupational Safety and Health, 5600 Fishers Lane, Rockville, Maryland 20857.

The institute will make a hazard evaluation for you if it proves necessary.

Hazards on the Industrial Job

Workers in many industries make use of equipment that exposes them directly to the risks of serious accidents. Among these safety hazards are machinery with fast-moving parts; equipment used to move heavy materials from one place to another; chemicals and pressurized containers that may explode; improperly grounded and defective wiring; mechanical operations such as cutting or grinding that throw off chips and particles that may get into the eyes; and liquids or mists that may damage the skin, eyes, or lungs. If your job brings you into contact with any of these potential dangers, your employer is required to supply you with the instructions and equipment necessary to reduce the risks you face.

Other equally serious safety hazards do their damage less directly by affecting the worker's concentration and alertness—thus increasing the possibility of accident. Noise, heat, and vibration are the most common of these hazards. People who work in excessively noisy places are known to have unusually high accident rates. Moreover, a sudden loud noise can rupture the eardrum; and continued loud noise leads eventually to hearing loss.

Such workers as firefighters, glassblowers, iron smelters, foundry workers, and steelworkers fol-

Health and safety on the job

If you want more information about the health and safety standards of your own job—legislation, workplace requirements, occupational diseases—write to the regional office of the Occupational Safety and Health Administration (OSHA) nearest you. All inquiries should be addressed to OSHA Regional Administrator, at one of the following regional offices:

16–18 North Street
One Dock Square, 4th floor
Boston, Massachusetts 02109

Room 3445
1515 Broadway
New York, New York 10036

Suite 2100
Gateway Building
3535 Market Street
Philadelphia, Pennsylvania 19104

Suite 587
1375 Peachtree Street NE
Atlanta, Georgia 30309

Room 3263
230 South Dearborn Street
Chicago, Illinois 60604

Room 602
555 Griffin Square Building
Dallas, Texas 75202

Room 3000
911 Walnut Street
Kansas City, Missouri 64106

Room 1554
Federal Building
1961 Stout Street
Denver, Colorado 80202

11349 Federal Building
P.O. Box 36017
450 Golden Gate Avenue
San Francisco, California 94102

Room 6003
Federal Office Building
909 First Avenue
Seattle, Washington 98174

low occupations that are, by their very nature, risky. The risk is increased by the high temperatures associated with their work because heat accelerates fatigue, decreases coordination, and increases irritability. In addition, overexposure to high temperatures can lead to heat stroke which, in some cases, can be fatal.

Continued exposure to vibration creates a safety hazard for an estimated 8 million American workers—truck and forklift drivers, operators of pneumatic tools, construction workers, railroad workers, drivers of intercity buses. Constant vibration and noise put the body under stress, thus increasing the risk of accidents. Vibration and noise also heighten the chance of an accident by making communication among workers difficult, and by affecting vision.

Materials used in many industries expose the workers who handle them to serious health risks. The primary dangers come from dusts; toxic gases, metals, and chemicals; carcinogens (substances or agents that can cause cancer); infectious diseases; and abnormal air pressure.

Dusts. Industrial dusts usually come from the grinding, crushing, cutting, or drilling of such materials as metals, stone, or coal. They most commonly enter the body through the respiratory system—that is, they are breathed in. The damage they do usually has its primary effect on the lungs. Its extent depends on a number of factors, among them the size of the particles, their concentration in the air, and the length of time the worker is exposed to them.

Workers exposed to dangerous dusts should be protected by the use of exhaust systems or suction devices that catch the dust at its place of origin, by systematic covering of the dust to keep it from rising, by good ventilation, and by the use of respiratory masks. Workers exposed to dangerous dusts should have periodic medical examinations, including chest X rays.

The types of dust that have been implicated most strongly in occupational diseases are silica, cotton, coal, asbestos, and beryllium.

Silica dust. More than 1 million American workers are exposed to silica dust through their work in the mining, quarrying, glassblowing, and stonecutting industries, and in foundries and in granite and brick works. The disease most commonly associated with prolonged exposure to silica dust is silicosis, an illness that shows itself in shortness of breath, coughing, chest pain, and physical weakness. Silicosis may take years to develop, but once the symptoms have become

manifest, there is little likelihood that the patient will survive for long. Tuberculosis is a frequent complication of silicosis. (For further information, see the entries SILICOSIS; TUBERCULOSIS in the encyclopedia section.)

Cotton dust. About 800,000 workers in the textile industry come into contact with cotton dust and are therefore exposed to the possibility of developing byssinosis, more commonly known as mill fever, or brown lung disease. The symptoms and effects of brown lung disease are similar to those of silicosis, and the prognosis is equally gloomy.

Coal dust. Some 200,000 workers in the coal mining and processing industries are exposed to the possibility of contracting anthracosis, commonly known as black lung disease. The symptoms and effects of this illness are also similar to those of silicosis.

Asbestos dust. About 350,000 American workers—asbestos miners, insulation and construction workers, sheet-metal workers, and automobile mechanics—are regularly exposed to asbestos dust. Breathing in these particles over a period of time can cause asbestosis, a lung disease that produces coughing, weight loss, and breathing difficulties. The disease does not reverse itself even when exposure to the dust is discontinued. Prolonged exposure to asbestos particles can have even more damaging results. It is known to cause mesothelioma, a type of chest tumor, and it can cause lung cancer, cancer of the pleura (the membrane that lines the chest cavity and covers both lungs), and cancer of the intestine.

Beryllium dust. A chronic lung disease associated with prolonged inhalation of beryllium dust, berylliosis is a threat to workers in the metallurgical, ceramic, and fluorescent-lamp business, and in industries where the metal is extracted from ore. Fortunately, berylliosis can be treated and cured, often within six months, and the number of workers risking berylliosis is relatively small—about 30,000. On the other hand, workers who come into prolonged contact with beryllium dust run a higher risk than average of developing lung cancer and cancer of the liver, gallbladder, or bile duct.

Toxic Gases, Metals, and Chemicals. The gases, metals, and chemicals used in many industrial processes can present a serious risk to the health of workers who come into contact with them. Toxic materials that enter the body through the respiratory system in the form of fumes can cause a wide range of medical problems. Benzene, for example, is widely used in the rubber, oil, and insecticide industries. Inhalation of large quantities of benzene vapor can cause headaches, dizziness, and fatigue; breathing in the vapor at sufficiently high levels can cause convulsions and death.

Fumes from the materials used in some hair sprays and hair dyes are dangerous to hairdressers and cosmetologists, who are regularly exposed to them. Constant inhalation of these fumes can lead to chronic lung disease and even to lung cancer. Workers whose jobs bring them into constant or frequent contact with chemical and gas fumes should be protected by efficient ventilation systems and, if necessary, by the use of respiratory masks.

Toxic materials can also enter the system through the skin. Dermatitis, or skin disease, is one of the most common of all occupational diseases. The chief troublemakers are petroleum products, solvents, and alkalis. Several important precautions can be taken to prevent dermatitis. Gloves, sleeves, and aprons offering protection against skin disease should be worn, kept clean, and often changed. Soap and water should be used generously and frequently during the working day, and especially before eating lunch and before leaving the job. Your doctor can recommend special ointments to be used to cover the skin before contact with an offending agent. If, in spite of all precautions, you develop a skin disease that seems to be related to the work you do, consult your doctor. Your problem may require a prescription drug.

Carcinogens. It is now widely accepted that environmental factors play a major role in the development of many forms of cancer. Substances used by workers in many industries may cause certain forms of malignancies. For example, workers in the plastics industry, where vinyl chloride is commonly used, run a higher risk than the rest of the population in developing liver cancer and brain cancer. Exposure of workers to coal combustion products increases their chances of developing lung cancer, bladder cancer, and cancer of the scrotum. Workers in the rubber and dye industries, where benzidine is commonly used, may develop urinary bladder cancer. Some workers in chemical processing plants, coke ovens, mines, and smelters are exposed to arsenic, which can lead to lung cancer, liver cancer, or cancer of the lymphatic system.

Asbestos dust and tar are especially dangerous because they are carcinogens. As well as being a health hazard for smokers, tar is an occupational health hazard for professional fishermen, who, statistics show, have a higher incidence of lip cancer than the rest of the population. Apparently this phenomenon occurs because tar is used to keep fishing nets from rotting, and fishermen often put mending needles in their mouths when they repair nets, thus inadvertently exposing their lips to tar.

Radiation can also be a carcinogen. Prolonged exposure to X rays is associated with incidence of leukemia. Welders, glassblowers, steelworkers, foundrymen, and electricians are often exposed to high intensities of ultraviolet light—a form of radiation associated with the development of melanoma, or skin cancer. (For further information, see the entries CANCER; LEUKEMIA in the encyclopedia section.)

Workers in industries that use known or suspected carcinogens should take care to observe all the industry rules for health and safety. It is especially important for the employees to have regular physical examinations.

Infectious Diseases. Workers who handle cattle may get brucellosis, or undulant fever; those who work with animal hides may contract anthrax; and those working in slaughterhouses should guard against tetanus. Dog-pound workers must beware of rabies. Barbers and beauticians should guard against ringworm and other fungus infections. (See the entries on these diseases in the encyclopedia section.)

Abnormal Air Pressure. Divers and sandhogs—men who build tunnels—do their work under unusually high air pressure. If the pressure is decreased too quickly, the blood supply from various parts of the body may be blocked off. This condition, known as the bends, caisson disease, or decompression sickness, is dangerous; it can even cause death. (See the entry BENDS in the encyclopedia section.)

Hazards for Agricultural Workers

Safety Hazards. The machinery used by farmers and agricultural workers presents a serious safety hazard. The most dangerous piece of farm machinery is the tractor, which can crush, mangle, and kill. A tractor should be equipped with ROPS (Roll Over Protective Structures), which prevent injury in case it turns over, and all farm vehicles should carry first aid kits. (See the FIRST AID section.)

Occupational accidents in 1974

Between 1912 and 1978 accidental work deaths in the United States were reduced by 71 percent, from 21 to 6 per 100,000.

Industry	Workers	Deaths	Death rate per 100,000	Disabling Injuries
Mining, quarrying	800,000	500	63	40,000
Construction	4,600,000	2,600	57	240,000
Agriculture	3,500,000	1,900	54	190,000
Transportation and public utilities	5,100,000	1,500	29	170,000
Government	15,400,000	1,700	11	310,000
Service*	22,900,000	1,700	7	360,000
Manufacturing	20,300,000	1,800	9	490,000
Trade†	22,200,000	1,300	6	400,000

* Finance, hospitals, insurance, lodging, real estate etc.
† Wholesale and retail

Even small wounds suffered by farm workers should be treated immediately because of the danger of infection. Everyone living in rural areas—particularly children—should be innoculated against tetanus (lockjaw), which is a far greater danger in the country than it is in the city. (See the entry TETANUS in the encyclopedia section.)

Heat stress can be as serious a safety hazard for farm and agricultural workers as for industrial workers. Strenuous, prolonged work in the open sun can lead to heat exhaustion or to sunstroke. The constant vibration associated with heavy farm machinery is also a hazard.

Health Hazards. Animal bites are always a health hazard for farm workers. The wounds should be washed with soap and water, then reported to a doctor. The animal should be examined for rabies. A number of other diseases can also be passed from infected animals to human beings, among them brucellosis, dysentery, tuberculosis, and tularemia (rabbit fever). In areas where sanitary facilities are inadequate, hookworm disease and typhoid fever are serious menaces. (See also the entries on these diseases in the encyclopedia section.)

The pesticides used in agriculture can be a major health hazard for workers who come into contact with them. Extreme caution should be taken when spraying pesticides and when entering a field that has recently been sprayed. Chemicals used on tobacco, cotton, citrus fruits, peaches, and apples can be lethal. These organophosphate insecticides are virtually nerve gases; if they have not been given sufficient time to dissipate before a worker comes into contact with them, they can produce serious illness.

Hazards for White-Collar and Professional Workers

The relationship between emotional stress and disease is now well established. The emotional stress associated with certain managerial and professional jobs presents a real health hazard to men and women in these occupations. For instance, it is known that administrators, who often work under severe pressure, are far more likely to develop coronary disease than are scientists or engineers. Other illnesses associated with job-related stress are gastric ulcers and hypertension. (For further information about emotional stress and disease, see Chapter 8.)

VACATIONS—HEALTH RULES AND SAFETY HAZARDS

A regular vacation is a necessary part of any plan for maintaining good physical and mental health. But to get the most from your vacation, there are important health and safety rules you should observe and major precautions you should take.

If you are going to some distant or exotic place, visit your doctor before making your vacation plans final. He will advise you as to necessary inoculations and prophylactic procedures. If you are going abroad, you may need a series of immunizations. Visits to some areas require protection against amoebic and bacillary dysentery. If you are going to a region where the anopheles mosquito is found, your doctor will supply you with chloroquine phosphate in 500-milligram doses to be taken once the week before you leave and continued weekly during your vacation and for six weeks after your return. Typhoid and tetanus shots may be advisable. If you have hay fever, your doctor will be able to advise you about conditions in the area you are planning to visit. (See also the entries HAY FEVER; TETANUS in the encyclopedia section.)

If you are planning to camp in the woods, you should take with you a complete first aid kit (see FIRST AID section) and the following medicines and supplies:

Aspirin, for headaches, fever, muscle aches and pains

Antiseptic, such as hydrogen peroxide or tincture of iodine

Skin lotion, for protection against sunburn and windburn

Antacid, for mild stomach upset

Pectin-kaolin compound for diarrhea

Decongestants, for the common cold

Antinauseant, for motion sickness (to be recommended by your doctor)

Broadband antibiotic, effective against a wide range of bacteria, in case of serious illness (Because antibiotics require a doctor's prescription, have your physician select the antibiotic you should take with you.)

Container of small bandages

Sterilized gauze squares

Adhesive tape, one-half inch wide

When you arrive at your vacation spot, do *not* plunge immediately into a full program of strenuous activity—especially if you normally lead a sedentary life; overexertion is bad for the heart. Work up to full activity gradually. Whenever you find yourself short of breath or panting, cut down on that activity or eliminate it entirely.

Be careful of what and how much you eat or drink. An overly rich diet, or unfamiliar foods, or contaminated water can cause diarrhea. (To find out how to handle this problem, see the entry DIARRHEA in the encyclopedia section.) If there is doubt about the purity of the water supply, be sure to boil your drinking water for 10 minutes. If you object to the flat taste of boiled water, aerate it by pouring it back and forth between the container and the glass several times. If pasteurized milk cannot be obtained, boil your milk before drinking it. Children sometimes object to the taste of boiled milk, but it can be disguised by chocolate or vanilla syrup.

Exposure to the Sun

Although sunshine helps psoriasis and some other skin diseases, overexposure can be dangerous. Sunshine can be harmful to people with tuberculosis of the lungs, nephritis, or lupus erythematosus, and overexposure can lead to melanoma (cancer of the skin). So be careful of the amount of sunshine you expose yourself to on vacation, both in sunbathing and in the normal course of your outdoor activities. Remember that the most sensitive areas of your body—the face, forearms, and legs—are the parts that normally receive the greatest exposure.

Watch out for the noonday sun because it can give you a serious burn. Sunburn can also be caused by reflected glare, even when the sky is overcast. This problem is particularly acute at the beach and on snow-covered mountains.

If you sunbathe, use a suntan lotion and plan your sunbathing time carefully. For the average person 15 minutes is long enough for the first exposure; thereafter, the amount of time can be increased daily.

Babies under two years of age and people with fair or sensitive skin are especially vulnerable to too much sunlight. During the brief periods in the sun—not more than five or 10 minutes—they should wear protective hats or visors and should use a suntan preparation containing the chemical PABA, or zinc oxide, which acts as a sunscreen. Others who should be particularly careful of overexposure are the elderly and people with heart trouble or other serious diseases. They should check with their doctors to find out how much sun is safe for them.

Becoming overheated in the hot sun is dangerous for everyone. When you perspire be sure to drink plenty of water to make up for the fluid you are losing. Salt tablets, salty crackers, or tomato juice with salt in it are also helpful.

Swimming

Swimming is a healthy sport for most people, but if you suffer from a chronic illness, or if you have been ill recently, check with your doctor to find out if it is safe for you. Diving and underwater swimming are not advisable for people having a tendency to sinus or ear infections. Too much water in the nose washes away the protective secretions that help prevent infection. Germs can spread into the sinuses through the nose or reach the middle ear through the Eustachian tubes.

Swimming in polluted water is dangerous to everyone. You should ask the local health department about the pools, beaches, and rivers in your vacation area that are safe for swimming.

Safety Rules for Swimmers. Even the best swimmers can get into trouble if they take foolish risks. Drowning ranks third among the kinds of fatal accidents that occur in the United States each year. So play it safe and observe these six safety rules:

(1) Do not go into the water immediately after meals or when you are overheated or tired from other exercise. Always come out before you get tired or chilly.

(2) Do not attempt a long swim during the first few days of your vacation. Your swimming muscles may have lost much of their strength through long disuse. Give them time to get strong again.

(3) When you take a long swim, have someone row along beside you, or have another good swimmer go with you. Always swim parallel to the shore or within rescue distance.

(4) No matter how well you swim, stay close to shore if you are swimming in an isolated spot.

(5) Before diving in a new place, test the water for depth and for hidden logs or rocks.

(6) All swimmers should know how to apply mouth-to-mouth resuscitation (see FIRST AID section).

Poisonous Plants

Poison ivy, eastern and western poison oak, and poison sumac are commonly found plants whose sap can irritate the skin. These plants are easy to recognize. The leaves of poison ivy and poison oak always grow in clusters of three—one at the end of the stalk, the other two opposite each other. Poison sumac has from 7 to 13 leaves, one at the end of the stalk, the others opposite one another, becoming smaller as they grow farther from the base.

Most cases of poisoning from a plant result from direct contact with it, regardless of whether or not it is in bloom. Poisoning can also be caused by handling clothing, garden implements, or pets contaminated by the plant's oily sap. Although some people seem to be immune to plant poisons, other individuals are so sensitive that mere exposure to smoke from a brush fire burning the offending plant can create a severe inflammation of the skin.

If you have accidentally handled or brushed against a poisonous plant, you should immediately wash the part of your body that has come into contact with it. Use yellow laundry soap if available and lather several times, rinsing the contaminated place in running water after each sudsing.

The first symptom of plant poisoning is a sensation of burning and itching that may develop at any time from a few hours to a week after contact. Thereafter, the skin swells and breaks out into a rash, and blisters are likely to form.

If large blisters, severe inflammation, or fever develop, or if the inflammation is on the face or genitals, do not attempt to treat the problem yourself. Consult a physician. But if there are only a few small blisters on the hands, arms, or legs, try the following treatment: Gently wash the affected parts with soap and cold water as soon as possible. Then apply calamine lotion to soothe the itch, or use a compress soaked in a diluted Burow's solution (aluminum acetate, an antiseptic)—one part of the solution to 15 parts of cold water.

Stubborn cases of plant poisoning that do not respond to proper treatment may be owing to repeated contact with contaminated clothing. Any suspected garment should be dry-cleaned or thoroughly washed with soap. (For further information, see the entry POISON IVY in the encyclopedia section.)

Insects

Spraying with insecticides will help get rid of most insects. But *all* insecticides contain material poisonous to humans, particularly children. So follow the instructions on the insecticide label carefully. Do not spray foods, dishes, or anything else that infants or children are likely to touch or put into their mouths. Do not use insecticides around open fires; many of them are flammable. Wash your face and hands after applying them.

Do not use a vaporizer, a device that gives off insect-destroying vapor for hours at a time. The constant presence of the vapor may be dangerous to both children and adults.

Insect repellants applied to the skin will usually keep insects away for about two hours. The U.S. Department of Agriculture recommends the following: dimethyl phthalate; dimethyl carbate; Indalone; 2-ethyl-1, 3 hexanediol (Rutgers 612). These chemicals may be used separately, but they do provide greater protection against a larger variety of insects if they are used in combination. Your druggist can supply you with a formula that is sometimes called 6-22 and is marketed by several firms; it contains 60 percent dimethyl phthalate, 20 percent dimethyl carbate, and 20 percent Indalone. These repellants are normally safe, but you should test them on a small area of your arm or leg before using them liberally, to see whether your skin is unduly sensitive to them.

Insect Bites. Most insect bites are relatively harmless annoyances rather than real threats. But the bites of certain spiders are extremely dangerous, and bee and hornet stings can endanger people who are especially sensitive to bee venom. Try to keep children away from holes in trees or other places where bees and hornets may gather. (For further information, see INSECT BITE in the encyclopedia section.)

Ticks, which fasten their heads into the victim's skin and suck the blood, can be disease carriers. You should carefully remove a tick by covering it with petroleum jelly. This will make the tick release its hold, and you can then remove the entire insect with a pair of tweezers. Destroy the tick—but not with your bare hands—and apply iodine to the tiny wound. (See also ROCKY MOUNTAIN SPOTTED FEVER in the encyclopedia section.)

Minor insect bites can be relieved by applying a paste made of baking soda and cold water. Never scratch insect bites. This only irritates them and may cause infection.

Snakes

Poisonous snakes are found in most of the warmer parts of North America. If you are going to a snake-infested part of the country, take a snakebite kit with you. Your doctor will be able to suggest its contents. (For information about emergency treatment of snakebite, see the FIRST AID section.)

Poisonous Foods

A number of types of poisonous berries and dozens of kinds of poisonous mushrooms grow in the woods and countryside. Although it is possible to learn to identify poisonous mushrooms and berries, the task is not easy. It is much wiser to play it safe by staying away from unfamiliar berries and mushrooms that are growing in the wild. Children are frequently tempted by poisonous holly berries and the berries that grow on privet. Train them not to eat anything they find in the woods or fields, and set a good example by following the same rule.

Mussels, clams, and certain other shellfish are dangerous during some seasons of the year, after they have fed on microscopic organisms that appear in the ocean during the warm months. Industrial wastes and other toxins have so polluted some waterways that their fish have become contaminated and unfit to eat. If you plan to fish during your vacation, do not eat the catch until you have made sure that it is safe. (For further information about food poisoning, see the FIRST AID section.)

CHAPTER 8

Your Mind and Your Emotions

When doctors use the word "mind," they do not mean it as a synonym for the word "brain." The brain is an organ of the body—a crinkled, folded mass of grayish tissue that serves as the center for intellectual functioning. The mind is something more than intellect. It includes the emotions and all the other qualities that we associate with the word "personality" and that are summed up in the Greek word psyche (life, spirit, soul), the prefix for virtually every word that has to do with the study or treatment of the mind.

But although it is not an organ of the body, the mind is profoundly influenced by the body's state. A cold or an upset stomach can make a normally cheerful person irritable and morose. A number of serious mental abnormalities are known to be the direct results of malfunctioning body chemistry, and others are the result of damage to the brain. But the mind is also a product of each individual's personal history—his childhood experiences, his cultural heritage, the events of his daily life. All these play major roles in establishing and maintaining his mental health.

THE NORMAL PERSON

When we discuss psychological functioning, the word "normal" is particularly difficult to define. The range of variations in human personality is enormous—from quiet to hearty; from serious to playful; from home-loving to adventurous. And even within the same individual, there are variations from one time to another and from one situation to the next. Moreover, different cultures set down different standards for normal psychological functioning. Behavior that is perfectly acceptable in Des Moines might be considered very peculiar in Tokyo. Even the same culture defines normality differently at various periods in history. Americans today regard as normal any number of behavior patterns that would have been labeled strange a mere 10 years ago.

Perhaps, then, the best definition of "normal" is also a fairly broad one. Most psychiatrists would agree that a person's psychological functioning is normal when he is able to perceive his environment realistically and is able to conduct himself in a fashion that enables him to find reasonable satisfaction in his work and his personal life. This does not mean that the normal

person does not experience mood swings or that he is always satisfied with his personal life or with his job. Nor does it mean that he assesses every single situation entirely realistically. What young man does not idealize the woman he loves? But just as no internist would describe as unhealthy someone with a minor cold, so no psychiatrist would describe as mentally ill the person whose boss or children occasionally tax his patience. Only when an individual's emotions cause him great pain or when he is unable to function adequately in the various roles his life calls on him to play, can he be described as mentally or emotionally ill.

CHARACTERISTICS OF THE NORMAL PERSONALITY

The normal adult has control over his impulses. He is not overwhelmed by sudden feelings of violent anger or rage. This does not mean that he never feels or expresses anger, but that his anger is moderate and that it does not arise for merely trivial reasons.

The normal adult does not demand that his every wish be fulfilled immediately. He is not stoically self-denying, but he is able to put off gratification today for the sake of tomorrow's goals. Moreover, those goals are realistic: the normal person has a clear sense of himself and his abilities. He is neither a loner nor a clinging vine. He is able to act independently and to take responsibility for his own behavior. At the same time, he recognizes his dependence on others and knows how to cooperate as well as to compete. He is at home with his conscience and is able to relax as well as to work hard.

Finally, the normal person has the capacity both to give love and receive it. This applies not only to sexual love, but to love of his children, family, and friends.

FIRST AID FOR EMOTIONAL UPSETS

No one, no matter how normal, is immune to emotional stress and upset. We live in a tense and fast-changing society, and pressures mount up for all of us in our daily lives—sometimes to the point of threatening our psychological equilibrium. Such feelings of tension should not be permitted to persist or to become chronic. They can generally be dispelled through one or another of the first aid suggestions that follow and that, indeed, you may already be using:

° Talk your worries over with a sympathetic friend, relative, doctor, or clergyman—or with anyone else whose judgment you respect.
° Get away from the immediate task or problem for a while—even if only for a walk.
° Deal with one thing at a time, especially if you feel overwhelmed by the pressure of too much to do.
° Give in sometimes in discussions or disputes, even if you are certain that you are right. It is just possible that you are not.
° Help others. Preoccupation with your own troubles can become a vicious circle.
° Be slow with criticism. Awareness of others' shortcomings is no excuse for harsh criticism.
° Above all, develop a capacity for contentment. Take pleasure in your physical well-being, in your surroundings, in the small gratifications of your daily life. Learn to enjoy your own company as well as the companionship of the people you really care for.

THE ABNORMAL PERSON

Medicine does not yet have all the answers to the problem of mental abnormality. But research in recent years has made it increasingly clear that some mental problems have a purely physical basis; others have their origin in unhappy childhood experiences; and still others result from a combination of the two. Mental retardation, for example, is known to be the consequence of physical factors—either faulty body chemistry or brain damage.

Some of the psychoses—the serious mental illnesses—are similarly organic in their origin. Other psychoses appear to be connected with both a genetic predisposition and with a psychologically unhealthy childhood. This combination of genetic predisposition and childhood experience also lies at the root of peptic ulcers and the other diseases that are described as psychosomatic. On the other hand, the neuroses (for example, phobias, depression, and persistent anxiety) and the so-called personality disorders (such as antisocial behavior) seem to be related entirely to the nature of the childhood history.

Most mental and emotional illnesses can be treated, and many can be cured. But because the same forms of therapy are used for different illnesses, the treatments available for these problems will be described at the end of the chapter.

Mental Retardation

The term "mental retardation" covers a wide range of conditions, from those associated merely with slower-than-average mental functioning to others so severe that their victims are totally unable to take care of any aspect of their lives. The degree of retardation is measured by the IQ score. Anyone with a score lower than 85 is considered to be a retardate; those whose scores are below 50 are generally too retarded to be able to care for themselves. (See the entries IN-TELLIGENCE QUOTIENT and MENTAL RETARDATION in the encyclopedia section.)

Whatever the degree of the retardation, the cause of the problem is biological—a defect in body chemistry, or brain damage of some kind, usually inflicted during fetal development or the process of birth.

A number of forms of mental retardation are associated with illness or other medical problems in the mother during her pregnancy. It is therefore important for every woman who wants to have a baby to check carefully with her doctor before becoming pregnant. Chapter 13, "Pregnancy and Childbirth," discusses some of the maternal conditions that can lead to defects in the unborn child and, therefore, make pregnancy inadvisable, or, at best, a calculated risk.

Some conditions that lead to mental retardation can be corrected if they are caught early enough. All of these cases develop while the fetus is still in the womb; all are the result of a faulty metabolism; and all can be corrected by diet. The most common of these illnesses are phenylketonuria, or PKU (see the entry PHENYLKETONURIA in the encyclopedia section), maple syrup urine disease, and galactosemia. Each of these has its own set of symptoms, and all are relatively easy to diagnose. The modern pediatrician is constantly on the alert for them.

But most forms of mental retardation cannot be reversed. If the infant's brain is damaged during the birth process, for example, that damage cannot be undone. For this reason, the parents of retarded children face special problems that should be discussed fully with the family doctor or with an expert in the problems of mental retardation.

If the retardation is so severe that the child will never be able to care for himself, the best solution—for the child as well as the rest of the family—may be early institutionalization. On the other hand, if the retardation is less serious, the child can and should be helped to make the most of the abilities he has. His parents' love and acceptance are most important in this regard. They can make a real contribution towards his development if they are warm and patient with his slowness and the difficulty he experiences in concentrating. Help is also available from the outside: a number of communities have special programs for retarded children, including special schools and classes, day-care centers, summer camps, and halfway houses.

The Neuroses

Everyone experiences conflict—the inability to make up his mind—at some time or another, and everyone finds that the experience produces anxiety. But the psychologically healthy person is able to tolerate the anxiety and to resolve the conflict by making a decision and acting on it. The neurotic cannot do these things. He cannot make up his mind, he cannot act, and he cannot tolerate the anxiety his feelings of conflict produce. His neurosis is his way of holding his conflict and his anxiety in check and of defending himself against awareness of them.

The conflicts from which neurotics suffer usually arise in childhood. If parents give their child the impression that his feelings are "bad" or "naughty"—if, for example, they do not permit him to express anger or love—the child will tend to view these perfectly normal feelings as dangerous. He will simply repress them, pushing them so far out of his consciousness that he does not need to feel the conflict between wanting to do something and fearing to do it. Instead, he will develop a neurosis, a set of symptoms he cannot control and does not understand and that impede his ability to function in one or more important areas of his life. Not only are his symptoms painful to him, they are also frightening—so frightening that he may even believe he is losing his mind. But neurosis is a far cry from psychosis. The neurotic is in good touch with reality; the psychotic is not. (See the entry PSYCHONEUROSIS in the encyclopedia section.)

Anxiety Neurosis. This form of neurosis often shows itself in one or more of the physical symptoms—sweating, dizziness, diarrhea, difficulty in breathing, pain near the heart—that are associated with the "fight or flight" reaction, the series of physiological changes that take place when the body prepares itself to deal with danger. Sometimes there are no physical symptoms, but simply feelings of foreboding or apprehension or even panic—the sense that danger is near. But the danger is not in the outside world. It is within the sufferer, hidden even from him. (See the entry ANXIETY in the encyclopedia section.)

Hysterical Neurosis, Conversion Type. The physical symptoms of anxiety neurosis are associated with the involuntary nervous system. When a neurosis takes the form of hysterical conversion, it expresses itself through the voluntary nervous system. An arm or leg may become paralyzed for no physical reason, or the victim may become blind or deaf—again, with no organic cause. Conversion hysteria can also express itself in thrashing, or convulsive seizures, or in severe pain for which no organic cause can be found. But conversion hysteria is not malingering. The victim's affliction or pain are very real to him. (See the entry HYSTERIA in the encyclopedia section.)

Hysterical Neurosis, Dissociative Type. In this neurosis, parts of the memory or of the personality are split off from consciousness, so that the victim becomes totally unaware of them. He may suffer from amnesia (see the entry AMNESIA in the encyclopedia section), or may enter trancelike states. Multiple personality, that rare occurrence in which two or more distinct personalities inhabit the same body, most of them unaware of the existence of the others, is also an example of hysterical dissociation.

Depersonalization Neurosis. This neurosis is similar to hysterical dissociation, but different in that depersonalization involves a generalized sense of unreality, both about the world and about one's self. Someone in a depersonalized state feels that the world is not what it seems, but something strange and frightening. He also begins to doubt his own identity—his connection with his own body. These sensations are quite terrifying, and individuals who experience episodes of depersonalization are frequently convinced that they are going insane.

Phobic Neurosis. The individual with a phobic neurosis defends himself against his anxiety by attaching it to some object or situation in the outside world—often a perfectly harmless one. The phobic person may be terrified of insects, of heights, of open or enclosed spaces; any number of things or situations can set off a severe anxiety attack. If the phobia is attached to objects or circumstances that the individual encounters frequently, his neurosis can keep him in almost chronic anxiety. Therefore, he takes extraordinary steps to avoid the encounters and thereby avoid the anxiety. (See also the entry PHOBIA in the encyclopedia section.)

Obsessive-Compulsive Neurosis. To be obsessive is to go over and over a thought fruitlessly and even against one's will. To be compulsive is to be dominated by the desire to do something, despite the knowledge that the action is meaningless or foolish. The person with these symptoms is defending himself against his real feelings by so crowding his mind and life with his obsessions and compulsions that his true responses simply cannot emerge. Many aspects of his life become ritualized: he must put on his clothes in a certain fashion; he must wash his hands 15 or 20 times a day; he may insist on seeing a certain television show every week although the program now bores him. Often, the obsessive-compulsive neurotic dislikes his own behavior. But he cannot control it.

Depressive Neurosis: A severe loss always causes mourning and unhappiness. This so-called reactive depression is normal, and everyone suffers from it at various times and to varying degrees. But the normal person works through his grief, and is able to resume his usual activities after a period of time. The person with a depressive neurosis remains constantly miserable. He may, in fact, be in that condition whether or not he has suffered any loss. Generally, such a person has a poor self-image, low self-esteem, and extremely high standards for himself. Such a combination easily leads to depression: the victim finds it impossible either to set realistic goals or to meet the unrealistic ones the depressive establishes for himself. (See the entry DEPRESSION in the encyclopedia section.)

Neurasthenic Neurosis. People who constantly feel weak and fatigued for no physical reason may be suffering from neurasthenic neurosis. This psychological disorder is especially common among middle-aged women who previously gave themselves over almost entirely to the care of their families, and now, with their children grown, find themselves without occupation or purpose. If their self-esteem was low to begin with, as is the case with neurasthenics, this sense of uselessness can be devastating.

Hypochondriac Neurosis. This neurosis is an obsessive concern with one's body and health, and a constant fear that one is ill. Like neurasthenia, hypochondria is usually found among the middle-aged, both men and women, and it, too, is almost always associated with low self-esteem. (See the entry HYPOCHONDRIA in the encyclopedia section.)

Personality Disorders

The neurotic submerges his basic conflicts, holding down his anxieties by such means as ritualized behavior or compulsive perfectionism. In contrast, the individual with a personality disorder is driven to act out his conflicts in his total behavior patterns. Because their problems permeate their lives, the victims of personality disorders are more difficult than neurotics to treat successfully.

Antisocial Personality. The antisocial personality is just what the name implies: an individual, a man in the majority of cases, who shows no regard for the rights of others or the rules of society; who feels no guilt for this behavior; and whose only real concern is for himself. He is angry at the world and strikes out against it, indifferent to whom he hurts. Usually such an individual has had a bad childhood—separated from his parents, ill-treated by them, or subjected to no discipline at all. His antisocial behavior is likely to have begun when he was still a boy. Marriage and fatherhood occasionally change such a person, but fequently the pattern persists through life.

Drug Dependence and Alcoholism. A number of authorities now believe that alcoholism—as well as addiction to other drugs—is at least partly caused by a chemical or physiological abnormality within the individual. But addictions also have their psychological aspects. They are *prima facie* evidence of immaturity—low self-esteem, the fear of failure, and the inability to postpone gratification. These negative feelings the victim has about himself vanish under the influence of the drug and the sense of well-being it induces—thus the drug's powerful attraction. If addiction, either to alcohol or other drugs, persists long enough, it can occupy the addict's entire life. Work, family ties, human relationships—none of these have any call on him. His only concern is with his drugs. (See also the entries ALCOHOLISM and DRUG ADDICTION in the encyclopedia section.)

Sexual Deviations. Human sexuality is a complex mix of the biological, the psychological, and the social. The "normal" and "abnormal" in sexual behavior are defined differently by various cultures and may change from time to time. Scientists did not begin serious study of sexual behavior in the United States until relatively recently, and it is only since then that we have begun to realize that the range of "normal" sexuality—like the range of "normal" personality—is quite wide. Many psychiatrists now classify certain sexual deviations as mental illness only if they bring unhappiness to the person who practices them or if they impair that person's ability to function normally. Homosexuality, the preference for members of one's own sex as sexual partners, is now viewed in this light by many, but not all, psychiatrists. Supporters of this position now believe that homosexuality, while possibly a sign of emotional immaturity, is an indication of illness only in persons who are unhappy with themselves as they are and would prefer to be heterosexual. (See the entry HOMOSEXUALITY in the encyclopedia section.)

In rare instances, a person thinks of himself or herself as belonging to the opposite sex and voluntarily undergoes a series of long and complex chemical and surgical procedures that change sex. Such persons, who are known as *transsexuals*, were probably the victims of a hormonal prob-

lem from birth: their difficulty was primarily physiological. On the other hand, *transvestitism*—the derivation of sexual pleasure from dressing in the clothes of the opposite sex—seems to be related only to psychological factors.

A number of other sexual deviations also seem to be entirely psychological in origin. In all these cases the deviant behavior affords the individual more pleasure than he derives from heterosexual intercourse:

° *Exhibitionism:* The act of displaying the genitals for the sake of inflicting a shock on the unprepared viewer. (See the entry EXHIBITIONISM in the encyclopedia section.)

° *Voyeurism:* The derivation of sexual pleasure from watching others undress or perform sexual acts.

° *Sadism* and *Masochism:* The first is the derivation of pleasure from inflicting pain; the second is the opposite—the derivation of pleasure from being hurt. These two deviations often coexist in the same person. (See the entries SADISM and MASOCHISM in the encyclopedia section.)

° *Fetishism:* The derivation of sexual pleasure from contact with some inanimate object, such as a shoe or underwear.

° *Nymphomania* and *Satyriasis:* The first is sexual insatiability in a woman; the second is the same condition in a man. The nymphomaniac and the satyr are compulsive and promiscuous in their sexual activity. (See the entries NYMPHOMANIA and SATYRIASIS in the encyclopedia section.)

Some sexual deviations such as pedophilia—sexual abuse of children—and rape are so offensive and dangerous to society that they are recognized as criminal offenses and carry a heavy penalty in all civilizations.

Psychosomatic Disorders

A number of physical illnesses are closely connected with emotional stress. We describe them as psychosomatic. They generally develop in people who have a physical predispositon to the problem, and usually affect only those parts of the body that are under the control of the involuntary nervous system, such as the digestive tract, the endocrine glands, the heart, the lungs, the urinary bladder, and the skin. Like neurotics, victims of psychosomatic disease are incapable of dealing with their conflicts openly. Instead, the emotional turmoil manifests itself in malfunction of various parts of the body.

The peptic ulcer is perhaps the classic psychosomatic disorder. It arises when the stomach produces acidic digestive juices in response to emotional stress rather than to the presence of food. If there is no food in the stomach for the juices to work on, they attack the stomach lining, eventually producing an open sore, or ulcer. The disease is physical and requires medical treatment. But the problem that gives rise to the disease is psychological and it, too, must be dealt with if the ulcer is to heal and not recur. (See the entry ULCER in the encyclopedia section.)

Other psychosomatic disorders include ulcerative colitis, rheumatoid arthritis, migraine headache, hypertension, and asthma, all of which are discussed in the encyclopedia section.

The Psychoses

The psychoses are the hard-core mental illnesses, and hospitalization of the victims is frequently necessary. Some of these illnesses are entirely organic in origin, but most of the more common (or functional) psychoses are associated with psychological factors as well as a chemical and genetic predisposition. These so-called functional psychoses are described below. (See also the entry PSYCHOSIS in the encyclopedia section.)

Schizophrenia. This is the most widespread of all the psychoses, and the people who suffer from it seem to fall into a recognizable psychological pattern. As children they are generally shy, dreamy, and bored. When they complete schooling and go to work, they usually do badly on their jobs. Their illness is a statement of their inability to cope with the world: they simply withdraw from reality. Schizophrenics may hallucinate: they see and hear things that are not there. They may remain for hours in the same position; they may make bizarre gestures or movements.

Schizophrenia usually has its onset fairly early in life and in some particularly unfortunate cases afflicts young children, who are described as *autistic*, and for whom special education and treatment are necessary. (For a fuller discussion, see the entries AUTISM and SCHIZOPHRENIA in the encyclopedia section.)

Paranoid States. The victims of paranoid psychosis build their lives around delusions of persecution and sets of false beliefs, from which reason cannot dissuade them. Paranoics simply twist the facts of reality to suit their emotional needs. They become enraged and filled with hatred at any sign of disagreement. The response patterns paranoids erect are their defense against overwhelming childhood feelings of anger and help-lessness. For this reason the paranoid's delusions are extremely difficult to shake. (See also the entry PARANOIA in the encyclopedia section.)

Manic-Depressive Psychosis. Everyone experiences mood swings, but in manic-depressive psychosis, the mood swing is bizarre. During the "high," or manic state, the patient is constantly on the go—making grandiose plans, or talking constantly, or hallucinating. During the depressive phase, he broods, is filled with self-contempt, and may seriously contemplate suicide. (For further discussion, see the entry MANIC-DEPRESSIVE PSYCHOSIS in the encyclopedia section.)

Involutional Depression. This is a severe depression that is associated with the middle years of life. It undoubtedly has physical as well as psychological causes. In women, for example, it usually coincides with the menopause.

Psychotic Depression. The grief and sorrow we all feel in the face of unhappy events is grotesquely exaggerated in psychotic depression. It is far more profound than neurotic depression, and its onset is always tied to some specific unpleasant event.

Patients who are depressed often threaten suicide. These threats should be taken seriously. Anyone who speaks of taking his own life may well do so. He is in need of immediate help, and the threat is often a disguised way of asking for it. A person who suddenly begins giving away all his possessions may also be a potential suicide.

Organic Psychoses. Severe damage to the brain through drugs, fever, hardening of the arteries, and similar causes can bring about extensive changes in personality. A competent person can be reduced to complete incompetence, unable to comprehend or deal with reality. The atrophy and degeneration of parts of the brain that afflict some old people can result in *senile dementia*. Similarly, *alcoholic psychosis* is brought about by the damage that excessive and continual use of alcohol does to the brain. (See the entries DELIRIUM and DEMENTIA in the encyclopedia section.)

PSYCHIATRIC THERAPIES

Emotional and mental problems can be treated through any one of three general kinds of techniques, or by any combination of them. In psychological therapy, the patient is helped by talking out his feelings with a qualified professional.

Organic therapy involves the use of drugs and/or electroshock therapy. Milieu therapy requires the patient to live in—or associate himself with—a special group assembled to give understanding and support to persons with severe emotional problems.

Psychological Therapies

This general term includes several different forms of therapy, all of which are based on the assumption that, through talk, the patient can develop ways of behaving that will enable him to live his life more comfortably and successfully. The family doctor frequently practices this form of therapy—whether or not he or his patient is aware of it. Every time your doctor listens to your personal problems or gives you advice, he is practicing a type of psychotherapy. But in more serious cases, the services of a psychiatrist or psychologist are called for.

Psychoanalysis

This method of treatment was devised by Sigmund Freud, the great Austrian physician who first formulated many of the basic ideas of modern psychology and psychiatry. The psychoanalytic patient usually sees his doctor five times a week and verbalizes everything that comes to his mind. The talk enables him, with the guidance of the analyst, to understand the childhood roots of his unsatisfactory behavior, so that he can make the effort necessary to change it.

Psychoanalysis is a long and expensive process, and is less frequently practiced today than it was a generation ago. It is most effective in treating the neuroses. (See the entry PSYCHOANALYSIS in the encyclopedia section.)

Psychoanalytic Psychotherapy

This technique, widely used today, evolved from psychoanalysis. It generally requires fewer sessions per week with the psychiatrist, and treatment takes a shorter time to complete. The patient focuses his discussions on his current relationships and goals as well as on his childhood experiences. The help he derives from the experience comes from the ventilation of his feelings and from the support his therapist gives him. This combination enables him to look at his unsatisfactory behavior objectively and to begin to change it. Psychoanalytic psychotherapy can be used in the treatment of a wide range of disorders: neurosis, psychosomatic disease, personality disorder, and some psychoses. (See the entry PSYCHOTHERAPY in the encyclopedia section.)

Behavioral Therapy

Sexual deviants and people with phobias can often be helped by behavioral therapy. In this technique, the patient is conditioned, through a carefully designed series of exercises, to change his behavior in relation to the objects, persons, or situations that previously aroused an undesirable response in him. For example, the individual with a great fear of flying is repeatedly taken to an airport to watch numerous planes routinely taking off and landing with no more ado than buses leaving and arriving at a downtown terminal. He or she is given an explanation of how a plane flies and why it is a far safer means of transportation than the family automobile.

Hypnosis

Hypnosis alters the state of consciousness and permits intense concentration on specific ideas or suggestions. Persons who enter the hypnotic state can be taught to make use of hypnosis to change certain kinds of neurotic behavior or to break certain undesirable habits. The technique is useful, for example, in the treatment of conversion hysteria and in helping people to give up smoking. (See HYPNOSIS in the encyclopedia section.)

Group Therapy

Many of the difficulties experienced by people with mental or emotional problems are associated with their dealings with others. In group therapy, two or more patients work with the therapist to change their behavior by examining the interactions that occur among the members of the group. There are a number of different types of therapy groups, based on various psychological approaches. In addition to groups employing psychoanalytic principles, there are those based on the principles of behavioral psychology and other techniques. All of them can be helpful for people with neurotic or psychosomatic problems, or with personality disorders, and for some with psychoses. Group therapy may be the only treatment the patient receives, or it may be combined with individual therapy. (See the entry GROUP THERAPY in the encyclopedia section.) However, anyone with a mental or emotional problem should consult a psychiatrist or psychologist before enrolling in group therapy not under professional supervision.

Marital Therapy

If there is conflict in a marriage, both partners share at least some of the responsibility. In marital therapy, both partners meet with the therapist to investigate the role each plays in creating the problems and to clear up the psychological difficulties from which both suffer. If the stress between partners is primarily sexual, expressing itself in such problems as impotence or frigidity, the couple may be helped by sex therapy, in which they work with a team of therapists—one male and one female.

Organic Therapies

Even though medicine does not yet entirely understand the precise role physiological processes play in producing mental or emotional disorders, we *do* know that people's moods and behavior can be altered by organic treatments that affect these processes, and that such treatments can be helpful. A number of different drugs are used in the treatment of mental and emotional disorders. When these drugs were first developed, they were hailed as panaceas in some quarters. But although the drugs have made a major contribution, they are not miracle-workers, and they must be used only under the supervision of a careful and qualified psychiatrist or other physician. The milder drugs relieve anxiety or depression in the neurotic patient; the stronger ones can stop hallucinations, delusions, and violent behavior in the psychotic. One drug, lithium carbonate (see this entry in the encyclopedia section), has been found especially effective in the treatment of manic-depressive psychosis.

In some cases, the drugs alone are enough to enable the patient to function effectively and comfortably. But normally they are best used in conjunction with psychotherapy. By temporarily relieving the neurotic's anxiety or depression or by bringing the psychotic back into contact with reality, the drugs enable him to deal with his problems in words.

Convulsive Therapy

Suicidal patients and others who are severely depressed can sometimes be helped by the use of electroshock therapy. Like the drugs discussed above, the treatment often relieves the patient's symptoms and makes him or her accessible to psychotherapy.

Milieu Therapy

When the patient's environment is structured to perform a therapeutic role, the treatment he receives is described as milieu therapy. Such treatment takes place in many mental hospitals, where occupational and group therapy are of-fered and were the patient assumes a responsible social role, just as healthy people do in the everyday world. Patients and staff meet regularly to plan activities and to discuss problems, and the patient begins to feel a rise in self-esteem and to learn to trust his environment. When he leaves the hospital, he may continue with another form of milieu therapy at a halfway house—a place where he lives with others recovering from similar difficulties. From the halfway house he can be eased back into the outside world.

Milieu therapy has proved effective in the treatment of two major personality disorders— drug addiction and alcoholism. Alcoholics Anonymous (see entry in the encyclopedia section), an organization with an excellent record in the treatment of alcoholism, is a therapeutic community, led by laymen rather than professionals. Similarly, there are a number of centers throughout the country where drug addicts can live while they are being detoxified and until they are ready to return to the general society.

WHAT DOCTOR AND WHEN?

Because the mind is more than the brain, the treatment of mental and emotional problems has never been confined solely to the medical profession. Clergymen, for example, have traditionally played the role of counselors and psychotherapists to members of their flocks. Today, there are a number of trained professionals outside medicine who deal with psychological difficulties. Among them are clinical psychologists (men and women with PhD degrees in their field) and psychiatric social workers, who hold the degree of Master of Social Work. In addition, there are a number of organizations, such as the National Mental Health Association, that are concerned with emotional difficulties.

But the medical profession remains in the forefront in the treatment of mental and emotional disorders. In the event that you, or any member of your family, feels the need of help with a psychological problem, you should first consult your family physician. His examination will be able to determine whether or not the difficulty has a physical basis. If the problem is physiological, treating the physical condition may clear up the psychological disturbance. If, on the other hand, no physical cause can be found, the doctor will be able to refer you to a qualified psychiatrist whose training and approach will be most effective in dealing with your difficulties.

9 Selecting Your Doctor

The American doctor is one of the world's most highly trained professionals. Medical education is lengthier than that of any other calling and, ideally, continues throughout a physician's career. His credentials have been rigorously tested and certified. But while degrees and years of training may indicate competence, they cannot guarantee it. And for the layman, faced with the problem of choosing a doctor for himself, questions of personality, compassion, and patience sometimes seem more important than the diplomas of any particular physician. Although there is no foolproof method for finding the doctor who best suits your needs and problems, this chapter does offer some important guidelines that, if followed, will make your choice better informed.

A word of urgent advice: If you do not have a doctor now, don't wait until illness forces you to use the first physician with the time to see you. You will be doing both him and yourself a disservice—because your doctor functions best if he knows you and your family in health as well as in sickness.

PRIMARY CARE

For the majority of people the most important medical need is for a personal physician who will treat all the members of the family (except, possibly, the very young children). His goal will be to establish a continuity of care, so that he learns not only about the physical weaknesses and strengths of the various family members, but also achieves some insight into their emotional characteristics, their relationships, their jobs, their economic position. He will have the knowledge to treat most ailments himself and to choose the right specialist to treat diseases outside his field. Until World War II such a doctor was most probably a *general practitioner* (GP). Today only about 12 percent of all doctors are GP's; the others have spent a considerable part of their medical education in training for a specialty. The two types of specialists who are most likely to establish a family practice are the *internist* and the *family practitioner.*

The *internist* is a physician who has had training in the whole spectrum of fields that constitute internal medicine—almost everything with the exception of surgery, obstetrics, and pediatrics. He will be competent to deal with almost any aspect of disease and, in addition, he may have taken additional training in a subspecialty, such as cardiology, allergy, or endocrinology.

The *family practitioner* is similar to the general practitioner—except that the family practitioner has had considerably more training, with particular emphasis on preventive and internal medicine, minor surgery, orthopedics, gynecology, and pediatrics. He is therefore well qualified to take charge of the care of young children, for instance, or to perform the less complicated surgical operations or to deal with problems of the bones and joints. His training will probably also include psychology so that he can recognize when illness is emotionally caused.

Although any licensed doctor is legally entitled to undertake any treatment or surgical operation, few will attempt to work in fields outside of their own where highly specialized knowledge or techniques are needed. If your doctor encounters a problem with which he cannot deal adequately, he will refer you to the appropriate specialist.

THE SPECIALTIES

Back in the 1930's some two-thirds of all physicians were general practitioners. But because of enormous advances in medical science in recent decades, today's medical student will probably choose a special field in which to concentrate his efforts. His postgraduate schooling will include specialty training for from two to five years after he has completed his internship. When he has ended his training—usually as a resident in the appropriate department of a hospital—plus two years of full-time specialty practice, he must then pass rigorous certification examinations to become "board certified" and a recognized member of his specialty. Today there are 22 medical specialty boards, each responsible for overseeing the criteria for training and the certifying of all physicians who want to practice within a specialty. The boards and their fields of specialization are:

Allergy and Immunology—such diseases as hay fever, asthma, hives, allergic reactions to food.

Anesthesiology—administration of anesthetics during surgery and childbirth.

Colon and Rectal Surgery—malfunction of colon, rectum, and anus.

Dermatology—diseases of the skin and hair.

Family Practice—generalized practice of any of the specialties. (It is the youngest of the specialties; its board was not established until 1969.)

Internal Medicine—almost any aspect of medical treatment except surgery. Many internists choose to specialize in narrower fields such as:

Cardiovascular Diseases—diseases of the heart and circulatory system;

Endocrinology—problems of the endocrine glands;

Hematology—diseases of the blood;

Infectious Diseases;

Nephrology—kidney disorders;

Oncology—the causes and treatment of all tumors;

Pulmonary Disease—lung problems;

Rheumatology—joint and connective tissue problems, such as arthritis.

Neurological Surgery—surgical treatment of diseases of the nervous system, including the brain and spinal cord.

Nuclear Medicine—diseases, primarily cancer, caused by radioactive substances.

Obstetrics-Gynecology—diseases of women; pregnancy and childbirth.

Ophthalmology—the eye and its diseases. (An *optometrist,* on the other hand, is not an M.D.; he may examine the eye to prescribe eyeglasses— which an *optician* makes—but he may not treat eye diseases.)

Orthopedic Surgery—diseases and problems of the bones and joints.

Otolaryngology—ailments of the ears, throat, sinuses, and nose.

Pathology—disease-caused changes in body tissues.

Pediatrics—the care of children.

Physical Medicine and Rehabilitation—diagnosis and treatment of diseases through physical therapy.

Plastic Surgery—primarily involved with the reconstruction of the skin.

Preventive Medicine—the basic causes of disease, with a view to changing or removing them.

Psychiatry and Neurology—emotional and mental disturbances; all diseases of the nervous system.

Radiology—the taking and interpretation of X rays, and the treatment of disease with radiant energy.

Surgery—operations. General surgery, or specialized surgery in some particular field.

Thoracic Surgery—a separate surgical specialty, involving the heart and lungs.

Urology—the kidneys, and the special problems relating to the male genital organs.

OSTEOPATHS

Osteopathy was founded on the theory that most diseases are caused by a misalignment of the bones and should be treated primarily by manipulation. Osteopathic schools today, however, offer an education comparable to that of conventional medical colleges, and graduates are required to pass regular state medical examinations. Doctors of Osteopathy also specialize in most of the same fields as do other physicians.

CHIROPRACTORS

Chiropractors believe that diseases are caused by pressures on the nerves because of faulty alignment of bones, especially the spinal vertebrae. Often, the chiropractor will combine manipulation of the spine with treatment by physiotherapy and diet. Chiropractors usually have had only the four years of training provided by chiropractic educational institutions. If you go to a chiropractor, be sure to check beforehand whether your medical insurance covers payments to him. Many policies do not.

CHOOSING YOUR DOCTOR

Despite the variety of specialists available, you should have no hesitation about which type to choose for general care for yourself and your family. As we have already indicated, the best source of primary care will be the general practitioner, the internist, or the family practitioner.

Most people still choose their doctor by asking friends and family, assuming that the man with a good reputation must be a good doctor. A far better way, though, is to gather a list of physicians through the following methods, and then check out the list with a few knowledgeable friends.

* If you live near a medical school, or a hospital affiliated with a medical school, call to get a list of the family practitioners, internists, and general practitioners (and pediatricians, if you want special care for your young children) who are on the hospital staff and who accept private patients. The doctor who works at one of these "teaching" hospitals is likely to be abreast of the most advanced medical knowledge and techniques. See Chapter 10 for a description of a teaching hospital.
* Call your local hospital for the list of doctors on its staff. It is vital that the doctor you choose have some hospital affiliation. But check out the hospital, too, to make sure it has been approved by the Joint Commission on Accreditation of Hospitals. (See Chapter 10.) If the hospital is not accredited—and many small hospitals are not—search for another hospital in your area that is accredited.
* With your list of doctors in hand, go to your library for a copy of the *American Medical Directory* or the *Directory of Medical Specialists*, both of which list the professional credentials of all doctors practicing in the United States. (Your local medical society may also publish a listing.) You will be able to find out the age of each doctor on your list, where he went to medical school, what his specialty training is, what type of practice he has. (The *Directory of Medical Specialists* also reports the hospitals where each doctor has had his internship and residency. Work in a large medical school hospital is an additional plus factor in a doctor's background.)
* Public interest groups in various sections of the country have published local doctors' directories which contain a great deal more information. Check your library to see if there is one available for your area. It will contain such useful facts about each physician as his fees and billing procedures; whether he has X-ray machinery and a laboratory for doing standard diagnostic tests; whether he makes house calls;

whether he accepts Medicare and Medicaid patients. This is the kind of information you will need to help you make a decision. And if you cannot find such facts in a directory, call the offices of the doctors you are interested in and ask.
* Think about whether a medical group rather than an individual doctor practicing alone might be better for your family's needs. A large group practice might include specialists in almost every branch of medicine; a small one will probably cover the basic family health fields and will have as members an internist, a gynecologist, and a pediatrician. A group offers the patient the advantage of shared expertise and shared facilities.
* Health Maintenance Organizations (HMO) are a growing phenomenon on the American medical scene. An HMO is an organization of doctors that, for a flat fee paid either monthly or yearly, offers its members a range of health services—usually excluding only dental and psychiatric care. The fee includes hospitalization. For many people, membership in an HMO is an efficient and often less expensive way to have good, consistent medical care. If there is one in your area, you may want to investigate it.

EVALUATING YOUR CARE

Choosing your doctor is not, however, the end of your responsibility. Even a physician with top-notch training and background may be the wrong doctor for you—if you feel that he is unsympathetic, too rushed, or too expensive. And there are ways of judging the quality of care your doctor offers. Among the things to look for and consider are:

Record-Keeping. Complete records of your visits should be kept, and the doctor should consult them regularly.

The Doctor's Attitude. You should feel comfortable with him, trust him enough to confide in him, and expect to be treated as an adult with a right to participate in your own health care.

Length of Visit. If you feel rushed in and out of the office, your confidence in the physician probably falters. If your doctor cannot give you enough time for you to feel comfortable about spelling out the reasons for your visit, find another doctor who can.

Explanations. Are they full and sufficient? You should be told the root causes of your symptoms, for instance. You should learn what possible side effects to expect from the drugs prescribed for you, and what results and risks are to be expected from any special procedure—surgery or special treatments.

THE COMPLETE PHYSICAL EXAMINATION

Most doctors will want to perform a thorough examination on every new patient. The exam begins with the taking of your past medical history (often an assistant will do this). It should be as complete as possible. It should include, for your own benefit, even those things that may be embarrassing or painful to talk about—personal difficulties, emotional problems—because these can affect your health as much as disease or diet.

The physical examination itself should be conducted with your clothes off. It will involve checking your entire body. For men, it will include a rectal examination; for women, a pelvic exam, a PAP TEST (see encyclopedia section), and a manual breast examination. All patients will have routine blood and urine tests. In addition, if you are in your mid-forties or older, you may be given a rectal-colonic examination, done with a proctoscope.

PROBLEMS OF COMMUNICATION

Patients are sometimes too embarrassed or too fearful to tell their physician what is really troubling them. And doctors are often so rushed that they do not have time to explain their findings in layman's language. As a patient it is your responsibility to be completely open and trusting and to ask for explanations that you can understand. If you comprehend your problem, you are in a much better position to help solve it. Be certain that you understand not only the diagnosis, but the treatment your doctor recommends. And if you are not sure you will remember details, write them down in your doctor's office while they are fresh in your mind.

CHANGING DOCTORS

If you are dissatisfied with your present physician, examine the reasons why you want to change. You may find that at least some of them are your fault. Did you tell the doctor everything he needs to know? Did you follow his instructions to the letter? Did you fully understand what he told you? If you answer "no" to any of these questions, you haven't given him a fair chance.

But if you do decide to change, ask to have your records sent to your new doctor so that your past medical history will be available to him.

10 What to Expect When You Go to a Hospital

For many people, going to a hospital for the first time is like visiting a foreign country—they are entering a strange new region of the world, with its own customs, clothing, food; with seemingly arbitrary rules that govern every action; with a language that is comprehensible only to the initiated. To the novice patient, often the simplest hospital event may seem threatening. He doesn't know why it is happening, what it is intended to accomplish, how he should react to it. If he is determined, he can seek out someone to ask—but the busy, depersonalized hospital atmosphere discourages questions. And he feels apprehensive, uncertain, and worst of all, ignored. Yet what is happening to him would be understandable—although not necessarily welcome—if he knew a few facts about hospital routine.

This chapter presents a brief guide to basic hospital operation so that, if and when you become a patient, you will have some idea of what to expect. And, while hospitals differ, and each patient is unique, general procedures are much the same for all institutions and the great majority of patients. On these pages, we shall address ourselves primarily to the patient who has agreed with his physician to enter the hospital for medical treatment, diagnosis, or surgery; who chooses a date for his hospital admission; and who has had time to find out something about his illness.

WHAT KIND OF HOSPITAL WILL YOU GO TO?

Ordinarily, your doctor will send you to the hospital where he has "staff privileges" which allow him to practice within the hospital and to use its facilities. He may be attached to a local "proprietary" hospital—usually a small, privately-owned, profit-making institution. There are about 588 of these in the U.S. More probably, he will be on the staff of a "voluntary" hospital, a nonprofit institution run by a city or state, or by a private group—a church, a charitable organization, or a medical association. The federal government finances its own institutions, such as the veterans' hospitals it has built across the country. (And if you are a veteran, you might find out if you are eligible to be treated in one). Finally, there are "teaching" hospitals, which are affiliated with a medical school, or have training programs for medical students. There are almost 1,000 teaching hospitals in the country. (Some of these are also federal hospitals.)

Accreditation

Of America's 7,000 hospitals, some 5,200 have been inspected by the Joint Commission on Accreditation of Hospitals. They have met certain standards regarding organization, record keeping, nursing, dietary and other services, and have received certificates of accreditation. Although it is very difficult for a layman to judge the quality of the hospital, a certificate of accreditation will assure you that the hospital is up to standard. If you can possibly avoid it, do not go to a hospital that is not accredited.

Large or Small? Teaching or Nonteaching?

The large university-affiliated or city hospital offers a wide range of specialties and the complex equipment necessary to practice them. On the other hand, a small accredited community hospital has the capacity to handle every common illness and many uncommon ones as well. And if you contract a rare disease or require a particularly complex method of treatment, it is altogether proper for the hospital to transfer you to the nearest institution with the facilities you need.

A small local hospital may be more comfortable, simply because it *is* small. Patients tend to disappear inside the hugeness of a major hospital, and to lose track of who is doing what to them. But the large hospital does offer one definite advantage: a "house staff" who work exclusively within the hospital walls.

The typical teaching hospital is traditionally divided into the four major services: medicine, surgery, pediatrics, and obstetrics-gynecology. Each service is headed by a chief physician who supervises a staff of medical students, interns, and residents. All are considered to be to some degree "in training": the students, who have not yet received their M.D.'s; the interns, who are in their first year of service after medical school; and the residents, who have completed their one-year internship, and are now finishing their specialized training—a process which may last up to seven years. The interns and residents comprise the "house staff." The "senior staff" is made up of the academic physicians who teach as well as practice medicine, and the private doctors with the privilege of admitting patients. In addition, the hospital has available the services of a range of specialists in such fields as radiology, pathology, anesthesiology, dermatology, ophthalmology, and plastic surgery.

As a patient at a teaching hospital, you can expect excellent medical care. But you may also become "the disease in the body in the bed" to the medical students who will receive a lecture at your bedside, if your illness is of sufficient medical interest. Interns and residents may argue about the diagnosis of your case. All this attention is exciting to some patients, disturbing to others. If you do not like it, you have the right to demand that you be seen only by the people who are actively involved in your treatment.

The nonteaching hospital, too, may or may not have a staff of interns and residents. But it will have a staff of private physicians who are available to the hospital "on call," plus consultant specialists.

The Nursing Staff

Despite the large number of doctors on the typical hospital roster, it is the nurses who provide most of the patient care. Nurses administer your medicine, change bandages, sometimes draw blood for lab tests, watch over the diet ordered by your doctor, monitor your temperature and blood pressure, and keep constant note of your condition. The Nursing Supervisor usually directs all care in a particular service—surgery or gynecology, for example—and if you have any complaints, you should speak first to her about them. A Head Nurse is in charge of your floor and supervises a staff of registered nurses (R.N.'s) who have been graduated from a three- to four-year nursing program, and usually a group of licensed practical nurses (L.P.N.'s) who have at least one to one and a half years of training and experience. In addition, there are nurses' aides and orderlies, who bathe and move patients, make beds, collect bedpans, give back rubs, and distribute meal trays. And occasionally you will meet nursing students who are in training.

THE DECISION TO GO TO THE HOSPITAL

Before you and your doctor decide that you should enter a hospital, you should have had your illness explained, its course of treatment charted, the prognosis clearly stated, and the risks laid out for you to understand. By knowing all this, you can become an active participant in your own treatment. Not knowing it, you are incapable of giving your "informed consent" to treatment.

The Consent Form

This is a written agreement between you, your physician, and the hospital. It is written proof that the patient understands the nature of his illness and agrees with the doctor on the necessary treatment. Often the form is signed in the doctor's office—before hospital admission— where its terms can be discussed at leisure. You should read the consent form carefully and make sure you understand it. If there are portions you object to (such as consent to the photographing or televising of the operation, or the admittance of observers to the operating room), you have the right to delete those portions before signing. Clauses releasing the hospital or a physician from liability are not binding. All such matters are covered in the "The Patient's Bill of Rights," released by the American Hospital Association (AHA) in 1972. Your hospital probably has copies available. If not, write to the American Hospital Association, 840 North Lake Shore Drive, Chicago, Illinois 60611.

Arrangements for your hospital admission will be made by your doctor. You will be mailed an admission form, or be asked to fill one out when you first enter the hospital. The form is a simple questionnaire which asks such questions as what church, if any, you belong to; who is your next of kin; what kind of hospital insurance you carry; and, often, whether you smoke. If you do not, you may ask to room with nonsmokers.

Private vs. Semiprivate Room

Hospitals have found that patients respond well to other patients, that being in a room with congenial occupants may pass the time more pleasantly and often hasten recovery. "Semiprivate" means two, three, or four beds in a room. (Very few hospitals still have open wards—the relics of the age of "charity" institutions.) But if you do not relish the idea of sharing your symptoms with strangers, you can ask for a private room—and expect to pay the extra charge yourself. Health insurance plans rarely cover the additional cost.

Private nurses, too, are becoming a rarity—expensive, as well as somewhat redundant in most well-staffed hospitals. But if your doctor feels that you will need constant supervision, he will arrange for private nurses or tell a member of your family what steps to take.

Lab Tests

If your condition does not require immediate hospitalization, and if your insurance covers "outpatient" costs, you can usually save money and time by having the hospital perform certain tests—blood, urine, X ray, electrocardiogram—before your admission. Otherwise, you can expect to have some of your tests immediately after your hospital admission. You will be directed to the lab, where a technician will ask you to give a urine sample and where a small quantity of blood will be drawn by syringe from your arm—a process almost everyone dislikes, although it is usually painless. Urine and blood analyses can indicate a diverse range of diseases, from diabetes to anemia to subtle chemical imbalances. The electrocardiograph registers your heart impulses, via electrodes held against your skin. You won't feel a thing.

If you have been scheduled for diagnostic X rays (other than a routine chest X ray), either as an inpatient or outpatient, you will be given explicit instructions about what you must do or not do to prepare yourself. It is essential that you follow them to the letter; otherwise you may have to repeat the whole procedure. X-ray departments are notoriously slow. The reason: the necessity for taking perfect pictures while the

patient is perfectly prepared. Thus, you may find yourself lying flat on an X-ray table for long, lonely minutes, while the technician develops the film he has just taken, to make certain it is right before he lets you go.

ENTERING THE HOSPITAL

Take pajamas, slippers, robe, toilet articles, books, and—this is essential—your insurance identity cards. The front desk will direct you to the admitting office, where you will fill out an admission form, if you have not already mailed one in. The admitting officer will explain the hospital rules (most of them are concerned with visiting hours), and will discuss methods of payment. (If you are not covered by private insurance, Medicare, or Medicaid, read the section in this chapter on the hospital's social service department.) You will be presented with a consent form, if you have not yet signed one. Remember that you have the right to object to any clause, and the right to receive a full explanation of the terms of your consent.

YOU BECOME A PATIENT

You have been admitted, you have had a few basic diagnostic tests, and you are now a patient. Your new status is certified by the plastic hospital bracelet snapped around your wrist. It identifies you by name, hospital, and room number; and, if you are diabetic, will distinguish you by the color of the plastic—red, for instance, rather than the usual green.

In your room, you'll be greeted by a nurse who will introduce you to your roommates, show you how the television set operates, how to raise and lower your bed, and where to find the button that will call her. She will also hand you a short and flimsy nightgown—in hospital parlance, a "Johnny"—and instruct you to slip it on and tie it, if you can, in the back. You will probably begin by insisting on wearing your own pajamas. However, sooner or later (probably sooner, if you are going to have surgery or special tests) you will find yourself in a Johnny. Its open back makes your anatomy much more accessible; and you will very quickly learn to ignore, along with everyone else, what may seem at first like indecent exposure. At this point, though, you will be very glad to have remembered your bathrobe. (In case you have forgotten, the hospital will usually supply a robe, and slippers too.)

Now you try out the bed, which is hard; the

sheets, which are coarse; the air, which is usually conditioned; and the general atmosphere—noisy. A hospital corridor has its own special clatter. Yet, although your room has a door which can be closed, you may find that you prefer the hustle and bustle. Once you are settled, a nurse will take your temperature, pulse, and blood pressure, and record them on your chart. Also on the chart: an order form, detailing the medication and diet you are to be given; and a "bedside" form, which will be used to record how well you have eaten, when you passed urine or evacuated, and in general, how you are responding to treatment. You may read these forms, if you wish; but unless you are familiar with hospital jargon, you will probably not understand them. If you want to know what your temperature is, or the name of the medicine you are being given and what it is supposed to do—ask.

The Hospital Day

It begins some time in the early hours of the morning, when nurses, with their briskly cheerful reveille manner, rouse the entire hospital population from sleep. No other hospital convention evokes such outrage as this wholesale awakening. The reason for it is primarily tactical: Night nurses end their shift at 7 a.m. (day nurses at 3 p.m., evening nurses at 11 p.m.), and custom requires that all patients will have had their faces washed and their temperatures recorded before the day shift comes on. By 7 a.m. the hospital day is well under way. Doctors are making rounds, surgery patients are on their way to the operating rooms, and, if you are in a teaching hospital, the first group of medical students are looking at medically interesting cases. The patients, now wide awake, lie in bed dreaming of breakfast, which begins to arrive about 7:45.

After the breakfast trays have been removed, the morning pace picks up: Beds are made, back rubs and baths administered, bedpans distributed and retrieved as requested. (On back rubs: Never refuse one. They refresh, soothe, and generally make you feel good. On bedpans: icy-cold and uncomfortable as they are, they are indispensable if you cannot get out of bed. And you will learn quickly enough that a bedpan embarrasses nobody but you.) About 11:45, lunch trays begin to rattle down the halls. After lunch, a universal, dozy quiet prevails, interrupted in mid-afternoon for visiting hours—usually from 2 to 4 p.m. Visitors are shooed out in advance of the dinner hour, which begins at 4:30; and after the evening visiting hour ends (usually at 7 to 8 p.m.), bedtime has

arrived. More temperature and pulse readings, more medications, and for almost all patients, a sleeping pill. Because hospital activity continues around the clock, patients often have difficulty sleeping. Hence the pill. You are *not* required to take it.

Hospital Food

Sometimes it's great, sometimes just . . . food. All hospitals must face the daily task of preparing three meals a day for hundreds of patients, many of whom are likely to be on specialized diets. Postoperative patients are given liquid meals: broth, jello, apple juice. When they are feeling a bit better, custard and eggnog are added. For a while they may eat a soft diet—eggs, grilled cheese, hamburger. Finally, if all goes well, they graduate to the regular "house" diet, and can take their choice of menus. In addition, there are salt-restricted diets, low-fat diets, low-cholesterol diets, diabetic diets . . . *and* special foods for you if you are an Orthodox Jew or a vegetarian.

Visiting

There are, of course, posted hours for visiting, and you should expect your family and friends to observe them. Hospitals impose only one visiting prohibition—children under 14 (in some hospitals, the minimum age is 16) may not enter the adult areas. The reason: children are often carriers of infectious diseases which, in sick adults, might prove dangerous. However, in special circumstances, exceptions to the child-prohibition can be made—as they will be, too, if your husband can visit only at 6 in the evening, or your aged aunt has to catch an early plane.

SURGERY

In the minds of many people, the operating room is the hospital's center and reason for being. And, in fact, about half of a hospital's annual population are surgery patients.

Although procedures differ slightly for different kinds of surgery, the basic pattern remains the same for almost everyone. You are expected to enter the hospital some time before the operation is scheduled, so that your diet can be controlled and your physical condition monitored. You will be given a chest X ray and an electrocardiogram; lung congestion or heart problems may indicate the need for a special anesthetic. You will also undergo any other lab tests your doctor has ordered.

On the night before surgery, the anesthe-

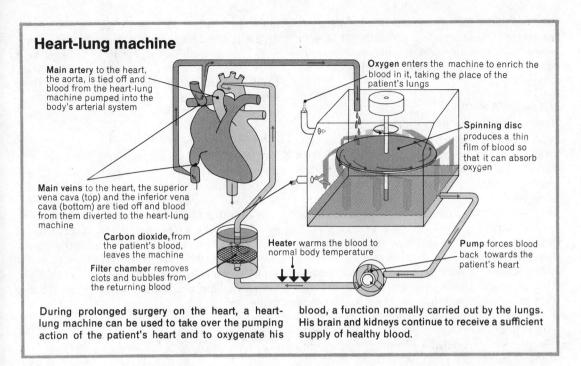

Heart-lung machine

Main artery to the heart, the aorta, is tied off and blood from the heart-lung machine pumped into the body's arterial system

Oxygen enters the machine to enrich the blood in it, taking the place of the patient's lungs

Spinning disc produces a thin film of blood so that it can absorb oxygen

Main veins to the heart, the superior vena cava (top) and the inferior vena cava (bottom) are tied off and blood from them diverted to the heart-lung machine

Carbon dioxide, from the patient's blood, leaves the machine

Heater warms the blood to normal body temperature

Pump forces blood back towards the patient's heart

Filter chamber removes clots and bubbles from the returning blood

During prolonged surgery on the heart, a heart-lung machine can be used to take over the pumping action of the patient's heart and to oxygenate his blood, a function normally carried out by the lungs. His brain and kidneys continue to receive a sufficient supply of healthy blood.

siologist assigned to your operation will probably visit you. (Smaller hospitals may not have an anesthesiologist on their staff; instead they may use a nurse anesthetist, working with your doctor. For major operations, it is probably a good idea to use a physician-anesthesiologist, and to have the surgery performed in a larger hospital.) He will discuss the kind of anesthetic he plans to use, and ask you about any previous operations you have had, and your reaction to anesthetics. If you have any special problems—allergies of any kind, or diabetes, epilepsy, high blood pressure—tell him. He should already know, of course, because this information will be in your records. But remind him, nevertheless. You may also be visited by your doctor, if he is going to do the surgery, or by the surgeon you have selected.

Except for a sleeping medication, you will be given nothing to eat or drink after midnight to insure that your digestion doesn't interfere with the anesthesia. The area of surgery may also be shaved, for hygienic reasons. Early on the morning of the operation, you will be given an injection which has a double purpose: to reduce the amount of saliva produced in your mouth, making the administration of anesthetics safer; and to relax you. Some 15 minutes before surgery is to begin, you will be moved from your bed to a "trolley"—a narrow bed-on-wheels—and taken to an area next to the operating room, while everything is made ready for you. At this point,

you may discover that despite the injection, you are completely aware of everything that is going on; not everyone reacts in the same way to the preoperative shot. If you are still awake, have a good look at the operating room as they wheel you in. You will see a white table under a battery of ceiling lights, and several green-gowned and masked figures, who will address you casually by your first name. You won't have time to answer. You may not even realize that the anesthesiologist has connected your arm to an intravenous solution (a soporific, and a muscle relaxant). And now you are definitely and completely "out."

Anesthetics

Basically, there are two types of anesthetics: general and regional, or local. A general anesthetic is the kind that puts you completely to sleep; gas is administered through a face mask or a throat tube, or for shorter operations the anesthetic is given as an intravenous injection. A common type of regional anesthetic is the spinal, in which the anesthetic is injected between the vertebrae into the space surrounding the spinal cord, producing loss of sensation throughout the lower part of the body. Spinals are often used for operations such as appendicitis and hernia. The process does not hurt, because the injection area is first deadened with another type of regional anesthetic, the local anesthetic. This is a solution, such as that used in dentists' offices, which is injected under the skin or mucous membrane to desensitize the operation site only. It is used when the operating area is small and near the skin surface, and the operation itself can be finished quickly.

Recovery Room

If you have been given a general anesthetic, you will wake up, very gradually, in a strange dim area called the "recovery room." You will have a blood-pressure cuff on one arm, which you can move; and an intravenous tube (containing a solution that is replacing lost fluids) in your other arm—which you cannot move. You may also be vaguely aware of a mask on your nose or a set of prongs in your nostrils. These supply you with oxygen, and are routinely used as an adjunct to your recovery. A nurse will probably be checking your pulse and blood pressure. She will tell you that your operation is over, ask how you feel and if you hurt anywhere. If you do, she may give you painkilling medication. She will continue to observe your condition, reading your "vital signs" (pulse, pressure, respiration) every 15 minutes or so, until you show full awareness of your surroundings, and your vital signs are stable. Length of time in the recovery room varies according to operation and patient—perhaps two to two-and-a-half hours after abdominal surgery, much less for less serious operations. Every surgical patient, except those who have had only local anesthesia, spends some time here. When you have fully emerged from the effects of the anesthesia, and the nausea that often accompanies it, you will be wheeled back to your room for more sleep.

Recovery Begins

Your recovery is just beginning. Despite your need for sleep and your feelings of weakness and lethargy, as early as the evening after your surgery you may be asked to sit on the edge of your bed for a few minutes, or to take a few steps with the help of a nurse. This kind of movement increases your blood circulation, preventing formation of blood clots. You will also be required to cough and take deep breaths to clear your lungs completely of the anesthetic, and to prevent postoperative complications such as pneumonia. Cough and breathe deeply, even if you are sure you will split your stitches. You won't.

Postoperative convalescence is always tedious, and sometimes painful. If you have pain, it is important that you tell your nurse or doctor. You can be given sedatives, although the amount will depend on your condition. With some kinds of operations, too much sedation obstructs the healing process, so do not expect to be drugged out of all pain as a matter of routine. On the other hand, you are not required to put up with prolonged severe pain; that obstructs the healing process, too.

Special Hospital Personnel

For breathing problems, you will see a respiratory therapist. He will have you breathe into a lung-capacity machine to determine the volume of air your lungs can hold; check your general lung condition; and recommend inhalation therapy if he thinks you need it. If your muscles need rebuilding after surgery, you will meet the physical therapist, who can teach you how to walk again after an accident, restore muscles that may have atrophied, and help to rebuild injured body tissues.

OTHER HOSPITAL FACILITIES

There are three other areas of the hospital that may be of concern to you at various times: the intensive care unit, the children's section, and the maternity ward.

The Intensive Care Unit (ICU)

Here, the most sophisticated medical machinery and a battery of nurses and physicians monitor acutely ill patients. A typical ICU will probably have a cardiac monitor—an electrocardiograph which can be attached to the heart-attack patient to provide a running graph of his heart activity; a ventilator, to help the patient's breathing if he has difficulty; a defibrillator, for shocking a stopped heart into starting; and piped-in oxygen and suction facilities. More extensive ICU's will also have automatic blood and urine analyzers, computer-controlled systems for intravenous injections, kidney machines, and facilities for treating badly burned patients. Whether the ICU is large or small, the ratio of patient to nurse is usually one to one; and in addition there will be respiratory therapists, mechanical and electronics technicians, and physicians in constant attendance. Most ICU patients are heart-disease or accident victims, or have had severe illness combined with extensive surgery. (Some hospitals now have separate coronary care units, or CCU's, however.) You probably will not need either the ICU or the CCU facilities, but it is comforting to know they exist.

Electrocardiogram

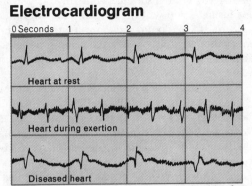

A doctor can learn much about the health of a patient's heart by taking an electrocardiogram, a tracing which records the electrical activity in the heart muscle. For example, any increase in size of one of the heart's chambers causes a change in the shape of the electrocardiogram.

Electroencephalogram

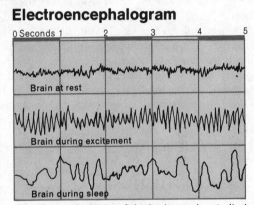

The electrical activity of the brain can be studied by electrodes taped to the skull, and recorded on an electroencephalogram. The shape of the tracing depends on the mental activity of the patient, and changes from the normal pattern can reveal disorders such as epilepsy.

Children's Ward

The very young child who enters the pediatrics section of a hospital finds himself in an incomprehensible and often seemingly hostile world. Despite the warmth and sympathy of the adult professionals who surround him, he is separated from the one person he wants most—his father or mother.

If your child must spend time in a hospital, find out if you may "room in" with him throughout his hospitalization. Rooming-in (which can be as minimal and spartan as a cot next to your child's bed) has proved to be an asset to the hospitals that permit the arrangement. With a parent present at all times, the child is happier and more relaxed, and the burden of ordinary day-to-day care is shifted off the shoulders of the pediatrics staff. Many hospitals—especially those in large cities—now have rooming-in facilities, and if your local hospital does not welcome the presence of parents, perhaps your doctor can help you find one that does.

Even if you can arrange to stay with your child, it is a good idea to tell him beforehand what he will experience. Ask your doctor to rehearse the procedures with you, so you can explain them to your child. Begin with basics. Describe a stethoscope (or borrow one to show him), and tell him why it is used. Talk about drawing blood for a test, and do not pretend he will like it. Show how temperatures are taken rectally, and assure him that it does not hurt. Talk about what he'll find in his room: a high crib with bars, so he can't fall out; a bedpan; the Johnny-gown. Tell him about the meals he'll eat in bed, the different people who will come to see him, the different sounds he'll hear. If he is going to have surgery, describe the process. If he is going to be X-rayed, assure him that the table and machinery are nothing to be afraid of, and that there is no pain. Tell him that you will come to see him, and how often, and for how long. Most important, find out what scares him most, and try to talk it through. Above all, be truthful. Do not pretend that going to the hospital is fun and games. It isn't, and your child knows it.

The Maternity Floor

Quite early in your pregnancy, your obstetrician will reserve space on the maternity floor for you. This is the time to discuss choices with him. For example, if you are planning a "natural" (without anesthetics) childbirth, you will want a hospital that conducts birth-preparation programs for prospective parents. If there is a certainty or even chance that you will have a cesarean operation, you may feel more secure in a university-affiliated or teaching hospital, with its superior resources. If it is important to you to have your baby with you at all times, you should ask for a hospital that allows babies to "room in" with their mothers. Remember, also, to inquire about the hospital's rules concerning the father's visits.

The hospital is aware that the date set is approximate, and your doctor—or sometimes nature—will tell you when it's time to head there. When you sign in, the routine is generally the same as for any other type of admission except that instead of going to an ordinary private or semiprivate room, you may be taken directly to a labor room. It is much like any other hospital room—with a bed, chairs, some form of communication with the nurses' station, and a private bathroom. You may even find a television set. In the labor room, a nurse's aide helps you undress and slip into a hospital gown, stows away your street clothes, takes your temperature, pulse, and respiration, and asks for a urine sample. At some point either your own physician or a resident in obstetrics will examine you. Later you will be shaved in the genital area and given an enema. In most hospitals, your husband is permitted to join you in the labor room; but unless you are having natural childbirth, he will be asked to wait in the "fathers' room" when the time comes for you to go to the delivery room.

Do not be surprised to find that the delivery room resembles an operating room, or that, to prevent infection, the doctor and nurses scrub and dress as they would for an operation. If you request relief from pain, your doctor will give you some form of anesthetic when he deems it safe for the baby. (In some instances, anesthetics are administered in the labor room. For details, see chapter 13, "Pregnancy and Childbirth.") After you have given birth to your baby, and perhaps held him in your arms for a moment, you may spend some time in a recovery room. But before long, elated and exhausted, you will be wheeled to your bed on the maternity floor.

Revolving as it does around the care of infants as well as their mothers, maternity floor routine usually differs from that of the rest of the hospital. At four-hour intervals your baby is brought to you for feeding, whether you breast- or bottle-feed. To protect the babies against infection, visitors are not allowed on the maternity floor at those times, although in most hospitals, father, garbed in a sterile gown and mask, is permitted to spend some time each day with his child and you. After about five days, you will be ready to take your baby home.

YOUR BILL

Expect the worst. Hospital costs soared about 100 percent just between 1975 and 1978. The rate for a hospital bed is, on the average, almost $200 a day, and all other costs are proportionately as high. For most people, insurance covers most of the expenses, and bills are usually sent directly to your insurance company. If you are not insured, you will be handed your bill on departure. If you do not have the money to issue a check immediately, you should arrange a method of payment with the business office before you leave.

Although a few hospitals now itemize every charge, most hospital bills are incomprehensible without an interpreter. If you have questions, ask to have your bill explained to you. You may challenge any item on it, but unless you have kept a written record of every test and telephone call (not an easy thing to do when you're sick), you will have difficulty proving that the hospital has made the mistake.

THE SOCIAL SERVICE DEPARTMENT

Not every hospital has one, but even the smallest employs at least one person who knows his way through the tangle of outside agencies that exist to help people in trouble. If your illness is going to create financial difficulties or problems with family care, ask to see the person in charge of social services. He can help to arrange welfare payments, if hospitalization has put you out of work. He can find visiting homemakers to replace hospitalized mothers, set up home-nursing care for the elderly, arrange outpatient treatment if it is needed after hospitalization.

LEAVING THE HOSPITAL

You and your doctor agree that you are now healthy enough to see after your own convalescence, and you have arranged for transportation home. Before the hospital doors close behind you, make sure (1) that you know precisely how you are to take care of yourself until your next doctor's appointment. (2) If you are going to be an outpatient in one of the hospital clinics, schedule appointments now. (3) If you expect to need help at home, arrange for nursing or homemaker care before you leave the hospital.

A FINAL WORD

Hospitals are enormously complex institutions, into which patients must fit themselves as best they can. But, knowing something of what is likely to happen to you can be of enormous help in making your hospital stay more comfortable.

CHAPTER **11** A Happy Marriage

Unless they are incurably romantic or hopelessly naive, no engaged couple today believes that "wedded bliss" is a permanent state. They know that the new relationship will require compromises and adjustments, many of them difficult, that a marital partnership, like one in business, will flourish only if both parties devote thought, effort, and understanding to the enterprise.

This awareness of the problems of marriage is manifested by the large numbers of young men and women who seek guidance. They want to lose their fears of and misconceptions about sex. They want to anticipate the difficulties that may arise because of differing values, religious attitudes, concepts of rearing children, and other areas of potential disagreement.

There is, of course, no valid blueprint for a happy marriage. But the chances of achieving that desirable state can be enhanced if one is conscious of the conditions that affect, favorably or adversely, the husband-wife alliance.

SOME GUIDELINES FOR CHOOSING A MARRIAGE PARTNER

No matter how much your pulse beats at the sight of your beloved, do not rush into marriage. Take the time to know each other. It will save a lot of trouble later on. Do *not* marry anyone with the idea of reforming him or her. Remember, you are marrying an adult whose tastes and habits are well fixed. Questions such as the following should be faced before marriage: Will the wife work? For how long? Can both of you live on just the husband's earnings? Who will manage the family income? How many children, if any, should you have?

The following questionnaire will serve as a helpful guide.

Answer Yes or No:

1. Do you like to spend most of your leisure time together?
2. Do you agree on whether or not to have children? If children are wanted, do you agree on their upbringing?
3. Do you both enjoy the same friends?
4. Do you have similar tastes in books, movies, art, and the kind of home you want?
5. Do you both have the same basic philosophy of life? Do you share religious attitudes?
6. Do you like, or share his (her) attitude toward, his (her) parents? Is there agreement on ways you behave toward them?

Some comments on the above questionnaire are necessary. "Yes" answers to all the questions would indicate a rare situation; danger exists only if there are basic antagonisms. Certain questions are more important than others. There should be a positive Yes on the questions 1, 2, 3 and 6. In regard to Question 5, it has been found that religious disagreements play some small part in disturbing a marriage. These differences tend to be worked out satisfactorily during the courtship. After marriage, the problem is usually centered on the religious upbringing of the children. Question 6 involves in-laws, who, over the centuries, have been the cause of many marital upsets. The courtship period is the ideal time to get to know them and to make every attempt to establish a good relationship.

LOVE VERSUS INFATUATION

An adequate definition of love has troubled poets and philosophers from time immemorial. However, for the practical purposes of a successful marriage, ask yourself these questions:

1. Do you feel a sense of oneness, each with the other? That is, do you consider the other person a part of yourself?
2. Do you feel you can trust the other person? Does he or she give you a sense of security?
3. Are you concerned about his or her welfare and well-being? Do you try in all ways to make the other person happy?
4. Have you found that when you are apart from the person for a period of time, you still feel the same emotional attachment?
5. Do you find that as you know each other longer, the desire to stay together grows stronger and that you do not grow bored as time goes by?

If you have answered Yes to these questions, you may safely say you are in love. If you look over these questions again, you will also notice that they describe true companionship. A physical attraction is not enough to guarantee a happy marriage. But as one authority puts it, sex is the sturdy foundation upon which the house must be built.

WHAT IS THE BEST AGE FOR MARRIAGE?

Generally speaking, the best age to be married is the age when one has reached physical and mental maturity. Naturally, this will vary with each person, but experts put it between the ages of 22 and 30, with the husband older than the wife. Here again, numerous exceptions are found. In many a happy marriage, the wife is the older partner. The point is that the couple should be emotionally stable and mentally mature enough to withstand the stresses and strains of marriage.

Many people postpone marriage past these "ideal" ages. However, we can assume that in the majority of cases a man or woman who has passed age 35 without marrying has remained single from choice. This may indicate character traits that are not compatible with becoming a good spouse and parent. It is unwise and usually unprofitable to try to force a confirmed single person into marriage.

Do not neglect to consider the marital history of a prospective partner. Do not dismiss the fact that he or she has been divorced; be certain you have a good reason for believing that history will not repeat itself. Men and women who have been married and divorced several times are not good marital risks.

Determination to make the marriage a success is one of the most important weapons against divorce. As one authority says, "Tolerance, understanding, and good humor are more valuable assets in marriage than a starry-eyed idealization of the other partner."

Before discussing the emotional attitudes and sexual adjustments that contribute to a good marriage, let us deal with some basic questions of physical health.

THE PREMARITAL CHECKUP

When two people marry, they promise to live together in sickness and in health. To start off in good health, a couple owe it to themselves and, possibly, to their children to come, to have a checkup, preferably by the same doctor. A thorough physical examination will determine whether either is suffering from any ailment that should be corrected before the wedding, or whether for the sake of their health, they should modify some of their plans for their life together.

Ruling Out Venereal Disease

Before issuing a marriage license, many states require a blood test, such as the Wassermann, to detect syphilis. If either party has this venereal disease, marriage should be postponed until a cure has been effected. Whether or not a syphilis test is mandatory in your state, your physician should be asked to give it; for undetected and untreated, syphilis leads to serious physical and mental disabilities and even to death. What is worse, the infected mothers may give birth to blind, deaf, and deformed babies. Fortunately this dread disease is curable in any but its most advanced stages. (For a detailed discussion, see the entry SYPHILIS in the encyclopedia section.)

Another venereal disease that should be ruled out before a couple marry is gonorrhea. Unlike syphilis, gonorrhea cannot be discovered by a routine blood test. It starts as a local infection of the genital organs, and its detection requires inspection of these areas and perhaps a microscopic examination of their secretions. Though not transmitted to unborn offspring, it may infect a baby's eyes in the course of delivery and can cause blindness. Gonorrhea, too, is curable. (For further discussion, see the entry GONORRHEA in the encyclopedia section.)

Family Health Planning

The premarital examination is a good time to discover other health factors that may affect a couple's future life together. Certain heart conditions, for example, make it foolhardy for a man to hold down some jobs, although he could do other kinds of work without endangering his health. Some illnesses, such as diabetes, make it dangerous for a woman to have a baby, although she could safely do so after the disease has been brought under control. Knowing of such conditions, if they exist, before you marry will enable you to avoid later disappointment and even grief.

Considerations for Future Parents

At some point during the checkup the physician will probably ask you both to give him all the information you have concerning the physical and mental illnesses from which members of your families have suffered. This knowledge will help him determine whether there is a risk that you may pass on to your children any of a number of genetic, or hereditary, diseases. If the family history reveals the presence of one of these diseases, you will benefit from genetic counseling before starting your family. (Genetic counseling is discussed in detail in Chapter 12, "Family Planning.") In all likelihood, however, your doctor will be able to set your mind at rest immediately regarding the probability of your having healthy children.

For Women Only

In some virgins, the hymen—the membrane at the opening of the vagina—is tough or inelastic and does not rupture easily. This may make intercourse at the beginning of the marriage extremely painful or even impossible. In the premarital physical examination the doctor can determine whether the prospective bride has this condition and, if she has, correct it. He can either stretch the hymen or remove it by a surgical procedure so minor as hardly to be called an operation. (For further discussion, see HYMEN in the encyclopedia section.)

MARRIED LOVE AND SEX

If we were to define married love in its simplest terms, we would say it has three parts: (1) a sexual attraction; (2) a deep feeling of companionship; and (3) a desire for parenthood. The first two are essential; the third is vital to many couples for emotional fulfillment.

Most of us have experienced the joys and the difficulties of companionship. We have been close to our parents, our brothers and sisters, and our friends. These experiences are vitally important in preparing us to make good homes of our own.

We have also had the opportunity to discover some of the things that go into making a good marriage. But the regular day-to-day life together and the sexual intimacy between two people of the opposite sex are the factors in marriage for which people have unfortunately been the least prepared by their own relationships and observations.

Is Sex Education Necessary?

From the questions that are asked them, doctors know that a great deal of ignorance and misinformation still becloud the subject of sex. Young and older couples frequently ask whether their sexual relations are "all right."

There are some people who feel that too much emphasis on sex education is a mistake. For example, one young married woman said to her doctor, "I'm sorry Bill and I ever read that book about sex in marriage! It just made him feel guilty because he can't live up to what it says a man should do to satisfy his wife; and I feel guilty because I'm upsetting him! I'd rather be ignorant than become self-conscious trying to follow a lot of blueprints!"

It is true that, because matters concerning sex techniques and skills were taboo for so long, some writers tend to go too far in the other direction, exaggerating the importance of mechanics and minimizing the importance of the physical attraction existing between two people who love each other.

The Purposes of Sex

Biologically, reproduction is the purpose of sexual intercourse—the means by which new life is created. There has been some tendency in recent years to pass over this aspect of the sexual act, perhaps because at one time it was regarded as the only purpose of sexual intercourse. Today, most people feel that sexual intercourse is also the most intimate way of expressing love. Giving and receiving the greatest pleasure and experiencing the release that accompanies it are natural and healthy desires.

Satisfactory Sexual Relations

In discussing this subject, we do not attempt to deal with the moral aspects of some of the questions that follow, for these are matters of individual conscience or the dictates of one's religion.

1. *Should a couple have sexual intercourse (coitus) before marriage in order to find out*

whether they are compatible? This is a matter for each couple to decide. However, it seems naive to believe that one can successfully test so subtle and delicate a matter within a relatively brief period and under less than ideal circumstances. Sexual adjustment is seldom achieved immediately. Far more often it is developed gradually.

2. *Does the size of the respective organs of man and woman play an important part in the success of their relationship?* No—at least, far less often than is generally imagined, because of the possibility of employing techniques that will minimize any difficulties.

3. *Does having practiced masturbation affect the ability to have successful sexual relations?* The harmful effects of this practice are owing to the fears and guilts associated with it. Physically, no damage is done by it. Almost everyone has practiced some form of masturbation. (See also the entry MASTURBATION in the encyclopedia section.)

4. *Does youthful petting interfere with satisfactory sex relations later on?* Most normal young people engage in some sort of lovemaking that does not terminate in intercourse. It is the usual way for them to discover or demonstrate their physical attraction for each other. Prolonged or habitual petting, which requires the constant exercise of great self-restraint, may have a temporary adverse effect. For example, a girl who is accustomed to being constantly on guard against premarital coitus may find it difficult when she is first married to relax and enjoy the sexual act.

5. *Is sexual experience with others in the past helpful or harmful to the establishment of successful sex relations with one's spouse?* Past experience is certainly not necessary. But it is important to realize that loving someone requires an understanding of the fact that even past relationships have contributed to creating the person one loves. On the other hand, promiscuity, as well as the coldness that comes from long repression of sexual desire, are indications of a neurotic attitude toward sex.

6. *Does a past homosexual experience mean that a person cannot have normal sex relations?* According to the Kinsey report, a great many men and an appreciable number of women have had some sort of homosexual experience that did not interfere with normal sexual relations later on. However, everyone who is concerned about such an experience should discuss it frankly with a physician or a competent counselor. (See also the entry HOMOSEXUALITY in the encyclopedia section.)

7. *Is the wedding night crucial in the establishment of satisfactory sexual relations?* It can be. The bride is usually tense and overwrought, especially if the wedding was a large one. She requires the utmost consideration from the groom, who is usually nervous himself.

Some of the difficulties of the wedding night can be avoided if the bride has had a preliminary medical examination. Before the wedding night, also, the marriage partners should discuss birth control with each other. Their doctor or the bride's gynecologist will advise them about various types of contraception. (For further information, see Chapter 12 and the entry CONTRACEPTIVE METHODS AND DEVICES in the encyclopedia section.)

8. *Will the bride enjoy sexual intercourse?* She may or may not. Some young women derive no more pleasure from coitus than they do from any intimate caress. They may not reach sexual maturity—i.e., full enjoyment of intercourse—until they have been married for quite a while.

Generally speaking, women are less quickly and spontaneously aroused than are men. Both partners should realize this fact.

Many women need a warming-up period before they feel a desire to have intercourse—in many cases, before they are physically ready for it. When a woman is sufficiently aroused, her vagina is well lubricated and naturally receptive to the insertion of the penis. Many women respond best to lovemaking that begins with verbal expressions of affection, kisses, and gentle caresses, and proceeds to stimulation of the breasts, the nipples, the clitoris (the small projection outside the vagina, which is composed of erectile tissue similar to that of the penis), and the vagina itself. Each husband should learn to know the degree to which his wife is excited by caresses of different parts of the body.

9. *Will a wife always achieve sexual satisfaction if her husband is sufficiently skillful, considerate, and gentle?* A number of women do experience an orgasm—in some instances multiple orgasms—almost every time they have intercourse. Other women do not have an orgasm even under the most favorable circumstances. Some experience an orgasm only after they have been married for some time. There are women who experience this climax only occasionally, perhaps at certain periods of the month; their desire may be of a cyclical nature, reaching its peak before, during, or after the menstrual period. In a man the orgasm is clearly defined; it may be vague or diffuse in a woman. Its degree of

intensity varies. It may be centered in the clitoris or it may involve the internal portion of the vagina; some women experience both types of orgasm. Failure to achieve an orgasm does not, in itself, prevent a women from having great pleasure in the sexual act. Nor does failure necessarily cause her to become tense and to feel frustrated.

Men often reach the climax of their sexual excitement more rapidly than women do. The man can usually compensate for this discrepancy in timing by making certain that the woman is highly stimulated before intercourse actually begins. As a general rule, a woman's desire fades slowly after she has had an orgasm, whereas that of a man is apt to vanish immediately.

If a man is young or greatly excited, he may occasionally have an orgasm immediately upon beginning the sexual act—this is called premature ejaculation. However, if it occurs habitually, he should consult a doctor. Failure to have an orgasm during coitus is rare in men—except when they are under the influence of alcohol—and should be discussed with a doctor.

10. *What causes frigidity in women?* Failure to have an orgasm does not necessarily mean a woman is frigid. Doctors speak of true frigidity in women as the inability to derive pleasure from sexual relations. This may be caused by insufficient lubrication or lack of adequate stimulation—i.e., precoital play. More likely, frigidity is the result of conscious or unconscious feelings of guilt, inferiority, or fears. In such cases, professional help is usually required to remove the underlying cause.

11. *What is impotence in men, and what causes it?* By impotence, doctors mean the inability of a man to have or maintain an erection. It does not mean sterility, which is the inability to have children. A physical condition can be, but rarely is, the cause of impotence. In most cases, it is related to such psychological difficulties as hostility to women, guilt, and fears—for example, the fear of impregnating the woman, or of inadequate sexual performance. Some men are impotent with women they admire or love, and can have intercourse only with women whom they do not respect. Usually this situation develops because the man subconsciously divides women into two groups: madonnas (good mothers), with whom sexual intercourse is forbidden, and harlots, with whom it is permissible. In most cases, psychiatric help is required to solve such problems causing impotence.

12. *How often should a couple have intercourse?* If both partners feel well, if coitus does not cause discomfort or fatigue and is followed by physical and emotional relaxation, there is no need to worry about frequency. Repeated failure to be satisfied after experiencing an orgasm should be discussed with a physician or trained counselor.

The desire to have intercourse usually declines as people approach middle age. Yet some women reach the height of sexual vigor quite late in life, even after they have passed the menopause; and some men retain virility into their old age.

Whether or not to have intercourse while the woman is menstruating is a matter for each couple to decide. It may cause the wife some discomfort, especially if she has cramps during her period; but it will do no physical damage to either the man or the woman. (Intercourse during pregnancy is discussed in Chapter 13.)

Having intercourse does not use up one's potency, and abstaining from it does not increase virility. However, having sexual relations several times a day regularly may decrease the amount of sperm a man produces, thus lessening the chances of conceiving a child. Excessive interest in sex or a marked lack of interest in it are both indications of difficulties that require expert help.

Never take any medicine, pill, or injection in order to increase or decrease sexual desire, unless a competent physician has discovered a physical condition that requires it. Potency pills that contain hormones can be extremely dangerous. Aphrodisiacs such as cantharides (Spanish fly) are actually poisonous irritants. (See the entry APHRODISIAC in the encyclopedia section.) Alcohol does not increase desire, although it may appear at first to do so because it releases inhibitions. Occasionally, a tense or shy person finds it easier to relax after having a glass or two of an alcoholic beverage. But anyone who remains dependent on such artificial aids will probably find some form of psychotherapy a far wiser way of getting rid of repressions.

13. *Is intercourse ever harmful or dangerous?* It is extremely dangerous when either partner is suffering from a venereal disease. Intercourse and all other forms of close contact should be avoided in cases of contagious illness. Certain noncontagious diseases make intercourse inadvisable or even dangerous. Anyone who is not in good health should discuss this matter frankly with his or her physician.

Positions During Intercourse

The majority of people in our culture habitually assume a single position during coitus. But this is only a matter of custom. There is no reason to believe that any position is the right one if another is desirable because of health, relative size of the genitals, or individual preference.

Man above woman. In our Western culture, this combination is considered the normal or standard position. The woman lies on her back and spreads her thighs until there is room between her legs for the man's thighs. By bending her legs, she allows for deeper penetration. The man lies upon his partner's abdomen, supporting his knees and elbows as far as possible on the bed so that he will not be too heavy a burden. If the woman holds her thighs together after entry, it will be helpful in cases where the penis is too small or the vagina too large. It will also increase friction against the clitoris. By holding the thighs tightly together, the woman can prevent the penis from entering too deeply, if this is needed to prevent pain.

Woman over man. The woman can assume a kneeling position over the man and let herself down gradually until the penis is inserted. The advantage of this position is that the woman has full control of the movements, quickening or slowing down as she pleases. It also enables her to adjust herself to the penis by bending forward so that full contact with the clitoris is made. Properly carried out, this position can lead to heights of sexual delight. It is advantageous if the man is tired. Its disadvantages are that it requires a good deal of exertion on the part of the female while the male is passive. The position is not recommended if the vaginal passage is unusually short or if the male is sick or convalescent, because it is apt to be more stimulating than the position described in the next paragraph.

Lying on side, face to face. The man and woman lie on their sides, facing each other. The woman raises her upper thigh, resting it on the man's upper thigh. This is an excellent position during pregnancy, as there is little pressure on the woman's abdomen.

Rear entry. This method is also recommended especially for pregnant women or in any other case where deep penetration and weight on the abdomen are not safe. The woman places herself with her back to the man, usually in a kneeling position. The man enters the vagina from behind. This position does not give the woman as much pleasure as some others, as the clitoris is not touched by the penis during the union. The man

can correct this by fondling her clitoris and her breasts with his hands.

What Are Abnormal Sex Practices Between a Man and a Woman?

Broadly speaking, a couple is sexually normal if each derives the highest sexual pleasure and satisfaction from the insertion of the male genital organ into that of the female. This does not preclude experimenting in obtaining satisfaction by other means. For example, there is certainly nothing abnormal for a man who has reached his climax rapidly and his wife has not yet reached hers, to make it possible for her to do so by manual manipulation. In the foreplay preceding coitus, there is nothing abnormal about any caress that both partners find pleasurable.

In adults the oral zone (mouth, lips, and tongue) is, to a greater or lesser extent, a sexual one. Some couples find the genital kiss important for the fullest realization of sexual satisfaction. Without attempting to draw an exact line defining the normal limits of this practice, today's psychiatrists tend to agree that maladjustment is indicated only when actions involving the mouth rather than the genitals are the main or only source of sexual pleasure and climax.

HOW TO GET HELP IN SOLVING MARITAL PROBLEMS

As indicated earlier in this chapter, some sex problems arise from ignorance or misinformation; these often clear up readily in the light of truth. Others are more complicated. If you need any information that has not been given here, or if you are worried about yourself, your spouse, or your marriage, be sure to talk things over with a trained person. Discuss the matter with your doctor first. If that is not possible, consult a marriage counselor, who will probably be able to help you, or may advise you to see a psychiatrist.

Marriage counselors concern themselves with all aspects of marital and premarital problems. Every large city has a Family Service Association that provides marriage counseling. If one is not available in your community, write to the Family Service Association of America, 44 East 23rd Street, New York, New York 10010, for suggestions. The American Association for Marriage and Family Therapy, 924 West Ninth Street, Upland, California 91786, will provide the names of trained accredited marriage counselors in or near your community.

CHAPTER **12** Family Planning

Married couples usually want and expect to have children. The final decision about the number to have and the intervals at which to have them is, of course, theirs to make. Nevertheless, there are some commonsense facts and some medical findings which may be helpful to know while planning a family. Bear in mind that the medical findings are statistical, based on studies of large groups of people, and cannot be applied with any degree of certainty to a specific individual.

THE FIRST CHILD

Many authorities advise that a couple wait until each has become adjusted to the other before having the first child. That time may be a few months or a few years. It depends on the couple, and on the time it takes them to get their home settled and to prepare themselves financially and emotionally for the arrival of a child. At the same time, it should be borne in mind that both men and women tend to become less fertile as they grow older, and that the risk to health, for both mother and child, is lowest when the mother is between 20 and 35 years old.

Similarly, the health risk for both mother and child is lowest if the period between the end of one pregnancy and the beginning of the next is between two and five years. Such spacing also has commonsense advantages. A child has usually reached a comparatively settled stage of development at about three years of age, so this is a good time to add a younger brother or sister.

How many children should a woman have? As many as she and her husband want and feel they can afford—financially, physically, and emotionally. In the matter of family size, their wishes and their doctor's advice are the important considerations. Some couples, concerned with population problems, may want to have no children at all, or to have no more than two. Others, in whom the maternal and paternal drives are strong, may want to have large families.

Notice the word "want." It reflects the central thought in this discussion. All children should be wanted. The medical evidence indicates that unwanted children face greater health risks than those their parents want to have. Your doctor can help you plan for your future family, as can the professionals at a local family-planning clinic or at your local chapter of the Planned Parenthood Federation of America. (If there is no local chapter in your community, write to the national office, at 810 Seventh Avenue, New York, N.Y. 10019, to find the address of the chapter nearest you.)

METHODS OF BIRTH CONTROL

Conception can be controlled by mechanical or chemical means and by the rhythm method, and it can be prevented by surgical procedures performed either on the woman or on the man. Although some birth control methods can be used without any medical supervision, the most effective of the ones used by women require a medical examination.

Methods Available Without Medical Supervision

The Condom. This is a thin, flexible sheath worn by the man over his penis in order to prevent the sperm from entering the woman's vagina. Condoms can be purchased without a prescription and do not require a visit to the doctor. The government has set standards which assure that the products available in reputable pharmacies are not defective.

The condom should be put on after an erection but before the penis first enters the vagina. It is

151

risky to wait until just before the male orgasm, because some sperm may leak out before ejaculation actually occurs. The condom should be rolled on, leaving about a half inch of loose space at the tip of the penis to collect the ejaculated semen. Both to facilitate entry into the vagina and to guard against possible breakage of the condom, it should be lubricated with saliva or vaginal jelly. (Petroleum jelly should never be used as a lubricant. It causes deterioration of the rubber.) Prelubricated condoms can also be purchased. Each condom should be used no more than once.

Used properly, the condom provides a good means of preventing conception. For additional safety the woman should use a spermicidal jelly, cream, or foam (see below) at the same time the man is using the condom. The condom is the best device to use during intercourse with a virgin partner who is not ready to employ the medically supervised methods available to women.

Spermicidal Preparations. Various creams, foams, and jellies are available without prescription for use by women during intercourse. Tablets and suppositories can also be purchased at the drugstore, but they are less popular and less effective. All these products work on the same principle, i.e., they prevent conception both by blocking the entrance to the uterus and by immobilizing the sperm. They must be inserted into the vagina less than an hour before intercourse; if more time elapses, they become ineffective and must be applied again.

But none of them is as reliable as the medically supervised procedures for preventing pregnancy. Spermicidal preparations are most effective when used in conjunction with other methods of birth control, such as the condom.

Methods Requiring Medical Supervision

All the birth control devices listed below require a medical examination of the woman, and all of them are far more effective than the nonprescription methods previously described. There are several of these more effective devices available and the woman and her doctor can choose among them to find the one most appropriate for her to use.

The Pill (Oral Contraceptives). This form of contraception was developed in the 1950's and officially released for sale in the United States in 1960 after extensive testing. Since then, it has become the most popular form of birth control among American women. A major part of the reason for its popularity is its effectiveness: short of sterilization, the pill is the most reliable method known for controlling conception. Moreover, the pill requires only swallowing, and its use involves no interruption of lovemaking at any stage. Nevertheless, the pill has its drawbacks and dangers. It must be taken on a regular basis: careless usage can undo its effectiveness. It is not medically safe for all women and it may cause unpleasant or undesirable side effects in others. It has also been known to cause serious illness. Finally, it is still relatively new, and all its long-range effects are, therefore, not yet known. Some pills, such as the so-called sequential type which contain a heavy concentration of estrogen, have already been withdrawn from the market because they have been found to be a risk to health.

Although various types of pills are available, all of them contain chemicals similar to the natural female hormones that control ovulation, and they work by preventing ovulation from taking place, thus keeping the woman infertile for as long as she takes the pill. To remain effective, therefore, it must be taken on a rigid schedule. The most commonly used pills (the so-called combination pills) are taken one a day for three weeks; for the next week either no pills or pills without hormones are taken. On the fifth week, the cycle begins again. The so-called mini-pills, which are somewhat less effective because they contain no estrogen, are taken daily, with no interruption. (Estrogen is the hormone responsible for more serious complications of oral contraceptives.) On first use, some women experience unpleasant side effects from the mini-pill such as nausea, weight gain, and headaches, but these generally wear off once the body has become adjusted.

Your doctor will determine, after a medical examination and a review of your medical history, whether it is advisable for you to use the pill, and which of the many types available is best for you to use. He will also supply a list of symptoms which may develop and tell you which of these indicate that you should stop the medication. He will not recommend the pill at all if you have had thrombosis (blood clots), a stroke, a liver disorder, a cancer of the breast or reproductive system, or certain kinds of cardiac difficulties. And he may not recommend it to sufferers from high blood pressure or migraine headaches.

Women who take the pill must have a medical examination at least once a year to make sure no problems have arisen. This is vitally important.

Intrauterine Devices (IUD's). Of all the methods of protection against unwanted pregnancy, the IUD is the least troublesome to use. Once the device is put in place, it remains there for a year or more—depending on the type—or until contraception is no longer wanted. No further steps are necessary to prevent conception.

Several types of IUD are available, but all are similar in the most important respect. They are small metal or plastic devices with nylon thread tails. The device is placed inside the uterus; the tail hangs down into the vagina. The IUD, which prevents conception by making the lining of the uterus unreceptive to pregnancy, is second only to the pill in effectiveness and reliability. Most doctors recommend that, for the first few months after the IUD has been inserted, a spermicidal jelly, cream, or foam should also be used in mid-menstrual cycle.

Although the IUD was first developed in 1909, it has not been in use in this country much longer than the pill. Some IUD's have been withdrawn from the market because they present a health hazard. Moreover, not all women can tolerate the IUD. Some experience uncomfortable side effects, such as spotting, increased mentrual flow, and/or cramps. Others spontaneously expel the device. A few women have experienced serious complications following its use.

The IUD is inserted by a trained professional, whose examination has determined that the woman is a likely candidate to use the device successfully, and what type of IUD is best for her to use. She will also be instructed in ways of making sure she is tolerating it well and that it is remaining in place. A woman using an IUD should have yearly examinations to be sure no problems have arisen.

The Diaphragm. Until the advent of the pill and the IUD, the diaphragm was considered the most reliable method of birth control available to women. It is a simple mechanical device that blocks the sperm from entering the uterus and thus prevents fertilization of the egg.

The diaphragm itself is a shallow cup of soft rubber stretched over and around a flexible ring, which is inserted into the vagina to cover the cervix—the entrance to the uterus. Because women's internal measurements differ, the diaphragm must be fitted by a medically qualified person, who can determine, on examination, the type and size required and who can instruct the woman on the correct method of inserting and removing it.

The diaphragm should be used in conjunction with a spermicidal cream or jelly applied both on the rim and on the diaphragm itself. It should be inserted no more than six hours before intercourse and should be kept in place for at least six hours thereafter. After a year, or after the birth of a baby, it is advisable for the woman to have another examination to be sure the diaphragm still fits properly. If it has been carefully fitted, if directions are followed exactly, and if it is regularly inspected for holes and tears, the diaphram should prove quite reliable in preventing conception and should cause no discomfort to either partner.

The Rhythm Method. Couples with religious scruples against other methods of birth control may wish to make use of the so-called rhythm method, which is based on abstinence from sexual intercourse during that period of the woman's menstrual cycle when she is fertile and therefore likely to conceive.

The disadvantage of the rhythm method lies in the difficulty of calculating the woman's "safe" period. Very few women have absolutely regular menstrual cycles; the greater the irregularity, the greater the likelihood that the rhythm method will not work. Therefore, although a visit to the doctor is not absolutely necessary to make use of the method, getting medical advice is prudent.

To discover her "safe" period, the woman must first keep track of the length of her menstrual cycle for at least eight months, in order to discover the longest and the shortest interval she can expect between her periods. Because ovulation generally occurs approximately two weeks before the menstrual period begins, this will help her determine the time range—usually about 10 days—when she is probably fertile and pregnancy is, therefore, likely to occur.

As a further check, the woman should also take her temperature every morning, immediately after awakening, because the body temperature usually drops several tenths of a degree just before ovulation and rises even more sharply about 24 hours thereafter. Some women have still other clues to rely on. At the time of ovulation, they experience a peculiar, sudden cramp followed by a heavy feeling in the lower abdomen that may last several hours. They may also notice an unusual amount of mucous secretion at this time.

Contraction

28-day menstrual cycle

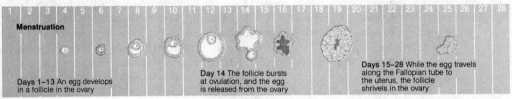

Menstruation

Days 1–13 An egg develops in a follicle in the ovary

Day 14 The follicle bursts at ovulation, and the egg is released from the ovary

Days 15–28 While the egg travels along the Fallopian tube to the uterus, the follicle shrivels in the ovary

Rhythm method

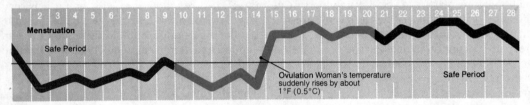

Menstruation

Safe Period

Ovulation Woman's temperature suddenly rises by about 1°F (0.5°C)

Safe Period

Oral contraceptives

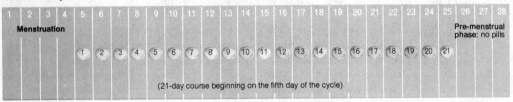

Menstruation

Pre-menstrual phase: no pills

(21-day course beginning on the fifth day of the cycle)

Diaphragms   Coils

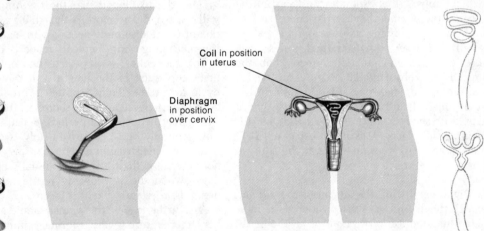

Coil in position in uterus

Diaphragm in position over cervix

Two types of contraception, the rhythm method and the pill, are related to a woman's menstrual cycle. The success of the rhythm method depends on avoiding intercourse around ovulation, the time at about the middle of the cycle when an egg is released from an ovary. Ovulation can be recognized by a sudden slight rise in body temperature (about 1°F or ½°C). Hormones contained in oral contraceptives—the pill—act by interfering with the cycle: they prevent ovulation from taking place. Menstruation still occurs, generally some time in the seven days when no pills are taken. The diaphragm, or cap, and the intra-uterine device (IUD), or coil, are contraceptive devices for use by women. The diaphragm fits temporarily over the mouth of the uterus and acts as a physical barrier against the entry of sperm. An IUD coil is fitted inside the uterus, where it prevents a fertilized egg from being implanted.

Illness or emotional upset may hasten or delay ovulation even in women whose periods occur with great regularity. If this should happen, the calculations will be in error. Because of this possibility, the rhythm method cannot be considered as reliable a means of preventing pregnancy as the other medically supervised methods.

Unsatisfactory Methods

Coitus Interruptus (Withdrawal). In *coitus interruptus*, the man withdraws his penis from the woman's vagina just before the semen is ejaculated. This method is unsatisfactory for several reasons. It places a heavy responsibility on the man at a time when he is highly excited and finds it difficult to control his actions. And even if withdrawal seems to be successfully practiced, it is not an adequate safeguard against conception; sperm may leak out before the actual ejaculation takes place. Moreover, the fear that the man will not withdraw soon enough puts both partners under tension and may interfere with the enjoyment of the sex act.

Douche. Used immediately after intercourse, the douche is designed to flush out or inactivate all the sperm remaining in the vagina. It is an extremely unreliable method. First of all, it is almost impossible to inactivate all the sperm. In addition, the faster moving sperm enter the neck of the uterus only seconds after the man has ejaculated.

If for any reason the woman *does* want to use a douche, plain warm water, possibly with the addition of a little salt or vinegar, is the best thing. Neither commercial douches nor those nonprescription "feminine hygiene" products which hint at contraceptive properties are any more effective.

VOLUNTARY STERILIZATION

A couple who decide that they will never in the future want any children may want to look into the possibility of voluntary sterilization for one or the other of them. It should be borne in mind, however, that these procedures—which are legal throughout the United States—are, for all practical purposes, irreversible. Once they are performed, a man who has been sterilized can never again impregnate a woman, and a sterilized woman can never again conceive a child. For this reason, the decision for sterilization should not be taken lightly. But women whose health may be endangered by pregnancy and couples whose families have already reached the size they desire, or who do not wish to risk transmitting hereditary disease, may wish to join the more than 10 million men and women who have chosen voluntary sterilization.

The sterilization operation for men is called vasectomy, and it consists in cutting and tying the ends of the *vas deferens,* the two small tubes through which the sperm pass. This breaks the connection between the testicles, where the sperm is produced, and the seminal vesicles, where the secretion that carries them is manufactured. It thus prevents any sperm from entering the semen and renders the ejaculation sterile.

Vasectomy is a safe, reliable, and simple procedure, usually performed under local anesthetic in the doctor's office or a clinic. The operation takes very little time; it does not incapacitate the patient, and it has no effect on his ability either to perform the sex act or to derive pleasure from it.

The sterilization operation for women is called tubal ligation. It, too, involves cutting and tying off the ends of two small tubes, in this case the Fallopian tubes, through which the egg is carried from the ovaries to the uterus. By preventing the egg from reaching the uterus, tubal ligation makes conception impossible.

Tubal ligation is more complex and somewhat more risky than vasectomy. It is most easily and safely performed in a hospital, soon after the woman has given birth to her last child. Like vasectomy, tubal ligation has no effect on sexual desire or on the ability to enjoy the sexual act.

ABORTION

Since 1973, early abortion has been legal in the United States. During the first 12 weeks, a woman has the right, in consultation with her doctor, to decide to terminate her pregnancy. During this first trimester, as it is called, abortion is a relatively safe and simple procedure. Thereafter it becomes more complicated and more risky, and in some localities there are state-imposed restrictions. Therefore, if a woman decides to have an abortion, she should have it done as early as possible. The procedure usually employed in early abortion is called vacuum aspiration. It involves the insertion of a thin, hollow tube into the uterus and the gentle withdrawal of its contents by the use of a pump at the other end of the tube. Obviously, contraception is preferable to abortion as a way of dealing with unwanted pregnancy, but current methods of early abortion are safe and appear to leave no permanent physical aftereffects.

There are, of course, many women who, for religious, ethical or moral reasons, could never accept abortion under any circumstances.

WHEN TO AVOID PREGNANCY

Women who have the following disorders should avoid becoming pregnant unless they have their doctor's approval:

Heart disease	Diabetes
Kidney disease	Tuberculosis
High blood pressure	Venereal disease

Some of these illnesses can be completely cured. Others, if they are not too severe or can be controlled, will not necessarily endanger the life of either mother or baby. If proper care is taken, even heart disease does not necessarily constitute an overly serious problem. But only a doctor can decide whether pregnancy will be dangerous in each individual case.

In addition, some conditions in the mother during pregnancy can have a very serious effect on the unborn child. If the woman contracts certain viral diseases, particularly rubella (German measles) while she is pregnant, her baby is likely to be abnormal in some way. She may wish, therefore, to terminate her pregnancy. Toxoplasmosis, a disease transmitted in the handling of cat litter or by the eating of contaminated raw meat, produces such slight symptoms that the victim is usually unaware of them. But if toxoplasmosis strikes a pregnant woman, her infant may be deformed or stillborn. A blood test, now made routinely by many obstetricians, reveals the presence of the infection. Another procedure, called amniocentesis (described below) determines whether the fetus has been affected. Women who are drug-addicted during pregnancy give birth to addicted babies whose survival is jeopardized. It also seems unfair to bring a child into the world if either parent is mentally ill or alcoholic. Similarly, it is poor judgment to have a child in the hope that its arrival will patch up a damaged relationship. Children are not therapy for an ailing marriage. On the contrary, they usually become its victims.

Genetic Diseases and Genetic Counseling

A number of diseases are passed on by parents to their children even though the parents show no symptoms of the illness. These so-called genetic diseases, carried in the egg and/or sperm which join to create life, can pose a serious hazard. They are the cause of some 40 percent of all infant deaths in the United States and often of handicaps, of severe suffering, and of early death for those infants who survive. Among the genetic diseases are hemophilia (the bleeding disease) and Down's syndrome (mongolism), a form of mental retardation which is most likely to affect a child whose mother is over 35 when she becomes pregnant. A number of disabling conditions are found more commonly in one or another population group: cystic fibrosis among whites; sickle-cell anemia among blacks; Tay-Sachs disease among Jews of Eastern or Central European origin; thalassemia among people of Italian and Greek origin; PKU (phenylketonuria) among people of Irish or North European descent.

Treatment for some of these conditions is now available, and the search is under way to find treatment for the others. Moreover, couples from families with a history of these diseases can usually discover, through a simple test, whether they are carriers of the illness and likely to pass it on to their children. (Blood tests for sickle-cell anemia and Tay-Sachs disease are advisable even for couples whose family history does not include the illness.) If the woman is already pregnant, the amniocentesis procedure can be used to discover defects in the unborn child. Amniocentesis involves withdrawing and analyzing a small sample of the amniotic fluid, the liquid which surrounds the developing fetus. If the defect is found to be present, the couple can then decide whether or not to continue the pregnancy.

Obviously, however, it is far better to make the decision in advance of pregnancy about whether or not to have a child. Couples who have reason to be concerned about possible birth defects in their children can be helped by genetic counseling—professional advice about the risks and alternatives open to couples who are concerned about hereditary disease. Genetic counseling only provides information; the decision is, of course, made by the prospective parents. If you do not know of a counseling service in your area, write to the National Genetics Foundation, 555 West 57th Street, New York, N.Y. 10019.

CAUSES OF CHILDLESSNESS

Miscarriages. Some women have no difficulty in conceiving, but are unable to carry a baby to term and repeatedly experience miscarriage, or spontaneous abortion. Emotional stress, general ill health, malnutrition, illnesses (including infections), and glandular disorders are among the causes of miscarriages.

Some doctors think that many miscarriages can be avoided by refraining from coitus during the days on which the woman's first three menstrual periods would normally occur. Sometimes a week's rest in bed at these periods, especially during the first months, may save the baby.

Do not be alarmed or discouraged by a miscarriage, especially if it is your first pregnancy. An estimated 15 to 20 percent of known pregnancies end in a miscarriage. Also remember that a miscarriage is often nature's way of expelling a defective embryo, one that could not develop into a healthy fetus or infant.

Low Fertility. One out of every six couples who want children have difficulty in conceiving them. In 50 percent of these cases, however, this problem can be solved. The solution is a joint responsibility of both man and woman: contrary to the popular notion, the problem lies with the husband in about a third of all cases, and in many instances it is shared by husband and wife.

Causes of Infertility. There are a number of causes of infertility. A man may not produce a sufficient number of sperm cells, or the sperm may be inadequate in quality or vitality. An obstruction in the vas deferens may block the passage of the sperm to the seminal vesicle. Neither condition interferes with the man's ability to perform sexually. A woman may not be producing any egg cells, or the eggs may be deficient in some way. A defect in the vagina or an unstretched hymen may keep the sperm from entering the birth canal. The Fallopian tubes may be closed, usually the result of a pelvic infection, thus blocking the passage of the egg and its union with the sperm. The fertilized egg may be unable to attach itself properly to the uterine wall. All these conditions can be discovered by a physician, and he should be consulted if, after a reasonable period of time (about a year), a couple are still unsuccessful in achieving pregnancy.

Reverse Rhythm. But you should give yourselves a chance first. This means that you should have intercourse at the time when it is most apt to result in conception. In other words, study the rhythm method of birth control, discussed earlier in this chapter, and practice it in *reverse*. Many couples have difficulty in conceiving simply because they never have intercourse at exactly the time conception could occur. The act of intercourse should be performed in such a way as to allow the semen to reach, and be retained in, the inner portion of the vagina. This will be facilitated if the woman elevates her legs and keeps them raised for a short time after the act is completed. No douches of any kind should be used. It is not necessary for the woman to have an orgasm in order to become pregnant. Some men fail to produce a sufficient number of sperm cells to impregnate a woman if intercourse is frequent. It is therefore advisable to refrain from coitus for a week before the calculated day of ovulation. On that day, the couple should have intercourse in the morning and again at night.

Fertility Clinic. If these suggestions do not work, husband and wife together should consult a physician or clinic specializing in the problem. Your doctor or your nearest hospital, medical center, or medical school will help you locate the help you need, as will the Planned Parenthood Federation of America. Do not be discouraged.

Treatment. Because tension may be a cause of low fertility, discussion with a sympathetic doctor can often solve the problem. Some cases of low fertility can be eliminated simply by a change in diet or a period of rest and relaxation. Others may require no more than minor surgery or hormone medication. Under certain specific circumstances, the physician may prescribe fertility pills for the woman. Remember, however, that the use of these pills increases the chance of multiple births. If the husband's sperm cells are too weak or too few in number to make conception possible, the physician may place the sperm deep within the vagina. This is the same procedure as is used in artificial insemination, which the couple may decide on if it is found that the husband has no sperm or has sperm of such poor quality that conception is considered impossible.

Artificial Insemination. Artificial insemination is medically safe and no one, other than the couple involved and the doctor who performs the procedure, need ever know it has been used. The donor remains unknown to everyone, including himself, and the baby's birth certificate will list the husband as father. But artificial insemination can present difficult emotional, medical, and legal problems, all of which should be thoroughly discussed before it is undertaken.

13 Pregnancy and Childbirth

During the last several decades remarkable strides in medical science have dramatically reduced the mortality of childbearing women. In 1940 the death rate of mothers during childbirth was 376 per 100,000. By the late 1970's that figure had dropped to 11.2 per 100,000. One of the major factors in this sharp decrease has been the recognition by physicians and laymen alike of the vital importance of prenatal care. During pregnancy, regular examinations by the doctor, his advice, and his supervision play a large role in the health of the prospective mother and her unborn child. But the main responsibility is the mother's. It is she who must maintain a healthful diet, control her weight, avoid harmful drugs and medicines, get the right amount of rest and exercise, and prepare herself physically and psychologically for the birth of her baby. This chapter provides guidelines to be followed from the early determination of pregnancy to actual childbirth.

SIGNS OF PREGNANCY

For most women, the first clue to pregnancy is the cessation of menstruation. However, missing a period is not infallible proof. Other factors—such as illness, malnutrition, rapid weight loss, and emotional upset—may delay menstruation. On the other hand, a pregnant woman may, in rare instances, experience vaginal bleeding during the early months of pregnancy. Although this bleeding resembles menstruation, there is a scantier flow and fewer days of it.

If you miss a menstrual period and suspect that the cause is pregnancy, there are other obvious signs to look for. Your breasts will become noticeably enlarged; they may feel tender or tingling, and the nipples may become hypersensitive, larger, and darker. You may experience nausea, usually called "morning sickness," although it may occur at any time during the day. Sudden lack of appetite, frequent need to urinate, and excessive desire for sleep are other symptoms. Any one of them is sufficient cause to send you to your doctor for a determination.

How a Doctor Determines Pregnancy

It is possible to determine pregnancy as early as three weeks after conception through laboratory analysis of a small quantity of the patient's urine or blood. The results can be read immediately, and are almost always accurate.

Even without tests, a doctor can usually make an early diagnosis of pregnancy from the symptoms you describe to him and by checking your breasts for enlargement and for darkening of the nipples and surrounding areolae. At about the 10th week of pregnancy, he can feel the enlarged uterus when he presses your abdomen. A pelvic examination at this time will show bluish-tinted tissues at the entrance to the vagina and a considerably softened cervix (the mouth of the uterus). If the doctor has any doubt about his findings, he can take a picture of your abdomen by means of a sonograph—a machine that uses sound waves instead of X rays to reveal structures inside the body. A sonograph will show the presence of a fetus as early as the eighth week of pregnancy.

The Unmarried Mother

Every prospective mother, unmarried as well as married, has the right to good care for herself and for the child that she is carrying. Many unhappy situations could be avoided if pregnant unmarried women, who are often very young, realized that good care is available to them in most communities. The local Salvation Army often has facilities for providing—or helping the mother to find—prenatal and hospital care, as well as counseling. Ministers, priests, and rabbis are prepared to direct unmarried pregnant women to agencies that will help them. Information about help for unmarried mothers can also be obtained from local health departments.

MEDICAL CARE DURING PREGNANCY

Although women throughout the world carry and give birth to their children essentially alone and without medical care, many of these mothers die or deliver stillborn or deformed infants. In this country the science of obstetrics offers the vast majority of women the virtual certainty of a normal pregnancy, a good delivery, and a healthy baby. It is important to select a doctor with whom you are compatible.

The Doctor's First Examination

By far the greatest number of pregnancies are free of serious complications, but your doctor will want to find out as soon as possible whether there is any likelihood that you will encounter difficulties. After he has confirmed your pregnancy, he will ask you many questions about your medical history. If you have previously had a miscarriage, for example, he will want to investigate the causes. He will want to watch you especially carefully if you are either very young (under 16) or, in obstetrical terms, "elderly" (over 35) when you conceive your first child; if you have had four or more children; or if you have conceived within two months after a previous delivery. Heavy smokers and women who are addicted to alcohol or other drugs are of special concern to him.

After taking your history, he will give you a complete physical examination to determine your general health. But he will concentrate especially on the pelvic examination—learning the size, shape, and position of your uterus, finding out whether it harbors any tumors such as fibroids (see the entry FIBROID TUMOR in the encyclopedia section), and looking for signs of venereal or other diseases. If a marked abnormality, such as a tubal pregnancy (discussed later in this chapter), should exist, he will discover it. He will probably measure your pelvis in order to determine whether the hard bony structure is large enough to let an average-sized baby through without undue difficulty.

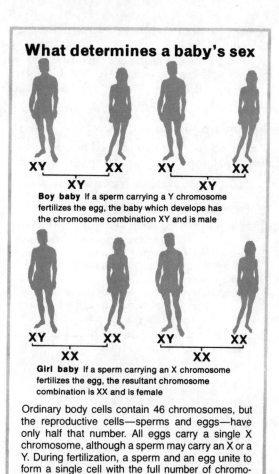

What determines a baby's sex

XY   XX   XY   XX

XY   XY

Boy baby If a sperm carrying a Y chromosome fertilizes the egg, the baby which develops has the chromosome combination XY and is male

XY   XX   XY   XX

XX   XX

Girl baby If a sperm carrying an X chromosome fertilizes the egg, the resultant chromosome combination is XX and is female

Ordinary body cells contain 46 chromosomes, but the reproductive cells—sperms and eggs—have only half that number. All eggs carry a single X chromosome, although a sperm may carry an X or a Y. During fertilization, a sperm and an egg unite to form a single cell with the full number of chromosomes. A baby's sex depends on whether the sperm involved carries a Y chromosome or an X chromosome. The combination XY results in a boy baby, whereas XX results in a girl.

Later in your pregnancy he will make an estimate of the probable birth size of the baby. If your pelvis appears too small in relation to the baby's size, he may recommend a cesarean operation. (See the entry CESAREAN SECTION in the encyclopedia section.)

Laboratory Tests. Several laboratory tests are usually performed at the first visit. The doctor will test your urine, mainly to discover whether it is free of sugar and albumin. Sugar may indicate diabetes, and albumin is sometimes a sign of kidney damage. He will test your blood for syphilis and anemia. He will also type your blood to find out to which blood group you belong (see the entry BLOOD TYPE in the encyclopedia section), in the event that you will need a blood transfusion at some time during your pregnancy or delivery. He will also determine whether or not you are

RH-negative (see the entry RH FACTOR in the encyclopedia section).

During your first visit, your doctor will probably give you a tentative delivery date. In general, gestation lasts 280 days from the first day of your last period.

Follow-up Visits

If your doctor finds you in good health on your first visit, he will set up a follow-up schedule that will probably look like this: a visit every four weeks during your first six months of pregnancy; a three-week interval during your seventh month; biweekly visits through your eighth month; and a weekly visit throughout your ninth month—about 14 visits in all. Each time you come to your doctor's office, he will feel your abdomen to see how the fetus is growing, take your blood pressure, weigh you, and check your urine. At later visits, he will also listen to the

How an egg is fertilized

Fertilization is the union of a sperm with an egg. Of the 500 million or so sperms introduced into the vagina during sexual intercourse, only one can penetrate and merge with the egg. This union usually takes place in the upper part of the Fallopian tube. Sperms live for about 24 hours, so pregnancy occurs only if the egg is fertilized within 24 hours of leaving the ovary.

Movement of the sperms

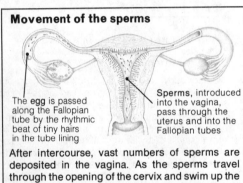

The egg is passed along the Fallopian tube by the rhythmic beat of tiny hairs in the tube lining

Sperms, introduced into the vagina, pass through the uterus and into the Fallopian tubes

After intercourse, vast numbers of sperms are deposited in the vagina. As the sperms travel through the opening of the cervix and swim up the cavity of the uterus, many die or are eliminated, and only a few reach the Fallopian tubes.

Moment of fertilization

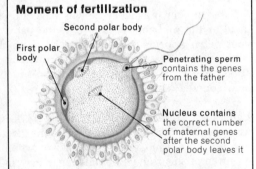

Second polar body

First polar body

Penetrating sperm contains the genes from the father

Nucleus contains the correct number of maternal genes after the second polar body leaves it

To penetrate the egg, the sperms release enzymes—chemicals which digest the barrier around the egg, and allow one sperm to enter it. Once inside, the sperm joins with the egg to form the fertilized egg. When this occurs, the barrier around the egg hardens, forming a membrane which is impenetrable to all other sperms.

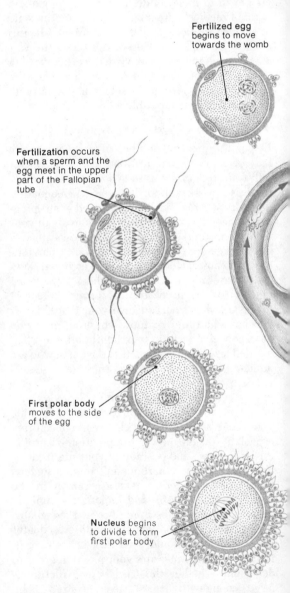

Fertilized egg begins to move towards the womb

Fertilization occurs when a sperm and the egg meet in the upper part of the Fallopian tube

First polar body moves to the side of the egg

Nucleus begins to divide to form first polar body

fetal heart and check the baby's position in your uterus.

PREPARATIONS FOR CHILDBIRTH

Long before your baby is due to arrive, you and your doctor will make arrangements for its birth. Discuss with him all aspects concerning the delivery, including the financial ones. If your finan-cial situation is strained, your physician may be able to offer alternatives—such as a less expensive hospital or participation in a maternity clinic.

Uppermost in your mind will be the birth itself—labor and delivery. No woman can fail to be apprehensive about the pain connected with having a child. On the other hand, newspaper and magazine articles about adverse effects of anesthesia on the fetus may make you fearful that any medication given to you for pain relief dur-

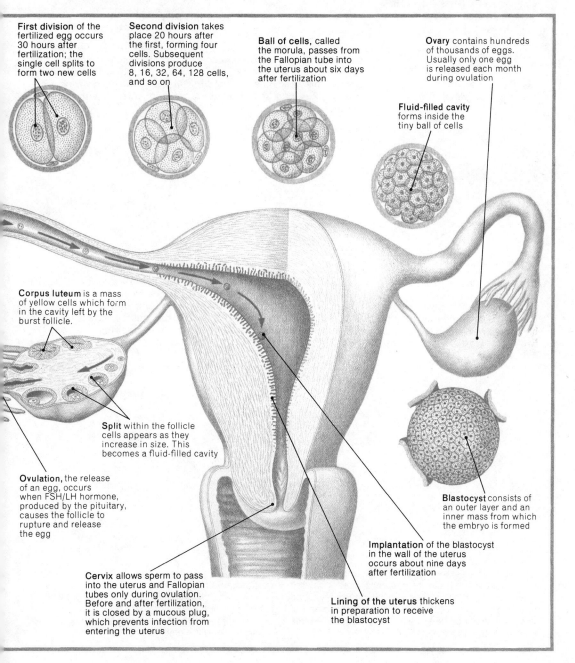

First division of the fertilized egg occurs 30 hours after fertilization; the single cell splits to form two new cells

Second division takes place 20 hours after the first, forming four cells. Subsequent divisions produce 8, 16, 32, 64, 128 cells, and so on

Ball of cells, called the morula, passes from the Fallopian tube into the uterus about six days after fertilization

Ovary contains hundreds of thousands of eggs. Usually only one egg is released each month during ovulation

Fluid-filled cavity forms inside the tiny ball of cells

Corpus luteum is a mass of yellow cells which form in the cavity left by the burst follicle.

Split within the follicle cells appears as they increase in size. This becomes a fluid-filled cavity

Ovulation, the release of an egg, occurs when FSH/LH hormone, produced by the pituitary, causes the follicle to rupture and release the egg

Cervix allows sperm to pass into the uterus and Fallopian tubes only during ovulation. Before and after fertilization, it is closed by a mucous plug, which prevents infection from entering the uterus

Blastocyst consists of an outer layer and an inner mass from which the embryo is formed

Implantation of the blastocyst in the wall of the uterus occurs about nine days after fertilization

Lining of the uterus thickens in preparation to receive the blastocyst

How the egg is implanted in the uterus

After fertilization, an egg is transformed into an embryo. The first stage of this process occurs in the Fallopian tube, and involves the division of the fertilized egg into a tiny ball of cells, called the blastocyst. In the second stage, which begins when the blastocyst enters the uterus and continues after its implantation there, these identical cells develop in various ways. In three weeks, the ball of cells changes into a sac about ½ inch across, containing a ¼-inch embryo.

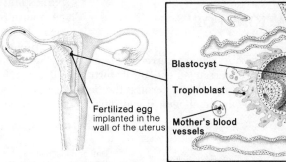

Fertilized egg implanted in the wall of the uterus

Blastocyst

Trophoblast

Mother's blood vessels

Day 4 to 5 after fertilization The blastocyst reaches the womb. This hollow ball of cells has an outer ring and an inner mass.

Day 6 Blastocyst implants itself in the thick, soft wall of the uterus. "Roots" growing from the trophoblast absorb nutrients.

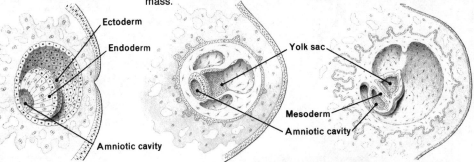

Ectoderm

Endoderm

Amniotic cavity

Yolk sac

Mesoderm

Amniotic cavity

Day 9 Inside the blastocyst there are two cavities. Between these, the inner mass of cells divides into layers—the upper ectoderm and the lower endoderm. This two-layered disc becomes the embryo.

Day 13 to 15 The endoderm grows beneath the disc to form the yolk sac, which soon shrinks away. However, the fluid-filled amniotic cavity expands to provide protection for the embryo.

Day 16 A new layer of cells, the mesoderm, appears between the ectoderm and the endoderm. These cells specialize to form bones, muscles, nerves, the brain, and other organs.

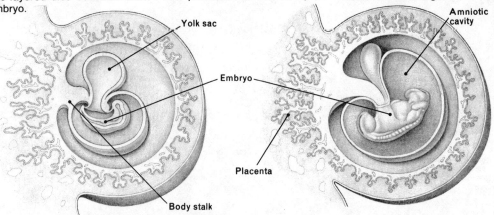

Yolk sac

Embryo

Placenta

Body stalk

Amniotic cavity

Day 20 The embryo, which consists of a curved three-layered disc, slowly detaches itself from the trophoblast. But, at its lower end, the embryo remains linked to the surrounding mass by a growing band of tissue, called the body stalk. Through it nutrients pass from the trophoblast to the embryo.

Day 28 By this time the embryo begins to show recognizable organs. The amniotic cavity is still expanding, but its outer layer gradually merges with the inner layer of the trophoblast. The body stalk develops into the umbilical cord, which contains blood vessels linking the embryo to the placenta.

ing labor and delivery will harm your baby. Express both your fears and your opinions about the subject to your doctor. He will be able to reassure you that anesthetics and analgesics (substances that lessen the sense of pain) are given to mothers only at the time and in the amounts that will have no harmful effect on the child. (For a further discussion of anesthesia in childbirth see ANESTHESIA in the encyclopedia section.) Nevertheless, you may want to have what is popularly called "natural childbirth," which requires some active preparation on your part.

Natural Childbirth

The number of women attending birth-preparation classes to receive instruction for "natural childbirth"—or, more accurately, childbirth without anesthetics or painkilling drugs—has increased enormously in the past decade. And greater numbers of obstetricians and the hospitals at which they work are offering mothers the choice between this and the conventional method of delivery.

Most women will have an uncomplicated delivery. Natural childbirth is based on the belief that if these women are educated in the physiology of pregnancy and are physically and psychologically prepared for labor, no drugs, or almost none, will be needed. The mother who is thus readied is fully conscious during labor and delivery, and is a full participant in the birth of her child. In the United States the natural childbirth system most commonly used is the Lamaze method, named after Fernand Lamaze, the French obstetrician who perfected it. This method is also referred to as psychoprophylaxis.

To facilitate labor and lessen its pain, the expectant mother attends classes where she learns exercises that strengthen the muscles used in labor, and breathing techniques that will help her to relax and control the birth contractions. Usually her husband also attends the classes in preparation for his role as understanding helper and comforter during his wife's labor and delivery. Of course, not all prepared mothers have their babies without any pain-relieving medication; and doctor and patient should agree that if the need arises, analgesics or anesthetics will be used.

If you decide that you want natural childbirth, it is essential that you find a doctor who knows the method, is convinced of its value, and can help you to prepare yourself. If your husband wants to be present throughout your labor and delivery, be sure that the hospital as well as the doctor will allow it.

Even if you do not intend to give birth without the aid of medication, learning the Lamaze technique can be a great help to you during labor.

Nurse-Midwife

In many large and middle-sized cities today, the healthy woman who wants a natural childbirth has a relatively new option. Instead of going to an obstetrician, she can opt for a nurse-midwife—a registered nurse with a specialist's degree in prenatal care and the delivery of babies. Working in a hospital or clinic as part of a medical team that includes an obstetrician, the nurse-midwife has expert assistance and all the technology of obstetrics available to her should the need arise. But for the majority of births, which are free of complications, her special skills are wholly adequate. Nurse-midwife programs are now in operation in about 200 hospitals and have proved highly successful. The cost for prenatal care and a normal delivery by a nurse-midwife is usually considerably less than that charged by an obstetrician.

Home Versus Hospital

Some few women now choose to have their babies at home. Although there are advantages in doing this (the minimal cost is one of them), there is as yet no system that will assure sufficiently prompt transportation to a hospital if difficulties arise at the time of delivery. Nurse-midwives—the only nonphysicians licensed to assist at childbirth—may *not* perform deliveries outside a hospital or clinic. There are a small number of clinics, however, that deliver babies in a home-like atmosphere, with arrangements for emergency back-up from a hospital. But again, if the birth involves complications—and they can occur suddenly and unpredictably—the safest place to be is still in the hospital.

YOUR LIFE DURING PREGNANCY

Because pregnancy is a normal condition, a healthy woman need experience few, if any, marked changes in her daily life. For most women a simple, commonsense regimen of diet and exercise is enough to assure a happy, comfortable pregnancy and a thriving newborn baby. Following are a few "do's" and "dont's" that apply, generally, to all pregnant women.

Activities During Pregnancy

Your activities will remain essentially unchanged and be limited only by your energy level. In general, it is wise to moderate strenuous activities during the first three months of pregnancy when the danger of miscarriage is greatest. Throughout pregnancy, give up those sports where there is a great risk of falling—skiing, for instance. But by and large, you will feel happier about your pregnancy if you continue to maintain your regular work and recreational activities. Unless you want a few days or weeks of leisure, there is no compelling reason why you should leave your job until you are ready to go to the hospital.

CLOTHING, PERSONAL HYGIENE, SEXUAL RELATIONS

You will probably want to wear maternity clothing during the latter stages of pregnancy, and perhaps a maternity girdle or brassiere if your doctor advises it or if it makes you feel more comfortable. Do not wear anything that restricts circulation—such as tight knee-high stockings. Wear sensible shoes; high heels are a hazard, and do not give proper support. You can continue to take showers or tub baths, as you prefer, but

Early development of the baby

Starting as a minute cluster of cells embedded in the wall of the womb, an embryo takes on a human form during the first two months of life—the most critical stage of its development. Initially the embryo is an elongated disk which has no external parts, only swellings. Within these swellings the major organs of the body, such as the heart and the brain, begin to grow. They start as simple tubes, in

	25 days	28 days	32 days	34 days
Drawn actual size				
Drawn to constant size				
	The embryo is a soft, bulging piece of tissue. It lacks a skeleton, but it has a few rudimentary parts. A swelling at the head-end contains the brain, which consists of a simple tube. Other bulges in the head region eventually become the jaws and mouth. The mid-section of the embryo contains a primitive, pulsating heart. At the end, a tail starts to form	At this stage the largest organ in the embryo is the heart. Through a simple system of vessels, the heart pumps blood around the body and into the placenta along the umbilical cord. The nervous system and the brain begin to grow in complexity. The stomach starts to form. The embryonic tail develops	The period of limb development begins. Segments of tissue, called somites, are found in 25 pairs down the trunk of the embryo. From these segments the bones and muscles eventually develop. Each somite has its own nerve supply. At this stage the embryo is particularly sensitive to harmful external influences, such as drugs or germs, which are in the mother's bloodstream	During the fifth week, rudimentary eyes appear on each side of the head, and the nose begins to take shape. The brain has become more elaborate and the cranial nerves, which control the head, have started to form. Arm buds, leg buds, and tail continue to develop

164

check with your doctor about douching. As for sexual relations, most doctors allow them until the last two weeks of pregnancy when intercourse might introduce an infection. However, if you notice any staining or bleeding after intercourse, consult your doctor before you resume sexual relations.

Emotional Reactions

Especially during the early months of pregnancy, you may be unusually sensitive and irritable. Try to take this in your stride. Our bodies and emo-tions are influenced by certain chemicals called hormones, which are discussed in Chapter 5. During pregnancy, a woman's body has more of some hormones and less of others than it had before. This imbalance may cause exaggerated emotional reactions. Remind yourself that they are only temporary, but if they cause you concern, consult your doctor.

Diet and Weight

The fact that you are "eating for two" does not mean that you must eat twice as much during

---

which kinks and folds appear. But in a few weeks, the different systems of the body are sufficiently well formed that they start to function. Externally, the legs and the arms appear in the sixth week of development; the eyes and the ears, slightly later. By the end of eight weeks, the embryo is almost fully formed, and subsequent development involves mainly growth and a gain in weight.

5–37 days	40–42 days	46–49 days	60 days (2 months)

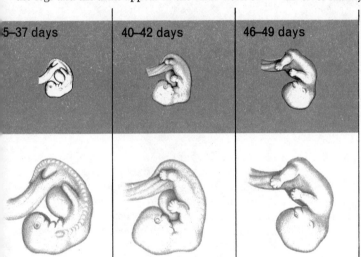
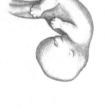
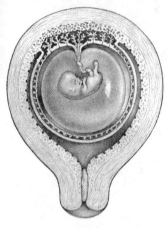

At five weeks the arms have become paddle-shaped buds, and are longer than the leg buds. The head grows, but there is no neck. Cartilage starts to appear in positions which will later have bones	The head grows rapidly. The retinas of the eyes take shape, and cradle the newly formed lens; the external ear begins to develop. The hands show outlines of fingers and the lower limbs are vaguely divided into thigh, leg, and foot. The role of blood production begins in the liver, which bulges above the umbilical cord. The heart is also located in this prominent swelling	The head continues to grow and, for the first time, the neck is established. The external ear and the opening to the ear canal are apparent. The eyes are open, and the eyelids start to grow over them. The mouth has lips and, inside it, the tongue forms and 20 milk-teeth buds appear. The heart is no longer visible, and the tail recedes and vanishes	By the end of the second month, the growing baby has almost all its organs and tissues. After this stage, its name changes from embryo to fetus. During the next seven months, the baby grows bigger, and its organs become much more intricate. Inside the body, the brain has developed its major subdivisions. The nervous system and muscles have also formed; and the skeleton—originally made of cartilage—begins to turn to bone. The face has recognizable features. The limbs are partly formed, but the fingers and the toes are well developed. The primary sex organs have formed

Nourishment for the fetus

Nourishment and oxygen from the mother's blood system are passed to the growing fetus through the placenta. This disk-shaped organ is attached to the surface of the uterus and is connected to the fetus by the umbilical cord.

Section of the placenta

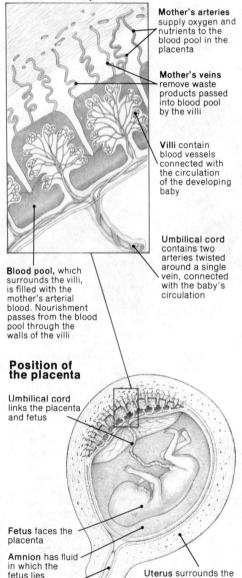

Mother's arteries supply oxygen and nutrients to the blood pool in the placenta

Mother's veins remove waste products passed into blood pool by the villi

Villi contain blood vessels connected with the circulation of the developing baby

Umbilical cord contains two arteries twisted around a single vein, connected with the baby's circulation

Blood pool, which surrounds the villi, is filled with the mother's arterial blood. Nourishment passes from the blood pool through the walls of the villi

Position of the placenta

Umbilical cord links the placenta and fetus

Fetus faces the placenta

Amnion has fluid in which the fetus lies

Mucous plug seals the cervix

Uterus surrounds the placenta and the fluid-filled amnion, which contains the fetus

Exchange of nourishment and wastes takes place through the walls of the villi which penetrate the blood pool in the placenta, but the circulations of mother and fetus are entirely separate.

Changes in the mother's figure

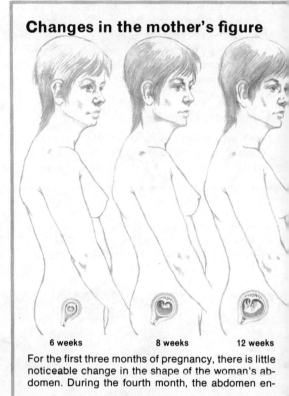

6 weeks 8 weeks 12 weeks

For the first three months of pregnancy, there is little noticeable change in the shape of the woman's abdomen. During the fourth month, the abdomen en-

pregnancy. If your prepregnancy weight was normal, you should expect to gain only about 22 pounds, averaging some two and one-half pounds per month. Underweight women should try to gain more. The overweight have to be careful not to gain so much that they become awkward and breathless.

A diet of not more than 2,000 calories is adequate for the average woman. But if weight is not a problem, you should be more concerned with the quality of what you eat than with the number of calories consumed. Your meals should consist mainly of meats and other protein foods, vegetables, fruits, fruit juices, and milk. About a quart and a half of fluids a day is sufficient, and this amount includes everything liquid—soups, coffee, juice, water, milk. To be sure that you get the proper nutrients, however, your doctor may recommend a vitamin supplement.

Chapter 2 discusses healthful diets and the nutritional value of various foods. Following is a typical diet for an average-sized, pregnant woman. Note that in addition to three moderate-sized regular meals, there are three between-meal snacks—and plenty of all types of foods except starches, fats, and sugars.

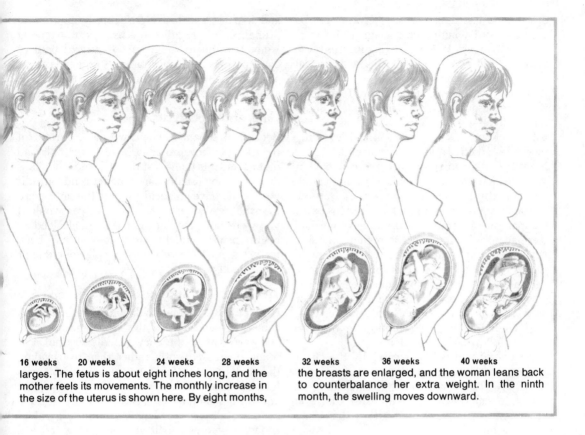

16 weeks   20 weeks   24 weeks   28 weeks
larges. The fetus is about eight inches long, and the
mother feels its movements. The monthly increase in
the size of the uterus is shown here. By eight months,

32 weeks   36 weeks   40 weeks
the breasts are enlarged, and the woman leans back
to counterbalance her extra weight. In the ninth
month, the swelling moves downward.

Sample Menus for Meals During Pregnancy

Breakfast
Fruit or fruit juice
2 eggs
1 slice whole wheat
  toast
Beverage

Mid-Morning
1 cup whole grain cereal
½ cup milk
Stewed fruit

Lunch
2 oz lean meat (or 2 oz
  cheese)
½ cup cooked vegetable
½ cup salad greens
½ glass milk

Mid-Afternoon
1 oz cottage cheese
1 slice whole wheat bread
1 glass milk

Dinner
6 oz lean meat, fish or,
  poultry
1 potato
½ cup cooked vegetable
½ cup salad greens
Simple dessert, such as
  fresh fruit, gelatin,
  or junket
Beverage: coffee, tea,
  or milk

Bedtime
1 oz Cheddar cheese
Whole wheat crackers
1 glass milk

PROTECTING YOUR UNBORN BABY'S HEALTH

A pregnant woman should not "eat for two" in terms of quantity, but she does need extra amounts of certain kinds of nutrients. For example, if she does not get enough calcium in her diet, she will probably lose some of her body calcium to her fetus. The same deprivation occurs for many other substances—iron, for instance. But protein deficiency is a more serious matter: a mother whose diet is extremely deficient in protein may produce a child whose brain responses are below normal. The sample menus we suggest contain numerous protein foods.

In addition, it is becoming increasingly evident that many things besides foods may adversely affect the unborn child. Among them are:
* Certain medicines, including some antibiotics and tranquilizers, aspirin compounds in large quantities, certain diuretics, excess vitamins.
* Drugs such as LSD, heroin, amphetamines, barbiturates, marijuana. The question of cigarettes remains controversial. There is evidence that a mother who smokes heavily will have a baby whose birth weight is about three-fourths

167

of a pound less than normal. Nicotine is also suspected of having other damaging effects.

° Alcohol in excess. Heavy drinking increases the chance of self-injury and will cause withdrawal symptoms in the newborn child.

° Artificial substances in food. Many food additives are suspected of having harmful, long-range effects on the fetus as well as on the mother. Many doctors recommend avoiding food with additives during pregnancy.

° X rays. Avoid radiation during pregnancy. If you must have an X ray, make sure the technician shields your stomach with a lead apron.

° Certain virus diseases, the most notorious being German measles (rubella). If you have not had German measles, mumps, or regular measles, try to stay away from children who have any of these diseases. It is important to have a rubella vaccination *before* you become pregnant (see Chapter 12), but do *not* get one if you know or even suspect that you are already pregnant. And do not attempt conception in the two months following vaccination.

Your doctor will consider carefully the effect of any medication he prescribes during your pregnancy. He may ask you to stop smoking, or at least to cut down. He will *insist* that you refrain from taking any medicine without first consulting him.

MINOR PROBLEMS OF PREGNANCY

There are a number of discomforts that seem to be fairly common to pregnant women. You may experience none of them, but if you do undergo any of the complaints described below, be assured that they are normal.

Backache

Backaches have a variety of causes unrelated to pregnancy, as explained in Chapter 23. But if a backache is caused by unusual strain because your heavy abdomen is pulling on unused muscles, the condition will be relieved by rest, a maternity corset, and sensible shoes.

Constipation

Often a woman's first experience with constipation occurs during her pregnancy, although not all, or even most, pregnant women suffer from this complaint. Diet is the most effective treatment. Eat coarse cereals such as oatmeal and substitute whole wheat for white bread. Eat plenty of leafy vegetables, such as salad greens and spinach, and fruits, particularly apples and prunes. A mild laxative such as milk of magnesia is not harmful to relieve an occasional bout of constipation. But never take a stronger laxative or an enema without consulting your doctor. (See also CONSTIPATION in the encyclopedia section.)

Falls and Accidents

Because pregnant women are more careful of themselves, they probably have fewer falls and other accidents than most people. And when falls do occur they usually cause the fetus no harm. If you should have an accident, take the same steps to make sure you are not injured as you would if you were not pregnant. But if vaginal bleeding begins, or if the fetal movements you have been feeling seem to have stopped, call your doctor immediately.

Heartburn or Indigestion

Heartburn has nothing to do with your heart; it is a burning sensation in the esophagus (see the entry PYROSIS in the encyclopedia section). Eat small meals frequently rather than overloading the stomach with large heavy ones. Omit gas-forming foods, such as cucumbers and cabbage, and cut down on desserts and rich foods. If these measures do not prevent discomfort, a table-spoonful of cream half an hour before a meal may help. To relieve heartburn or indigestion, take a teaspoonful of milk of magnesia rather than bicarbonate of soda (baking soda), which most physicians do not recommend for a pregnant woman.

Hemorrhoids

Hemorrhoids, enlarged veins in the anal region, often develop during pregnancy. One of the causes is constipation, which can be avoided or alleviated by proper diet. Your doctor will prescribe treatment for hemorrhoids, which usually disappear after childbirth.

Insomnia

Many pregnant women have difficulty falling asleep, especially during the last months when the fetus seems to stay up all night. A relaxing bath often helps. If it does not, your doctor may prescribe a mild sedative. But remember—*never* take any medication without his permission.

Leg Cramps

Spasms of the leg occur most often during sleep. Massaging and kneading the cramped muscles until they relax is the best method of treatment.

Nausea and Vomiting

"Morning sickness," the nausea and vomiting that usually, but not always, occur in the morning, is common in the early months of pregnancy, although more than a third of all pregnant women escape it completely. Sometimes it consists of little more than a mild intestinal uneasiness or indigestion. In severe cases, the pregnant woman vomits and feels miserable. It seldom lasts beyond the third month, but in rare cases it can persist or become so extreme that hospitalization is required.

Here are some suggestions for preventing or minimizing morning sickness:

1. Have some dry crackers, a thermos of weak tea, or whatever appeals to you, at your bedside table ready for you to eat or sip before arising. Then, after lying still for a while, get up and have breakfast. Or, if possible, have breakfast in bed.

2. Eat six or seven small meals a day instead of three big ones.

3. Eat dry foods first, then sip fluids in small quantities.

4. Rest after eating. Lie down for 20 minutes or so after even a small meal. If nausea recurs every day, try getting more rest.

5. Greasy foods, butter, and fat are likely to cause distress. Cucumbers, cabbage, cauliflower, spinach, and onions may also cause trouble. But wheat germ, found in whole wheat bread and some cereals, often alleviates nausea.

Shortness of Breath

As the uterus expands and exerts pressure on your diaphragm, and as you gain weight, you may develop some shortness of breath. If it interferes with your sleep, try propping yourself up with several pillows until you are half sitting, half lying. If you still cannot sleep, tell your doctor, who may prescribe a mild sedative. But if the breathlessness is more severe—if, for example, you are unable to climb a short flight of steps without becoming winded—be sure to report the fact to your physician.

Swelling of the Feet, Ankles, and Fingers

Swollen feet, ankles, and fingers are caused by the increased fluid which the body retains during pregnancy and which gravity pulls to the extremities. Putting up your feet while you are relaxing in a chair helps reduce the swelling of feet and ankles, and overnight rest usually restores their original contour. Swollen fingers can be reduced by soaking them in cold water. If swelling persists or spreads to other parts of your body, consult your doctor. (See also EDEMA in the encyclopedia section.)

Varicose Veins

Varicose veins, enlarged, knotted blood vessels that usually occur in the legs, may develop or grow worse during pregnancy. Fortunately, they tend to shrink again after childbirth. If you should develop varicose veins, sit or lie as much as possible with your legs raised, and do not wear anything, such as knee-high stockings, that restricts circulation. If the veins are especially large or troublesome, your doctor may recommend an elastic bandage or stockings. (For a fuller discussion, see the entry VARICOSE VEIN in the encyclopedia section.)

DISORDERS THAT MAY ACCOMPANY PREGNANCY

The possibility of complications during pregnancy exists for every expectant mother. She is also unusually susceptible to certain illnesses. A brief discussion of these malfunctions and diseases follows.

Cystitis and Pyelitis

Cystitis is a bladder infection manifested by bacteria, pus, and sometimes blood in the urine. The symptoms are a frequent urge to urinate, and a burning sensation while urinating. Cystitis responds quickly to sulfa compounds or specific antibiotics and to the patient's drinking large quantities of fluid. The illness should be treated immediately, for it may lead to pyelitis, an infection of the kidney. The symptoms of pyelitis are chills and fever, back pain in the region of the kidneys and, again, the frequent urge to urinate. Pain often accompanies urination. This malady, too, is treated with sulfa drugs or antibiotics.

Ectopic (Tubal) Pregnancy

This condition, in which the fertilized ovum is implanted in the Fallopian tube instead of in the wall of the uterus can be diagnosed early in the pregnancy. Occasionally, the tube ruptures before the condition has been discovered, causing vaginal bleeding and severe pain along one side of the body and in the shoulder. If you have any of these symptoms report them to your doctor at once. An ectopic pregnancy necessitates immediate surgery: either the tube is removed, or the pregnancy is terminated and the tube repaired.

Removal of one tube does not rule out other pregnancies, but the woman may have more difficulty in conceiving.

Placenta Previa and Premature Separation of the Placenta

These complications are rare, and little is known about what causes them. Both occur in the last three months of pregnancy, and are accompanied by vaginal bleeding.

In placenta previa, the placenta, instead of being attached high up on the uterine wall, is down near the cervix, the mouth of the uterus. If some of the placental tissue is torn by the expansion of the cervix, pain and premature labor will result, with bleeding that can be dangerous to the baby.

Premature separation of the placenta is caused by a hemorrhage just below its point of attachment. A blood clot forms and loosens the placenta from its mooring. In both these conditions, immediate medical care is necessary.

Toxemia and Eclampsia

These conditions are rare and little is known about their cause. Toxemia of pregnancy is identified by hypertension, albumin in the urine, and edema. Eclampsia is an advanced stage of toxemia. The treatment varies in individual cases, but usually the doctor recommends rest and reduction of salt intake.

Because these conditions can be serious, it is important to notify your doctor immediately if you observe any of the following symptoms: puffiness about the face and hands, persistent vomiting, severe and persistent headache, disturbances in vision, and rapid gain in weight.

DANGER SIGNALS IN PREGNANCY

You should definitely notify your doctor if you have any sickness more severe than a mild cold or stomach upset, or if you experience any of the following:

° Vaginal bleeding
° Loss of water from the vagina
° Severe swelling of your face, eyes, fingers, or feet
° Severe vomiting, dizziness, headache, or blurred vision
° Severe abdominal cramps or pains
° Fever over 100° F
° Pain or burning with urination
° Absence of fetal movement lasting for more than 24 hours

LABOR AND DELIVERY

And now your time of delivery is near. The doctor has confirmed or adjusted your "due date" and told you approximately when to expect your baby. Approximately, but not exactly. How, then, will you be able to tell when your labor begins?

The new mother is usually worried that she will not recognize when her labor begins. To complicate matters, there is such a thing as "false labor," which is sometimes hard to distinguish from true labor. False labor consists of irregular contractions of the uterus, sometimes accompanied by the passage of blood-tinged mucus, and it can occur at any time during the last months of pregnancy. You will be able to identify true labor by one of the following signs:

1. Breaking of the bag of waters (the fluid surrounding the unborn child). This rupture of the membranes is indicated by a gush of liquid from the vagina or by a slow leakage. If it happens as the first step in your delivery (and it may not), labor pains usually start within a few hours of the rupture.

2. Recognizable, describable pains that are characteristic of true labor only. Though the labor pains may be slight, you can identify them because they usually increase to a peak and then fade away. At the beginning the pain is cramplike and seems to be located at the small of the back. In a few hours it moves to the front. Even at first, true labor pains are regular and rhythmical, with a pain-free period between them, and are accompanied by a contraction of the uterus. When such pains arrive every 10 minutes or so, call your doctor. He will tell you when to go to the hospital.

Induced Labor. Occasionally, for the well-being of either the mother or the baby, the doctor may decide to speed up the beginning of labor. He will do this by rupturing the membranes of the bag of waters or by using a contraction-stimulating drug.

The Three Stages of Labor

The Dilation Period. The womb, or uterus, which holds the baby, is like a large rubber bottle with a very small neck, almost closed. The neck (the cervix) is about a half-inch in diameter. In order for birth to take place, the mouth of the "bottle" must stretch to a diameter of about four inches to allow for passage of the baby. The walls of the uterus constitute a powerful set of muscles.

At a certain time, the muscles begin to contract and force the baby downward. Gradually, the mouth of the uterus (the cervix) is stretched until there is room for the baby to pass through.

While this is happening, you will experience labor contractions. At first, they are fairly far apart and last for a very short time. As labor progresses, they occur more often, are more intense, and last longer. Being relaxed during the intervals between pain encourages the cervix to dilate more rapidly.

If you are restless during this stage of labor, walk around a little. The breathing exercises taught in childbirth-preparation classes also prove invaluable now. They help reduce tension, ease pain, and give a positive feeling of control.

The Expulsion. After the cervix is fully dilated, the baby must be pushed out through the narrow and resistant birth canal. Here you can help by holding your breath and bearing down as though you are having a bowel movement. Even though the doctor gives you a whiff of gas to lessen the pain, you are usually conscious enough to bear down.

Many doctors routinely use low forceps at the last moment to guide the baby's head gently through the opening of the vagina. This is entirely safe for the baby.

The doctor may also perform an episiotomy. Between the vagina and the rectum there is a strip of tissue called the perineum, which the baby's head stretches and often rips in the final moment of birth. To prevent a tear and to protect the infant's head from injury if the vagina is not sufficiently enlarged, many doctors cut the perineum. (For a fuller discussion, see the entry EPISIOTOMY in the encyclopedia section.)

Delivery of the Afterbirth. Technically, the third stage of childbirth is the expulsion of the afterbirth—the placenta and the umbilical cord. What takes place in this stage of delivery, which is virtually painless, is discussed below in the section "After the Delivery."

How Long Does Labor Last?

The duration of these three stages of labor varies greatly. A woman having her first child is likely to be in labor as long as 15 or 16 hours, although a period as brief as three hours is not uncommon. For subsequent labors, 8 to 10 hours is about average. The dilation period is the longest. The expulsion period usually lasts about an hour and a

Problem pregnancies

Complications that may arise during pregnancy involve the positioning of the baby in the uterus, or the presence of twins or triplets. Normally a baby lies head-downwards, but in one in 25 pregnancies, the baby lies head-up in the breech position, which may cause a difficult birth. With multiple pregnancy, delivery usually follows the normal course, although the babies may be premature.

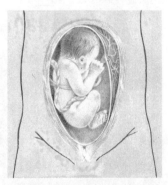
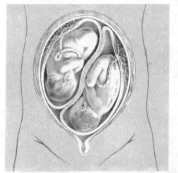
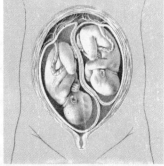

In the breech position the baby sits in the uterus, with the buttocks downwards and the head uppermost. This position is fairly common up to the sixth month of pregnancy, after which the baby may turn over in the uterus.

One pregnancy in about 86 results in twins. Identical twins come from the same fertilized egg, which divides into two. The resulting babies resemble each other closely, are of the same sex, and share the same placenta (right). Fraternal, or nonidentical, twins develop when two eggs are fertilized by two different sperms. Each twin has its own placenta, and may or may not be of the same sex as the other one. Of all the twins born, two-thirds are the fraternal kind.

half for the first child, and half an hour for subsequent children. The third period, delivery of the afterbirth, lasts about 15 minutes or less.

COMPLICATIONS OF CHILDBIRTH

Complications occur when the baby's position is not normal and when, for this or other reasons, instruments or surgery must be resorted to.

Breech and Transverse Presentations

Most babies are born head first—the so-called *head presentation*. In about four out of 100

births, however, the child may emerge feet or buttocks first, in the *breech position*. This is not too serious a problem for the mother, but the baby can be hurt during delivery. Fortunately, many techniques have been developed in recent years to protect breech babies from injury during birth, and the doctor chooses the best one for each situation.

Less than one baby in 100 will lie crosswise in the womb—the *transverse presentation*. In this case, the doctor will almost always perform a cesarean operation. The doctor knows beforehand the type of delivery he faces.

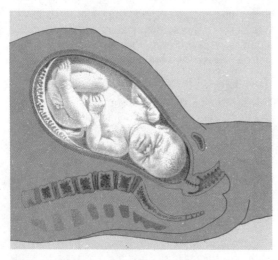

1 By the ninth month of pregnancy, the baby is usually lying upside down in the uterus. The head sinks down firmly into the mother's pelvis, ready for birth.

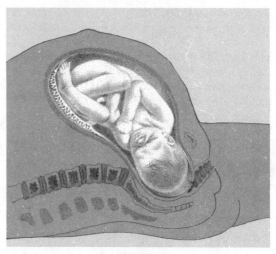

2 In the first stage of labor, which lasts about nine hours, the muscular walls of the uterus contract, pressing the head of the baby against the cervix.

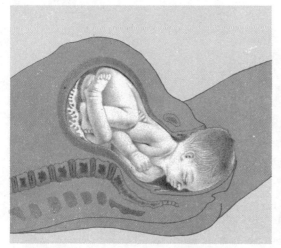

5 The head is forced into the vagina. Once it passes between the bones surrounding the birth canal, the mother is generally told to begin to bear down to push the baby outward.

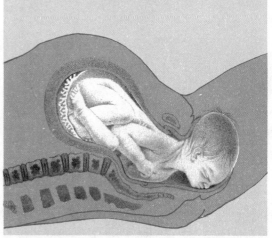

6 In the second stage of labor, which lasts half an hour to two hours, the baby is born. As it leaves the birth canal, its head faces the mother's back. Her backbone is forced down to let the baby pass.

High-Forceps Delivery

In some rare instances it is necessary, for the safety of the baby or of the mother, to hasten delivery before the head has appeared at the opening of the birth canal. The doctor will then reach into the birth canal and draw the baby out with forceps. This procedure has been almost entirely replaced by use of cesarean section.

Cesarean Delivery

If, for some reason, the baby cannot be born through the vagina—because the mother's pelvic structure is too small or because complications have occurred—the doctor will perform an operation to remove the infant through the abdomen. (For a fuller discussion, see the entry CESAREAN SECTION in the encyclopedia section.)

AFTER THE BABY IS BORN

As soon as the baby is born, the doctor holds him upside down to allow the amniotic fluid, with which the baby's lungs have been filled in the uterus, to run out, and also to allow the blood in the umbilical cord to flow back into your body.

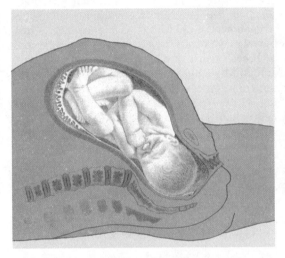

3 As contractions continue, the pressure of the head of the baby slowly stretches the cervix open. These contractions grow longer and more intense.

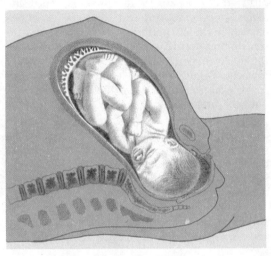

4 At the end of the first stage, the cervix is open. The amniotic sac breaks, releasing fluid. This is "the breaking of the waters."

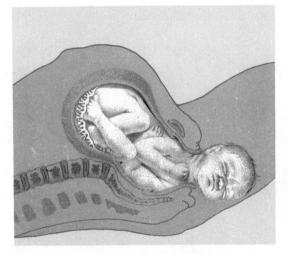

7 After the head of the baby has emerged, the shoulders, which are turned, slip out easily. The rest of the body is quickly delivered. With the baby's first cry, breathing begins. The umbilical cord is cut.

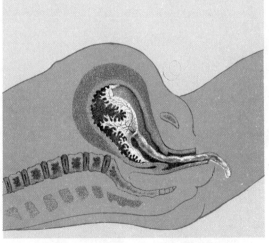

8 In the final stage of labor the uterus discharges the placenta and the remains of the umbilical cord, which are forced out through the vagina. The uterus returns to normal size about 10 days after birth.

While the cord narrows and whitens as it is emptied of blood, the doctor suctions the mucus out of the baby's nose and mouth, wipes the baby clean, and watches for the first breaths. If your delivery has been unmedicated, he may put the infant on your stomach while he clamps the umbilical cord, and cuts it. The stump of the cord, about two inches long, is bandaged. Then the baby's eyes are treated with an antibiotic solution or silver nitrate to prevent any possibility of gonorrheal infection.

The doctor now returns his attention to you. While he waits for the expulsion of the afterbirth—the placenta, with umbilical cord attached—he sutures any tears that may have occurred. If he has performed an episiotomy, he repairs that cut. If you are awake at this stage, the doctor may give you the baby to hold for a moment. To aid in uterine contraction, the doctor or a nurse will massage the abdominal wall until the uterus feels firm and hard.

The baby is now weighed, measured, and examined. If the baby is premature, it will probably weigh less than if it had been born at the end of the nine months' gestation. While weight is important, it is not the only factor in determining the condition of a premature baby. Babies whose weight falls below some "normal" figure (5½ pounds is usually considered normal) are not necessarily treated as premature. If the baby at a lower weight is fully developed and healthy, he or she can be treated like any other newborn.

CONVALESCENCE AFTER CHILDBIRTH

Today, a woman who has had a normal delivery with little or no medication is usually capable of walking, talking, and eating just a few hours after her child has been born. Many women experience some "afterpains" for several days after childbirth. This is caused by the contractions of the uterus, which is rapidly shrinking back to its original size. If the pain is particularly troublesome, it can be alleviated with aspirin. Some women need a mild laxative to encourage a first bowel movement. Those who have had a forceps or breech delivery may have trouble urinating, and will be catheterized until the opening leading from the bladder resumes normal functioning. The episiotomy incision may also cause soreness, which can be relieved by a warm sitz bath, a heat lamp, or an ointment if recommended by your doctor.

The four or five days you spend in the hospital should be a time for renewing your strength and making friends with your baby. The maternity section of any hospital is usually a happy place to be. Enjoy it while you prepare yourself for a long life together with your new baby.

CHAPTER 14

Giving Your Baby a Good Start in Life

You are at home with your baby. The moment you have looked forward to has at last arrived. And then, either gradually or suddenly, you may discover that you feel quite overwhelmed by your new responsibility, and that your situation is not the heaven you imagined it would be. This chapter tells you how to cope with your new circumstances, what to expect, how to care for your newborn infant, and when you need—and do not need—help from your physician.

THE FIRST DAYS

Two things are useful to remember when you return to your home. The first is: *Trust yourself.* Even if you are a mother for the first time you know much more than you imagine, and in an amazingly short time you will find yourself responding instinctively and correctly to your baby's needs. You will get more than enough advice from friends and relatives. Take only what seems sensible to you. The care and love parents naturally give their babies are infinitely more valuable than checking the exact temperature of the bath water or knowing the best way to fold a diaper.

The second thing to remember is that you should get all the help you can for the first month or two, and especially during the first two weeks. If you can afford to hire a practical baby nurse from a reputable agency, or a dayworker to clean and cook so that you can concentrate on the baby, by all means do so. But first make sure that anyone you hire is in good health. Ask for proof of a recent medical checkup or, at the very least, insist on a chest X ray.

If you cannot find or afford paid help, arrange to have a visiting nurse or public health nurse come in and show you the fine points of preparing formulas, diapering, bathing the baby, and whatever else you need to know. The nurse may make one or several visits, depending on your needs, usually at minimal cost to you. Arrangements can be made through the hospital where you have your baby, through local or state health departments, or through the Visiting Nurse Service in your town. You may be able to get other help—and a lot of moral support—from any friend or relative who has some free time and with whom you feel comfortable.

Above all, get help from your husband—he is just as much a parent as you, and he may be feeling a little left out and is simply waiting to be asked. If he can take some time off from work to help with baby care, meals, shopping, or cleaning—or just to *be* there so you can have an afternoon nap or go out for a walk—it will certainly make the first days easier, and he will be part of things instead of feeling in everyone's way.

THE NEW MOTHER'S HEALTH

Conserving Your Energy. Pregnancy and childbirth are normal, natural events, but they are also trying, both physically and psychologically. Even if you feel marvelous when you come home from the hospital (and you probably will), do not overtax yourself. You will need daytime naps during the period that the baby wakes for night feedings. It's difficult to limit visitors, but do it; an endless parade of well-wishers can be tiring. If you feel uncomfortable about putting visitors off, just tell them you're acting on your doctor's advice. If you have no help for such jobs as shopping, cooking, and cleaning, keep the meals *very* simple and let the dust collect. Heavy housework can certainly wait.

Bathing. You may take a shower or sponge bath as soon as you want, and a tub bath in two or

Postnatal exercises: getting your figure back

Soon after childbirth a mother should think about regaining her normal figure through postnatal exercises. During pregnancy, a woman's posture changes because of the added weight that she has to carry. Normally, the expectant mother gains about 24 pounds, half of which disappears at the birth of her child. Once this weight is lost, the woman has to pay special attention to the way in which she moves and stands in the weeks following childbirth. After she has decided on the correct posture for herself, she has to practice this stance. This involves remembering to keep the stomach muscles contracted and to stand without slumping. Postnatal exercises make it possible to maintain

Day 1

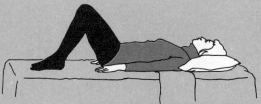

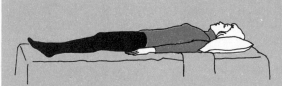

Lying in bed, deep-breathing exercises should be practiced several times each hour. Breathe in deeply, expanding your stomach muscles. Then breathe out again, drawing in the stomach muscles tightly.

Repeat the breathing exercise, but with your knees drawn up and your feet flat on the bed. Also stimulate circulation in the legs by occasionally moving the feet, ankles, and legs.

Day 2 add:

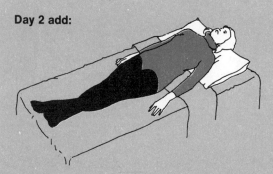

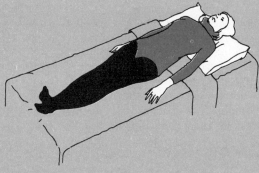

Cross your ankles, and point your toes downward. Press the buttocks and thighs together, tighten the stomach muscles, and pull up inside, as if trying not to

pass urine. Repeat. Then cross the ankles the other way, and again do the exercise twice. This helps to tone up muscles stretched during childbirth.

Day 3 add:

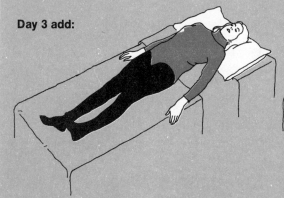

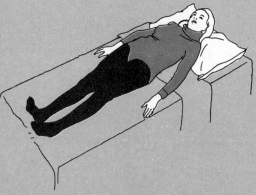

Lie on your back in bed, with the legs stretched out. Keeping your knees straight and flat on the bed,

shorten first one leg and then the other by tightening the muscles of the thighs and hip joints.

correct posture without too much difficulty. They also help to tone up muscles that have become overstretched and flabby during pregnancy, and they speed up the circulation in the legs, which may be sluggish for a short time after childbirth. Continuing the relaxation techniques, such as the breathing exercises which have been learned during pregnancy, should also be a part of any set of postnatal exercises. Before starting to exercise, a woman should get her doctor's confirmation that she can begin; usually she can start the day after the birth. But she should do the exercises gradually and avoid overtiring herself. She should get help with shopping and routine housework.

Day 5 add:

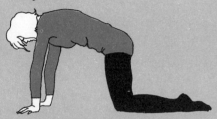
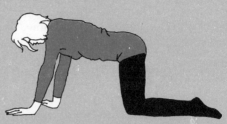

Kneel on all fours either on the floor or on the bed. Your hands should be slightly in front of the shoulders, with your arms straight. Raise your back upward so that it forms a hump, and then lower it so that it is hollowed. This is a good exercise for strengthening the muscles in the back and in the abdomen.

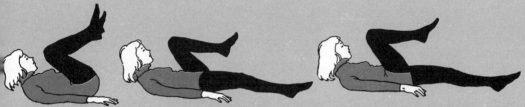

Lying on your back in bed, raise your head and draw up one leg toward it, as if to kiss the knee. Repeat this exercise with the other leg. Then, still lying on your back, do the exercise with both legs raised and drawn back at the same time. This postnatal exercise tones up the muscles at the front of the abdomen, which were stretched during pregnancy, and helps to flatten the stomach and return it to its normal shape.

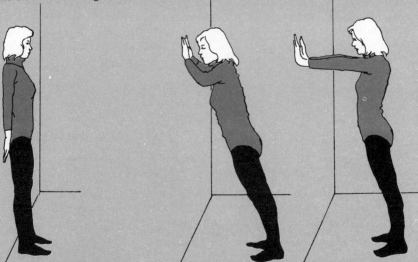

Stand 4 in. from a wall, with your feet 9 in. apart. Press shoulders, back, and buttocks against the wall. Face a wall with outstretched arms and palms against it. Relax your arms, turning the elbows outward.

three weeks. Ask your doctor before you use a douche. You may wash your hair whenever you like.

The Blues. You may have heard a good deal about the so-called "post-partum blues" or "new-baby blues"—sudden feelings of weepiness or depression, or perhaps a loss of self-confidence coupled with excessive anxiety about the baby's welfare. Such feelings are fairly common, especially after the birth of the first child. They usually occur a few days or even weeks after the mother's return from the hospital and are nothing to be ashamed of. Women go through considerable physical and glandular changes after childbirth, and it can be a shock to make the transition from the hospital—where new mothers are pampered and waited on—to the normal responsibilities of a household *plus* the care of a brand-new baby. If you are troubled by the "blues," remember that the feeling is temporary. This is a good time to ask someone you trust to look after the baby for a few hours while you go out—for a movie, some pleasurable shopping (new nonmaternity clothes are a special delight), a lunch or dinner with good friends. If, as sometimes happens, the feeling persists and you can't shake it on your own, or if it gets considerably worse, ask your doctor or clinic to refer you to a psychiatrist or community mental-health center for counseling.

Intercourse. Delay sexual intercourse until you have had a checkup, usually about six weeks after childbirth. At this time, your doctor will examine you to make sure your tissues have healed thoroughly. If you use a contraceptive, discuss this with your doctor now; if you wear a diaphragm, you will definitely need a new fitting. If intercourse is painful, take a hot bath first, and then use a vaginal jelly to lubricate the vagina. If the pain persists, consult your doctor.

Menstruation. Menstruation usually returns within four to eight weeks. The first menstrual period is almost always unusual in some way. The flow may be profuse, there may be clots, or it may stop and start again. The second period should be normal or nearly so. Menstrual periods are often irregular, or postponed altogether while a mother is nursing her baby—but this does *not* mean that nursing mothers cannot get pregnant again.

Muscles. It may take a while for your muscles to recover their springiness and your figure to re-turn to normal, especially if you gained excess weight during pregnancy. Whether or not to wear a girdle is up to you and your doctor. If you suffer from back pain, a well-fitted girdle may be helpful, even if you do not normally wear one. Exercises also help, but consult your doctor before starting them. Most new mothers can start an exercise program within two weeks, but those whose babies were delivered by cesarean section may have to wait considerably longer.

See suggested exercises in this chapter.

THINGS YOU SHOULD HAVE ON HAND FOR THE BABY

You should have the following items ready when you come home with the baby. Not everything need be new. Ask friends or relatives with small children for good equipment and clothes they are no longer using; the baby doesn't care about fancy cribs or nightgowns—just comfort. Buy clothes in the six-month or one-year size; the three-month size is outgrown too quickly.

Clothing

° Four to six dozen cloth diapers, or a two-week supply of infant-size disposables (you will use about 10 a day), or one or two dozen diapers to supplement diaper service. Prefolded diapers save time, and you can get extra-small ones for newborns.
° A half-dozen diaper pins with safety guards.
° Two or three pairs waterproof pants, preferably silk or nylon. Rubber pants cause sweating.
° Four to six shirts, long- or short-sleeved according to weather and house temperature. (Snap-closed shirts are easier to put on the baby than pullovers.)
° Four to six cotton knit nightgowns or kimonos.
° Four to six terry stretch suits that snap down the front. These can be used instead of nightgowns if you prefer, but it is handy to have both.
° Two sweaters.
° A hooded wrap, bunting, or outdoor pram suit—how warm depends on the weather.
° A heavyweight blanket sleeper—for a cold bedroom or for an active baby who wiggles out of blankets.
° Bootees or socks (optional).
° Three or four bibs.

Bedding

° A crib with a firm, waterproof mattress. Be certain that only unleaded paint has been used on the crib's sides. You can also improvise a bed from a sturdy box, basket, or bureau drawer, using a foam pad or smoothly folded blanket for a mattress. Carefully cover any sharp or rough edges on the sides of the bed, and make sure sides are secure and spaces between crib rails are narrow enough so the baby's head cannot get wedged. Do *not* use a pillow.

° A waterproof case for the mattress or pad, and two or three pieces of waterproof flannelette sheeting large enough to cover it. (Smaller waterproof pads to place directly under the baby's body in the crib, or to use as lap pads, are also handy.)

° Three or four fitted crib sheets.

° Three or four quilted pads (optional), to place between sheet and waterproof pad if weather is hot or the baby's skin is especially sensitive.

° Three or more cotton flannel "receiving" blankets to use as towels, as summer blankets, and as bundling for the baby.

° One or two warm blankets of wool or acrylic.

° Crib bumpers, to keep the baby's head from pressing against the crib rails.

Furniture

° A table or wide-topped bureau on which to dress and change the baby. (Make sure the height is convenient for you—about hip-level is usually best.) You can secure a pad on top of it for the baby to lie on and hang a sturdy shelf above it, out of his reach, for diaper pins, lotion, cotton balls, etc.

° A comfortable rocker or armchair for the parent to sit in during feedings.

° A playpen (preferably with mesh sides) and pad. Used judiciously, a playpen will not thwart your baby's need to explore but will provide a safe place for him to play while you work or relax for a while.

Feeding Equipment

Note: If you nurse your baby, you will need only a few bottles, for the "relief" bottle and for water or juice.

° Eight to ten 8-ounce bottles and three or four 4-ounce bottles (for water or juice); or a disposable nurser kit and refills. Get plastic or Pyrex bottles. They should come with nipples, caps, and bottle covers or disks.

° Extra nipples.

° Bottle and nipple brush.

° Feeding dish and spoons for solid foods.

° Long-handled stirring spoon (for mixing powdered formulas).

° Formula: You can buy prepared infant formulas

in powdered, concentrated liquid, or ready-mixed form.

° If you prepare your own formula at home, you may want a sterilizer kit, glass measuring cups in 8-ounce and 32-ounce sizes, measuring spoons, a funnel, and a stirring spoon. Ask your doctor to give you a suitable formula. Buy the necessary ingredients ahead of time.

Bathing Equipment and Toilet Articles

° Three to four soft towels and washcloths.

° A plastic baby tub with a wide rim on which you can rest your arm.

° A tray to hold bath supplies (optional).

° Pure, unmedicated soap and a soap dish.

° Baby shampoo (optional).

° Cotton balls (not cotton-tipped sticks).

° Baby brush and comb.

° Baby nail scissors with safety points.

° Diaper-rash ointment.

° Baby lotion or premoistened baby wipes for cleaning diaper area after changes.

° Bath apron to protect parent's clothes.

Other Supplies and Equipment

° Mild laundry soap for soaking and washing diapers and baby clothes.

° A rectal thermometer.

° Petroleum jelly for use on thermometer.

° A one- or two-gallon, rustproof diaper pail.

° Mosquito netting to place over the crib if there are insects in the baby's room.

° A room thermometer.

° For outings: a baby carriage, a sling carrier, or a reclining infant seat-carrier (also useful as a baby's feeding chair) in which the child can be securely strapped.

° A car seat, if you take a lot of automobile trips. Get one that anchors securely to the car's back window shelf.

° A diaper bag to hold diapers, bottles, lotions, etc., during trips.

° Night-lights for hallway and baby's room.

° Baby record book, for keeping records of weight, immunizations, new teeth, etc.

° Cold-water vaporizer to keep air from getting too dry in the baby's room, especially when he has a cold.

DECISIONS TO MAKE IN ADVANCE

There are a number of things you may want to decide before the baby is born, so that you will not use up your energy making decisions after you get home—when everyone is giving you solicited and unsolicited advice.

Diapers: Service, Disposables, or Home-Washed?

Diaper services and disposable diapers are great time-savers, but using them will cost you more than buying and laundering your own. If you do plan to use home-laundered diapers, remember that harsh detergents, bleaches, and insufficient rinsing can irritate the baby's skin. (Disposables also irritate some babies because of their plastic coverings.) Diapers from a service are usually sterilized. If you use the service, you will probably need about 80 diapers a week—about 70 for the baby and the rest for lap pads, "burp cloths," and similar uses.

Breast-Feeding vs. Bottle-Feeding

Breast milk is easy for babies to digest and is unsurpassed in nutritional value. Breast-fed babies benefit from temporary or partial immunities to certain diseases; they develop fewer and milder infections of every type in the early months (colds included) than formula-fed babies. They also enjoy an especially warm and pleasant contact with their mothers.

The mother benefits as well. Nursing contracts the muscles of the uterus, hastening its return to normal size. Nursing also makes many mothers feel needed and extremely close to their babies. In addition, it is convenient, cheap, and a time-saver—there are no formulas to be prepared or to sterilize.

Breast-feeding does not ruin a woman's figure—although she should wear a well-fitting brassiere for support during the nursing period. Nor need this method cause any weight gain. You should be able to eat a normal diet and drink a quart of skim milk each day without gaining. Also, you may smoke and drink alcohol in moderation (though neither is recommended) without affecting the milk. But check with your doctor before taking any medicines. Certain types of drugs can be harmful to the baby. (Incidentally, many doctors feel that nursing reduces a woman's chances of getting breast cancer in later life.)

There are, however, certain disadvantages to breast-feeding for the mother. Her freedom is restricted. It is, for example, difficult for a working mother to nurse a baby. But if she returns to her job when the baby is about two months old and on an approximate four-hour schedule, she may be able to manage things so that she misses only one feeding, which can be given in a bottle. (But she should start giving a "relief" bottle during the first two months, so the baby can get used to the idea.) If you wish to learn more about nursing before you decide on it, you can write La Leche League International, 9616 Minneapolis Ave., Franklin Park, Illinois 60131. This voluntary organization has many local branches and can give you advice on how to manage breast-feeding successfully.

Some women simply do not like the idea of breast-feeding; others want to nurse but have difficulty for various reasons. In either case, there is no reason for anyone to feel inadequate or guilty for choosing bottle-feeding instead. There are many excellent formulas available, and a mother who bottle-feeds her baby can give him just as much love and security as one who nurses. Bottle-feeding also gives the father and other family members a chance to be close to the baby.

Schedule

Most doctors today favor "modified demand" feeding—a flexible, self-regulatory schedule based primarily on the baby's own hunger patterns. The old-fashioned rigid schedules, in which feedings were given at precise four-hour intervals, often meant that the baby was fed either when he was half asleep or when he was tense and miserable from prolonged crying—a situation that benefited neither baby nor parents. You do not have to respond like a robot to the baby's first peep, or assume that every cry necessarily means hunger. But in general you can trust a young baby to know when he is hungry; most of them soon develop fairly regular hunger patterns which you will quickly get to know. (A few very placid babies who are gaining slowly may need to be wakened for some feedings.) Feeding a hungry baby will not spoil him. What young infants want and what they need, in the way of food, love, and comfort, are virtually the same thing.

Be very flexible about the "2 a.m." or late-night feeding; your baby will sleep through the night as soon as he is able to go that long without food. Leaving him to cry will not hasten the process. If your baby is sleeping, it may help to delay the feeding that precedes the late-night one until just before you are ready for bed. With a little luck, the infant will not waken quite so early next time. Except for breast-fed babies before the mother's milk has "come in" fully, most infants do not get truly hungry oftener than every three hours.

If your baby cries an hour after a feeding, he may be having digestive problems; infants cannot distinguish between hunger pangs and other pains. If you are extremely groggy during the late-night feeding, do not be tempted to lie down with the baby; sit up and stay awake! (Or, if the baby is getting formula, ask the father to give this feeding.)

It is advisable to let the baby have his own room—at least after the first few weeks—if your space permits. A young baby can be surprisingly noisy when he sleeps. In any case he should definitely be out of your bedroom by the time he's six months old. (If you do not have a spare bedroom and the baby's crib is on casters, you can roll it out of your room and into the living room when *you* go to bed.) A baby's room should be well ventilated, have screened windows, and be fairly easy to keep cool in summer. Get simple, easily cleaned furniture, and washable rugs. Also, a washable linoleum or tile floor is better than wood. Avoid expensive carpeting.

Your Baby's Doctor

Decide ahead of time who is going to look after the baby's health, whether you choose a family doctor or a children's specialist (a pediatrician). For further information on choosing a good doctor, see Chapter 9.

For the first six months your baby should be taken regularly to a doctor or clinic for checkups and immunizations. *Follow your doctor's advice,* and remember that a relationship of frankness and trust between you and your physician is extremely important. If you feel you have not chosen a suitable doctor, you probably are not going to follow his instructions. Find another one.

Circumcision

If your baby is a boy and you wish to have him circumcised, ask your doctor for a thorough explanation of the pros and cons of the operation before you make your final decision. Circumcision consists in cutting off the sleeve of skin (foreskin) covering the head of the penis. It is not usually a medical necessity, but is often done for religious reasons, or for reasons of cleanliness and convenience. It should always be done in early infancy, because it is frightening to an older child. Many people feel that the foreskin is natural and should remain, but it is sometimes difficult to retract it in order to clean the baby's penis. If the foreskin is unusually tight, circumcision may be advisable. If your baby is circum-

cised in the hospital and the wound has not yet healed when you bring him home, keep a layer of gauze saturated with petroleum jelly wrapped around his penis to keep it from being irritated by the diaper.

CARING FOR YOUR BABY

Because each baby is a unique individual, all babies cannot be treated the same way. They are active or placid, tense or easy-going, jolly or subdued by nature—though most babies, like the rest of us, have a combination of traits both pleasing and otherwise. All babies, however, have the same basic need for security and affection. They should be accepted as they are and given a loving, relaxed atmosphere—as well as attention to their physical requirements—in order to develop their full potentialities.

Here are some of the things you can do to create such an atmosphere:

Training

Be careful about trying to "train" the baby. Most babies fall into good habits with the proper encouragement as far as eating, sleeping, and amusing themselves are concerned. Toilet training should not begin before 18 months at the earliest. True, a baby who wants to sleep all day and stay awake all night will require extra patience from you. A fretful baby can drive new parents frantic, especially if he has colic. Try not to let fatigue, resentment, or guilt upset you unduly. Make certain you get some time off, and keep in touch with your doctor or clinic for advice.

Avoiding Needless Worry

Don't worry about your baby's being fragile. He is not. The soft spot, or fontanel, on top of his head is safe to touch and wash; the membrane covering it is quite tough. The odd shape of the newborn's head will soon improve, as will the loose, "cottony" look of his skin as he fattens up. The baby's navel may have a raw spot on it when the stump of the umbilical cord first drops off; it should be kept dry and gently cleaned with soft cotton and alcohol. Notify your doctor only if the area becomes swollen or red. A slight puffiness or enlargement of the breasts or genitals, in both boy and girl babies, is normal in the first week or two. A girl may also have a slight discharge from the vagina and may even pass a small amount of vaginal blood. Mild inflammation of the eyes in the first days (caused by the medication given in the hospital to prevent infection) will also disappear in a short time.

Nor is your baby fragile emotionally. He or she will not be warped for life if you are human enough to be occasionally preoccupied, irritable, or overattentive. It is his basic security that counts.

Father's Role

A baby needs a father as well as a mother. Although the mother is usually considered the most important figure in the infant's life, today's father plays an increasingly active role. Contemporary fathers often attend child-rearing classes, are present during childbirth, and take part in the baby's daily care. Some fathers, however, still feel wary of small babies. It may take tact and time to persuade the father that caring for a baby is not "unmasculine" but a natural part of *parenthood*. It is worth the effort, however, to insure that the relationship between father and baby is close and easy from the beginning—especially in a time when many mothers go to work.

Calling the Doctor

If you think your baby is sick, call your doctor or clinic immediately. (Do not delay simply because you're not sure what is wrong—parents are not expected to be expert diagnosticians.) Your best guide is your own feelings. If he *looks* sick or *acts* sick—if he is feverish or unusually cold, if he is abnormally restless or listless or loses his appetite, if he has difficulty breathing or has prolonged vomiting or diarrhea—call! Take the time to make a list of all your questions beforehand, and *write down* the instructions the doctor gives you.

Do not give your baby any medicine or treatment on your own or try to force him to eat. If he is not vomiting or having diarrhea, let him have his milk as usual. If he is, try to get him to take a little boiled water frequently, unless he vomits it; in that case, wait an hour or two before trying again. Keep him quiet and let him sleep as much as possible. Do not let him cry if rocking or some similar motion will help soothe him.

The General Routine

A healthy baby does not need heavier clothing than anyone else in the family. He will be far more comfortable in his gown or stretch suit (add a sweater in a cold house) when he is out of bed. Avoid uncomfortable fancy clothes. If he wears a cap, it should be a light knitted one so that he can breathe if it slips over his nose, and it must not have the kind of drawstring that can accidentally tighten under his chin. *Never put a pillow in his bed or carriage.* In general, the house temperature should be about 68°–72°F in the daytime and can be kept at 60°F at night if the baby is wearing a warm sleeper.

Sleep. Let the baby sleep on his stomach most of the time; it is the safest position in case he spits up. If he always turns his head in a certain direction, face him first one way in the crib, then the other so that his head won't flatten on one side. Incidentally, when the baby is asleep is a good time to clip his nails. Get nail scissors designed for babies. In general, do not make any special effort to keep the house quiet while the baby sleeps. Most babies can get used to an ordinarily noisy house as easily as a quiet one.

Diapers. Change his diapers as soon as possible when they are soiled; when they are wet, change them if he fusses or if you are picking him up anyway. Get all traces of the bowel movement off his skin, especially in the creases. Baby lotion and cotton balls, or premoistened wipes designed for babies, can be used to clean his bottom. (Wipe *back*, away from the genitals, especially with a female infant.) If the baby's navel is not yet healed, fold the diaper below it so that the navel stays dry. In case of diaper rash (red pimples and rough, red patches), you may need to wash the skin gently after each change. Ask your doctor to recommend a good, protective diaper-rash ointment. If the rash persists, discontinue plastic-covered disposable diapers or waterproof pants until it clears up. If it still does not heal or you suspect infection, call your doctor. He may suggest that you leave the diaper area uncovered for several hours each day.

Shake soiled diapers into the toilet before you put them in a covered pail of water; you can add some mild laundry soap to the water for soaking. If you launder the diapers, wash them in very hot water with mild soap and rinse them thoroughly; dry them outdoors or in a dryer.

A baby's normal bowel movements often seem quite loose and odd-looking to first-time parents. Young babies usually have between one and six bowel movements a day. Breast-fed babies have a light yellow or greenish-yellow stool which may be watery. Babies usually pass their stool quite easily, even if they move their bowels relatively seldom. Bottle-fed babies tend to have a more pasty, moist movement which is yellow or brownish.

Heat Rash. For prickly heat (tiny pimples that usually start around the neck in hot weather) you can rub on a little cornstarch, which is cheaper and as effective as talcum powders. *Never shake any powder over a baby; he may inhale it.* Put a little in your hand (away from his face) and then rub it on the skin. Do not be afraid to keep the baby lightly dressed in very hot weather.

Handling the Baby. When you pick your baby up, support his head as well as his body. When you carry him, hold him with his head leaning over your shoulder a little so that it will not bob backward. He will need this kind of support until he is about three months old when he can hold up his head by himself.

Some fresh, cool air is good for him. By the time he weighs eight pounds, he can go out when the temperature is 60°F or above, and a 10-pounder can stay out about two hours if it is above freezing and the wind is not too strong. Larger babies can go out in even colder weather if they are kept in a sunny, sheltered spot.

Germs. Every baby is bound to be exposed to some germs, but do not expose yours unnecessarily. There should be *no kissing from visitors and no contact with older children who have colds, sore throats, or contagious diseases of any kind.* If you have a cold, buy some disposable sterile masks to cover your nose and mouth while you tend the baby, and wash your hands often. A sick baby, even one with only a cold, is a worry to everyone, the doctor included.

Safety. Observe safety rules carefully. Never leave any baby, however small or placid, alone for a second on a changing table, chair, or bed, or in the bath. If you must answer the door or phone, pick him up and hold him or put him in his crib or playpen. Do not leave babies alone with young children; they may be feeling jealous or experimental. Do not leave anything around that the baby might swallow. Beware, especially, of open pins or other small objects on the changing table or around the bath. He may choke on one of them. If he swallows a small, smooth object that goes down easily, tell your doctor; but such things often pass readily through a baby. An open pin or other sharp object can be quite dangerous, so take him to a doctor or hospital immediately if he swallows one. Do not hang toys or other objects from strings inside the crib or playpen; the baby could get tangled up in them.

Bathing the Baby

Your doctor will advise you how soon your baby may have a real bath—probably when he is two weeks old, though some doctors prefer having babies sponge-bathed for the first month or so. Any convenient time when you are not rushed by other duties—provided it is not immediately after a feeding—is all right for his bath. Any draft-free, warm room (75°F or so) is suitable. Use a plastic baby bath or a similar soft tub with a wide rim to rest your elbow on. Wear an apron to protect your clothes. Be sure to wash your hands and have everything you need ready before you start. Put about two inches of warm water in the tub, about 90°–100°F (test it with your wrist or elbow; it should feel comfortably warm *but not hot*), and line the bottom of the tub with a clean diaper or small towel so the baby won't skid around.

You will soon learn how to hold the baby: your left hand under his left arm, with your thumb over and your fingers under it, so that your wrist supports his head. (Reverse this if you are left-handed.) Use a mild, unscented soap and a soft washcloth; but do not soap the baby's face. If a little mucus stays in his nose, twist a bit of cotton (do not put it on a stick), moisten it in water, and insert it gently a little way into the nostril, holding onto it as you twist so that the mucus sticks to it when you pull it out. Wash the baby's scalp once or twice a week, tilting his head back so that no soap gets in his eyes. If he has any "cradle cap" (infant seborrhea of the scalp) and daily shampooing does not help, consult your doctor about the use of a suitable ointment. You may need to apply it several times a day and use a fine-toothed comb to loosen the scales until the condition clears up.

Soap his body lightly with your hands or the cloth, paying special attention to the folds and creases behind the ears, under the chin, and around the genital organs. (Again, do not use cotton-tipped sticks, and do not try to clean his eyes or the insides of his ears—use a corner of the washcloth for the creases.) If a boy's penis needs special cleaning, your doctor or the hospital nurse will show you what to do. You may find it easiest to place the baby on a towel in your lap for the soaping and then—slowly—lower him into the tub for rinsing. Let the baby splash about a little, and then lift him out carefully (wet babies are slippery), wrap a towel around him, and gently but thoroughly pat him dry, especially in the creases.

Nursing the Baby

Your breasts require little care. Just before each feeding, wash your hands. (Some mothers also sponge their nipples with cotton moistened in clear water.) If your breasts leak milk between feedings or just before you nurse, you can place cotton (not plastic-coated) nursing pads inside your brassiere, but make sure no wisps of cotton remain on your nipples when you feed the baby.

As a rule, babies are nursed at both breasts during each feeding, with one breast being offered first at one feeding, and the other first at the next. Make sure the baby gets the entire areola (the dark area around the nipple) into his mouth as well as the nipple; it is the action of his gums as they compress the areola that makes the milk flow. (Also make sure the baby's nose is not pressed against your breast so as to interfere with his breathing.) If your baby does not empty the breasts completely, your doctor may instruct you to empty them by hand after the feeding in order to encourage the supply of milk. Some babies nurse rapidly and some slowly, but in general they take the greatest part of the milk from each breast in the first five to seven minutes. The average feeding is about 15 to 20 minutes, with 30 to 45 minutes considered the maximum time a baby should be left to nurse.

Once or twice during the nursing period, and just afterward, burp the baby by holding him over your shoulder so that any air he has swallowed will be expelled. (You can also sit him up or lay him face down in your lap, and gently rub or pat his back.) Protect your clothing with a clean diaper. If he positively will not burp and he is old enough to sit in an infant seat, you can strap him in there until the bubble comes up. If nursing makes your nipples sore, ask your doctor or clinic what to do.

Many nursing mothers worry about how to tell whether a baby is getting enough, especially if the infant is fussy after feedings. In general, as long as the baby is gaining well and seems happy, he is probably getting what he needs. The *average* weight gain is about one and a half to two pounds a month during the first three months; by six months the weight increase is down to about one pound a month, and by nine months, about two-thirds of a pound per month. The average baby also doubles his birth weight in approximately five months. But, of course, many healthy babies are not "average," and most of them don't need to be weighed except when they visit the doctor. If your doctor is concerned about poor weight gain, excessive crying, or possible digestive difficulties, you can buy a baby scale to use at home; but do not weigh the baby more often than the doctor advises.

The Bottle-fed Baby

A formula is milk that has been modified to make it resemble mother's milk as much as possible. Most people today prefer to use commercially prepared, ready-mixed formulas, either in concentrated liquid or powdered form. Preparing your own is cheaper, however. Be sure you have a refrigerator in good working condition and a pure water supply. Even though sterilization of bottles and equipment is no longer as widely practiced as it once was, to be on the safe side, boil the water used in mixing the formula for 20 minutes and keep it in a clean, covered jar in the refrigerator. If your house has a well or cistern and a septic system, you *must* boil the water because of possible contamination.

To prepare the formula, carefully follow the directions on the container. Clean the top of the can with soap and water, then rinse, before opening it with a clean punch-type opener. It is easier to use up the entire can and prepare a number of bottles for storage in the refrigerator, rather than to prepare one bottle at a time and cover the can for refrigeration.

Use bottles, caps, and nipples that have been washed in clean, hot water with detergent and a brush. Before washing, squeeze nipple holes to be sure they are open. Rinse everything well and let stand in a rack to dry. Bottles—but not nipples—can also be washed in an automatic dishwasher; nipples tend to get baked dry in the drying cycle. If you have a disposable nurser kit, follow the directions for cleaning and preparing bottles that come with it.

If your refrigerator stops working, prepare each bottle just before a feeding from boiled water and powdered formula. (The usual proportion is one tablespoon of powder for each two oz. of water.) Throw out *any* unrefrigerated formula that isn't used within 30 to 40 minutes, especially in hot weather; germs multiply rapidly in unchilled milk. The powdered formula need not be refrigerated before mixing, but it should be kept well covered. Do not give any added vitamins or iron unless they are prescribed by a doctor. If your baby proves to be sensitive to milk, there are nonmilk formulas available; many have a soybean base.

A baby's bottle can be given warmed, at room temperature, or straight out of the refrigerator if he doesn't mind, but try to be consistent about this. You can warm the bottle in a saucepan of water on the stove. Test it by squeezing a few drops on your wrist, and if it feels hot, cool it down to body temperature.

Few people nowadays take the trouble to make their own formulas, but if you wish to do so, ask your doctor for a suitable "recipe."

When you give the feeding, cradle the baby in your arm in a semi-sitting position and hold the bottle so that its neck is always completely filled with milk and the baby does not suck in air. If the baby takes more than 20 minutes to empty the bottle, the nipple holes may be too small or the nipple may be collapsed. (Holes can be enlarged; follow the directions that come with the nipples). If the baby takes the milk too fast, the hole may be too large, and a new nipple should be used. Remember, babies do not necessarily need the same amount at each feeding, so do not urge a balky baby to take more than he wants. Burp him as you would a breast-fed baby, making sure to get the burp up before you put him back to bed. During both breast and bottle feedings sit in a comfortable armchair or rocker. *Never* prop a newborn's bottle in his crib, and avoid doing so with an older baby's unless you absolutely must, i.e., if you are trying to feed twins at the same time. The bottle can fall over, causing the baby to suck in air, or the milk can flow too fast and choke him.

Water

Both breast-fed and bottle-fed babies occasionally need drinking water, especially when they are sick or during hot weather. You can offer a few ounces of boiled water between (but not just before) feedings. Do not worry if the baby sometimes refuses it. Most babies get enough fluid in their milk and many do not like plain water.

Vitamins

Babies need vitamins. Vitamins A and D are already added to whole and evaporated milk; vitamins A, C, and D, as well as other vitamins and minerals, are usually added to commercial formulas. (Breast milk contains little vitamin D, however.) Strained orange juice, which can be given whenever your doctor so recommends, is rich in vitamin C. If your doctor prescribes vitamin-supplement drops, remember to tell him what formula you are using. He may also suggest fluoride drops to strengthen the baby's teeth if you live in an area where the water is not fluoridated.

Your doctor or clinic will give you a list of new items to add to your baby's diet. Do not be distressed if the baby rejects them at first. It is wise to introduce new foods, such as cereals and strained fruits, one at a time and in very small servings. If allergic reactions develop or a particular food disagrees with the baby, you will then be able to pinpoint the cause.

DIGESTIVE PROBLEMS

Vomiting

Most babies vomit, or "spit up," from time to time—usually in relatively small amounts just after being fed. This kind of vomiting generally does not mean anything—not even if it happens daily—provided the baby is obviously healthy and gaining weight. If your baby does not seem well to you, if he vomits a large amount more often than once a day, or above all if he vomits with great force (projectile vomiting), be sure to consult your doctor or clinic. In some cases, vomiting accompanied by mild indigestion can be helped by a change in the formula.

Colic

The regular, painful attacks of colic that plague many strong, healthy babies until the age of three or four months are also very hard on parents, who may be quite upset when their efforts to soothe the baby do not help. During a colic attack, the baby's abdomen is distended and the pain makes him pull up his legs and scream loudly. He may also expel gas by rectum. Some babies have colicky periods at the same time each day. Attacks usually come soon after a feeding, yet most colicky babies eat and gain very well, and changing the formula seems to make little difference. If you have a colicky baby—or one who is unusually tense, or cries irritably without definite signs of pain—experiment with various ways of comforting him. A pacifier helps with some babies. Simply being placed on their stomachs and given a back rub quiets others. You can also try rocking the baby in his cradle or carriage. Keep in close touch with your doctor, who will help manage the attack and determine if it has a more serious cause. In some rare instances, he may prescribe a sedative.

Diarrhea

The *kind* of stool a healthy baby has, even if it seems strange to you at first, is less important than a sudden or drastic *change* in his bowel habits. Consult your doctor or clinic immediately if the number of movements increases greatly, or if the stools smell different, become unusually watery or greenish, or are expelled suddenly or explosively. Do not be alarmed, however, if the color of the stool changes after you have given the baby a new vegetable—beets or spinach, for example. Also, a stool that has been in the baby's diaper for some time may become greenish from exposure to air.

Constipation

A breast-fed baby is almost never constipated. If he should be, give him a little strained prune juice. Try a teaspoonful at first, increasing the amount to two teaspoonfuls the next day if the first dose has not been effective.

A bottle-fed baby who is badly constipated— that is, one whose movements are hard, formed, and perhaps painful as well as infrequent— should also be given prune juice. Do not do anything else about constipation without your doctor's advice.

WEANING

Most authorities recommend that you begin weaning a baby before the age of one year. But this change of feeding should take place gradually, so that the infant does not feel that he is being deprived of anything essential. (Delay the process if the baby is not feeling well or the weather is very hot.) Praise your baby's efforts with the cup, do not get upset by his resistance and spilling, and do not be afraid of forcing the issue. Reluctance on your part will encourage the baby to cling to his bottle.

TEETHING

In Chapter 4 you will find a schedule of the ages when a baby's teeth usually appear. Teething can be uncomfortable, and some babies are quite upset by it, losing their appetite or suffering from digestive disturbances. Teething may cause a slight fever, but not over 101° F. You can help your baby by giving him something hard and safe to chew on, such as a clean rubber ring—but nothing that might crack or splinter.

THUMB-SUCKING AND GENITAL PLAY

Thumb-sucking and handling of the genitals (sometimes referred to as infant masturbation)

are nothing to be disturbed about in infants. (You will find a discussion of MASTURBATION in the encyclopedia section.)

IMMUNIZATIONS

Your child will need certain immunizations to protect him against diseases. Be sure to follow the schedule your doctor or clinic recommends, and keep a record of immunizations at home. The following is a standard schedule:

At two months, four months, and again at six months, babies are given the DTP, or DPT, immunization, which protects them against diphtheria, tetanus, and pertussis (whooping cough). At these times they are also given the TOPV (trivalent oral polio virus vaccine). Measles vaccine is given at or shortly after the age of one year, and may be combined with rubella (German measles) vaccine or with both rubella and mumps vaccines. A tuberculin test is also made at one year. The DTP and TOPV immunizations are given again at one and a half years and at four to six years (school age), and an adult-type TD (tetanus-diphtheria) inoculation is given at 14 to 16 years. Doctors no longer recommend routine smallpox vaccinations, and extra tetanus boosters need rarely be given.

YOUR BABY GROWS OLDER

The following list includes a very few of the things the "average" baby does at certain ages. It is intended only to give you some idea of what you can anticipate and be prepared for.

° *4 to 8 weeks:* The baby begins to smile and make small throaty noises. He watches his mother's face for brief periods, and his feeding and sleeping schedule becomes more regular.

° *16 weeks:* He chuckles, watches moving objects, turns his head in the direction of someone's voice, holds up his head when lying on his stomach, and can roll from stomach to back.

° *28 weeks:* The baby sits up for fairly long periods with some support. He grasps objects, puts them in his mouth, and shifts them from one hand to the other. He is very sociable, recognizes family members, and makes "talking" sounds.

° *40 weeks:* He sits up well on his own, gets on hands and knees and pulls himself up to standing position; he may also begin creeping. He grasps objects between thumb and forefinger, understands "No," and makes word-sounds like "da-da" and "bye-bye."

15 Your Child's Early Growth and Emotional Life

Parents—especially those with only one child—usually have many questions. "What is the average child like at this age?" "What should he be able to do?" "How should he behave?" "How big should he be?" "How much should he eat and sleep?" This chapter answers these and other questions concerning the physical growth and emotional development of not only the "average" child—but of your own child. Among the topics discussed are the proper methods of discipline, toilet training, dealing with children's nervous habits, answering a child's questions about sex, coping with sibling rivalry, starting school—even children's television programs.

THE "AVERAGE" CHILD

At two years of age, the average child weighs 28 pounds and is 34 to 35 inches tall. He has about 16 teeth. He sleeps about 14 to 16 hours of the 24. He has been able to walk (holding on) since he was a year old, and by himself since he was 18 months. Now he can run, after a fashion, as well as walk. When he was 18 months old his vocabulary included some dozen or so words; now it has increased to about 200. He has a fair degree of bowel and bladder control in the daytime.

By the time he has reached age three, the child has passed through a certain amount of turmoil manifesting itself in temper tantrums, negativism, and other traits trying to parents. Now he is in a relatively stable period. He has all his baby teeth (20), speaks in short sentences, practically dresses himself, is fairly well toilet trained.

At five, having passed through some additional stormy stages, he is once again in a relatively stable period. He is quite competent and independent, having reached the end of his early childhood; and he is getting ready to go out into the world of kindergarten or school. He sleeps about 12 hours a day, with a quiet period and occasionally a nap after lunch.

THE "AVERAGE" CHILD VERSUS YOUR CHILD

The child described above is the average child as portrayed by statistics. Your child, however, is an individual. It would be remarkable if he happened to be average in every detail. What is more likely is that he is above average in some respects, below it in others, and will alternate from one side of the statistical mean to the other at various periods during his development.

Physical Growth

It is a good idea to keep a record of your child's weight and height and the arrival of his teeth, so that your doctor will know whether the growth rate is within normal limits. In general, leave concern about normal limits to the physician and do not worry unduly about your child's physical development. Comments by well-meaning relatives on his size and accomplishments, particularly when compared with those of other members of the family, should be discouraged.

Sleep

Give your child the opportunity to obtain the average amount of sleep. It will not hurt to keep him up late once in a while on special occasions, but do not make a habit of depriving him of sleep to suit your own convenience. Provide a comfortable place for his bed or crib where he will be relatively free from disturbance.

Sleep should not be a major problem. If there is any trouble, do not assume that your child is being contrary, but try to find and eliminate the cause of the difficulty. For example, your child may be afraid of the dark, but is unable or too embarrassed to tell you about his fear. Try to remember that his fear—however unfounded—is real to him. You will not be able to cajole him out of it; nor should you try to make him feel ashamed for being afraid. You can help him, however, by providing a dim light in his room, or by leaving his door open just a little. A cuddly doll or teddy bear may be comforting company for him. Soft music may be restful and relieve his tension.

A youngster usually goes to sleep more readily if the evening meal is a simple one and he is not too stimulated at bedtime. A tapering-off period of quiet relaxation and perhaps a soothing story will be helpful.

Do not punish a child by putting him to bed earlier than usual. Be fair and considerate; make going to bed as pleasant as possible, but also be firm about it.

Eating

Self-regulation, which is described in Chapter 14, usually gets a youngster off to a good start; but at some time or other, most children fail to eat as well as their mothers would wish. Eating habits

Stages in a baby's growth

The heights, weights, and stages of development described here and the other illustrations in this chapter are average ones. There is no cause for alarm just because the timing of a child's development is slightly different, although marked departure from the average timetable should be discussed with a doctor.

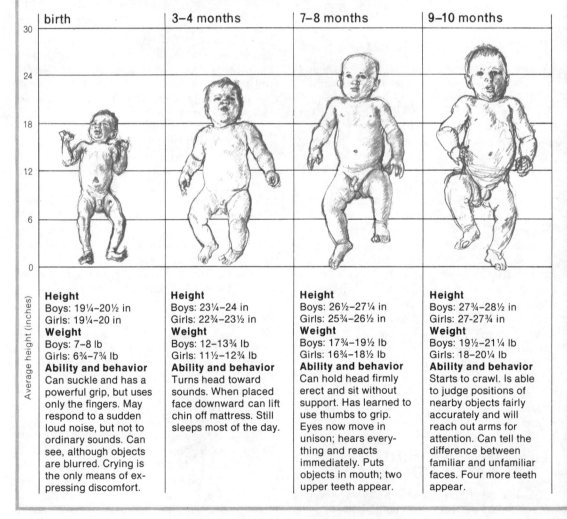

	birth	3–4 months	7–8 months	9–10 months
Height	Boys: 19¼–20½ in Girls: 19¼–20 in	Boys: 23¼–24 in Girls: 22¾–23½ in	Boys: 26½–27¼ in Girls: 25¾–26½ in	Boys: 27¾–28½ in Girls: 27–27¾ in
Weight	Boys: 7–8 lb Girls: 6¾–7¾ lb	Boys: 12–13¾ lb Girls: 11½–12¾ lb	Boys: 17¾–19½ lb Girls: 16¾–18½ lb	Boys: 19½–21¼ lb Girls: 18–20¼ lb
Ability and behavior	Can suckle and has a powerful grip, but uses only the fingers. May respond to a sudden loud noise, but not to ordinary sounds. Can see, although objects are blurred. Crying is the only means of expressing discomfort.	Turns head toward sounds. When placed face downward can lift chin off mattress. Still sleeps most of the day.	Can hold head firmly erect and sit without support. Has learned to use thumbs to grip. Eyes now move in unison; hears everything and reacts immediately. Puts objects in mouth; two upper teeth appear.	Starts to crawl. Is able to judge positions of nearby objects fairly accurately and will reach out arms for attention. Can tell the difference between familiar and unfamiliar faces. Four more teeth appear.

Average height (inches) — 30, 24, 18, 12, 6, 0

should not become an issue in the household. Pediatricians advise placing the food in front of the child and removing the plate without comment if the food is not eaten. The child is usually ready to eat by the next meal.

If a child has a poor appetite, either regularly or at certain stages of his development, the mother should try to discover the circumstances under which he eats best. Often eating alone in quiet surroundings where he will not be distracted helps. Sometimes he does well with small portions but not with large ones. A full plate can loom very large to a small child, and he will wonder how he can ever finish such a mass of food. He may prefer food that is easily chewed and simple to handle. He may want food that is all one color—such as mushroom soup, rice, breast of chicken, mashed potatoes, and vanilla ice cream. Sometimes he prefers to be fed, even though he is old enough, according to the timetable of averages, to feed himself.

In regard to eating (and sleeping) there are four main points to remember:

1. Don't worry. Children do not starve them-

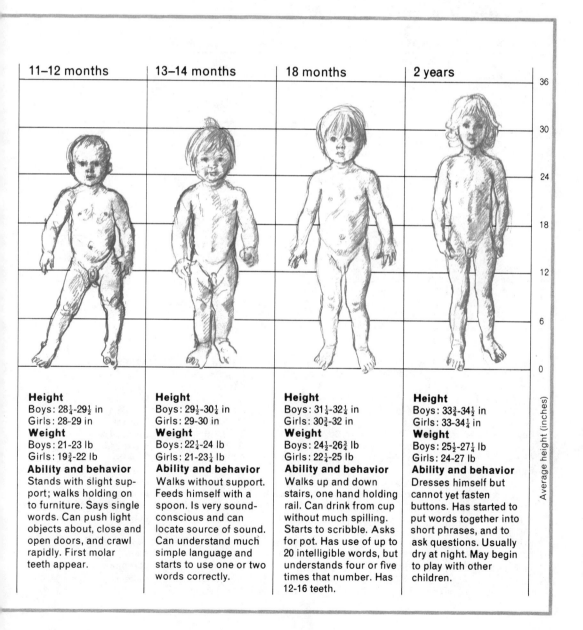

11–12 months	13–14 months	18 months	2 years
Height Boys: $28\frac{1}{4}$-$29\frac{1}{2}$ in Girls: 28-29 in	**Height** Boys: $29\frac{1}{2}$-$30\frac{1}{4}$ in Girls: 29-30 in	**Height** Boys: $31\frac{1}{4}$-$32\frac{1}{4}$ in Girls: $30\frac{3}{4}$-32 in	**Height** Boys: $33\frac{3}{4}$-$34\frac{1}{2}$ in Girls: 33-$34\frac{1}{4}$ in
Weight Boys: 21-23 lb Girls: $19\frac{3}{4}$-22 lb	**Weight** Boys: $22\frac{1}{4}$-24 lb Girls: 21-$23\frac{1}{4}$ lb	**Weight** Boys: $24\frac{1}{2}$-$26\frac{3}{4}$ lb Girls: $22\frac{1}{4}$-25 lb	**Weight** Boys: $25\frac{1}{2}$-$27\frac{1}{4}$ lb Girls: 24-27 lb
Ability and behavior Stands with slight support; walks holding on to furniture. Says single words. Can push light objects about, close and open doors, and crawl rapidly. First molar teeth appear.	**Ability and behavior** Walks without support. Feeds himself with a spoon. Is very sound-conscious and can locate source of sound. Can understand much simple language and starts to use one or two words correctly.	**Ability and behavior** Walks up and down stairs, one hand holding rail. Can drink from cup without much spilling. Starts to scribble. Asks for pot. Has use of up to 20 intelligible words, but understands four or five times that number. Has 12-16 teeth.	**Ability and behavior** Dresses himself but cannot yet fasten buttons. Has started to put words together into short phrases, and to ask questions. Usually dry at night. May begin to play with other children.

Average height (inches)

selves. Some carefully controlled investigations have shown that even very small children who are allowed to choose their foods select a reasonably well-balanced diet. They do not limit themselves only to ice cream and candy.

2. Feeding problems usually involve something other than, or in addition to, just eating. A general atmosphere of love and relaxation will be helpful until you can find out what the other factors are and deal with them.

3. Your child is not the "average" child. He may eat less or more than usual at times because that is what he needs at some stages.

4. Your child constantly grows and changes. At one time he may eat or sleep well; at another time he may not. Most children eat less in hot weather, when they are teething, and during the second year of life.

Emotional Development

Behavior is the result of complicated feelings. The development of reasonable behavior and

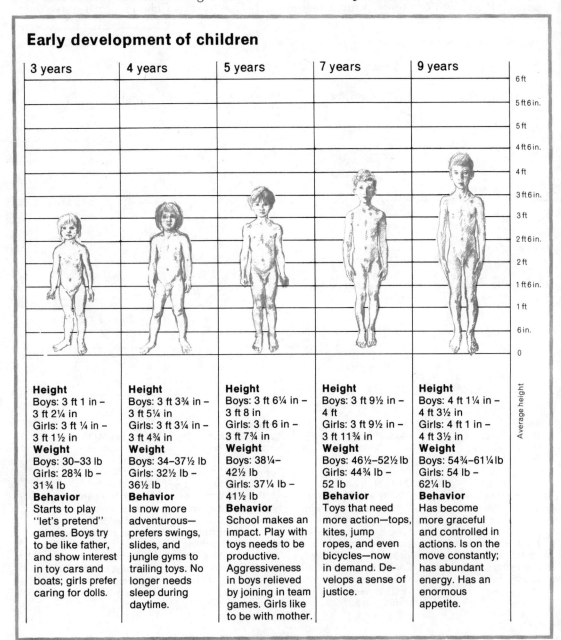

Early development of children

	3 years	4 years	5 years	7 years	9 years
Height	Boys: 3 ft 1 in – 3 ft 2¼ in Girls: 3 ft ¼ in – 3 ft 1½ in	Boys: 3 ft 3¾ in – 3 ft 5¼ in Girls: 3 ft 3¼ in – 3 ft 4¾ in	Boys: 3 ft 6¼ in – 3 ft 8 in Girls: 3 ft 6 in – 3 ft 7¾ in	Boys: 3 ft 9½ in – 4 ft Girls: 3 ft 9½ in – 3 ft 11¾ in	Boys: 4 ft 1¼ in – 4 ft 3½ in Girls: 4 ft 1 in – 4 ft 3½ in
Weight	Boys: 30–33 lb Girls: 28¾ lb – 31¾ lb	Boys: 34–37½ lb Girls: 32½ lb – 36½ lb	Boys: 38¼–42½ lb Girls: 37¼ lb – 41½ lb	Boys: 46½–52½ lb Girls: 44¾ lb – 52 lb	Boys: 54¾–61¼ lb Girls: 54 lb – 62¼ lb
Behavior	Starts to play "let's pretend" games. Boys try to be like father, and show interest in toy cars and boats; girls prefer caring for dolls.	Is now more adventurous—prefers swings, slides, and jungle gyms to trailing toys. No longer needs sleep during daytime.	School makes an impact. Play with toys needs to be productive. Aggressiveness in boys relieved by joining in team games. Girls like to be with mother.	Toys that need more action—tops, kites, jump ropes, and even bicycles—now in demand. Develops a sense of justice.	Has become more graceful and controlled in actions. Is on the move constantly; has abundant energy. Has an enormous appetite.

Average height

good judgment comes only with growing up physically. Therefore, we should expect children to be governed more by their feelings than by reason. When children act in ways that are puzzling, inconsistent, or just plain obstinate, it is incumbent upon the parents to try to discover the cause of the behavior. Acceptance and understanding of the child are important in providing him with confidence in himself as a human being, even at an early age. But he should not be confused by a lack of, or an inconsistency in, guidance or discipline, so that he is unable to know what to expect from his parents.

Letting Children Express Emotions

Children often express their emotions extravagantly. They say, "I love you," "I hate you," or "I will kill him dead," when an adult would say, "That's nice of you," "I wish you wouldn't," or "I'd like him to go away."

Do not be shocked by this. If Johnny says, "I hate you," take it in your stride, perhaps making some noncommittal remark to the effect that everyone feels like that sometimes. As soon as the child's frustration or hostility is over, he will be in a loving mood again. On the other hand, if you show that you are horrified, the child will feel guilty and repress his reactions. It is natural to have some feelings of hostility, even hatred.

While children should be encouraged to act out and talk out their natural feelings of hostility, they should not be allowed to hurt other people physically. When youngsters go too far, they seem to welcome being restrained.

Discipline

The problem is one of balance, and every parent faces it. Obviously the child cannot be permitted to grow up without restrictions, free to do whatever he pleases regardless of consequences to others and to himself. But the necessary discipline must be employed thoughtfully and judiciously to avoid curbing his spirit and natural energy and smothering his curiosity. This combination of sensible restraint and the greatest possible freedom is described by Dr. Arnold Gesell, noted specialist on child development, as "informed permissiveness." Parents who adopt this concept try to understand what they can reasonably expect from their children, always keeping in mind their age and basic personality. Mother and father keep their demands on their children within reason, so that they can be guided consistently and in kindly ways, and still be permitted to grow at their own pace.

During the child's first year he is wholly dependent. It is unwise to put any responsibility on him for either his cleanliness or his safety. Babies and toddlers are not willful; they are just eager to explore the world. We must help and encourage them in their explorations and not frustrate them whenever they want to handle an appealing object. But it is up to adults to protect them from danger.

At the beginning of the child's second year, he should be taught that certain things must be avoided. He must be met with a firm "No" when he plays near the stove, climbs on a table, or starts to pick up a sharp knife. However, we must inhibit his exploration as little as possible.

By the time he is three, he is ready to accept a limited amount of discipline as far as his own safety and that of other people—and of some objects—are concerned.

To discover whether you are demanding too much of your child, count the number of times you and the other adults in the household say "No," or discipline him in other ways. If there is a continual chorus of "No's" and "Dont's," you can be reasonably sure the discipline is too strict. You are training your youngster to move acceptably in an adult world, rather than "childproofing" the surroundings so that he can enjoy them.

Punishment. Your child does not "need" to be punished. When a good relationship exists between parents and child, most difficulties can be resolved without resorting to punishment. Watch how a good nursery school teacher or camp counselor handles a number of children! The trouble is, however, that parents have many other things to attend to in addition to their children, and punishment is often a shortcut. It is, however, unrealistic to suggest that you should never punish a child. If, for example, your firm "No" does not prevent him from reaching for a forbidden, dangerous object, a slap on the hand will probably stop him. In most cases it will cause him little more than momentary discomfort and may even make him remember not to touch the object again.

Punishment frequently results in more harm than good. It is almost impossible to find a punishment that will accomplish what you want without creating another problem. Nagging, threatening, or shaming a child can have a bad effect on him by undermining his fragile sense of self-esteem. Never punish a child for things that are not his fault, or for acting like a child instead of like an adult. Remember that a child has to learn or be taught most of the things grown-ups think everyone should know instinctively. He is not born with a code of ethics or morals, nor can he judge the consequences of an act or see the relationship between one set of circumstances and another. Most important of all, whatever disciplinary measure you take, make it clear that the child has not lost your love. He must understand that you disapprove of what he *does,* but not of him.

Toilet Training

Parents frequently attempt to toilet train their children too early and too strictly. As a result,

their children may become unsure, timid, worried about dirt, or ashamed of parts of their bodies. The most important thing to remember is that if left to himself, the child will usually stop wetting and soiling when he is ready to do so. Parents should be willing to let nature take its course, with just a little guidance and understanding encouragement.

Toilet training is disapproved of for all children in the first year and for most children during the second. Parents who insist on attempting it early should be prepared for many failures, especially if the child becomes ill or has an emotional upset. At such times the parents should assume a relaxed rather than a punitive attitude toward

How bones grow

Bones develop from pieces or rods of cartilage (gristle), or from membranes. The bone-forming process begins before birth and continues throughout childhood and adolescence until the age of about 19 in women and 21 in men. Most long bones, such as thigh and shin bones, initially grow at both ends; some short bones, such as those in the fingers and toes, grow mainly at one end.

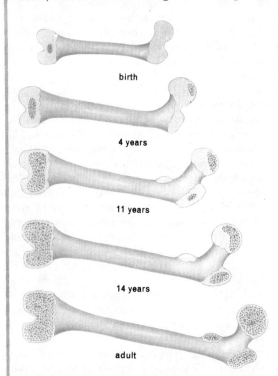

birth

4 years

11 years

14 years

adult

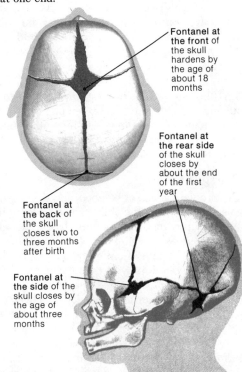

Fontanel at the front of the skull hardens by the age of about 18 months

Fontanel at the rear side of the skull closes by about the end of the first year

Fontanel at the back of the skull closes two to three months after birth

Fontanel at the side of the skull closes by the age of about three months

The long bones of the limbs

Long bones, found in the arms and legs, begin by growing at both ends, but by adolescence most of the growth takes place at the lower end (left) only. This illustration shows the femur (thighbone).

The baby's skull

At birth, hardening of the skull bones is incomplete. During a baby's first 18 months, the soft areas between the bones, called fontanels, gradually harden and fuse. After this age, the skull is entirely bone.

the child's lapses and be willing to start the training all over again.

It should be noted here that the flushing of the toilet after a bowel movement can sometimes create an odd, emotional problem for a young child. If he does not understand that he is eliminating waste matter, he may sometimes be concerned that he is flushing a part of himself down the toilet. It should be a simple matter for the parents to explain, remembering always not to laugh at him for being anxious.

Thumb-Sucking

Almost all children suck their thumbs at times. It is a perfectly harmless way in which they obtain gratification or reassurance. Babies generally suck their thumbs when they are going to sleep or when they are frightened or lonely, when they are hungry, and when they are teething. Thumb-sucking needs no treatment.

Older children who still suck their thumbs may do so because they are bored, tired, or sleepy; or because they have been scolded, are lonely, or feel tense. Usually, children stop sucking their thumbs by the time they are four or five years old, although the habit may persist after that age. It is not anything to be overly concerned about.

Nervous Habits

It is important for parents to realize that children have periods of increased tension in their development. These occurrences will vary according to age, home situation, and the temperament of the child, and will manifest themselves in different ways.

Some babies will bang their heads against the crib or rock it violently. An older child may bite his nails, make grimaces, or twitch his lips. A child may stammer in an effort to use the new words he is learning so rapidly.

From infancy through childhood the youngster is bombarded with new sensations and experiences—sights, sounds, people, words, happenings—that he is constantly being called upon to deal with successfully. For some children this can be an enormous burden. Involuntary nervous mannerisms indicate that the child is under stress.

Nagging, scolding, or shaming him will only increase the child's tension and establish the habit more firmly. Ignore the symptoms and attempt to discover their cause so as to eliminate it. If you listen attentively to a stammering child, he will relax because he does not have to work so hard to put his ideas across. Make a mental note of what triggers a child's nervous activity and, whenever possible, try to relax him in that particular situation.

Usually time will take care of nervous habits. As the child grows more confident, the need for them subsides. If tensions still persist, describe them fully to the child's doctor.

Interest in Sex

Sooner or later, the child will be interested in the sex organs, where babies come from, pregnancy, and even sexual intercourse. If his relationship with his parents is a good one, he will ask these questions just as freely as he asks why the sky is blue.

It is best to tell the truth, but not with more

1 year Growth areas, or epiphyses, start to appear, not joined to the finger bones, or phalanges

6 years Epiphyses in the fingers are still separated, but most of the wrist bones have hardened

17 years All the epiphyses in the fingers are united with the phalanges

The bones of the hand
The hand has three main areas: carpal or wrist bones, metacarpal or palm bones, and phalanges or finger bones. The areas of cartilage between the bones harden into bone by the mid-teens.

details than the child wants or can understand. Tell the facts simply, without analogies about the birds and the bees.

The first thing most children want to know—often when they are only two years old—is where babies come from. The answer can be that they grow inside their mothers. Next—perhaps immediately, but sometimes not for a while—a child is apt to ask how the baby got there. An adequate answer is that it grew from a little seed that was there all the time. When the child asks how the baby got out he can be told: "Through a special opening that mothers have." When the child wants to know whether daddies have anything to do with it, he can be told that the father's seed is needed, too. Volunteer this information by the time the child is three or four.

Similarly, give your child truthful answers to questions about the sex organs. It is sometimes necessary to volunteer a little information because children are not always able to make their curiosity or concern known to their parents. The fact that a boy has a penis and a girl does not is often a source of worry to both of them. The girl may feel deprived, while the boy may fear that something can happen to him and he will be like the girl. It often makes sense to take the lead and explain that boys and girls are made differently because they are going to be different when they grow up: a boy will be able to be a father and a girl to be a mother.

Although parents should avoid false modesty, most experts in child psychology advise them not to expose their naked bodies to children, even very young ones. Adults and children should not take baths together. It may be disturbing to children to be reminded so vividly of the great physical differences between themselves and their parents.

It is also important to take precautions against having children witness or hear the sexual act. Children are apt to mistake passion for violence and become frightened by seeing, or listening to, ardent lovemaking.

Remember that sex is more than reproduction. Nothing you tell your child about the "facts of life" can be as important as seeing and knowing for himself—from your example—what a good relationship between a man and a woman means in terms of mutual respect, loyalty, teamwork, and tenderness.

Masturbation

Take it for granted that your child is going to masturbate. Babies play with their genitals just as

they play with their toes. Unless their attention is concentrated in this area—because of an inflammation or irritation, or because of the disapproving attitude of their parents—no bad habits or physical or emotional harm can result. (For a fuller discussion, see Chapter 17 and the entry MASTURBATION in the encyclopedia section.)

The Only Child

There is no reason why an only child should have special problems—unless you help create them by feeling guilty because you do not provide a brother or sister. From the time he is about two years old he should, of course, have contact with other children, if only to watch them play. As the child grows older, make your house a pleasant place to visit, and permit him to play at other homes. A good nursery school can be very helpful. Make a particular effort to see to it that your child has companionship during the preschool period.

Jealousy (Sibling Rivalry)

Parents should remember that jealousy is painful and that pain can have bad effects. Of course, jealousy between brothers and sisters cannot be prevented entirely, and under no circumstances should children get the impression that they should conceal their feelings to avoid parental disapproval. Sensitive parents can help their children overcome reactions of jealousy, which are, after all, quite natural.

The first child is always going to have to adjust to sharing the limelight when a second child is born. Make the situation as easy for the first child as you can, while at the same time respecting the rights of the second. The new baby will not be emotionally harmed if you refrain from talking about him constantly in front of his older brother or sister. Let your children know that they are not alike and that you would not want them to be, because you love them both, just as they are.

Incidentally, this is good advice for parents of twins, too. While it is a great time-saver for the parents to buy two of everything, it is really a denial of the individuality of each twin to dress them alike. Identical twins will discover for themselves the "which-is-which?" games that they can play on strangers. In the meantime, it is more helpful for them to explore their natural differences.

The Adopted Child

Even more than your natural child, an adopted child needs to know that you love him. Should you tell him he is adopted? By all means. Let him know about it indirectly at first, mentioning it casually and happily in his presence even before he is old enough to understand fully. When he does ask questions, answer them freely. Adopted children have enormous curiosity about their real parents. This is a natural curiosity so do not be evasive. And yet, within that framework, do try to convey to the child the assurance that the natural parents liked him or her but, for good reasons, felt that it would be better for the child if they let him or her be your little boy or girl, an arrangement that makes you very happy.

The Handicapped Child

Most handicapped children will grow up to associate with people who are not handicapped. Therefore, the handicapped should not be segregated. But the special treatments and/or additional schooling that they often require should, in most cases, be started when they are very young.

Often a parent will understandably go too far to make everything easier for a handicapped child. Some years ago an experiment was conducted with a group of handicapped children. They spent the morning playing with each other and with toys that they managed to manipulate quite successfully. For lunch they were served foods that had to be cut with knife and fork, and most of the children were able to perform the task without difficulty. The youngsters who needed help were aided either by the other children or by staff members. When dessert was served, the children's mothers were allowed into the room. As each parent ran to her child, the youngsters' voices changed: the babble of a bunch of happy kids turned into the whining of dependent cripples. Many who had been feeding themselves moments before now needed their mothers to hold their glasses of milk. There is a fine line between being helpful and being over-solicitous.

SCHOOL AND YOUR CHILD'S HEALTH

A good school keeps an eye on the child's physical progress. Records are kept of his height, weight, general health, eyesight, and hearing that are useful to the school and also to the child's regular physician. A good school is also aware of the child's intellectual and emotional development, and of any problems that may arise. The school should either supply or recommend competent assistance when necessary.

The school is an adjunct to the home. Wise parents will cooperate with teachers to make it a beneficial place for the child.

Nursery School and Kindergarten

Most children between the ages of three and six benefit from a good nursery school and later on from kindergarten. They give children a sound introduction to the world around them and a start in playing and being with other children and associating with adults other than their parents. The preschool classes also give the mother a needed respite from the constant demands of her children.

Unfortunately, there are relatively few good, inexpensive nursery schools in most communities. Many mothers have formed cooperative groups and have created excellent schools. With your neighbors you may be able to start a good nursery school in your own area if one does not already exist.

Special Classes

Many children derive great pleasure from attending classes in music, art, crafts, dance, or exercise. These are usually offered as part of cultural enrichment programs by community organizations such as the YMCA and YWCA. Museums also have children's workshops. The specialists who conduct these classes can often inspire a child's imagination, uncover a hidden talent, and possibly provide him with a lifelong interest.

If these kinds of programs are not available in your community, you may want to learn if any of the adults in your community have special skills and would be willing to devote time to such children's activities.

TELEVISION

No discussion of child-rearing today is complete without some reference to the place of television in the child's development. While there is much that is good in children's programming, the unselective use of television to keep the child out of the mother's way is deplorable and dangerous. We are only beginning to learn the effects of a constant diet of TV on our children; but we already know that it adversely affects attention span, reading level, and emotional development. In short, carefully select the programs you allow your child to see, limit the time he is permitted to spend in front of the TV set, and do not use the tube as an electronic baby-sitter.

16 Sicknesses of Infants and Children

Sickness in infancy and childhood cannot be avoided; even the healthiest child will have his share of ailments. Therefore, all parents should be well acquainted with the various childhood illnesses and their symptoms. Such knowledge will not only keep you from needlessly panicking at the unknown, but will help you protect your child from some illnesses and avoid complications in others. This chapter is a guide to the sicknesses common to infants and children. It tells you how to recognize when your child is ill, at what point you should call the doctor, and what you should or should not do until you reach him. Some ailments, such as the common cold, need only a "tincture of time" and proper parental care—but you still must be able to tell when a cold may be developing into something more serious, such as bronchitis. Other sicknesses—such as croup, convulsions brought on by high fever, and an ordinary nosebleed—come on so fast that you will have to deal with them before you can take time to call the doctor.

HOW TO TELL WHEN YOUR CHILD IS ILL

Babies cannot tell us that they are sick. Children under the age of three cannot be relied on to call our attention to their symptoms of illness. Even older children may become so frightened or drowsy at the onset of sickness that they fail to alert us to their condition. It is the responsibility of parents and others who take care of children at home and at school to learn to recognize the sick child by certain changes in his behavior or his appearance.

Signs of Illness in Infants

Not only are infants unable to tell us they are ill, but parents have more difficulty in spotting their symptoms than those of older children. An infant, for example, can be quite sick and not have fever, which in older babies and children is often one of the surest signs of a problem. It is also harder to diagnose diarrhea in an infant, whose stools may normally be quite loose or frequent. (For a discussion of diarrhea in infants see chapter 14.)

But there *are* ways to tell whether your infant is ill. For instance, you may notice a difference in his cry—cries of hunger or for attention are different from cries of pain. He may become lethargic or lose interest in feeding. His spitting up of milk may have turned into true vomiting, or his diaper may be dry for a long period of time. He may have difficulty in breathing. If you even *suspect* that an infant is displaying any one of these symptoms, call your doctor. Do not wait to be sure that the infant is really ill and do not attempt home medication. Let your doctor decide on a course of action based on your description of what is happening.

Symptoms in Babies and Older Children

You should suspect illness in an older baby or a small child if he shows any of the following symptoms:

- He is drowsy at a time of day when he is usually alert.
- He is irritable or loses his appetite. He has repeated episodes of vomiting or diarrhea.
- He is pale and cold, or flushed and hot.
- He has nasal congestion, a cough, or breathing difficulties.
- His output of urine decreases markedly.

Any one of these signs should be reported immediately to your doctor.

Reporting Symptoms to the Doctor

When you call the doctor, he will ask you for specific information. For example, if there is diarrhea, he will ask about the frequency, color, and consistency of the stools. Be prepared to answer his questions. Also, before you call, undress the child and inspect his skin for rashes, and take his temperature. Your report can be a valuable aid to the doctor in deciding whether or not he should see your child immediately.

In older babies and small children the onset of an infection is usually accompanied by fever, a useful "early warning system" for detecting illness. An accurate reading of your child's temperature is therefore important to both you and your doctor. In the following sections we will discuss the various methods of taking a temperature, at what point a rise in temperature is a signal for you to call the doctor, and how to care for a child with a fever.

When you report a child's temperature to the doctor, tell him whether you took an oral, rectal, or axillary (armpit) reading, because the rectal temperature will be slightly higher than the oral—about half a degree, or 0.5° F—and the axillary temperature about a half a degree lower.

THE THERMOMETER

There are two kinds of thermometer, *oral* and *rectal*, which are distinguished only by the shape of the bulb: the rectal thermometer has a shorter, blunter bulb than the oral type. The rectal thermometer is also less fragile and has the advantage of being suitable for oral use as well. But do not use a mouth thermometer in the rectum.

How to Read a Thermometer

The thermometer bulb is filled with mercury that moves up the tube as the temperature rises. When you read the thermometer, hold the end opposite the bulb and turn the tube until you see the column of mercury. Each long line on a Fahrenheit thermometer represents one degree, while each short line measures two-tenths of one degree. The point at which the top of the column stops registers the child's temperature. For example, if it stops at the first short line after the longer line marked 100° on a Fahrenheit thermometer (see the entry FAHRENHEIT in the encyclopedia section), the temperature reading is 100.2° F.

At one place on the thermometer, three short lines above 98° F, there is an arrow that points to 98.6°. This is considered to be the "normal" temperature. Above this point, most thermometers continue the markings in red.

Taking the Temperature

Until a child is about six years old, it is safer and more reliable to take rectal or axillary temperatures because most young children—especially those with upper respiratory infections—can't keep their mouths closed properly around an oral thermometer. There is also the danger that very young children may bite the thermometer.

Before taking the temperature, hold the thermometer tightly at the end opposite the bulb—and shake it with a strong twist of your wrist, until the mercury is below the 97° mark. (Shake it over a bed or pillow, so that it won't break if it slips out of your hand.)

Taking a Rectal Reading. Cover the bulb with petroleum jelly or cold cream so that it can be inserted into the rectum easily. The best way to take an infant's temperature is to place him on his abdomen across your knees. Push the thermometer gently into his rectum—no more than one inch—and hold it in place between two fingers with your palm flat across the buttocks, so that you can pull it out quickly if the child moves suddenly. Never let go of the thermometer. Leave it in about two minutes if you can, but if the child is struggling, one minute is enough. An older child can lie in bed on his side, with his knees drawn up to make it easier to insert the thermometer.

Axillary (Armpit) Temperature. Axillary readings are not quite as accurate as rectal ones, but sometimes a child is frightened and will put up a struggle at having his temperature taken rectally. In such a case, unless the doctor instructs you otherwise, take the temperature by the axillary method.

Use a rectal thermometer. After removing the child's shirt, place the bulb end in the deepest part of the armpit. Hold his arm tightly against his chest, and keep it closed over the thermometer for five minutes.

Mouth Temperature. When a child is able to hold a thermometer properly in his mouth, take oral temperatures unless your doctor specifically requests another method. Keep the thermometer in the mouth for at least three minutes. Do not take an oral reading immediately after the child has eaten or drunk anything hot or cold.

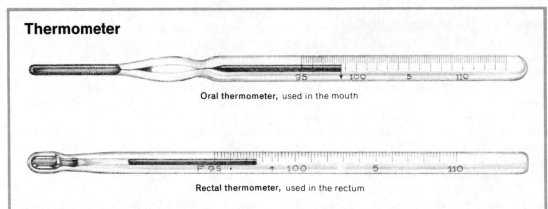

Thermometer

Oral thermometer, used in the mouth

Rectal thermometer, used in the rectum

There are two types of clinical, or medical, thermometers: the oral type, used for taking the temperature in the mouth, and the rectal type, used by inserting it into the rectum. A rectal thermometer should be employed only by someone skilled in its use. Before using a clinical thermometer, shake it briskly so that most of the mercury returns down the stem and into the bulb.

What Your Child's Temperature Means

Do not worry if the temperature in an otherwise healthy child is either a little above or a little below the 98.6° F reading. Temperatures in both children and adults vary according to such factors as physical exertion and time of day. Immediately after running or other violent exercise, a child may have a temperature of 100° F with no sign of illness. Ordinarily, most people's temperatures are lowest in the early morning and highest in the late afternoon.

By itself, fever is not necessarily an indication of the gravity of a particular disease. A child can be quite sick with a low fever or have a relatively high fever during a mild, passing illness. But most sicknesses in babies and small children do have fever as a symptom. If your child has a temperature of 100° or 101° F with no other signs of illness or discomfort, you can wait before calling the doctor. Take the temperature every three hours, and notify the doctor if it rises above 101° F. However, if a low fever persists for more than a day, or suddenly returns in a child who has apparently been recovering from an illness, call the doctor. Always record the time when the temperature was taken and the method used— oral, rectal, or axillary—as well as the temperature itself.

Until the doctor sees your child, keep him quiet, in bed if possible, and away from other people in case his illness is contagious. If he has lost his appetite, do not try to make him eat, but *give him liquids frequently, in small amounts.* (What you give will depend on whether he has been vomiting and/or has diarrhea. See the sec-

tion on "Vomiting, Diarrhea, and Dehydration" later in this chapter.) Keeping the child from becoming dehydrated is extremely important. Small amounts of water, cola, ginger ale (or diluted skim milk for infants), given frequently, are usually well tolerated. Do not bundle up a feverish child, but make sure his room is comfortably warm (about 70° F) and draft-free. If he has a respiratory infection, use a vaporizer to humidify the room.

FEBRILE CONVULSIONS

Although most children never have febrile convulsions—seizures brought on by a rapid rise in temperature or by a very high fever—they are not uncommon. They occur mainly in babies and in children under four, and often accompany otherwise harmless viral diseases such as roseola (see that entry in the encyclopedia section).

A febrile seizure is extremely frightening to parents, but it is not usually dangerous. Just before the convulsion, the child is likely to be trembly and irritable. Suddenly he stiffens, his eyes roll back, and his muscles tense and move spasmodically. He may pass urine and feces, his breathing is temporarily impaired, and his jaws clamp tightly together. The seizure lasts only a few seconds to a few minutes, but they seem like hours to the child's parents. As recommended in the FIRST AID section of this book, put the child on the floor or on a wide bed, placing him on his side. Force his mouth open and insert a rolled handkerchief or washcloth between his teeth on one side of his mouth to keep him from biting his tongue and to keep his mouth open, so that in case he vomits or gags he won't choke. You need not restrain his body in any other way, as long as you keep him from falling or bruising himself. Do not leave the child alone while he is having the seizure, but call the doctor as soon as possible. If you cannot reach him immediately, cool the child's body when the seizure is over. An alcohol rub, sponge bath, or cool tub bath will help. Once you have brought the fever down, put the child to bed in light pajamas and cover him with a sheet. Bundling him up may make the fever rise again.

Occasionally, fevers as low as 102° F have been known to trigger convulsions in sensitive children, especially if the temperature has risen rapidly. All children who have had a seizure should be examined by the doctor as soon as possible. He may want to prescribe an anticonvulsant such as phenobarbital to help prevent a recurrence. (See the entry PHENOBARBITAL in the encyclopedia section.) But whatever treatment is prescribed, it is important for the parents to treat the child calmly, not to show fright, and not to make the child feel like an invalid. He is not.

A seizure that occurs when no fever is present is another condition entirely and requires even more careful investigation by the child's doctor. It may be an indication of epilepsy (for further discussion, see both EPILEPSY and CONVULSION in the encyclopedia section). Immediate action—preventing the child from biting his tongue or otherwise injuring himself—is the same as for a febrile convulsion.

A WARNING ABOUT MEDICINES

When a doctor examines a sick child, he immediately tries to determine whether the disease was caused by bacteria or viruses. An estimated three-quarters of all childhood respiratory infections, including the common cold, are viral. Because viruses are rarely affected by an antibiotic, your physician will probably not prescribe the drug even if a fever is present. He will employ such a medicine only if he knows, or strongly suspects, that a bacterial infection is present. Moreover, certain antibiotics can produce allergic reactions or other harmful side effects and must be used only when they are needed to combat a serious bacterial infection, such as strep throat. But when the doctor does prescribe an antibiotic, make sure your child completes taking the prescribed amount. If you stop giving the medicine as soon as he begins to feel better, the infection is likely to recur.

Never use any medicine left over from a previous illness, without consulting the doctor. The penicillin or cough medicine that was good for one illness or one person can be harmful for someone else. Laxatives, cathartics, and enemas should never be given without a doctor's advice. Aspirin should never be given in a dosage greater than the doctor recommends, and you must make sure you understand his instructions—"grains" of aspirin are not the same as "tablets."

CHILDREN'S ACCIDENTS

The leading cause of death in the age group up to 14 years is accidents, and the only way to help protect your child against them is to remove the hazards. (Safety measures for infants are described in Chapter 14.) As soon as your child is old enough to move around on his own, start "baby-proofing" your house or apartment. Install secure gates at the top and bottom of all open staircases. Keep electric cords out of the child's reach and cover all unused outlets with a heavy plastic tape. Install tight-fitting screens or protective grates on all windows, especially on high floors, or insert screws that prevent the windows from being raised more than a few inches. Remove sharp, breakable, or otherwise dangerous objects from low tables. Make sure your home is free from lead-based paints. Interior house paints have not had lead in them for years, but in some old houses there may still be layers of lead-based paints under recent coats. Keep all medicines, polishes, cleaning fluids, and other potentially dangerous substances in securely locked cabinets that a child cannot possibly open—not on open shelves, no matter how high. Above all, always keep a baby or small child in sight, unless he is in a secure crib or playpen. Other measures you can take will occur to you as you watch your own child in action; and when he is old enough to understand, you can start teaching him how to avoid dangerous situations. (For information on what to do if an accident does occur, see the FIRST AID section.)

Poisoning

A young child's curiosity often takes the form of putting objects into his mouth and of tasting things—no matter how unlikely or repulsive they may seem to an adult. Children will ingest all kinds of medicines, vitamins, pills, household cleaners, poisonous plants and berries, even cigarette butts and the dregs of alcoholic drinks. All these things can be dangerous for a child, and it is your responsibility as a parent to keep them out of his way.

In the event that poisoning does occur, have on hand—securely locked away—these two items: syrup of ipecac, to induce vomiting, and charcoal suspension, an all-purpose emergency antidote. Keep the telephone number of the nearest poison-control center or hospital emergency room next to the telephone. If you suspect your child has ingested any poisonous substance, call for help immediately. You *must* try to find out what the child has swallowed, because it is vital for anyone treating the child to know what he has taken. With some poisons, such as aspirin, vomiting should be induced; but it must *not* be done with others, such as caustics and petroleum products. If you cannot get immediate advice by telephone, take the child to the nearest doctor or emergency room without delay, and be sure to bring along the container and any remaining poisonous substance. (For further information on the treatment of poisoning, see the FIRST AID section.)

CANCER IN CHILDREN

Although cancer is rare in children, it accounts for more deaths up to the age of 14 than any other single disease. Leukemia, Hodgkin's disease, and cancer of the kidney are the most common types occurring in children. But great advances have been made—and are continuing to be made—in treating these afflictions. An important factor in the success of treatment is early diagnosis.

The cause of *leukemia* is a disorderly, widespread overproduction of white blood cells which results in anemia, easy bruising, fever, loss of weight and appetite, and nausea.

A child with *Hodgkin's disease*—which affects the lymph nodes, especially those of the neck—experiences loss of appetite, fatigue, fluctuating temperature, and sometimes an enlarged lymph node.

The primary symptom of *Wilms's tumor*—the most common type of kidney cancer in children and one that usually develops before a child is three—is a firm mass that causes the abdomen to swell. In reading about these symptoms, remember that many of them are also the symptoms of other, much less serious illnesses—such as mononucleosis and anemia—and that the odds are strongly against a child's getting cancer. The important thing is to report promptly any of the symptoms to your doctor.

UPPER RESPIRATORY INFECTIONS

Upper respiratory infections—a group of illnesses that includes the common cold and viral and bacterial infections of the ear, nose, and throat—are the most common afflictions of youngsters. Children are usually far more susceptible to these infections than adults, and, unfortunately, can build up resistance to them only through repeated exposure. As most parents know, a child seems to be sick as often as he is well during his first year or two of school—usually his initial experiences with crowds of children in close quarters.

Colds

Colds are not much of a problem in themselves, but they can lead to more serious respiratory infections. If a child's cold is persistent or suddenly gets worse, consult the doctor. Be especially alert for earaches, sore throat, persistent cough, increased or recurrent fever, swollen eyes, a thick or greenish nasal discharge, or a stiff neck. Any of these symptoms may mean that a more serious infection is also present.

You can help reduce the frequency or severity of colds by not letting your child get overtired or chilled. However, it is a mistake to put too much clothing on him or to keep him indoors in an overheated room. Not only is hot, dry air irritating to the nasal passages, but the ability to adjust to temperature changes decreases when a child spends most of his time in an overheated house. (In general, a good indoor temperature is 68° F to 70° F in the daytime and 60° F at night.) All healthy children, except very young infants, should be outdoors several hours a day in good weather so that their bodies become accustomed to colder air.

Treating a Cold. Keep a child with a cold in a comfortably warm, draft-free room, in bed if possible, at least for the first day. A vaporizer or humidifier (safely out of reach) will help him breathe more comfortably. If he is feverish, make sure that you encourage him to drink small quantities of fluid often.

Older children with colds usually respond well to the simple routine of rest, plentiful fluids, and aspirin for fever and discomfort. Unless fever is present, the child need not be confined to bed. Consult your doctor before administering decongestants or nose drops to shrink swollen mucous membranes. Drops can be severely irritating to the nasal passages. With older children, too, you must watch for signs—such as high fever and persistent coughing—which may mean secondary infections.

Colds in Infants. An infant with a cold is especially uncomfortable because he breathes primarily through his nose. He snorts, gasps, and has considerable difficulty feeding. Two simple measures will relieve a baby's mucus-plugged nose: (1) Set up a vaporizer. It works best in a small room with the windows closed. (2) Loosen the mucus by putting in the nostrils a few drops of warm sterile water. After a few minutes, gently draw out the mucus with a rubber-tipped nasal syringe: Compress the bulb of the syringe, insert it into the nostril, and then slowly release it.

Infants with colds may be so fretful that their parents rush them to the doctor. While the trip may be unnecessary, it is usually prudent to let the doctor take at least a brief look at the baby. And be sure to see the physician if there are signs of a secondary infection, such as fever over 101° F, persistent vomiting, high-pitched fretful crying (which may indicate earache), a severe cough, unusual pallor or listlessness, or rapid heavy breathing.

Sore Throats

A sore throat may be caused either by a virus or by streptococcal bacteria. Sore throats accompanied by other respiratory symptoms, such as nasal congestion, are likely to be viral; whereas an uncomplicated sore throat with fever is more likely to be caused by strep bacteria. The only way to be sure of the cause, however, is for the doctor to make a throat culture. If persistent, even the mildest sore throat should be so tested, as should the more painful cases and those in which fever or swollen glands are present. If there is a strep infection, the doctor will probably prescribe penicillin or another antibiotic. If you give your child the entire dosage for the prescribed number of days, the infection should readily clear up. The doctor may then want to take another culture to be sure that the infection has been cured. Early diagnosis and prompt treatment of strep throats are vital because the possible complications, rheumatic fever and nephritis, are extremely dangerous.

Tonsillitis. The tonsils, located in the back of the mouth at either side of the entrance to the throat, have the same purpose as lymph glands—to waylay and destroy germs. But sometimes the

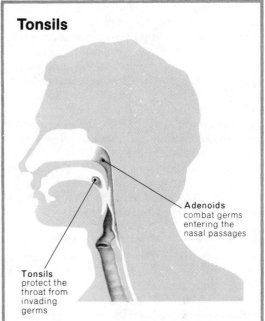

Tonsils

Adenoids combat germs entering the nasal passages

Tonsils protect the throat from invading germs

The tonsils are a pair of glands at the back of the throat. Together with the adenoids, they play a part in guarding the body against germs entering by way of the nose and mouth. Infection and inflammation of the tonsils cause the sore throat of tonsillitis. If a child's tonsils become repeatedly infected, a doctor may advise that they be removed surgically by the operation called tonsillectomy. Often the surgeon takes the opportunity to remove the patient's adenoids at the same time, if they are diseased.

tonsils get overloaded by a heavy invasion of germs and become infected. When this happens, the tonsils may cause a high fever that may last for several days, vomiting and headache, and a throat so sore that the child can hardly swallow. Like other sore throats, tonsillitis can be caused by either bacteria or viruses and must be treated by a doctor.

Adenoidal Infection. The adenoids, located in the throat behind the nasal passages, guard these passages against germs as the tonsils do the throat. When adenoids become infected and enlarged, they partially block the outlet from the nose and the child is forced to breathe chiefly through his mouth. Enlarged adenoids may also block the Eustachian tubes to the middle ear, causing swelling, pain, and middle-ear infection, as well as temporary interference with hearing.

Tonsillectomy and Adenoidectomy. The popularity of these operations—usually performed simultaneously and known as a "T&A"—was at its height a number of years ago when it was thought that such surgery would prevent recurrent colds and other respiratory infections. Today, however, physicians are aware that any operation, no matter how simple, carries with it a certain risk. Also they recognize that removal of the tonsils or the adenoids cures only those problems directly related to them, such as recurrent tonsillitis and middle-ear infection. Neither procedure prevents respiratory infections. Therefore, doctors usually recommend surgery only for children who have serious and recurrent infections in the tonsils and adenoids. (See TONSILLECTOMY in the encyclopedia section.)

Earaches and Middle-Ear Infections

Earaches in young children are both common and extremely painful. Germs from colds, sore throats, and infected adenoids or tonsils can travel from the throat region through either Eustachian tube to the middle ear, just behind the eardrum. Infections in the middle-ear chamber, in turn, produce pressure on the eardrum, causing the pain. Because the Eustachian tube in a young child is relatively short, the infection hasn't far to go in order to reach this chamber. Any child who has had a cold or other respiratory infection followed by acute pain in, or discharge from, the ear (often accompanied by fever, vomiting, and headache) should see a doctor immediately. Treatment may include aspirin and/or eardrops for the relief of pain, decongestants to reduce inflammation, and antibiotics to combat the infection itself, if it is bacterial. Children who experience recurrent or chronic middle-ear infections sometimes suffer a temporary hearing loss because of them. In such cases, the doctor may recommend surgical draining of the ear (myringotomy) to rid the middle-ear chamber of fluids.

A baby or young child with an ear infection often cannot tell the parents where the pain is coming from. Therefore, notify the doctor if the boy or girl cries without letup or shows other signs of acute or prolonged discomfort, or if the child experiences loss of appetite, vomiting, and diarrhea.

Swimmer's Ear. Another type of infection, common in summer, is "swimmer's ear." It affects the external ear canal and can be fungal, bacterial, or both. The warmth and wetness of the ears of children who swim a great deal give such infections an ideal breeding ground. Consult the doctor if your child complains of a persistent sensation of water in his ear, or if his ear hurts when you gently wiggle it.

Swollen Glands. Swelling of glands in the neck often accompanies other kinds of viral or bacterial infections. If the swelling comes and goes, if the glands are not tender and do not make the child uncomfortable, there is likely to be no immediate problem. But if the glands are large and very firm, or if the area is painful and the child has fever, notify the doctor. In the case of mumps, for instance, the parotid glands—lying in the areas beneath the earlobes—become swollen and acutely painful. Swollen glands that persist for a week or more, even if they cause no discomfort, should be checked by the doctor.

Sinusitis

The nasal sinuses are air-filled hollows in the skull near the nose. They are tiny in a very young child, but enlarge as he or she grows. The sinuses are highly subject to infection, although less so in children than in adults. A small opening connects each sinus with the inside of the nose. During a cold, infection may spread from the nose to the sinuses, which become clogged with mucus that can drip down from the back of the nose into the throat. This postnasal drip may cause a dry, hacking cough, especially when the child is lying down. Severe sinusitis may result in fever and a headache, which is often felt just behind the eyes and which may respond better to the use of decongestants than to aspirin. Ask your doctor. (See SINUS and SINUSITIS in the encyclopedia section.)

FOREIGN BODIES

Young children like to experiment, and many of them push foreign objects—bits of crayons, buttons, anything—into their noses, ears, and other body openings without telling their parents about it. If your child discharges pus from *one* nostril or ear, take him to the doctor. If the cause is a foreign object, it is risky to try to get it out yourself.

NOSEBLEEDS

Nosebleeds are quite common in children whose nasal passages have been irritated by infection or by dry, hot air. A poke of the finger into the irritated nostril may set off the bleeding. Nosebleeds can usually be stopped by simple pressure.

Have the child sit up, with his head thrown back, and gently but firmly hold his nostrils pinched shut for at least 10 minutes (preferably 20) while he breathes through his mouth. Repeat if necessary, and if the treatment does not work the second time, call the doctor. A doctor should examine a child who has frequent, severe nosebleeds with no apparent cause.

LOWER RESPIRATORY INFECTIONS

The lower respiratory tract resembles a tree turned upside down. On top of the main trunk sits the voice box (larynx). Beneath it lies the windpipe (trachea), which divides into left and right branches (the main-stem bronchi), and then into smaller branches (bronchioles) before reaching the "leaves" (alveoli) of the lungs. Lower respiratory diseases may be more serious than are infections of the upper respiratory tract. But illnesses of the lower tract usually respond well to treatment, and a number of them are entirely preventable. As with all children's illnesses, it is important to recognize symptoms early.

Coughs and Other Symptoms

Like a fever, a cough is a symptom of illness, not a disease in itself. The forceful expulsion of breath is the body's attempt to rid itself of something that is irritating the air passages. Just as fevers vary in degree, coughs vary in kind; learning to recognize the different kinds of cough is important in deciding when to call the doctor.

The dry, hacking cough that accompanies the common cold is usually caused by mucus dripping from the nose to the back of the throat and either irritating the throat or blocking the passageway. You can relieve this kind of cough by propping the child up with extra pillows and by using a vaporizer and, if recommended by the doctor, decongestant cough medicine.

Much more serious is a severe, deep cough that comes in spasms and may be followed by vomiting. Such a cough can indicate an infection in the bronchial tubes or lungs. You should also be suspicious of a brassy, echoing, barking cough, especially if there is a labored intake of air. It may signal the onset of croup (see following description). Any severe, persistent, or painful cough requires prompt treatment by the doctor.

A child with one or more of the following symptoms—especially if accompanied by a fever—should be checked for possible infection of the bronchi or lungs: severe, deep cough; chest pain; shortness of breath or labored breathing; poor color.

Cough Medicines. Parents often ask why the cough medicine prescribed for their child does not stop the cough. The answer is that in ridding the lower respiratory tract of foreign matter, such as mucus, the cough serves a useful purpose. Most cough medicines are meant not to stop this natural reflex but to loosen and thin the mucus, to shrink swollen membranes, and to limit the production of new mucus. But if a cough is severe enough and interferes with a child's sleep, for example, the doctor may prescribe a suppressant.

Croup

Croup involves an inflammation and obstruction of the larynx. It is usually caused by viruses but sometimes results from bacterial infection. In a typical case of acute spasmodic croup (the most common kind), the child starts off with a mild upper respiratory infection and low-grade fever, followed by the hoarseness that characterizes laryngitis. Then, usually late at night, the characteristic ringing, barking cough begins. The child usually awakens in fright because he has trouble catching his breath between coughs.

Croup most often occurs in winter and spring and usually attacks children between two and four years of age. A child is naturally terrified by his inability to breathe properly, so *it is most important to keep calm yourself and to help him breathe by getting him into humid air at once*. If possible, have someone else set up a vaporizer in the child's room and call the doctor, while you take the youngster into the bathroom, close the door, and turn on all the hot-water taps to humidify the air quickly. Sit with the child and talk to him quietly, or read him a story, until his breathing improves. If it doesn't, or if his color turns bluish from lack of air, call the doctor immediately or take the child to the hospital.

Most children are sufficiently relieved by the "steam room" treatment to go to bed comfortably afterward. In fact, many of them—except during the attacks themselves—do not seem very sick. But you should keep the humidity high in the child's bedroom until the infection is gone; and for two or three nights a parent should stay in the room with him, in the event of another attack.

If the croup is severe, accompanied by fever of 103° F or higher, and the attack persists into the next morning, the cause may be bacterial and the
(continued on page 208)

KEEPING A SICK CHILD AMUSED

A child getting over an illness can find the day seems extremely long as soon as he or she is well enough to sit up. Concentration is not as lasting when a child is sick as when he is well, and he soon gets bored unless his occupations are varied. But do not give the child everything at once: give him only one thing at a time. Sick or convalescent children occupy themselves best with things they can manage easily: give them toys and games normally suitable for a slightly younger age group than their own. Jigsaw puzzles, if not too complicated, are popular with most children. But if the child is very young, you will have to tell him stories and read to him; and he will take up even more of your time playing with him. Make the periods you spend with the child each day as regular as you can. Bricks and kits suitable for all ages from two-and-a-half upward can be bought at most toy shops, but many simple items can be made at home with little expense. All require some parental participation—even if only at first. Give the child a surface to work on, such as a piece of hardboard or a large tray. Older children can be given materials for scrapbooks.

Paper-chain figures

Fold a piece of paper into a concertina shape. Draw half the shape on the top surface of the concertina folds with the connecting piece of the shape at the edge of the paper. If a curved chain is required, draw the shape at a slight angle. Remember when cutting out the shape that the connections between the figures are at the folds of the paper, so ensure that any cuts you make do not meet there.

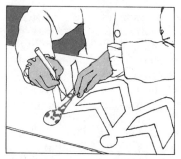

1 Use a piece of paper about 30 centimetres long. Seven concertina folds make four complete figures.

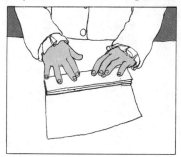

2 Draw half the shape with the narrow connecting parts at the edge of the paper, not the fold.

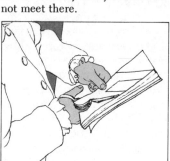

3 Cut around the drawn outline through all the paper. Do not let the cuts meet at the folds.

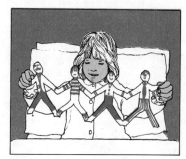

4 Unfold the pattern to reveal the chain. Lay it on a flat surface to color the figures.

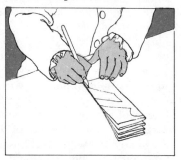

5 In addition to human figures, trees, flowers, birds and animals are suitable shapes for cutting.

Pipe-cleaner figures

Amusing human and animal figures can be made from pipe cleaners. Buy several packets, including colored ones. Twist two cleaners around each other to form a body. Arms and legs are made by separating one pair of ends or by adding more cleaners. Make the heads from modeling clay, and clothes from colored paper. Support the figures by gluing or fixing with thumbtacks to matchboxes.

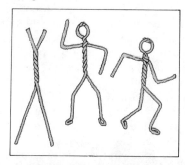

1 Twist two cleaners to form the head, body and legs of a person. Arms are shaped from a third one.

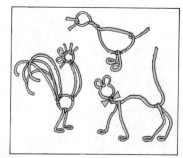

2 Twist the ends only and open out the centers to form the rounded bodies of animals.

Thread patterns

Fix 12 small nails or panel-pins in a circle 12 inches across on a piece of plywood or hardboard. Nail them in the positions of the hours on a clock to get them evenly spaced. Give the child a good supply of cotton or wool, and show him how to stretch it from pin to pin, around the circle and across it, to form patterns and shapes. Use short lengths of different-colored wools to make colored patterns.

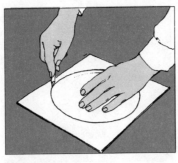

1 Draw a circle around a plate or tin lid about 12 inches across on a piece of hardboard.

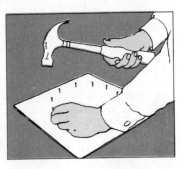

2 Remove the plate and hammer in 12 panel-pins around the drawn circle (a parent should do this).

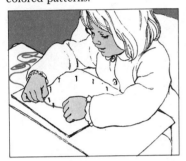

3 Tie one end of the cotton or wool to any one of the pins and push the knot down to the base.

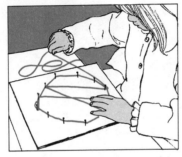

4 Take the thread from pin to pin; keep it continuous unless different colors are used.

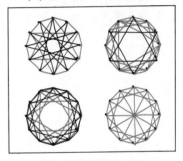

5 More intricate patterns can be formed by joining crossings of the thread already made.

Pom-pom balls

Pom-poms for sewing onto hats or the ends of scarves are easily and quickly made with two cardboard rings and some wool. The diameter of the rings determines the lengths of the wool in the pom-pom—the wider the rings, the bigger will be the pom-pom; and the more wool you wind around the rings, the denser it will be. Secure the end of the wool under one of the windings if changing to a different color, but do not tie.

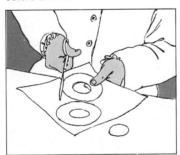

1 Cut two disks out of cardboard and make a half-inch hole in the center of each.

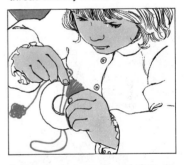

2 Put the two cardboard rings together and wind wool around and around through the hole.

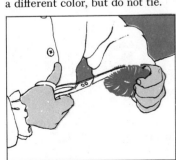

3 Cut the wool with a knife or scissors all around between the outer edges of the two rings.

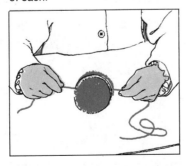

4 Tie the pieces tightly at the center, between the cardboard rings, with string or thread.

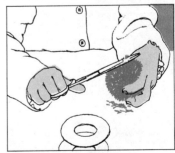

5 Remove the cardboard rings and trim any long lengths of wool to make a regular ball.

Telephone

Most young children are fascinated by a telephone and take every opportunity to answer and use it. Improvise one for a sick child from two 3-inch cans that have lids, such as soup cans. If lidded cans are not available, cut one end off two other cans and bind the cut edges with adhesive tape. With tight string between the two cans, a child can speak into one while another listens in the other.

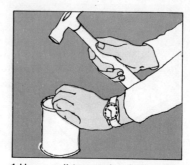

1 Use a nail to punch a hole in the bottoms of the cans, large enough for the string to go through.

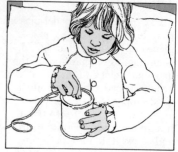

2 Thread the string through the hole in the base of one can and knot it on the inside.

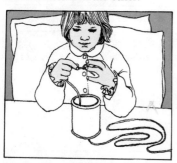

3 Thread the other end of the string from outside to inside of the second can and knot it.

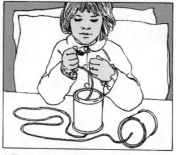

4 The string can be any length required, and the can should be held close to the mouth or ear.

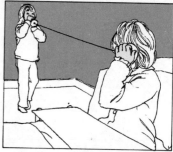

5 Each unit can be used as mouthpiece or receiver when users change from speaking to listening.

Ball puppets

A finger puppet can be made out of a hollow ball—a ping pong ball is ideal. You will need a square piece of cloth, large enough to cover the hand and wrist, for the puppet's dress, which can be decorated around the hem with an odd piece of lace or embroidery. Cut two small "hands" from a light-colored material and sew them onto the dress, and stick small buttons or pieces of cloth onto the ball for the ears.

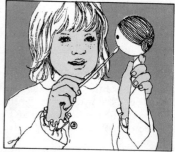

1 Cut a hole in a ping pong ball, large enough to take the end of the first or second finger.

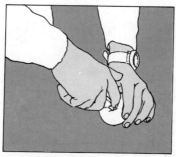

2 Hold the ball on a stick while a face and hair are painted on it; glue on buttons for the ears.

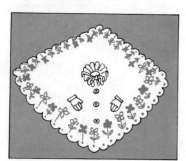

3 Sew a diagonal row of buttons on the dress, and attach a "hand" on each side of the buttons.

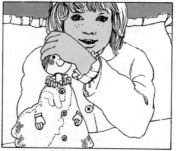

4 Remove the stick, drape the dress over the child's hand and get her to push her finger into the ball.

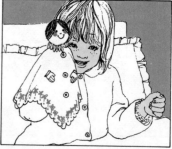

5 The child can then manipulate the puppet by moving her hand and finger inside it.

Potato prints

Scrub two or three large potatoes clean, cut them in two and draw patterns with a soft pencil on the smooth surfaces. Then cut away the potato so that the patterns are raised by about one-eighth of an inch. Remember that they will be reversed when reproduced on paper: irregular patterns such as numbers should be in reverse on the potato. The cutting can be done by the child if he or she is old enough to handle a knife.

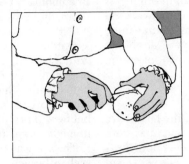

1 Cut the potatoes across so that the two pieces are an easy size for a child to handle.

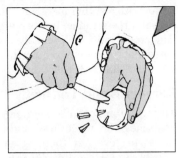

2 Draw patterns on the smooth surfaces and cut around them so that the patterns stand out.

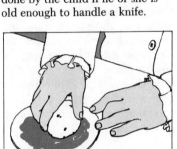

3 Mix some watercolors, or use poster paint, and dip the raised patterns in the coloring.

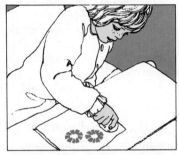

4 Shake off any surplus paint and press the pattern firmly onto a sheet of paper.

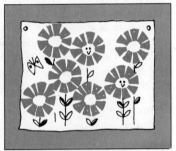

5 One shape, or different shapes, in various colors can produce any pattern required.

Mobiles

Use thin cardboard or stiff paper for the mobiles and draw the shapes required (fish are usually popular with children). Suspend each shape on a separate piece of thin string. Make a hole near the center top of the shape, thread the string through it and knot the string. Alternatively, fix the string to the shape with adhesive tape. Two or three strings can be taped to a coat hanger with the mobiles at different heights.

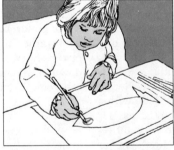

1 Draw the shape of the mobile onto a piece of thin cardboard, postcard, or stiff paper.

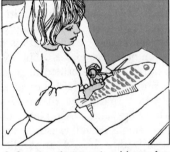

2 Cut the shape out, add any features such as eyes, and color both sides of the shape.

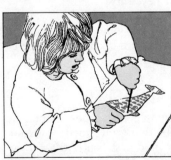

3 Thread thin string through a hole near the top of the center and knot the string.

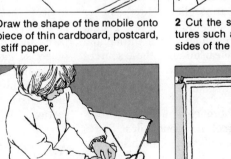

4 Cut the strings to different lengths to vary the heights of the mobiles; tie to a coat hanger.

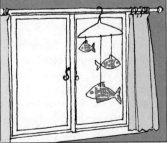

5 Hang the mobiles where there is a draft of air and where they have room to rotate.

207

doctor *must* be consulted. Viral croup often gets better with no other medicine than humid air and parental reassurance, but bacterial croup can be dangerous and will probably require antibiotic treatment. (For more on the treatment of croup, see the FIRST AID section.)

Laryngitis and Tracheitis

The symptoms of inflammation of the larynx are hoarseness or voice loss and sometimes sore throat or fever. If there is an infection, it is usually viral. Have the child rest his voice, keep him in a humid atmosphere, and be alert for symptoms of croup. As noted above, laryngitis is often a forerunner of croup. Sometimes laryngitis is caused or aggravated by an allergy, and then it responds to antihistamine treatment. A hacking cough and voice loss may also indicate tracheitis, usually a viral infection of the windpipe. The condition usually clears up in a few days with rest and a humid atmosphere.

Bronchitis

A cold, flu, or other respiratory infection may spread down into the bronchial tubes and cause bronchitis. Although the child may not feel especially sick, he usually develops a loose, "juicy" cough and brings up a lot of mucus. Often his breath sounds squeaky. Parents cannot always pinpoint a cough as bronchitis, but the doctor can diagnose the illness easily when he listens to the child's chest with a stethoscope; the accumulation of mucus makes a bubbly sound. Antibiotics are often prescribed for bronchitis.

Bronchitis may also be caused by an allergic reaction. In this case the child will exhale with a wheezing sound. Asthmatic bronchitis, as this condition is called, is usually treated with antibiotics and a humid atmosphere. Frequent or chronic bronchitis may be the result of repeated infections in the sinuses, adenoids, or throat, and the problem will not clear up until these sources of infection are properly treated.

Bronchiolitis

There is one type of bronchial infection, bronchiolitis (inflammation of the bronchioles), that is associated with severe difficulty in both inhaling and exhaling. It usually attacks infants and can cause such acute breathing problems that the child has to be hospitalized.

Pneumonia

Like bronchitis, pneumonia, an infection of the lungs' alveoli, may have a variety of causes.

Pneumonia is usually of bacterial origin and can normally be treated effectively with antibiotics, but it is still a serious disease. The commonest symptom is a fever of 101° F to 104° F combined with a hacking cough and chest pain. Twitching or convulsions may also occur when the fever is high. Even with these symptoms, it may be a few days before the doctor can make a firm diagnosis, but he will probably begin appropriate treatment immediately if pneumonia is suspected.

There are a number of "atypical" pneumonias, such as bronchopneumonia and viral pneumonia that are not usually as severe as the bacterial kind. However, they may actually last longer because they are more difficult to treat. If a child has a cold and fever which seem to get better, but he then develops a persistent loose cough, a return of fever, and unusual fatigue, call the doctor promptly. If even a very mild pneumonia is present, the child must rest frequently and keep his activities to an absolute minimum until his chest is completely clear.

Pulmonary Tuberculosis

Tuberculosis is now rare in children, thanks to improved methods of prevention and early detection, notably the TUBERCULIN TEST described in the encyclopedia section. Many schools require this test along with the standard immunizations (see Chapter 14). When the disease does strike children, it often affects the glands of the neck rather than the lungs. Any child with an obviously swollen neck gland that does not go down in a couple of weeks should be checked for tuberculosis infection.

Foreign Bodies in the Lungs

A sudden onset of choking and wheezing may indicate that a child has inhaled a particle of food or some other substance into his lungs. He must be examined by the doctor, who will remove the object surgically if necessary.

For further information on specific lower respiratory ailments, see individual entries such as BRONCHITIS and PNEUMONIA in the encyclopedia section.

ABDOMINAL PROBLEMS

There are many simple bellyaches, caused by eating too much of the wrong foods, by emotional stress, or by mild gastroenteritis—the so-called "24-hour virus." More severe abdominal pain may be owing to any of a number of causes—such as acute bacterial gastroenteritis, appendicitis, intestinal obstruction, or chronic constipation—and should be investigated carefully by the doctor. He should, in fact, be consulted about any persistent abdominal pain.

Signs of Intestinal Obstruction

If a child vomits, has abdominal pain and distension, or swelling, of the abdomen combined with constipation, he may have some form of intestinal obstruction. He requires immediate medical care; the condition is serious and cannot be treated at home. The prolonged absence of bowel movements is a clue, because obstruction blocks the flow of matter through the intestinal tract. Surgery may be necessary. (For further discussion see INTESTINAL OBSTRUCTION in the encyclopedia section.)

Appendicitis. Another condition that requires surgery is appendicitis. The appendix, a tube-shaped appendage in the lower abdomen, becomes infected, and when it does, there is some pain and tenderness in the abdomen—usually in the lower right side but often starting around the navel. Often nausea and vomiting occur, and sometimes diarrhea as well. In a young child, the pain may not be severe enough or other symptoms obvious enough to make the diagnosis certain. Your physician may recommend surgery even if appendicitis is not proved. In this instance, the risk of leaving the condition undetermined is greater than the risk of an operation. (See also APPENDICITIS and APPENDIX in the encyclopedia section.)

Ruptured Spleen

If the spleen, an organ in the upper left section of the abdomen, is injured in an accident, there will be persistent pain and tenderness in the area, followed by symptoms of shock—pallor, sweating, and clamminess of the skin. Should your child have such symptoms, get him to the hospital fast. A ruptured spleen always requires emergency surgery.

Vomiting, Diarrhea, and Dehydration

Infections of the intestinal tract that cause vomiting and diarrhea can range from mild to severe. Viral infections, for example, are usually relatively mild. The bacterial infections such as salmonella and shigella can be quite severe, but they are rare. In general, if the upper part of the intestinal tract is most affected, the child will vomit; if the lower part is, he will have diarrhea. In severe cases there is trouble at both ends, and

often fever as well. Any child who passes watery stools more than once an hour requires immediate medical help, especially if there is vomiting. The younger the child, the sooner he must be treated, because of the possibility of dehydration.

The chief signs of dehydration are: (1) a decrease in the amount of urine and/or a darkening of its color; (2) a doughy look to the skin; (3) sunken eyes; (4) listlessness or extreme drowsiness; and (5) rapid breathing. Consult your doctor promptly if any of these symptoms are present. The younger a child or infant, the more fluid he needs per pound of body weight in order to survive. Therefore, if you cannot reach the doctor immediately, you must take certain measures yourself. For diarrhea alone, give an infant his usual formula, diluted to half strength with boiled water. Offer it frequently in small amounts. An older child may have clear liquids such as ginger ale, cola, or sweetened weak tea, as well as crackers or plain toast. However, if the signs of dehydration worsen, or if the child seems to be seriously ill, do not delay. Take him to the hospital.

If a child is vomiting frequently, you may be able to help him overcome his nausea by giving him a lollipop or cracked ice to suck (not to chew), and then offering plain water or ginger ale in very small amounts. But do not try to treat severe vomiting, especially in an infant, without medical advice. Consult the doctor *at least* within 24 hours of the onset of illness. He will try to pinpoint the cause of the trouble, which may sometimes be food sensitivity rather than infection, and advise you on proper diet as the child gets better.

Chronic Bellyaches

Persistent bellyaches, without severe pain or clear-cut symptoms can have a variety of causes. One of the most common is constipation, which is often experienced by a young child who is upset by toilet training. Under such circumstances, halt the training until the problem clears up. In an older child constipation is often caused by his improper bowel habits—such as getting up late and rushing to school without taking the time to go to the toilet. Nagging bellyaches can also be caused by a parasitic infection (see the discussion of "Worms and Other Parasites" later in this chapter), urinary-tract infections, and emotional stress. The "school-morning" bellyache, for example, occurs in children who are nervous about going to school, but the condition usually clears up magically on weekends.

Urinary-Tract Infections

Any female child who has persistent abdominal pain or pain when urinating should be checked for urinary-tract infection. This type of infection is common in little girls because their urinary tracts are extremely short, and infection can easily pass up through them into the bladder. (See BLADDER in the encyclopedia section.)

ALLERGIES

Some people are highly sensitive to certain substances that have no adverse effects on most of us. Children of allergic parents are likely candidates for allergic reactions, although not necessarily to the same substances. In general, infants and children under two are most apt to be allergic to certain foods; cow's milk, eggs, and wheat are common causes of allergies in this age group. Older children are likely to be allergic to things they inhale, such as pollen or cat's hair.

Allergic reactions take many forms. Among them are skin conditions such as eczema (discussed later in this chapter) and hives (see that entry in the encyclopedia section). Runny and itchy nose and eyes (hay fever) or chronic nasal and chest conditions may also indicate allergy; but because these symptoms can also be caused by infection, the diagnosis is harder to make. Even vomiting and diarrhea may indicate an allergy. Be suspicious if either or both occur just after your child tries a new food, especially if the symptoms are accompanied by wheezing, stuffy nose, or other respiratory distress. Probably the allergic reaction most feared by parents is asthma, a condition that causes wheezing, coughing, breathing difficulty, and a constricted feeling in the chest.

Very mild allergies may require little or no treatment. The child builds up his resistance as he gets older and "outgrows" them. For severe allergies the doctor may prescribe such measures as eliminating the allergy-causing foods from the diet, getting rid of household pets, conducting an all-out battle against dust, and maintaining a constant effort to keep the child away from all substances to which he is known to be sensitive. If allergic attacks interfere greatly with a child's activities, the doctor may recommend skin tests and a series of desensitizing injections.

Some allergies, such as those to certain medicines, are frequently difficult to diagnose. If, for instance, a child has been given penicillin for a disease that turns out to be viral and then a rash develops, the doctor may find it hard to determine whether the rash was caused by allergy or by the virus itself. But penicillin reaction in children is less common than many people suppose.

CLASSIC CHILDHOOD DISEASES

Many contagious diseases, once considered threats to all children, have been nearly eliminated. A properly immunized child should never have to suffer from poliomyelitis, diphtheria, whooping cough, tetanus, measles, German measles, or mumps. (For a full discussion of these diseases see the relevant entries in the encyclopedia section.) There have been no recorded cases of smallpox in the United States since 1949. The American Academy of Pediatrics now recommends against smallpox vaccination. It is important, however, for your child to receive other innoculations at the right time in order for him to get full immunity. The schedule of immunizations recommended by the American Academy of Pediatrics is given in Chapter 13. Communicable diseases are the subject of Chapter 6.

Infants may still carry some of their mothers' antibodies, which help protect them if they are exposed to any of these diseases before immunization. But if an uninoculated infant has been exposed to a contagious disease, report that fact to his doctor.

Chicken Pox

One common childhood disease for which no reliable vaccine has yet been developed is chicken pox. Your child will probably get it sooner or later; but if he is otherwise in good health, getting the illness may be actually beneficial in the long run. The disease is often far more serious in adults than in children, and an attack in childhood confers lifelong immunity.

The time between exposure to chicken pox and onset of the disease (the incubation period) is about two weeks. The rash starts with small red pimples that quickly develop clear blisters; when these dry up, the pimples crust over. Successive crops of pox appear during the illness and the rash is very itchy. Chicken pox is contagious from the day *before* the rash appears and remains so until all the pox scabs have fallen off. (For a full discussion see CHICKEN POX in the encyclopedia section.)

Roseola Infantum

The viral disease known as roseola, which seldom strikes children over the age of three, is charac-

Rash

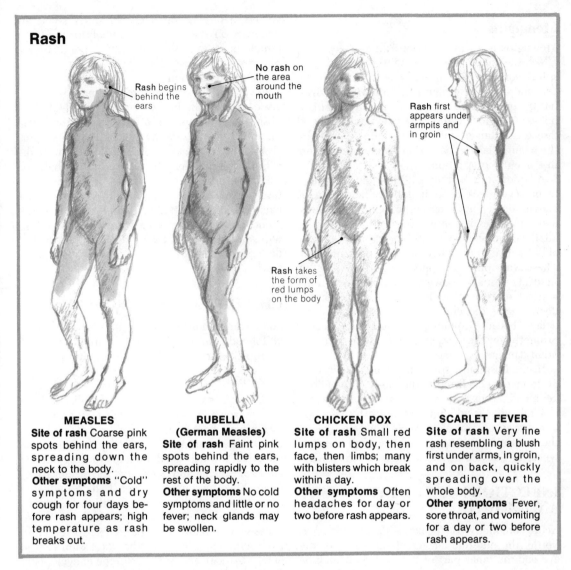

Rash begins behind the ears

No rash on the area around the mouth

Rash first appears under armpits and in groin

Rash takes the form of red lumps on the body

MEASLES
Site of rash Coarse pink spots behind the ears, spreading down the neck to the body.
Other symptoms "Cold" symptoms and dry cough for four days before rash appears; high temperature as rash breaks out.

RUBELLA
(German Measles)
Site of rash Faint pink spots behind the ears, spreading rapidly to the rest of the body.
Other symptoms No cold symptoms and little or no fever; neck glands may be swollen.

CHICKEN POX
Site of rash Small red lumps on body, then face, then limbs; many with blisters which break within a day.
Other symptoms Often headaches for day or two before rash appears.

SCARLET FEVER
Site of rash Very fine rash resembling a blush first under arms, in groin, and on back, quickly spreading over the whole body.
Other symptoms Fever, sore throat, and vomiting for a day or two before rash appears.

terized by a sudden high fever (103° F or more) which lasts for four or five days. At first there are no other definite symptoms. After the fever disappears, the child develops a red, measlelike rash that disappears again in 24 hours. The disease is not dangerous, but the high fever may bring about convulsions.

Lesser-Known Viral Rashes

There are at least two viral diseases, caused by the so-called ECHO and Coxsackie viruses, that may bring on symptoms similar to those of scarlet fever—i.e., sore throat, fever, and a rash. A child with these symptoms should have a throat culture made to determine whether the infection is caused by the scarlet fever streptococcus or by a virus.

Protection for Nonimmunized Infants

An infant is sometimes exposed to chicken pox or some other contagious disease when an older child in the family develops the ailment. Always report such exposure to your doctor as soon as possible.

LESS COMMON INFECTIOUS DISEASES

Some relatively uncommon infectious diseases that can strike children are meningitis, encephalitis, infectious hepatitis, mononucleosis, and Rocky Mountain spotted fever ("tick fever"). All of these diseases are discussed in the encyclopedia section.

Meningitis

Meningitis is always a serious illness because it affects the membranes (meninges) enveloping the spinal cord and the brain. The disease can be brought about by either a bacterium or a virus, but the former is usually the cause. Meningitis is not as contagious as the more common childhood diseases, although spinal meningitis, caused by the meningococcus bacterium, sometimes occurs in epidemic proportions.

A typical attack of meningitis will cause a high fever, severe headache, irritability (and perhaps convulsions), plus vomiting, extreme drowsiness, and sometimes unconsciousness. Most telling of all, the child will have a stiff neck and will probably be unable to touch his chest with his chin. These symptoms can appear either gradually or suddenly. Usually, however, the child will look and act extremely ill. If you cannot reach the doctor, take the child to the hospital without delay, because meningitis must be treated promptly or the disease can cause permanent brain damage or even death.

In the hospital a spinal tap will probably be performed to confirm the diagnosis. The child is kept in isolation, and antibiotic treatment (except in viral cases) is administered until the infection has cleared up completely—as it usually does if the treatment is begun early enough. Several weeks of convalescence at home are necessary.

INFECTIONS OF THE EYES AND MOUTH

Acute conjunctivitis ("pinkeye") is an inflammation of the outermost layer of the white of the eye and the inner part of the eyelids. It may be caused by bacteria, viruses, or allergy, and can be highly contagious. One or both eyes become reddened, and mucus collects in the corners. Sometimes a child wakes up frightened because his eyelids are stuck together by the dried mucus. Antibiotic ointments or antiseptic drops (depending on the cause) are usually prescribed. If the symptoms involve one eye only, the doctor may want to examine the child to determine whether a speck or cinder has caused the problem. (For further discussion of causes and treatment see CONJUNCTIVITIS in the encyclopedia section.)

Two other fairly prevalent eye problems are swelling of the areas around the eyes and sties. The former may be caused by allergies, sinus infections, or insect bites. If just one eye is in-volved, a bite is the likely cause. A sty is an infection on the eyelid, commonly around the follicle of an eyelash. It usually responds to applications of moist heat. (See also STY in the encyclopedia section.)

Fever blisters, or cold sores, around the mouth are caused by the herpes simplex virus. Clusters of small blisters appear, often between the lower lip and chin or inside the mouth itself. The sores are painful, but they usually heal without medication. The pain may be relieved by lip balm or calamine lotion. Fever sores are sometimes confused with a more serious condition, impetigo, a bacterial infection that requires antibiotic treatment. If you are not sure what you are dealing with, take the child to the doctor. (For further discussion, see FEVER SORE in the encyclopedia section.)

CHILDHOOD SKIN PROBLEMS

Some skin conditions occur more commonly in childhood than in later years, or present more of a problem for a child than for an adult.

Eczema

Red, rough, swollen skin with fine blisters indicates eczema, an itchy rash that may be caused by a fungus, bacterium, or an allergy. The blisters may ooze and form scabs, and they easily become infected. You will need a doctor to pinpoint the cause of eczema and determine the proper treatment. Make certain, however, that the affected areas stay clean. Keeping the child's fingernails short and scrubbed will help in this effort, because you probably will not be able to keep him from scratching. (For a further discussion see the entries ECZEMA and ALLERGY in the encyclopedia section.)

Impetigo

This bacterial skin infection is usually caused by a staphylococcus or streptococcus germ and is most common in hot weather. Small clusters of yellowish crusted sores or pimples appear, often starting around the nostrils. When the child picks at them, he spreads the infection. Impetigo is extremely contagious, so an infected child's clothes, towels, hairbrush, etc., should not be used by anyone else. Clothing and linens should be boiled when laundered. Impetigo responds readily to treatment, including antibiotics, but it is not a "harmless" rash. Untreated impetigo caused by a strep infection can lead to serious complications such as erysipelas and kidney disease. (For further discussion see IMPETIGO in the encyclopedia section.)

For this condition, proper hygiene is the best preventive. Instruct your child not to use other people's towels or washcloths and to wash often *with soap*, especially in summer.

Warts

Warts are thought to be caused by viruses. They are annoying but seldom uncomfortable, except for plantar warts on the sole of the foot, which should be treated by the doctor. Most other warts can be left alone, provided they do not become irritated; they usually go away by themselves.

Ringworm

Ringworm is not a worm but a fungus. Itchy eruptions form on the scalp (and sometimes on other parts of the body) and then heal at the center, after which the infection spreads outward in a ring. Frequently the hair in the infected areas is weakened and breaks off. The disease can be acquired from humans and sometimes from animals. It is stubborn and contagious and should be treated under medical supervision.

For those skin problems not described in this chapter—poison ivy, boils, fungus infections, for example—see the encyclopedia section.

WORMS AND OTHER PARASITES

Contrary to popular belief, children do not get convulsions because of intestinal worms, and they do not get worms from animals. Roundworm and hookworm disease, which are described fully in the encyclopedia section, are spread through contaminated foods and infested soil. Both illnesses are now relatively rare in the United States.

Pinworm

Pinworm, or seatworm, is the most common worm infection in American children today. The tiny pinworms are less than a half-inch long and lodge in the large intestine. Their presence may cause little abdominal discomfort, but when the worms emerge around the anal region to lay their eggs at night, the child will complain of violent itching around his rectum. If he scratches, the eggs will be deposited on everything he touches, and the rest of the family may well pick up the infection. The doctor can diagnose the condition by means of a stool sample, and he is the one to treat the problem. Do not try to get rid of it

yourself with over-the-counter "worm" medicines. Although the idea of your child having "worms" is upsetting, pinworms are not dangerous. Approximately 50 percent of children have pinworms at one time or another.

Head Lice

Unfortunately, this pest is making a comeback in school classrooms and dormitories, especially among children who are casual about hygiene. The head louse is a tiny wingless insect that lives on the scalp and hatches its eggs, or "nits," there. Infestation can cause intense itching, secondary scalp infections, and inflammation of the lymph glands in the neck. If you see evidence of lice or their eggs on your child's head, don't make him feel ashamed of the condition. Consult your doctor about the use of special shampoos and other effective preparations (not insecticides). The child's hair need not be cut off unless it is very long and tangled.

HEADACHES

Children often complain of a headache when they have a fever, sinusitis, toothache, or an ear infection. Vision problems such as nearsightedness or farsightedness can also cause headaches, and so can emotional stress or muscular tension.

Recurrent or extremely severe headaches can be serious. Any child with a recent head injury followed by a persistent headache should be watched carefully for signs of concussion. (See that entry in the encyclopedia section, and "Head Injury" in the FIRST AID section.) Migraine headaches, which are discussed in Chapter 23, are extremely painful and should be treated by a doctor. They often occur in children who suffer fairly constant emotional tension or who come from a family with a history of migraine.

OTHER PROBLEMS OF CHILDREN

Besides actual illness brought on by infections or allergies, some children suffer from other kinds of problems, such as obesity, poor posture, defects of vision or hearing, various kinds of learning disabilities, and hyperactivity. The earlier these kinds of difficulties are brought to the attention of the doctor, the better off the child will be. A child who cannot see or hear well may be labeled "slow" in school, while a hyperactive child is often condemned as being deliberately "bad" or disruptive. Such labels are obviously unfair.

Much of the damage they do to a child's self-esteem can be avoided if the problem is spotted early and treated with sympathy and tact. If a child is examined regularly by his doctor, many malfunctions of this kind will be noticed before they cause difficulties in school and consequent emotional damage to the child.

Child Abuse

Few parents ever intend to hurt their children. But some adults lose control easily, especially if they themselves are under severe stress or if they expect too much of their children. Any parent who finds himself growing increasingly abusive with his children—either verbally or physically—should seek immediate help. Counseling is available through local or state child welfare agencies and through a nationwide organization known as Parents Anonymous. In California call (800) 352-0386 toll-free. In all other states call (800) 421-0353. These numbers can be called 24 hours a day for help and advice.

Crib Death (Sudden Infant Death Syndrome)

An infant is placed in his crib or carriage to sleep. The next time someone looks in on him, he is dead. Neither his parents nor the child's physician had any reason to believe that the baby was ill, and he did not suffocate. There is no evidence that the infant suffered pain. What caused his death? No one knows. But each year some 7,000 to 8,000 infants in the first year of life die in this mysterious fashion. Intensive medical research into "crib death" or "sudden infant death syndrome," has not yet revealed the cause or causes of this strange phenomenon.

Such a tragedy usually has a devastating effect on the parents. They not only mourn the loss of their baby; but because of the unex-plained nature of the death, they tend to blame themselves or each other. They may also feel censure, real or imagined, from relatives or friends.

This sense of guilt is understandable but baseless. *The one thing that is known about crib death is that it is not preventable.* If you have relatives or friends whose child has died in this mysterious way, you can do much to comfort them with the reassurance that neither they, nor any doctor, could have done anything to avert the tragedy.

For further information write to the National Sudden Infant Death Syndrome Foundation, 310 South Michigan Avenue, Chicago, Illinois 60604.

17 The Healthy Teenager

If a child has been physically and emotionally healthy during the first decade or so of life, he or she is likely to go through adolescence with a minimum of problems. But there still will be problems. Even under the best of circumstances, adolescence is a turbulent period when the body and psyche go through profound and often rapid changes. The period is usually trying—although in different ways—for both youngster and parents.

This chapter deals with the physical and emotional difficulties of the teenager. Growth, diet, body hair, skin eruptions, sex, peer-group conformity, drugs, smoking, and driving are among the subjects discussed.

GROWING UP

Unfortunately, the body and mind of a teenager do not mature at the same rate. Many boys and girls are sexually mature by the time they are 13 to 15 years of age. Physically, they are ready for mating. But teenagers are not ready for marriage with all of its responsibilities, including parenthood. They are not yet adults emotionally.

The events leading to healthy maturity do not occur according to a predictable timetable. Like members of any other age group, adolescents vary greatly from person to person; their physical growth and emotional development do not always proceed at the same pace. The "average" teenager may or may not bear a strong resemblance to the one who lives in your home.

All of this means that some young people will seem to be out of step with their peers. For example, shortly before puberty or in early adolescence, boys and girls pass through a period of preferring to be with members of their own sex. This is a natural and valuable phase of life that soon gives way to the development of an interest in members of the opposite sex.

The age of adolescents in a group, such as a class in school, may vary by as much as two years, and boys usually reach maturity two years later than girls. Therefore, some young people may be attracted to members of the opposite sex while the rest of their group are not. Or others may wish to remain with members of their own sex, while the "crowd" has gone on to conventional dating.

The influence of the group is particularly strong at this period. Not wanting to be "different," adolescents will try hard to be like others of their own age. Sometimes this means that they rush through or even miss an important phase of their emotional development, or that they will be forced to remain in it too long.

THE HEALTH OF ADOLESCENTS

Teenagers' diets tend to be poorly balanced. If a mother provides a well-balanced diet at home, however, there will be no great harm done if her adolescent children gorge themselves with French fries, cokes, and hamburgers when they eat out with their friends. Remember, adolescents' appetites are enormous; they often eat more than their parents do.

The Right Foods for Teenagers

As explained in Chapter 2, human beings must have proteins, minerals, vitamins, and iron. Protein foods include meat, fish, eggs, and milk, and are essential for growth. Two good sources of protein should be served at every meal—for example, an egg and a large glass of milk for breakfast, or bacon and a slice of ham instead of the egg. For lunch there should be meat or fish or a cheese dish, plus a large glass of milk. Dinner should include a main course of fish, meat, eggs, or cheese, with another glass of milk. Between meals, milk should be drunk to make a total of four glasses a day. Milk not only supplies protein, but is the best source of calcium and phosphorus, which are essential for building bones.

Vitamins should be provided by serving fruits and vegetables; both green and yellow vegetables should be included. Liver, which is an excellent source of all the vitamin B group, should be eaten once a week. A daily addition of vitamins A and D is helpful during this active growth period. Some margarine is fortified with vitamin A, and milk usually supplies vitamin D. In addition, many parents supplement the diets of adolescents with one or two USP (United States Pharmacopoeia) multivitamin capsules a day. Ask your doctor about this.

Iron is needed to ensure rich red blood. Girls who are beginning to menstruate may require additional iron to replace what is lost in the menstrual blood. Some foods rich in iron are: lean meat (especially liver, heart, and kidneys), leafy green vegetables, egg yolk, whole grain and enriched bread and cereals, potatoes, oysters, dried fruits, peas, and beans.

Overweight and Underweight

Being underweight to the point of impaired physical well-being is not an important problem among the vast majority of American teenagers. On the other hand, being overweight is more prevalent and more serious, both physically and emotionally. (See the accompanying table for the ideal weights of boys and girls according to their age and height.)

Getting young people to gain or lose weight requires the tact of a diplomat. The following five suggestions apply not only to matters pertaining to health but to other situations in which the parent must exert authority:

1. Never ridicule an overweight child. Ridicule is always cruel, and adolescents are particularly sensitive.

2. Do not nag. This defeats its own purpose, especially with adolescents who are usually impatient with parental badgering.

3. Give the problem serious attention, with special consideration for the particular youngster involved. Remember that teenagers should be treated as individuals, even though they tend to travel in herds and dress alike. If your child needs to gain or lose weight, decide which of the tips given in Chapter 2 will work best for him.

Average weight for teenage boys and girls
(in schoolroom clothing, without shoes)

Boys' average weight in pounds for each specified age

Height in inches	12–13 years	13–14 years	14–15 years	15–16 years	16–17 years	17–18 years
52	64	—	—	—	—	—
53	68	—	—	—	—	—
54	71	72	—	—	—	—
55	74	74	—	—	—	—
56	78	78	80	—	—	—
57	82	83	83	—	—	—
58	85	86	87	—	—	—
59	89	90	90	90	—	—
60	93	94	95	96	—	—
61	97	99	100	103	106	—
62	102	103	104	107	111	116
63	107	108	110	113	118	123
64	111	113	115	117	121	126
65	117	118	120	122	127	131
66	119	122	125	128	132	136
67	124	128	130	134	136	139
68	—	134	134	137	141	143
69	—	137	139	143	146	149
70	—	143	144	145	148	151
71	—	148	150	151	152	154
72	—	—	153	155	156	158
73	—	—	157	160	162	164
74	—	—	160	164	168	170

Girls' average weight in pounds for each specified age

Height in inches	12–13 years	13–14 years	14–15 years	15–16 years	16–17 years	17–18 years
53	71	—	—	—	—	—
54	73	—	—	—	—	—
55	77	78	—	—	—	—
56	81	83	—	—	—	—
57	84	88	92	—	—	—
58	88	93	96	101	—	—
59	92	96	100	103	104	—
60	97	101	105	108	109	111
61	101	105	108	112	113	116
62	106	109	113	115	117	118
63	110	112	116	117	119	120
64	115	117	119	120	122	123
65	120	121	122	123	125	126
66	124	124	125	128	129	130
67	128	130	131	133	133	135
68	131	133	135	136	138	138
69	—	135	137	138	140	142
70	—	136	138	140	142	144
71	—	138	140	142	144	145

SOURCE: Bureau of Education, Department of the Interior

4. Do not gloss over the problem of over-weight. While your teenager may indeed be unduly concerned about what is a purely temporary condition, it is real, distressing, and painfully important to him. Give him the respect and consideration he deserves.

5. Fall back upon an authority your child will respect, such as a doctor or dietitian.

Skin Troubles During Adolescence

Always consult a doctor if an adolescent suffers from severe acne. The doctor may want to refer the young person to a dermatologist (a skin specialist) or to the skin-diseases department of the nearest medical center or hospital.

Frequent boils may be a sign of diabetes. This disease, which you may associate only with adults, frequently strikes young people.

Freckles can be a source of worry to adolescents. Although there is no safe way to remove them at home, they can be prevented from getting worse by reducing exposure to the sun or by using protective ointments or lotions. (See also the discussion of common skin troubles in Chapter 3 and the entry ACNE in the encyclopedia section.)

SPECIAL PROBLEMS OF GIRLS

Breasts

Some adolescent girls feel shy, or even ashamed, because of their breast development. Mothers should encourage them to be proud of their emerging womanhood. Mothers should not only emphasize the fact that breast development is a normal part of puberty, but should also explain that shortly before or during menstruation, some tenderness and swelling of the breasts are apt to occur and should cause no concern.

The adolescent girl who despairs because of a relative absence of breast development can also suffer, and great care must be taken to ease her anxiety. Her mother should reassure her that small breasts in no way diminish her femininity or potential charm. (For a fuller discussion, see also Chapter 19 and the entry BREAST in the encyclopedia section.)

Body Hair

The adolescent girl may develop an excess of hair over the thighs and legs or under the arms. Facial hair can sometimes become disfiguring. Parents should take this condition seriously; it can be a source of great worry to a sensitive young girl.

Bleaching or shaving is usually a satisfactory solution. If applied carefully, a depilatory may be used—but *never* on the face. Wax preparations, which pull out the hair, are sometimes employed, but the treatment is usually painful. Your daughter may want to have some of the hair permanently removed by electrolysis. This can be dangerous if it is attempted by anyone but an expert. (See the entry HAIR REMOVAL in the encyclopedia section.)

Menstruation

Usually, menstruation begins at 12 to 14 years of age, but it may start as early as 10 or as late as 18. Maturing early or late often runs in a family. However, if a girl's menstrual periods begin at 10 or earlier, or if they have not started by the time she is 17, a doctor should be consulted. See a doctor also if the characteristic changes of puberty—the development of the breasts and pubic hair—occur unusually early or late.

All girls—and boys as well—should be told about menstruation, preferably by their mothers, before the youngsters and their friends reach the age of puberty. Tact and sensitivity are needed. Parents should not give their children information which they cannot understand or in which they are not interested. The possibility of the child's learning about menstruation from other sources, possibly poorly informed, must be considered in determining the age at which each child should be told. The attitude of the person giving the information is all-important.

Menstruation is not a sickness, nor is it something to be ashamed of—it should *not* be called "the curse." Mothers should explain to their teenage daughters that many females experience some discomfort or cramps in the lower abdomen, usually at the onset of a menstrual period, and that menstruation may be a nuisance for the first few days, especially if the flow is profuse. However, it should cause no real difficulty. (See also the entry MENSTRUATION in the encyclopedia section.)

Menstrual flow can be absorbed by either a pad or a tampon; both are safe from a health standpoint. If the flow is profuse, pads may be required to absorb it. Most virgins can use the small-size tampon.

Feminine Hygiene

Aside from ordinary washing and bathing, no other feminine hygiene measures, such as douching, are necessary. Baths or showers may be taken during menstruation, although extremely hot or cold water should be avoided. Women and girls who prefer not to bathe during their periods should wash the outer genital parts with warm water and soap at least once or twice a day.

If strong odors persist or if there is a discharge from the vaginal passage between periods, be sure to see a doctor. These discharges and odors usually result from an infection that should be attended to. (See also the entry DOUCHE in the encyclopedia section.)

SPECIAL PROBLEMS OF BOYS

On the average, boys arrive at puberty between the ages of 14 and 16, about two years later than girls. Some boys, however, mature as early as 12 and others as late as 20. If a boy matures at an exceptionally early age, a doctor should be consulted. And medical advice is especially important if a boy is unusually late in maturing; there may be a glandular deficiency requiring treatment. Even if nothing is wrong, a doctor's reassurance may be necessary to prevent emotional problems for the boy.

Boys grow rapidly during this period, and their appetites are often enormous. Hair appears on the face and the pubic region, the genitals become larger, and the boy is able to have erections and ejaculations.

Nocturnal Emissions

Nocturnal emissions (wet dreams) start in this period. It is nature's way of relieving sexual tension. The fluid containing spermatozoa (see the entry SEMEN in the encyclopedia section) is discharged at night and is usually accompanied by a sexual dream. This physiological event should not be a cause for shame, pride, or concern; it is a natural part of adolescence, about which boys should be informed in advance. Parents should not comment upon finding seminal stains on the bedclothes or pajamas. Young girls, especially if they have brothers, should also be told about nocturnal emissions so that they will not be shocked by accidentally discovering evidence of the phenomenon or by getting misinformation from other youngsters.

PROBLEMS OF BOTH SEXES

Masturbation

Almost every individual, male and female, has been confronted with the urge to masturbate and must work out his or her own solution to this question. Masturbation is a problem in the sense that sexual desire is not purely physiological; the physical aspects are normally associated with the desire for intimacy with a member of the opposite sex. During masturbation, this intimacy exists only in the form of fantasy.

In most instances, this is the only real problem of masturbation. Nearly all the others have been created out of whole cloth by misinformed adults, including parents, who have frightened children with old wives' tales of the physical harm resulting from the practice, and shamed youngsters into believing it is an especially obnoxious perversion. Countless heartaches—and even tragedies—have resulted from such baseless fear and guilt.

If a boy or girl becomes addicted to masturbation, the problem is an emotional one and should be discussed with a doctor or counselor. Excessive preoccupation with masturbation is a sign, not a cause, of the emotional difficulty.

Homosexual Practices

Many boys and girls indulge in some form of homosexual play with companions. Here the parents should be on the alert. Usually such practices are harmless and cease as the boy or girl matures. However, it is at this time that an older, confirmed homosexual may exert an unfortunate—and possibly lasting—influence. If such a situation arises, the parents must exercise a great deal of skill and tact. In many cases, they should discuss the situation with a psychologist.

Talking It Over With Your Children

We do not propose that you lecture your children on these subjects under discussion. It is far better to make the points as the opportunities present themselves. Some parents find it difficult to talk about these matters. Are you one of them? Do you feel embarrassed about discussing masturbation, nocturnal emissions, or any similar subject with your children? If you do, you may wish to seek help from your doctor, a psychologist, or an expert in the field of child guidance. Such a talk will either increase your self-confidence or make you decide to let some professionally trained person discuss these topics with your children.

A SANE LOOK AT SOME DELICATE SUBJECTS

Adolescence is a time for experimenting with new ideas, experiences, and bodily sensations. If your teenage children can depend upon you to tell them the truth about danger to their health and safety, rather than to threaten, exaggerate, or mislead them, you have established a healthy atmosphere in which to thrash out some of the problems that inevitably arise.

Driving

Most teenagers are impatient to get behind the wheel of a car and drive off to freedom. From the moment a boy or girl gets a driver's license and the occasional use of the family car, he or she must be made to understand that a car can be a lethal weapon if mishandled.

First, make certain that the youngster receives expert driving instruction. Next, keep in mind that the best insurance against recklessness by the young person is the parents' example. Father and mother must show that they respect traffic laws and exercise good judgment when they drive.

But if you sincerely believe that your teenager is not mature enough for the responsibility of driving, tell him that it is out of concern for his safety as well as that of other people that he will have to wait another year or so. Your stand will be difficult to maintain, but you must be firm.

Drinking

Studies of alcoholism show that children are least likely to abuse alcohol when they grow up in households where alcoholic beverages are an accepted part of meals or of special occasions, and where drunkenness is equated with foolishness rather than with maturity.

Remember that it is not the end of the world if Junior reels home after his first beer binge, or if your teenage daughter announces that she drank a glass of wine with her spaghetti dinner at a friend's house. A more serious problem is the adolescent who rebels against family rigidity by drinking in secret and glorying in his sinfulness. Do not let the matter get out of hand. Alcoholism is a grave and widespread problem among adolescents of all classes.

Smoking

There is no doubt that the children of parents who smoke are likelier to take up smoking than are the children of parents who do not smoke. What good are health warnings and hygiene instruction to a teenager who is confronted day in and day out with a parent who smokes fairly constantly?

If neither you nor your spouse smokes and your youngster begins the habit on his own, you might suggest that smoking is neither sophisticated nor grown-up—it is, in fact, more akin to thumbsucking!

Drugs

The use of drugs among youngsters is increasing. No longer confined to the ghetto, drugs have moved to the so-called good neighborhoods and are now used by many middle-class teenagers in the cities, suburbs, and rural areas.

Statistics show that there is an even chance that your child will experiment with drugs at some time or other. The habitual use of a psychochemical drug is a means of avoiding the problems of reality. Drug addiction is a disease like alcoholism; in fact, alcohol *is* a drug. Because so many adults use alcohol for social purposes, they find its use (or even abuse) by their children more acceptable than, say, marijuana or amphetamines. But the use of any drug is harmful to the health and growth of the adolescent. Parents should be aware of this and should be honest enough to admit it and take action when and if their child is a user. Drugs, including alcohol, are dangerous, and it is the duty of parents to protect children from danger.

Most young people who misuse drugs are not going to become addicts. But it is conceivable that drugs may become a constant part of their lives.

Laymen often do not recognize the symptoms of drug use. But a parent can tell that something is wrong if a child suddenly does badly in school, if he becomes hideously sloppy, if he inexplicably loses a lot of weight, if he is unusually lethargic or hyperenergetic, if his complexion changes, or if his eyes become red and swollen. These signs do not necessarily imply drug use, but they definitely indicate that there is something to be concerned about.

Drugs used by today's adolescents fall into three main types: stimulants such as amphetamines; depressants such as tranquilizers and alcohol; psychedelics such as marijuana, hashish, peyote, or LSD. Most middle-class youngsters tend to choose drugs in the last category. Insecure, frightened, and vulnerable as they are, these children find the psychedelic distortion of time and distance a seeming aid to what they believe is social interaction.

The peer group is a necessary element in the youngster's life. A child needs to have friends who share the same feelings of awkwardness, the same fears and frustrations, and the same victories. A child requires a peer group to fulfill his need for rebellion and approval, and the group may introduce him to drugs as part of the search for adventure. The seriously troubled child is likely to become the problem user.

The physical danger of drug use is less important than the potential mental damage it can cause. Drugs offer the illusion of security from adolescent anxiety. Their use signifies the avoidance of the pain that goes along with growing up. And regular drug users do not grow up into healthy, mature adults.

Parents should know where they can go for help. A drug problem cannot be handled by the parents alone. Check out the resources in your community: schools, churches, hospitals, and private counseling agencies.

Many parents react more quickly to the noises from their car's engine than to the distress signals from their children. The adults worry that being realistic and demanding—and making clear that they are prepared to do *anything* to stop their children from using drugs—will somehow damage the relationship with the children. But parent and child are not equals, peers, or friends—at least not at this time in their lives. The parent must be understanding and at the same time let the child know that there are no choices at all where drugs are concerned.

For further information, contact Phoenix House, Public Information Department, 164 West 74th Street, New York, N.Y. 10023. If you think the drug problem is a serious one in your community, try to get together with other parents and ask an adult leader respected by teenagers to lead open discussions on the subject.

GROWING UP TO SEXUAL MATURITY

No one knows the complete answer to the difficult question about petting and sex relations during adolescence. In *The Happy Family* by psychiatrist John Levy and Ruth Munroe, Dr. Levy presents an attitude that many parents find helpful:

"Advising adolescents about their sex life is a highly personal and individualized problem. You cannot recommend the same behavior for all of them indiscriminately. I rather hope that my own daughter will pet or neck, or whatever the proper term may be, preferably with boys she knows well and likes, and only with her contemporaries. Lovemaking of this type is a healthy preparation for marriage. I hope that she will not have intercourse or end up merely a tech-

nical virgin. Quite aside from any moral implications, such a step is risky. If she does have a complete relationship, though, I most earnestly hope that she will know what she is about, that she will not go into an affair because she happens to be tight, or thinks it's "the thing," or wants to prove that she can carry it off. These are my hopes. They are based on my observation of the kind of behavior least likely to cause trouble in our particular social group. But she may order her life quite differently and be none the worse for it. If she is neither afraid of sex nor bamboozled by its glamor, I shall be very content."

Note particularly the points Dr. Levy makes, which apply equally to boys and girls: (1) Adolescent lovemaking should be with friends who are approximately the same age. (2) A certain amount of petting and necking is a good thing as a preparation for the fuller, richer love of marriage. (3) If the young person prefers some other way, accept the decision with the hope that it will be realistic and not cause unhappiness.

HOW YOU CAN HELP YOUR TEENAGER

As a parent, try to recollect your own reactions and desires during adolescence. If you remember how you resented the authority of your parents, you will understand why your children object to strict rules. If you remember your own fantasies, daydreams, and grandiose plans, you will listen with tolerance, rather than derision, when your children plan to remake the world or to become poets, missionaries, or explorers. Parents must realize that their children's adolescence may be stormy while theirs was quietly miserable, or vice versa.

Dr. Benjamin Weininger, a psychiatrist, points out that adolescents frequently have the correct attitude toward living. They are idealistic, intense about life, and hopeful that they can participate in making life better for everyone. The adolescent may not be very practical in his attempts to attain his ideals, but his idealism is worth our consideration and respect.

Our job is to help the adolescent reach the goal of maturity. We have already talked about how to help the child reach sexual maturity. There are a number of things you can do to help him attain social maturity:

1. Let the teenager feel he has a place in the family. Discuss family decisions.

2. Give him the details of the family budget.

Present a true picture of what things cost in terms of the parents' outlay of time and energy. Let him see that his share of the income is a reasonable one, and not the result of an arbitrary decision.

3. Encourage a sense of adult responsibility about money. Give the teenager a regular allowance—once a month for those 16 or over. If it is possible, provide older children with a personal checking account, which makes them realize that they are being treated as responsible individuals.

4. Do everything you possibly can to enable an adolescent boy or girl, or one who is approaching adolescence, to have friends.

5. Give the adolescent a chance to leave home. Younger children can first go to camp or visit relatives. Then let them visit friends. Older and more mature adolescents should be permitted to take jobs away from home during the summer vacation. These breaks from home life give the adolescent valuable training in self-confidence. The experience also helps reduce the tensions that adolescents generate in their rebellion against home rules and restrictions. The adolescent soon learns that there are rules everywhere he goes.

6. Let the teenager decide on his own career, and try to get expert guidance for him. If your daughter wants to enter a profession rather than marry at the age that her mother did, let her work it out in her own way. Do not add to the social pressure that often makes a girl marry before she is ready for it. Similarly, if your son is willing to give up a lucrative family business for the lesser financial return of some other work, let him follow his own interests.

7. Help your children learn to know you and your spouse as individuals—not just as parents, but as human beings who may make mistakes but want to do the best for their children because they love them. It is better to show your love than it is to talk about it.

One way you can show your love is by remembering that the growing egos of adolescents need psychological nourishment as much as their growing bodies need food. But be careful not to praise your children for qualities they do not possess. They will either suspect you of being insincere or think you believe what you say, which will make them feel inadequate and insecure. Surely you can find many good things you can truthfully say about your children.

18 The Middle Years

When does middle age begin, and when does it end? These questions are difficult to answer, because life alters so subtly and constantly. In our society, the changes that characterize the middle years occur roughly from the mid-thirties to the mid-sixties. In this chapter we shall explore some of these physical and emotional changes that take place during these years.

CHANGING PATTERNS

The beginning of the middle years is usually a period of settling down. In most cases, men have attained a certain level of achievement in their work and are beginning to have an idea of what other goals they can look forward to. For most women, it means that the dependency of young and growing children has been or will soon be supplanted by the special problems of the relatively independent adult. And as middle age progresses, attention begins to turn toward retirement with its implications of greater freedom in the use of one's time, the possibility of solving financial problems, and a realistic assessment of life's accomplishments.

Changes occur in the body in middle age. Loss of a youthful figure and the appearance of wrinkles are external signs. New ailments may develop that are likely to remain with you for a long time, such as arthritis, glaucoma, and heart disease. Other ailments that once could be coped with easily may become more of a problem.

Because our culture tends to place so much emphasis on youth, we forget that middle age, like any other period of life, is dynamic and offers new opportunities and challenges. It is important, therefore, to do everything possible to remain fit.

EXERCISE

Paul Dudley White, the noted cardiologist, helped to popularize the concept that the risks of heart disease could be lessened through regular exercise. Although the attitude of most cardi-

ologists at present is that the onset and severity of coronary heart disease are probably influenced by many variables such as age, heredity, the presence of other ailments, and eating habits, exercise also plays an important role.

Regular exercise also helps to control overweight, avoid sag and middle-aged spread, tone up muscles, and improve your figure.

Given a state of reasonable health, the middle-aged person can easily engage in and enjoy walking, bicycling, tennis, swimming, bowling, and many other activities. However, a sedentary person should not embark suddenly upon strenuous exercise. This is especially true for males from about age 35 on who run the greatest risk of coronary attack. It is wise to have a physician test your capacity for exercise and then prescribe an individually tailored program of gradually increasing physical activity. (See "Exercise and Sports" in Chapter 1; also PHYSICAL EXERCISE in the encyclopedia section.)

ACCIDENTS

For the middle-aged person, a "minor" accident may have serious repercussions, because bones tend to be more brittle and healing is not as rapid as it once was. Shock and slow recovery may, in turn, lead to the worsening of illnesses that the body had been able to keep under control until the accident. (Advice on accident prevention is given in Chapter 21.)

In addition to alcohol with its well-known effects, there are many medicines that can slow down a person's reactions and make driving or any hazardous activity even more dangerous.

Particular care should be exercised in the use of antihistamines and tranquilizers when alertness and physical coordination are vital. Always ask your physician about what restrictions you should observe when taking such medicines.

Psychiatrists feel that in many cases accidents do not just happen. They may be unconscious wishes to gain revenge or sympathy, or even to commit suicide. Therefore, it is sound advice not to drive or engage in hazardous activities when in a state of severe emotional upset, depression, or agitation.

DIET

Throughout life the quality and quantity of the food we eat are of tremendous significance. In the younger years, proper growth and maturation depend on a balanced diet; in the middle years, a diet that is well balanced helps to maintain a healthy body and prepare it to resist mental and physical strain. (For an explanation of a well-balanced diet, see Chapter 2 and the entry DIET in the encyclopedia section.)

Overweight is a significant health problem in the middle years. Life insurance mortality tables show that in the age group of 45 to 60, the death rate climbs sharply for both men and women who carry excess fat.

Some of the problems caused by overweight are an increased incidence of arteriosclerotic heart disease, blood-vessel disease, high blood pressure, and the possible aggravation of a latent diabetic condition. Also, convalescence from surgery is prolonged and there is an increased risk of surgical and anesthetic complications.

Of particular interest at this time of life is the role of cholesterol and other fats in the diet. (This is discussed in the entry CHOLESTEROL in the encyclopedia section.)

OTHER HEALTH PROBLEMS

During the middle years, one can reasonably expect a transition from relatively good health to a certain amount of medical trouble. Some of the more important and more common ailments are discussed below.

Diabetes Mellitus

The form of diabetes that begins in middle life is often characterized only by a high incidence of sugar in the blood and urine. It carries a lesser risk of coma than the juvenile form of diabetes does and can usually be treated by diet or by insulin and other drugs. (See also the entry DIABETES in the encyclopedia section.)

Diabetics, in general, run greater risks of heart disease, high blood pressure, and blood-vessel problems. They should, therefore, be under constant medical supervision.

Cancer

While cancer does strike the young, it is a particularly dread disease of the late middle and older years. Good preventive health practices, such as regular physical examinations, decrease its dangers because the earlier the disease is discovered, the better is the prospect of cure. (Cancer is discussed further in Chapter 22 and in the entry CANCER in the encyclopedia section.)

Emphysema and Bronchitis

These are usually diseases of middle-aged persons with histories of smoking. Shortness of breath, owing to destruction of lung tissue, and frequent colds and pneumonia characterize these ailments. (See also the entries BRONCHITIS and EMPHYSEMA in the encyclopedia section.)

Coronary Heart Disease

The arteries supplying the heart with blood become narrowed because of arteriosclerosis (hardening of the arteries) as we grow into middle age, and this may lead to angina pectoris (severe chest pain on exertion) and heart attack. The risk of heart attack may be lessened by a low-fat diet, exercise, relaxation, and not smoking. (See Chapter 3 and CORONARY HEART DISEASE in the encyclopedia section.)

Rheumatic Heart Disease

Rheumatic fever in childhood frequently does not show its destructive effects on the heart until adulthood. In rheumatic heart disease the valves of the heart become misshapen, and the heart is unable to function efficiently. Medicines and surgery are helpful for most of those who suffer from this ailment.

Hypertension

High blood pressure (hypertension) imposes an extra strain on the heart in particular. Its causes are often not known, but it is frequently associated with diabetes. Hypertension, if not treated adequately, can severely damage the heart, the brain (as in a stroke), the kidneys, and the blood vessels. Treatment of hypertension has been one of the great advances in modern medicine. (Risks, prevention, and treatment of hypertension are

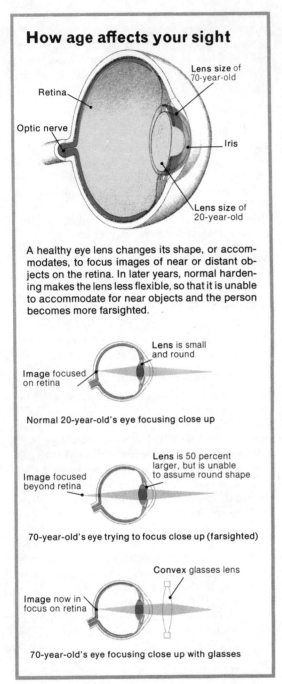

How age affects your sight

Lens size of 70-year-old

Retina

Optic nerve

Iris

Lens size of 20-year-old

A healthy eye lens changes its shape, or accommodates, to focus images of near or distant objects on the retina. In later years, normal hardening makes the lens less flexible, so that it is unable to accommodate for near objects and the person becomes more farsighted.

Lens is small and round

Image focused on retina

Normal 20-year-old's eye focusing close up

Lens is 50 percent larger, but is unable to assume round shape

Image focused beyond retina

70-year-old's eye trying to focus close up (farsighted)

Convex glasses lens

Image now in focus on retina

70-year-old's eye focusing close up with glasses

discussed in Chapter 22 and under HYPERTENSION in the encyclopedia section.)

Congestive Heart Failure

Heart failure is a sign that the heart is working inefficiently. This may be due to coronary heart disease, valvular damage from rheumatic fever, or other disorders. Congestive heart failure is characterized by fluid accumulation in the body and shortness of breath, during even the mildest exertion.

Glaucoma

Increased pressure of the fluid in the eyeball (glaucoma) may eventually lead to blindness. Through regular eye examinations, glaucoma can be detected early, and cure effected. (See GLAUCOMA in the encyclopedia section.)

Presbyopia

Almost all middle-aged persons gradually become more farsighted. This results from the lens of the eye becoming less elastic and, therefore, less able to change its focusing characteristics. Corrective eyeglasses are the only remedy. (See PRESBYOPIA in the encyclopedia section.)

Presbycusis

The aging process in the ear leads to a variable degree of hearing loss, particularly for higher and lower tones.

Ulcers

Peptic ulcers (those of the stomach and duodenum) cause abdominal pain and discomfort. Diagnosis is most frequently made by X ray (gastrointestinal series). Heredity and emotional stress are two important factors in the development of ulcers. They usually can be treated by diet and medicines, but in some cases surgery may be necessary. (See ULCERS in the encyclopedia section.)

Hernia

As the body tissues age, they become weaker. A particularly weak part of the body wall, and one frequently subjected to stress, is the groin area. The bulging of the underlying intestines through an opening in this wall is called a hernia. Treatment is usually by surgery. (Hernias are discussed further in Chapter 23.)

Gallbladder Disease

Stones and chronic inflammation irritate the gallbladder and prevent it from releasing bile properly. Because the bile that the gallbladder stores is needed for digestion, particularly of fatty foods, indigestion is a frequent symptom of gallbladder trouble. Emotional upsets as well as excess fatty foods may cause an acute inflammation of the gallbladder, characterized by abdominal pain, fever, and vomiting. Recurrent attacks are an indication that the diseased gallbladder may have to be removed by surgery. (See GALL-BLADDER and GALLSTONES in the encyclopedia section.)

Varicose Veins

Distended, tortuous veins in the legs are a rather frequent problem of middle age, particularly in women. Varicose veins may be a site for blood clots. In the most severe types, the blood is not adequately drained from the lower extremities, and the overlying skin may become swollen and irritated and break down, forming an ulcer. People with varicose veins frequently complain of pain and fatigue of the legs. Treatment varies from the wearing of support stockings to surgical removal of the veins. (See VARICOSE VEINS in the encyclopedia section.)

Disease of Blood Vessels in the Extremities

Arteriosclerosis tends to narrow blood vessels in the brain, heart, and extremities. When the vessels conducting blood to the legs become narrowed sufficiently, there are usually such symptoms as the inability to walk several blocks without severe calf pain. Sudden occlusion (blocking) of the vessels to the leg by a blood clot may occur. This results in severe pain and is often an emergency that must be treated surgically by removing the clot. (See HARDENING OF THE ARTERIES in the encyclopedia section.)

Arthritis

Arthritis is an inflammation of the joints. The causes vary and the joints are affected in different ways. Osteoarthritis is caused by the wear and tear of the joint tissues. It usually is not severe or disabling and develops after age 40. Rheumatoid arthritis is a more serious form of the disorder, and may produce deformities and major disabilities. (Both forms are discussed further in Chapter 23 and under the entry ARTHRITIS in the encyclopedia section.)

Prostate Gland

In many men over 50, the prostate gland becomes so enlarged that it interferes with the normal passage of urine. Symptoms of this enlargement are frequent urination, decreased stream, difficulty in beginning to urinate, and a feeling of incomplete urination. If symptoms become severe enough, the gland has to be removed surgically, a major but relatively safe operation. (See PROSTATE GLAND in the encyclopedia section.)

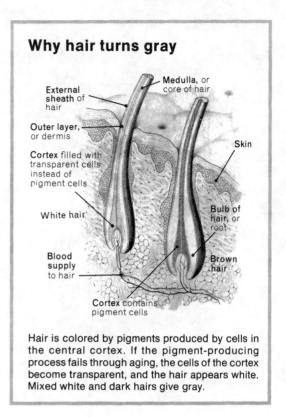

Why hair turns gray

External sheath of hair

Medulla, or core of hair

Outer layer, or dermis

Cortex filled with transparent cells instead of pigment cells

Skin

White hair

Bulb of hair, or root

Blood supply to hair

Brown hair

Cortex contains pigment cells

Hair is colored by pigments produced by cells in the central cortex. If the pigment-producing process fails through aging, the cells of the cortex become transparent, and the hair appears white. Mixed white and dark hairs give gray.

Menopause

For most women, the menopause occurs sometime in the forties or fifties. The menstrual flow may stop suddenly, taper off gradually, or it may stop temporarily, restart, and then taper off. Menopausal symptoms vary. Some women have none at all; many, if not most, experience hot flashes, or flushes, in varying degrees of discomfort; and some may suffer from vertigo or a sudden rise in blood pressure. Severe symptoms may be treated with estrogens (female sex hormones), but their use should be discussed thoroughly with a physician; estrogens have proved to be extremely hazardous for some women. Bodily changes may take place after the menopause, such as redistribution of fat, sagging breasts, coarsening of the skin, and weakening of the bones. These changes may also respond favorably to estrogen therapy. (For a fuller discussion, see Chapter 19 and the entry MENOPAUSE in the encyclopedia section.)

SEX IN THE MIDDLE YEARS

For both men and women, there is good evidence that there is a decline in—but not a termination of—sex-hormone production in the forties and fifties and later. This does not mean, however, that there is an accompanying decline in sexual activity. Sexual function depends only partly on the level of hormone production, and probably is influenced mainly by emotional factors such as psychological makeup, marital relationship, and previous satisfactory or unsatisfactory sexual experiences. Some diminution in sexual drive and capacity can be expected in the middle years, but not to an extent that precludes an active sex life.

Some women may experience an increase in sexual drive in the late forties and early fifties. This may be related to release from fear of pregnancy or a searching for outlets of energy formerly expended in raising and caring for children. Other women may be plagued to an ever-increasing extent by unsatisfactory sexual relations, most often a manifestation of previously unresolved inner conflicts regarding sexuality. Such problems are best handled by a qualified physician such as a gynecologist or a psychiatrist. In general, sexual interest and satisfaction are more likely to continue for many years beyond the menopause in those who have had a happy, well-adjusted marriage with a healthy attitude toward sex.

Sexual adequacy in men tends to take a sharp drop after the age of 50. However, according to recent findings, it need not do so. Many cases of impotence can be treated successfully through good guidance in sexual practices. Given reasonable health, men can enjoy adequate sexual performance into the seventies and eighties—as can women. What is needed to maintain effective sexuality in the aging male is a constant interest in sex and active sexual expression.

There are several factors that tend to inhibit sexual responsiveness in men. Overindulging in food and drink can lead to a transitory decrease of intensity of sexual interest and desire; alcohol, in particular, can cause an inability to maintain an erection.

The types of physical activity that have an unfavorable effect on male sexuality are usually associated with excessive strain or fatigue. Maintaining good physical condition helps prevent the letdown in sexual tension associated with physical fatigue.

But mental fatigue has a greater detrimental influence on sexual interest than does physical fatigue. Whether it be a strenuous day at the office or family difficulties or financial emergencies, the expenditure of energy on such concerns lessens the energy available for sexual responsiveness—often for days beyond the immediate emergency. This sensitivity of sexual desire to mental strain is significantly greater in middle-aged than in younger men.

Sexual capacity and performance can be affected either transiently or for long periods of time by physical illness. But heart disease, for example, need not mean an end to sexual relations. Medical guidance as to how and when to have sexual relations after any kind of serious illness is important and should be discussed frankly with your physician. He often can give you good advice or refer you to a specialist.

The key to sexual responsiveness in the middle years lies in regularity of sexual expression. Lack of sexual performance leads to a reduction of sexual desire, while active sexual expression combined with adequate physical health and a positive attitude toward the changes of the middle years can provide a satisfying sex life well into the later years.

19

Special Health Problems of Women

The female reproductive system is a truly remarkable mechanism, and its functioning is an integral part of every woman's life, whether or not she bears children. The special health problems associated with this system are discussed in this chapter. It also deals with the health problems associated with the main activity of many women—housework, which, like any other job, has its own risks to health.

MENSTRUAL DISORDERS

For about 35 years of her life—the childbearing period—every normal woman menstruates. (See the entry MENSTRUATION in the encyclopedia section for a fuller discussion of this physiological function.) At some point during this long span of years, one or another menstrual disorder may arise. Most such disorders are trivial and, in fact, usually correct themselves. Nevertheless, they should not be ignored. If your menstrual period is abnormal in any way, consult your doctor.

This is especially important if you bleed between periods or after the menopause. The symptom may mean nothing: women who take the birth control pill sometimes experience this so-called "break-through" bleeding. But it can also be a warning sign of cancer, and it should therefore be reported to the doctor immediately. (For a fuller discussion of cancer of the reproductive system, see Chapter 22.)

Absence of Menstruation (Amenorrhea)

Sometimes a girl who has reached the age of puberty fails to begin menstruating. This condition is known as *primary amenorrhea*. In rare cases, it is caused by malformed or underdeveloped organs. For example, the hymen (see the entry HYMEN in the encyclopedia section) may block off the entrance to the vagina completely, instead of only partially, thus causing retention of the menstrual blood. The condition may also be caused by glandular disorders, which can be treated and corrected. If the *menarche* (onset of menstruation at puberty) seems unduly delayed, it is wise to consult a physician.

The term *secondary amenorrhea* is used to describe cases in which menstruation begins and then quickly ceases. Secondary amenorrhea normally accompanies pregnancy, and women who breast-feed their babies may find that it continues intermittently for as long as they are nursing. It is also quite common in the period immediately following menarche and the period preceding menopause.

Primary and secondary amenorrhea can also be associated with other factors—general poor health, a change in climate or living conditions, or emotional difficulties, such as stress, or the fear or hope of being pregnant. All these can affect the hormone balance and, therefore, the menstrual periods. These same factors can sometimes reduce the menstrual flow to little more than staining. A severely reduced menstrual flow may also be caused by anemia (see the entry ANEMIA in the encyclopedia section).

Excessive Menstruation (Menorrhagia)

The term *menorrhagia* is used to describe the condition that exists when the regular menstrual flow is exceptionally heavy. It is not easy to describe the amount of menstrual flow that constitutes menorrhagia. However, if your regular means of sanitary protection are not adequate to absorb the menstrual flow, or if the menstrual blood forms into large clots, you are likely to be suffering from this condition and should consult your doctor immediately.

Irregular Menstruation

For some women, the menstrual cycle is extremely regular; they can predict within 24 hours when their next period will begin. In other women, the cycle is far less predictable; the interval between periods varies from month to month. Women in both groups may occasionally experience cycles that are irregular for them. Such irregularity may be caused by a harmless variation in nature's timing, by changes in climate or living conditions, or by emotional factors. The irregularity will usually correct itself spontaneously.

On the other hand, menstrual irregularity can be the result of a medical problem that requires the doctor's help. For example, irregularity may be associated with disease in some part of the body, such as the thyroid gland, or with a tumor of the uterus or the ovaries. A doctor should be consulted if menstrual irregularity persists. This is particularly important in the case of bleeding between periods, because this can be a sign of cancer somewhere in the reproductive system.

Painful Menstruation (Dysmenorrhea)

Many women experience discomfort and mild cramps at the onset of their periods—a condition known as *dysmenorrhea*. Usually the pain will yield to an aspirin and a brief rest.

Dysmenorrhea is almost never found in women who have had a number of children. Often it cannot be accounted for by any organic condition, and in many cases there is conclusive evidence that it is caused by emotional factors acting on the body. Your doctor can prescribe medications—antispasmodics, analgesics, and sedatives—to relieve severe menstrual pain.

Intermenstrual Pain

Some women experience pain approximately midway between their periods, at the time of ovulation. (See the entry OVULATION in the encyclopedia section.) The pain may be accompanied by a slight show of blood, or by a nonbloody vaginal discharge. Although the pain is sometimes quite severe, in most cases there is only mild discomfort, which lasts for only a short time.

Premenstrual Difficulties

A number of symptoms—headache, depression, irritability, slight nausea, and puffiness of the abdomen, skin, and other parts of the body—may precede the menstrual period. The reasons for these symptoms are not fully understood, but it is known that they are associated with a disturbance of the body's salt balance and a consequent accumulation of water in the tissues. Sometimes these symptoms can be relieved by the use of a

The menstrual cycle

Menstruation is the monthly loss of blood from the uterus which takes place throughout a woman's childbearing years. It is just one event in the series of changes known as the menstrual cycle.

The female reproductive system

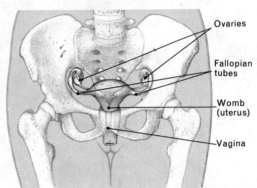

- Ovaries
- Fallopian tubes
- Womb (uterus)
- Vagina

The average cycle lasts about 28 days, although in some women it is several days longer or shorter. Menstruation begins during puberty, usually when a girl is 12 to 14 years old, and ends at the menopause by about the age of 50. During the menstrual cycle, an egg cell develops in an ovary and passes along a Fallopian tube into the uterus; at the same time, hormones cause changes in the lining of the uterus. If the egg is not fertilized, it and the lining of the uterus are discarded in the monthly flow of blood. After menstruation, the structure of the uterus heals, and another cycle begins. If the egg is fertilized, the process ceases and does not start again until the end of pregnancy. The regularity of the cycle is controlled by hormones secreted by the pituitary gland at the base of the brain.

How the egg reaches the uterus

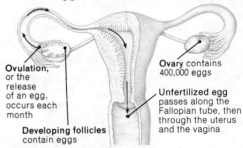

Ovulation, or the release of an egg, occurs each month

Developing follicles contain eggs

Ovary contains 400,000 eggs

Unfertilized egg passes along the Fallopian tube, then through the uterus and the vagina

An egg released from the ovary is picked up by fringes at the end of the Fallopian tube. Inside the tube, the egg is carried along to the uterus by tiny hairlike cilia and by muscular contractions.

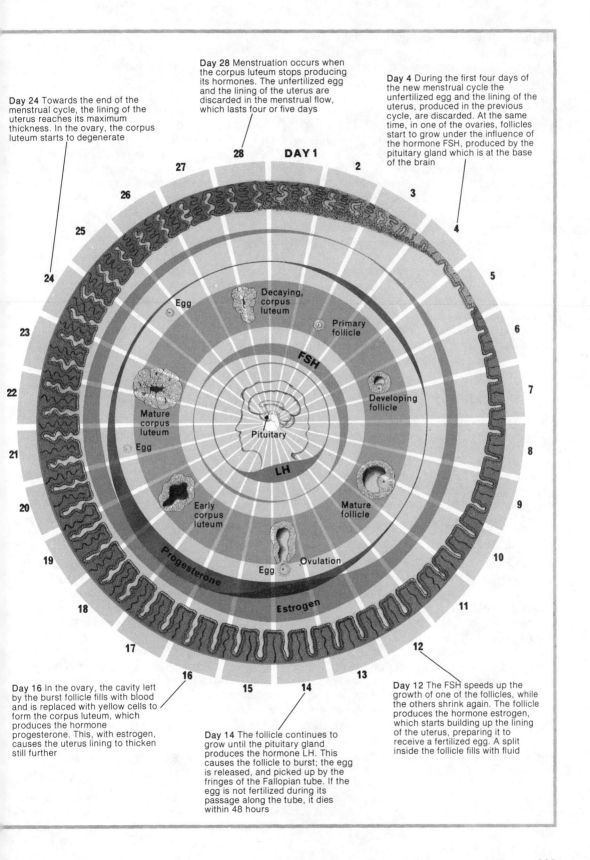

Day 28 Menstruation occurs when the corpus luteum stops producing its hormones. The unfertilized egg and the lining of the uterus are discarded in the menstrual flow, which lasts four or five days

Day 4 During the first four days of the new menstrual cycle the unfertilized egg and the lining of the uterus, produced in the previous cycle, are discarded. At the same time, in one of the ovaries, follicles start to grow under the influence of the hormone FSH, produced by the pituitary gland which is at the base of the brain

Day 24 Towards the end of the menstrual cycle, the lining of the uterus reaches its maximum thickness. In the ovary, the corpus luteum starts to degenerate

Egg

Decaying, corpus luteum

Primary follicle

FSH

Developing follicle

Mature corpus luteum

Pituitary

Egg

LH

Mature follicle

Early corpus luteum

Egg

Ovulation

Progesterone

Estrogen

DAY 1

Day 16 In the ovary, the cavity left by the burst follicle fills with blood and is replaced with yellow cells to form the corpus luteum, which produces the hormone progesterone. This, with estrogen, causes the uterus lining to thicken still further

Day 14 The follicle continues to grow until the pituitary gland produces the hormone LH. This causes the follicle to burst; the egg is released, and picked up by the fringes of the Fallopian tube. If the egg is not fertilized during its passage along the tube, it dies within 48 hours

Day 12 The FSH speeds up the growth of one of the follicles, while the others shrink again. The follicle produces the hormone estrogen, which starts building up the lining of the uterus, preparing it to receive a fertilized egg. A split inside the follicle fills with fluid

diuretic (see the entry DIURETIC in the encyclopedia section), which your doctor can prescribe, or by the elimination of salt from the diet.

THE MENOPAUSE

The years during which a woman can conceive and bear children are limited to those during which she ovulates and menstruates—that is, the years of her regular monthly cycle. At the end of this period, ovarian function declines and finally ceases, and menstruation ends. This is the menopause. It begins when ovarian function begins to decline, and it ends when ovarian function has ceased—a period which may last anywhere from six months to three years.

Menopause can occur prematurely as a result of certain diseases and hormonal disorders or as a consequence of hysterectomy—the surgical removal of the uterus, or womb. However, the average American woman normally enters the menopause at the age of 48 years. In general, the younger she is when she begins to menstruate, the older will she be when her menopause begins.

Adjusting to the Menopause

Menopause is a perfectly normal event, like menstruation, and for many women it is a liberating experience. No longer do they need to worry about unwanted pregnancies, or take precautions against them. If they are mothers, their children are likely to be grown up, or close to it, and well on the road to independence. This means that women have more time to pursue interests that the responsibilities of motherhood may have compelled them to drop. If the woman has been working, she can go back to her interrupted job or career. She can enjoy her newfound freedom in any one of a number of rewarding ways.

Unfortunately, however, a number of superstitions have grown up around the very idea of menopause, and these have brought misery and suffering to women who might otherwise be enjoying this time of their lives. It is *not* true that menopause brings mental instability, or that it lessens a woman's attractiveness or her ability to give and receive pleasure in sexual relations. These are dangerous misconceptions with absolutely no medical support, and they should have no place in your mind. Nor should you feel embarrassed or hesitant to discuss with your doctor or some other qualified health professional any other questions or fears you may have about menopause.

Physical Symptoms of the Menopause

The physical symptoms that are associated with the menopause are caused by a slowing down in the production of estrogens (see the entry ESTROGEN in the encyclopedia section). These female sex hormones are produced chiefly in the ovaries, but in far smaller amounts once menopause has begun. The symptom this reduction most commonly produces is the series of vasomotor disturbances familiarly known as "hot flashes." These are frequently the first sign that the menopause is occurring, and they disappear gradually after the menstrual periods have ceased. Hot flashes may be limited to the face and neck or they may extend over the entire body. They may be accompanied by flushing, by excessive perspiration, or by a sensation of closeness of the air that makes a woman feel uncomfortably warm on even a cold day. Hot flashes may also bring on headaches or a coldness of the hands and feet. Some women experience these symptoms only a few times during the entire course of the menopause, while others experience them several times a day.

In addition, some women have other physical difficulties. They may be easily fatigued, or they may suffer from a nervous irritation of the bladder that leads them to urinate frequently. They may have backaches, or feel a kind of dizziness or giddiness (vertigo), occasionally associated with nausea or loss of appetite. Sometimes the blood pressure rises sharply.

It is important to consult your doctor during this period in your life, whether or not you have any of the symptoms described above. Your symptoms, if any, may require no treatment at all, or be helped by some form of medication. In the past, estrogen therapy was frequently used to relieve some of the more unpleasant symptoms of the menopause and to help women whose ovaries were removed before the menopause normally would have begun. However, recent studies have shown an increased incidence of uterine cancer in women given estrogen therapy, and your doctor is likely to prescribe it only if the symptoms are severe and if there are no contraindications. If he does prescribe it, he will also insist on frequent gynecological checkups.

OTHER DISORDERS OF THE REPRODUCTIVE ORGANS

In the past, infections of the ovaries, Fallopian tubes, and uterus were extremely common, causing considerable suffering for many women. But such infections no longer need pose a threat because all of them can be successfully treated with antibiotics. Similarly, improvements in obstetrical methods have drastically reduced the number of injuries that in the past were often associated with pregnancy and childbirth.

Relaxed tissues or muscular injuries can cause disorders of the reproductive system, all of which can be treated either medically or surgically. Among these problems are: *cystocele,* a bulging of the bladder owing to weakness of the vaginal wall; *rectocele,* a bulging of the rectum into the vagina; *prolapse* of the uterus, which pushes the cervix far down into the vagina; and displacement of the uterus.

Leukorrhea

Leukorrhea—sometimes called "the whites"—is a persistent, nonbloody vaginal discharge. The condition is both common and troublesome. It is not a disease, but a symptom of a number of different illnesses, ranging from the trivial to the serious. So if you have leukorrhea—or any persistent discharge that is not colorless and that is accompanied by vaginal itching or irritation—consult your physician.

Among the possible causes of leukorrhea are gonorrhea, polyps, lacerations of the cervix that sometimes occur during childbirth, or the irritation caused by an improperly fitted diaphragm. Occasionally leukorrhea is caused by some condition outside the genital tract—malnutrition, for example, or even pelvic congestion associated with heart disease.

One of the most common causes of leukorrhea is a one-celled microorganism known as *Trichomonas vaginalis,* which produces a yellowish discharge with an unpleasant odor. *Trichomonas* also causes itching of the external genitals and sometimes leads to chronic inflammation of the cervix. It can be treated and cured. Because the organism can be passed on to the woman's sexual partner, it may also be necessary for the doctor to prescribe medication for the man.

Leukorrhea may also be a symptom of moniliasis, a fungus disease that may affect other areas of the body besides the vagina. (For a full discussion of MONILIASIS see the encyclopedia section.)

Inflammation of the Cervix

A number of conditions can cause the cervix—the mouth of the uterus—to become inflamed. As mentioned above, an inflamed cervix may be associated with injuries during childbirth. Various kinds of irritations can also lead to cervical in-

flammation, or *cervicitis.* Chronic cervicitis can be treated either by cauterization, which with only slight discomfort removes or destroys the inflamed area, or by cryosurgery, which accomplishes the same result equally painlessly by the application of extreme cold. An inflamed cervix should be treated promptly, because it is a fertile area for the development of cancer. Cervical polyps, a type of small tumor, should always be removed and examined under the microscope to see if they are malignant.

Fibroid Tumors

Sometimes harmless growths called fibroid tumors develop in the wall of the uterus. These growths may produce no symptoms whatever and may be detected only during a gynecological examination. On the other hand, they sometimes cause menstrual difficulties, and if they grow large enough, they may interfere with the functioning of organs adjacent to the uterus. Small fibroids, which cause no trouble, can usually be left alone. Larger ones may require surgery. (For a further discussion of this subject, see the entry FIBROID TUMOR in the encyclopedia section.)

Senile Vaginitis

Elderly women frequently develop vaginal infections as a result of the aging of the tissues; these infections manifest themselves by the appearance of a discharge. If you have such a discharge, consult your doctor. It can be relieved by treatment with a vaginal suppository, available by prescription.

Pruritus Vulvae

Itching of the genitals (*pruritus vulvae*) is frequently caused by leukorrhea and vanishes when it is corrected. But the itching can have other causes. It may be owing to irritation from urine (especially in diabetics), to skin diseases, or to irritation caused by chafing or nervous scratching of a minor inflammation. Itching may also be connected with an allergic reaction. Your doctor can help you discover and eliminate the cause. Phenobarbital or other sedatives can reduce the nervous tension the itching creates.

Endometriosis

The special kind of mucous membrane that lines the walls of the uterus sometimes develops in other organs inside the pelvic cavity—for example, in the ovaries. This condition is known as *endometriosis.* It may lead to the creation of cysts—called "chocolate cysts"—which are

231

formed from the blood produced in the tissue. Endometriosis is frequently accompanied by pain in the lower abdomen, especially at the time of menstruation. In some cases, hormone therapy may cure the problem; in others, surgery may be necessary.

SURGICAL PROCEDURES

Dilatation and Curettage (D and C)

This surgical procedure involves dilation of the cervix and the scraping of the internal walls of the uterus. It may be performed for a number of reasons. It is one accepted method of abortion. It is sometimes performed after a miscarriage to remove any embryonic tissue that may have remained. If a woman experiences bleeding between her periods or excessive bleeding—especially after she has entered the menopause—dilatation and curettage may be used to relieve the condition and to obtain a tissue sample for further study. Uterine tumors and polyps may also be removed by curettage. (See also the entry DILATATION AND CURETTAGE in the encyclopedia section.)

Hysterectomy

Hysterectomy means removal of the uterus, or womb. It is the only effective procedure for treating certain life-threatening conditions. But once the uterus has been removed, a woman is no longer able to bear children. Hysterectomy should therefore never be performed unless it is absolutely necessary. It is imperative for the woman to have at least two medical opinions—including the opinion of a gynecologist—before undergoing the procedure.

Depending on the necessities of the individual case, one or both of the ovaries may be removed along with the uterus. Removal of the ovaries is likely to bring on premature symptoms of menopause. But if the ovaries remain intact, normal hormone production may continue after the operation, and no menopausal symptoms will appear until the normal age. (See also the entry HYSTERECTOMY in the encyclopedia section.)

THE BREASTS

The breasts, or mammary glands, have three main components: the milk glands, the milk ducts, and fatty tissue. The milk glands are arranged in a complicated pattern of lobes, somewhat in the form of a wagon wheel, at the center of which is the nipple, into which the milk duct

feeds. The fatty tissue gives the breasts their shape and size; the amount of fatty tissue varies considerably from one woman to the next.

The breasts are vulnerable to a number of disorders. Benign tumors and cysts occur fairly frequently, as do various forms of *mastitis* (inflammation of the breast). Mastitis can develop for a variety of reasons, and it can become chronic. Chronic interstitial mastitis and chronic cystic mastitis are the chief types of breast inflammation; although usually not serious, they can be quite painful, especially before the menstrual period. Mastitis is sometimes caused by an injury, and this is one of the reasons it is important to give the breasts proper support and protection. Mastitis can also follow childbirth. A cracked nipple can permit germs to enter the breast, thus producing an infection that leads to an abscess. Do *not* attempt to treat any breast disorder by yourself. Report it to your physician.

The most serious disorder of the breasts is cancer, which is discussed in detail both in the encyclopedia section and in Chapter 22. Read these two sections to learn the symptoms of the disease and the correct method of self-examination. A rare type of cancer of the breast is known as Paget's carcinoma, which frequently involves the nipples, causing itching and burning until the nipple becomes ulcerated.

The earlier breast cancer is detected, the more effectively can it be treated. It is therefore urgent for every woman to examine her breasts carefully at least once a month and to consult with her physician in the event there is any lump, pain, injury, or change in the shape of the breast, and any discharge from the nipple. The development of mammography—X ray of the breasts—makes it possible for the doctor to discover breast cancer at any early stage. The use of this technique may be indicated for women over 50, who run a higher risk of breast cancer than younger women, and for women whose breasts are large and difficult to examine accurately by touch.

HOUSEWORK AND HEALTH

As most women are aware, housework is hard labor, involving much physical exertion and long hours. Even with modern labor-saving devices, the job can put a considerable strain on the health of anyone who engages in it.

In the past, the form of bursitis known as housemaid's knee (see the entry HOUSEMAID's KNEE in the encyclopedia section) was the best-known and most common condition that could

Checking the breasts

A lump in the breast is not necessarily a symptom of cancer, but it could be—the earlier it is found and diagnosed, the greater are the chances of a complete cure. A growth can be discovered in its earliest stages by a routine monthly self-examination. This is best done by a woman just after a menstrual period, because harmless lumps in the breasts are common just before a period starts. Begin by looking at your breasts in the mirror for any changes in their appearance. Then lie on your back and examine each breast. If there is anything unusual, see your doctor.

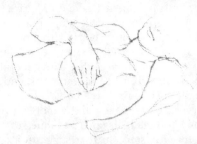

1 Lie down to check the breasts. Put padding, such as a pillow, under one shoulder and feel tissues extending into the armpit.

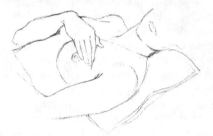

2 With the flats of the fingers, not with the tips, examine the upper, outer quarter of the breast. Give this area special attention.

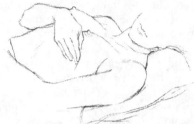

3 Next examine the remainder of the outer half of the breast by feeling round the edge to the area at the center near the nipple.

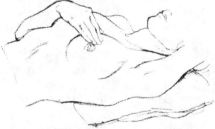

4 Press the inner half of the breast against the wall of the chest, moving the fingers from the breastbone to the middle of the breast.

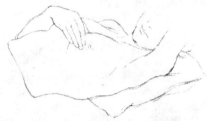

5 Feel the nipple area, then the remainder of the inner half of breast. Put the pad under the other shoulder, and examine the other breast.

properly be described as an occupational disease of housewives. Today it occurs much less frequently because most women no longer spend many hours on their knees scrubbing the floors. But there has arisen a new occupational disease associated with housework that many doctors call housewives' dermatitis. This is a chronic skin irritation caused by the very soaps, detergents, and cleansers that have made housework easier. Not only do these cleansing agents dissolve grease and dirt, they dissolve the natural oils and fats needed to lubricate the skin.

But most of the health hazards involved in housework are far less direct than this. Like most other occupational health hazards, their ill effects come on slowly. It is chronic or too-hasty exposure to the hazard that does the damage. Many housewives, for example, have trouble with their reproductive organs, trouble that is directly traceable to their having resumed work too soon after giving birth, and to having attacked that work with too much vigor. Especially in the period immediately following childbirth, a husband should give his wife all the help he can.

Similarly, housework can seriously aggravate a preexisting chronic illness or disability. All housewives with chronic illnesses should consult with the organizations associated with the particular disability from which they suffer. Groups such as the American Heart Association and the

Arthritis Foundation can provide useful help and advice to supplement the doctor's care.

There are a number of things that the housewife can do to protect her health. Some of them have already been discussed in this book, especially in the chapters dealing with general care of the body (Chapter 1), the functions and care of the individual parts of the body (Chapter 3), diet (Chapter 2), pregnancy and childbirth (Chapter 13), and household hazards and illnesses (Chapter 21). Here are some further suggestions:

1. *Make a job study of your work.* Unlike work in business and industry, housework has seldom been the subject of investigations designed to increase efficiency and reduce strain, and most housework is done in a rather random manner. Observe the way you perform your various household tasks, especially those which you find distasteful or tiring, and see if you can find a way of doing them that will eliminate, or at least reduce, their negative aspects.

2. *Consider yourself in relation to your work.* Household appliances and tools were designed for the average woman of a certain height, weight, and strength. If you differ from that average, adjusting to the "norm" may be putting a strain on you. But it may not even be necessary for you to make the adjustment. Reaching and stooping are often unnecessary evils. Whenever you buy something new—whether a stove, a sink, or an ironing board—find out what can be done to make it the proper height for you. If you are going to make do with the equipment you already have, there are still ways to make things easier. If you are too tall for the sink, for example, place something under the dishpan to bring it to a more comfortable height. If you are too short, you can make yourself taller by sitting on a high stool. Many household objects—chairs, couches, cabinets—are heavy and difficult to move; putting casters under them can help.

3. *Become posture-wise.* Poor posture is responsible for many of the strains and injuries, as well as the aches and pains, from which many housewives suffer. Consult Chapter 1 for illustrations that show the correct and incorrect ways to sit and to stand, and the exercises to take to strengthen your back. Guard against back injuries by avoiding sudden twisting or moving when you are off balance. When you lift things, bend your knees and keep your back straight—this puts the work load on your legs, and not on the delicate muscles of your back. When you are vacuuming the baseboards, or performing other tasks close to the floor, follow the same rule: straight back, bent knees.

Posture begins with the feet. The average housewife spends from 80 to 90 percent of her working day on her feet, which means that she is standing for about eight hours. It is therefore especially important that her feet be in good condition. (For information about the care of the feet, see Chapter 3.)

4. *Take care of your hands.* Rubber gloves are a good protection against housewives' dermatitis. If you do not like to wear them, you should observe the following precautions. Use only as much soap or detergent as is absolutely necessary to do an efficient cleaning job. Be sure that the water you use is not too hot, because heat removes the natural oils from the skin and causes irritation. Dry your hands thoroughly, and use a lotion, especially in cold or dry weather. Use an oily lotion before going to bed. An air humidifier helps to keep the skin from becoming too dry. It is a good idea to use one, especially during the winter months, and all year long in desert areas. Be careful of the skin under your rings; always dry it thoroughly and be on the alert for sores or inflammations that may start there. Never neglect cuts or sores of any kind. Wear a rubber finger or glove to protect any injuries.

5. *Give yourself some time off.* Workers in offices and factories expect to have some time off during the day and at the end of the work week. Housewives also need time away from their jobs. It may not be possible for you to take off an entire day, but you can usually arrange for a few free mornings or afternoons during the week. During that time, do something that is a complete change from housework. Remember that it is important for you to be able to get away from your housework routine.

Just as office and factory workers have regular coffee breaks during the day, housewives should have rest breaks. You will be able to accomplish more in less time if you take a complete recess both morning and afternoon. Try to make the breaks fairly long ones, but take at least two 15-minute periods each day to rest and relax.

CHAPTER **20** Retirement and the Later Years

No matter what your age, you would be wise to consider the advantages and problems of what have been called—ironically by some—"the golden years." Whether or not these are happy years depends largely on the individual. Careful attention to your health, especially from age 40 on, can eliminate many of the common "old-age" complaints. Most of the medical problems associated with elderly people actually start in the middle years. Guarding your health and planning your finances from the ages of 40 to 65 are the best ways to assure yourself of a satisfactory retirement.

This chapter discusses not only the problems but the more rewarding aspects of old age, stressing the mental, emotional, and physical assets available during the later years of life. It deals with the major diseases and minor discomforts that often afflict the elderly, and gives valuable health-care tips on how to live to a ripe old age. The chapter concludes with helpful advice on planning your own successful retirement.

OUR EXPANDING LIFE SPAN

The average life span has increased remarkably over the years. In ancient Rome life expectancy was about 23 years. The typical colonial American lived to about the age of 35. By 1900 the average life span in the United States was 47 years. But today an American can expect to live to about 73.

The tremendous increase in life expectancy during the present century is owing in great part to the conquest of diseases such as cholera, smallpox, and diphtheria. The largest drop in mortality rates has been among infants. However, many more people are living much longer than they did in the past, and the number of retired persons increases greatly each year. Clearly, good nutrition and improved health care do make a difference—for the group and for the individual. (See also the entries AGING; GERIATRICS in the encyclopedia section.)

ASSETS OF THE LATER YEARS

Most people tend to think only of the liabilities of aging. It makes sense to consider the physical, mental, and emotional assets of the elderly as well.

Mental Assets

Here the ledger shows many assets and very few liabilities. It is encouraging to know that the mind, at least, does not wear out from use or even from overuse. The more a physically and emotionally healthy person uses his brain, the better it will be in the later years.

Learning tests have proved conclusively that there is no truth to the saying, "You can't teach an old dog new tricks." It all depends on whether the old person wants to learn. These tests have shown that older people tend to learn a trifle more slowly, but they also learn more thoroughly, so that they actually master a new subject in about the same time as younger students.

We used to believe that memory faded with age. Now we know that memory is directly related to interest. Older people do, indeed, forget recent events, because many of them are concerned only with the past.

Older people have a natural advantage when it comes to judgment, which depends not only on the ability to reason, but on experience.

Emotional Assets

The well-adjusted older person approaches true freedom because he has overcome the self-consciousness that causes so much pain in earlier years. He gains in poise and self-control, becoming more tolerant of himself and others. Although emotional experiences are less acute and intense, they are richer, deeper, and more subtle.

Fear, anxiety, and feelings of insecurity are probably more damaging to the emotional health of old people than they are to the young. The irritability common to some aged men and women is often caused by the inability to sleep well. The dislike of change and the suspicious attitude toward anything or anyone new is frequently rooted in a lack of self-confidence. However, these are *not* characteristic responses of old people who are emotionally secure.

It is true that elderly people have special emotional difficulties. Some of these problems, as well as common ailments, are discussed in Chapter 18.

It is only after we reach middle age that many of us first face the fact that we are mortal. Some of us accept the idea with equanimity. But to a great many others of us, the reaction is profoundly disturbing. It is not at all abnormal or a sign of weakness to feel uncomfortable at the thought of death. Sometimes it is helpful to talk about the meaning of life and death with members of your family or your close friends. If there are things in the past that weigh heavily on your conscience, or if you fear death excessively, you should discuss the matter with your clergyman or with your doctor or a psychiatrist.

Physical Assets

The organs and tissues of an elderly person often compare favorably with those of his juniors. The process of aging is usually uneven. For example, the thymus gland atrophies and disappears after puberty, and the tonsils are senile at the age of 50. In most individuals certain organs will show signs of impairment, while others remain young. In fact, every adverse condition found in elderly people is usually evident in individuals one or even two generations younger.

As people age, they are less apt to suffer from infectious diseases. This is true not only because they are immune to certain diseases they had in the past, but also because they have acquired a partial immunity to other infections without ever being ill—and even some immunity to colds.

When older persons do develop an infectious illness, it is usually less severe than it would be in a young adult. For example, tuberculosis endangers elderly persons less than adolescents.

Many people worry about the effect of aging on their sexual lives. This anxiety usually troubles men more than women. True, there is a gradual decline in sexual capacity after age 40, but experts state that the period of full potency in the male extends into the fifties and sixties. Many older couples, including those 90 years of age, continue to enjoy normal sexual relations. There is some evidence that sexual activity tends to maintain normal endocrine balance, and that this in turn may help inhibit the aging processes.

DISEASES IN THE ELDERLY

There is no disease actually caused by old age. Medical studies clearly show that the majority of fatal diseases in elderly people originated when the patients were in their middle years. This is one more strong argument for regular medical examinations and health education.

Certain chronic disorders, progressing into the advanced years, form a general pattern of diseases commonly found in the elderly. The highest toll is taken by heart diseases, cancer, and cerebral hemorrhage (or stroke). Other common afflictions of old age are arthritis, rheumatism, diabetes, prostate trouble, kidney ailments, and nervous and mental disorders, along with problems of the arteries and high blood pressure. The symptoms of these diseases are discussed in Chapters 22 and 23. It is important to minimize their threat by having regular medical checkups.

Senility, once considered an inevitable result of old age, is now viewed as no great threat. The majority of men and women who reach the later years are neither feeble nor confused. Poor mental health, along with poor physical health, can be averted in most cases. Once again, a healthy attitude and regular medical care can make a major difference. (For a discussion of morbid senility, as contrasted with normal aging, see SENILITY in the encyclopedia section.)

Surgery for the Aged

Older people are able to withstand operations extremely well in these days of improved surgical techniques. It is now possible to carry out a four-hour operation on an 80-year-old with minimal danger.

Among the disorders of old age that can be corrected surgically are enlargement of the prostate, hernia, cataracts, and a prolapsed, or fallen, bladder, rectum, or uterus. For an old person to break a bone—especially in the hip or thigh—once spelled disaster, but today successful operations to set and promote healing of fractured bones in elderly people are routine.

Old people must be thoroughly reassured about impending surgery. All possible details should be explained, even those that seem insignificant. (See Chapter 10.) If at all feasible, the person should visit the hospital to see the room he or she will occupy and to meet the nurses. When the family doctor is calling in a surgeon, the elderly person should, if possible, become acquainted with the surgeon well in advance of the scheduled operation.

Partial Restoration of Bodily Functions

For an old person, the partial restoration of a normal bodily function may be enormously important. Physicians understandably hesitate to take money from elderly people for prolonged therapy that may produce only minimal results. The older person should make it clear to the doctor that even a small improvement will be deeply appreciated. For example, an elderly person may be quite miserable when confined to bed, whereas being able to get up for meals and go for an occasional drive or a short walk will make life far happier.

An elderly person, especially one who does not have children and grandchildren nearby, will find a trusted doctor one of the greatest comforts of old age. Like a clergyman, the physician can always be depended upon. The older individual should stick to one doctor and get to know him well and be known by him, not only as a patient but as a person.

DISCOMFORTS AND MINOR IMPAIRMENTS OF OLD AGE

Old age does bring some inevitable changes in the body, which can result in discomfort and minor impairments. Because the bone joints and bursas are not as well lubricated as they are in younger people, certain forms of rheumatism and arthritis frequently occur. Usually these are not the crippling types, but they do cause pain. The symptoms of these ailments, as well as many other discomforts, such as buzzing in the ears, insomnia, and dry skin, can be greatly relieved by a doctor.

A number of elderly persons suffer from constipation. Mineral oil is probably the remedy most recommended by doctors, but taking it should not become a habit. The important thing is to watch for a sudden change in established bowel habits. For example, the onset of constipation in someone who has always been "regular" warrants an immediate examination because it may indicate an obstruction due to a tumor. (For a fuller discussion of CONSTIPATION, see that entry in the encyclopedia section.)

Skin and facial changes occur as old age approaches. The skin may sag or wrinkle. If a number of teeth are missing and have not been replaced by dentures, the face is frequently disfigured.

Facial massage, lubricating cream or oil, and exposure to fresh air and sunshine will help keep the skin in a more youthful condition. If wrinkles and sagging cause serious concern, they can be helped by a skin specialist. It is even possible to remove or stretch badly sagging or wrinkled areas of the skin on the face and neck, but this must be done only by a qualified expert in plastic surgery. Actors, actresses, and other theatrical performers have been using the services of plastic surgeons for years. (See also the entry COSMETIC SURGERY in the encyclopedia section.)

Good foot care is a basic, but often overlooked, factor in maintaining active, healthy later years. Weight loss and bone changes can produce aching feet and back pains unless attention is given to selecting comfortable shoes that give proper support.

As for diet, some old people develop finicky appetites, partly because they actually need less food, but often because of trouble with their teeth. They may avoid meat if chewing is difficult. But it is important for them to maintain an adequate diet, especially one containing plenty of proteins and minerals, rather than one high in starches and sugars. (See also the discussion of diets in Chapter 2.)

Some doctors prescribe extra vitamins for people over 60. Usually a capsule or two of multivitamins a day is sufficient. If supplementary vitamins cause troublesome intestinal gas, natural foods can be substituted for them: whole-grain cereals, liver, and pork chops for the B vitamins; orange and tomato juice for vitamin C; and cod liver or halibut oil for vitamins A and D.

Most of the problems connected with digestion do not arise from eating too little but from eating too much. In fact, many of the illnesses that are called diseases of old age could be more accurately labeled diseases of overweight. Life-insurance statistics show that obese people are much more apt to suffer from disorders of the circulatory system (the heart and blood vessels), which cause half of all deaths in the elderly. (See the discussion of overweight in Chapter 2; and the entry OBESITY in the encyclopedia section.)

Aids for the elderly

In old people, the simple everyday activities that were done without exertion in their earlier days can become difficult tasks. Even getting out of a seat, especially a low one, becomes a laborious action perhaps involving pain and taxing the strength. To make this easier, special chairs with adjustable seats and extended arms can be bought. In the bathroom, fix a higher seat to the toilet with a handrail at the side, and another rail at the side of the bathtub. Rising from a sitting position transfers the weight of the body to the feet: avoid the risk of slipping on a polished surface by fitting nonslip or foam-backed mats. Minimize stooping by fitting brushes and dustpans with long handles, by keeping items in daily use off the floor and on shelves, and by providing a device for putting on stockings. If an elderly person has difficulty in gripping with one hand, buy a combined knife and fork for his meals and rubber suction bases for plates and cups.

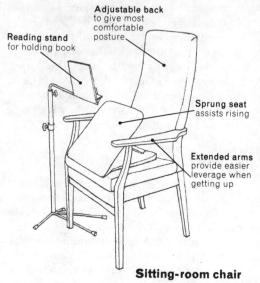

Reading stand for holding book

Adjustable back to give most comfortable posture

Sprung seat assists rising

Extended arms provide easier leverage when getting up

Sitting-room chair

In the bathroom

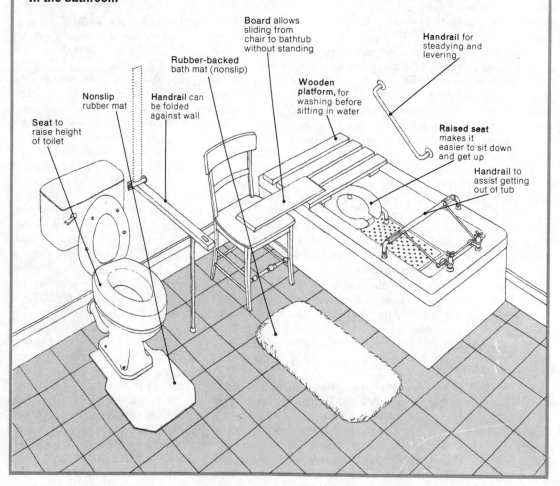

Board allows sliding from chair to bathtub without standing

Handrail for steadying and levering

Rubber-backed bath mat (nonslip)

Wooden platform, for washing before sitting in water

Nonslip rubber mat

Handrail can be folded against wall

Raised seat makes it easier to sit down and get up

Seat to raise height of toilet

Handrail to assist getting out of tub

LIVING TO A RIPE OLD AGE

There is much truth to the joking remark that one way to live a long time is to choose the right ancestors. Statistical studies show that almost 87 percent of the people who live to be 90 had either one parent or two grandparents who reached a ripe old age.

Many other reasons have been offered by aged people who felt they knew the secret of long life. Some, like Luigi Cornaro, a famous Venetian who lived for almost a hundred years, recommended leading a sober and unemotional life. On the other hand, Titian was an intensely emotional man, and he lived until his late nineties. George Bernard Shaw, who lived to be 94, adhered to a vegetarian diet. Connie Mack, who managed a major-league baseball team when he was in his eighties, urged people to eat small meals and to get nine hours of sleep each night.

Despite all their contradictory secrets of longevity, most of these people had one thing in common: an interest in life coupled with great enthusiasm.

This combination is at the head of the list. The remaining precepts are mostly common sense: Be especially careful to avoid accidents; see a doctor regularly so that minor illnesses do not become major; observe the general rules of good health and good hygiene.

Exercise

Vigor is desirable, but older people should always avoid strain and exhaustion. Regularity of exercise is the primary concern. One major benefit of regular exercise to the elderly is the maintenance of good digestion. The digestive process is closely connected with the circulatory system, so that moderate exercise that promotes good blood circulation benefits the entire gastrointestinal tract, as well as all other organs of the body.

By the time an individual is 40, he should have established the custom of consulting his doctor before undertaking any new form of exercise. This procedure should continue.

An older person should always stop exercising as soon as he is tired—and long before he feels exhausted. He should try to be a philosopher, not a sprinter, when he is tempted to chase after a bus—or anything else.

Rest and Sleep

In the later years, rest for a half-hour after meals and at intervals during the day is a sound practice. Older people whose work does not permit them to lie down should take advantage of breaks or rest periods to relax completely, with their feet elevated when possible. But the older person should avoid inactivity. If he happens to be ill and the doctor says he should get up, the patient should make every effort to do so. A prolonged stay in bed can be harmful to the aging.

It is not true that older people require less sleep than younger ones. Research shows that most elderly persons who sleep eight hours or more have fewer complaints than those who sleep less. In fact, some problems of the aged may be caused by lack of sleep, resulting in tension, crankiness, and nervous exhaustion. There is no need to suffer from sleeplessness, because consultation with a doctor can usually find a solution to the problem.

Weight-Watching

People tend to require less food as they grow older. If an individual puts on too much weight, he should talk it over with his doctor. Older people should diet only under a doctor's supervision. If the person is overweight, the only thing safe for him to do on his own is to cut out sweets and starches between meals, and make certain he is eating well-balanced meals. (For further information on a balanced diet, see Chapter 2.)

Generally it is better for the elderly to eat three meals a day of about the same size, rather than to have smaller breakfasts and lunches, with large dinners in the evening.

Alcohol and Tobacco

Those who drink in moderation generally do not have to stop in later years, provided they are healthy. In fact, there is some indication that light drinking can aid digestion and perk up the appetite. Tobacco, however, is apt to cause distress, such as dizziness and indigestion. It is best to avoid smoking at any age, and it is frequently forbidden by doctors when an older person has relatively minor illnesses such as a tendency toward bronchitis or high blood pressure.

Climate

Older people should be particularly careful not to exert themselves when the cold or, more important, the heat and humidity lower their vitality. For instance, shoveling snow is terribly taxing, and most people past middle age are not conditioned for that level of strain. If snow must be shoveled, it should be done in several installments; the elderly should never work to the point of fatigue.

An elderly person should carefully weigh the pros and cons before pulling up stakes to find a more moderate climate in which to settle. Some older people find it difficult to adjust to new surroundings. Their old friends and the sight of their own street are often better medicine than anything a warmer climate can offer. But if the individual still has a desire for new experiences, he should not hesitate to move.

Medical Insurance

New medical insurance programs, private and public, have taken much of the financial worry about illness out of old age. The federal government's Medicare program (see the entry MEDI-CARE in the encyclopedia section) offers financial assistance with hospital, nursing home, and private medical care.

Anyone approaching age 65 who has not received Medicare information from the Social Security Administration should go to his district office to apply for it. He should be sure to get a Medicare Handbook, if he did not receive one automatically with his Medicare card.

Other medical insurance plans, such as Blue Cross and Blue Shield, have special provisions for the elderly. An older person should investigate these carefully, so that he knows he will be able to afford the special medical attention often required in the later years.

PLANNING RETIREMENT

In order to retire successfully, one must have more than money in the bank. A healthy reserve of personal interests that make life worth living is vital. That is why many doctors urge young people to cultivate hobbies and recreational activities that they can continue in their later years.

Clubs of all kinds for elderly people are springing up throughout this country and abroad. The town hall, church, community center, or library can provide information about those in the community. If there is no Day Center, Golden Age, or Old Timers group in the area, one can be organized. The local department of social services should be able to help or provide advice on where to go for assistance and advice.

For additional information, get in touch with the National Retired Teachers Association/American Association of Retired Persons (NRTA/AARP). This organization as well as the National Council of Senior Citizens have local organizations affiliated with them. The federal government also supplies information: write to the Administration on Aging, Office of Human Development, U.S. Department of Health, Education, and Welfare, Washington, D.C. 20201.

Living Arrangements for the Elderly

Difficult family situations often arise when older people must live under the same roof with their children. That is one reason it is usually best for the elderly to maintain their own homes as long as possible. Often a room in a light-housekeeping hotel or boarding house will prove satisfactory if it is not possible for the older persons to maintain a house or apartment because of the expense or the housework involved.

Apartment houses and entire communities are now organized to meet the special needs of the elderly. Older people should investigate these places, because many of them offer excellent facilities—physical, social, and medical. Before agreeing to anything in writing, however, the individual should consult his doctor to be sure that he is in sufficiently good health to settle in a new apartment or community, and to ascertain that the medical facilities and staff are adequate for most needs. The advice of a lawyer should also be sought before signing away property or income, or assuming a heavy financial obligation.

When aging parents must live with their children, it is usually best not to separate them by putting the mother with one child and the father with another. It is not easy for elderly people to divide their time among their various children, although this is usually considered the only fair arrangement. The difficulties can be minimized by establishing definite dates of residence. Having a room of their own awaiting them, with some of their cherished possessions in it, adds immeasurably to the older couple's feeling of security and independence.

Achieving Independence and Usefulness

Many of the emotional difficulties of old age will not occur, and the older person's enthusiasm for life will be sustained if he or she remains independent, useful, and interested.

Every effort should be made on the part of both generations living under one roof to achieve a degree of independence. Older men and women can be genuinely helpful in a household. They should be allowed and encouraged to do whatever they can.

Projects outside the home can help to foster a feeling of independence by the elderly and also help to prevent irritations caused by the generations spending too much time together. Attending church, participating in charitable affairs, and taking part in other outside activities such as visiting friends—if possible, on a regular basis— are stimulating breaks in what otherwise could be a monotonous routine.

Volunteer programs such as "telephone reassurance" and "friendly visiting" are important services older people can give to others of their own age. In the telephone programs, elderly people call others daily to check on their well-being and to talk. Under visitation programs, regular visits with an older person are arranged solely for social reasons. Doctors, clergymen, and social service workers can often find volunteer work for the older person to do. This is particularly important for those who have no family or friends whom they can help.

It is possible to provide a cheerful, stimulating atmosphere for both the elderly and their juniors if everyone regards older persons, not as problems, but simply as people.

When you need a nursing home

Guidelines for selecting a hospital when one is needed are given in Chapter 10. Frequently, however, older people who cannot be cared for at home need professional nursing attention but not the specialized services of a hospital. A nursing home is the obvious answer. Then the dilemma arises—how to choose a good nursing home. The checklist below will help you rate such institutions. As a rule the best one is the home that gets the most "yes" answers, but if the answer to any of the first five questions is "no," keep looking.

1. Do both the home and its administrator have a current license from the state?

2. If the patient is eligible for financial aid, is the home certified to participate in government programs that provide it?

3. Does the home provide special services that the patient may need, such as individualized diet and physical therapy?

4. Does the home meet federal and/or state fire-safety codes, with exit doors clearly marked, unobstructed, and unlocked on the inside, and with a written evacuation plan and frequent fire drills?

5. Is a registered nurse responsible for the nursing staff, and is a licensed practical nurse on duty day and night?

6. Is the location of the home convenient for the patient, his or her doctor, and family?

7. Is the home near a hospital?

8. Is the interior well lighted, and are there handrails in the hallways?

9. Does each bedroom open onto a hallway?

10. Does each bedroom have a window, call bell by every bed, at least one comfortable chair for each patient in the room, reading lights, and clothes closet and drawers for each patient?

11. Are toilet facilities convenient to the bedrooms, easy for a wheelchair patient to use, and equipped with a call bell and grab bars?

12. Do bathtubs and showers have nonslip surfaces?

13. Is the home clean and free of unpleasant odors?

14. Does the lobby or lounge have a welcoming atmosphere, with comfortable furniture and attractive decor, and is it used by the residents?

15. Is the dining room pleasant and easy to move around in, even for the wheelchair patients?

16. In the kitchen, are food preparation, dishwashing, and garbage areas separate, and is food requiring refrigeration not carelessly left out on counters?

17. Are there rooms and equipment for patient activities, and are the residents using them?

18. Does the home organize outside trips for patients able to go on them?

19. Do volunteers from the community visit and work with the patients?

20. Is there an isolation room for the use of a patient with a contagious illness?

21. Is there an outdoor area for residents?

22. Are there ramps to enable the handicapped to move about the home and grounds?

23. Is regular medical attention available, and a physician on call in emergencies?

24. May the patient have a private physician?

25. Is a thorough physical examination required before or immediately upon admission of every patient?

26. Does the home keep medical records and a plan of care for each patient?

21

CHAPTER

Coping With Hazards and Illness in Your Home

The size and condition of your house or apartment are extremely important to the general health and safety of you and your family. Adequate space and good sanitary conditions hinder the spread of infectious disease. Elimination of safety hazards around the home make serious accidents far less likely. There are probably more dangers in your home than you realize. According to the National Safety Council, more than 3½ million Americans are victims of home accidents annually, and about 23,000 of these are fatal.

In all probability, your residence will serve periodically as a convalescent home for a member of the family recovering from illness, an accident, or an operation. Knowing how to care for the patient and how to make the most efficient use of your own time and effort will make the experience less a burden for everyone concerned.

This chapter is filled with helpful hints in all these areas.

MINIMUM REQUIREMENTS OF GOOD HOUSING

When looking for a house or an apartment, or in evaluating the housing you now occupy, several important points should be kept in mind:

1. Every home should contain enough rooms to accommodate all the members of the family without discomfort or crowding. An adequate number of bedrooms is essential. Ideally, every child should have his or her own room. If this is not possible, no more than two children should be asked to share a room, and these two should be close in age and of the same sex. Under no circumstances should a child be required to sleep in the same room with adults.

2. All rooms should be well ventilated and well heated, and should be kept free from dampness. Roofs, walls, and ceilings should be rainproof.

3. All plumbing should be in good repair, as should stoves, refrigerators, and furnaces.

4. The house should be free of pests. Because flies and mosquitoes can be disease-carriers as well as annoyances, window screens should be in good repair, and screen doors should close tightly. Because rats are a serious health hazard, all homes should be rat-proofed.

5. Children need fresh air, sunshine, and outdoor space to play in. A back yard or a nearby park or playground will contribute to maintaining your children's health.

PREVENTION OF HOME ACCIDENTS

Falls

More than one-third of the deaths from home accidents are the result of falls. There is a direct relationship between the state of repair of stairs and railings in a house and the number of sprains and broken bones suffered by the people who live there. Stairs and railings, both inside and outside should be kept in good condition, and any defects should be corrected immediately. In cold weather, icy or slippery steps should be scraped and protected, if necessary, by sprinkling with ashes, sand, or rock salt. Cellar stairs should be sturdy and kept in good condition; they should have at least one steady handrail.

Stairs are not the only hazard. Tools, toys, and other objects left lying on lawns, driveways, and floors are invitations to a fall, as are loose rugs and slippery floors. Spills on exposed flooring should be wiped up immediately. Slippery floors

242

should be carpeted, and small rugs should be anchored so that they do not slide around. Tears in carpeting and on stair runners should be repaired as soon as they are discovered; heels and toes can catch in them and lead to a tumble.

Electric light switches should be so positioned that members of the household can light their way from one room to another. Keep a light burning all night near the bathroom.

Windows in upper-floor rooms used by children and elderly people should be protected by heavy screens or guards. If they are not, they should never be opened from the bottom.

Fire Hazards

Matches and Smoking. Keep matches and lighters out of the reach of small children. If you or any other member of your family smokes, be sure there is an ashtray near at hand. And *never* smoke in bed or when lying on a sofa or reclining in a chair that invites you to go to sleep.

Electricity. If you do not have circuit breakers in your home, make certain that all fuses are of the correct wattage for the lines. If a fuse blows, it should never be replaced with one of greater wattage. And *never* use a penny as a temporary substitute for a blown fuse; you are asking for a fire.

Wall outlets should not be overloaded with lines to too many appliances. If you do not have enough outlets, have an electrician install additional ones. Unused outlets should be protected with dummy plugs to make it impossible for children to harm themselves by pushing metal objects into the sockets. Frayed wiring or damaged plugs should be replaced immediately.

Keep an air space behind and around your television set, because it can build up heat and pose a fire hazard. Unless you are an expert, do not attempt to repair the set yourself.

Flammable Liquids. All flammable liquids should be stored in tightly closed, clearly labeled metal containers and should be kept in a cool, well-ventilated place away from anything that might catch fire. Cleaning fluids should be used only in a well-ventilated area, far away from any flame, lighted cigarette, or electric spark. Aerosol containers should also be stored away from heat, and when they are empty they should not be thrown into an incinerator or fire of any kind.

Never use kerosene or any other cleaning fluid to start a fire in the furnace, wood stove, fireplace, or outdoor grill.

Rooms with Special Hazards

The hazards that lead to falls can be found in virtually every room in the house. Similarly, bad lighting, which can lead to all kinds of accidents, is a safety hazard that can occur anywhere, as is loose electrical wiring along the floor. All radiators should be covered; when exposed, they can cause burns. Young children who are just learning to walk can hurt themselves on sharp-edged furniture, which should either be padded or removed from the places where children are likely to be. Because it is easy to walk into a clear glass door or wall, those in your home should be made of safety glass, with an eye-level decal on each pane.

Kitchen. Kitchens with gas or coal stoves should be equipped with vents or flues to take away the gases, or they should have windows that can be kept partly open when the stoves are in use. Never light a gas stove if there is an odor of gas in the air; if the odor persists, call a repairman.

Asbestos pads, tongs, and pot holders are needed to prevent burns and scalds when you are cooking. Turn all pot handles toward the back of the stove; if they face front, you could get a serious burn by brushing against a handle and overturning the utensil.

Hot fat and grease require special precautions. Never pour water or flour on grease that has caught fire, because these substances will only spatter the flame. Such small fires can be extinguished by pouring salt, sand, dirt, or ashes on them, or they can be smothered with heavy wet cloths or asbestos pads. A home fire extinguisher, which can be purchased at reasonable cost, is a worthwhile investment.

Be sure to disconnect your toaster before cleaning out crumbs or dislodging a piece of bread that has become stuck.

Kitchens are a special hazard to children. Teach them to stay away from the stove at all times, even when it is not in use. Remember that it takes a long time for the heat from any stove—coal, gas, or electric—to dissipate. Knives, forks, and all other sharp implements should be kept locked up, or out of the reach of children. This same advice applies to all harmful substances frequently found in the kitchen—lye, ammonia, acids, insect and rodent poisons, and cleaning solutions.

Bathroom. Some electrical equipment used in the bathroom—an electric toothbrush, for example—is meant to be used in conjunction with water; and such equipment, if it is in good repair, is perfectly safe. But because tap water is an excellent conductor of electricity, such electrical appliances as heaters, hair dryers, razors, and hair curlers should not come in contact with moisture. You should never use these appliances, or touch an electric socket or switch, while you are taking a bath or when your hands are wet.

Grab rails are available for bathtubs and toilets to minimize the danger of falls, especially for older people. A rubber mat in the bathtub will also help prevent falls and slips. Make certain that the thermostat on the water heater is not set too high. An unexpected stream of scalding water from the shower can give a serious burn and cause a fall as the victim tries to escape the spray.

Many medicines now come in child-proof containers. Even so, all medicines should be kept locked up or at least out of the reach of children, as should razor blades, aerosol containers, and other contents of the medicine chest.

Cellar. Whether you heat your home and your water by oil, gas, coal, or electricity, have the entire system checked by a repairman each year before the cold weather sets in. Flues and chimneys should be examined. The central air-conditioning unit should also be checked annually.

Because the ashes from a coal furnace retain heat for a considerable period, they should be kept in metal containers.

If you chop wood for your furnace or your fireplace, be sure the ax is adequate and that you know how to use it. When not in use, the ax should be kept under lock and key. The same is true for all household tools and equipment with which children might hurt themselves.

An ill-lit or cluttered cellar is a danger. Every part of the cellar should be well lighted, and clearly defined areas should be set aside for tools, equipment, screens, and other household paraphernalia. If your children use the cellar as a playroom, these storage areas should be separated by walls from the space used by the youngsters. A few two-by-four wood studs and some inexpensive pressed-board partitions will make a perfectly adequate wall. Do not, however, let your children go into the cellar by themselves for any reason until they are old enough to be trusted alone for an hour or more.

Safety Tips on Yards and Gardens

Keep children away from outdoor cooking equipment. Remember that it is as easy for them to burn themselves in the yard as in the house.

Power lawn mowers can be dangerous, especially those with rotary blades that can send loose rocks flying. If you use this type of mower, be sure to rake up all rocks in the yard before starting to mow. Gasoline-powered mowers can easily get out of control and must be guided by a firm hand.

Garden tools—especially rakes—should never be left lying on the lawn. Anyone who accidentally steps on them is likely to suffer serious injury.

Do not let children play in the yard immediately after you have used an insecticide or a weed killer on the lawn, because these contain toxic substances particularly dangerous to children.

CARING FOR A SICK PERSON AT HOME

Some diseases and medical problems require hospitalization for proper diagnosis and treatment, but many can be handled as well—or even better—at home. Many patients who previously would have been hospitalized are now being cared for at home. It can be virtually guaranteed that at some point you will have to care for an invalid—whether a youngster who has come down with one of the childhood diseases, a postoperative patient, or a chronic invalid.

Home care has its difficulties, but it has its benefits, too, both for the patient and for the patient's family. The home is a comfortable and natural environment for the patient—a factor of particular importance in the case of young children and elderly people, for whom hospitalization can create a serious emotional upset. Care at home can be individualized to take into account the patient's food preferences, sleeping habits, and desire for company. Home care has equally significant advantages for the rest of the family. The most important are the satisfactions of being useful and contributing to the care of a loved person.

In addition, home care can have important financial advantages. Hospitalization is extremely expensive today, and not all medical insurance covers protracted hospital stays. Moreover, many health insurance plans—including Medicare—now cover certain expenses involved in home care, such as the rental of equipment and the services of therapeutic and nursing agencies that minister to home-bound invalids.

In any case where there is a choice between hospitalization and home care, the entire question should be seriously discussed by all the members of the family—including the patient, if he or she is able to participate—in consultation with the family physician. The following factors should be considered:

1. *The family situation:* Will one family member have to carry the entire burden of care, or can several family members share it? How willing are the various members of the family to put up with the inevitable inconveniences to which they will be subjected?

2. *The patient's situation:* How complex is the illness? How much can the patient participate in his or her own care?

3. *The home:* Is the home safe? Will the patient have easy access to the bathroom? Will he—or the person who is taking care of him—be required to climb stairs frequently? Can the home be rearranged, if necessary, to make things easier for both the patient and the family?

4. *Back-up services:* Is there a hospital nearby? Is a doctor readily available? Are there home service agencies in the vicinity that can be called on to help?

5. *The financial situation:* Can your family afford protracted hospitalization? Does your health insurance cover any aspect of home care?

Qualities Needed for Home Nursing

Caring for a patient at home requires more than willingness, patience, and the mastery of such basic nursing skills as making the bed, taking the patient's temperature and pulse, and administering medicine. Home nursing calls for the ability to make plans and to change them if necessary. It calls for empathy—the ability to put yourself in the patient's place—and objectivity, so that you can observe the patient carefully to see how he or she is getting along. Invalids should not be overtaxed, but neither should they be overprotected. It is important for you to know what the patient can and cannot do for himself, and to encourage him to make as much contribution toward his care as his condition will permit. Patients who are acutely ill can generally do very little for themselves, but many chronically ill patients are able to participate to some degree in their own care.

It is equally important for you to be aware of your own abilities and limitations. Home nursing is a tiring and demanding task. Conserve your time and energy by keeping records and by planning your daily activities in advance. This will save unnecessary steps and contribute to your confidence in your ability to help. And be sure to arrange for some time away from your nursing tasks while someone else assumes the duties and responsibilities.

What to Ask the Doctor

There are several things you will need to know from your doctor:

1. The amount of activity the patient can and should engage in. Should he go to the bathroom and wash and bathe himself?

2. The proper diet for the patient. How often should he eat? What kinds of food should he have, and how much? What kinds of fluids should he have? How often? How much?

3. The patient's medication schedule. You need to know the dosage, the times the medicine should be taken, and the way it should be administered. In addition, it is helpful to know the purpose of the medication and its possible side effects. You should have this same information about any treatment—whether or not it involves taking medicine—that the doctor prescribes.

4. Here are some questions you may want to ask the doctor: Should the patient's temperature be taken? If so, how often? And should it be taken by mouth, rectum, or armpit? Should his pulse be monitored? Should you watch for his reaction to his medication and the treatments that have been prescribed? How carefully should you observe the amount and quality of the patient's activity? The color and condition of his skin? His mental state? His elimination? The kind and amount of pain he has? What changes in the patient's condition should cause you to call the doctor?

If you do not understand something that the physician tells you, do not be embarrassed to say so. If you feel more comfortable with written instructions, ask to have them given to you. If you need more than one demonstration of a technique you will need to apply—giving an injection, for example—do not hesitate to ask. If any specific problems come up that you want to discuss with the doctor or visiting nurse, write them down. The nurse and doctor can give you much better advice about a pain, for instance, if they know its precise location, duration, and character—dull, throbbing, or sharp.

The Patient's Room

Because both you and the patient are likely to spend considerable time in his room, it should be as cheerful and as conveniently located as possible. If you live in a house with more than one story, using a room on the ground floor will save you a great many trips up and down stairs. The closer the room is to the kitchen and the bathroom, the better. If the patient cannot make the trip to the bathroom, buy or rent a commode.

Keep the temperature of the room as even as possible, around 72° to 76° F during the day and 68° to 72° F at night. To ventilate the room without creating a draft, place a screen or a blanket-draped chair in front of the open window, or open it from the top. Use blinds or shades to protect the patient from the glare of direct light. If the air is too dry, put a large shallow pan of water on the radiator, or use a humidifier.

The room should be kept clean and odor-free. If it is necessary to use sharp-smelling antiseptics or disinfectants, you can mask their odors with a pleasant smelling deodorizer or odor neutralizer.

Depending on the patient's condition, it may be advisable to rent a hospital bed or guard rails for the sides of the patient's own bed. Both of these are available through surgical supply houses and are reimbursable expenses under many health insurance policies, including Medicare. You will need a bed tray in the event the patient takes his meals in bed.

The room should have chairs for visitors and should also have a comfortable armchair for the patient. The chair should not be too deep; it should be cushioned at the back and under the patient's buttocks, and there should be no pressure at the back of his knees when he is sitting in it. If his feet do not reach the floor, you will need to provide a footstool for him.

If the patient is able to walk, be sure there are no throw rugs on the floor. The patient who can walk unaided may trip on them, and a walker or a cane can get snarled in them. If the patient uses a walker, be sure that it is the right height for him, is not too heavy, and has rubber tips on its legs. A cane, too, should be the right height, should have a rubber tip, and should be strong enough to support the patient's weight.

The Bedridden Patient

Protracted bed rest is not desirable for any patient, and the doctor will probably not advise it except under very special circumstances, such as an injury to the spine. A long period in bed is less harmful to younger patients than to older ones, but it always carries with it the danger of numerous complications, among them bedsores, constipation, and respiratory difficulties. To protect against these and other problems, several things should be done in caring for a patient who is confined to bed.

1. The patient's position should be changed at least every two hours. His body should be kept in good alignment, so that the weight is distributed evenly. The patient's skin should be kept clean and dry. All bony protuberances should be protected from pressure. Sheep-skin padding is available, which can be placed between the mattress and the bottom sheet. Foam rubber cushions to relieve pressure can also be obtained.

2. The patient's diet should contain adequate amounts of bulk and protein, and he should be given adequate amounts of fluid. The doctor or visiting nurse will prescribe a proper diet.

3. Even in bed, the patient needs a certain amount of exercise. This may be either passive exercise (such as massage) or active exercise (movements that the patient himself can make). The nurse or doctor can advise you about the appropriate exercise for your patient.

4. The bedding should be kept clean and smooth and free of crumbs or other irritants to the patient's skin. The mattress should be firm.

Making the Bed. It is less difficult than you may think to make a bed with the patient in it. There are two important things to remember. The first is that the under part of the bed is always made from side to side—not from top to bottom. The second is that when you move the patient, you should always move him toward you. See the illustrations on pages 248 and 249.

Using the Bedpan. Usually the patient will go to the bathroom at least once daily, or use a commode in his room if the bathroom is too far away. Underpants are available that can be used for incontinent patients. But if the patient needs to use a urinal or a bedpan, here are some things that you should know:

1. A male patient can probably use a urinal without much assistance if it is placed on a towel beside him under the covers. Warm the urinal slightly, either by putting it on or near the radiator or by rinsing it with hot water and drying it quickly, just before you bring it to him.

2. A bedpan should be warmed in the same way. Most patients can raise themselves, or help to raise themselves, onto it by flexing their knees and pressing with their heels and the palms of their hands on the mattress. Place the bedpan under the patient's buttocks, its flattened end just below the hip bones.

Washing and Bathing. Cleanliness and neatness contribute to the patient's well-being, but be guided by the patient's wishes and the doctor's suggestions, rather than by a fanatical desire for an ideal condition.

The patient's hair should be combed or brushed once or twice a day. If the hair is long and snarled, a little alcohol will make it easier to manage. The hair should be combed or brushed in small strands. Long hair should be braided. Dry shampoos are available to clean the hair.

Rubbing the patient's back once or twice daily usually makes him feel better, and it is good for the skin. Use a lotion that the nurse or doctor recommends, and rub with long, gentle, firm strokes.

If the patient must remain in bed for his bath, he should nevertheless do as much to help himself as possible. A bedridden patient does not need a daily bath. His baths should be given before making the bed and after the patient has relieved himself. You will need a bath blanket, a fairly small cotton blanket that is easy to handle and dry; two bath towels; a face towel; a washcloth; soap; a basin of warm water; and clean pajamas or nightgown. Change the water at least once, especially if it becomes cool.

Begin by removing the top bedding and covering the patient with the bath blanket. Then his nightclothes are removed. Next, place a towel underneath the patient to protect the bedclothes, and put paper under the basin when you set it on the bed. The patient should wash himself—or be washed, if necessary—in sections, always drying each section of the body thoroughly before going on to wash the next.

Giving Fluids. If the patient is unable to sit up and drink by himself, raise his head, either by using pillows or by slipping one arm under the pillow and lifting it while you hold the glass in your other hand. Have the glass less than half full and, if necessary, use flexible plastic straws. Always hold the glass for the patient, and make certain that the straw is in the liquid so that he does not suck air.

Taking the Patient's Temperature and Pulse

The proper way to take the temperature by mouth, rectum, and armpit is described in Chapter 16. If the doctor wants you to take the patient's pulse, have him demonstrate the procedure to you several times, and then practice it on a well person before trying to take the invalid's pulse. Place the tips of two or three fingers—not your thumb, because it also has a pulse—on the

artery just inside the patient's wrist and above his thumb. Press just hard enough to feel the pulse. Count the pulse for one minute, using a watch with a second hand for accuracy. The patient's pulse should be taken when he is relaxed, not immediately after he has exerted himself. The important things to note about the pulse beat are its rate and whether it is strong or weak, regular or irregular.

Administering an Enema

Stool softeners and rectal suppositories are available to help constipated patients, and an enema should not be given unless prescribed by the doctor. Prepackaged enemas in disposable containers are available. If the doctor does not recommend their use, he will instruct you about the proper solution to use in an enema bag.

If possible, the patient should administer his own enema while sitting on the toilet seat. If the enema must be administered in bed, have the patient lie on his left side, his back toward you and his legs flexed—the upper leg slightly more flexed than the lower. If you are not using a prepackaged enema, test the water with a thermometer—it should be about 105° F—or by letting a little of it run on the inside of your wrist. With a piece of tissue, apply petroleum jelly to the rectal nozzle. Open the stopcock and let some water run out into the bedpan to make certain there is no air in the tube. If the patient cannot himself insert the nozzle, insert it very slowly and gently for about three inches. Hold the bag about 18 inches above the bed; if the enema flows too rapidly, lower it. Stop the flow if the patient complains of pain. When the bag appears empty, remove the nozzle carefully, have the patient turn on his back, and place the bedpan under him.

Applying Heat or Cold

A hot-water bag or an electric heating pad can be used to provide heat if the patient is cold or if the doctor orders it for treatment of an affected part. If you use a hot-water bag, be sure to check it first for leaks. A hot-water bag should never be more than half full. If you use an electric pad, be sure the patient's skin is completely dry.

Neither a hot-water bag nor an electric heating pad should be used directly on the patient's skin. It is not advisable to let a sick person go to sleep with an electric heating pad operating. Heating pads or hot-water bags should be removed immediately if the patient complains of

(continued on page 254)

247

CARING FOR THE SICK

Make a sick patient's room as cheerful as possible. He has to lie there all day, and boredom and despondency can soon settle in if the atmosphere is drab and colorless. Merely moving some of the furniture around can give a room a new look and create a new interest for the patient. Do not leave a patient on his own for too long: loneliness can be one of the most depressing aspects of convalescence at home, especially for the bedridden. Just putting your head in the door occasionally and asking the patient if he wants anything can help to relieve the monotony. Place a table near the bed—large enough for the patient's medicine, drinking water, and a small bell he can ring if he needs attention. Give him a radio, and put it within easy reach (a TV set is of little use unless it can be switched over, and on and off, by remote control); and see that he gets a good supply of newspapers, books, and magazines.

When he is well enough, let him have visitors, but not too many or too frequently, and do not allow their visits to be too long—talking with a sick patient can become dull and tiring for both patient and visitor. Food at all stages of convalescence plays an important part in recovery after an operation or an

Making a bed

When possible, a bed should be made by two people, especially when it has to be done with the patient still in the bed. Have two chairs at the side of the bed: on one place the clean bed linen, on the other the blankets and bedspread removed from the bed. To make an empty bed, cover the mattress with a mattress pad, and over that put the bottom sheet, right side uppermost and with its center crease down the middle of the bed. Tuck in the ends and sides and make mitered folds at the corners. Make sure it is firmly tucked in, so that the patient cannot wrinkle it into uncomfortable creases. If the patient is likely to wet the bed, put a plastic or rubber sheet on top of the bottom sheet so that it will be under the patient's buttocks. Next fit a drawsheet whether or not a rubber sheet is fitted. This is about 3 feet wide and 6 feet long, and fits lengthwise across the bed with only the ends tucked in. Place the pillows at the head of the bed, then put the top sheet in position, with its wrong side uppermost and center crease down the middle of the bed. Only about 18 inches of the sheet should lie on the pillows. Make a pleat about six inches wide at the foot of the bed, to allow sufficient room for the patient's feet when his toes are pointing upward. Tuck in the sheet at the foot of the bed, make mitered corners, and tuck in the sides. Fit each blanket in a similar manner but without any lying on the pillows. Place the bedspread over the blankets, miter the corners and leave the sides hanging free. Fold the head of the sheet down. You will require the following: mattress pad, top blankets (1 or 2, depending on the temperature of the room), top and bottom sheets, drawsheet, plastic or rubber waterproof sheet (if necessary), bedspread, pillows, chairs (2), and a bag to hold the soiled bed linen.

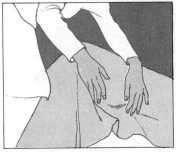

1 Lift up the mattress at the foot of the bed and tuck the end of the sheet underneath it.

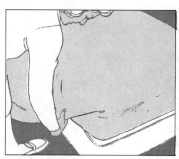

2 Repeat at the head of the bed so that the sides of the sheet are left hanging down.

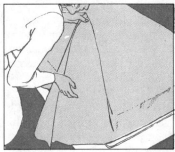

3 Pick up the edge of the sheet about 18 inches from the end and tuck the corner under the mattress.

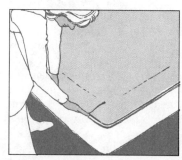

4 Release the edge of the sheet and let it fall so that it hangs at the side of the bed.

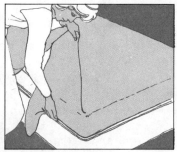

5 Tuck in and repeat at the other side. Make mitered corners at the other end and tuck in.

illness. At first, the patient may be on a special diet; but when the doctor tells you that the patient can have what he likes, remember that he needs ample amounts of protein, which is provided by meat, fish, eggs and milk. Fresh fruit and vegetables supply all the vitamins he needs.

Let the convalescent start to do things for himself as soon as he can, to prepare him for his return to normal life as well as dispel the idea that he must rely upon someone else for everything he wants. An adult after some days in bed may be too weak to stand on his own feet immediately and should sit on the edge of the bed for a few minutes for the first few days. He can then sit in a chair for a short while each day—he may need a helping hand to reach and

get into it at first—until the doctor is satisfied that the patient is strong enough to be more active.

A sick child will take up more of your time than an adult will. When he is resting, the child must be looked at frequently; he may slip down in the bed in an uncomfortable position and stay like that because he cannot be bothered to move. When he is well enough to sit up, his zest for activity will test even the most imaginative mind; be prepared for calls for attention many times an hour throughout the day.

A child, by the time he is well enough to get up, will have had sufficient exercise moving about in bed to go to the bathroom unaided, but the wise parent will be on hand in the early days to give a helping hand if required.

Making a bed with a patient in it

To change bedclothing while a patient is still in bed involves making first one half, then the other. This sequence shows how to change a bottom sheet only. If more than one item is to be changed underneath the patient, remove them together but rolled up separately. The fresh items can be put in position together, but again separately rolled. Remove all pillows except one.

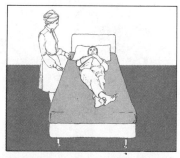

1 Cross the patient's arms and legs so that he can more easily be turned onto his side.

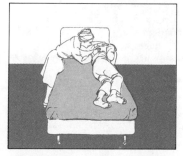

2 Turn him over onto the side of the underneath leg and move the pillow over to that side.

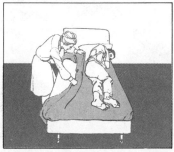

3 Roll the whole length of the sheet to be changed right up against the patient's back.

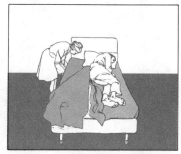

4 Roll up half of the clean sheet and place this roll close up against the other.

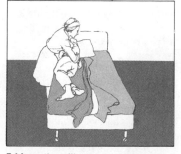

5 Move the pillow over and turn the patient onto his back and then his other side.

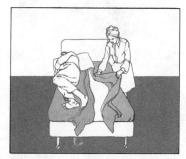

6 He is then on the other side of the rolled bedding. Remove the old sheet completely.

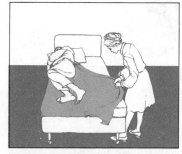

7 Unroll the fresh sheet and pull it tightly over the bed so that there are no creases.

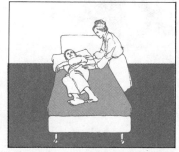

8 Tuck the sheet in, turn the patient onto his back, and put the pillow in the center.

Moving a patient

Every effort should be made to get the patient out of bed as soon as he is fit enough, even if only to sit in a chair while his bed is being made. If the patient is too weak to walk or to move himself into a sitting position in bed, he needs two people to lift him. To avoid strain when lifting, bend your knees and hips and keep your back straight, then straighten the knees and hips to lift. Clasp each other's wrists—not the hands—so that if one releases a hand, the support is still maintained by the other. The patient should also keep his back straight and firm against the supporting arms, keep his head well forward and, if being lifted into a sitting position, cross his arms over his chest. If the chair in which he is to be placed is fitted with casters, put something firm behind it so that it cannot move. Put a blanket over the chair seat, and then wrap it around the sitting patient.

Making a footrest

Most sitting patients in bed find that they slip down into the bed after a time. This can be prevented by using a footrest in the form of a bolster made from a hard pillow and a drawsheet, securing it in position by tucking the ends of the sheet under the mattress. The footrest has an additional benefit in keeping the feet at right angles to the legs and preventing the arch muscles from wasting.

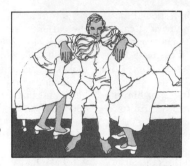

1 Lift patient's legs over side. Let him rest his arms around your neck and on your shoulders.

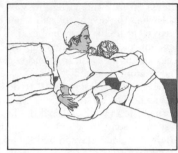

2 Clasp your wrists under the patient's knees and in the small of his back.

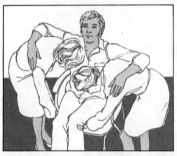

3 Lift and carry the patient to the chair. Cover him with blankets to keep him warm.

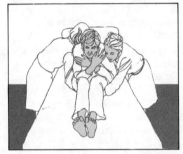

Sitting up a patient Place your arms low on patient's back and under legs near his buttocks.

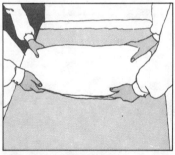

1 Lay the drawsheet (it is usually 6 feet long and 3 feet wide) lengthwise on the bed.

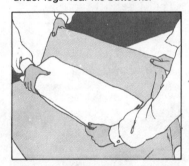

2 Put the hard pillow in the center of the sheet and fold one side of the sheet over it.

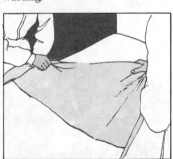

3 Fold the other side of the drawsheet over so that the pillow is enveloped.

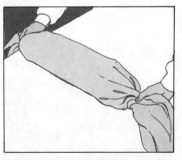

4 Twist the ends of the drawsheet, or tie them, so that the pillow is secure inside it.

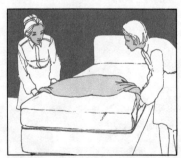

5 Place the footrest in the required position in the bed and tuck in the twisted ends.

Washing a patient in bed

Although he may be inactive, a bedridden patient needs frequent washing: the skin continues to function and sweat during illness. Keep the patient covered with a bath towel or thin blanket except for the part being washed, and put a second one underneath him to protect the bed from splashes of water. The top covers of the bed can either be removed (put a towel over them and let the patient hold it in position while they are being taken off) or they can be protected by a towel and be folded back as required. Let the patient wash himself where he can, especially in the groin and between the legs. Change the water if it becomes cool or dirty. You will need: bath towels or thin blankets (2), bowl and jug of hot water, soap, face and body washcloths, towels (2), and clean pajamas or nightgown. Make sure there are no drafts in the sickroom.

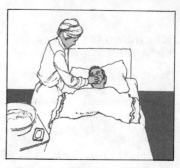

1 Remove pajamas or nightgown. Wash, rinse, and dry eyes (clear water), face, neck, and ears.

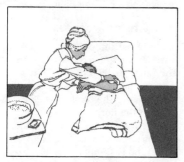

2 Wash, rinse, and dry one arm, then the other, working from the armpit to the fingers.

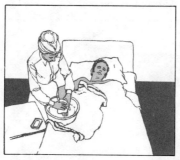

3 While arms are being washed, the patient may find it refreshing to put his hands in the water.

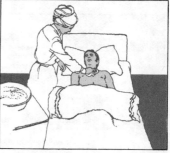

4 Fold the towel down to the waist: wash and dry the patient's chest and then his abdomen.

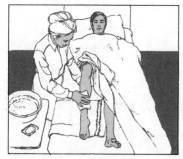

5 Cover the patient up to his chin: wash, rinse, and dry each leg in turn, working from thigh to ankle.

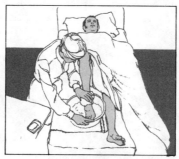

6 Wash the feet in the bowl. Wash groin and between legs if patient cannot do it himself.

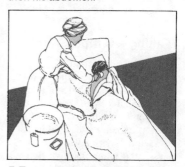

7 Turn patient onto his side, being careful he does not roll too far; wash and dry his back.

Washing a patient's hair

If the patient is well enough to lie face downward with his head over the side of the bed, wash his hair in that position. Otherwise remove the pillows and use one to support his shoulders high enough for the bowl to be placed under his head. Cover the shoulders and chest with a bath towel and use it for the initial drying. Finish drying with an electric hair dryer or by rubbing the hair gently with warm towels.

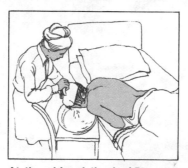

At the side of the bed Place the bowl on a stool or low table so that it is below the bed.

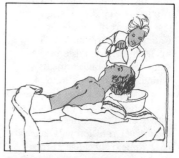

On the bed Move the patient down the bed so that a bowl can be placed underneath the head.

251

Recording the patient's progress

The doctor may need a daily record of the patient's temperature and pulse—and possibly his respiration rate. These details can be kept in graph form or listed, day by day, under separate headings. Make a note of all observations at the time they are made; and keep them where they cannot be studied—and possibly worried about—by the patient. Do not take readings more frequently than required: additional ones will not be significant, and any variations may cause you unnecessary concern. Keep the equipment required on a tray and under a cover. You will need the following equipment: paper (lined or graph), watch or clock with second hand, pen or pencil, paper handkerchiefs, thermometer, cold water, jar containing weak solution of antiseptic, and cotton.

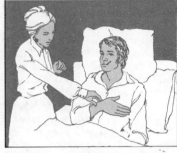

Pulse and respiration can be counted while the thermometer is registering the temperature.

Body temperatures

The normal temperature differs in various parts of the body within the range 97-99°F (36-37°C). The normal oral temperature, taken under the tongue, is 98.6°F (37°C); the normal skin temperature, usually taken under the arm, is about 1°F(0.5°C) lower. Body temperature can also be taken in the rectum, but only by someone trained in the method. For comparison, always use the same method.

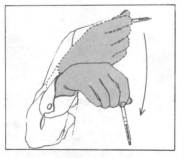

Oral thermometer, used in the mouth

Rectal thermometer, used in the rectum

Clinical thermometers, whether graded in Celsius or Fahrenheit, are usually triangular in section to give a magnifying lens effect for easier reading. Normal body temperature is indicated by an arrow.

Taking a temperature

Do not take a patient's temperature immediately after he or she has taken a bath or had a meal or drink. After taking the thermometer out of the jar of antiseptic, rinse it in cold water and wipe it with cotton (it is essential when taking a skin temperature that both the skin surface and the thermometer be dry). To read the thermometer, hold the end opposite the bulb and look through one angle of the glass toward the opposite base. Rotate the thermometer slowly until the small bubble in the stem near the bulb appears to widen. The silver column of mercury should then be visible. If it is not, rotate the thermometer slowly until the column can be seen. Over-rotation will cause it to disappear, because of the angles of the glass. After reading, rinse the thermometer in cold water, dry it, and replace it in the jar of antiseptic.

1 Shake mercury down into bulb by holding other end firmly and giving sharp downward flicks.

2 Place bulb of thermometer under patient's tongue for two minutes. Ask him to close mouth.

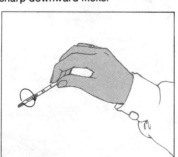

3 Remove thermometer, hold it up to a good light, and read off temperature at end of mercury.

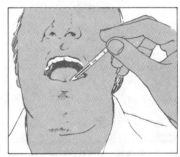

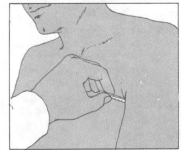

Skin temperature Put bulb of thermometer under armpit for two minutes with arm across chest.

Taking a patient's pulse

The rate, regularity and strength of the pulse, which results from heartbeats pumping the blood through the circulation, are indications of a patient's health. The pulse can be felt anywhere an artery crosses a bone near the surface of the skin; the most convenient place is just below the base of the thumb. The best time to take a patient's pulse is while the thermometer is registering his temperature.

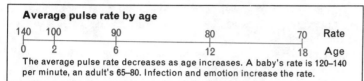

Average pulse rate by age					
140	100	90	80	70	Rate
0	2	6	12	18	Age

The average pulse rate decreases as age increases. A baby's rate is 120–140 per minute, an adult's 65–80. Infection and emotion increase the rate.

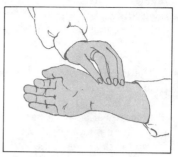

Pulse Feel with tips of the fingers, not the thumb: count number of beats in a minute.

Respiration

The rate of respiration—breathing in and out—is counted by the rise and fall of the chest. It is easily altered by emotion, and it is difficult for a patient not to cause a change from the normal rate of breathing when he is aware that his respirations are being counted. It is, therefore, best to measure it while he is asleep or after counting the pulse and while you are still holding his wrist.

Average respiration rate at rest					
50	40	25	20	15	Rate
0	2	6	12	18	Age

The normal rate of respiration also decreases with age. In a newborn baby it is 40–50 times per minute; in an adult, it is 15–18.

Dealing with vomiting

Being sick is not only unpleasant but it usually frightens the patient, especially a young one. Reassure him, support his head, and hold the bowl for him. Encourage him to breathe deeply. When the attack is over, let the patient rinse his mouth out with water. Then wash his face and change any bedding or nightclothes that have become soiled. If intense pain follows vomiting, tell the doctor immediately.

Preventing bedsores

Confinement to bed with little movement can lead to bedsores. These are mainly caused by prolonged pressure from weight of the body on those areas where it is in contact with the bed. If the pressure is not relieved, the tissues in these areas start to lose their blood supply, and the skin covering them gets sore. Sores can also be caused by bedclothes pressing on the knees and toes. Moisture and friction help to form the sores more quickly, and once they have formed, they take a considerable time to heal. Every effort should be made to prevent bedsores; and if the patient is likely to be confined to bed for some time, it may be worthwhile obtaining a sheepskin for him to lie on. Turn or lift him into a different position every two hours, or relieve the pressure with pads or pillows under the parts likely to be affected. Rub pressure points or any tender spots with rubbing alcohol.

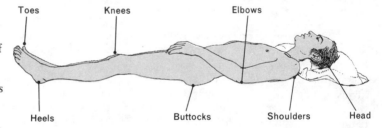

Toes   Knees   Elbows   Heels   Buttocks   Shoulders   Head

Bedsores Friction and unrelieved pressure of the body on skin tissues can result in bedsores. If one does develop on a patient, consult the doctor about the best method of treatment to follow.

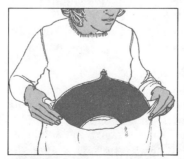

Inflatable rings used to protect pressure points should be enclosed in pillow slips.

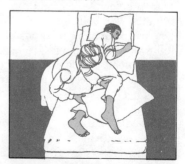

Pressure A pillow between the legs of a patient lying on his side prevents them pressing together.

the heat. In dealing with an elderly patient, it is advisable to test the heat yourself. The skin of older people is particularly sensitive to heat, but if the patient is exposed to it for long periods, he may become unaware of its intensity.

The doctor may order hot, moist applications to an affected area. To keep from burning your hands while you prepare the compress, put a Turkish towel across a basin and place the compress in the middle of it. Pour on very hot water. Grasp the dry ends of the towel and twist them in opposite directions until no more water can be wrung out. Untwist the towel and lift out the compress with your fingers; if you cannot pick it up, it is too hot for the patient. Before putting the compress in place, lubricate the affected area. When the compress is in position, cover the compress with a dry towel. Change the compress when it cools or as often as the physician has requested.

If an ice bag or an ice collar has been prescribed to relieve pain or inflammation, be sure to check it for leaks before using it. Crush the ice so there will be no sharp edges, and fill the bag no more than half full. Dry it carefully and put a cover over it before applying it to the effected area.

CARING FOR A CHILD WITH A COMMUNICABLE DISEASE

Preventive measures can be taken against many of the communicable childhood diseases, and there is no reason your child should suffer from them. But children still pick up a number of highly contagious diseases against which so far there is no protection. (See Chapter 16 for a detailed discussion of childhood illnesses.)

Precautions

In caring for a child with a contagious illness, you must protect yourself and others from catching it, unless you and they are immune. The necessary precautions depend on the disease, but the following steps should be observed for every communicable childhood illness:

1. Keep the patient away from others for as long as your doctor says it is necessary. Keep the sick child in a room by himself; and if you have other children, be particularly careful not to let them go into his room. Ask the doctor about preventive shots for the other children, because they were probably exposed to the illness while the sick child was coming down with it.

2. Many diseases are spread by saliva. Always turn your face away from the patient when he coughs or sneezes, and be sure that he covers his mouth and nose at those times.

3. Keep your hands away from your mouth when you are with the sick child.

4. Leave a smock or long apron in the patient's room and slip it on over your clothes when you are with him.

5. When you leave the patient's room, be sure to wash your hands thoroughly with soap and water.

6. Dispose of the cleansing tissues the child has used either by throwing them into the toilet or by burning them. It is a good idea to keep a bag for soiled tissues at the side of the child's bed.

In the case of most children's diseases, the patient's linens and dishes can be washed with the rest of the family's. After the child has recovered, his room should be thoroughly cleaned. If the toys he has played with cannot be cleaned, it may be necessary to throw them away.

Nursing a Sick Child

Most children sleep a great deal and are generally quiet when they are very ill. That quietness and lassitude can be frightening to a parent. But once the worst of the illness is over, and the child has begun to recover, you may miss the previous peace. As youngsters begin to recover, they often become demanding, irritable, and restless. They will tax your strength as well as your patience, and you should make every effort to take especially good care of yourself during this period.

Get the child some special, inexpensive toys which you can dispose of when he has recovered. Put a radio or record player in his room for his listening enjoyment. Sick children also enjoy looking at picture books. Do not allow the child to tire his eyes watching television while he is feverish.

Devote some time to playing with him. He will demand less unnecessary care that way and will be more willing to rest when he should. This is particularly important, because rest is essential for a child recovering from illness.

Sick children are usually not much interested in eating or drinking, but adequate nutrition is important for their recovery. Try giving your child a number of small meals, rather than three large ones. Colored, flexible plastic straws can make liquids more interesting to him.

If your child resists taking medication, report this to the doctor. He may be able to provide the same medication in a different form—a liquid, for example, rather than a pill—and the child will probably find the medicine to be less objectionable this way.

Finally—and most important—never blame your child for his illness. This is not the time to drive home any lessons about wearing his rubbers or his hat.

CARING FOR AN ADULT WITH A SERIOUS ILLNESS

The problems of caring for an adult with a serious and possibly chronic medical problem—a stroke, heart failure, or a kidney condition, for example—are very different from those of caring for a child with a contagious disease. Nursing care will probably be needed for a longer period of time. The patient's condition may vary sharply from one period to the next: it may become worse for a time, and then there may be long periods of remission. In cases where there is no likelihood of permanent improvement, the care of such a patient can be a discouraging experience for his family.

On the other hand, the adult is far less likely than the child to need constant nursing attention and is far more likely than the child to be able to participate in his own care. To the extent that he can help himself, he should do so. It is good for his morale and the morale of the rest of the family.

A calm atmosphere and a fairly regular routine will help reduce the patient's anxiety to a minimum. Visitors—if he wants them—can be as therapeutic as medicine. But use your own judgment; on some days the patient may not feel up to the demands of sociability.

You should learn as much as you can about the nature of the patient's illness and the course it is likely to take. Do not hesitate to ask the physician questions about the patient's care. If the patient asks you about his condition, be honest with him—he is not a child and should not be treated as one. But remember that you are not a physician and are in no position to offer a prognosis for the patient.

GETTING HELP FROM OTHERS

A number of organizations are dedicated to helping in the home care of invalids—both with nursing problems and with the emotional difficulties that patients and their families may experience. There are visiting nurse services and home health agencies available in most communities. Your doctor and local social agency can help you get in touch with these groups.

CHAPTER 22 The Killer Diseases

For purposes of this chapter, the "killer" diseases are defined as those that attack the largest numbers of Americans and cause the greatest numbers of deaths. (The leading "killer" diseases vary, sometimes greatly, from country to country.) This chapter describes these dangerous diseases, identifies the warning signs by which you can recognize them, and gives some precautions you can take to protect yourself. The kinds of information presented here may help to reduce the toll these diseases exact and—perhaps at some time in the future—may even help to eliminate some of them as our most serious illnesses.

THE MAJOR CAUSES OF DEATH

Evidence of the way that medical science has alleviated the fatal effects of some diseases in this century is shown in the marked changes in the identity or the relative positions of the five leading causes of death in 1900, as compared with the first five in the late 1970's. Their rankings, numbers of fatalities, and death rates for 1900 and 1977 are shown in the table below.

FIVE LEADING CAUSES OF DEATH	
1900	
Five Leading Causes	*Deaths per 100,000*
Pneumonia–Influenza	202.2
Tuberculosis	194.4
Diarrhea, Enteritis	142.7
Heart Disease	137.4
Stroke	106.9
1977	
Five Leading Causes	*Deaths per 100,000*
Heart Disease	332.3
Cancer	178.7
Stroke	84.1
Accidents	47.7
Pneumonia–Influenza	23.7

PREPAREDNESS AND PREVENTION

Here are some general health rules to help protect you against serious illness or at least make it possible for you to recognize the onslaught of a deadly disease early enough to keep the damage to a minimum:

1. The best single weapon against the killer diseases is the periodic medical checkup. The increased expertise and growing sophistication of medical science permit a complex battery of examinations and tests that will reveal vital information to your physician and thus offer a promise of continued good health for you.

2. It is your responsibility to learn to recognize and promptly report to your doctor the warning signs and symptoms of disease.

3. Keep your weight either normal or slightly below normal after you reach middle age. Also, you should avoid smoking, should have a well-balanced, nutritious diet, and should get adequate exercise.

4. Should you have a disease or have reason to be concerned about contracting one, study the information about it given in this book. Do this to become a good patient, but *not* in order to treat yourself. When you understand better what your doctor tells you about an illness, you can be more effective in carrying out your share of the treatment so that a cure will be more prompt and more successful.

5. Avoid quacks, faith healers, and "guaran-

teed cures." Patients who suffer from chronic diseases for which there is no "cure" are particularly susceptible to the frauds who prey on unfortunate sufferers—for instance, cancer victims. Moving outside recognized medical channels may waste precious time desperately needed for truly effective help.

CARDIOVASCULAR DISEASES

The cardiovascular (from the Greek *kardia*, or heart, and the Latin *vasculum*, the diminutive of *vas*, or vessel) diseases are two of the three leading causes of death in the United States today. Heart disease is first by a wide margin, causing more than twice as many fatalities as cancer, and stroke is third. Another cardiovascular disease, arteriosclerosis, ranks eighth among the first 10. The cardiovascular diseases, in fact, cause more than half of all deaths in the country each year. It therefore is only logical that our chief concern should be with this large group of diseases.

For your own protection it is essential to know when to seek prompt help from either your doctor or a hospital. The chances of surviving a heart attack improve immeasurably when the victim goes to the hospital immediately; yet there is often a delay because people do not know what symptoms signal a heart attack. See the chart on page 258 for the early signs of a heart attack as given by the American Heart Association.

Symptoms of Heart Disease

Spotting heart disease or disorders in time may well prevent either a heart attack or serious heart damage later on. There are certain general symptoms that indicate something may be wrong with your heart, and these are sufficiently important to warrant seeing a doctor at once if you discover any of them.

1. *Dyspnea* is a feeling of breathlessness or shortness of breath and is common following such physical exertion as a hard game of tennis or a long run. But, should breathlessness occur after ordinary, everyday activities which you could previously do without ill effects—for instance, walking a short distance or climbing a few steps—be sure to consult your doctor.

2. *Nocturnal dyspnea* is an acute shortness of breath that occurs suddenly at night—usually after an hour or two of sleep—and wakens the sufferer with a choking sensation. This often happens when the person has congestive heart failure, and it calls for a prompt visit to a doctor.

3. *Orthopnea* is breathlessness that takes place when the sufferer is lying down; it is relieved by sitting or standing up. This, too, is usually connected with a heart problem and also demands a prompt medical consultation.

4. *Edema*, or swelling, of the body tissues—the ankles in particular—may be another warning sign. You can determine whether it is edema by simply pressing your finger into the area; indentation of the skin that persists after you take your finger away indicates edema.

5. *Angina pectoris* is literally a strangling pain in the chest. It is characterized by paroxysmal pain behind the breastbone, accompanied by a feeling of suffocation. The distress is usually brought on by hard exercise, unusual excitement, or even a heavy meal. It lasts only a minute or two and is relieved by a few minutes' rest or special medication. Tell your doctor about it at once because it indicates serious heart problems.

6. Other symptoms that may warn of heart disorders include dizziness, fainting spells, blueness of the lips, asthmalike attacks, extreme fatigue, and spitting or coughing up blood. Such symptoms demand a medical examination.

Palpitation or fluttering of the heart and the episodic rapid beating of the heart (paroxysmal tachycardia) are not necessarily danger signals. Many healthy people sometimes have extra heart beats or suddenly feel that their hearts have flopped over or have stopped for a moment. The spells of rapid heart beating that certain nervous or worried people experience may last for hours or even days without causing serious heart trouble, but they do warrant a medical consultation and opinion.

Preventing damage to the heart beforehand is obviously better than trying to minimize the effect of heart disorders afterward. This is why identification of the risk factors in heart disease is important. By recognizing these, doctors can single out persons who may be susceptible to heart trouble and treat them now with the intention of preventing later problems. (For further information about the heart, see Chapter 3.)

Kinds of Heart Diseases

Coronary Artery Disease. The coronary arteries supply blood to the heart muscle. Because the muscle is being used continuously, it needs an uninterrupted full blood supply or it suffers irreparable damage known as *myocardial infarction*, the death of tissue in the heart muscle. Most commonly, coronary artery disease is either coronary occlusion or coronary thrombosis.

In *coronary occlusion* the bore of the artery is narrowed by arteriosclerosis, or hardening of the arteries, which reduces the volume of blood supplied to the heart muscle. This choking off of blood flow can even reach the point of total occlusion in which no blood comes through.

In *coronary thrombosis* a blood clot either forms locally or is brought to a particular spot by the bloodstream from elsewhere in the body. Sometimes after major surgery part of a blood clot may break loose and be carried through the body until it sticks in a vessel too narrow to let it pass through. When either of these conditions cuts off the blood supply to the heart muscle, the tissues no longer supplied with blood will die. If the blockage affects a large part of the muscle, a massive coronary attack occurs and the patient may die.

About 60 percent of the victims of myocardial infarction survive the initial attack, although some 650,000 Americans die of heart attacks annually. The first hour after the attack is the critical period. The American Heart Association estimates that 350,000 victims die each year before they reach the hospital. It is vital to call a doctor immediately and to move the victim to a hospital that has an emergency coronary care unit. Modern ambulances and their personnel are well equipped to care for the heart attack victim while transporting him to the hospital. The lives of many heart attack victims have been saved by means of cardiopulmonary resuscitation, a combination of mouth-to-mouth breathing and closed chest massage. (For further information, see the FIRST AID section.)

The heart attack victim is usually given an injection of morphine or other powerful pain-killer to relieve his severe agony. Oxygen is supplied through a mask or by an oxygen tent to relieve the work burden of the heart and to supply extra oxygen to the vessels around the blood-starved heart muscle.

While at least four weeks of bed rest were once considered mandatory after a heart attack, there is a growing tendency today to get the patient up and about as soon as possible. The survivor of a heart attack is gradually brought back to nearly normal activities within about three months. However, there may be curtailment of certain activities such as strenuous sports. Smoking is forbidden, and the person must keep his weight down, but alcohol may be allowed in moderation. With the growing knowledge about all aspects of medicine, it is best to depend on the doctor for the specifics of treatment—for example, the use of anticoagulant drugs. (See also the entries HEART ATTACK; HEART FAILURE in the encyclopedia section.)

Angina Pectoris. In a sense angina pectoris is the result of the heart's enormous activity. A muscle that is used constantly needs a large, uninterrupted blood supply to bring oxygen and food and to take away the burned-out by-products. When coronary artery disease or arteriosclerosis, and the resulting coronary occlusion cut down on this blood supply, any additional demand leaves the heart muscle short of oxygen and triggers the frequently agonizing pain of angina pectoris. Medication to increase the blood supply—such as nitroglycerin tablets—or even a few minutes of rest are usually sufficient to end the pain. An operation may relieve the condition by bringing additional blood supplies to the heart muscle. (See also the entry HEART DISEASE in the encyclopedia section.)

Congestive Heart Failure. This is the inability of the heart to carry out its function of pumping the blood in adequate quantities. Almost any kind of heart disease can lead to this failure, which increases venous pressure and may lead to edema in tissues in the ankles, lungs, liver, or other parts

---

Early warning signs of heart attack

Symptoms vary but these are the usual warnings of heart attack:

- Prolonged, oppressive pain or unusual discomfort in the *center* of chest, behind the breastbone.

- Pain may radiate to the shoulder, arm, neck or jaw.

- The pain or discomfort is often accompanied by sweating. Nausea, vomiting and shortness of breath may also occur.

- Sometimes these symptoms subside and then return.

Minutes count when heart attack strikes. Act promptly. Call a doctor and carefully describe the symptoms. If no doctor is immediately available, get the victim to a hospital emergency room at once. Be prepared to use emergency measures.

(Source: American Heart Association Inc.)

of the body. Restriction of salt in the diet and the use of diuretics to cause the kidneys to rid the body of salt and water have materially brightened the outlook for patients who suffer from this disorder.

Rheumatic Heart Disease. This results from rheumatic fever and accounts for more than 90 percent of all heart problems in persons under 30 years of age. About half of the rheumatic fever patients suffer heart complications that commonly leave permanent scars. The damage may later cause congestive heart failure. The introduction of penicillin and other antibiotics to treat rheumatic fever has vastly reduced the dangers of rheumatic heart disease. Modern surgery has made possible the relief of some types of heart valve damage and even the replacement of defective valves with artificial substitutes. Often the patients are able to lead long, healthy lives, thanks to new medical and surgical techniques. (See also the entries HEART SURGERY; RHEUMATIC FEVER in the encyclopedia section.)

Bacterial Endocarditis. This is an infection of the thin membranes that line the inside of the heart. The disease is caused by bacterial infections, which can now be successfully treated with antibiotics. Persons with heart defects or rheumatic hearts should ask their physicians what precautions to take to prevent bacterial endocarditis.

Heart Rate Disturbances. Cardiac arrhythmias are variations in the normal rhythmic heartbeat. The range is enormous. For example, most children have normal variations that coincide with different phases of their breathing. At the other extreme are the ineffectual heart-muscle contractions that can lead to sudden death. Mild variations in heartbeat are often benign and occur frequently to elderly people. *Paroxysmal tachycardia* is a fast, regular heartbeat of over 100 beats a minute and is usually harmless. But the speedup can be dangerous if it is a complication of a heart disease, occurs to an aged person, or lasts longer than a few days. Heart flutter and fibrillation can cause as many as 300 beats a minute; depending on which part of the heart is involved, it can be tolerated for many years, or it can lead to death.

Heart Block. This condition occurs when the nervous impulses that control the heart's beating are slowed or brought to a virtual halt. The heart slows down and, in extreme cases, can suffer cardiac arrest or heart stoppage. When the heartbeat rhythm is too erratic, an electrical pacemaker can be surgically implanted to keep the heart beating at its correct rate. Cardiac arrest can be treated with cardiopulmonary resuscitation to keep the victim alive, then with an electrical defibrillator to restart the heartbeat. Upon recovery the patient may be virtually normal in every way. (See also the entry HEART BLOCK in the encyclopedia section.)

Treatment of Heart Disease

Drugs and surgery are used today to treat heart disease, although there is still considerable controversy and disagreement over their use and value. Heart patients should always question the use of new medications because the interaction of several drugs has caused major problems, and certain medications can induce adverse reactions in some patients. Rely on your doctor's judgment about any new medicines on the market.

Many forms of surgery—including open-heart operations and even an occasional heart transplant—are used today for a variety of heart problems. These ailments range from heart murmurs (remedied by the implantation of artificial valves) to angina pectoris (often helped by the transplantation of blood vessels to supply an ailing heart). If you have a heart disorder, it pays to consult your doctor about possible new developments in the treatment of heart disease.

Hypertension

High blood pressure, or hypertension, is often a hidden illness. An estimated 35 million Americans, or one in every four adults, suffer from it, but about 30 percent are not aware they have the disease. It has been called the "silent killer" because there are no characteristic symptoms. Often the cause is not known, and there is no known cure; but if hypertension is not controlled, it can be the direct cause of heart attacks, strokes, and kidney failures.

Hypertension is usually discovered when the blood pressure is taken during a routine physical examination. The pressure is highest when the blood is being forced ahead by the heart—the systolic pressure—and is lowest between beats when the heart relaxes—the diastolic pressure. In normal children the systolic pressure usually ranges from 75 to 100; in young adults, from 100 to 120; and in older people from 120 to 140.

An abnormal increase in blood pressure is believed to be caused by the body's need to force the blood through a constriction, or narrowing, of the smaller blood vessels, but why this constriction occurs is not fully understood. Nervous strain certainly plays a part, and probably hereditary factors as well. The outlook is bright for cooperative patients, however, because enough is now known for doctors to be able to treat hypertension successfully. Depending on the patient's condition, the doctor may forbid smoking, reduce the salt in the diet, eliminate consumption of alcohol, bring body weight down to normal, try to reduce stress and nervous tension, and utilize one of the many drugs now available.

There is still much to be learned about this condition, but doctors are gaining knowledge steadily. If you have hypertension, it may be worth your life to follow your doctor's instructions faithfully and to have regular checkups. In a rare form called malignant hypertension, the disease rapidly produces serious complications and sometimes an early death. With proper care, however, many people with high blood pressure are able to live long, satisfactory lives.

Hypotension

The opposite side of the coin is low blood pressure, or hypotension, which usually causes no symptoms and disappears once the underlying problem is cleared up. (For further information about hypotension, see Chapter 23.)

Arteriosclerosis

Arteriosclerosis, or hardening of the arteries, starts with the depositing of fatty materials in the walls of the arteries. This is accompanied or followed by calcification, which is common in middle and old age. With the loss of elasticity in the arteries and the thickening of their walls, less blood flows through them and symptoms of poor blood circulation occur. If the blood vessels in the arms or legs are involved, movement can produce cramps or aching pains. If arteries to the brain are affected, there may be a partial loss of intellectual powers. And if the coronary arteries harden, angina pectoris or another serious heart condition may result.

Because knowledge about and treatment of arteriosclerosis are changing rapidly, your doctor is the best source of information about the problem. In most cases low-cholesterol diets and special medication are prescribed. In certain cases the affected arteries are literally reamed out so that blood flow is restored, or blood vessels from other parts of the body are surgically implanted in order to bypass the blocked vessels and restore blood circulation.

Stroke

Strokes occur when the blood supply through an artery to the brain is markedly reduced or cut off entirely—from arteriosclerosis, by a blood clot that lodges in a blood vessel, or by a burst vessel that hemorrhages. The result is commonly paralysis of an arm or leg, but can also result in other symptoms such as the loss of speech. Often the condition clears up later, in part or completely. Strokes are so individual that few generalized statements can be made about them, but a massive stroke or one affecting a vital area of the brain can cause death quickly.

The outlook is better for patients who suffer strokes caused by blood clots or embolisms. (See the entries THROMBOSIS and EMBOLISM in the encyclopedia section.) Persons totally paralyzed by this kind of stroke often recover completely. In cases of paralysis, the paralyzed muscles must be treated early and the joints moved, so that when the brain recovers its function, the joints and muscles will not be too stiff and weakened to respond. Institutes of rehabilitation are available in large medical centers, and most doctors and nurses have had training in rehabilitating patients. (For further information, see the entry STROKE in the encyclopedia section.)

Phlebitis and Thrombophlebitis

Phlebitis occurs when the wall of a vein becomes inflamed from trauma or infection. It sometimes occurs after surgery or childbirth. Phlebitis causes redness, swelling, and pain, and may last for years. Phlebitis often leads to a blood clot formation called thrombophlebitis, which is common but not very serious if the vein is a superficial one. If the vein is a deep one, however, there can be complications: the whole leg can swell; and should the clot break loose, it can eventually lodge in the lung, heart, or brain and even be fatal. Doctors now employ a variety of medical and surgical methods to deal with thrombophlebitis.

Aneurysm

Aneurysms are balloonlike outpocketings in the wall of an artery. They are dangerous because they threaten to burst the stretched artery and cause hemorrhage. Should this occur in the brain or the aorta, the body's major artery leading directly from the heart, the effect can be fatal. Treatment of such an aneurysm is by surgery; the diseased arterial section is removed and replaced by a synthetic tube.

CANCER

Cancer is greatly feared because of the terrible torment that most people associate with this killer disease. However, great strides have recently been made to alleviate the ravages of cancer. Whereas in 1900 few cancer victims had any hope for long-term survival, today about one-third of all people who suffer from this dread disease are expected to live at least five years after beginning treatment.

Cancer is actually a large group of diseases rather than one single disorder. It is basically an overgrowth of cells which spread to other parts of the body and result in death if not stopped or at least controlled in time. Many cancers today can be cured when detected promptly and treated properly.

Why do cells suddenly start to proliferate and multiply, spreading to distant parts of the body at rates of speed as different as the cancers themselves? The answer is not really known even today. What is known is that smoking does cause lung cancer, that excessive radiation can cause other types of cancer, and that factors in the environment—too much sun, for example—are carcinogenic, or cancer-causing. But why these factors cause cancer, or why they do so in one person and not in another, is not fully understood. There is still much to learn about cancer, but at least there are ways of preventing some cancers and of stopping others when they are detected in time.

A word of warning is in order: *only a doctor can tell whether a tumor is malignant or benign.* He has to examine a bit of the growth under a microscope in order to know whether or not it is cancer. Never decide for yourself that a tumor is only a harmless growth. Once a cancer has spread, the chances of a cure diminish rapidly.

Fortunately, cancer is not contagious. No cancer has ever been transmitted from one person to another. It is therefore perfectly safe to visit, associate with, or care for an individual who has cancer.

Types of Cancer

Cancers are divided into two large groups: sarcomas and carcinomas. Sarcomas usually affect the bones and muscles, and are apt to grow rapidly and be very destructive. The carcinomas make up the great majority of the cancers of the breast, stomach, lungs, uterus, skin, and tongue.

At first most cancers grow only in the site where they originated. Even then, the cancer may invade neighboring cells and tissues and perhaps destroy vital structures. It is far more dangerous, however, when it sets up new growths in other parts of the body. When cancer enters this stage, it becomes very difficult to cure; yet in some cases it can still be held in check. Obviously, the time when cancer can best be cured is in the early period of its growth—before it destroys neighboring tissues or spreads to other parts of the body.

Lung Cancer. The American Cancer Society estimates that about 117,000 people will be stricken annually by lung cancer, and that 101,000 will die of this disease in 1980. This is one cancer for which the chief cause is usually clear—smoking. Lung cancer is prevalent among heavy smokers who use more than one pack of cigarettes a day. Constant smoking of cigarettes, pipes, or cigars is a medically risky habit. (See the entry SMOKING in the encyclopedia section.) But in some cases lung cancer can also strike non-smokers as well.

The chief indications of lung cancer are:

1. A cough that does not let up after two weeks, or a change in an old cigarette cough. Also, wheezing or other noises in the chest.

2. Coughing up blood or bloody sputum—any sputum that looks rusty, pink, or blood-streaked.

3. Shortness of breath without a cause such as running or climbing.

4. Chest ache or pain.

Breast Cancer. This is the most common type of cancer in women. The chances of a woman developing breast cancer are one in 11, and the disease is found most often in those over the age of 40. The value of early detection cannot be overemphasized.

The value of prevention has been shown by research projects which found that almost 50 percent of women with breast cancer had negative armpit lymph nodes, which indicated that the cancer had not spread. By catching breast cancer before it had spread to the lymph nodes, a woman's chances of survival increased to the point where 85 percent of these early cases were alive five years later. The American Cancer Society urges self-examination of the breasts at least once a month (see the illustration on page 233) and an annual examination by a physician. (See BREAST CANCER in the encyclopedia section.)

Early warning signs of breast cancer are:

1. Painless lumps in the breast.

2. Bleeding or discharge from the nipple.

Colon–Rectum Cancer. This common form of cancer affects about 114,000 Americans each year. About 45 percent of its victims are alive five years later, but the American Cancer Society estimates that when the cancer is detected early enough the percentage rises to 70 percent. The key to diagnosis is a proctoscopic examination which should be taken every 3–5 years by people over the age of 50. (See Chapter 20.)

Signs and symptoms of colon-rectum cancer are:

1. Periods of constipation that mark a change from usual bowel habits, sometimes followed by episodes of more frequent elimination.

2. Cramps in the abdomen and a sensation of incomplete elimination, or a feeling that there is a lump in the rectum.

3. Rectal pain and rectal bleeding—for example, blood spots on the toilet tissue or in the feces. (Remember that hemorrhoids also cause rectal pain and bleeding. A thorough physical examination by a doctor will determine whether the condition is hemorrhoids or cancer.)

Skin Cancer. More than 400,000 new cases of skin cancer are reported in the United States annually, but most can be prevented by avoiding excessive exposure to the sun. The American Cancer Society estimates that some 95 percent of the victims can be cured if the following warning signals are heeded in time:

1. Sores and ulcers that do not heal.

2. Moles, warts, blemishes, scars, or birthmarks that suddenly change in color, size, or texture.

3. Growths constantly exposed to irritations—such as from tight-fitting brassieres or from shaving.

Cancer in Children. Although usually thought of as an adult disease, cancer ranks second only to accidents among the causes of death in children under the age of 15. Cancer kills more children between the ages of three and 14 than any other disease, with leukemia accounting for about half of these deaths. Fortunately, death rates for all types of childhood cancer have declined from more than 8 per 100,000 in 1950 to 5 by 1977. This decline was caused in part by the increasing medical success in dealing with leukemia, lymphoma, and kidney cancer. The most common forms of cancer in children are leukemia and lymphoma, brain and central nervous system cancers, cancer of the kidney, and bone cancer.

Treatment for Cancer

Treatments vary but have met with encouraging success either singly or in combination. Surgery is the most common means of attack. Increasingly, radiation treatment by means of X rays or such radioactive substances as cobalt is being used either by itself or in conjunction with surgery. Chemotherapy is also finding an exciting place in cancer therapy and offers considerable hope in the case of blood cancers. Some new drugs have been used with great success. Hormonal therapy—notably in prostate cancer—is another approach. The newest of all is immunotherapy, which is actually too recent for final evaluation as yet. There is much hope for successfully treating cancer victims today, and success still lies primarily with prevention and early detection. (See the accompanying chart for cancer's warning signals and safeguards.)

LUNG DISEASES

Your very life depends on your lungs. If the average person were to stop breathing for more than four minutes, his brain would be irreparably damaged. Your two lungs have 300 million air sacs, each with its cobweb of blood vessels through which red blood cells pass single file to discharge carbon dioxide and pick up oxygen. The lungs are subject to dangerous infections such as pneumonia, tuberculosis, and influenza, and to chronic, obstructive pulmonary diseases such as emphysema, chronic bronchitis, and asthma. (For further information, see the entries on these diseases in the encyclopedia section.)

Pneumonia

Pneumonia is an infection of the lungs caused by a large variety of germs. There are three general kinds: bacterial, viral, and mycoplasmal—their names reveal the type of infecting germs. Prompt medical care is essential because pneumonia is one of mankind's oldest killers. Antibiotics are effective against bacterial and mycoplasmal pneumonia, but not against viral pneumonia. Victims generally develop coughs, fever, and chills. Always call the doctor, for though pneumonia is no longer fatal for one out of four victims as it once was, it still kills about 51,000 Americans each year.

Emphysema

One of the most common disabling diseases of the respiratory tract is emphysema. In recent years, deaths from emphysema have almost tripled; about 25,000 Americans now die from it annually. It commonly strikes men between the ages of 50 and 70. A high percentage of its victims have long been heavy smokers, and they frequently live in places where air pollution is a problem.

Emphysema sufferers often have a long-standing history of coughs and shortness of breath after physical exertion. As the disease develops, just walking or carrying out common activities causes breathing difficulties, finally reaching the point where every breath demands hard effort. Inside the lungs the walls of the tiny air sacs, the alveoli, stretch and finally rupture; the cobweb of blood vessels in the walls of some air sacs may disappear, leaving less contact between blood and air—thus making the exchange of carbon dioxide for oxygen much more difficult.

Its actual cause is unknown, but it is thought that emphysema is often a later result of chronic infection or irritation of the bronchial tubes, which connect the windpipe with the lungs. Although there is no absolutely known preventive, it is generally believed that smoking should be avoided. Today doctors can give emphysema sufferers some relief and improve their lung function. Early recognition and treatment of the disease are essential, for emphysema can eventually lead to heart failure.

Tuberculosis

Tuberculosis is an infectious disease caused by a bacterium that can strike the body anywhere, but most frequently hits the lungs. In 1900 tuberculosis was the second leading cause of death in the United States, killing 200 out of every 100,000 persons, but by 1960 it ranked only 16th, causing but six deaths per 100,000 population. Prevention and control measures have made the difference. Modern sanatoriums, by providing specialized care and isolating tubercular patients who might otherwise spread the infection, have been an important factor in reducing the incidence of the disease. Antibiotics and chemotherapy have been very helpful as well. The widespread use of chest X rays and the tuberculin test to identify the disease have also helped.

An estimated 15 million Americans today have live tubercle bacillus germs in their bodies. The American Lung Association therefore advises that everyone have at least one tuberculin test during his or her lifetime. Tuberculosis is most likely to be found among people with inadequate nutrition who live under crowded, generally poor conditions.

Chronic Bronchitis

Another serious disease, chronic bronchitis, affects an estimated 7 million people annually and costs some 4,000 people their lives. It causes coughing and spitting up of heavy mucus, or phlegm. It affects both men and women, and the disease is likely to start in middle age. The initial bronchial irritation may begin with a bacterial infection, infected tonsils, or some other disease. But the most common causes of the irritation are heavy smoking and air pollution. Chronic bronchitis has often led to emphysema. Prompt medical care is essential.

Influenza

The "flu" is a highly infectious disease of the respiratory system. The tissues swell, become inflamed, and may even crack, causing nasal or throat discharges to be streaked with blood, and this may spread to the lungs. Although the tissues do heal in a week or two, they are then susceptible to other types of infection, particularly in the lungs. Medical care should be sought when you come down with the flu because it may prove fatal. However, modern vaccinations have been about 70 percent effective in preventing this debilitating disease. (See also Chapter 23.)

OTHER MAJOR CAUSES OF DEATH

Diseases of the Liver

The liver is such an indispensable organ that its total destruction is followed by death in a very short time. However, it has been estimated that more than 80 percent of the organ can be damaged or destroyed before symptoms of liver insufficiency will appear.

The liver removes some of the waste products from the bloodstream and disposes of them in the bile. If the liver becomes diseased, the bile may then pile up in the bloodstream, causing the whites of the eyes and the skin to become yellow. This yellowing is called jaundice. A particular type of liver disease that causes jaundice is the result of a virus infection of the liver. Called infectious hepatitis, or viral hepatitis, the disease attacks chiefly young people.

Another symptom of liver disease may be a gradual enlargement of the abdomen. Vomiting blood or passing bloody, black, or clay-colored stools is also a symptom of liver disease. Other symptoms include constant fatigue, loss of weight, nausea, poor appetite, anemia, and hemorrhoids. These warnings should immediately send you to a doctor for an examination.

Liver ailments can develop from a number of causes, including viral infections, nutritional deficiencies (sometimes related to alcoholism), diseases of the gallbladder, and injuries caused by exposure to noxious chemicals. Puncture wounds of the liver, such as that caused by a fall on a pointed object, must be operated upon immediately. The liver may also be injured by a blunt impact, and anyone having an abdominal pain resulting from such an injury should see a doctor at once.

Cirrhosis is a chronic disease of the liver; its cells are destroyed and replaced with fatty or fibrous tissue. The symptoms are the same as those of other liver diseases. (See also the entries CIRRHOSIS; HEPATITIS; JAUNDICE; LIVER in the encyclopedia section.)

Kidney Disease

Bright's disease and nephritis are different names for a group of kidney ailments that can be fatal when both kidneys are involved. Because the kidneys remove liquid wastes from the body, their improper functioning can result in death because no other organ can do the job.

Glomerulonephritis, often referred to as nephritis or Bright's disease, is a widespread inflammation of both kidneys. The delicate membranes of the filtering units of the kidneys are affected, and proteins and blood cells pass out into the urine. The presence of the blood proteins, especially albumin, and of red blood corpuscles in the urine suggests nephritis, especially if the physician finds certain other microscopic structures called *casts* in the urine. An acute attack of Bright's disease affects the blood capillaries of the entire body so that water leaks out into the tissues. In a typical attack, the eyes look swollen and puffy, and the ankles may be distended with painless accumulations of edema fluid.

One form of nephritis called nephrosis affects children. It may last for years and then clear up completely, provided infections and complications can be avoided. In adults, nephrosis is a stage of Bright's disease that tends to become irreversibly chronic. (For further information, see the entries KIDNEY DISEASE; NEPHRITIS; NEPHROSIS; UREMIA in the encyclopedia section.)

Diabetes

A widespread metabolic disorder, diabetes is characterized by excessive amounts of sugar in the blood and urine. Despite its long history, diabetes is still not fully understood; it has been blamed on a lack of sufficient insulin (a hormone produced by the pancreas) or on no insulin at all. It has been estimated to occur in about 10 million Americans, and more than 600,000 new cases are diagnosed annually. Diabetes and its complications claims over 300,000 lives each year. (See also the entry DIABETES in the encyclopedia section.)

Accidents

Accidents rank fourth as a leading cause of death in the United States, accounting for more than 104,000 fatalities each year. They occur mainly in the home, on the job, and on streets and highways. (Prevention of accidents in the home is described in Chapter 21, and on the job in Chapter 7.) Highway accidents kill many young people who are just on the threshold of life. The death and disability rate among teenagers in automobile accidents is horrifying.

What can parents and doctors do about the deaths from highway accidents? Chiefly, we must set an example for our children by being safe drivers ourselves. This means observing the legal speed limits and all other rules for good driving. It also means not drinking alcoholic beverages when driving.

Every driver should have good vision and good hearing and be in good health. Anyone with a chronic illness should discuss the hazards of his driving with a doctor. (For information about emergency first aid measures in case of an automobile accident, see the FIRST AID section.)

23 The Disabling Diseases

People who suffer from the disabling diseases—those in which disability, either total or recurrent, is a chief feature—are apt to become the forgotten segment in modern medical care. This chapter discusses the important disabling diseases, pointing out their causes and symptoms so that you can recognize them as soon as possible and be able to escape or alleviate their crippling effects. Modern diagnosis and treatment of each disease are also described. These illnesses, which affect millions of Americans every year, include such common and well-known disablers as arthritis, backache, peptic ulcer, neuritis and neuralgia, asthma, and even alcoholism.

ARTHRITIS

The nation's number one crippler, arthritis plagues more than 30 million Americans. Arthritis is defined as an inflammation of a joint, but the term is widely misused and is frequently applied to vague aches in almost any part of the body. Arthritis occurs in the knees, wrists, elbows, fingers, toes, hips, and shoulders. The neck and back have joints between the bones of the spine that may become arthritic. If you do feel a pain in a joint, however, it may not always indicate arthritis, because other parts such as ligaments and tendons also make up the structure of the joint.

Symptoms of chronic arthritis are pain, swelling, stiffness, and deformity in one or more joints. The signs may appear suddenly or come on gradually. Victims feel aches and pains that vary from a sharp, burning sensation to grinding pain. Moving the affected joint usually hurts, although sometimes it is only stiff.

The underlying cause of many cases of chronic arthritis is unknown. Attacks of arthritis are set off by exposure to cold and dampness, a poorly balanced diet, infections, an injury to a joint or constant strain upon it, hard physical labor that is too much for your age or strength, constant fatigue, and acute nervous tension. These factors also aggravate the painful symptoms of the disease. A doctor will look for these conditions when arthritis symptoms appear. But he will consider other causes, because occasionally a case

of arthritis may result from such diseases as gout or undulant fever. In younger people, arthritis may be caused by rheumatic fever. The latter fortunately does not cripple the joints.

The two commonest types of arthritis are rheumatoid arthritis and osteoarthritis. More than 6 million Americans suffer from rheumatoid arthritis, and some 16 million suffer pain from a severe form of osteoarthritis, which most often attacks the body joints that carry weight—such as the knees, hips, and fingers. Therapy for arthritis includes aspirin and a host of other drugs. Rest, heat treatments, and judicious exercise are usually prescribed, and in some cases surgery is recommended. Treatments for some 100 different arthritic diseases naturally vary—which is why a doctor must be consulted. Nevertheless, many people with arthritis can go about their lives as usual. (See the entries ARTHRITIS; GOUT; SPONDYLITIS in the encyclopedia section.)

BACKACHE AND OTHER AILMENTS OF THE JOINTS AND BONES

The backache may have replaced the common cold as the most frequent malady of Americans. The problem began in prehistoric times when man started to walk upright; his spine had not been designed to carry his weight in this manner. The spine, or backbone, is flexible because of the way the bones and disks are loosely strung to-

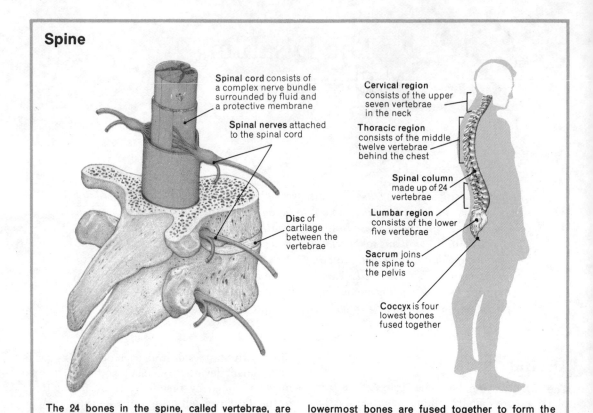

Spine

Spinal cord consists of a complex nerve bundle surrounded by fluid and a protective membrane

Spinal nerves attached to the spinal cord

Disc of cartilage between the vertebrae

Cervical region consists of the upper seven vertebrae in the neck

Thoracic region consists of the middle twelve vertebrae behind the chest

Spinal column made up of 24 vertebrae

Lumbar region consists of the lower five vertebrae

Sacrum joins the spine to the pelvis

Coccyx is four lowest bones fused together

The 24 bones in the spine, called vertebrae, are separated by discs of cartilage which allow the spine to bend and cushion it from shocks. The lowermost bones are fused together to form the sacrum and coccyx; the sacrum attaches the spine to the pelvis.

gether, and this structure permits bending and other kinds of bodily movements.

Backaches may be the result of a slipped disk, sacroiliac strain, sciatic neuritis, arthritis, poor posture, or emotional tension. If you have a backache that persists, you need a medical checkup. (See also the entries BACKACHE; VERTE-BRAL DISK in the encyclopedia section.)

Causes of Backache

If you are otherwise healthy but develop frequent backaches, the cause may be:

1. Your mattress may be soft and sagging, thus curving your spine when you sleep. If you do not want to get a new mattress, use a bed board between the mattress and the bedsprings.

2. Your posture may be wrong. Incorrect posture is one of the commonest causes of backache. When your back is distorted by poor posture or strained from carrying too much weight, the bones, ligaments, nerves, and muscles are either pressed closely together or stretched too far apart, causing pain. (For illustrations of good and bad posture, see Chapter 1.)

3. You may be carrying too much at one time—for instance, a heavy shopping bag in one hand. This tends to curve your spine to the right or left, causing the back muscles and ligaments to be strained.

4. Your work habits may be wrong. If you must sit at a typewriter or desk all day, don't slump—sit upright. When you sit or stand correctly, you tend to develop a strong, pain-free back. If your job requires that you do a lot of bending over, make sure you take time out at regular intervals to stretch and straighten up.

5. Watch out for drafts. Try to avoid sitting with your back exposed to drafts from hallways, open doors, or windows.

6. Backaches in women may be caused by abnormalities in the position of the female pelvic organs. These are sometimes related to past pregnancies, but women who have not been pregnant may also have such backaches.

7. Emotional tension creates muscular tension. Pain from stress is just as real and severe as pain attributed to any other cause.

When you get a backache that persists, go to

your doctor for a checkup. The pain may be caused by a minor condition such as poor posture, or by a more serious disorder such as a tumor.

A serious type of backache is caused by a ruptured vertebral disk (slipped disk). The disks, made of cartilage that lies between the bones of the spine, sometimes slip out partially from between the spinal bones and press on the nerve roots emerging from the spinal cord. The condition was not fully understood until recently, and the symptoms were mistakenly attributed to sciatica, lumbago, or other ailments.

Treatment of Back Conditions

Improvement of posture, operations for slipped disks and tumors, massage, and X-ray treatment for certain tumors are among the kinds of treatment the doctor will prescribe, depending on the cause. For the occasional, mild backache, a simple home treatment may help greatly. Relief from pain may be had by taking two aspirin every four hours, resting on a hard mattress, and applying moist heat—such as from a shower or tub of water—at a temperature only slightly above that of the body. The doctor may prescribe drugs such as muscle relaxants to stop acute pain by relieving associated muscle spasms. (See also the section in Chapter 1 on ways of avoiding back trouble.)

Bursitis

Bursitis is an inflammation of the lubricating parts around joints. Our joints would creak and wear out if there were no efficient "oiling" system. Sometimes the smoothly working bursas around the joints become inflamed. When they do, there is severe pain.

Bursitis may occur in an acute or chronic form. In an acute attack the inflamed bursa may be felt as a tender swelling near the shoulder or whichever joint is affected. Chronic bursitis may follow the acute attack. There is continued pain and limitation of motion around the joint. In the shoulder an X ray will usually reveal calcium salts that have been deposited in one of the important bursas around the joint. If rest, heat, and medicines do not relieve the condition, surgery may be required to remove the deposits or free the area of chronic inflammation. (See also the entries BUNION; BURSITIS; ELBOW; HOUSEMAID'S KNEE in the encyclopedia section.)

Bursitis can lead to a condition called frozen shoulder, a disabling limitation of motion of the important shoulder joint resulting from bands of

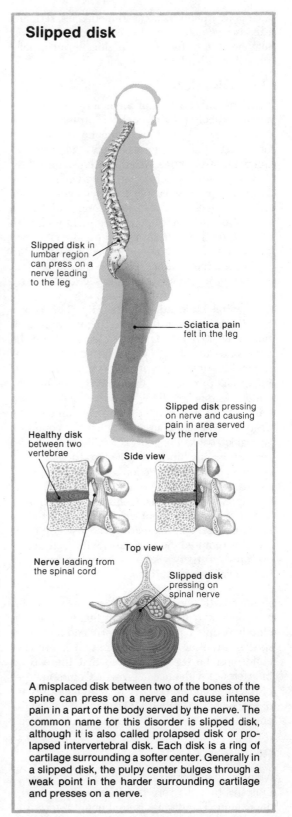

Slipped disk

Slipped disk in lumbar region can press on a nerve leading to the leg

Sciatica pain felt in the leg

Slipped disk pressing on nerve and causing pain in area served by the nerve

Healthy disk between two vertebrae

Side view

Nerve leading from the spinal cord

Top view

Slipped disk pressing on spinal nerve

A misplaced disk between two of the bones of the spine can press on a nerve and cause intense pain in a part of the body served by the nerve. The common name for this disorder is slipped disk, although it is also called prolapsed disk or prolapsed intervertebral disk. Each disk is a ring of cartilage surrounding a softer center. Generally in a slipped disk, the pulpy center bulges through a weak point in the harder surrounding cartilage and presses on a nerve.

adhesions around the joint. If medicines, rest, and exercises do not relieve the condition, the doctor may be able to free the adhesions by manipulation of the shoulder under anesthesia.

Bone Disorders

Until the introduction of medicines that destroy staphylococci and streptococci, prolonged disability frequently resulted from bone infections produced by these germs. They can cause an infection of the bone called acute osteomyelitis. This infection, which creates sudden pain and fever, generally strikes at the long bones of the arms and legs. Children and young adults are most often affected. Prompt treatment with penicillin and other antibiotics will usually eradicate the infection. If not, surgery may be required to drain the affected area. (See also the entry OSTE-OMYELITIS in the encyclopedia section.)

Congenital Dislocation of the Hip. This condition is present at birth, more frequently in girls than in boys, but it may not be evident until the child starts to walk. Then it will be noticed that the child's movements are not symmetrical. It is important to diagnose the condition before the child does much walking with the weakened hip joint. At this time proper treatment can cure the dislocation without surgery, but if the condition is neglected for long, surgery will be needed to reconstruct the hip joint. (See also the entry HIP in the encyclopedia section.)

Clubfoot. This is a congenital condition that seriously affects the foot. It can be corrected by early treatment, and sometimes only strapping or a cast is required. Serious cases will need expert orthopedic surgery. (See also the entry TALIPES in the encyclopedia section.)

Fractures. If a broken bone does not heal properly, there may be disability for life. Fractures in elderly people tend to knit poorly and may need special attention. Bone fractures in a growing child must be set correctly so that there is no interference with normal growth. Common types of fractures and emergency first aid measures are described in the FIRST AID section. (See also the entry BROKEN BONE in the encyclopedia section.)

PEPTIC ULCER

An ulcer is simply a sore, and the word "peptic" indicates that the sore is in the stomach or the duodenum. The disease is commonly referred to as ulcers and affects an estimated 4 million Americans.

Its cause is not fully understood, but it is associated with the presence of an excessive amount of acid gastric juices secreted by the stomach for purposes of digestion. People with ulcers have excessive secretions, not only after eating but also between meals and at night during sleep. Because worry and anxiety can increase these secretions, ulcers are considered to be primarily a psychosomatic disease. (See the entry PSYCHOSOMATIC in the encyclopedia section.)

Symptoms

The most common symptoms of peptic ulcer are:

1. *Pain and discomfort:* The victim of an ulcer feels either pain, a burning sensation, or discomfort in the upper abdomen. These symptoms are usually felt about two or three hours after meals or in the middle of the night; sometimes the distress occurs sooner after eating. Nausea and vomiting can also occur. These so-called hunger pains generally subside promptly upon eating, drinking milk, or taking bicarbonate of soda or other antacids.

2. *Bleeding:* Untreated peptic ulcers can cause a slow seeping of blood, resulting in anemia and the loss of health and strength. The bleeding may be in the form of a sudden hemorrhage that threatens life itself. Blood is sometimes vomited and appears brownish because of the effect of the stomach acids. Blood in the bowel movements may be responsible for black or tarry stools. In the case of a massive hemorrhage, the person becomes weak, faint, and thirsty. He requires immediate medical attention and hospitalization. Full recovery often is a slow process.

3. *Perforation:* An ulcer may perforate the wall of the stomach or duodenum. This causes excruciating pain in the upper abdomen. Patients have described it as "the worst pain of my life." The victim must be rushed to the hospital for immediate surgery to prevent possibly fatal consequences.

Diagnosis

In order to diagnose peptic ulcer, the stomach acids are tested after a sample of the stomach contents has been obtained by passing a tube through the mouth and esophagus. X rays of the stomach and duodenum are also taken. A gastroscopic examination, in which the doctor looks into the stomach by means of an instrument resembling a periscope, is especially important in many cases.

Anyone with symptoms suggesting a peptic ulcer should see a doctor promptly. An ulcer that has caused only mild discomfort can suddenly threaten the victim's life. Other potentially dangerous diseases can resemble a gastric ulcer; some of these require immediate treatment.

Treatment

Ulcers can be successfully treated, but there is no quick and easy cure. The fundamentals of the treatment are a bland diet and medications to neutralize excess stomach acid. An ulcer that has been healed by medical treatment may return if emotional tensions persist. Therefore, every effort should be made to help the person relax. Medicines such as barbiturates and other sedatives are sometimes given for this purpose.

Various operations have been attempted for the relief of ulcers. In an operation called a gastroenterostomy, the stomach contents are bypassed from the duodenum into the jejunum, that portion of the small intestine that extends from the duodenum to the ileum. The procedure is not as successful as some doctors once hoped it might be, because the ulcer may recur at the new opening between the stomach and intestine. This marginal, or jejunal, ulcer can be fully as troublesome as the original one. In another operation called subtotal gastrectomy, the acid-producing part of the stomach is cut away. It is a drastic operation and must be performed by an experienced surgeon. Still another operation, vagotomy, cuts the vagus nerves leading to the stomach and thus reduces the flow of acid in the stomach. (For a fuller discussion, see the entry ULCER in the encyclopedia section.)

NEURITIS AND NEURALGIA

When pain accompanies an illness, the condition is usually created by the disease that has inflamed an organ and irritated the ends of the pain nerves, or pain fibers. However, there are certain circumstances in which the nerves themselves become inflamed. Such nerve inflammation is called neuritis. If the irritation affects a nerve that carries pain fibers, severe pain will be perceived by the brain, and this pain is usually referred to as neuralgia.

The peripheral nerves connecting the brain and spinal cord with the muscles, organs, skin, eyes, and other parts of the body may be affected by a variety of diseases and injuries. When a peripheral nerve is involved, the condition may be either neuritis or neuralgia. Because these nerves generally contain both pain and motor fibers, a disease that affects them would be expected to—and usually does—cause painful symptoms plus some paralysis of muscle power. (See also the entries NEURITIS; NEURALGIA in the encyclopedia section.)

Facial Palsy (Bell's Palsy)

Frequently, only one nerve may be affected. For example, a person who sleeps in a cold draft that blows on the one side of the face may find that the side of the face that is "powered" by muscles controlled through the facial nerve may be temporarily paralyzed. This type of paralysis is called facial palsy, or Bell's palsy. Most often, such a paralysis will clear up after a few days or weeks.

Sometimes a tumor presses on the nerve and causes facial palsy, or the nerve may be injured by a blow, a cut, or a bullet. In such cases the results of treatment will depend on the success in treating the tumor or injury. If the cause of facial palsy is not apparent, or the condition does not improve, your doctor is justified in sending you to a neurologist.

Sciatica

The sciatic nerve is the widest and longest nerve in the body; it runs from the spinal column to the lower leg, where it divides into two branches. It is exposed to many kinds of injury in the back, the pelvis, and even the lower legs. Injury or inflammation of the sciatic nerve causes pain that travels down the leg from the thigh or the back into the feet and toes. Certain muscles of the leg may be partially or completely paralyzed.

The cause of sciatica may be a back injury or irritation from arthritis of the spine, or pressure on the nerve that occurs during some types of work. Certain diseases such as diabetes or gout may be the inciting factor. If the cause has been located, the cure will be facilitated by correcting the underlying trouble. In addition, sedatives and physiotherapy may be required to relieve the pain or disability. Unfortunately, some cases of sciatica will turn out to be the idiopathic variety—that is, without known cause. (See also the entry SCIATICA in the encyclopedia section.)

Shingles (Herpes Zoster)

Shingles, or herpes zoster (*herpes* means "creeping," and *zoster* means "girdle"), is a painful inflammation of the sections of nerves emerging from the spinal cord. The illness is caused by the same virus that causes chicken pox. Fever and prostration may accompany the pain when shingles first develops. Small blisters, or vesicles, usually appear on the skin along the course of the affected nerves. The chest is frequently the site of the affliction. A form of shingles that inflames the nerves leading to the face and eyes is especially dangerous because it may damage vision.

An ordinary attack of shingles runs its painful course in a few days or weeks and does not leave residual difficulties. In some cases, most frequently in elderly people, there is a persistence of pain that may be disabling. (See also the entry SHINGLES in the encyclopedia section.)

Other Spinal Nerve Ailments

Any of the many nerves traveling out from the spine may be affected by injury or disease. For example, the nerves that lie between the ribs may become inflamed and cause pain in the chest that may resemble pleurisy or even a heart attack. This form of nerve ailment is called intercostal neuritis or neuralgia. Similarly, the nerves traveling down the neck to the arm may be subject to various injuries and diseases. For example, a chronic pain in the hand or arm is sometimes traced to the irritation caused by the pressure of an extra rib in the neck—the cervical rib syndrome. Sometimes too vigorous pulling on the nerves in the neck—such as might occur in infants during difficult obstetrical deliveries—causes the condition known as brachial nerve palsy, which may lead to paralysis of the arm.

Cranial Nerve Ailments

The 12 pairs of important nerves leading directly from the brain are called the cranial nerves. The fifth cranial, or trigeminal, nerve that runs to the face and jaws may be the source of a neuralgia that causes spasms of pain on one side of the face. This trigeminal neuralgia is also called *tic douloureux*. It may be set off by a draft of cold air, by chewing, or by other factors.

The nerves leading to the retina of the eye may be involved in various ailments. This condition is called optic neuritis and, because of its potential danger to vision, requires immediate treatment. The other cranial nerves may be damaged by infections, tumors, and toxins. Any disturbance of vision, hearing, balancing, swallowing, taste, or speech may be a signal of trouble in the cranial nerves and should be reported to your doctor.

Injuries to Nerves

The peripheral nerves may be cut, bruised, or torn by fractured bones, blows, or gunshot wounds. But they have a capacity to heal and regenerate. A torn or cut nerve should be treated by a surgeon in order to avoid possible paralysis and other serious consequences of nerve injuries.

ASTHMA

Asthma, technically called bronchial asthma, is a disease of the bronchial tubes that lead from the windpipe, or trachea, into the lungs. These tubes normally do not furnish any marked resistance to the entrance or exit of air, but in asthmatic attacks they tend to close down, causing asthmatic wheezing. If the attack is severe, the sufferer seems almost to be suffocating. He apparently uses all his strength just trying to breathe. He becomes pale and bluish and often perspires. This spasm of the bronchial tubes can usually be relieved quickly by an injection of adrenaline. Fortunately, most attacks are mild and do not last long. Many of them can be prevented or stopped by medical treatment.

Bronchial asthma is a chronic illness marked by these attacks. In severe cases the bronchial tubes become swollen and offer greater resistance to treatment. Plugs of clinging mucus may form in the tubes and cause chronic irritation and coughing. They are dislodged and brought up as sputum. If the attacks are frequent, prolonged, and severe, the lung tissue is damaged. This puts a strain on the heart.

The average case of asthma is mild and is more of a recurrent nuisance than a real threat to health. But it is always important to get competent medical advice, especially in the cases of young people, before asthma can damage the heart or lungs.

Causes of Asthma

Allergies. One type of bronchial asthma is definitely allergic. During ragweed season a victim may suffer from asthma alone or from hay fever and asthma simultaneously. Other allergens include the dander from animal fur and feathers, face powder, and certain foods.

Infections. Many cases of bronchial asthma are associated with bacterial infections, especially of the sinuses, throat, and nose. Sometimes these improve markedly when the infection clears up.

Nervous Tension. Some cases of bronchial asthma appear to be caused by nervous tension. A victim's condition often improves tremendously when his emotional problems are solved. In some cases, treatment requires the help of a psychiatrist.

Even asthma that has a physical cause is apt to become worse if the patient is emotionally disturbed or tense. For this reason asthma is usually included among the psychosomatic diseases. (See also ALLERGY; ASTHMA; PSYCHOSOMATIC in the encyclopedia section.)

UROGENITAL SYSTEM DISORDERS

The urogenital system—sometimes called the urinary tract—consists of the kidneys, the ureters that connect the kidneys with the bladder, the urethra that carries off the urine from the bladder, and—in men—the prostate gland as well. It is estimated that more than 13 million Americans suffer from kidney-related diseases. (For information about diseases of the kidneys, see Chapter 22 and the encyclopedia entries KIDNEY DISEASE; KIDNEY STONE.)

Bladder Diseases

Cystitis. An infection of the bladder called cystitis is the most common of the bladder diseases, particularly in women. Normally, cystitis is only a nuisance, but if neglected it can lead to kidney infection. Prompt medical care is essential.

Symptoms include a frequent and urgent need to urinate, although little urine is passed; burning or pain during urination; and the presence of blood in the urine. Diagnosis involves urine tests and a cystoscopy—an examination with a cystoscope, a periscopelike device that is passed through the urethra and allows the doctor to see into the bladder. The problem may be cleared up with antibiotics or sulfa drugs. Victims may have to drink at least two quarts of fluid a day while avoiding coffee, tea, alcohol, or highly seasoned foods. The patient may have to eat certain foods to make the urine either acidic or alkaline.

Bladder Tumors. These tumors can be malignant (cancerous) or benign, and polyps may occur. Bladder tumors are often caused by such substances as aniline dyes, nicotine, or other products that are passed in the urine. The symptoms are similar to those of cystitis, and treatment is the same as that for other tumors.

Bladder Stones. These stones form in the bladder or enter the bladder from the kidney. Symptoms

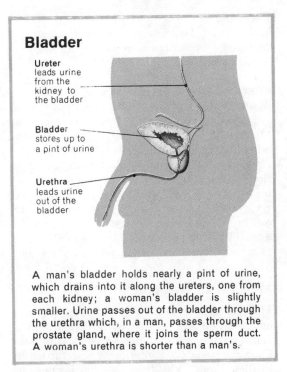

Bladder

Ureter leads urine from the kidney to the bladder

Bladder stores up to a pint of urine

Urethra leads urine out of the bladder

A man's bladder holds nearly a pint of urine, which drains into it along the ureters, one from each kidney; a woman's bladder is slightly smaller. Urine passes out of the bladder through the urethra which, in a man, passes through the prostate gland, where it joins the sperm duct. A woman's urethra is shorter than a man's.

of bladder stones are generally similar to those of bladder tumors, but if the urinary canal is blocked by a stone, the pain is intense. A stone can be removed through a cystoscope or crushed internally so that the pieces are passed in the urine. Sometimes the formation of additional stones can be prevented by means of diet or medication.

Prostate Troubles

The prostate gland, situated at the base of a man's bladder, causes problems for about half of all American men over the age of 50. The warning signs of prostate trouble are blood or pus in the urine, a weak or defective urinary flow, the frequent urge to urinate—often waking sufferers at night—along with difficulty in starting or stopping the flow, and painful urination.

Prostatis. This is an inflammation or congestion of the prostate gland that seems to occur when the gland is under- or over-active. The symptoms are similar to those mentioned above. A medical consultation is necessary.

Benign Prostatic Hypertrophy. This noncancerous enlargement of the prostate gland is common in middle-aged men. The symptoms are the same as those given above, and they occur because the gland, which enfolds the urethra, enlarges and squeezes the urethra shut. Treatment is by means of a variety of surgical operations, including reaming out or removing the gland in whole or in part.

Prostate Cancer. Prostate cancer is as mysterious as it is deadly; its cause is unknown, its symptoms not fully understood, and its treatment uncertain. Methods of treatment include surgery, therapy with female sex hormones, irradiation, and chemotherapy. Discovery of prostate cancer is possible through a simple examination—the doctor inserts a gloved finger into the rectum to feel the gland. Experts advise this examination annually for men over the age of 40—and semiannually for those over 50. (See also the entry PROSTATE GLAND in the encyclopedia section.)

MULTIPLE SCLEROSIS

Multiple sclerosis is a slowly progressive disease of the central nervous system. Hardened patches, called scleroses, form on the nerve sheaths of the brain and spinal cord, interfering with the nerves in these areas. Why these patches become inflamed and hardened and why they come and go is still unknown. The symptoms depend on the portion of the nervous system that is affected. Because the location, extent, and duration of the damage vary, it is difficult to describe a typical case of multiple sclerosis.

The most common symptoms are:

1. A tremor or shaking of the limbs, often weakening the victim and interfering with fine movements such as sewing or writing. Speech may become slow and toneless.

2. Unsteadiness in walking and inability to maintain balance.

3. Stiffness in walking, the knees failing to bend.

4. Difficulties with vision. The victim may see double or lose part of the visual field.

5. Paralysis, which may occur in any part of the body.

(See also the entry MULTIPLE SCLEROSIS in the encyclopedia section.)

CEREBRAL PALSY

Cerebral palsy is caused by damage to one or more of the three main areas of the brain. The damage usually occurs at or just prior to birth, and chiefly because of a lack of sufficient oxygen. Injuries or diseases can also cause the disorder. In only a small percentage of cases does the damage cause mental deficiency. Instead, it generally interferes with the nerves controlling the muscles. As a result, the victim of cerebral palsy may appear to be an imbecile—for example, by drooling, grunting, and making strange gestures even though his intelligence is normal.

There are three different types of victims:

1. The *spastic* moves stiffly and with difficulty because of impaired movement of the muscles. Such a person walks with a scissorslike gait.

2. The *athetoid* has involuntary, uncontrolled movements of the limbs and the head, which may be accompanied by bizarre grimaces.

3. The *ataxic* has poor coordination and a disturbed sense of balance and depth perception.

Indications of cerebral palsy can be detected when a baby is only a few months old. The infant should be examined at a medical center that specializes in the disease. It is important for parents to realize that it is not kindness to do everything for such a child; they must encourage him in the difficult task of doing things himself. Help may be obtained from such national organizations as the United Cerebral Palsy Associations and the American Academy for Cerebral Palsy and Developmental Medicine. (See CEREBRAL PALSY in the encyclopedia section.)

POLIOMYELITIS (INFANTILE PARALYSIS)

Polio, short for poliomyelitis, is a serious, crippling, occasionally fatal disease that usually claims the young. The introduction of polio vaccines and widespread immunization in the 1960's, however, has brought the disease under control. Polio is an infection of the central nervous system that attacks the cells of nerves that control the muscles. Most commonly, it affects the arms and legs. Less frequently, it paralyzes the muscles of breathing or swallowing. Actually, it can affect any muscle, but it does not affect the mind.

Most cases that are reported occur in young children, but polio attacks persons of all ages. Although it may strike at any time of the year, the highest incidence is in the summer. The best preventive is to make sure that you and your children are immunized with the Sabin oral polio vaccine. The first dose of the vaccine should be given to an infant at the age of six weeks; the second dose, four to six weeks later; and the third, in about a year. Do not put off polio immunization just because the disease has appeared less frequently in recent years. Many physicians fear a recurrence because people have grown careless about immunization.

Early symptoms of polio include fever, headache, vomiting, fretfulness, drowsiness, sore throat, change in bowel habits, and stiffness and pain in the back and neck. These signs do not necessarily mean polio, but do not ignore them. Many diseases of childhood start in this way, but they, too, can be serious, and it is best not to dismiss such symptoms as just a cold or upset stomach. Call your doctor promptly, for early treatment can prevent the disabling effects of polio and other diseases. (For a fuller discussion, see POLIOMYELITIS in the encyclopedia section.)

DISEASES OF THE MUSCLES

In poliomyelitis and other diseases that affect the nerves or the brain, the muscles are disabled because the nerves leading to them have been injured or destroyed. When these nerves no longer stimulate them, the muscles waste away (atrophy) from lack of use. In addition to the nerve type of muscle illness, there are diseases of the muscles themselves that can cause severe disabilities. Of these, the two most important are *muscular dystrophy* and *myasthenia gravis*.

Muscular Dystrophy

The term "muscular dystrophy" actually refers to a whole group of diseases that cause progressive degeneration of the body's voluntary muscles— such as those of the arms and legs. Muscular dystrophy is a particularly sad disabling disease because it strikes chiefly young children and teenagers. The muscles are weakened and gradually shrivel away. The childhood type usually manifests itself by the time the child reaches age six. The pseudohypertrophic type occurs much more frequently in boys than in girls. The disease affects important muscles, even those of the trunk of the body. As it progresses, it may incapacitate the person so completely that he cannot even stand or sit.

A less extensive form of muscular dystrophy that usually appears between the ages of 10 and 20 is apt to involve the muscles of the face and shoulders. Because of the particular muscles that the disease affects, it is referred to as the facio-scapulo-humeral type. Afflicted persons generally live out their years, and the fortunate ones have rather mild disability.

Although at the present time there is no really effective treatment for muscular dystrophy, physical therapy and orthopedic devices are helpful. Muscular dystrophy patients should be in touch regularly with a doctor, a clinic that treats the illness, or the Muscular Dystrophy Association, (810 Seventh Avenue, New York, New York 10019), to keep informed about developments in research and treatment. (See MUSCULAR DYSTROPHY in the encyclopedia section.)

Myasthenia Gravis

Myasthenia gravis is a chronic neuromuscular disease apparently caused by a defect in the transmission of nerve impulses to the voluntary muscles. As a result, the muscles do not function properly. It can start at any age but most commonly attacks women in their twenties and men past 40. Persons with this illness feel a general muscular weakness and are aware that certain muscles tire quickly with exertion. Muscles of the face, eyes, larynx, and throat are frequently affected. A victim may first detect the onset of the disease because his eyelids droop, or he may have trouble swallowing a drink of water, or he sees double.

There is no true paralysis of the muscles, and they do not usually shrivel away. But in severe forms the disease can be disabling or even fatal because it may involve the vital muscles of swallowing or breathing. Fortunately, there are both medical and surgical treatments that are helpful to a large number of victims.

Other Muscle Diseases

A less common muscular condition is familial periodic paralysis, in which the muscles undergo temporary, intermittent paralysis. It has been found that this is a disease associated with a low content of the vital chemical potassium in the blood serum. Administration of potassium will alleviate or prevent the attacks.

Myotonia dystrophica is a familial muscle disease that causes weakness and wasting of the muscles. Cataracts of the eyes may accompany this illness. Another muscle disabler that tends to run in families is peroneal muscular atrophy, also called Charcot-Marie-Tooth disease. It can spread slowly to other areas from the leg muscles where it starts. Sometimes there are associated nerve disturbances in the spinal cord.

EPILEPSY

The word "epilepsy" means "seizure." Epileptics often suffer from a loss of consciousness, momentary or prolonged, and involuntary, convulsive movements. An epileptic seizure, or fit, is the result of a temporary disturbance of the brain impulses. No one knows exactly why epilepsy occurs, although it can be caused by brain damage or defects, poor nutrition, infectious diseases, and other factors.

Minor seizures, called *petit mal*, last only five to 20 seconds, and the loss of consciousness is momentary. Although the victim suffers a twitching about the eyes or mouth, his posture does not change and he appears to have had no more than a moment of absentmindedness.

In major seizures, or *grand mal*, the victim falls to the floor unconscious for a moment or more, often foaming at the mouth, biting, and shaking his limbs violently. Involuntary bowel movements or the passage of urine may occur. The person may hurt himself during such a seizure. Fortunately, people with epilepsy frequently experience a warning, called the aura, before a major attack occurs, and this enables them to lie down and avoid falls.

Ordinary epilepsy is also called genuine epilepsy or idiopathic epilepsy, which means the cause is unknown. This is the most common type, and it is what most people have in mind when they speak of epilepsy. It usually begins early in life and is not directly inherited, although a predisposition to it may run in families.

Some 80 percent of epilepsy cases can be fully or partially controlled with proper medication. Individuals with epilepsy can hold responsible positions and lead practically normal, restriction-free lives.

PARKINSONISM

Parkinsonism, or Parkinson's disease, affects the brain. It is characterized by stiffness of muscles and tremors of the body. At first the person may be troubled by mild tremors of the hands and nodding of the head. Then his face seems not to have its usual mobility—for instance, the capacity to smile may have disappeared. This is called the masklike face of parkinsonism. As the disease advances, the shaking tremors of the muscles progress and may involve the entire body. The back tends to become bent forward. Yet the mind is unaffected.

In recent years new surgical techniques and a new drug, levodopa, have helped to relieve the symptoms of parkinsonism. If a victim is fortunate enough to have a job that requires chiefly mental effort, he can frequently continue working for many years. (See also the entry PARKINSONISM in the encyclopedia section.)

ALCOHOLISM

Alcoholism is one of the greatest disabling diseases. It is hard to draw a line between drinking in moderation, drinking to excess, and habitual drinking, or chronic alcoholism. (For information on these forms of drinking and the effect that alcohol has on the body, see Chapter 1.) Alcohol is a depressant, not a stimulant. The habitual drinker craves alcohol, is dependent on it, and drinks regularly and excessively. As a result, alcohol seriously interferes with his or her work, home life, and normal relationships with other people. All accepted patterns of behavior are ruthlessly sacrificed to satisfy the addiction.

Recent medical research indicates a physical basis for the real causes of alcoholism, which is now regarded by experts as more an illness than a form of antisocial behavior. Group therapy, especially by the national organization Alcoholics Anonymous, has proved enormously successful in rehabilitating alcoholics. (See also the following entries in the encyclopedia section: ALCOHOLISM; CIRRHOSIS; DELIRIUM TREMENS; DEMENTIA; HANGOVER.)

HYPOTENSION (LOW BLOOD PRESSURE)

Low blood pressure seldom causes true illness. Diseases in which chronic low blood pressure occurs are rare. Yet many people consider themselves disabled because their blood pressure is low, and arrange their lives accordingly. Their worry is baseless.

Although the average blood pressure of young men is about 120, a certain number will have systolic arterial pressures below 100. In most cases, they are perfectly healthy people who just happen to have low blood pressure. In fact, they are apt to live longer than most people with normal blood pressure.

Cases of low blood pressure with symptoms such as dizziness or faintness are very rare. In other rare instances, low blood pressure may be associated with definite diseases such as Addison's disease and inadequate thyroid function. (See also the entry ADDISON'S DISEASE in the encyclopedia section.)

INFLUENZA

Because influenza, usually called the flu, often resembles a common cold, many people fail to take it seriously. This is a grave mistake, because it may go hand in hand with the killer disease pneumonia. Influenza is caused by a virus. Its symptoms include fever, sore throat, cough, runny nose, a feeling of malaise, chills, sweats, and aches, especially in the head, back, and legs. Like a cold, it is spread from one person to another, most often through coughing or sneezing. It is so contagious that health authorities are seldom able to prevent it from becoming an epidemic, but fortunately, a flu epidemic usually lasts no longer than a month or so.

Prevention

The following precautions will help you avoid catching influenza:

1. Get plenty of rest and avoid becoming overtired or chilled.

2. Avoid crowds and unnecessary contact with people who may have the flu. It is highly contagious during the early stages. Regard every cold as potential influenza.

3. If someone in your house has the flu, keep him isolated from other members of the family. His dishes, towels, and similar items should be kept and washed separately, and rinsed in scalding water.

Do not count on being immune from the flu because you have recovered from an attack. It is true that temporary immunity does follow the flu, but there are a number of different strains of the virus, and having had one kind does not protect you from another. Vaccines give protection for some months, but only against certain influenza viruses.

Treatment

The best way to get well quickly and avoid dangerous or disabling complications is to give yourself all the possible odds in fighting the flu virus. When there is influenza about, go to bed if you have symptoms of a cold or the flu, or even if you just do not feel well. Do not overtreat yourself with nose drops, sprays, or antihistamines. If you have aches and pains or fever, call the doctor immediately. He will prescribe the medication you need. (See also the entry INFLUENZA in the encyclopedia section.)

THE ANEMIAS

Anemia (from the Greek word meaning "without blood") indicates that the number of red blood cells is below normal. These vital cells contain the pigment hemoglobin, which carries oxygen from the lungs to the body tissues. In anemia the hemoglobin is reduced, too. (See the entries ANEMIA; BLOOD; BLOOD COUNT in the encyclopedia section.)

You can recognize more serious cases of anemia by the pallor of the palms of the hands, the fingernails, and the inner parts of the eyelids (the conjunctivas). Mild degrees of anemia are not detectable visually, but your doctor has, or has access to, instruments for testing the blood for anemia.

Symptoms

Mild anemia may be indicated at first by a lack of energy, and by a tendency to fatigue. More severe anemia causes shortness of breath during exertion. This may be accompanied by pounding of the heart (palpitation), and a rapid pulse and heart action (tachycardia). In addition, there may be severe headaches, loss of appetite, dizziness, ringing in the ears, and even fainting spells. In advanced cases of anemia, swelling of the ankles may occur.

Causes

There are many causes of anemia. The most important are described below, and brief mention is made of most of the others.

1. *Sudden loss of blood:* If there is a massive hemorrhage from a wound, the body may lose enough blood to cause severe anemia and, frequently, shock. Immediate transfusions are generally required to replace the blood that has been lost.

2. *Chronic blood loss:* The slow leakage of blood from an ulcer of the stomach may create a severe anemia. It may also result from the loss of blood brought about by hemorrhoids. Excessive menstrual flow may act in the same way. A cancer of the stomach or intestine may cause sufficient bleeding to produce anemia.

These anemias will usually clear up if the cause can be found. Because iron is necessary to build hemoglobin, medicines and foods containing iron are helpful in these cases. In addition to iron, hemoglobin production requires protein, vitamin B_{12}, and other minerals and vitamins; therefore the diet for this type of anemia should be rich in these elements. (For more information on diet, see Chapter 2.)

3. *Deficient diet:* Diets deficient in iron, protein, vitamins, and minerals such as copper and cobalt can cause anemia. The production of hemoglobin and the formation of red blood cells will also be impaired by these deficiencies.

Pernicious Anemia

Pernicious anemia produces all the usual symptoms in the victim, plus a pale yellow skin, sore and reddened tongue, and difficulty in swallowing. Changes in the nerves and spinal cord frequently cause the sensation of "pins and needles" in the fingers and toes. The victim's gait may be unsteady.

In treatment of pernicious anemia, injections of vitamin B_{12} result in dramatic improvement. The blood becomes normal again; pallor, weakness, and shortness of breath disappear. Symptoms attributable to the nerves and spinal cord are generally improved, too. However, these medicines cannot cure pernicious anemia—they merely replace some substance the body lacks to make normal red blood cells. Therefore, treatment must be continued regularly and throughout life in order to control the anemia and its symptoms.

Hemolytic Anemias

Anemias caused by the destruction of red blood cells are known as hemolytic anemias. Some are congenital in type, others are acquired; some are chronic, others acute. They differ from other anemias, too, in that jaundice may be present, because the destroyed red cells release hemoglobin that is converted into the jaundice pigments.

Sickle-Cell Anemia. This is a serious, inherited form of anemia that appears almost entirely in the black population. The malady is so named because of the shape of the diseased red blood cells. Few victims live beyond the age of 40 because of infection and blood clots in vital organs. There is no cure for sickle-cell anemia. Treatment is chiefly an attempt to relieve the ill effects of the disorder by means of highly skilled and specialized medical care.

Cooley's Anemia. This is another inherited hemoglobin defect, with many of the same effects as sickle-cell anemia. It is also called thalassemia, or Mediterranean anemia, because it is found in people living in Mediterranean lands or in their descendants who have migrated to other countries. Cooley's anemia may be a fatal disease in some young children. In others, it is compatible with a long adult life.

Aplastic Anemias

Because the red blood cells are manufactured chiefly in the red marrow of the bones, any disease and a chemical or radioactive substance that invades, destroys, or depresses the activity of the bone marrow can cause anemia. Known as aplastic anemia, this bone-marrow illness damages the blood platelets and the white cells. There will usually be other symptoms besides those of anemia, such as bleeding from the nose and mouth, and black-and-blue spots on the skin. Infections and fever may accompany the debilitation following aplastic anemia. It is a serious condition and should be treated in a hospital.

Other Anemias

Anemias often arise in the course of other diseases. In chronic kidney disease, there is usually a severe and persistent anemia. In hypothyroidism, or myxedema, anemia may be persistent until thyroid medication is given. Intestinal parasites cause various kinds of anemia. And sprue, a chronic disease of the small intestines, may be accompanied by anemia. (See the entry SPRUE in the encyclopedia section.)

IRRITABLE COLON AND ULCERATIVE COLITIS

Ulcerative colitis is sometimes confused with a milder, troublesome functional disease called either irritable colon, functional bowel distress, colitis, or mucous colitis. The terms "colitis" and "mucous colitis" are misleading; therefore the expression "irritable colon" is used here to describe the milder forms of functional illness of the large intestine.

Irritable Colon

Irritable colon is distinct and different from ulcerative colitis. It is a functional disorder in that nothing is wrong with the large bowel, or colon, except the way it acts. No organic disease can be found, and the lining of the rectum and colon appears normal. X rays, however, may reveal minor disturbances of movement—for example, spasm. People who have irritable colon almost never get ulcerative colitis. Because these diseases are quite different, it is particularly important to follow the advice of your doctor.

Ulcerative Colitis

Ulcerative colitis is a serious disease that can be disabling. Its cause is still unknown. The initial attack of ulcers in the colon can be so severe that the resulting hemorrhage, intestinal perforation, debility, and toxemia may cause death. Usually, however, the disease appears as recurrent attacks of bloody diarrhea, with symptomless periods between. The victim may become a partial or total invalid who suffers from nutritional disturbances, loss of weight, extreme weakness, and numerous other complications.

Careful medical examination and tests are required to diagnose the condition. These include X rays of the large intestine after it is filled with barium, a compound that is employed as an enema in the form of a milky white liquid. The rectum is also examined with a proctoscope or sigmoidoscope through which the lining of the bowel can be seen. Marked redness and sometimes actual ulcers, or sores, are observed.

Prompt medical treatment can prevent the disabling effects of ulcerative colitis, which otherwise may make the life of its victim miserable. The cornerstones of the treatment are bed rest and a bland, low-residue diet without fruits and vegetables, but with plenty of vitamins, minerals, and other essential nutritional requirements. Medicines, including ACTH and cortisone, are helpful in treating certain cases. In many instances, this is sufficient to cure the disease. Some victims of ulcerative colitis, however, may be unable to relax and rest properly because of nervous tension; in such cases psychiatric help may be extremely valuable. (See also the entry COLITIS in the encyclopedia section.)

HERNIAS

"Hernia" is the medical term for a rupture or tear, although nothing is actually torn by a hernia. What usually happens is that a weak spot develops in the bands of muscle tissue in the abdominal wall, and the intestines begin to bulge through to form a soft lump. When the victim lies down, the intestines slide back to their proper place, and the bulge usually disappears entirely, especially if the hernia is of fairly recent origin.

Types of Hernias

The most common type is the inguinal hernia, which occurs in the groins of males. The weakest spot in the male's abdominal wall is located in the groin, where the cord leading to the testicles passes. Unfortunately, in some male infants the wall fails to shut tightly around the cord at this spot, leaving it especially weak. In later years a strain—such as lifting a heavy object—may cause the wall to give way suddenly, or constant straining may force it out gradually. At first, the intestinal bulge may be hardly noticeable, and there

may be little pain. As time passes, the bulge may become as large as, or larger than, a hen's egg. Hernias may extend downward into the scrotum.

Hernias in women are most frequently located on the upper thigh, just below the groin, and are called femoral hernias. In umbilical hernia, the navel protrudes. This type is most common in new babies and is unusual in adults. Among other types of hernias are those that follow operations in which the scar does not heal properly, permitting bulging to occur. Hernias may be aggravated by coughing, sneezing, or, especially in constipated individuals, straining to effect bowel movements.

Anyone with a hernia should see a doctor without delay because strangulation may develop. When this happens, a loop of intestine becomes caught in the bulge, and its blood supply is cut off. This results in gangrene of the strangulated loop of bowel, a condition that is as serious as a ruptured appendix and can cause death. If you have an untreated hernia that suddenly becomes painful, see a doctor at once.

Treatment

The best treatment for hernia is a minor, safe operation to repair the weakness in the muscles responsible for it. No one with a hernia should avoid or delay the operation if it has been recommended. With the modern advances in surgery, there is no reason to use a truss or other support except in unusual circumstances. Trusses are inconvenient, frequently uncomfortable, and may add to the injury by enlarging the weak spot. (See also the entry HERNIA in the encyclopedia section.)

MONONUCLEOSIS

Mononucleosis, also called infectious mononucleosis and glandular fever, can cause a surprisingly prolonged degree of disability for what may seem to be a mild illness. Because it can temporarily damage the liver, medical care and adequate bed rest are essential in order to prevent permanent damage to this vital organ. The disease appears to be caused by a virus, which is spread primarily by oral contact—thus the popular name, "the kissing sickness," for mononucleosis. About three-fourths of its victims are students, soldiers, nurses, and other young people between the ages of 15 and 30 who live in groups. The symptoms are fever, sore throat, swelling of the glands of the neck, and weakness and fatigue. There may be skin rashes. Jaundice will occur if the liver has been sufficiently involved. A special blood test can make the diagnosis more definite. Usually the disease clears up in a few weeks, but it may leave the victim weak and easily tired for months thereafter. (See also the entries JAUNDICE; MONONUCLEOSIS in the encyclopedia section.)

VENEREAL DISEASES

Venereal disease is no longer the fearful killer it once was, thanks to modern treatment with antibiotics, but it is still widely prevalent. Gonorrhea and syphilis are disabling diseases for which there are prompt and sure cures—if they are detected and treated immediately. Herpes simplex of the genitals is a common venereal disease for which a cure has not yet been found. In recent years scientists have tended to discard the term "venereal disease" and to use instead the expression "sexually transmitted disease" to define infections that are spread not only by sexual intercourse but also by other sexual practices.

Gonorrhea

An infection caused by the germ *Neisseria gonorrhoeae*, or gonococcus, gonorrhea attacks the sex organs of men and women. It is almost always contracted by sexual contact—rarely by kissing or handling contaminated objects. Sometimes infections of the eyes may be contracted in other ways.

The first symptoms of gonorrhea usually appear from five to seven days after sexual exposure. In men, there is a whitish discharge from the penis and/or a burning sensation upon urination. Women may develop pain in the lower abdomen with or without a period of burning urination and/or a whitish vaginal discharge. Never disregard any symptoms of gonorrhea.

While it is now possible to cure gonorrhea with injections of penicillin, prevention is still the best and safest method of coping with it. Briefly, this includes avoiding intercourse with an infected person; using a rubber condom during sexual intercourse; and giving the genital area a thorough washing after coitus. (See also the entries GONORRHEA; VENEREAL DISEASE in the encyclopedia section.)

Syphilis

Syphilis results from infection by a pale, corkscrew-shaped germ, a spirochete called *Treponema pallidum*. It is a rather delicate microorganism that thrives in the moist mucous membranes of the genital tract, mouth, or rectum. Syphilis is transmitted chiefly through sexual contact. In very rare cases, it has been contracted by drinking from a glass previously used by a syphilitic person.

Any sore on or near the sexual organs should be examined and tested by a physician immediately. If it is not a hard chancre of the primary stage of syphilis, a great deal of needless worry will be avoided. If it is syphilis, treatment can be started at once with assurance of a prompt cure.

If undetected and untreated with antibiotics, syphilis may continue for many years before there is obvious harm to the body. Syphilis may eventually cause blindness or severe disease of the bones and joints, skin, or internal organs, because the unchecked spirochetes can invade every cell of the body. The forms of syphilis most often resulting in death are those that damage the nervous system and the heart. An infected woman can pass the disease on to her unborn child, but this congenital syphilis in an infant can be prevented by treating the pregnant woman. (See also the entry SYPHILIS in the encyclopedia section.)

Herpes Simplex of the Genitals

Another common venereal disease in the United States is a type of herpes simplex that is usually spread by sexual contact. The disease has proliferated rapidly in recent years; in the mid-1970's it was estimated that 300,000 new cases occur annually, chiefly among young people. A genital infection, it is caused in 90 percent of the cases by herpes simplex virus type 2 (HSV-2); about 10 percent of the cases are caused by herpes simplex virus type 1.

A symptom of genital herpes is the appearance of painful, fluid-filled blisters on the genital organs; in women the infection often appears within the vagina or on the cervix. Victims sometimes suffer blistering of the thighs and buttocks, fever, enlarged lymph nodes, and a general feeling of malaise. Although the blisters dry up, crust over, and disappear within a few weeks even without treatment, the infection may recur within months or even years.

Herpes simplex is the first venereal disease to be identified as a possible cause of cancer in women. Research has indicated that a woman with HSV-2 is more likely to develop cancer of the cervix than a woman who has not been infected. In the case of a pregnant woman who is infected with genital herpes at the time of delivery, it is possible that her child will be affected and perhaps seriously damaged. Her baby might be protected if the delivery is done by cesarean section.

There is no established treatment for genital herpes. Like all viruses, HSV-2 is unaffected by antibiotics. Several types of anti-herpes drugs and vaccines are being developed.

BRUCELLOSIS (UNDULANT FEVER)

There are several forms of undulant fever, a worldwide infectious disease that is known by various names. The word "undulant" indicates that the fever comes in waves or undulations instead of being constant. Recently, all forms of the disease have been given the name "brucellosis," because they are all caused by infections of the germ family Brucellaceae (named for Dr. David Bruce, the English bacteriologist who discovered it in 1887).

The symptoms of brucellosis usually come on slowly and are rather indefinite, consisting of irregular fever, chills, sweating, and aches and pains in the joints and muscles. It is rare for a person to recover after only one attack. As a rule, another attack follows after an interval, and this may be repeated almost indefinitely.

Brucellosis is rarely carried from one person to another, but it is constantly carried from animal to animal, and from animal to human. The animals that harbor the germ are chiefly domesticated goats, cattle, and hogs. It is possible to acquire brucellosis from contact with diseased animals or their carcasses. Farmers, veterinarians, slaughterhouse employees, and butchers are exposed to the infection, as are housewives who handle infected meat in the kitchen.

The best way to prevent brucellosis is to eradicate the disease in animals. The danger of brucellosis is a powerful argument for universal pasteurization of public milk supplies. Infection by contact with diseased animals or their carcasses is less easy to prevent and is essentially a matter of industrial hygiene. Persons exposed to brucellosis in their jobs should be fully informed of the dangers and should take precautions against unnecessary exposure. Treatment is by antibiotics alone or in combination with sulfonamides. They are more effective in the early, acute stages than in the chronic form of the disease.

LEPROSY

Leprosy is one of the least contagious of the infectious diseases. Usually, it is not a particularly severe disease, but it is a disabler. Most people have a natural immunity to leprosy, and the disease is rare in the United States. The psychological disability it causes can be as serious as the physical, affecting not only the sick person and those in contact with him, but others who only imagine they have been exposed.

Leprosy is caused by Hansen's bacillus (*Mycobacterium leprae*), which generally attacks the skin and nerves. It does not affect the brain. It is not inherited. There are several types of leprosy, one of which often arrests itself even without treatment.

The most common symptoms include the typical leprosy patches on the skin, small nodules on the face and legs, and a loss of feeling in limited areas of the body, such as the fingers. The disease develops slowly and is difficult to recognize. Doctors use specific tests to diagnose leprosy, which can then be inactivated by a variety of drugs. (See also the entry LEPROSY in the encyclopedia section.)

TROPICAL DISEASES

Millions of people, especially in the tropical countries of Africa, Asia, and South America, are completely or partly disabled each year by the so-called tropical diseases. These include cholera, typhus, yellow fever, and sleeping sickness, but malaria is the most important. Tropical diseases can be prevented by vaccinations, medicines, and the vigilance of health officers. If you visit a tropical country, be sure to ask your doctor about its health hazards and follow his instructions. Remember also that maids and other domestic workers coming from tropical countries may bring diseases with them—a good reason for having a medical checkup of anyone working in your home. (For information about protection against these diseases, see the entry TROPICAL DISEASE in the encyclopedia section.)

Malaria

Malaria is still one of the most prevalent diseases in the world, especially in Africa, Asia, and South America. It has been practically eliminated from North America, but some U.S. military personnel and civilians who have lived in tropical regions may have contracted the disease, which can recur long after they return home. Malaria does not kill very frequently, but it is disabling because of its high fever, severe chills, and long duration. The disease is caused by a parasite in the red blood corpuscles; it is carried from a person with malaria by the female anopheles mosquito. The mosquito, after biting an infected person, transmits his blood to a healthy human being on whom it subsequently feeds. About two weeks later, that person will develop characteristic symptoms: chills, shaking, and a high fever. The fever subsides in several hours, leaving the sick person drenched in sweat, exhausted, and very sleepy. The types of malaria are named according to the interval between the fevers—for example, tertian, every third day; quatran, every fourth day.

If the disease is not treated, the chills and fever may continue for months before the body overcomes the acute stages. Even then, malarial symptoms can recur if the person's resistance is lowered by strenuous activity, alcoholic excesses, or exposure to cold. Persons chronically ill with malaria suffer from anemia, headaches, muscle pains, and general poor health.

A doctor diagnoses the illness by examining a drop of blood under the microscope. Malarial parasites are generally abundant and easily recognized. Treatment with drugs such as chloroquine have proved effective. (See also the entry MALARIA in the encyclopedia section.)

AMEBIASIS

Formerly regarded as a tropical disease, amebiasis is caused by a parasite that invades the intestines. A considerable number of cases of even the severe form, amebic dysentery, are found in temperate climates, and it is widespread in its mild form. About one of every 20 Americans may harbor the parasitic ameba in the intestines.

Infection from this organism can be prevented by taking proper sanitary precautions with food and water in areas where public sanitation is poor. The disease can also be passed on by someone who handles food, and who may not know that he is harboring the invisible cysts of this parasite. This can happen because individuals with the mild variety may experience only minor symptoms such as headache, fatigue, occasional nausea, flatulence, and bowel irregularity.

It is most important not to neglect any symptoms of amebiasis. You are apt to give the disease to someone, perhaps a child, who may develop it in its severe form. In addition, mild cases may develop into amebic dysentery, with abdominal pain and diarrhea, often accompanied by blood-streaked stools and, in severe cases, chills and fever. Severe amebic dysentery can cause death. There is also the risk that the parasite may travel to the liver and produce an abscess, which can be fatal.

Amebiasis is usually treated successfully. Medicines have been developed for all types of the disease. Even people who have had chronic, resistant cases should not be discouraged, but should again consult their doctors, as they can probably benefit from new treatments. (For further information on amebic dysentery, see the entry DYSENTERY in the encyclopedia section.)

SARCOIDOSIS (BOECK'S SARCOID)

Sarcoidosis is a long illness that can be considerably disabling at times, but fortunately is often a mild disease. It is more prevalent in dark-skinned races than in white. In North America, more cases are found in the southeastern rural areas of the United States than elsewhere.

In this disease, little fleshy lumps invade the tissues. Most frequently the lungs, skin, and lymph nodes are affected. However, it has been known to occur in almost every part of the body, including the eyes, liver, and bones. Because the disease produces lung lesions similar to those of tuberculosis, it has been confused with that illness. Unlike tuberculosis, however, sarcoidosis is not communicable. The sick person may live with his family.

Few if any symptoms appear in mild cases of sarcoidosis. In more severe forms, there may be fever, loss of weight, coughing, and other distressing symptoms. It is possible to relieve these symptoms by the use of cortisone and ACTH.

(For information about diseases of the eye and ear, see Chapter 3; see also the entries DEAFNESS; EARACHE; EYE INFECTIONS; GLAUCOMA; MÉNIÈRE'S DISEASE in the encyclopedia section.)

CHAPTER 24   The Nuisance Ailments

The so-called minor illnesses rarely disable people or result in death, but they do cause pain and emotional upset—most of it unnecessary, because the illnesses can usually be cured or alleviated by proper medical care. Too many people seem to feel that nuisance ailments such as headache, constipation, hemorrhoids, and varicose veins are not worth the bother of seeking treatment, but doctors are interested in relieving these troublesome aches and pains, because they may interfere with your sleep, appetite, and general good health.

This chapter discusses some of the most common of the nuisance ailments. Others are dealt with in earlier chapters—for example, "Taking Care of Your Teeth and Gums" (Chapter 4), "Special Health Problems of Women" (Chapter 19), "Retirement and the Later Years" (Chapter 20).

ACHES, PAINS, AND NUISANCES

Everyone is troubled at times by aches and pains that, although not serious, are certainly bothersome. Many of the nuisance ailments—such as the common cold—are diseases caused by germs, but others—such as indigestion—are not diseases themselves but may be symptoms of disease. Still other everyday aches and pains are caused by the condition of our teeth and gums, skin, hair, or even the posture of our bodies. And women sometimes suffer pain and discomfort from such natural bodily functions as menstruation, pregnancy, and menopause.

Keep in mind that what starts out to be little more than a nuisance ailment can frequently end up a serious problem if it is not treated early. Never assume that a continuing nuisance ache or pain can be ignored unless you first receive competent medical diagnosis.

The common nuisance ailments discussed in this chapter are listed below.

Headaches
Insomnia
Common cold
Postnasal drip
Sinusitis

Smoker's cough
Allergies
Constipation
Hemorrhoids and other
  rectal troubles

Psoriasis
Varicose veins
Motion sickness
Leg cramps

Earache
Low back pain
Ingrown toenails

HEADACHES

Tension Headaches

About 70 percent of all headaches are tension headaches, so called because they result from excess tension of the neck and shoulder muscles. This type of headache is often easy enough to diagnose: the muscles at the back of the neck are exceptionally rigid. Anything that causes a person involuntarily to tighten the muscles of his neck can produce the headache. Long hours of uninterrupted driving can do it, as can intense concentration—such as viewing a suspenseful film or reading an engrossing book.

Usually, of course, it is the emotional stress of our daily lives that causes us to become tense. Sometimes a gentle massage of the muscles helps to relieve the tension, as do moist, warm compresses. Aspirin relieves some of the pain, but usually not all. Muscle-stretching exercises such as those practiced in yoga can often bring at least temporary relief, but such exercises must be done gently to prevent damaging a muscle.

The ideal solution is to eliminate the problem causing the tension in the first place. Because the source is usually emotional, it may mean seeking psychiatric help.

Migraine Headaches

Migraine attacks plague more than 4 million people. They are profoundly unpleasant experiences, often starting with visual disturbances—a flickering before the eyes, flashes of light, or blind spots in the field of vision. The pain is localized to either the right or left part of the head—almost never both. Often nausea and vomiting accompany the severe head pain.

Today the migraine sufferer has potent drugs on which he can rely for prevention of or relief from attacks. These include ergotamine tartrate, alone or combined with caffeine or phenobarbital. If taken early enough, they can prevent an attack; if not, they can relieve one within an hour. Physicians sometimes prescribe methysergide maleate to reduce the frequency of attacks. It is effective, but some patients react violently to it, so that a doctor's close supervision is essential.

Many doctors find that the migraine patient also requires some form of psychotherapy to modify the tense personality that is predisposed to migraine attacks.

Common Headaches

About one in four headaches is neither migraine nor caused by tension. A great variety of factors are responsible. For example, some women develop headaches a few days before menstruation. The headache appears as regularly as the electric bill each month.

Other people find that if they drink too much alcohol they develop a headache, which is frequently an allergic response to the drug. Also, long hours of driving often produce tense muscles and the resulting headache. But headaches may develop for another reason on long drives: Carbon monoxide may seep into the car, replacing some of the oxygen, and a prolonged minor deficiency of oxygen can induce a headache. Blocked sinuses can also be responsible for excruciatingly painful headaches.

Usually headaches, though uncomfortable, pose no serious threat to health. On occasion, however, they go beyond the aches, pains, and nuisances category and require immediate medical attention. It's essential to seek help when the headache:

1. Follows a fall or blow to the head.

2. Is accompanied by a fever, along with nausea, vomiting, and blurred vision.

3. Occurs with steadily increasing frequency and severity.

INSOMNIA

Just about everyone has difficulty falling asleep now and then. Sometimes the enthusiasm of planning a vacation or building a new home will be responsible—daydreams far too fascinating to be abandoned for something as mundane as sleep. Such causes are easy to recognize. But some people, chronic insomniacs, lie awake tossing and turning for hours night after night with no idea why sleep eludes them. As a result, they grow sluggish and fretful. If you are one of these individuals, the following questions may help you to help yourself:

How much sleep do you need? Some people, particularly those who find the routine of their lives boring, try to sleep more than necessary. While it is true that many people need eight hours of sleep, some people require as little as five or six hours, and a great many require no more than seven. If you need no more than five to seven hours, but insist on going to bed at 10 p.m. and awakening at 7 a.m., you will understandably have at least two hours of wakefulness. Probably, you will be awake even longer than that, for you will make yourself tense by trying to force yourself to sleep. (For further discussion of sleep, see Chapter 1 and the entry SLEEP in the encyclopedia section.)

Are you too tired to sleep? It is hard to relax if you are, and relaxation must precede sleep. Try not to overdo things during the day. Even more important, slow down as evening approaches.

Is there a physical cause for your inability to sleep? Poor sleeping conditions, such as noise, light, or someone moving around, may make it impossible to sleep well.

Do you drink too much coffee, tea, or cola? Caffeine in these beverages keeps some people awake. Do you eat heavy meals before bedtime and toss around because of gas and "indigestion," or drink fluids that make your bladder feel distended? Have you any illness or nuisance ailment causing pains or discomfort?

Is there any emotional cause for your insomnia? Problems, worries, and fears—real or imaginary—will make you tense, whether you are conscious of them or not. They may also cause nightmares that make you resist the idea of going to sleep.

Methods of Getting to Sleep

1. Do not be afraid of staying awake. Many people can simply relax or doze and be perfectly rested the next day. Most persons suffering from insomnia actually sleep more than they think they do.

2. Make the two hours before you go to bed peaceful ones.

3. Go to bed half an hour to an hour sooner than you expect to go to sleep. Read something soothing until you feel drowsy. Then turn off the light.

4. Relax physically. Try to let your muscles "go." Some people take warm baths because heat helps muscles to relax; others drink warm milk or eat a light snack to induce relaxation. Another good way to encourage release of muscle tension is exercise—not immediately before retiring, but a few hours before.

5. Relax mentally. Try to find something soothing to think about when you start courting sleep.

6. If you do not go to sleep, and lying quietly disturbs rather than relaxes you, begin again by reading for a while or listening to soothing radio music.

7. If sexual tension is a major factor in your insomnia, read Chapter 11.

8. Sometimes you can trick your mind into seeking sleep as an escape. If you cannot sleep, you might force yourself out of bed and begin doing something you simply hate to do: read an utterly boring book, shampoo the rug, trim the poodle. Soon enough you will find yourself falling asleep against your will—as an escape.

If none of this helps after a few days of experimenting, it is time to see your doctor.

THE COMMON COLD

More accurately referred to as an upper respiratory infection, the common cold is the most frequent of all medical maladies. At this moment, an estimated one in every eight people throughout the country has a cold. It will last from four to seven days, unless complications set in. Colds often lead to middle-ear infections, laryngitis, bronchitis, and sometimes even pneumonia.

Recent findings by medical researchers have put to rest some myths concerning the common cold. For example, there is no benefit in "starving" a cold. In fact, to fight the microbes causing the infection, the body needs its full complement of essential nutrients. Another myth is that sneezing and coughing are the primary means by which most colds are spread. In fact, although colds are highly contagious, the beads of moisture in which germs are expelled during coughing and sneezing usually fall to the ground unless they are immediately inhaled by other persons. Studies have found a much higher number of infection-causing microbes on the hands of people suffering from colds than in the air into which they have been coughing or sneezing.

A third myth is that penicillin and other antibiotics can cure, or at least relieve, the symptoms of a cold. In fact, they are completely ineffective; a cold is not caused by bacteria which antibiotics destroy, but by viruses. Only when cells damaged by viruses become infected by bacteria, can the antibiotics help cure the secondary infection.

Nor can antihistamines bring relief from a true upper respiratory infection. Often, what is mistaken for a cold is actually an allergy, and the symptoms can be relieved by antihistamines. These drugs have several side effects of which the public is generally unaware, though, and should be taken only upon a doctor's advice.

Preventing Colds

Colds are a special problem in children, not only because of the potential complications, but also because many childhood diseases start with the symptoms of a cold. (For a discussion of colds in infants and children, see Chapter 16.)

Colds *can* be prevented—but the responsibility rests heavily on the person who already has a cold to keep others from contracting it. People who have a cold virus in its active form spread it to others. It can be transmitted by close contact, by handling contaminated objects such as handkerchiefs, and by using contaminated drinking glasses or utensils. People who are clustered together in crowds can easily inhale cold germs from those carrying them.

It has long been the consensus among physicians that vitamins could not prevent a cold. But in recent years many responsible and respected researchers and physicians have contended that high doses of vitamin C may prevent common colds or at least reduce their severity. There is still no proof one way or the other. Advocates of vitamin C recommend very high doses at the very first sign of a cold—from 1,000 to 8,000 milligrams a day, divided into doses taken every three hours.

Chilling lowers the body's resistance to colds. This varies a great deal in people, some of whom become chilled very easily. Put on warm, dry clothes as soon as you can after becoming wet or chilled.

Unfortunately, most people cannot afford to—or do not want to—call the doctor for an ordinary cold. However, *there are certain people who must see a physician* because even mild colds can represent a severe threat to their health, possibly to their lives. A pregnant woman should report a cold to her doctor. So should anyone with one of the following diseases:

Tuberculosis
Rheumatic fever or rheumatic heart disease
Chronic bronchitis or bronchiectasis
Bronchial asthma
Kidney disease, especially Bright's disease and chronic pyelonephritis
Severe liver disease
Severe diabetes
Heart disease severe enough to cause shortness of breath
Asthma
Severe sinusitis

What to Do for an Ordinary Cold

If you possibly can, go to bed as soon as you feel that you are coming down with a cold. Stay there, or at least keep warm and avoid chilling temperatures, until you are past the "runny" stage. Drink plenty of liquids and eat moderately. Be careful about blowing your nose so hard that you force infection into the sinuses and ears. If your nose is badly stopped up, ask your doctor to tell you what kind of nose drops to use. Plain aspirin (or buffered aspirin if ordinary aspirin upsets your stomach) brings the quickest and safest relief for general discomfort. Take one or two tablets every two to three hours, if necessary.

Protect the other members of your family: smother all coughs and sneezes in a handkerchief or tissue. Put all tissues into a paper bag after using them. The tissues can then be easily disposed of without contaminating anyone else.

See to it that no one handles the objects you have contaminated. If someone must, see that he handles them as little as possible and washes his hands immediately afterward. Your eating utensils, dishes, and so on, should be washed separately and rinsed in scalding water.

Be sure to see a doctor if:

1. You have a fever that lasts for more than two days or goes above 101°F.
2. You have a severe headache that does not respond to an aspirin.
3. You have chills, a severe cough, chest pains, or blood-stained or rusty-looking sputum.
4. Your back, neck, or bones ache.
5. You "ache all over."
6. You have an earache.
7. Your cold symptoms do not clear up. (You may have hay fever or some other allergy.)

POSTNASAL DRIP

The mucous membrane lining the nasal cavities normally secretes a watery substance that has a very important function: it traps dust, germs, and other foreign particles, and keeps them from entering the lungs where serious infections could develop. This fluid, along with mucus, then flows into the throat on its way to the stomach—this flow is called postnasal drip. Sometimes it becomes excessive, causing a sore throat or a gagging sensation. If you do not have these unpleasant symptoms, you need not worry about postnasal drip.

Excessive postnasal drip is much more common in cold weather than in warm. It can be avoided by taking the following precautions:

1. Avoid cold and dry air and cigarette smoke. Keep pans of water in the room, preferably on or near the heating units. Better yet, get a humidifier.
2. Stay indoors, if possible, on a cold, raw day; if you go out, wear warm clothing and do not get chilled.
3. Blow your nose gently to avoid irritation and the spread of germs.

SINUSITIS

Quite frequently the person suffering from a stuffy nose and headache will conclude, "My sinuses are acting up." Actually, true sinusitis is relatively rare, and the sufferer usually is experiencing an uncommonly bad common cold or an allergy. A case of genuine sinusitis is extremely painful, and could require surgery.

The normal human head has eight sinus cavities through which mucus drains into the nasal passages. Sinusitis occurs when the passages become blocked, causing the mucus to back up in the sinuses, creating pressure. Symptoms vary among the following:

1. Hoarseness and sore throat; a decrease in hearing ability.
2. Headache, minor to very severe; sensitivity around the cheek bones; stuffy nose.
3. In very serious cases, a high fever, restlessness, delirium; pus and blood flecks from the nose.

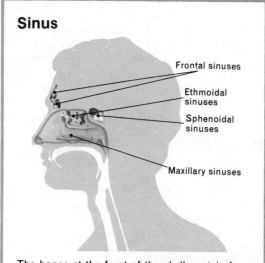

Sinus

Frontal sinuses

Ethmoidal sinuses

Sphenoidal sinuses

Maxillary sinuses

The bones at the front of the skull contain four sets of hollow cavities called the paranasal sinuses. If they become infected and inflamed, they cause the painful condition sinusitis. A minor operation to drain the cavities generally prevents repeated attacks.

Sinusitis is almost always the result of a viral or bacterial infection of the nose. It can be triggered by vigorous nose blowing, sneezing, or swimming and diving while one has an upper respiratory infection. A rapid change in barometric pressure such as occurs frequently in airplane flights can damage the membranes lining the sinuses and thus invite infection.

The sinusitis sufferer must seek medical help. Nose drops and sprays may make breathing easier temporarily, but in the long run they contribute to the problem through what doctors call "rebound engorgement": The sensitive sinus membranes react to the medication by swelling, thus increasing the blockage. Only a physician, preferably a specialist, will know what drugs to prescribe and for how long—or whether surgery is essential.

SMOKER'S COUGH

Many—perhaps most—smokers awaken in the morning to violent coughing. That is the result of an irritated throat and larynx, and there is no medication that can prevent it. The smoke from cigarettes is a very potent abrasive, and the damage cannot be avoided as long as the sufferer continues smoking.

If a sore throat accompanies the coughing, the pain can be relieved somewhat by gargling with a third of a glassful of water in which two aspirin tablets have been dissolved. Swallow a small amount of the thick suspension; aspirin is a mild local anesthetic and helps to soothe the irritated mucous membranes. If the solution gags you— and it may, especially in the morning when the victims are most in need of relief—try plain warm water as a gargle, or chewing gum followed by a soothing throat lozenge. Avoid breathing through the mouth.

The most sensible treatment, of course, is to stop smoking, or at least to cut down on it drastically. If that is not possible, switch to filter-tipped cigarettes, or a holder with a filter in it, to screen out at least some of the irritating substances in the smoke.

ALLERGIES

An allergy is an unusual or exaggerated reaction to a substance most people find harmless. Allergens—the substances causing the reaction—abound. Sensitive people may be affected by the food they eat, the air they breathe, their pets, their clothing, the climate, sunlight, moisture—the list is practically endless.

Hay Fever

The allergic response is believed to be a case of mistaken identity. When an allergen contacts or enters the body, most people do not react to it. They may not be conscious of breathing the pollen dust of trees, plants, and weeds, but that same dust will cause misery for the hay fever sufferer. When the pollen comes in contact with his mucous membranes, his body will mistake it for an invading enemy, just as it does bacteria. It will set about sending large quantities of mucus to the "invasion site," and this will clog the sinuses, stuff the nose, and possibly produce a sore throat. Antibodies will rush to the area, the sneeze mechanism may be activated, and the tear ducts may work overtime to wash the pollen from the eyes.

It is a false alarm, but the body is unaware of that, so the sensitive person suffers. If particularly susceptible to hay fever, he will have only a few weeks to recuperate during the summer before the country air is laden with ragweed pollen and once again his body begins "defending" itself. Eventually, the chronic hay fever victim may develop nasal polyps, growths blocking the nasal cavity, and he may also suffer asthma. Those are serious problems, and asthma particularly can be life-threatening.

The only truly satisfactory solution for the hay fever sufferer is to relocate in an area where pollen does not exist. An allergist can give advice in helping to choose the right location.

Skin Allergies

It has been said, "The skin is the mirror of the body's health," and that is particularly true regarding allergies. Whether you are allergic to certain foods (strawberries, dairy products, eggs, and chocolate are among the more common), plants (poison ivy, oak, sumac), wool, synthetic fabrics, medicines, or a host of additional substances, the chances are good that the symptoms will include a skin reaction. One common response is the white fluid-containing blisters that produce violent itching—a condition known as hives. Emotional turmoil can also cause hives.

Drug Allergies

Among the most dangerous allergies is that to penicillin, experienced by 5 to 10 percent of those who receive the drug. The body reacts violently; sometimes the more common allergic symptoms are followed by a severe drop in blood pressure, coma, and possibly death. Doctors call this potentially fatal response anaphylactic shock, and penicillin is not the only drug which can cause it in susceptible people. Other drugs causing severe allergic reactions include sulfa compounds, tetracyclines, insulin, local anesthetics, tranquilizers, and even aspirin.

Any allergic reactions to drugs may be serious, and a doctor should be consulted at once.

Insect Allergies

The sting of bees, wasps, hornets, yellow jackets, and ants can also produce anaphylactic shock. In extreme cases, the throat swells, breathing difficulty develops, unconsciousness follows, and death can result. The reaction often ensues rapidly, and prompt medical attention is imperative.

Those allergic to insect bites should carry a special medical kit containing adrenaline and antihistamine at all times. If a kit is not available and a sensitive person suffers an insect bite, a tourniquet should be promptly applied between the bite and the heart, to prevent the allergen from circulating throughout the body. Then the victim should be rushed to the nearest doctor.

Diagnosis

Allergies are medicine's great imposters. Sometimes they are mistaken for a common cold, but, in addition to puffy eyes, runny nose, and a multitude of aches and pains, they can often mimic specific diseases.

Because allergens often produce skin reactions along with other symptoms, your doctor can often determine whether or not you are suffering from an allergy, and what is producing it. He'll perform what is known as a patch test, applying a series of common allergens to your skin. If a rash develops, he knows he has found the culprit.

What to Do If You Have an Allergy

If you have an allergy, you should take the following steps:

1. See a doctor, the sooner the better. Allergies very seldom vanish by themselves. More often, they get worse.

2. Keep in good health. Get plenty of rest and fresh air, and maintain a balanced diet. This will help you to avoid the infectious diseases that may make you more susceptible to nose and bronchial allergies.

3. Avoid tensions and emotional disturbances. We do not know the exact connection between allergies and emotions, but we know that a relationship does exist between them.

4. Remember, you can become allergic to practically anything. Even if the cause of your allergy has been discovered, do not assume you need not look for a different allergen if your attacks return.

5. Take special precautions if you have an allergy, however trivial. Make sure you are tested before taking medicines, vaccines, or serums. You might have a serious reaction to a medicine.

If allergic attacks are severe, you should carry a card stating clearly what you are allergic to (for example, insect stings), followed by instructions from your doctor saying what should be done for you. Tell people about your allergy whenever it is necessary. Do not be sensitive about your sensitivity! (For further information, see the entries on specific allergies in the encyclopedia section.)

CONSTIPATION

Constipation can be organic—that is, the result of actual physical change in an organ. It can be caused by a tumor or cancer that is obstructing the intestines, a stricture that narrows them, or some disorder such as a hypothyroid condition. That is why it is important to consult a doctor if you have constipation, especially if it has come on fairly suddenly and lasts for more than a day or two.

Movements that are hard to pass and require

straining can bring about rectal problems such as hemorrhoids and fissures, or they can aggravate hernias or the tendency to a hernia. Constipation can cause a number of uncomfortable symptoms that include nausea, heartburn, headache, and distress in the rectum or intestines, continuing until the stool is passed.

Sometimes the bowel movements are not difficult to pass and cause no unpleasant symptoms, but simply do not occur as the individual thinks they should. The average person has a movement every day, usually right after breakfast, but countless people are perfectly normal even though they have more than one movement a day, or a movement every other day—or every third, fourth, fifth, or even eighth day!

Causes

Self-induced constipation is caused by one or more of the following factors:

1. Improper diet: eating the wrong things or eating too little.

2. The habitual use of laxatives, cathartics, and other medication.

3. Irregularity in habits of elimination.

Functional constipation can also be caused by sluggishness. After food has been digested in the stomach and intestines, the residue is passed along in the form of watery material. The water is absorbed in the colon; that is why the feces become hard and difficult to pass if they remain there too long before being eliminated. The stools are pushed along by a series of wavelike, peristaltic movements. These waves are irregular; usually they are strongest in the morning. Therefore, it is easiest to have a bowel movement before or just after breakfast.

In some people, peristalsis is weak. This is apt to happen with increased age; elderly people may need treatment to help elimination.

How to Prevent or Cure Functional Constipation

If you actually have constipation, there are certain things you can safely do to cure it. These same methods will also prevent you from becoming constipated.

1. *Cultivate regular habits of elimination.* Choose a regular time shortly before or after breakfast every morning for going to the toilet, and attempt to defecate—without straining—whether or not you have the urge. Allow 10 minutes. Relax and be comfortable. If you go before breakfast, it will help to drink a glass or two of fluid upon getting out of bed; it can be

warm or cool water, fruit juice, tea, or coffee. Teaching your bowels to move regularly can be done with patience, and once acquired, the habit persists.

2. *Diet.* The residue of the foods you eat is easier to eliminate if it contains some roughage in the form of fibers, lubricants in the form of fats or oils, and fluids. These should be included in the diet of healthy people. However, persons suffering from certain diseases will not be able to tolerate roughage. (See Chapter 2 for menus listing normal food requirements.) To cure or prevent constipation, make sure that your diet also includes the following foods and beverages:

For breakfast: One half to one glassful of juice—tomato, grapefruit, prune, or orange. Also, one item from each of the following categories:

　　Mixed dried fruits: prunes, apricots, or stewed figs
　　Cooked, whole-grain cereals with milk: barley, brown rice, oats, or wheat
　　Butter or margarine
　　Whole-grain bread
　　Beverage

For lunch, dinner, or supper, some of the following:

　　Green leafy vegetables—beet greens, spinach, escarole, lettuce, turnip greens, dandelion greens, or mustard greens
　　Baked potatoes (eat skins)
　　Butter or margarine; salad oils
　　Dried or stewed fruits, especially for dessert at the evening meal

Drink two glasses of fluid between meals, and at least eight glasses during the day. Take an extra amount of water in summer, because part of it is lost in perspiration.

3. *Exercise.* Strong abdominal muscles are helpful in aiding the bowels to eliminate gas and stools. If you do not have a firm, well-toned abdominal wall, be sure to start the exercises described in Chapter 1. If your job requires much sitting, you should indulge in regular sports or other forms of exercise.

4. *Live sensibly.* Try to avoid the strains and stresses of modern living. Get some relaxation. Do not worry about your constipation. If your doctor gives you a clean bill of health on your periodic checkups and you follow the suggestions in Chapter 9 for home checkups between visits, your constipation is not going to harm your health. But if failure to move the bowels causes real discomfort, you may carry out the suggestions in paragraphs 5 and 6.

5. *Take an enema.* It should consist of a pint of warm water containing a level teaspoonful of table salt. If an enema does not help, your doctor can show you how to insert olive oil into the rectum at night through a catheter; this will soften the stool and make it easier to pass in the morning.

6. *If you cannot take an enema, take a mild laxative,* such as mineral oil, petrolatum and agar, or milk of magnesia. (For a discussion of laxatives, see the entry LAXATIVE in the encyclopedia section.)

Do not take enemas or laxatives until you have given your bowels a chance to work by themselves. The first step in curing constipation is to stop taking all laxatives and cathartics. Laxatives are frequently the cause of your constipation, and seldom necessary in its cure. Suppositories can be irritating and cause rectal fissures, or increase their severity. Bulky substances such as bran can produce irritation of the colon.

A final word of warning: Do not give a laxative to a child, and do not take any cathartic or laxative yourself, if there is any fever, nausea, pain, or general feeling of illness associated with the constipation. It can result in death if the condition is caused by appendicitis.

PSORIASIS

Skin ailments are among the more annoying nuisances, and while most of them are allergies, one very troublesome skin disease is not—this is psoriasis. Even today its cause is unknown. It is produced by neither a parasite nor a germ, and it is completely noncontagious. Perhaps it is inherited in some cases, although probably not in all. It seems to have no relationship to diet. Lack of sunlight may play a part in its development; it is less common in the tropics and rarely appears on the parts of the body exposed to sunlight, such as the face and hands. What is more, it usually gets worse in winter.

In psoriasis, rounded or scalloped red patches, with sharp borders, appear on the skin. They are covered by layers of shiny, silvery, dry scales resembling the scales of mica. They appear most frequently on the elbows, knees, lower back, and scalp. The hair is apt to fall out in the affected scalp areas, but, fortunately, it usually grows in again. The soles of the feet and folds of the body—in fact, any place—can be covered with these patches, and often they must be bandaged to prevent the clothing from sticking to them. Psoriasis does not affect the body's general health—there is no fever, weight loss, or any other symptom. Still, it can be an intolerable nuisance because the patches often itch (*psora* is a Greek word meaning "to itch"), and the scaly patches are unsightly and can cause severe emotional trauma. Some sufferers refuse to go swimming or appear before others in situations that would reveal the unattractive scales. Victims may be so self-conscious that they will not involve themselves in a romantic relationship that might lead to intimacies.

Several courses of treatment have proved quite effective. One involves complete exposure to sunlight regularly until the skin tans. When sunshine is not available, sun lamps can be used with the same result. Also effective are ointments containing coal tar chemicals or ammoniated mercury. Corticosteroids have been used effectively, but one must keep in mind that these drugs are particularly potent and sometimes produce harmful side effects. If used, the physician must check regularly for adverse reactions.

No one need suffer the discomfort and embarrassment of severe psoriasis today, because proper, aggressive treatment can dramatically improve or often eliminate the condition.

HEMORRHOIDS AND OTHER RECTAL TROUBLES

Hemorrhoids, or piles, are enlarged, dilated veins situated inside or just outside the rectum. They cause itching, discomfort, and pain, and are frequently accompanied by bleeding.

Aside from the fact that they are a nuisance, you should see a doctor promptly if you think you have hemorrhoids because they may be caused by something potentially serious, or they may have dangerous complications. Usually, the cause is a local one, such as the hard, dry stools and straining that accompany constipation; this irritates the veins and slows the flow of blood. In pregnancy, the enlarged uterus sometimes presses on the veins. However, the pressure can be caused by a disease of the liver or even the heart, or by a locally situated tumor or cancer.

For emergency treatment of painful hemorrhoids, apply very cold water on cleansing tissues or a cloth directly to the anal area. Continue for five to ten minutes, until the pain is allayed. Witch hazel can be used instead of water.

A hot bath morning and night may also bring relief. A soothing rectal ointment or suppository is worth trying, too, and in some cases proves very effective.

Rectal Fissures

A rectal fissure—that is, a tear in the surface of the rectum—may accompany hemorrhoids, and is extremely painful. It may be caused by the straining and irritation resulting from constipation. If it does not heal promptly, see your doctor without delay.

Pruritus Ani (Anal Itching)

This is a common and very bothersome condition. It can be brought about by worms and allergies, contact with irritating chemicals, and by many other causes. Sometimes emotional factors are responsible for the problem. Be sure to give your doctor a chance to help you, because pruritus ani can result in infections or even interfere with your general health by disturbing your sleep or by making you tense.

Anal Fistula

Anal fistula is a most annoying ailment. Because of some diseased condition, an opening develops inside the anal canal, or rectum, and a small tunnel forms, which leads out to the skin or adjacent organs. Such a fistulous tract will permit the passage of fecal matter. This in itself is unpleasant and painful because of the associated irritation and infection. In addition, the fistula may be the result of tuberculosis, actinomycosis, or other serious disease that also can destroy tissue. Sometimes, a rectal fistula results from an injury that may tear the rectal and anal tissues.

When there is a discharge of any sort from the skin near the anal area, it should be mentioned to your doctor. It may be the beginning of an anal fistula, and exact diagnosis is required to establish the cause. On that basis, the doctor decides between medical and surgical therapy.

VARICOSE VEINS

Varicose veins are knotlike, twisting enlargements of the veins, usually just beneath the skin of the legs. They result from a breakdown of the valves that are found at regular intervals in the veins. It is through these valves that the blood flows back to the heart, after having been pumped to the extremities through the arteries. These valves divide the veins into sections, each valve forming a floor to support the blood above it. When a valve is faulty or degenerates, it cannot support the blood; when a number of valves in a surface vein break down, the weight of the column of blood can distend the vein.

Varicose veins are seen most frequently in persons whose work requires them to stand or to sit upright for long periods. A tendency toward valves that break down easily has been found to run in families. Any increase in the internal pressure of the blood in the veins also strains the valves. This can be caused by heavy lifting, abdominal tumors, and pregnancy. There may also be a connection between the endocrine glands and the valves, which tend to degenerate with age.

In addition to being unsightly, varicose veins usually cause some trouble eventually, generally in the form of dull, nagging aches and pains. The ankles may swell. The enlarged veins can become the site of infection; and because the resistance of the surrounding tissue has decreased, a bruise or injury can become serious. The resulting varicose ulcers are not easy to clear up, especially in elderly people or diabetics.

In mild cases, varicose veins can be handled adequately by such measures as eliminating tight shoes and tight garters that restrict the circulation; elevating the feet at intervals; and walking about occasionally instead of standing or sitting still for long periods. Sometimes wearing an elastic stocking or bandage for even part of the day will support a varicose vein and prevent it from becoming more distended.

In severe cases, or with individuals to whom appearance is especially important, varicose veins can and should be eliminated. There are two ways in which this can be done. One method is surgical: the distended veins can be cut or else ligated (tied off). Afterward, the blood will flow through other veins. The other method is medical: a fluid is injected into the varicose vein, causing it to harden, after which the blood can no longer flow through it and will seek a new course. However, very large veins or other considerations may make the surgical treatment the better one.

Varicose veins can safely be treated by injections in old people, or in pregnant women if they would otherwise suffer pain for some months before childbirth. It should not be done in those rare cases where an infection of the blood vessels has injured the deep veins, because the circulation in the leg would then be interfered with. Of course, eliminating one or more varicose veins will not prevent other valves from breaking down or other varicose veins from developing. People who have to work in certain occupations or who have a marked tendency toward faulty valves in the veins are apt to have to contend repeatedly with this nuisance disease. (See also VARICOSE VEINS in the encyclopedia section.)

MOTION SICKNESS

Why seasickness, one of the forms of motion or travel sickness, should be considered humorous is a mystery to anyone who has ever suffered from it. There are few experiences that compare with the misery its victims endure. Nausea, dizziness, headache, and vomiting can be so severe that prostration results. Fortunately, however, it usually vanishes quickly, leaving no ill effects.

The exact cause of seasickness is not fully understood. We do know that it is related to visual stimulation as well as to the labyrinth of the ear, which is an organ of balance as well as of hearing. Psychological factors can also be important.

If you go on a cruise, there are countless ways to help ward off seasickness. Here are some useful suggestions:

Be sure you are rested and in good condition.

Get plenty of fresh air; avoid stuffy rooms and unpleasant smells. Sit on deck with your eyes facing the ship, not the ocean.

Get some exercise unless you become actively ill; in that case, lying down with the head low often helps.

Keep warm.

Do not overload your stomach. Small amounts of food taken frequently are usually better than a large meal.

Avoid rich, indigestible food.

Alcoholic beverages make some people feel less nervous, and in that way help to ward off seasickness. Also, iced crème de menthe and other pleasant-tasting drinks may help "settle the stomach." Alcoholic drinks in excess, however, can upset the digestion.

There are other things your doctor can do to help. Be sure to consult him if you know from experience, or if you are afraid, that you are going to have motion sickness on a boat, car, train, or plane. He may give you a sedative such as phenobarbital for a few days before the journey. He may prescribe certain medicines that help in preventing or curing seasickness and other types of motion sickness. These must not be taken except on a doctor's orders. (See also MOTION SICKNESS in the encyclopedia section.)

LEG CRAMPS

Leg cramps are among the more common aches and pains. The pain is caused by excessive, un-relieved contraction of muscle fibers. Usually leg cramps result from a deficiency of one or more of the following: calcium, sodium (salt), potassium, vitamin B, and water. If you suffer leg cramps, the first thing you should do is to be sure you are getting sufficient amounts of these nutrients.

People who exercise a lot, particularly in the summer, develop leg cramps because they lose in their sweat the sodium and potassium essential to maintain proper electrolytic balance, which is needed for efficient functioning of the nervous system. If the balance is off, the nerves may overreact. You may attempt to move your leg slightly, but the nerves will stimulate the muscle to contract violently. That is a cramp.

The ideal way to avoid such cramps is to eat well-balanced meals, including tomatoes and tomato juice, broccoli, chicken, poached eggs, liver, milk, and dark green, leafy vegetables— foods rich in the nutrients mentioned above. But once a cramp strikes, it is too late to run to the refrigerator.

The immediate treatment is slowly to stretch the muscle out fully, and at the same time to massage above the cramp so that you push blood into the painful fibers. This fresh blood will supply the electrolytes that the nerves need.

People who find themselves disposed to getting cramps should do warm-up exercises before and after strenuous activity. This will increase circulation and stretch the muscles. Hot baths before bedtime also help many chronic cramp sufferers.

EARACHE

Earwax, or cerumen, is one of nature's great blessings. It lubricates the skin, preventing a dry, crusty, infection-prone ear canal. It traps bacteria, dust, and even insects, then rolls the debris into a little ball that finally falls out of the ear while we sleep or chew or talk. But sometimes earwax causes problems such as deafness and tinnitus, a buzzing, ringing, or roaring sound in the ears. It can cause severe earaches, and if lodged in the isthmus of the ear, can induce violent coughing. Another occasional symptom is dizziness.

The worse possible approach to earwax is probably the most commonly used: the cotton-tipped swabs which some mothers jab into their children's ears. There is much wisdom in the old injunction, "Never put anything smaller than your elbow into your ear." According to one study, more damage is done to the inner ear by swabs and similar devices than by any other means. What is more, the swabs are ineffective. If the wax can be dislodged by them, it is already working its way out of the ear anyway. If it is not coming out, the swab will only pack it in tighter.

Normally, earwax can be dislodged by chewing. If your food is usually soft and your teeth are in good shape, switch to foods such as raw vegetables or chewy meats that let your jaws do some work at mealtime. The constant action of the jaw muscles massages the ear canal and is nature's method of dislodging the wax. But if that fails, ask your pharmacist for a preparation containing glycerol, one of the few substances that can soften the wax without causing it to swell. There are several such preparations available without prescription.

If you are not sure earwax is responsible for a hearing loss, dizziness, or any of the other symptoms mentioned, by all means have a specialist examine your ears. The checkup should include exploration of the inner ear with an otoscope, for a cerumen plug cannot be detected otherwise. (For further information on earaches, see Chapter 3 and the entry EARACHE in the encyclopedia section.)

LOW BACK PAIN

The amazingly flexible and mobile spine can withstand relatively enormous stress and serves as a protective armor for the nerves of the spinal cord. The necessarily complex structure consists of a series of bone segments, or vertebrae, which are divided into five distinct sections: the neck (cervical), upper back (thoracic), lower back (lumbar), lower spine (sacral), and the final segment (coccyx). The great majority of backaches occur in the lumbar area, and the problem is usually referred to as low back pain.

Sometimes back pain is caused by damage or degeneration of the spine itself. If the vertebrae do not develop properly, they may slide against each other when the back is moved, instead of resting comfortably on the "cushions" separating them. The result may be not only a painful wearing away of these important segments, but an actual pinching of nerves between the vertebrae themselves.

A related ailment is the ruptured disk, which has undoubtedly received more publicity than any other back condition. But the fact is that a "slipped" disk is probably the least common of all back disorders, and only surgery can offer permanent relief from its great pain. If someone who thinks he has suffered a slipped disk has been

relieved by nonsurgical means, he probably did not have a ruptured disk in the first place.

The wear and tear of daily life can compound the damage from defective or ruptured disks; so seek a doctor's advice if you find yourself suffering from chronic backache. On occasion, backache is a symptom of a serious ailment—for example, kidney or bone disease. Careful examination can detect such problems before they get out of hand.

Causes and Diagnosis

Fortunately, the great majority of backache sufferers need not be bothered with slipped or damaged disks or serious diseases. An estimated 80 percent of low back pain is muscular in origin, usually the result of poor posture or lack of flexibility or strength in the back muscles. Of these, poor posture is the greatest culprit. Many physicians can predict which of their patients will develop low back pain simply by watching them walk into the office: the future sufferer will have lumbar lordosis, or "swayback," a condition in which the abdomen hangs forward, the buttocks protrude rearward, and the spine is twisted more or less into a "C" shape. That posture is responsible when pain eventually develops in the lower back, for the spine is intended to be rod-like, not C-shaped.

Ordinarily, we have great flexibility in our hip and pelvic areas. Not only can we tilt our hips left and right, but we can tilt our pelvic area outward and inward—forward and back. We accomplish a forward tilt by contracting our abdominal muscles, which lift the front of the pelvic bone upward. But there are three reasons the person with a swayback can not easily accomplish that movement:

1. The abdominal muscles are too weak to lift the pelvis.

2. The various muscles at the front of the thigh to which the lower part of the pelvis is attached are not sufficiently flexible and hold the pelvis down.

3. The back muscles are, like the thigh muscles, too short and inflexible. They continue to tug the rear of the pelvis upward, which tilts the front downward.

If you are not sure whether you have swayback, there is a simple test you can take. Lie on the floor on your back, with legs stretched out and knees straight. Now, slip your hand under your back. With your palm on the floor, the upper part of your hand should be resting firmly against your spine. If your back does not touch your hand, you have at least some degree of lordosis.

What to Do for Low Back Pain

Once your doctor has eliminated the possibility of structural defects in your spine, you might practice two simple exercises to strengthen abdominal muscles and stretch the back and thigh muscles.

1. Lying flat on your back with your arms across your chest and your knees bent slightly, curl your head and shoulders up toward your knees. It is an ordinary sit-up exercise except that the bent knees make the abdominal muscles do all the work.

2. Lying on your back, lift the buttocks off the floor until your body makes a straight line from your neck up to your knees. This stretches the thighs and strengthens the gluteal muscles (buttocks), which help the abdominal muscles to tilt the pelvis forward.

Sometimes emotional tension causes back muscles to tighten, resulting in back pain. Anything that would loosen those muscles—gentle stretching, a vacation, tranquilizers—will ease the back pain. An excessively soft bed can also cause an aching back, because as the body sinks into it, muscles that are being stretched have a tendency to contract against the stretching. After hours of such tension, the muscles will begin to ache. One common solution is to place a bed board between the springs and the mattress to keep the back straight.

The consensus today is that surgery, while required on occasion, is neither necessary nor helpful in most cases of low back pain and should not be undertaken lightly. The wise backache sufferer will get several professional opinions and try simpler methods of relief before consenting to an operation.

INGROWN TOENAILS

This ailment is almost always caused by improper toenail clipping or ill-fitting shoes. A toenail clipped too close sometimes splinters deep in the toe's flesh where it is not visible. Still partly attached to the main nail, the splinter continues to grow, jutting into the sensitive flesh. The longer it grows, the more painful it becomes until, in severe cases, even walking is virtually impossible. Eventually the pierced tissue begins bleeding, and infection frequently sets in.

Very tight shoes can also cause ingrown toenails by irritating the nail to the point where it splinters as it does when too closely clipped. In addition, the shoe actually forces the flesh against the nail, rubbing it back and forth across the sharp edge.

As long as an ingrown toenail is attached at one point to the main nail, it is not likely to vanish. The splinter must be cut away by a doctor; tinkering with an ingrown toenail yourself might lead to serious hemorrhaging and the spread of infection. The physician can usually perform this minor surgery in his office, using a local anesthetic.

To prevent ingrown toenails, do not cut the nail shorter than the end of the toe; particularly at the nail's corners, do not cut close to the flesh. In selecting shoes, do not let fashion override common sense. The toe of the shoe should be rounded, just as your foot is, and there should be plenty of room for the toes.

Part 2

FIRST AID

What First Aid Is

There are two kinds of first aid: the emergency, life-saving measures you must take to aid a seriously ill or injured person before you can get medical help; and the home treatment of minor injuries. This section covers both types.

What you do or don't do in critical situations—when, for example, a person has a heart attack, is badly injured in an automobile accident, or is choking—can mean the difference between life and death to the victim. You owe it to yourself, your family and your neighbors to know the simple procedures that can be applied, quickly and intelligently, until the doctor or ambulance arrives or you get the victim to the nearest hospital emergency room. The following pages give you this vital information in concise, convenient form.

The First Aid section also describes the proper home treatment of less serious injuries that usually do not require professional medical help—minor cuts and bruises, slight burns, insect bites and stings. The entries are listed alphabetically.

Study this part of the book carefully—before an emergency situation arises. Then keep your *Family Health Guide* in a convenient place where it will be handy for reference when it's needed.

Where to Find:

FIRST STEPS
IN
FIRST AID

1. The thing to think of when you approach a seriously injured person is the ABC's:

A is for Airway. Make sure the victim's airway has not been blocked by the tongue, secretions, or some foreign body (see page 299).

B is for Breathing. Make sure the person is breathing. If not, administer artificial respiration (see page 299).

C is for Circulation. Check for bleeding. Make sure the patient has a pulse. If no pulse is felt, administer cardiopulmonary resuscitation—CPR (see page 300).

2. Act fast if the victim is bleeding severely (see page 298), or if he has swallowed poison (see page 310), or if his heart or breathing has stopped. Every second counts.

3. Although most injured persons can be safely moved, remember that it is vitally important not to move a person with serious injuries of the neck or back, unless it is necessary to save him from further danger (see pages 297 and 308).

4. Because life-and-death emergencies are rare, you can usually start first aid with this step: Keep the patient lying down and quiet. If he has vomited—and there is no danger that his neck or back is broken (see page 302)—turn his head to one side to prevent choking. Keep him warm with blankets or coats, but don't overheat him or apply external heat.

5. Have someone call an ambulance and a doctor while you apply first aid. The doctor should be told the nature of the emergency and asked what should be done before he or the ambulance arrives.

6. Examine the victim gently. Cut clothing, if necessary, to avoid unnecessary movement or added pain. Don't pull clothing away from burns (see page 303).

7. Reassure the victim and try to remain calm yourself. Your calmness can allay his fear and panic, and convince him that everything is under control.

8. Don't force fluids on an unconscious or semiconscious person; they may enter his windpipe and cause strangulation. Don't try to arouse an unconscious person by slapping, shaking, or similar physical means.

Note on Cardiopulmonary Resuscitation

This lifesaving technique requires skill, training, and practice. To be prepared for emergency, at least one member of every family should seek instruction (see page 300). The untrained person who attempts it may cause serious damage to the patient.

Appendicitis (see Stomach Pain)

Artificial Respiration (see Breathing Stopped)

Automobile Accidents

Nothing is likely to test one's knowledge of first aid more than accidents suffered on the highway. Injuries may be severe; you may be a great distance from professional help. The American Medical Association recommends that you carry the following equipment in your car in case of emergency:

- Wooden splints (obtainable from surgical-supply stores or lumber dealers)—several measuring 1 by 4 by 30 inches and several 1 by 3 by 14 inches.
- At least six bandages and a supply of four- by four-inch sterile dressings.
- Blanket to keep an injured person covered and

to serve as a stretcher when moving him (see page 308).

- A good flashlight, with fresh batteries; and warning lights or flares to be used if car is stalled.

In giving first aid, remember that moving the victim or making a hasty attempt to get him out of the car may do untold harm, particularly if spinal injuries or leg fractures are involved.

Give first aid at once, *inside the vehicle whenever possible*, before attempting to move the injured person. Exceptions: (a) when the vehicle is on fire; (b) when gasoline has been spilled and fire hazard is great; (c) when you are in a congested high-speed area where there is danger of a second accident. Follow these rules:

1. Be sure that the victim is breathing and has a pulse (see pages 299, 300).

2. Check for hemorrhage (see page 298).

3. Examine for injuries, particularly fractures.

4. Apply first aid measures appropriate for the type of injury (see Index).

5. In case of fractures, wait for medical help. Or, if the patient must be moved before assistance arrives, follow the suggested procedures for dealing with fractures (see pages 301, 302) and for moving injured persons to a safe area (see page 308).

Bites—Animal

Wash the wound immediately with water to flush out the animal's saliva. Then cleanse the wound for five minutes with plenty of soap and water. Rinse thoroughly and cover with a dressing or clean cloth.

Consult a doctor immediately. He will treat the wound more effectively and decide what measures are necessary to guard against rabies and tetanus infection.

If the bite is from an unknown dog or cat, try to have the animal caught and turned over to the police or health department for observation. If the animal disappears or shows rabies symptoms, the victim may need antirabies injections.

Bites—Ant, Chigger, Mosquito

Wash the affected parts with soap and water. Apply a paste made of baking soda and a little water, or use calamine lotion. (Chiggers don't attach themselves firmly to the skin for an hour or more. Scrubbing with a brush and soapy water promptly after exposure should remove them.) If there is swelling, cover the bite with a cloth saturated with ice water.

Bites—Snake

1. Have the victim lie down. This should slow blood circulation and the spread of the venom.

2. If the bite is on an arm or leg, tie a constricting bandage (necktie, belt, or shoestring) close to the bite. The bandage must be placed between the bite and the victim's heart. Tie it tight enough to retard blood flow in the surface vessels, but not tight enough to shut off deeply-lying vessels. If the bandage is properly adjusted, you should see some fluid oozing from the wound.

3. Stop and think for a moment: Is this bite poisonous? The bite of any one of the three commonest poisonous snakes—rattlesnake, copperhead, moccasin—causes immediate stinging pain, swelling, and discoloration, followed by rapid but weak pulse, pallor, and weakness, and perhaps nausea and vomiting. The bite of the only other poisonous snake in the United States—the coral snake—may cause only slight pain and mild swelling, but other symptoms

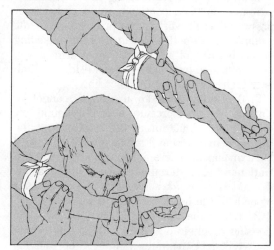

In treating snakebite, first place a constricting bandage about 2 to 4 inches above the bite. With a sterilized knife or razor blade, make a ½-inch cut lengthwise, slightly lower than each fang mark. Then suck the venom from the wound.

(shortness of breath, rapid pulse, dimming vision, nausea, and weakness) come within minutes.

4. If no doctor is available, and if the bite is of a poisonous snake, sterilize a knife or razor blade in a flame (that of several matches will suffice). Taking care to cut only the skin, make an incision lengthwise along the axis of the limb (don't make X-shaped incisions), $\frac{1}{8}$ inch deep and $\frac{1}{2}$ inch long, slightly lower than each fang mark.

5. Using your mouth (or the suction cup from a snakebite kit), suck the venom from the wound. (Although the venom is not a stomach poison, rinse it from your mouth with water, if possible.) Continue suction for about 30 minutes. Do not use ice packs or cold compresses.

6. Get medical aid as soon as possible after the bite occurs. If you have killed the snake, take it with you to be identified.

Bites—Tick

Don't try to tear an embedded tick loose. Usually you can dislodge it from the skin with a few drops of heavy oil or petroleum jelly. This closes the tick's breathing pores, which will often cause it to disengage itself within a half hour. Turpentine will work, but it is liable to sting.

If this doesn't work, remove the tick with tweezers, working gently and slowly so that you don't crush the insect and so that all parts of its head come loose. (Avoid touching ticks with your hands.) Then scrub the area with soap and water for five minutes. Ticks can transmit several diseases, but usually don't if removed soon after they've become attached. If the bite becomes inflamed and swollen, or if the patient develops a fever, notify a doctor.

Bites (see also Stings)

Bleeding—Severe

1. Have victim lie down to prevent fainting. To stop the bleeding, press a sterile gauze dressing (or the cleanest cloth item at hand) firmly over the wound. It is important to apply constant pressure. Do not dab at the wound, or lift the gauze every few seconds to see if the bleeding has stopped. If the dressing becomes saturated with blood, lay a fresh dressing directly over the saturated one and continue pressure. If direct pressure doesn't work, often pressure *above the wound* will stop the bleeding. If the bleeding occurs because of a deep cut in an arm or leg, uncomplicated by other injuries, raising the limb very high helps to control bleeding.

2. If bleeding from an arm or leg cannot be stopped by direct pressure over the wound, try shutting off circulation in the artery supplying the blood by pressing firmly against it with your hand or fingers. There are four points (see illustration) where arterial pressure is practical for first-aiders. But *don't* try arterial pressure for wounds of the head, neck, or torso.

3. When the bleeding stops, bandage the dressings firmly in place—but not so tightly that you can't feel the pulse below or beyond the wound. Call the doctor, and leave the cleaning and treatment of the wound to him. Watch carefully for signs of *shock* (see page 311).

4. If direct pressure on the appropriate pres-

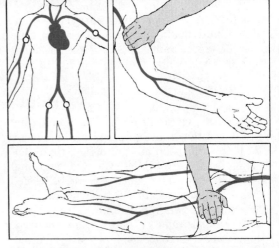

Arterial pressure can be applied at four points on the body to someone with severe bleeding from an arm or leg. Press hard on one of the spots shown above.

sure point fails to stop severe bleeding, you may use a tourniquet as a last resort. A tourniquet is a hazardous first-aid measure; you run the risk of causing the eventual loss of the limb or finger from which you are cutting off the blood.

When you make a tourniquet:

a. Tie the tourniquet around the limb between the wound and the heart, and don't allow it to touch the wound. (Use a cloth strip at least two inches wide and long enough to wrap around the limb twice).

b. Wrap the tourniquet tightly around the limb, and make a simple half knot as shown.

c. Put a strong stick (or similar object) on the half knot, and tie two additional half knots on top of the stick.

d. Tighten the tourniquet by twisting the stick. Don't twist too hard. You will know that the tourniquet is tight enough when the bleeding stops, as if a faucet had been turned off.

e. Tie the tourniquet-stick to the injured limb with the loose ends of the cloth strip, and make a written note of the time. This last step is important; the physician will want to know how long the blood flow has been stopped.

f. Don't loosen the tourniquet at all, and treat the victim for shock (see page 311).

To prevent infection, avoid, if possible, touching any wound with an unsterilized covering or your unscrubbed hands. But in an emergency you

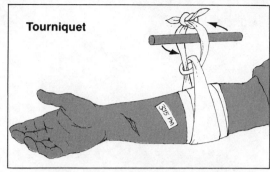

Tourniquet

The tourniquet should be used only when all other efforts to stop severe bleeding have failed.

may have no choice. The average adult has five to six quarts of blood; loss of more than a pint can be serious. So, you may have to act fast and use whatever covering is available.

If you can estimate how much blood has been lost, the information may help the doctor in treating the patient.

Blisters

The unbroken skin covering a blister affords the best protection against infection. If a blister is accidentally broken, wash the area gently and cover with a sterile dressing.

Boils and Sties

Don't squeeze or puncture boils; this may drive the infection deeper. Apply warm, wet compresses several times daily. When the boil breaks, wipe the pus away with a sterile pad, wet with saline solution, and cover with a sterile dressing. *Sties* are small boils on the eyelids. Follow the same procedure. If sties or boils are numerous, persistent, or painful, see your doctor.

Breathing Stopped—Artificial Respiration

First, make sure the airway is clear. (Do this by looking into the mouth and throat and removing any obstructing substance, solid or liquid.) Watch the patient's chest, and test the air in front of his nose and mouth with your fingers for any signs of breath. Check his wrist for a pulse.

If the victim is not breathing as a result of drowning, electric shock, chemical fumes, or any other cause, but the airway is clear and his heart is still beating, apply mouth-to-mouth breathing. In electric shock, make sure that contact with the current has been broken before you touch the patient (see Electric Shock, page 306).

(*Caution:* Check the front of the victim's neck. Some 25,000 Americans have had their larynxes surgically removed and can breathe only through openings, called stomas, in their necks. With these people, artificial respiration must be applied mouth to stoma, not mouth to mouth.) If

gas or smoke is present, move the victim into the fresh air. For mouth-to-mouth breathing:

1. Lay the victim on his back. Wipe any foreign matter out of his mouth with your fingers. Place one hand under his neck. Lift up on neck and partially tilt the head back.

2. Pull his chin upward.

3. Place your mouth firmly over the victim's open mouth, pinch his nostrils shut, and blow hard enough to make his chest rise. If the victim is a small child, place your mouth over his nose and mouth when blowing.

4. Remove your mouth. Listen for the sound of exhaled air and look for the fall of the chest. Repeat the blowing effort. If there is no air exchange, recheck the victim's mouth. His tongue may be blocking the air passage. Try again.

5. If you still get no exchange of air, turn the victim on his back. Facing him, kneel astride his

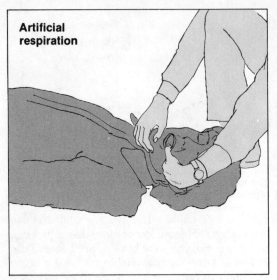

Artificial respiration

1 Lay the victim on his back, turn his head to one side, and clear his mouth of any obstruction. Then turn his head upward.

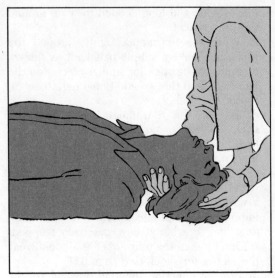

2 Put one hand under the victim's neck and lift the head. Put the other hand on the victim's forehead and tilt the head backward.

hips. With one hand on top of the other, place the heel of the bottom hand on the abdomen slightly above the navel and below the rib cage. (See illustration on page 304.) Press into the victim's abdomen with a quick upward thrust. Repeat the thrust several times. Wipe victim's mouth clear once you establish air exchange. (This technique for expelling an obstruction on which a person is choking is called the Heimlich Maneuver and is described further beginning on page 304.)

6. Resume mouth-to-mouth breathing. For adults, blow one vigorous breath every five seconds. For small children, blow shallow breaths every three seconds. If you prefer, place a handkerchief over the victim's mouth (or nose) and blow through it.

Don't give up until the victim begins to breathe. Many persons have been revived after hours of artificial respiration.

7. Call a doctor or ambulance as soon as possible. Place blankets or coats under and over the victim for warmth. When he revives, don't let him get up.

Breathing Stopped, No Pulse—
Cardiopulmonary Resuscitation (CPR)

If the patient is not breathing, make certain there is no airway obstruction (see page 299). Feel his wrist for a pulse.

If there is none, his heart has stopped. You and a helper—or you alone, if necessary—must now apply cardiopulmonary resuscitation (CPR). This includes intermittent mouth-to-mouth respiration plus closed-chest heart massage. (See illustration on opposite page.)

To administer CPR, first stretch the victim flat on his back on the ground or floor. Kneel at his side and with your fist strike his breastbone sharply. This may start the heart beating. If it does not, feel the victim's chest to locate the lower tip of his breastbone. Put one finger of your left hand on the cartilage. Move the heel of the right hand (never use the palm) to the spot located by the finger. Place the left hand atop the right.

With a quick firm thrust, push down. Use sufficient force to press the lower one third of the breastbone down 1½–2 inches, letting your back and body do the work. Now lift your weight. Repeat compression smoothly and rhythmically once per second: press . . . release . . . press . . . release. Each time you bear down, you squeeze the victim's heart, forcing blood out to his body, literally substituting for his heartbeat.

If you are alone with the victim, stop after each 15 compressions and give him two deep breaths mouth-to-mouth, continuing this 15-to-2 rhythm until help comes. If someone can assist

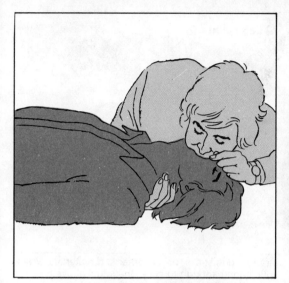

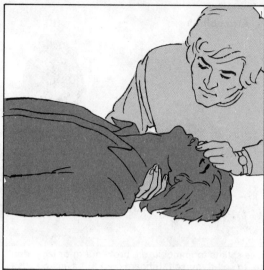

3 Pinch victim's nostrils with the hand on his forehead. Take a deep breath, cover the victim's mouth with yours, and give four quick breaths.

4 After his chest rises, remove mouth and look for exhalation of air. Repeat blowing procedure 12 times a minute (for a child, 20 a minute.)

you, have him kneel at the victim's head and give mouth-to-mouth respiration at the rate of 12 times a minute—one breath for each five compressions of the heart that you perform.

Continue complete CPR until the victim revives—pupils constrict, color improves, breathing begins, pulse returns. A person can be kept alive this way for at least an hour.

Caution: Even when done correctly, CPR may cause cracked ribs. When done incorrectly, the tip of the breastbone or a broken rib can puncture the liver or a lung. Hence, proper training in the technique is urged. (Instruction may be obtained at the local Red Cross or fire department or Heart Association. Ask your hospital where to go in your community.) But in a crisis, even if you aren't trained, give CPR; without it, anyone whose heart has stopped will die.

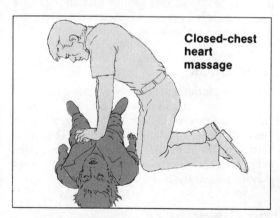

Closed-chest heart massage

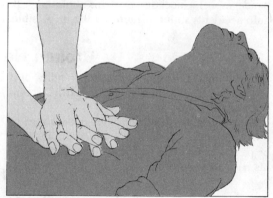

To administer closed-chest heart massage, lay the victim flat on his back and place the heel of your right hand above the lower tip of the breastbone. Put the left hand on top of the right. Press down firmly, then release pressure. Repeat press-and-release motion until the heart begins to beat.

Broken Bones

Keep the patient warm, and treat for shock (see page 311) if necessary. Apply an ice bag to the painful area. If a broken bone protrudes through the skin and there is severe bleeding, stop the bleeding (see page 298), but do not attempt to push the bone back in place. Make no attempt to

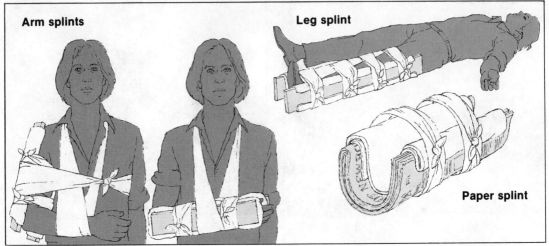

Arm splints

Leg splint

Paper splint

Use splints to immobilize a broken arm or leg—don't try to set it yourself. If boards are not available, use rolled-up newspapers or magazines, cardboard strips, broomsticks, or any other stiff materials. Make splints long enough to cover the joints above and below the break. Pad splints with cotton or cloth.

clean the wound; call an ambulance, or get the patient to a doctor.

If the victim *must* be moved to receive medical aid, the fracture should be immobilized with splints to prevent further damage. For splints, use anything that will keep the broken bones from moving—rolled-up newspapers or magazines, broomsticks, or boards for arms or legs. Make the splints long enough to reach beyond the joint both above and below the break. Pad improvised splints with cotton or clean rags and tie them snugly (but not too tightly) in place with bandages, belts, neckties, or strips of clothing. In auto accidents splint a fractured leg, if possible, before moving the victim from the car. Using bandages or other material, tie the injured leg to the uninjured leg above and below the fracture site, and immobilize it as much as possible with an improvised short splint.

Do not attempt to straighten a broken limb. Arm or leg splinting is done merely to immobilize the break. Leave bone setting to the doctor. If the break is in the back, neck, pelvis, or skull, *do not* attempt to move the patient. (See "Broken Neck or Back," below, and "Head Injury," page 307.) Don't assume that no bones are broken merely because the victim can move the injured joint or limb.

Broken Neck or Back

If the victim cannot move his fingers readily, or if there is tingling or numbness around his shoulders, his neck may be broken.

If he can move his fingers but not his feet or toes, or if he has tingling or numbness in his legs, or pain when he tries to move his back or neck, his back may be broken.

Loosen clothing around the victim's neck and waist. Cover him and summon a doctor or ambulance. Don't move him or let him try to move. Don't lift his head to give him water. The spinal cord extends from the head down through the neck and back vertebrae, and any movement may cause paralysis.

Bruises—Including Black Eye

Place an ice bag or cold compress (a small towel soaked in ice water and wrung out) over the bruise. This should reduce both the pain and the swelling. If the pain persists, consult a doctor.

Burns—Chemical

Flush the burned area copiously with water for at least five minutes to dilute and remove the chemical. Then treat as you would a comparable burn from any other cause (see "Burns and Scalds" on the following page).

If an eye is burned by a chemical, especially by

302

an acid or a basic substance such as lye, flush it gently but thoroughly with water toward the outside of the face. Cover both eyes with gauze and have the injured eye checked by a doctor.

Burns and Scalds—Major

1. If clothing or hair is on fire, rapidly smother the flames with a coat, blanket, or rug. Do not pour water, milk, or other liquid on the victim unless you are certain the fire is not oil-based.

2. Keep the victim lying down.

3. Cut clothing away from the burned area. If cloth adheres to the burn, don't pull it loose; leave it and gently cut away the fabric around it.

4. Carefully scrub hands to prevent contamination. Cover the burn with a thick pad of dressings. This excludes air and reduces pain and contamination. If dressings are not available, use freshly laundered sheets or towels. Don't apply burn ointments or oil or antiseptic of any sort, and don't attempt to change the dressings.

5. Call ambulance.

6. If a large area of the body is burned, administer first aid for shock (see page 311). If the victim is conscious, dissolve a half-teaspoonful of baking soda and one teaspoonful of salt in a quart of water. Give him half a glass of this solution every 15 minutes to replace lost body fluids. Discontinue fluids if victim vomits.

Burns and Scalds—Minor

Submerge the burned skin immediately in cold water. On burns that cannot be immersed, apply ice wrapped in cloth; or apply cloths soaked in ice water, and change them constantly. Continue treatment until pain is gone. Avoid ointments, greases, and baking soda, especially on burns severe enough to require medical treatment. Doctors must always scrape off such applications, which delays treatment and can be extremely painful. If the skin is blistered, cover the burn with sterile dressings. Don't break blisters.

Caution: Even superficial burns or scalds may be dangerous if large areas are involved. Consult a physician.

Carbon-Monoxide Poisoning

Carbon monoxide is a colorless, odorless gas that kills without warning. A car engine left running in a closed garage can swiftly produce a lethal dose of carbon monoxide. The gas is also generated by wood, coal and charcoal fires, faulty oil burners, etc. In poorly ventilated rooms, the hazard of poisoning is always present.

Symptoms of carbon-monoxide poisoning are: headache, dizziness, weakness, labored breathing, possible vomiting, followed by collapse and unconsciousness. Skin, fingernails, and lips may be pink or cherry-red.

First aid: Get the victim into the open air immediately, or open all windows and doors. Begin artificial respiration promptly (see page 299) if he is not breathing or is breathing irregularly, and cardiopulmonary resuscitation (see page 300) if his heart has stopped. Keep him lying quietly to minimize his oxygen consumption. Cover him for warmth. Call the doctor, hospital, fire department, or police emergency squad. Be sure to state the nature of the trouble and *specify the need for oxygen* because of carbon-monoxide poisoning.

Childbirth—Emergency

This Childbirth—Emergency entry is adapted from the American Medical Association's First Aid Manual.

Childbirth is natural and normal. Let nature take its course. Do not hurry the birth; do not interfere with it. Wash your hands; keep the surroundings as clean as possible. During the birth process, touch and support only the emerging baby. Keep hands out of the birth canal.

• When the baby has been delivered, place him between the mother's thighs, his head slightly lowered. Cover him to keep him warm.

• If the infant is not breathing, use mouth-to-mouth breathing. Be gentle.

• Gently massage the mother's abdomen to help her uterus contract and expel the afterbirth.

• Immerse scissors in boiling water, or clean them with alcohol. Tie a clean tape or strip of cloth in a square knot around the umbilical cord about four inches from the baby to stop circulation in the cord. Tie a second tape around the cord six to eight inches from the baby (two to four inches from the first knot). If no tapes are available, shoestrings may be used.

- Do not hurry to cut the cord; wait until the afterbirth has been expelled. Then cut the cord between the two tapes with the sterilized scissors. Do not wash white material off the baby; it protects his skin.
- Do nothing to the baby's eyes, ears, nose, or

mouth unless he is gurgling or breathing with difficulty, in which case there is probably mucus collected in the nose and mouth. It is important to clean out this mucus. Try to suck it out somehow, with a straw or similar apparatus, or wipe it out with a cloth (or even your finger if necessary). Keep baby and mother warm. Notify the mother's physician, and transport the mother and child to the hospital or to a clinic.

Choking on an Obstruction—The Heimlich Maneuver

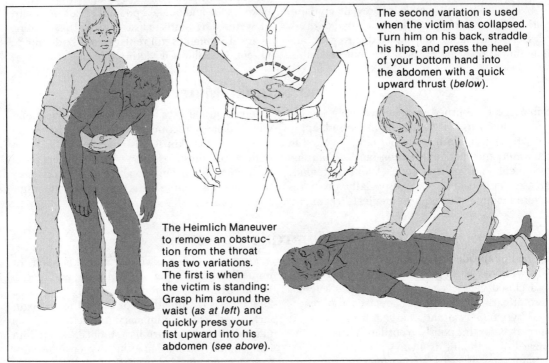

The second variation is used when the victim has collapsed. Turn him on his back, straddle his hips, and press the heel of your bottom hand into the abdomen with a quick upward thrust (*below*).

The Heimlich Maneuver to remove an obstruction from the throat has two variations. The first is when the victim is standing: Grasp him around the waist (*as at left*) and quickly press your fist upward into his abdomen (*see above*).

Choking victims are usually incapable of speaking or breathing while they are choking. If someone collapses while eating, the first thing you must do is to establish whether he is choking or having a heart attack. To rule out a heart attack, ask the victim if he can talk. If he cannot, then in all probability he is choking. You must then take immediate action.

The Heimlich Maneuver for removing an obstruction that causes choking has two variations—one for use when the victim is standing, and one to use if the victim is lying down—and they are both simple and effective. For a choking infant or small child, perform maneuver as usual, but *reduce the amount of pressure used in the upward thrust.*

1. *Standing Maneuver:* When the victim is

standing, stand behind him and wrap your arms around his waist. Make a fist with one hand and place it, thumbside in, against the victim's abdomen, slightly above the navel and below the rib cage (see illustration). Grasp your fist with the other hand, and press into the victim's abdomen *with a quick upward thrust.* Repeat the thrust several times if necessary. When the victim is sitting, the rescuer stands behind the victim's chair and performs the maneuver in the same way.

2. *Lying-Down Maneuver:* If the victim has collapsed and the rescuer is unable to lift him, turn the victim on his back. Facing him, kneel astride his hips. With one hand on top of the other, place the heel of the bottom hand on the abdomen slightly above the navel and below the rib cage (see illustration). Press into the victim's abdomen *with a quick upward thrust.* Repeat the thrust several times if necessary. (Should the victim vomit, quickly place him on his side and clear out his mouth.)

3. *Self-Administered Maneuver if You Are Alone:* If you are alone and unable to find quick assistance, you can perform the Heimlich Maneuver on yourself, by pressing your fist (thumb-side in) against your abdomen (slightly above the navel and below the rib cage), and dropping down hard on your fist against the edge of a sink or a chair, or pressing your fist or a firm object into the area below the diaphragm.

Cold—Overexposure and Frostbite

Overexposure symptoms are: numbness, drowsiness, staggering, failing vision, unconsciousness. Place the patient in a warm room. Wrap him in blankets. Give him warm, nonalcoholic drinks if he is conscious. Watch for stoppage of breath; apply mouth-to-mouth breathing if necessary (see page 299).

Frostbite: Just before frostbite occurs, the victim's skin may be flushed; but, as the freezing progesses, the skin turns white or gray-yellow. There may or may not be pain. Cover the frozen area with a warm hand, clothing, or blanket. Do not rub the frozen members or apply snow. Do not apply hot-water bottles or heating pads or keep the victim near a stove; excessive heat increases tissue damage. Instead, give the victim a warm (not hot) bath. When he is warm, encourage him to exercise the affected parts.

Convulsions

In convulsive attacks, the victim's lips turn blue, his eyes roll upward, his head is thrown back, his body is jerked by uncontrollable spasms.

Don't try to restrain convulsive movements. Place the victim on the floor, and turn his head to one side to allow saliva to drain. Move furniture so that he can't injure himself. Put a rolled handkerchief between his teeth to keep him from biting his tongue. If he has fever, place cool, wet cloths on his forehead and sponge his body with alcohol or cool water. When the spasms subside, make him as comfortable as possible and call a doctor. Convulsions usually last only a few minutes, but the victim should have immediate medical attention. Be certain that his airway remains open.

Croup

An attack of croup—which usually afflicts children—is an infection of the larynx (voice box) and is apt to be very upsetting to both child and his parents. The child coughs in a harsh, strangled manner and gasps for breath. Usually the attacks come late at night. Croup generally follows a cold, and it may occur for two or three nights in succession. To give emergency relief, place the child in a location where there is warm, moist air. Sit with the child for a time in the bathroom with the door closed. Turn on the hot water in the shower or tub—full blast—until the room is filled with steam. Keeping the door closed, sit with the child in the bathroom until his breathing becomes easier. Then set up a vaporizer in his room. (See also Chapter 16.)

Cuts, Scratches, Abrasions

1. To minimize the possibility of infection, wash your hands thoroughly before treating any wound. Clean the skin around the wound with soap and water. To avoid contamination, wash away from the wound, not toward it.

2. Then, wash the wound itself with soap. If it is necessary to use tweezers to remove debris, boil them for 10 minutes, or sterilize them in the flame of several matches and wipe the carbon away with sterile gauze.

3. Cover the wound with sterile gauze, or the cleanest cloth available, held in place by a bandage or adhesive tape.

4. Remember that with any wound there is always danger of tetanus (lockjaw); in deep, extensive, or dirty wounds, the threat is serious. Try to find out whether the victim has been previously immunized with tetanus toxoid and whether immunity has been maintained with booster shots, so that the doctor can determine proper treatment.

5. Watch carefully for these signs of infection

(which may not appear for several days): (a) a reddened, hot, painful area surrounding the wound; (b) red streaks radiating from the wound up the arm or leg; (c) swelling around the wound, accompanied by chills or fever. If infection should appear, see a doctor at once.

Diabetic Coma and Insulin Reaction

If someone becomes confused, incoherent, or unconscious for no apparent reason, he may be a diabetic who is either having an insulin reaction or developing a diabetic coma. The two situations are treated differently. (Be sure to check the victim for a card, bracelet, necklace, etc.—identifying him as a diabetic.)

Insulin reaction is the result of a too rapid drop in the diabetic's blood-sugar level. Symptoms come on rapidly. The diabetic sweats profusely and is nervous; his pulse is rapid, his breathing shallow. He may be dazed and shaky. If he is conscious and can swallow, give him some form of sugar—candy, lump sugar, fruit juice, or a sweet soft drink. If he cannot swallow, or if recovery is not prompt, summon a doctor or an ambulance.

The symptoms of *diabetic coma* come on gradually. The diabetic's skin becomes flushed and dry, his tongue dry, his behavior drowsy, his breathing labored; his breath develops a fruity odor (like that of nail-polish remover). Diabetic coma requires prompt medical attention and emergency hospitalization if life is to be saved. (See also Chapter 5, "Your Endocrine Glands and Their Hormones.")

Dislocated Joints

Do not move the joint. If the dislocation is in a hand, arm, shoulder, or jaw, and the patient can be moved safely, get him to a doctor or hospital as quickly as is consistent with his safety and comfort. If the patient has a hip dislocation, call an ambulance or move him on a stretcher to a hospital emergency room. Do not attempt to set a dislocated joint yourself. To reduce swelling and relieve pain, apply an ice bag to the injured part.

Drowning

Clear the airway first by turning the victim onto his abdomen or lowering his head. Then start mouth-to-mouth respiration (see page 299). Give complete CPR (cardiopulmonary resuscitation) if the heart has stopped (see page 300). If debris or any other obstruction prevents mouth-to-mouth respiration, perform the Heimlich Maneuver for choking on the drowning victim (see page 304).

Earache

Proper treatment requires diagnosis of the underlying cause. Consult a physician. For temporary relief, have the person lie down and elevate his head on several pillows. Place a hot-water bottle or heating pad over the affected ear and the side of the head.

Do not let the patient blow his nose hard or with one nostril closed. Do not use ear drops, ointments, or heated oil unless prescribed by a doctor. Nose drops (aqueous, *not* oily) may reduce nasal swelling and thereby help relieve ear distress.

Electric Shock

Every second of contact with the source of electricity lessens the victim's chance of survival. Break the victim's contact with the source of current in the quickest *safe* way possible. Indoors, disconnect the plug of the offending appliance, or pull the main switch at the fuse box. Outdoors, remove the victim's body from contact with current, using a tree branch, a *dry*, nonmetallic pole, a *dry* rope or *dry* clothing to push or pull the wire off the victim—or the victim off the wire. Stand on a *dry* surface, and touch only *dry*, nonconductive materials. Don't touch the victim until contact with current has been broken. Then check to see if the victim is breathing and has a pulse. If necessary, apply mouth-to-mouth breathing (see page 299) or complete cardiopulmonary resuscitation (see page 300). Send for medical aid at once.

If it is necessary to move the victim again, check to be sure the accident has not caused bone fractures or internal injuries. (See "Moving an Injured Person," page 308.)

Epileptic Seizure

In a major epileptic seizure (*grand mal*), the person screams and falls unconscious to the floor, often frothing at the mouth and thrashing his limbs about. Lower him to the floor at the beginning of the attack, and remove all furniture and other objects on which he might hurt himself. Put a rolled handkerchief or washcloth between his teeth on one side of the mouth to keep him from biting his tongue. Because there is danger of strangulation, do not force him to swallow any liquid while he is unconscious. Unless the person has a series of seizures within a short period of time, it is not necessary to rush him to a hospital. However, anyone who has seizures or brief spells of loss of consciousness (*petit mal*) should have medical care.

Eye—Something In

First, examine the eye by pulling down the lower lid and turning back the upper lid. If the speck is on either lid, try to remove it by touching it lightly with the *moistened* corner of a clean cloth as shown in the illustration at right. If the speck is on the eyeball itself, *don't* attempt to remove it. Place a bandage over both eyes and see a doctor.

If the substance in the eye is a strong chemical, such as an acid or lye, flush it away gently but thoroughly with water from nose outward. Cover with gauze dressing or a clean cloth and take the patient *at once* to a doctor or a hospital.

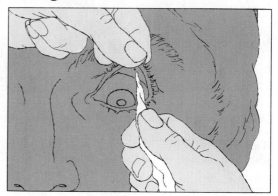

Fainting

Place the patient on his back, with his head low. Make certain that his airway is clear and that he is breathing. Loosen tight clothing; apply cold cloths to his face; allow him to inhale aromatic spirits of ammonia. When he revives, give him hot coffee or tea.

If the fainting lasts more than a minute or two, keep him covered warmly and call an ambulance or take him to the nearest hospital emergency facility. Fainting may be caused by fatigue, hunger, sudden emotional upset, a poorly ventilated room, etc. The patient's breathing is usually weak, pulse feeble, face pale, and the forehead covered with beads of perspiration. If the patient merely feels faint, have him lie down, with his feet raised higher than his head.

Head Injury—Fracture, Concussion

There is the possibility of head injury in any traffic accident, fall, or other incident of violence. Symptoms may include: victim dazed or unconscious; bleeding from mouth, nose or ears; pulse rapid but weak; pupils of eyes unequal in size; paralysis of one or more extremities; headache or dizziness; double vision; vomiting; pallor. Or the victim may appear quite normal and have a momentary loss of consciousness or a lack of memory of the event causing the injury—only to lapse into unconsciousness later, or to develop the other symptoms.

Even though the blow may not have brought unconsciousness, there is always danger of brain hemorrhage and serious trouble later. Lying quietly lessens the chance of hemorrhage. If the patient is unconscious or strangling, turn his head gently to the side so that blood or mucus can drain from the corner of the mouth. If the scalp is bleeding, place a dressing—sterile, if possible—over the wound and bandage it into place. Keep the patient lying down until you get medical help or can deliver him to a hospital emergency facility.

Heart Attack

Common symptoms of heart attack are extreme shortness of breath, pain in the center of the chest, sometimes radiating into the neck or arms, or occasionally pain in the upper abdomen. The patient may sweat and lose consciousness.

Call an ambulance and notify the patient's doctor. If the patient is having trouble breathing, do not force him to lie down. Help him take the position that is most comfortable for him. Loosen tight clothing (belt, collar, etc.) Don't attempt to lift or carry him. Don't give him anything to drink. Remain calm, and try to reassure him. Rehearse in your mind the steps in cardiopulmonary resuscitation (see page 300), in case the patient's pulse cannot be felt and he stops breathing.

Heat Exhaustion and Heat Stroke

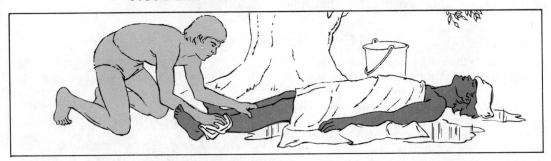

Lower the temperature of a victim of heat stroke by repeatedly sponging the body with cool water.

Heat stroke is a life-threatening emergency for which immediate medical care is needed. The victim of heat stroke stops sweating; his skin becomes red, hot, and dry. His temperature soars—to 106° F or higher. He may become unconscious. Cool the victim off immediately, which should bring his temperature down. Remove victim's outer clothes, and repeatedly sponge the bare skin with cool water or rubbing alcohol, or place the victim in a tub of cool water. Give him cool drinks but no stimulants. Call an ambulance, or get the victim to a hospital emergency facility as soon as possible.

Mild heat exhaustion (headache, extreme fatigue, dizziness, cold and clammy skin, perhaps fainting) can be treated by rest in a shaded area (or air-conditioned room) with cold towels on the patient's head. Put one teaspoonful of salt in a glass of water, and give the victim about half a glass every 15 minutes.

Hyperventilation

Hyperventilation is a common complication of emotional upset and most often affects anxious, high-strung persons who unknowingly breathe too rapidly. This disturbs the normal balance of oxygen and carbon dioxide in the blood. The result is tingling and spasms of the fingers and toes and a peculiar numbness around the mouth. These symptoms make the victim still more anxious, and still more hyperventilation results. The patient's color and pulse remain good.

Hyperventilation can usually be helped by reassurance and this simple measure: Have the person breathe slowly for 10 minutes, or longer, into a paper (not plastic) bag held tightly over his mouth and nose. If this does not work, take the patient to a hospital emergency room.

Moving an Injured Person

If an injury involves the neck or back, damage can be done by moving the victim. Get a doctor or ambulance quickly. Meanwhile, cover the patient with blankets or coats where he lies. Don't attempt to change his position until you determine the nature of his injuries—unless moving is absolutely necessary to prevent further injuries. If the victim must be pulled to safety, move his body lengthwise, not sideways. If possible, slip a blanket or long coat under him so he can ride on that. If he must be lifted, don't jackknife him by lifting his heels and head only;

How to move an injured person

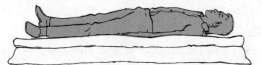

1 Half roll a blanket lengthwise and put the rolled edge alongside the victim.

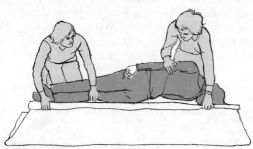

2 Turn him carefully toward you and slide the blanket up to his back.

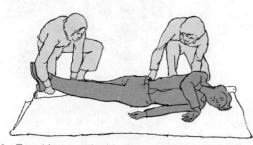

3 Turn him over the blanket, unroll it, and then turn him onto his back.

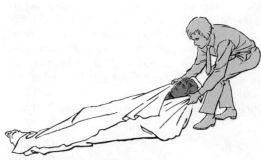

4 If the victim must be moved and you are alone, use the blanket to drag him headfirst, keeping his back as straight as possible.

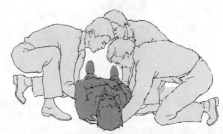

5 If there are others present who can help, be sure they support each part of his body as you lift him.

support each part of the body so that you lift it in a straight line.

Until you are certain that there is no neck or back injury, don't bundle a seriously injured person into an automobile and speed to the nearest town. If a victim *must* be transported, move him in a reclining position. Improvise a stretcher, if possible. The most desirable is a door, a wide board, or a leaf from a table. Lacking any of these, make a stretcher by wrapping clothing, a rug, or a blanket around two poles.

Be sure to support the victim's head firmly with an improvised pillow made by gathering more material from the blanket under the head or by using a folded jacket (or similar cushion). Use a straight chair (carried by two or more persons) to bring an injured person down narrow or winding stairs.

When reporting an accident, inform the doctor or ambulance service of the nature of the accident and injuries. Seek advice regarding the safest procedure.

Nose—Something In

If the object cannot be withdrawn easily, consult a doctor at once. Don't permit violent nose blowing. Don't probe the nose yourself; you may push the object deeper or injure the nostril.

Nosebleed

Have the patient sit quietly with his head thrown forward for 10 minutes. This may cause a clot to form over the ruptured blood vessels. If the bleeding continues, pack each bleeding nostril with a plug of sterile gauze (not absorbent cotton). Leave one end of each plug outside for easy removal. Lay the patient down, head raised, and place a cold, wet towel across his face.

Overdose of Medicine or Drug

One of the problems in recognizing poisoning by an overdose of a medicine or drug is that there may be no immediate symptoms. Your suspicion may first be aroused when you notice an open medicine or drug container. If this happens, call the doctor immediately and tell him what the substance is, how much was swallowed, and how much time has passed since it was taken. You may not know all these facts, but anything you can tell him will help.

If the person is conscious, try to induce vomiting by any of the methods described on page 311. Call a doctor. *Never* induce vomiting if the person is unconscious or is having convulsions. Do *not* give any alcoholic beverages. If he is drowsy or unconscious, he needs immediate medical help.

Poison Ivy, Oak, Sumac

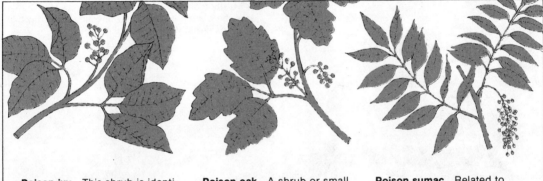

Poison ivy This shrub is identified by its glossy green leaves, growing in groups of three.

Poison oak A shrub or small tree, poison oak has downy leaflets and bears white berries.

Poison sumac Related to poison ivy, this tall shrub or tree sometimes grows 20 feet tall.

Wash exposed areas with soap and cold water as soon as possible, working up a thick lather and rinsing several times. *Do not scrub with a brush.* If itching and burning have already appeared, wash the affected areas gently with soap and cold water, and pat on calamine lotion to soothe the itch. If you are frequently or seriously bothered by poison ivy, ask your doctor about immunization, and go to a hospital emergency room for immediate treatment for each episode.

Poisoning, Food

Food poisoning is usually caused by bacterial contamination of food. It can also be caused by toadstools, poisonous mushrooms or berries, shellfish, or other foods that are dangerous to eat, have "spoiled," or have been improperly canned. The symptoms include pain or tenderness in the abdomen, nausea, vomiting, painful spasms, diarrhea, weakness, and in some cases, such as mushroom poisoning, dimness of vision and symptoms like those of alcoholic intoxication.

The stomach should be washed out with large quantities of water and emetics, as described below in "Poisoning, by Mouth," No. 5. Keep the person warm. Get the victim to a doctor as soon as possible, especially if he has eaten poisonous mushrooms or toadstools, poisonous berries, or contaminated shellfish. The symptoms of mushroom poisoning may not occur until some time after eating. Try to bring a specimen of the suspected food to the doctor.

Poisoning, by Mouth

1. Administer the antidote recommended on the container from which the poison came.

2. Call your doctor or a poison-control center immediately. Tell what the suspected poison is.

3. If you can't get medical aid, or the poison and antidote are unknown, dilute the poison in the stomach by giving the victim several glasses of milk or water. *Don't induce vomiting.*

4. And do not induce vomiting if the person is unconscious or is having convulsions, or if he has swallowed a corrosive substance such as acid, ammonia, cleaning fluid, drain cleaner, or lye; or a petroleum product such as kerosene, benzene, gasoline, turpentine, lighter fluid, or paint thinner. If possible, get the victim to swallow some milk or a glass of warm water. Wash the poison off the face and eyes, and rush the victim to the nearest medical help.

The petroleum products are not so dangerous if swallowed and retained in the stomach. They become very dangerous if drawn into the lungs. This may occur during vomiting. The victim should be taken to medical aid as soon as possible so that the doctor can decide how best to deal with potentially dangerous material in the stomach. *Always keep the container of poison and bring it with you to the doctor or the hospital.*

5. If the poison is neither a corrosive substance (acid or alkali), nor a petroleum product, induce the victim to vomit. Give one ounce of ipecac (for a child, give one-half ounce) followed by four or five glasses of water. If no vomiting occurs in 20 minutes, the dose may be repeated once only. If powdered, activated charcoal is available, and the poison is neither a corrosive substance nor a petroleum product, give the victim an ounce of the charcoal mixed in water. This highly absorbent material will take up large quantities of the ingested poison and conduct it through the intestinal tract. Activated charcoal will also absorb syrup of ipecac. Therefore, if the latter is used, give charcoal only after the ipecac has induced vomiting. If these antidotes are not at hand, stick your finger into the victim's throat to induce vomiting.

6. After the victim has vomited, again administer the antidote specified on the label of the poison container.

Puncture Wounds

1. Punctures that are caused by nails or other penetrating objects tend to "seal in" contamination. Do not squeeze or "milk" the wound. To do so would break this seal and encourage the spread of infection.

2. Wash your hands, then clean the wound with soap and water.

3. Cover the wound loosely with a sterile dressing. Apply an ice bag to reduce swelling, relieve pain, and slow absorption of toxicity.

4. Take the patient to a doctor who will clean the wound, opening it further if necessary, and will take steps to protect against tetanus.

Shock

In any serious injury (such as a bleeding wound, fracture, major burn), *always* expect shock, and act to lessen it before the symptoms appear. The symptoms: the skin is pale, cold, and clammy; the pulse is rapid; breathing is shallow, rapid or irregular; the injured person is frightened, restless, apprehensive, or comatose.

1. Keep the patient lying down with head lower than feet (except that in cases of head or chest injuries, when the patient has difficulty breathing, the head and shoulders should be raised so that the head is 10 inches higher than the feet).

2. Loosen patient's clothing.

3. Get the patient to a hospital emergency room, or call an ambulance paramedic service.

Splinters

Wash your hands and the skin around the splinter with soap and water. Sterilize a needle and tweezers by boiling them 10 minutes in water or by heating them in the flame of a match and wiping off the carbon with sterile gauze. Loosen the skin around the splinter with the needle, and remove splinter with the tweezers. Encourage slight bleeding by squeezing the wound gently. If the splinter breaks or is lodged deeply, see a doctor.

Sprains

Elevate the injured joint. Apply an ice bag or a cold compress over the sprain to reduce pain and swelling. Severe sprains should be examined by a doctor for possible bone fracture.

Stings—Bee, Wasp, Hornet

Remove the stinger if possible with a sterilized table knife. Run cold water over and around the sting to relieve pain and slow the absorption of the venom, or pack ice around it. Calamine lotion may relieve itching.

Soak a victim of massive stings (by a swarm of insects) in a cool bath in which baking soda (one tablespoonful per quart of water) has been dissolved. If antihistamines are available, these may be taken in the usual dose prescribed on the label. An allergic person reacts violently to insect stings; he should be taken promptly to the nearest hospital emergency room, and treated with antihistamines and cold compresses en route.

Stings and Bites—Poisonous Spiders and Scorpions

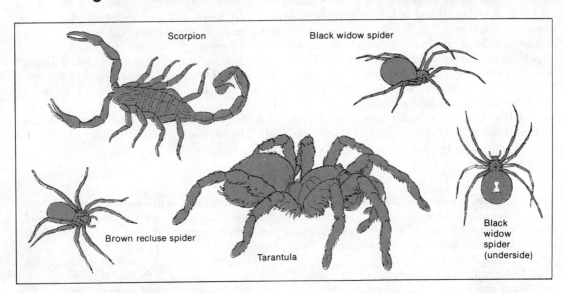

Scorpion

Black widow spider

Brown recluse spider

Tarantula

Black widow spider (underside)

Keep the victim lying quietly and warmly covered. There may be a redness and swelling around the sting, along with painful abdominal or muscle cramps, fever, sweating, and nausea. A tingling or burning pain may spread throughout the body.

Pack ice around the bite to slow the spread of the poison. Summon a doctor immediately or take the patient to a hospital emergency room as soon as possible.

The bite of a black widow spider is seldom fatal, except in the case of infants or elderly and infirm people. The bite of a brown recluse spider is more deadly, although it normally hides in dark corners and will not bite unless it is threatened. However, some babies have been bitten when they rolled onto this spider. Its bite causes intense pain some two to eight hours later, followed by nausea, cramps, and a high fever. The sting of a poisonous scorpion can be fatal, so take immediate action.

The U.S. tarantula is not seriously poisonous, but its bite is painful and can cause bacterial infection.

Stomach Pain—Appendicitis

Do not give the patient a laxative. Take his temperature. Feel his abdomen while he is lying down with his abdominal muscles relaxed. If there is any fever, even slight, and if the abdomen feels hard or tense and is sore or painful to the touch, especially on the lower right side, call a doctor at once or take the patient to a hospital emergency room. The trouble may be appendicitis. Other appendicitis symptoms: nausea, vomiting, persistent pain. When there is pain in the lower right side of the abdomen, *suspect appendicitis* until another diagnosis is proved. Meanwhile, don't let the patient eat anything: food or a laxative increases the possibility of the appendix rupturing. Also, do not permit the patient to drink anything.

Stroke

Strokes occur either because an artery in the brain has burst (cerebral hemorrhage) or because a blood clot or other material has blocked an artery (cerebral thrombosis and cerebral embolism). The victim's face may become very red and the eyeballs prominent. One side of the body may become paralyzed. Speech may be affected and the mouth drawn to one side.

Call a doctor or ambulance immediately. While you are waiting for medical help, place the person halfway between a lying and sitting position, or at least prop up his head. Loosen any tight clothing. It is important to maintain a calm attitude yourself. If the person should vomit, turn his head to one side to prevent his choking. Otherwise, do not try to move him.

Sunburn

If the skin is reddened but not blistered, apply cold cream or mineral oil. Do not use butter or margarine; either may irritate or introduce infection. If the skin is blistered or extensively burned, cover it with a dressing wet with cold water. Do not re-expose burned skin until healing is complete. Severe or extensive sunburn requires prompt medical aid.

Swallowed Objects

Small, round objects (beads, buttons, coins, marbles) swallowed by children usually pass uneventfully through the intestines and are eliminated. Do not give cathartics or bulky foods—just the normal diet. If there is pain, consult a doctor. For several days strain stool through cheesecloth to determine whether the object has been eliminated.

Sharp or straight objects (bobby pins, open safety pins, bones) are dangerous. Don't panic; consult a doctor. Special instruments may be required to locate and remove the object.

Throat—Something Caught in

If something is caught in the throat (pharynx), it may obstruct swallowing or breathing, or both. If only swallowing is obstructed, the person should proceed as calmly as possible to the nearest hospital emergency facility. If the object obstructs the airway, it should be removed immediately. (The technique is described in "Choking on an Obstruction," page 304.)

Toothache

A toothache may be temporarily relieved by aspirin or any of the other similar mild painkillers. If the toothache is due to a cavity or the loss of a filling, put some oil of cloves on a tiny bit of cotton and pack it firmly into the cavity with a toothpick.

Unconsciousness—Cause and Victim Unknown

If you encounter an unconscious person, and the nature of the trouble is unknown:

1. Apply artificial respiration (see page 299)—*only if the victim is not breathing or is breathing with great difficulty.* If his pulse has stopped, apply cardiopulmonary resuscitation (see page 300).

2. Examine effects (pockets, wallet), preferably before witnesses, for a card stating that the victim is a diabetic (see page 306) or an epileptic.

3. If the victim's *face is pale, his pulse weak,* lower his head slightly and give no stimulants.

4. If his *lips are blue,* check his breathing and pulse. Apply artificial respiration or complete CPR if necessary.

5. If an unconscious person vomits, turn his head to one side to prevent him from choking.

6. Get as full a report as possible as to what happened; ask everyone present.

Have someone call an ambulance. Do not move victim unless absolutely necessary to prevent further harm. (See "Moving an Injured Person," page 308.) Do not disturb or remove an unconscious stranger's personal effects or anything that may be evidence of a crime or attempted suicide.

WARNING
Discard Old Drugs and Keep Others Locked Up

Remember that drugs do not last indefinitely. They may lose their potency, or they may evaporate to concentrations that can be harmful.

To prevent deterioration, keep all bottles tightly stoppered. Keep medicines in a cool, dry, preferably dark place.

Don't keep any drugs left over from a previous illness unless advised to do so by the doctor.

Discard as unsafe any drug that has changed color or consistency or become cloudy. Especially avoid the use of old iodine, eye drops, eye washes, nose drops, cough remedies, ointments.

Keep all medicines, including nonprescription drugs such as aspirin, out of reach of children.

First Aid Kit

Assemble your first aid supplies now, before you need them. Don't add these items to the jumble in the medicine cabinet. Instead, assemble them in a suitably labeled box (such as a fishing-tackle box or small tool chest with hinged cover), so that everything will be handy when needed. Label everything in the kit clearly, and indicate what it is to be used for. Be sure *not* to lock the box—otherwise you may be hunting for the key when seconds count. Place the box on a shelf beyond the reach of small children. Check it periodically to restock used items.

Checklist of Supplies
(All items are obtainable without prescription)

- Sterile gauze dressings, 4x4 inches, individually wrapped, for cleaning and covering wounds
- Triangular bandages
- Roll of gauze bandage, two inches wide, for bandaging sterile dressings over wounds, etc.
- Box of assorted adhesive bandages
- Roll of inch-wide adhesive tape
- Roll of absorbent cotton
- Pint bottle of sterile saline solution (one level teaspoonful of salt to one pint of boiled water)
- Mild antiseptic for minor wounds (mild solution of iodine or mercurial antiseptic)
- Bottle of calamine lotion for sunburn, insect bites, rashes, etc.
- Bottle of ipecac syrup to induce vomiting
- Container of powdered, activated charcoal to absorb swallowed poisons
- Tube of petroleum jelly
- Box of baking soda (bicarbonate of soda)
- Small bottle of aromatic spirits of ammonia
- Scissors
- Tweezers
- Packets of needles and safety pins
- Sharp knife or packet of stiff-backed (one-edged) razor blades
- Medicine dropper (eyedropper)
- Measuring cup
- Oral thermometer
- Rectal thermometer
- Hot-water bottle
- Ice bag
- Box of wooden safety matches
- Flashlight
- Tourniquet

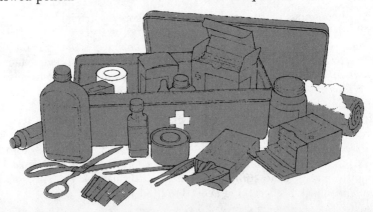

Part 3

MEDICAL ENCYCLO-PEDIA

How to Use This Encyclopedia

The entries in the encyclopedia section are arranged alphabetically, from **ABASIA** to **ZYGOTE.** To provide quick access to additional information about a given subject, references to other entries appear in small capital letters. For example, in the entry **ABDOMINAL PAIN** is the sentence:

> Some of the more common causes of recurring abdominal pain…are GALLSTONES, HEPATITIS, GASTRITIS, ULCER of the stomach or duodenum…COLITIS, and APPENDICITIS.

You will learn more about abdominal pain and its causes if you turn to the entries indicated by the small capital letters: GALLSTONES, HEPATITIS, GASTRITIS, ULCER, COLITIS, and APPENDICITIS. There are additional words in the sentence quoted above that have their own separate entries (stomach, duodenum), but the information in those entries is not so specifically concerned with abdominal pain as in the entries whose titles appear in small capital letters.

Another type of cross-reference is indicated by the entry:

ACID INDIGESTION See ACID STOMACH.

In this case, the information about acid indigestion will be found in the entry **ACID STOMACH.**

A third form of cross-reference is to this book's FIRST AID section, which precedes the encyclopedia. This reference always appears in large capital letters. Topics that you are referred to within the FIRST AID section are in small capitals, thus:

See POISONING in FIRST AID section for emergency treatment.

Be sure to examine carefully the illustrations that appear in the encyclopedia. Not only do they give a vivid representation of the text, but in many cases they furnish additional information.

Pronunciations are given for difficult medical terms within the encyclopedia articles. A "Pronunciation Key" follows the encyclopedia, on page 582.

A complete index to the entire book begins on page 607.

ABASIA The inability to walk because of a lack of muscular coordination or strength. Abasia (pronounced *a·bay′zhee·a*) is caused by damage to the brain or nervous system.

ABDOMEN The region of the body located below the chest and above the pelvis. The diaphragm, a muscular wall, divides the chest from the abdominal cavity. Inside this cavity are organs that play a key role in the vital processes of digestion or excretion: the liver, stomach, spleen, kidneys, pancreas, large intestine, small intestine, urinary bladder, gallbladder, and some of the sex organs. It also contains the vermiform appendix, regarded as a VESTIGIAL organ, or one that performed some necessary function in our very remote ancestors but appears to have no useful function in modern man. A membrane, the peritoneum, lines the abdominal cavity. A wall of muscle helps to hold the organs in place and give them support.

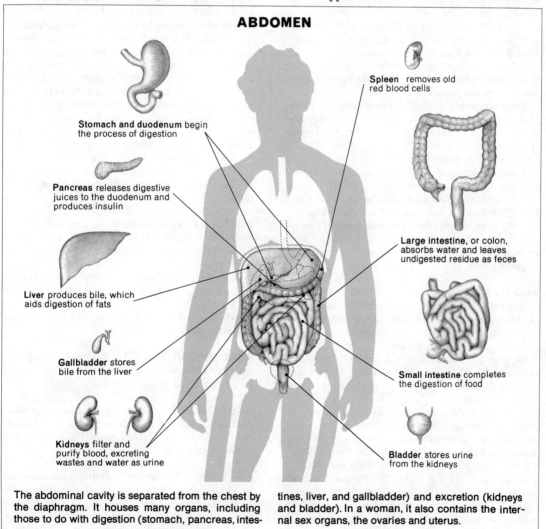

ABDOMEN

Spleen removes old red blood cells

Stomach and duodenum begin the process of digestion

Pancreas releases digestive juices to the duodenum and produces insulin

Large intestine, or colon, absorbs water and leaves undigested residue as feces

Liver produces bile, which aids digestion of fats

Gallbladder stores bile from the liver

Small intestine completes the digestion of food

Kidneys filter and purify blood, excreting wastes and water as urine

Bladder stores urine from the kidneys

The abdominal cavity is separated from the chest by the diaphragm. It houses many organs, including those to do with digestion (stomach, pancreas, intestines, liver, and gallbladder) and excretion (kidneys and bladder). In a woman, it also contains the internal sex organs, the ovaries and uterus.

317

ABDOMINAL PAIN indicates a disorder, not necessarily serious or lasting, of one of the internal organs that lie in the region between the chest and the pelvis. These organs include the stomach, liver, pancreas, spleen, gallbladder, urinary bladder, kidneys, appendix, and intestines; in women, the ovaries and the uterus.

If abdominal pain is severe or lasts more than a few hours or is accompanied by vomiting, fever, blood in the stool, or diarrhea, your doctor should be notified promptly. Do not take an enema, CATHARTIC, or LAXATIVE unless he instructs you specifically to do so.

Causes: Symptoms such as mild heartburn, belching, and a stuffed feeling in the upper part of the abdomen are usually a sign of no more than a slight case of INDIGESTION. This type of discomfort may often be relieved by taking an ANTACID. A dull pain and a "full feeling" unaccompanied by any other symptoms may be caused by CONSTIPATION. Mild cases can be treated with a laxative. If constipation continues, it may be the result of poor diet, insufficient exercise, emotional upset, or other causes. Your doctor's advice should be obtained.

A severe attack of indigestion combined with sharp pains in the chest may indicate heart disease. See also HEART DISEASE—SYMPTOMS.

FOOD POISONING or chemical poisoning will cause abdominal pain as well as nausea, vomiting, and diarrhea. See FIRST AID section for emergency treatment.

Some of the more common causes of recurring abdominal pain that require professional diagnosis and treatment are GALLSTONES, HEPATITIS, GASTRITIS, ULCER of the stomach or duodenum, kidney and bladder infections, COLITIS, and APPENDICITIS.

Some women suffer from lower abdominal cramps during MENSTRUATION. During pregnancy, such cramps may indicate a serious complication requiring immediate attention from a doctor.

ABORTION When a baby is born before it is sufficiently developed to live outside the uterus, doctors call the loss of the fetus an abortion. There are two types of abortion: (1) *spontaneous*, or natural, brought on by an accident or a defect in the fetus, and (2) *induced* abortion, which is produced deliberately. The term MISCARRIAGE is popularly used by laymen to describe a spontaneous, or natural, abortion.

In the past, the specific requirements for a legal, induced abortion varied from state to state. Since 1973 abortion during the first three months of pregnancy has been legal throughout the United States. During this period a woman, with her doctor's concurrence, has the right to terminate an unwanted pregnancy for any reason. After three months, however, the operation becomes increasingly complicated and risky and, in some states, is no longer legal.

If a woman wants to end her pregnancy, she should have this done during the first three months when an abortion by a licensed doctor under medically approved conditions is legal, simple, and usually not dangerous. See also DILATATION AND CURETTAGE; MISCARRIAGE.

ABRASION A skin scrape in which there is surface bleeding or oozing blood. Care should be taken to remove splinters or other foreign bodies that may be lodged in the skin. Clean tweezers that have been dipped in alcohol for five minutes are useful for this. Abrasions (pronounced *a·*bray′zhunz) tend to become infected easily and should be thoroughly cleansed with mild soap and water and then covered with a sterile dressing. Abrasions on the face may be left uncovered.

ABSCESS A localized area of infection in which there is pus formation. An abscess (pronounced ab′ses) may occur either internally or externally and is most often caused by BACTERIA. The bacteria may enter the body through a puncture or wound in the skin. Material containing pus-forming bacteria may originate in the mouth from infected gums, teeth, or tonsils, and spread internally. Abscesses of internal organs, such as lungs, liver, and kidneys, usually develop inconspicuously; the onset of symptoms may be abrupt, however. Elevated temperature and pain commonly develop. An external abscess is often accompanied by swelling and inflammation, and, if left untreated, may lead to GANGRENE or to BLOOD POISONING (septicemia). Thus, all suspected abscesses should be brought to the attention of your physician.

ACCIDENT For emergency treatment of accident victims, see the FIRST AID section. For advice on the prevention of accidents in and around the home, see Chapter 21.

In medicine, the term "accident" is used to mean any sudden event that is injurious to health. For example, a type of heart attack involving the blood vessels of the heart may be described as a cardiovascular accident.

ACCOMMODATION The change in the curve of the crystalline lens within the EYE which is necessary to bring an image into focus.

ACETANILID A compound, used in a number of medicines, that causes a lowering of the temperature in fever and brings relief from pain. (Pronounced as″*e·*tan′*i·*lid.)

ACETONE A colorless, volatile substance normally found in extremely small amounts in the blood and urine. In the absence of sufficient insulin in persons with DIABETES mellitus, large amounts of acetone (pronounced as″*e·*tohn) may develop in the blood and cause a condition, called diabetic acidosis, that can result in coma or death if untreated. A simple urine test will reveal the presence of abnormal concentrations of acetone. Its fruity smell may be detected on the breath of someone suffering from diabetic acidosis.

ACETOPHENETIDIN Another name for PHENACETIN. (Pronounced as″*e*·toh·*fe*·net′*i*·din.)

ACHALASIA Inability to relax the smooth muscle fibers of the gastrointestinal tract, so that food may pass into the stomach. Failure to relax and therefore to open the circular sphincter muscle, or cardia, at the entrance of the stomach, is called achalasia cardia. Achalasia (pronounced ak″*e*·lay′zh*a*) may be treated with muscle-relaxant drugs.

ACHE A pain that lasts for a while and, usually, is dull, in contrast to a pain that is sharp, or acute, such as a sudden twinge. An ache or pain that persists or becomes worse is nature's warning that something is wrong in the body, and a physician should be consulted. See also PAIN.

ACHILLES TENDON The large, strong tendon at the back of the ankle which connects the calf mus-

cles to the heel bone. Ill-fitting shoes may cause the Achilles (pronounced *a*·kil′eez) tendon to become strained, resulting in pain in the area of the heel.

ACHLORHYDRIA A stomach condition in which there is no hydrochloric acid in the gastric juice. Although it may produce no ill effects (in which case it needs no treatment), it is also a feature of pernicious ANEMIA and of stomach CANCER. (Pronounced ay″klor·hie′dree·*a*.)

ACHONDROPLASIA A type of DWARFISM in which the long bones of the arms and legs (but not the bones of the rest of the body) do not grow to full size. The condition is inherited and its cause is not known. (Pronounced ay″kon·dro·play′zh*a*.)

ACID A class of chemical compounds which have the distinctive property of tasting sour. (The Latin word *acidus* means "sour.") Technically, an acid may be defined as a substance that forms salts and water in reaction to a base, such as an ALKALI. Typical strong acids are nitric, sulfuric (used in storage batteries), and hydrochloric; weak acids are those such as acetic acid, found in vinegar. Acids can be manufactured and are widely used in industry. A number of strong acids, such as nitric and sulfuric, must be handled with great care since they can inflict serious ACID BURN.

Acids are produced in animals and plants as part of their normal life processes. Hydrochloric acid is secreted in the stomach and plays an important role in digestion. An acid may be neutralized (made to lose its acidity) by an alkali, such as sodium bicarbonate. See also ACID STOMACH.

ACID BURN A burn that is caused by a strong acid or caustic alkali, such as nitric or sulfuric acid or lye. Both acids and alkalies can cause serious damage to the skin and eyes, so instant action is called for. Bathe the burn immediately and continue to wash it with cool water. Be sure to remove all contaminated clothing. If large areas of the body are affected, get the victim into a shower, if possible, and keep him under the running water; otherwise, pour water over him.

Medical assistance is essential, so while you are giving first aid treatment, have someone telephone a physician (or do it yourself, but only after you have bathed the affected areas for 10 minutes). Keep applying water to the burned area for 30 minutes while awaiting the arrival of the doctor. If no doctor is available, take the person to a nearby hospital emergency room.

If an acid or alkali has come in contact with the eye, rinse it gently with water. Pull the eyelids back to hold the eye wide open so that all the acid is washed out. Keep up the treatment for 15 minutes. Telephone the doctor as quickly as possible.

For further details, see the FIRST AID section.

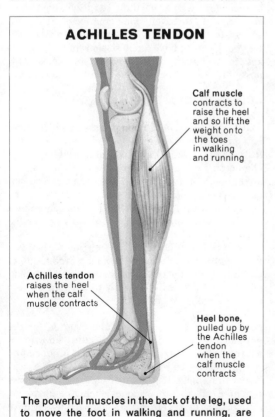

ACHILLES TENDON

Calf muscle contracts to raise the heel and so lift the weight onto the toes in walking and running

Achilles tendon raises the heel when the calf muscle contracts

Heel bone, pulled up by the Achilles tendon when the calf muscle contracts

The powerful muscles in the back of the leg, used to move the foot in walking and running, are attached to the heel by the Achilles tendon.

ACID INDIGESTION See ACID STOMACH.

ACIDOSIS A condition in which there is an insufficient amount of SODIUM BICARBONATE (alkali) in the blood, thus upsetting the blood's normal acid-alkali balance; also called acid blood. Acidosis (pronounced as"*i*·doh'sis) is a serious condition that may occur in DIABETES, KIDNEY DISEASE, and some other illnesses. The underlying cause must be treated to remedy the condition.

ACID STOMACH A term that, like acid indigestion and hyperacidity, is popularly used to describe stomach discomfort, or an upset stomach.

Mild stomach discomforts are often the result of stomach irritation produced by eating the wrong thing at the wrong time. Partaking of food that is too highly seasoned or fried in grease, overindulgence in alcoholic beverages, and eating in a hurry or to excess are common causes of stomach distress. Other possible factors are nervousness and dining in unpleasant, noisy surroundings.

If you avoid the cause of the discomfort, your stomach will normally right itself soon. Relief from mild discomfort may be obtained by taking an antacid, such as SODIUM BICARBONATE (from one half to a whole teaspoonful) in a glass of orange juice or water. You may prefer taking another type of antacid in tablet form.

If the condition does not clear up promptly or becomes more severe, you should consult your family physician. See also INDIGESTION.

ACNE An inflammation of the sebaceous (oil) glands just beneath the surface of the skin, causing pimples, BLACKHEADS, whiteheads, and, in extreme cases, infected cysts and scarred skin. Acne is a disorder that usually sets in at puberty. Cases may be brief and mild or chronic and severe, but, in one form or another, acne affects as many as 80 percent of all teenagers. Areas most frequently affected are the face, shoulders, chest, and back.

When adolescence begins, glandular activity increases. The sebaceous glands secrete a greater amount of the oil, called SEBUM, that lubricates the skin. The excessive oil clogs the pores, causing them to dilate. This increases the likelihood of further infection.

A mild case of acne will consist of no more than a few pimples and blackheads. If the sebum seeps under the surface of the skin instead of coming out to the surface, the surrounding tissue is irritated, and a CYST is formed. At this stage, your doctor should be consulted. He may recommend treatment by a skin specialist (DERMATOLOGIST), to prevent a more serious bacterial infection. In severe acne, the skin of the upper torso and the face may be so seriously damaged that permanent scars will result. Prompt medical attention to early symptoms is, therefore, extremely important.

What Not to Do: Young people with a tendency to skin eruptions should avoid chocolate, nuts (including peanut butter), fatty and fried foods, seafoods, spicy foods, cola and other sugar-rich drinks, and too much whole milk (skim milk is preferable). Sugary foods should also be kept to a minimum; cakes, pastry, pie, and alcoholic drinks should be eliminated. Because many persons who have acne are growing youngsters, it is preferable to have them obtain complete diet instructions from their physicians.

Hands should be kept away from the face; squeezing pimples, blackheads, or whiteheads with the fingers must be avoided, and a special effort must be made to stop any unconscious picking at scabs. Washing the skin too vigorously or with a washcloth that is not absolutely clean can inflame a sensitive area.

Treatment: Mild cases of acne are usually brief and are likely to disappear if proper care is exercised with regard to diet and cleanliness. More severe cases should be treated by a doctor. When the skin has been scarred by acne, there are medical and surgical techniques that can help repair the damage. Try not to let the acne reach that degree of severity.

Severe cases of acne can be emotionally upsetting to teenagers, who are acutely sensitive about their appearance. Moreover, since emotional upsets can aggravate the condition, it is sometimes advisable for youngsters to have a few sessions of psychotherapy to deal with such emotional problems. This possibility should be discussed with the doctor.

ACNE ROSACEA See RHINOPHYMA.

ACROMEGALY A chronic disease in which there is a gradual but conspicuous enlargement of the features of the face, the hands, and the feet. These characteristic symptoms are the result of exaggerated growth of bone endings and cartilage, brought on by excessive secretion of growth hormones in the PITUITARY GLAND. The condition is often caused by a benign TUMOR and may be treated by X ray, or the tumor may be removed by surgery.

Acromegaly (pronounced ak"roh·meg'*a*·lee) is a disease of adults. Excessive hormone production in children causes the condition known as GIANTISM, in which the individual may grow to a height of from six and a half to eight feet.

ACTH The commonly used abbreviation for the *a*drenocorticotrophic *h*ormone, also known as adrenocorticotrophin. The hormone is produced by the pituitary gland and stimulates the adrenal cortex of the ADRENAL GLANDS. It controls the release by these glands of hormones such as CORTISONE.

Injections of ACTH (pronounce each letter) have been found to have effects similar to those of cortisone. It is not effective, however, when taken orally or applied externally. It was once used for the temporary relief of pain in severe cases of rheumatoid arthritis, rheumatic fever, and asthma, but it is a symptom reliever and not a cure. Because ACTH can have serious side effects, including diabetes, personality changes, and other disorders, it has been largely replaced by STEROID hormones.

ACTINOMYCOSIS A disease caused by infection with the ray FUNGUS (*Actinomyces israelii*). Also called streptotricosis, actinomycosis (pronounced ak"ti·noh·mie·koh'sis) may involve the mouth or throat (in half of all cases), lungs, intestines, the skin, or other organs. The fungus tends to form abscesses which continuously drain to the surface. If untreated, actinomycosis may last for months or years. ANTIBIOTICS, SULFONAMIDES, and surgical measures may be used in treatment. The disease is widespread in cattle and swine, in which it is called lumpy jaw because it most commonly affects the jaws of these animals.

ACUPUNCTURE An ancient Chinese medical system in which needles are inserted at specific points under the skin to cure or alleviate pain or diseases. In recent years it has also been developed, in China, as a general ANESTHETIC for major SURGERY. Under acupuncture (pronounced ak"yoo·pungk'cher) anesthetic the patient can talk and eat and, in some instances, walk out of the operating room after surgery.

This needle therapy is based on the traditional Chinese theory that a form of "inner energy" endlessly circulates within the living body in a network of pathways, or meridians. By stimulating strategic points along the meridians, the acupuncturist is able to "tune up" a particular internal organ or physiological function. Such a theory has no known basis in orthodox Western medical science. In spite of this, acupuncture does work, especially in relieving pain and treating functional diseases such as INSOMNIA, NEURALGIA, and ASTHMA.

Although American physicians were initially dubious about acupuncture when a wave of interest swept over the country in 1971, the medical profession is now giving it careful study and some doctors are incorporating it into their own practice.

Acupuncture is no panacea; and if practiced by an inexperienced or incompetent person, it can be harmful. If a patient wants acupuncture in the United States, he should choose an acupuncturist who is also a licensed physician, or works in collaboration with one, or belongs to an acupuncture clinic, now licensed in some states.

ACUTE Sharp or intense, as, for example, an acute pain. When applied to a disease, "acute" means that the condition is marked by relatively severe symptoms and that it comes on suddenly and is of comparatively short duration. An acute disease is

not necessarily a serious one. Acute indigestion may be unpleasant, but the attack usually does not last long. By contrast, a CHRONIC disease is one that persists for a long period of time.

ACUTE YELLOW ATROPHY A serious disease of the liver, in which many of the liver cells are damaged or killed. It may be caused by poisons such as arsenic; by a large overdose of a drug such as acetaminophen, used to reduce fever and lessen pain; or by virus infections. Rarely, it may be a side effect of pregnancy. The liver shrinks and the victim suffers from JAUNDICE and TOXEMIA. The basic cause is treated, if possible.

ADAM'S APPLE A projection at the front of the neck, formed by the thyroid cartilage of the LARYNX. It is more prominent in men than in women.

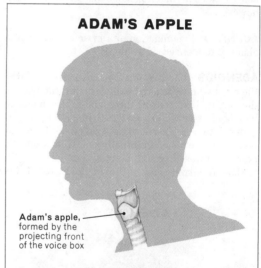

ADAM'S APPLE

Adam's apple, formed by the projecting front of the voice box

A pointed piece of cartilage at the front of the voice box, or larynx, sticks out on the neck and forms the Adam's apple. A man's Adam's apple is more prominent than a woman's because his larynx is larger to hold larger vocal cords.

ADDICTION The state of feeling compelled to take certain foods or drugs. Some drinks, such as alcohol, and some drugs and medicines, such as heroin and codeine, are addictive. The body becomes accustomed to them and may eventually become dependent on them. An addict experiences an intense craving for a particular drug and when deprived of it becomes physically ill and distressed.

Other drugs, such as marijuana, may be nonaddictive in the sense that the body does not develop a need for them, but the user can become dependent on them for the feeling of psychological comfort or escape they produce. Such nonaddictive drugs are thought by many medical authorities to be potentially dangerous because the persistent user may seek "bigger and better" relief by recourse to "hard," or habit-forming, drugs.

See also ALCOHOLISM; DRUG ADDICTION; NARCOTIC; and the names of individual drugs.

ADDISON'S DISEASE A disease caused by insufficient hormone production by the cortex (outer part) of the adrenal glands, one of which is located on top of each of the two kidneys. The insufficiency may be a result of ATROPHY or of infection.

The disease causes a loss of salt and water in the body and a decrease of fluid in the blood. Some of the symptoms are muscular weakness, darkening of the skin, weight loss, vomiting, diarrhea, and a drop in blood pressure. Since the development of purified and synthetic CORTISONE and other allied hormones, successful treatment of even the more serious cases has been possible, and afflicted persons have been able to lead a normal life. Some may need extra salt, however.

ADENITIS Inflammation of a LYMPH NODE or of a gland. (Pronounced ad·e·nie'tis.)

ADENOIDS The two small glands located behind the point where the nasal passages enter the back of the throat. Like tonsils, these glands are made of lymphoid tissue whose role it is to block the entry of germs into the RESPIRATORY SYSTEM and destroy them. The adenoids are usually enlarged when the nose and throat become infected.

Marked enlargement of the adenoids, which oc-

curs usually in children, blocks the escape of air from the nose and causes the child to breathe through his mouth. Enlargement can also block the Eustachian tubes, which connect the middle parts of the ears with the back of the throat, causing infection and pain in the middle ear. This may eventually interfere with hearing. Thus, repeated infections of the adenoids may cause your doctor to recommend their surgical removal, a relatively minor operation. It is sometimes performed together with a TONSILLECTOMY, or removal of the tonsils. This joint operation is often referred to as a T and A.

ADENOMA A benign TUMOR, which may produce pain or other symptoms by exerting pressure on neighboring tissues. An adenoma (pronounced ad"e·noh'ma) can occur anywhere in the body.

ADHESION A band of fibrous tissue that connects two surfaces within the body that are normally unconnected. Adhesions may result from inflammation or from abnormal healing of a lesion or a surgical wound.

ADIPOSE Fatty, or containing fat. Fat is stored in the adipose (pronounced ad'i·pohs) tissues of the body.

ADIPOSIS DOLOROSA A rare disease in which painful fatty nodules or swellings form throughout the body. The chief victims are women who have passed middle age, and sometimes it may be necessary for a surgeon to remove painful lumps. (Pronounced ad"i·poh'sis doh"lo·roh'sa.)

ADOLESCENCE The period of life during which a boy becomes a man and a girl, a woman. Roughly speaking, it embraces the teenage years, but usually begins earlier in girls. There are marked physical changes in the body, and with these come emotional changes and problems, as the adolescent prepares to play an adult role in life. Adolescence begins with puberty, the period when the child shows signs of sexual maturation.

The Adolescent Boy: In boys, puberty occurs commonly between the ages of 13 and 16. The genitals grow in size, and the boy exhibits the beginnings of a moustache and a beard. Hair appears in the genital region and the armpits. The boy's voice changes and assumes a deeper tone. His body grows rapidly, and his shoulders develop; sometimes he shoots up several inches in a relatively short period. He is also likely to exhibit a bigger appetite than his father.

In this period, the boy may have seminal emissions during the night. The TESTICLES have begun to secrete sperm cells (the male element in fertilization), and these are discharged in the nocturnal emission. Sometimes there is a dream, sexual in content, associated with the discharge. Nocturnal emissions are normal, natural happenings in adoles-

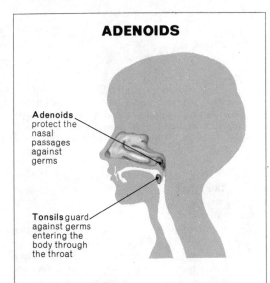

ADENOIDS

Adenoids protect the nasal passages against germs

Tonsils guard against germs entering the body through the throat

The adenoids are masses of lymphoid tissue lying at the back of the nasal passages where, with the tonsils, they guard against infection from germs in the air breathed in. Swollen adenoids can block the airways and prevent the patient from breathing through his nose.

cence. It is advisable to tell the youngster about them before they occur, so that he will not react with apprehension.

MASTURBATION is a common sexual outlet for boys at this age. In our grandparents' time, people believed that it would inevitably have serious consequences, such as insanity or deterioration of the body. Today, we know that it does not lead to mental or physical disease. Actually, masturbation's worst effect is the feelings of guilt it arouses, particularly when the child is severely reprimanded or punished by his parents. The wise parent ignores it.

The Adolescent Girl: The girl enters puberty earlier than the boy—as a rule, between the ages of 11 and 13. In some girls it may commence at 10 or 14 or later. The girl begins to lose her boyish figure; the breasts develop and the hips become rounder. Hair appears in the genital region and armpits, and MENSTRUATION begins.

Sometimes there is considerable delay in the first appearance of menstruation, or a girl may remain flat-chested long after her contemporaries have rounded out into buxom womanhood. This is no cause for alarm; some girls bloom later than others. However, if menstruation or any other feature of adolescence is long delayed, this should be brought to the attention of the family physician.

The mother should point out to her daughter that menstruation, when it comes, is not a "curse" or illness or anything nasty or dirty; that there may be cramps at the start of a period, and the girl may have to limit her activities during a heavy flow; but all of this is a normal, healthy part of womanhood.

Skin Troubles: Adolescence brings with it hormonal changes. These often lead to skin complaints, including ACNE, boils, BLACKHEADS, and pimples. With proper care and patience, most of these conditions will disappear, but if they do not, or if they are unusually severe, a doctor should be consulted.

Emotional Problems: Adolescence is usually accompanied by a variety of emotional problems. The child has grown to physical adulthood and wants to be treated as an adult. He wants to make his own decisions. He sees his parents in a new perspective and is conspicuously aware of their weaknesses and shortcomings. The girl may become her mother's worst critic; the boy will frequently be in conflict with his father. Parents may feel that all of their efforts in child-rearing have been for naught and wonder where they went wrong.

It is helpful to realize that adolescents have always been in rebellion against their elders. The "generation gap" is not a characteristic of just our own time; youngsters in the past may have had to conceal their feelings, but inwardly they reacted just as hostilely against the limitations and discipline imposed by their parents.

In this difficult period, parents would be wise to remember that while the adolescent is profoundly sensitive and insecure, he has at the same time a deep need to be recognized and treated as an adult. Psychological support can be provided better by sympathetic listening and friendly but firm advice now and then, than by authoritarian scolding or constant nagging. Praise should not be withheld if it is merited. Adolescents complain with some justification that their elders see only their faults and never their good points.

Many parents find it possible to allow their maturing sons and daughters increasing responsibility and independence, while continuing to offer them firm and sympathetic guidance. In such a family atmosphere, it may not be very long before a lasting, affectionate—and calmer—relationship is achieved.

ADRENAL GLANDS A pair of ENDOCRINE GLANDS, from one to two inches in length, located at the top of the kidneys. They secrete a number of hormones, including ADRENALINE and CORTISONE, which influence many processes in the body.

ADRENALINE A hormone that is produced by the adrenal glands. When the body is under stress, the glands increase their secretion of adrenaline and pour it into the blood, which carries it to every part of the body. The hormone speeds up the beating of the heart. It also causes an increase in blood pressure and enables the muscles to work faster and longer.

Adrenaline (or epinephrine, as it is also known) has extensive uses in medicine. It is used as a stimulant in certain heart conditions and is helpful in cases of bronchial asthma and shock. Adrenaline is produced synthetically or is extracted from the adrenal glands of animals.

AFRICAN SLEEPING SICKNESS See SLEEPING SICKNESS.

AFTERBIRTH The tissues that are forced out of the mother's body, normally without pain, by contraction of the UTERUS after childbirth. They consist of the PLACENTA, a mass of tissue that was attached to the wall of the uterus, and the UMBILICAL CORD, by which the infant was connected to the placenta. Both are rich in blood vessels; through them food passed from the bloodstream of the mother's body to the unborn child, and waste products were eliminated from the fetus.

AFTERPAINS (afterbirth pains) Pains that some mothers may experience for the first 24 to 72 hours, or somewhat longer, following childbirth. They are not unlike the pains associated with menstruation. The uterus is responsible: freed of the fetus, it begins to contract in the process of returning to its normal size. There may also be discomfort in the area of the perineum located between the vaginal opening and the rectum. (See EPISIOTOMY.)

Relief may usually be obtained by taking aspirin

or any similar mild analgesic three or four times a day. If the pain is severe, the physician will prescribe a more powerful pain reliever.

AGALACTIA The condition of being completely unable to produce milk after childbirth. This is a relatively rare occurrence; much more common is the condition of a mother being able to produce some, but not enough, milk. (See LACTATION.) In agalactia (pronounced a"ga·lak'sha), there may be pains in the breasts, and these pains occasionally spread to the back. Anemia, malnutrition, childbearing at a very late or at a very early age, and emotional disturbance are among the possible causes of this trouble.

AGAR A product obtained from red algae (tiny water plants) and seaweed. Its main uses are as a laxative and as a laboratory medium, or culture, on which to grow bacteria. It is also known as agar-agar (pronounced ay'gahr ay'gahr).

AGGLUTINATION TESTS Laboratory tests used to identify different types of BACTERIA, diagnose infections, determine blood groups, or establish pregnancy. "Agglutination" (pronounced a·gloo"ti·nay'shun) means "clumping." When certain types of cells, such as typhoid germs, are brought in contact with serum that has been immunized against them, the blood cells react by clumping together, thus providing a positive indication of the presence of typhoid fever. Urine is used in the agglutination test for pregnancy (see PREGNANCY SIGNS AND TESTS).

AGING Today, more people are surviving to an advanced age than ever before. Life expectancy has been spectacularly increased by medical science, which, in North America and Europe, has virtually wiped out such killers as diphtheria and smallpox. A newborn American baby now has a life expectancy of 71.3 years. This compares with a life expectancy of 63 years in 1940 and of 47 years in 1900. Furthermore, a woman who is between the age of 60 and 65 can nowadays look forward to 21.1 additional years of life; a man in the same age bracket can expect to have 16.3 more years.

Of course, old age has its discomforts. The arthritic ailments and digestive disturbances of the elderly are well known; eyesight, hearing, and the functions of other organs undergo changes. However, many of the physical problems of aging can be helped by prompt and thorough medical attention. For example, a HEARING AID can be worn to amplify sounds. Well-fitting dentures improve the appearance, besides being of help in eating. If an operation is needed to remedy a condition, such as osteoarthritis, it can often be performed even on quite an elderly patient. Surgical advances in recent years have greatly minimized the risks of operations.

Growing old has many compensations, physical and mental. Old people do not catch colds as often as most young people, and they have gained a degree of immunity to infectious disease. Most have a rich store of experience behind them and can bring a ripeness of judgment to bear on the problems of living. Contrary to popular belief, memory does not necessarily fade with age, but may hold up well if it is sustained by interest. See also GERIATRICS.

AGNOSIA A disorder of the brain in which a person cannot correctly interpret the information from his senses and understand what goes on around him. It may be caused by blocking of blood vessels to the brain by a BLOOD CLOT or by a TUMOR. Treatment of agnosia (pronounced ag·noh'zha) varies according to the cause of the condition.

AGRANULOCYTOSIS An acute disorder in which there is an extreme decrease in the number of granular white cells, or granulocytes, in the bloodstream. In most cases a chemical or a medicine is responsible. Certain ANTIHISTAMINES, ANTIBIOTICS, and SULFONAMIDES may produce agranulocytosis (pronounced a·gran"yool·oh"sie·toh'sis) in a person who is sensitive to them. Exposure to radioactivity may also be responsible.

The granulocytes play an important part in fighting infection. When they are missing, the mucous membranes and other susceptible areas may become infected. Common symptoms are sore throat, ulcers in the mouth, rapid pulse, and high fever.

Treatment includes removal of the toxic compound and the use of antibiotics to which the patient is not sensitive. Cortisone may be helpful. Transplantation of fresh, healthy bone marrow may prove to be an effective treatment in severe cases.

AGUE A chill. Ague (pronounced ay'gyoo) is also the fever associated with MALARIA.

AIR POLLUTION AND HEALTH Air pollution poses an increasingly serious health problem in the city of today. Everywhere in urban centers, burning is going on: oil, gas, and coal are burned in factories and homes; gasoline and oil are burned by cars and trucks; garbage is burned in city incinerators. The result is the release into the atmosphere around us of vast quantities of ashes, soot, gas, and other noxious substances. When these pollutants are held close to the earth's surface by special weather conditions, the problem of smog becomes a menace. In New York City, Los Angeles, London, and other major cities, severe smog has caused the deaths of hundreds of susceptible persons.

Air pollution appears to be contributing significantly to a rise in the incidence of a number of diseases. One of these is EMPHYSEMA, a serious disorder of the lungs. Chronic BRONCHITIS is also severely aggravated by air pollution. Increasingly, pollutants are implicated in cases of LUNG CANCER, which is more common among people living in the city than in the country. Pollution can also be a cause of ALLERGY. Further research over a period of time may reveal additional effects that prolonged exposure to air pollution has upon the health of our urban population.

There is only one solution to this grave problem: control of the wastes being poured into the air. Some cities now regulate the amount of burning that is allowed under smog conditions. Attempts are being made to persuade or compel industrial offenders to convert to nonpolluting burning processes, and new automobiles are being equipped with pollution-reducing devices. But the battle is a complex one that must be fought on many fronts. The struggle for air-pollution control merits the support of every citizen interested in his own health and the health of his children.

AIRSICKNESS See MOTION SICKNESS.

ALBINO A person lacking melanin, the dark pigment that gives color to skin, hair, and eyes. The albino (pronounced al·bie′noh) is characterized by naturally platinum-blond hair, pink skin (the blood flowing through the capillaries shows through the skin), and a pinkish tone in the eyes. Albinos' eyes, in particular, are extremely sensitive to light, and their vision is often defective. Albinism is not a disease, but a hereditary defect, which affects about one person in 10,000.

ALBUMIN A protein that is present in many plant and animal tissues. It occurs in the blood as serum albumin, in which form it helps to regulate the distribution of water in the body. When albumin (pronounced al·byoo′min) is present in the urine, it may be a sign of damage to the kidneys, though it is found occasionally in the urine of healthy persons. See also ALBUMINURIA.

ALBUMINURIA A condition in which there is ALBUMIN present in the urine. This is determined by URINALYSIS (microscopic or chemical examination of the urine). Albuminuria (pronounced al·byoo″mi·noor′ee·a) may be present for only a short time and may be of no particular significance. It may occur, for example, after strenuous exercise, or it may simply be a harmless peculiarity in some individuals. However, it can also be a symptom of kidney damage. Only a physician is qualified to determine what causes its presence in the urine. See also KIDNEY DISEASE.

ALCOHOL Any of a large group of colorless liquid compounds, all of which are toxic to some degree. When used alone, the term "alcohol" usually refers to ethyl alcohol.

Ethyl alcohol is less toxic than other alcohols. It may be taken internally in the form of alcoholic beverages. It is often used medically to stimulate the appetites of convalescent or elderly persons. It is also used as a skin disinfectant, as a cooling lubricant for rubbing, in TINCTURES and lotions, and to dissolve other ingredients in medicines.

Denatured alcohol is ethyl alcohol to which something has been added to make it unfit to drink. (The high taxes that make drinking alcohol so expensive do not apply to denatured alcohol.) Denatured alcohol should never be drunk, but it can be used on the skin.

Isopropyl alcohol is also used as a rubbing alcohol. It is too toxic for internal use.

Methyl alcohol, or wood alcohol, is used commercially as a fuel and a solvent. It is very toxic. Blindness and death have frequently resulted from drinking methyl alcohol.

Alcoholic Beverages: Ethyl alcohol is produced by the fermenting action of yeast on grains such as corn, barley, and rye, and on potatoes. Pure alcohol is obtained by distilling the fermented product. Beer is made by brewing and fermenting cereals such as barley, using hops for flavoring. It has a low alcoholic content, about 5 percent. Wines are produced by the natural fermentation of the juice of the grape or other fruits. When the fermentation process stops, the percentage of alcohol in the wine ranges from 7 to 15 percent. Some wines, such as sherry and port, are fortified by the addition of pure distilled alcohol, and may contain 16 to 18 percent alcohol or more.

Liquors, such as whisky, gin, and vodka, have a much higher alcoholic strength which is expressed as "proof." An 80-proof liquor is 40 percent alcohol by volume; a 100-proof liquor is 50 percent alcohol. To determine the alcoholic content, divide the proof by two.

How Alcohol Affects the Body: Alcohol is a food, something like sugar, furnishing energy (CALORIES) but no other nutrients required by the body. (These are called empty calories.) Alcohol begins to be absorbed into the bloodstream as soon as it enters the stomach. The blood carries it to the liver, then to the heart, the lungs, and the brain, where it usually has its most important effects. Alcohol acts as a depressant—that is, it slows down activity and impairs the efficiency of the central nervous system. The anxieties and inhibitions that reside in the higher brain centers are cast off, and the drinker goes through a stage when he feels carefree and happy.

Many states have established a blood-alcohol level of 0.1 percent as evidence of intoxication. In this concentration, alcohol acts like an anesthetic on the brain and nervous system. Perception and the thought process are further slowed down, and it becomes difficult to coordinate one's movements. The ability to react quickly is lost. A person who has been drinking is in no condition to drive.

Alcohol and Health: There is nothing unhealthy about taking one, or even two, average-strength (two-ounce) drinks of hard liquor per day. Taken this way, alcohol can serve as a relaxant and as a stimulant to appetite.

However, excessive indulgence in alcohol can produce the chronic condition known as ALCOHOLISM. There are many disorders in which alcohol should be avoided altogether. Among these are epilepsy, liver disorders such as hepatitis, and stomach or duodenal ulcers.

Alcohol has a high caloric content; persons who are overweight should not drink. Alcohol should be avoided by the person who is taking sedatives. Tranquilizers, antihistamines, and liquor also make a perilous combination. If you are called upon to give first aid, do *not* offer alcohol as a restorative or treatment for any condition.

ALCOHOLICS ANONYMOUS (AA)

An organization of men and women who have overcome the problem of chronic ALCOHOLISM and are helping others to do the same. Through meetings and discussion groups, the alcoholic or potential alcoholic can listen to, and learn from, the experiences of others who have faced alcoholism. He is also given the opportunity to air his own problems. If there is no listing for Alcoholics Anonymous in your phone book, write: P.O. Box 459, Grand Central Station, New York, New York 10017, the central address of Alcoholics Anonymous for North America.

ALCOHOLISM

The marked toxic effects of alcohol on the central nervous system and various organs; also, compulsive and excessive use of alcohol.

Acute alcoholism, or intoxication, is experienced by anyone who takes too many drinks, whether or not he is a habitual user of alcohol. The symptoms depend upon the amount of alcohol in the system, and they range from unsteadiness of gait to complete loss of muscular coordination, from impairment of mental processes to complete blackout, or COMA. Usually, the symptoms disappear as the alcohol is slowly burned up by the body's metabolism. In extreme cases of acute alcohol poisoning, death may result. Recovery from an episode of acute alcoholism is often accompanied by a HANGOVER—headache, nausea, and dehydration. Some of these effects stem in part from substances other than alcohol, called the congeners, which are responsible for the distinct differences in taste and effect between the various alcoholic beverages. In general, the effects of the congeners in an alcoholic drink are minor compared to the effects of the alcohol itself.

The pleasant initial effects of alcohol are well known. Drinking is a normal accompaniment of many social occasions. Social drinking is not commonly regarded as a hazard to health, but it should be remembered that a large number of highway accidents are due to drivers' drinking. Thus, even occasional use of alcohol may be regarded as a major cause of disablement and death in the United States.

Chronic alcoholism, the compulsive use of alcohol over a period of time, is generally regarded as a distinct disease. As with many psychiatric disorders, there is evidence that chronic alcoholism may be associated with a metabolic defect. That is, alcohol may be used in the body's system in a way that makes it more toxic to the potential alcoholic than to the average occasional drinker. Some groups of people, such as Northern Europeans and American Indians, seem to be especially prone to alcoholism, but this may be due to culture rather than to any basic physiological difference. In groups whose religion or culture frown on or prohibit the use of alcohol, chronic alcoholism is of course rarely seen.

Given the basic need for relief from anxiety and depression that characterizes the potential alcoholic, drinking produces a well-defined progression from social drinking to problem drinking to physical dependence (ADDICTION). As social drinking increases, an increased tolerance is developed, and the individual needs more alcohol than before to produce a given effect. Gradually, a compulsive need for alcohol develops. There are changes in personality. The problem drinker becomes suspicious and resentful, and these feelings are increased by criticism and rejection by family and friends. There is a loss of appetite, which leads to an unbalanced diet and vitamin deficiency. Health, in general, declines. The person may have a bloated appearance and suffer from digestive and circulatory disorders. Eventually the liver, the heart, and the nerves are involved. A sudden decrease in tolerance of alcohol may develop, along with episodes of DELIRIUM TREMENS, CONVULSIONS, and DEMENTIA. Death is also among the eventualities.

The physical effects of chronic alcoholism can be avoided or sometimes reversed only by abstinence from alcohol. Vitamin supplements and a careful diet are required to correct the effects of poor nutrition. If the physical condition of the person is poor, he is usually confined to a hospital for intensive treatment of the physical symptoms.

Various treatments have been tried to help the alcoholic abstain from alcohol. A treatment that is effective with one individual may be unsuccessful with another. SEDATIVES should be avoided. Drugs, such as ANTABUSE, which lead to extremely unpleasant effects when combined with alcohol, may help to create a decided distaste for it. It may be necessary to consult a PSYCHIATRIST for diagnosis and treatment of the underlying psychiatric disorder. Counseling of the immediate family is often needed as well, in order to counteract the adverse emotional climate of which the alcoholic may be both creator and victim. GROUP THERAPY has proved to be remarkably successful in treating chronic alcoholism.

ALCOHOLICS ANONYMOUS (AA), an organization of former alcoholics, offers effective and understanding support to compulsive users of alcohol who are seeking help. Another organization, Al-Anon Family Groups (and Alateen for its teenage members) offers self-help programs for families and friends who are adversely affected by somebody else's drinking problem. For information about an Al-Anon Group near you, write to the organization's international headquarters at P.O. Box 182, Madison Square Station, New York, New York 10010.

ALCOHOL RUB A procedure, sometimes recommended by a physician, in which alcohol is occasionally applied externally to reduce a high fever or, more frequently, to give a patient a sense of well-being during confinement in bed. Alcohol rubs also help prevent infection of the skin and bedsores.

The benefits of an alcohol rub are due partly to the alcohol itself and partly to the gentle massage used in applying it. Alcohol cools the skin as it evaporates; it also has a mildly antiseptic action. The massage stimulates circulation.

The best way to give an alcohol rub is to apply the liquid with a saturated sponge or the bare hand to various parts of the body, one at a time. Arms, legs, back, chest, and so on should be exposed individually for rubbing and then covered with a sheet. Remember that alcohol is very painful if applied, or permitted to drop, on the genitals. If the alcohol is used undiluted rather than in combination with water, precautions should be taken to protect the patient from overexposure to the fumes. It is useful to warm the bottle of alcohol to body temperature by putting it under hot water—but never near a flame!

Commercial preparations called rubbing alcohol are available in drugstores. They are usually ethyl (denatured) or isopropyl alcohol and must not be taken internally. See FIRST AID section for treatment of poisoning by alcohol.

ALIMENTARY CANAL The route along which food passes from the mouth to the rectum. (Pronounced al″i·men′ta·ree.) It is also called the digestive tract. See also DIGESTION.

ALKALI A substance that neutralizes an ACID by chemical reaction. Strictly, the word "alkali" (pronounced al′ka·lie) applies only to certain very active or corrosive substances, such as caustic soda, quicklime, and ammonia. In the body, the principal acid neutralizer, or base, is SODIUM BICARBONATE, which is manufactured from carbon dioxide and from sodium obtained from salt in the diet. It is alkaline (that is, it resembles alkali), but it is much gentler in its action than the true alkalis. Sodium bicarbonate helps to maintain the delicate balance between acidity and alkalinity that is necessary for the normal chemical activity in the body.

The blood of a healthy person is slightly alkaline. The digestive juices from the pancreas and the liver are alkaline. The gastric juice in the stomach, on the other hand, is decidedly acid. Thus stomach acidity is a normal, healthy condition. It is true that excessive acidity is found in some serious disorders, such as gastric ULCER. However, gastric ulcer and other serious stomach ailments cannot be cured simply by swallowing an ALKALIZER or ANTACID. If you have persistent stomach distress, do not waste time trying to treat yourself with medicines supposed to counteract acidity. Instead, have a doctor examine you and begin treatment related to the real cause of your trouble.

ALKALIZER A substance, such as sodium bicarbonate, that reduces acidity in the digestive tract. An alkalizer, when prescribed by your doctor, helps to neutralize excess acid in the body system. Usually it is taken for an upset stomach.

INDIGESTION and heartburn (PYROSIS) are among the commonest disorders, since the stomach is one of the most abused organs of the body. Perhaps the most readily available and least expensive remedy is SODIUM BICARBONATE, also known as bicarbonate of soda and baking soda. A level teaspoonful in a glass of water will usually provide relief for a mildly upset stomach. Do not make a habit of taking it, however, for if you do it may produce excess alkalinity—the opposite of acidity. Sodium bicarbonate should be avoided by persons on salt-restricted (low-sodium) diets.

ALKALOID A class of chemicals that includes many drugs. Most alkaloids occur naturally in plants, although some are now made synthetically. They include atropine (belladonna) from deadly nightshade, digitalis from foxglove, morphine and codeine from the opium poppy, nicotine from tobacco, and strychnine from nux vomica. Many alkaloids are NARCOTICS, and all are poisonous. (Pronounced al′ka·loyd.)

ALKALOSIS A condition in which there is a significant rise in the amount of alkali in the blood or the plasma (the fluid part of the blood). The disorder may develop when there is a heavy loss of acid from the body as a result of sickness accompanied by protracted vomiting. Alkalosis (pronounced al″ka·loh′sis) may also result when the person has been taking an antacid, or alkalizer, such as sodium bicarbonate in excessive amounts, usually for the relief of peptic ULCER or INDIGESTION. The person may experience a prickling feeling and a sensation of muscular weakness. Sometimes his breathing is shallow, and he may have cramps.

The condition can be relieved by treating the cause. For example, in cases of severe vomiting an infusion of a saline solution restores the loss of acid to the body.

ALLERGY A reaction, such as a running nose, rash, or breathing difficulties, in persons sensitive to certain substances. These allergy-producing substances, or allergens, are all around us. Animal dander, house dust, and the pollen produced by trees and flowers are examples.

Much publicity has attached to the death from bee stings of persons who are SENSITIZED to the venom of that insect, but relatively few people are aware that allergies may be produced by an endless list of seemingly innocent substances present in the air we breathe, in our food and drink, in the clothes we wear, and in the things we touch.

Common Kinds of Allergy: Everyone is familiar with the sneezing and red, teary eyes of the HAY FEVER sufferer. This reaction is triggered not by hay, as was once believed, but by pollen, the masses of tiny, dust-sized "seeds" (actually, male reproductive cells) produced by seed plants. Ragweed pollen as well as the pollen of other plants, flowers, trees, and grass can cause hay fever. Pollen grains are usually yellow, but they may also be red, blue, or green.

Pollen belongs to the class of allergens known as inhalants because they are breathed into the respiratory tract. Other allergens in this group are the airborne, free-floating spores of fungus plants (similar to those that produce bread mold and mildew), house dust (one of the commonest causes of allergic symptoms), animal dander, and cosmetics.

Foods are a frequent source of trouble. The commonest offenders are milk, eggs, wheat, fish, strawberries, chocolate, and pork. They may produce nausea, vomiting, rash, or hay-fever-like symptoms in allergic persons.

Contact DERMATITIS, or inflammation of the skin, is a condition that may appear when the skin comes in contact with such potential allergens as furs, leather, plants, flowers, dyes, cosmetics, industrial chemicals, and insecticides. Poison ivy and poison oak are also responsible for contact dermatitis.

HIVES (urticaria) is also an allergic reaction, as are many cases of ECZEMA and bronchial ASTHMA.

How Allergies Develop: Most allergic persons are sensitive not just to one substance but to a number of them. Allergies are among the commonest of disorders; surveys have shown that at least 10 percent of the population suffers from them in either acute or chronic form.

How does a person develop an allergy? Heredity appears to play a part in many cases. If there have been allergic persons in your family, there is a greater chance that you, too, will be allergic. That does not mean that you will have precisely the same allergy as your father or mother, but simply that you can inherit a tendency to develop some type of allergic response. Emotional factors may also contribute to some allergies.

Allergies can show up at any period in life, from childhood to old age. Usually, however, allergic tendencies will assert themselves before a person reaches his forties. Precisely when a person will develop a sensitivity to an offending substance is determined by how much of it he is exposed to and for how long. An allergy may be in a developmental stage for a period of years before the person becomes sufficiently aware of it to decide that he requires treatment. Some persons, even those with severe allergies, lose their sensitivities and recover spontaneously.

The mechanism by which a typical allergic attack takes place is a curious one. In hay fever, for example, the sensitive person breathes in the pollen or other offending substance. Because he is sensitive, his body finds it an irritant. In response, the tissues produce antibodies, similar to the agents that the body normally uses to combat bacteria, viruses, and other carriers of sickness. The next time the allergen enters the body, the antibodies are already present, and they unite with the invaders to neutralize them. As part of the process, however, histamine and other chemicals are produced. These toxic agents are responsible for many of the distressing symptoms of allergies, including the familiar ones of hay fever.

Treatment: The first need is to identify the substance provoking the allergic reaction. Sometimes it will be obvious, as in the case of a food that instantly makes the person sick. But usually a detailed case history and a series of skin tests are needed to determine the allergens or other responsible factors. There are several hundred potential allergens, and tests are undertaken only when the allergy is severe.

The doctor will ask many questions: Exactly when do the attacks occur? In what surroundings? Do other members of the family have allergies? He will usually give a physical examination and then will make the skin tests. Generally, these consist of a series of minute scratches on the back or arm, into each of which a different allergen is introduced. Injections and patch tests are also used. If the reaction is positive, it will appear in from 5 to 20 minutes; a wheal (small bump), surrounded by a reddish area forms at the site of the scratch, and there is itching—very much the same symptoms as occur after an insect bite. A large variety of allergens may have to be tried before the offenders are found. Often there will be a number of them rather than just one.

In the case of food allergy, the person tries different diets, each time eliminating one of the foods that may cause allergy. He keeps a diary in which he notes his reactions, both positive and negative, and in this way the offending items are identified.

The treatment for allergy, in many instances, consists simply in avoiding the cause. If it is animal dander, the pet responsible will have to depart. When the cause is a food, drug, or article of clothing, it must be avoided at all costs. In the case of dust allergy, the house must be vacuum-cleaned regularly and a foam-rubber mattress and pillow used. Air conditioning may help.

Often the allergen cannot be avoided, and a program of desensitization has to be undertaken. This consists of a series of injections, each containing an extract of the allergen or allergens—serums, various pollens, dusts, molds, or other substances—which are increased over a period of time. If the person shows an untoward reaction to any dose, the following one is smaller. Step by step, his resistance to the allergic invader is built up. In time, many individuals achieve partial or complete immunity.

For numerous allergies, medications provide relief. ANTIHISTAMINES have wide effectiveness, although they are not successful in all cases. Hormone therapy may be given in some severe cases of allergic dermatitis.

ALOPECIA The medical term for baldness. Most loss of hair occurs on the scalp, but sometimes other parts of the body are involved. The cause of alopecia (pronounced al″o·pee′shee·a) is most often hereditary, but hair loss, if it is sudden, may be due to a disease, such as scarlet fever. (Normally, when the disease has run its course, the hair begins to grow in again.) Some medicines may cause hair loss. Aging and emotional factors may be responsible. The balance of sex hormones is also important.

Hereditary Baldness: If a male's forebears were bald on either his mother's or his father's side of the family, the chances are that baldness will be his lot, too. It may show itself as early as the late teens, beginning as a thinning of hair at the sides of the forehead or as a bald patch on the crown. Generally, all the hair is not lost, and even in severe cases, a fringe is left around the sides and back of the head.

The hair may also thin out in women, but the thinning is less severe than in men, and cases of baldness are uncommon.

Although a wide variety of treatments and tonics for baldness have been advocated from time to time, these popular nostrums do not have the approval of medical science. Hormones are not recommended. It is possible to have hair transplants, but they are very costly and still in an early stage of development. If a bald person feels he should have a head of hair for business or cosmetic reasons, a toupee offers a sensible solution.

Alopecia Areata: In this disorder the hair may drop out in patches, usually from the scalp and, in men, from the region of the beard. If the case is not severe, the condition will cease in a short time. Tension or severe shock may be the cause.

ALTITUDE SICKNESS A condition that occurs at high altitudes, where the air is thin and the concentration of oxygen is low. This disorder is also called mountain sickness because it is common among newcomers to mountain regions. It is known to physicians as hypoxemia, which means an inadequate supply of oxygen in the blood. At higher altitudes there is less oxygen available, and the red blood cells cannot absorb it in the customary quantity as the blood travels through the lungs. Typical symptoms are difficulty in breathing, nausea, fatigue, and anxiety.

Visitors to such U.S. cities as Denver (altitude 5,130 feet) and Albuquerque (4,950 feet) or to some of the mountainous Western national parks may be afflicted thus. The same condition may produce a feeling of excitement or exhilaration in some persons. Athletes or tourists who overexert themselves are particularly vulnerable to altitude sickness, as was learned by many persons who attended the 1968 Olympic Games in Mexico City (altitude 7,440 feet).

To avoid or overcome the symptoms of altitude sickness, it is advisable to refrain from strenuous activity for 24 to 48 hours, or longer, until your circulatory system has become used to the altitude. Alcoholic beverages should be avoided or taken in moderation. If you do not have a health problem, you will soon become acclimatized and able to resume your normal activities. However, a person with a history of heart or circulatory trouble should not travel to a high altitude without first consulting his physician.

AMA Abbreviation for AMERICAN MEDICAL ASSOCIATION. (Pronounce each letter.)

AMALGAM A material used to fill cavities in teeth. Amalgam (pronounced a·mal′gam) is made of a mixture of silver, tin, and mercury.

AMAUROSIS Blindness caused by a disease or defect of the optic nerve, retina, spine, or brain. There are no outward changes in the eye's appearance. (Pronounced am″aw·roh′sis.)

AMBLYOPIA Dimness of vision, with no apparent impairment of the structures of the eye or the optic nerve. Amblyopia (pronounced am″blee·oh′pee·a) may be hereditary, or it may be produced by dietary deficiencies, by certain medicines, or by excessive use of tobacco or alcohol. It can occur in children where an uncorrected squint of the eyes does not allow normal vision to develop in the eye that deviates. Amblyopia generally responds to treatment of the basic cause.

AMEBA (amoeba) A microscopic form of life consisting of an irregularly shaped, fluid blob enclosed in a membrane. Amebas (pronounced a·mee′baz) live in the soil and in water. A few kinds are disease-producing PARASITES.

AMEBIASIS An alternate name for amebic DYSENTERY. (Pronounced am″e·bie′a·sis.)

AMEBIC DYSENTERY A form of DYSENTERY. (Pronounced a·mee′bik dis′en·ter″ee.)

AMERICAN MEDICAL ASSOCIATION (AMA)
A society to which many members of the medical profession in the United States belong. It was founded in 1847 and is dedicated to the improvement of public health and the development of medical science. It conducts continuing research on scientific equipment, medical techniques, drugs, foods, and other matters that have a bearing on health. The association also maintains a health education program, supports new health legislation that it considers worthwhile, and regulates the ethics of the medical profession.

Not the least of AMA's achievements are the improvements it has brought about in the standards of education in medical schools. A nonprofit organization, it issues an imposing number of scientific publications to keep the medical profession up to date on treatment and research.

AMINO ACID Any of about 20 complex substances that form the building blocks of protein. All amino (pronounced a·mee'noh) acids contain nitrogen, carbon, hydrogen, and oxygen. Some of them contain sulfur as well. When food is digested, the protein in it is broken down into amino acids, which are then put together again in various combinations to make the particular kinds of protein required by the muscles, red blood cells, and other body tissue. Any amino acids left over are broken down further to supply energy.

Some amino acids can be manufactured by the body (chiefly in the liver) if they are not supplied in the diet. However, there are eight amino acids that the body needs but cannot manufacture. They must be obtained from proteins in the diet. These so-called essential amino acids are isoleucine, leucine, lysine, methionine, phenylalanine, threonine, tryptophan, and valine. Arginine and histidine are included in this list by some authorities. Alanine, cystine, glycine, proline, serine, tyrosine, and other amino acids can be manufactured by the body.

A given protein food does not necessarily contain all of the essential amino acids. Gelatin, for example, is pure protein but lacks the essential amino acid tryptophan. In order to assure an adequate intake of all the essential amino acids, the diet should include a variety of animal protein foods such as meat, fish, poultry, eggs, milk, and cheese.

AMMONIA A pungent-smelling gas that, combined with other substances, occurs naturally in the human body. It is an ALKALI that plays a significant role in preserving the body's acid-alkali balance. In its manufactured form, this hydrogen-nitrogen compound has many commercial applications; it is used in making fertilizers, explosives, and medicines. Prepared in a solution known as aromatic spirits of ammonia, or "smelling salts," it is used as an inhalant to revive a person who feels faint. Household ammonia should be used with care because both the liquid and its fumes are poisonous. For emergency treatment of ammonia poisoning, see the FIRST AID section.

AMMONIUM CHLORIDE A white crystalline acid compound. Given orally, it is used as an expectorant (a substance that assists coughing) in BRONCHITIS. It may also be prescribed to increase the general acid content of the body and the acidity of the urine, as in the treatment of heart failure with a DIURETIC.

AMNESIA The technical term for temporary or permanent loss of memory and the inability to connect words with ideas. Amnesia may be *general*, the loss of a great portion of one's memory, or *partial*, for example, an inability to remember names, colors, or dates.

Amnesia can occur following brain damage caused by disease, injury, or ALCOHOLISM. It can also occur following a severe emotional shock, as the mind often chooses to forget an especially terrible or frightening occurrence. Psychiatric treatment (see PSYCHOTHERAPY) is advised when amnesia is caused by an emotional disturbance.

AMNION A thin, membranous sac that encloses the unborn infant in the uterus. The amnion (pronounced am'nee·on) is filled with a liquid known as amniotic fluid; the infant is immersed in this fluid. The bursting of the amnion, or bag of waters, is generally a sign that childbirth is beginning.

AMOEBA See AMEBA.

AMPHETAMINE A stimulant, usually taken in tablet form, popularly known as a "pep pill," or "upper." Among common varieties of amphetamine (pronounced am·fet'a·meen") are BENZEDRINE and DEXEDRINE.

Amphetamine produces a feeling of well-being or exhilaration, reduces the appetite, increases muscular efficiency, and causes a condition of extreme wakefulness. In any of the various prescriptions in which it is sold, amphetamine should be taken with care. It may eliminate the warning signals of fatigue and lead to dangerous overexertion. There is a constant danger that the user may develop a serious dependency upon it. Amphetamine should always be taken in strict accordance with your physician's directions.

AMPUTATION The removal of a part of the body, such as a limb or a section of a limb. It is undertaken only when there is serious damage to the part. Many cases of amputation arise out of accidents with industrial machinery or on the highway. But diseases and conditions such as cancer, hardening of the arteries, gangrene, or frostbite may also be responsible.

PROSTHESIS, or the addition of an artificial part such as a leg or an arm, has brought about a remarkable change in the status and outlook of the amputee. A prosthetic hand can lift objects, turn pages, or run a machine. Prosthetic legs have such supple joints that it is hard to tell, in many actions, that they are artificial. Prosthetic devices make it possible for many amputees to lead a completely normal life. In planning the precise type of operation, the surgeon will take into account the patient's occupation and habits and the type of device that will let him live normally. (See KINEPLASTY.)

Perhaps the greatest danger the amputee faces is emotional. It is important that he be well informed about the operation before it occurs. Some treatment and a rehabilitation program may be necessary afterward, and he should know about this. He should also be made aware that there is a prosthetic device available and that it will serve him in much the same way a real limb would. Presented in a reassuring manner, such forthright information can prevent much apprehension and worry.

AMYLOID DISEASE
A disorder of the kidneys, liver, and spleen in which a waxy material accumulates in the tissues. It may be associated with prolonged infections such as OSTEOMYELITIS and TUBERCULOSIS, but sometimes occurs without a known cause. (Pronounced am'i·loyd.)

AMYTAL
Proprietary name for a BARBITURATE drug, prescribed when a patient is in need of sedation or sleep. Amytal (pronounced am'i·tal) should be taken only as prescribed by the doctor, or a dependency on it may develop.

ANALGESIC
A medicine that relieves pain. An analgesic (pronounced an"al·jee'zik) does not cure the cause of the pain, but deadens the sensation or makes it more bearable. ASPIRIN is probably the most familiar of the analgesics.

PAIN is a natural alarm, warning us that something is interfering with the normal functioning of the body. Just as a toothache is a signal that we should pay a visit to the dentist, so persistent or severe pain in other areas is an indication that medical attention is necessary. However, there are many minor aches and pains which can be treated by an analgesic such as aspirin. Still, even aspirin should not be taken in excess. It is not recommended for persons suffering from peptic ULCERS.

There are many aspirin substitutes. One of these is PHENACETIN, which is the main ingredient in a large number of popular nonprescription medicines. In spite of the claims made for it, phenacetin has not been found more effective than ordinary aspirin, and it is potentially more toxic.

If an analgesic does not relieve pain within 24 hours, or if pain recurs periodically after treatment with an analgesic, check with your physician. When the pain is severe, he may recommend a stronger analgesic, such as DARVON or CODEINE, both of which are available only by prescription. Some analgesics are habit-forming, however, and the patient should take them only as directed—no more than the prescribed dosage and only for the period the doctor advises.

Aside from medicines, there are simple treatments that can have an analgesic effect. A hot-water bottle, an electric heating pad, or a warm bath is useful when there are muscular aches. An ice bag or cold compress may relieve the discomfort of a sprain. Simply going to bed and sleeping for a time will tide you over many day-to-day minor aches and pains.

ANALYSIS
Separating a substance into its various parts and examining them, usually to determine evidence of disease. Analysis of the blood and URINALYSIS are typical examples. The term "analysis" is also used to mean PSYCHOANALYSIS.

ANATOMY
The study of the body structure and how its various parts are related to each other. The term is also used for the structure of the body itself.

ANDROGEN
A male SEX HORMONE. Testosterone, the principal androgen, is secreted by special cells of the TESTICLES. Another type of androgen (pronounced an'dro·jen) is produced by the adrenal glands.

Androgens are the substances that bring about the physical changes in a boy during adolescence. If a boy has a deficiency of androgens, he will not acquire complete male characteristics, such as a deep voice, a beard, or fully developed sex organs. This condition is often helped by giving androgens. However, injection of androgens will not restore sexual powers when the loss is due to aging.

Male sex hormones are also produced in small amounts in the ovaries and adrenal glands of women. If the secretion is excessive, a woman may develop masculine characteristics—a condition known as VIRILISM.

ANDROSTERONE
An ANDROGEN, or male hormone, that, like testosterone, helps to produce masculine characteristics. Androsterone (pronounced an·dros'te·rohn) is produced in the testicles of men and, in extremely small quantities, in the adrenal glands of women. It is found in the urine of both men and women. See also SEX HORMONE.

ANEMIA
A disorder of the blood in which the red cells are fewer than normal or have less HEMOGLOBIN than normal. Hemoglobin is the pigment that gives the red blood cells their color. These cells are important in breathing, since they carry oxygen from the lungs to all the tissues of the body, and carbon dioxide to the lungs for elimination. The red

blood cells (ERYTHROCYTES) are manufactured in the bone marrow. Normally there are trillions of them in the blood.

Anemia is usually not a disease in itself, but a symptom of disease. In advanced stages of serious diseases such as cancer and kidney failure, anemia develops as the processes of blood production and purification become impaired. In its milder forms, anemia is not a serious disorder; many people have been anemic at one time or another.

Symptoms: Anemia may show itself in many ways, depending on its severity. The person may be pale; this is particularly noticeable in the fingernails, lips, palms, and the lining of the eyelids. There may be an almost constant feeling of tiredness. In serious cases, dizziness, pounding heart, short breath, and loss of appetite may occur. A blood test confirms that there is a deficiency of hemoglobin.

Iron-Deficiency Anemia: This, the commonest type, is most often found in pregnant women and in children. Foods containing iron are essential to health, and during pregnancy and the rapid growth of childhood the body's needs may not be satisfied. Increasing the amount of iron-containing foods in the diet (such as leafy green vegetables, kidney, heart, liver, lean meat, whole-wheat bread, dried peas, beans, and fruit) and taking doses of medicinal iron soon correct this type of anemia.

Blood-Loss Anemia: Heavy menstrual flow, bleeding hemorrhoids, peptic ulcers, and other chronic disorders that cause excessive loss of blood may bring on anemia. The first requirement is to locate and remedy the cause of the blood loss. Iron and iron-rich foods are prescribed.

Pernicious Anemia: This is usually a disease of middle or old age. In this condition the red cells fail to develop in the normal way, although vast numbers of immature cells are present in the BONE marrow. The person may have any or all the symptoms previously described. In addition, there may be gastrointestinal trouble or nervous symptoms such as numbness, tingling, and erratic gait, as well as bladder trouble.

This disease, which formerly was responsible for many deaths, is now fairly simple to control. The patient is given injections of vitamin B_{12}, and most of the symptoms disappear almost overnight. The injections must be continued through life.

Aplastic Anemia: This form of anemia results when the bone marrow is damaged or destroyed. Symptoms include dark spots on the skin, bleeding from the mouth and nose, and frequent infections. The cause may be sensitivity to certain medicines or chemicals, overexposure to radioactive substances or X rays, or the presence of a cancerous growth in the marrow. Immediate hospitalization and blood transfusions are required. The patient may recover if the cause is located quickly and eliminated.

Hemolytic Anemia: In this type the red blood cells are destroyed at a faster than normal rate. The condition may arise as a reaction to the SULFONAMIDES, QUININE, or other substances. It sometimes occurs in the child of an Rh-positive father and Rh-negative mother (see RH FACTOR) or in a person who has been given a TRANSFUSION of the wrong blood type. This is a dangerous disease requiring prompt hospitalization. The outlook is good, provided treatment is begun in time.

Sickle-Cell Anemia: A hereditary disorder in which the red blood cells become deformed into irregular, pointed shapes resembling a sickle. The deformed cells do not slip easily through capillaries and small veins and arteries, and circulation is impaired. Symptoms, including severe pain in the abdomen and the joints, develop when the affected person uses up much oxygen in strenuous exercise. In North America, sickle-cell anemia is found almost entirely in people of African origin. It occurs also in some parts of India and the Mediterranean area.

ANESTHESIA Loss of feeling or sensation, throughout the body or in part of it, produced by various methods, such as administration of certain medicines or gases. Anesthesia (pronounced an″is·thee′zha) means, literally, "without feeling"; ANESTHETICS make it possible for a person to have an operation without the slightest sensation of pain. In earlier times, surgeons had to operate as quickly as possible, because of inadequate measures for reducing pain. Now, as a result of the many types of anesthetics and other developments in painless SURGERY, operations may be conducted carefully and methodically, with a minimum of risk and suffering.

The anesthesiologist today is a medical specialist who is present at all but the most minor operations. He is in charge of special medical instruments with which he monitors the patient's heartbeat and breathing, in addition to supplying the anesthetics. The anesthesiologist also administers liquid nourishment and blood TRANSFUSIONS, and is responsible for other important phases of an operation.

ANESTHETIC A substance capable of producing loss of sensation or sensitivity to pain. There are two main types of anesthetics. The local, or regional, anesthetic produces lack of feeling in a limited area of the body, while the general anesthetic does the same for the whole body, producing total unconsciousness in the patient.

The use of anesthetics is a complex branch of medicine known as anesthesiology. Much more is involved than simply giving an injection or administering ether. (See ANESTHESIA.) A number of different chemicals may be used for general anesthesia during the same operation. One, for example, may be employed to produce unconsciousness quickly. Another may be needed to relax the muscles. Then, there is the substance which induces deep, prolonged sleep. All of these anesthetic agents must be kept in balance.

The anesthesiologist has a wide choice of anesthetics and methods of using them in surgical operations. He consults with the surgeon, and they choose those that are most likely to prove effective for the particular patient. It is customary, before the operation, to acquaint the patient with the anesthetics and the procedure that will be used.

General Anesthesia: ETHER was once the most universally used of the general anesthetics, although it has now been largely replaced by others. In the usual procedure, the patient breathes the ether, which is delivered to him through tubes to a mask. Another general anesthetic inhaled by the patient is NITROUS OXIDE (laughing gas). This is used in brief operations, such as in dentistry, and in childbirth, and may produce a feeling of exhilaration or put the patient to sleep. Ethylene, CYCLOPROPANE, and halothane are general anesthetics now in wide use. CHLOROFORM, which was developed well over 100 years ago, is not used extensively anymore because of undesirable side effects.

Anesthetics are also injected into the veins to produce quick, short-acting general anesthesia. PENTOTHAL is used in this way.

Local Anesthesia: Probably the most familiar local anesthetic is NOVOCAIN, used in dentistry. The nerves surrounding the injection are deadened for one to two hours. Some local anesthetics are applied to the surface of the skin or to mucous membranes. BENZOCAINE, for instance, is applied to wounds, and TETRACAINE HYDROCHLORIDE to the nose and throat membranes.

Spinal anesthesia is local, but it can deaden sensation in very large areas of the body. It involves injecting an anesthetic into the space between vertebrae so that the spinal cord at this point is affected. The entire body below the point of injection becomes insensitive to pain, because no "pain messages" can pass up to the brain. (See BLOCK.) When an anesthetic is injected in the lowest (caudal) area of the spine, the method is called caudal anesthesia.

Anesthesia in Childbirth: This presents special problems. First, there is a tendency for general anesthesia to induce some nausea and vomiting, with the danger of choking if the patient's stomach is not empty. Because women in childbirth have not always had 12 hours or more warning not to eat, the anesthesiologist has to anticipate these complications. Second, many forms of anesthesia enter the mother's bloodstream and cross the placenta to the unborn child; therefore, anesthetics must be of the kinds that do not seriously affect the baby. Third, anesthesia must not be so profound as to decrease birth contractions and so prolong labor unduly. For these reasons, doctors try to make minimal use of anesthetics for women in labor, reserving them for the relatively brief periods when pain is most severe and for repairs after delivery.

Demerol is the drug most commonly used to reduce first-stage labor pains. (See CHILDBIRTH.) It is an analgesic, which does not interfere with consciousness, but produces a mildly euphoric state. A more completely pain-eliminating anesthetic is the lumbar or caudal epidural block, an injection administered just outside the spinal canal, which removes almost all sensation in the uterus and vaginal region. A general or spinal anesthesia is used in CESAREAN SECTION deliveries, or where there are major complications.

During delivery, the vaginal area may be desensitized with a pudendal block, injections of anesthetic on either side of the vaginal opening; or with a local Novocain injection to deaden the tissue between the vagina and rectum before an EPISIOTOMY is performed.

New developments in anesthesia are being produced through continuous research. To name one advance, the temperature can be reduced in the part of the body to be operated on, so that the part loses its sensitivity. Similarly, the temperature of the entire body may be lowered by an ice blanket. This slows down the body processes, decreasing the risk of hemorrhage in operations involving the circulatory system.

ANEURYSM An abnormal weakening of the wall of a blood vessel (usually an artery). An aneurysm (pronounced an'ye·riz"em) forms a blood-filled, pulsating sac that protrudes from the vessel. The disorder may be accompanied by pain, which is caused by the pressure of the protruding sac. Aneurysms may result from injury, SYPHILIS, and HARDENING OF THE ARTERIES. They are most frequently found in the abdomen and chest, particularly in the AORTA. The rupturing of an aneurysm (that is, the breaking of the weakened wall) can be fatal because of the internal bleeding that results.

Surgical techniques for correcting aneurysms have made great progress. If an aneurysm is discovered by X ray in a small blood vessel, the damaged artery or vein is tied so that the passage of blood is directed to a healthy vessel. In more serious cases, grafting technique is used. This involves replacing the damaged area of the blood vessel with a portion of the patient's veins or of a synthetic material.

ANGINA Any type of spasmodic pain. Sometimes the spasms of angina (pronounced an·jie'na) produce a feeling of suffocation. ANGINA PECTORIS is a painful symptom of a heart disorder.

ANGINA PECTORIS A pain in the chest which is experienced ordinarily when there is an unusual demand for blood in the HEART muscle (myocardium), but the coronary arteries cannot supply it in adequate quantity. A susceptible person may feel angina pectoris (pronounced an·jie'na pek'to·ris) after eating a heavy meal, while engaging in some physical activity such as walking up a flight of stairs, or while in a condition of excitement.

The pain is usually, but not always, located in the chest over the heart. Sometimes it occurs in the shoulder or the neck, and it is not uncommon in the left arm. Generally it is not a sharp pain, but rather a feeling of being constricted or suffocated. It may be associated with palpitations or dizziness. The attack is usually short; often the worst of it is over in several minutes. NITROGLYCERIN, prescribed by a physician, will give relief.

Angina is not a disease as such, but a symptom. Generally it is an indication of atherosclerosis of the coronary arteries in the heart. (See HARDENING OF THE ARTERIES.) It is a warning to seek medical treatment and take the proper precautions. Prominent among these is the avoidance of excitement and unnecessary exertion. The overweight person should go on a diet, preferably one low in fats. Coffee should not be taken excessively, and the smoker should give up tobacco.

ANIMAL BITE The bite of an animal may lead to serious infection and should be treated immediately. If the bite breaks the skin:

1. Wash with soap and water for five minutes.
2. Cover with a sterile dressing and bandage.
3. Call a doctor.

Although RABIES is spread primarily by the bite of dogs (see DOG BITE), it may also be spread by many other animals, including cats, skunks, raccoons, foxes, horses, and even swine. If an individual is bitten, an attempt should be made to catch the animal so that it may be examined for rabies. If the animal is not caught and proved healthy, the individual may have to undergo a series of rabies-prevention injections.

Many bites are inflicted in self-defense, and not necessarily by mad dogs. To prevent bites, a child should be taught not to tease or taunt animals, whether the animal is his own pet or a stray.

ANKLE The joint between the leg and the foot, as well as the general region of that joint. The ankle is used in a great many actions, such as walking, running, and getting to one's feet from a sitting position. In an abrupt movement or in a fall, the ligaments, muscles, and tendons that support the ankle may be wrenched or torn. This is the condition known as a SPRAIN. If the sprain is severe it is best to see your doctor for its treatment; he may want it X-rayed to check on a possible fracture. For treatment of minor sprains, see the FIRST AID section.

Some persons find that their ankles tend to swell up. This happens particularly to individuals who have to be on their feet a good deal, who have VARICOSE VEINS or poor circulation, or who are overweight. Often, the condition can be corrected by simply "putting your feet up" on a footstool for half an hour or so at the end of the day. If the swelling persists for 48 hours, you should consult your physician.

Ankle swelling may also be a symptom of kidney disease, heart disease, or other potentially serious disorders.

ANKYLOSIS Immobility of a joint resulting from fusion of its bones. Ankylosis (pronounced ang″ki·loh′sis) commonly occurs as a consequence of rheumatoid ARTHRITIS.

ANODONTIA A condition in which one or more, or sometimes all, of the TEETH fail to appear. Anodontia (pronounced an″o·don′cha) may occur with the baby teeth or the permanent ones. The absence may be due to hereditary factors or to a malfunction of the ENDOCRINE GLANDS. In other respects, the person may be completely normal.

In cases of anodontia, the mouth should be X-rayed to make certain that the teeth are actually missing. Sometimes they are present but in such a position that they cannot push through without minor surgery by a dentist.

ANOREXIA The medical term for prolonged loss of appetite. (Pronounced an″o·rek′see·a.)
Anorexia nervosa is a condition, found mainly in adolescent girls and young women, in which the patient eats little or no food for psychological reasons. If expert advice is not sought, the severe wasting that results can eventually lead to death.

ANTABUSE A proprietary name for the drug disulfiram, sometimes used to treat ALCOHOLISM. When the person who has Antabuse in his system takes as little as half an ounce of whiskey, he experiences unpleasant sensations, such as nausea and vomiting.

ANTACID An alkaline substance that, when taken internally, neutralizes an excess of stomach acid which causes mild or severe discomfort. Foods such as milk and bland cheeses are natural antacids. SODIUM BICARBONATE is a common antacid that usually relieves light attacks of heartburn or INDIGESTION. For chronic excessive stomach acidity, which can lead to GASTRITIS or peptic ULCER, a combination of antacids in tablet or liquid form may be prescribed by a physician. Antacids are sold, without prescription, as chewable tablets, liquids, or fizzy powders, under dozens of brand names, but their habitual use can be dangerous to your health. If you are using antacids regularly, you should check with your doctor.

ANTHRAX A disease of cattle, sheep, and other animals that can be passed on to man by contact with the animals, their hides, or their carcasses. Symptoms include skin ULCERS and swelling of the LYMPH NODES. Anthrax is treated with antibiotics.

ANTIBIOTIC A substance that fights certain disease germs by inhibiting their growth and reproduction. The name "antibiotic" (pronounced an″ti·bie·ot′ik) literally means "against life." Common antibiotics include penicillin, streptomycin, and tetracycline. These medicines are made by harvesting substances produced by certain bacteria, molds, and other microorganisms.

Prolonged use of antibiotics, or their use for treating minor disorders, may weaken the body's natural defenses against invading germs and may have undesirable side effects. Bacteria once treatable by antibiotics may produce new, drug-resistant strains.

For these reasons doctors warn against taking antibiotics on your own or insisting on a penicillin shot, for example, when your doctor does not believe an antibiotic is really required. Antibiotics have no effect on most illnesses caused by viruses, including those that produce the common cold and influenza.

ANTIBODY A natural substance that protects the body against a specific disease or infection. Antibodies are part of the body's natural IMMUNITY system. They destroy harmful bacteria and counteract the poisons produced by disease germs. A specific antibody is usually produced by the body in response to a particular foreign protein, such as bacteria, allergens, or an organ transplanted from another person. (See ALLERGY; ANTIGEN.) Certain types of antibodies never disappear from the body, thus providing lifelong immunity to some diseases. Two examples of such antibodies are those that protect against second attacks of measles and of mumps. Most VACCINES work by stimulating the formation of antibodies against a particular disease. See also IMMUNIZATION.

ANTICOAGULANT A medicine that slows down the natural tendency of the blood to clot. HEPARIN and warfarin are two kinds of anticoagulants extensively used in the treatment of disorders of the heart and blood circulation.

The formation of clots is a particular threat in disorders such as HARDENING OF THE ARTERIES. The artery becomes thick and rough, and a clot, or thrombus, may form. It may block the blood vessel, producing a serious condition known as a THROMBOSIS. Sometimes a clot breaks off and is borne away to lodge in another blood vessel, causing an EMBOLISM. Anticoagulants are employed to prevent the formation of clots, or to prevent them from growing larger.

ANTICONVULSANT A medicine used to control CONVULSIONS in such disorders as EPILEPSY and TETANUS. By making the nervous system less reactive, the drug reduces the severity of the convulsions and makes them less likely to occur.

ANTIDEPRESSANT A substance that has the effect of bringing a person out of a deep DEPRESSION. The antidepressant, of course, does not correct the underlying emotional condition, but only temporarily relieves the acute feeling of depression.

Deep depression may be the symptom of an EMOTIONAL AND MENTAL DISORDER. The antidepressant puts the person in a more positive frame of mind, so that he can become responsive to psychiatric treatment. (See PSYCHIATRY.) For this reason, such medicines have played a significant part in helping medical science deal with emotional disorders.

The two main types of antidepressants used today are known scientifically as *monoamine oxidase inhibitors* (such as phenelzine) and *tricyclic antidepressants* (such as imipramine and amitriptyline). Both types are powerful drugs which are available only on prescription and which should be taken only under medical supervision.

ANTIDOTE A remedy that is used to counteract the effects of poison. In a case of poisoning, it is important to give first aid treatment at once, while you have someone call the doctor. For a full discussion of measures to take in the event of poisoning, see the FIRST AID section.

ANTIGEN A substance that stimulates the body's production of ANTIBODIES—substances that combat invading organisms. Common antigens (pronounced an′ti·jenz) are viruses, bacteria, pollen, dust, fungi, and other substances that may produce a physical reaction, such as an ALLERGY, or an infectious disease, such as a cold.

When antigens appear in the blood or a tissue, antibodies that are produced or that are already present move into action against them and neutralize them. This process helps to produce IMMUNITY to infectious diseases.

ANTIHISTAMINE A medicine that is used to counteract typical symptoms of colds and allergies, such as a runny nose, postnasal drip, and congested sinuses. In an ALLERGY, certain irritants known as allergens—for example, POLLEN, house dust, fungi, and animal dander—enter the body and trigger the production of HISTAMINE, which causes the foregoing symptoms as well as others such as HIVES and ECZEMA. An antihistaminic medication will sometimes, or to some extent, reduce or prevent these symptoms. However, it does not cure the cold or allergy.

An extensive array of antihistamines is sold over-the-counter (without a doctor's prescription) at your local drugstore. These have varying effectiveness, depending on the individual. However, your physician is best equipped to prescribe one that works best for you.

Antihistamines often have a variety of side effects. For example, they can produce sedation or sleepiness, much the same way that SEDATIVES do. It is important to take antihistamines with extreme caution—or not at all—if you are going to drive. Antihistamine preparations usually carry a warning to this effect. Often, bedtime is a good time to take antihistamines. Other side effects may include a dry mouth, dizziness, and a weak feeling.

ANTIPYRETIC Any medicine or treatment that helps bring down a fever. ASPIRIN and cold compresses are familiar examples of antipyretics.

ANTISEPTIC A substance that slows down the growth of or kills the microorganisms we call disease germs, which are so tiny that they can be seen only with a microscope. After the French bacteriologist Louis Pasteur had discovered that infections are caused by such germs, a primitive and very strong antiseptic, CARBOLIC ACID, was introduced by the English surgeon Sir Joseph Lister in the 1860's to cleanse operating rooms and instruments. Today, aseptic techniques—for example, sterilization to prevent germs from developing in the first place—have largely replaced antiseptics in surgery, but they still play a major part in general HYGIENE. See also ASEPSIS.

Physical antiseptics include sunlight and heat. Heat is usually applied by boiling objects to decontaminate them. *Chemical* antiseptics have numerous uses. They are employed as GERMICIDES to disinfect wounds, as food preservatives, to sterilize surgical instruments, and as household DISINFECTANTS.

Antiseptics for Home Use: It is important to remove foreign matter from a wound by washing it thoroughly with soap and water before you apply an antiseptic. MERTHIOLATE, HYDROGEN PEROXIDE, and mild tincture of IODINE are among the most widely used antiseptics for treating abrasions and infections. Both isopropyl alcohol and ethyl alcohol (70 percent solution) are also employed externally as disinfectants, but they should not be applied to open wounds or to the eye, as they can cause pain and permanent damage. Antiseptic solutions are available in aerosol (spray) forms, but these are considerably more expensive than ordinary liquid antiseptics. Zinc sulfate and boric acid ointments are mildly antiseptic and are useful in preventing a dressing from adhering to a wound. SULFONAMIDES and ANTIBIOTIC ointments are used on burns and wounds but must be prescribed by a physician.

ANTITOXIN A type of ANTIBODY that acts against a poison, or TOXIN, that has entered the body. Some antitoxins are produced naturally in the body during response to disease. Others are produced by injecting horses and other animals with the "human" disease. The animals' purified blood serum is then administered to confer "artificial immunity" against a specific disease-producing substance. Two examples are antitetanus serum and antibotulism serum.

The first gives protection against tetanus, and the second is used to treat botulism, a form of food poisoning.

ANTITUSSIVE See COUGH MEDICINE.

ANTROSTOMY An operation to make an opening in an ANTRUM, in particular the main SINUS in the upper jaw. It is a treatment to promote drainage in chronic SINUSITIS. (Pronounced an·tros'toh·mee.)

ANTRUM A cavity in a bone, particularly the SINUS in the upper jaw, and the cavity in the mastoid process behind the ear. (Pronounced an'trum.)

ANURIA A serious condition in which the patient's kidneys do not produce urine. It is different from retention, in which a person passes no urine because he cannot empty his BLADDER, perhaps because of an enlarged PROSTATE GLAND. See also KIDNEY; URINARY TRACT. (Pronounced an·yoor'ee·a.)

ANXIETY In psychiatry, a feeling of intense worry or fear in the absence of any obvious danger. Anxiety may cause tension and fatigue and, in extreme cases, profuse sweating and palpitations. Nearly everyone experiences rational, or *realistic,* anxiety when faced with a new job, financial difficulties, or even when about to take an examination. Such anxiety is usually short-lived and "cures itself" when the particular problem is solved. But more serious trouble arises with irrational, or *unrealistic,* anxiety, where the feeling of apprehension is out of proportion to the facts of the individual's situation. Prolonged anxiety can be a contributing cause of such illnesses as peptic ULCER, COLITIS, ASTHMA, and heart disease. Thus, a doctor may recommend some form of PSYCHOTHERAPY if he senses irrational anxiety in a person.

Children are particularly susceptible to attacks of mild irrational anxiety. They may become worried about their naughtiness or a loss of parental affection or an unpleasant situation at school. In youngsters, a short-lived attack of anxiety may produce bed-wetting, nightmares, stomach pain, vomiting, and diarrhea. When the specific cause of the child's anxious feelings is discovered, he can usually be reassured in a way that will put an end to his fears.

Deep anxiety that takes the form of an undefined dread or that produces physical symptoms may require prompt attention from a PSYCHIATRIST or other specialist in emotional disorders.

AORTA The great ARTERY that conducts the blood from the left ventricle of the HEART. Other arteries branch out of the aorta (pronounced ay·awr'ta) and carry the blood to every part of the body.

APHASIA Loss or impairment of the power to express oneself by speech, writing, or signs, or to comprehend spoken or written language. In milder cases, aphasia (pronounced a·fay'zha) can be overcome by speech therapy or psychological counseling. It is an organic condition caused by brain damage, often following a STROKE.

APHONIA Loss of the voice or of the ability to speak normally, although it may be possible to speak in whispers. Aphonia (pronounced a·foh' nee·a) may be due to excessive use of the voice, to paralysis of the vocal cords as a result of a brain tumor, to a STROKE, or to an accident. Sometimes aphonia occurs as a symptom of HYSTERIA.

Another cause of aphonia is cancer of the LARYNX, or voice box, a condition which has been on the rise in recent years, and often removal of the larynx is the only alternative. (See LARYNGECTOMY.) Techniques have been developed to retrain persons so that they can communicate understandably after such an operation. Detailed information about this training can be obtained from the American Cancer Society, whose national office is located at 777 Third Avenue, New York, New York 10017.

APHRODISIAC A food, drink, or other substance that is supposed to stimulate sexual ardor and power. (Its name is derived from Aphrodite, Greek goddess of love.) Many foods have been considered aphrodisiacs (pronounced af"ro·diz'ee·aks) or tried as cures for IMPOTENCE, none with any success. Oysters, caviar, hard-boiled eggs, wheat-germ oil, and celery are some notable and harmless examples. Spanish fly, which is a preparation of dried beetles (cantharides), is dangerous and should never be taken. Alcohol may initially serve as a stimulant, since it releases inhibitions, but it is a DEPRESSANT in the long run. Impotence and related sexual problems are often helped by medical or psychiatric treatment (see PSYCHIATRY).

APOPLEXY A STROKE, caused by a CEREBRAL HEMORRHAGE or the blocking of a blood vessel in the brain by a blood clot. Warning signals include headache, mental confusion, and a feeling of dizziness; but an attack may also occur abruptly, without warning. The usual consequence is that the person is paralyzed on one side of the body. There is often partial or complete recovery in time. Apoplexy (pronounced ap'o·plek"see) usually strikes persons with high blood pressure or arteriosclerosis who are 40 or older. For emergency treatment of stroke, see the FIRST AID section.

APPENDECTOMY Surgical removal of the appendix. This hollow, tubelike organ, located in the lower right part of the abdomen, sometimes becomes infected. (See APPENDICITIS.) It is important that the condition be diagnosed promptly and the inflamed appendix removed as quickly as possible, or serious disability or even death may result.

The removal of the appendix is a simple operation if it is performed before the appendix ruptures and spills germs into the abdominal cavity. The day after an appendectomy (pronounced ap"en·dek'to·mee), the patient may be allowed out of bed for a little while, and in a week or less, normally, he will leave the hospital. He can take up his usual activities from 14 to 21 days after the operation.

If appendicitis is not diagnosed in time, the inflamed appendix ruptures, and an abscess may form. When this happens, the abscess must be drained, and the operation may be put off for a month or longer.

Whenever there is pain in the abdomen that continues for three hours or longer, appendicitis should be suspected. Remember: A healthy appendix performs no function at all; a diseased one may be extremely dangerous.

APPENDICITIS An acute inflammation of the appendix. This is a narrow, tube-shaped appendage attached to the large intestine. (Its formal medical name is "vermiform appendix.") It has no apparent

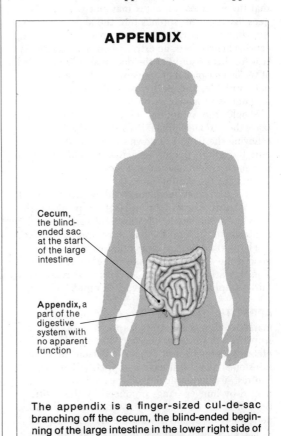

APPENDIX

Cecum, the blind-ended sac at the start of the large intestine

Appendix, a part of the digestive system with no apparent function

The appendix is a finger-sized cul-de-sac branching off the cecum, the blind-ended beginning of the large intestine in the lower right side of the abdomen. If it becomes inflamed, generally associated with infection and blockage of its opening into the cecum, the resulting appendicitis is treated by surgery to remove it.

function. Usually, but not always, it is located in the lower abdomen, on the right-hand side.

When the appendix is blocked by a swollen LYMPH NODE, a hard piece of FECES, or through some other cause, an infection is produced, and this brings on the inflammation. The infected appendix must be removed as quickly as possible, or there may be serious consequences. Appendicitis is usually, but not always, a disease of young people and occurs most frequently before the age of 30.

Symptoms: Appendicitis is often announced by pain or cramps in the region around the navel. Nausea and vomiting may also occur. Later, possibly after a few hours, pain may be felt in the lower right-hand part of the abdomen. It may be acute or dull, but it is fairly constant. There may be a high fever in a child, a mild one in an adult. A distinctive symptom is that *the area over the appendix feels tender* when it is pressed. However, the only person qualified to diagnose appendicitis is a physician. Call one immediately if you have any reason at all to suspect appendicitis.

What to Do: The great danger with appendicitis is that the inflamed appendix may burst. If this happens, fecal matter spreads into the abdominal cavity, and the peritoneum may become infected, causing PERITONITIS, an extremely serious condition. It is for this reason that the doctor should be called at the first suspicion of appendicitis. If a physician is not available, the person should be driven to a hospital as promptly as possible.

Should the symptoms of appendicitis appear, leave the abdomen alone. Do not knead it in hope of relieving the pain. Lie down on your bed and wait quietly for the doctor to come. Should the pain become excessive, have someone fill an ice bag and apply it to the painful area.

Do not take any medicine, food, or drink. Do not take a laxative of any sort; a laxative speeds up the activity of the small intestine and can cause the appendix to rupture. Enemas must also be avoided.

The outlook for the appendicitis patient is very good if the appendix is removed before it ruptures. The operation, known as an APPENDECTOMY, is a fairly simple one, and recovery is rapid.

APPETITE The desire for food or drink. There is a marked difference between appetite and hunger. Appetite expresses a craving that may be completely independent of hunger; a person can have a full stomach and still have an appetite. Hunger, by contrast, is the physical need for food. It is accompanied by hunger pangs produced by the contractions of the walls of the empty stomach. A healthy person has an appetite when he feels hunger.

The conditions under which you eat can have a good deal to do with appetite. If food appears inviting and is served in neat, cheerful surroundings, people are likely to approach a meal with relish. Noise, distasteful-looking food, or a bad frame of mind can banish any desire to eat. The dinner table is not the place to bring up money problems, Junior's misbehavior, or any subject in which strong feelings are involved. Do everything you can to make eating a relaxed, enjoyable occasion.

Undereating: If appetite is lacking over a period of time, it can be a warning signal. (See ANOREXIA.) Often lack of appetite is a result of emotional problems. It is also a common symptom in a wide range of diseases, including HEPATITIS and cancer. Lack of appetite usually corrects itself, but if it persists, a physician should be consulted.

Overeating: People who are unhappy sometimes have an exceptional appetite. The teenage boy or girl or lonely older person may become a compulsive eater to make up for the shortcomings of his emotional life. (Keep in mind, however, that adolescents normally eat heavily to supply the nutrients that their growing bodies need). Overeating can also be a sign of disease, particularly if it is accompanied by loss of weight. This can happen in cases of DIABETES and overactive THYROID GLAND.

ARCH, FALLEN See FALLEN ARCH; FOOT.

AREOLA (1) The colored area around the nipple. (2) The part of the iris bordering the pupil of the EYE. (Pronounced *a·ree'o·*la.)

ARM Either of the upper extremities, from shoulder to wrist. The arms are like the legs in structure and resemble basically the front legs of four-legged creatures. The arms can be regarded as forelegs that are no longer involved primarily in supporting and moving the body but have taken on the function of moving and manipulating things.

The humerus, or upper arm bone, corresponds to the femur (thighbone) in the leg. The shoulder joint, like the hip joint, can swivel in any direction, within certain limits. The elbow joint is hinged like the knee joint and can move freely in only one direction. The elbow lacks a protective plate corresponding to the kneecap, but it has something more important—a special arrangement of ligaments by which the radius and ulna, the two bones of the lower arm, can be twisted to cross over each other. This gives the lower arm much greater flexibility than the lower part of the leg. The lower arm can be rotated so that the hand turns inward or outward.

If the arm were not so well adapted to picking up things and bringing them into a good viewing position near the face, it is very probable that the human brain would never have reached its present state of development.

ARTERIES, HARDENING OF See HARDENING OF THE ARTERIES.

ARTERIOGRAM An X-ray picture of an ARTERY taken after an opaque dye has been injected directly into it. An arteriogram (pronounced ahr·tir′ee· oh·gram″) shows any disturbance in the supply of blood going to organs such as the brain or the kidneys.

ARTERIOSCLEROSIS Another name for HARD-ENING OF THE ARTERIES. (Pronounced ahr·tir″ee· oh·skle·roh′sis.)

ARTERY Any BLOOD VESSEL that carries oxygen-rich blood away from the heart to the various organs and tissues of the body. (A vein carries oxygen-depleted blood back to the heart.) See also AORTA.

ARTHRITIS Pain or inflammation of the joints and the tissues supporting them. This term, as well as rheumatism, is applied not to just one but to a whole group of diseases, including osteoarthritis and rheumatoid arthritis. GOUT and RHEUMATIC FEVER are related disorders.

According to the U.S. Public Health Service, arthritis is the most widespread crippling disease in the country. About 31 million Americans have arthritis of some kind; of these more than 7 million are partly or wholly disabled. Distressing as these figures are, they still indicate that most people who have arthritis are able to go about their business as usual.

Osteoarthritis: A typical disease of old age, osteoarthritis is caused by the wearing away of the cartilage on the bone endings. One end of a bone then rubs against another, and there is stiffness and sometimes pain. This condition involves the joints of the fingers, big toes, knees, hips, lower spine, and other joints exposed to great wear and tear. Osteoarthritis is not as severe as some other arthritic disorders. Most sufferers find the condition tolerable, but for those who do not, new drugs may alleviate the pain. Also, recently developed surgical techniques enable surgeons to replace old finger, knee, and hip joints with new, plastic ones.

Rheumatoid Arthritis: This disease is much more serious. Most often, it involves the joints of the fingers, wrists, and feet. However, any JOINT may be affected. The membrane that lines the joint becomes inflamed, and the joint swells up. Eventually the surrounding cartilage is worn away, causing the joint to become exceedingly painful and hard to move. Neighboring muscles are also affected. If the condition is not treated early, the joint may become immovable. Careful treatment, however, will prevent disability in most persons. The cause of this painful and crippling disorder has not been definitely determined.

Treatment: Various medications are used with good effect in treating different types of arthritis. Among these are phenylbutazone and sometimes cortisone and other hormones. Salicylate compounds, including aspirin, are beneficial when taken as prescribed.

Heat often brings relief when applied to the troublesome joint. An electric pad, hot compresses, hot tub baths, or an infrared tungsten bulb may all be useful. The arthritic should have a bed board under his mattress. Good upright posture, both sitting and standing, is most important. Exercise, as prescribed by the doctor, can help considerably in combating this disorder.

Arthritics are frequently taken in by quack remedies. There are no magic shortcuts to the control of arthritis. Strange electrical devices, special foods, vaccines, radioactive waters at home or abroad, and a thousand and one other "miracle cures" are often highly touted, but they will only waste your time and money. Always consult your physician for advice on treatment.

ARTIFICIAL INSEMINATION Depositing of semen (male sex cells) at the mouth of the UTERUS by artificial means to make conception of a baby possible. Usually this is performed by a physician, who transfers the semen with a syringe.

Artificial insemination is utilized in three types of cases. In the first, the husband may be fertile but unable to complete the sex act. If his semen is transferred into the vagina at a suitable time in the wife's fertility cycle, it is frequently possible to achieve a successful pregnancy. (See OVULATION.)

In the second type, the husband's semen is produced in smaller than normal amounts, making conception difficult. In such a case, the semen can be preserved over a period of time in a frozen state. When a sufficient amount has been collected, it is inserted into the vagina with a syringe.

In the third type, the husband cannot produce healthy semen, so it is obtained from another source by the physician. The doctor will make certain that the donor is in good health, of sound heredity, and of a blood type compatible with that of the future mother. The identity of the donor is always concealed. Certain legal requirements must also be satisfied. There are sometimes serious disadvantages in artificial insemination performed this way. The husband, for example, may have an unfavorable emotional reaction later, although he may be cooperative at the time. Frequently, adopting a child is a happier course.

ARTIFICIAL ORGAN A device that performs the work of an organ of the body for a short while or permanently. An artificial organ is frequently used to perform the function of a body organ while surgery is being performed on that organ, or while the organ is unble to do its normal work.

A number of important artificial organs have been developed in recent years. One of the most valuable is the artificial-kidney machine, which includes a selective filter that cleanses the blood of waste products in cases of kidney failure. The filter permits the poisonous materials to escape, but holds back the blood cells and proteins.

Among other devices of exceptional usefulness are the CARDIAC PACEMAKER, an electronic mechanism that restores a normal rhythm to a damaged heart; heart valves and blood vessels made of synthetic materials; and the heart-lung machine, which takes over the work of heart and lungs during an operation by removing the waste-laden blood from the circulatory system, purifying it, adding oxygen, and pumping the blood back into the body.

See PROSTHESIS for information on artificial external body parts.

ARTIFICIAL RESPIRATION

Any method of forcing air into and out of the lungs of a person who has stopped breathing. Because the very life of a person who has stopped breathing depends on artificial respiration, you must apply it *without delay*. The most effective method is mouth-to-mouth resuscitation, described in detail in the FIRST AID section. While you give artificial respiration, have someone call a hospital, the police, or the fire department for an emergency resuscitation unit. Continue treatment until the individual begins breathing or until help arrives.

Drowning, electrocution, suffocation, carbon monoxide inhalation, and overdosage with medicines such as barbiturates (sleeping pills) are among the emergencies that call for artificial respiration. If the cause is choking, the object that obstructs breathing should first be removed (see FIRST AID section). Cessation of breathing may also be caused by cardiac arrest. Treatment of this emergency is called cardiopulmonary resuscitation, also described in the FIRST AID section.

ARTIFICIAL SWEETENER

A synthetic compound used instead of sugar to sweeten foods and beverages. Artificial sweeteners, or sugar substitutes, have no food value. They pass through the body largely unchanged and are excreted in the urine. People with DIABETES, who cannot tolerate ordinary sugar, must use artificial sweeteners or eat their food without sweetening.

Relatively few people have diabetes, but a great many people try to control their CALORIE intake by not using sugar. Sugar is normally a minor item in the daily intake of calories, and using sugar substitutes is not by itself a very effective way of losing weight. Nevertheless, low-calorie "diet" foods and beverages find a ready market. During the 1960's, great quantities of the artificial sweetener known as cyclamate were used, not only in low-calorie foods but in general food processing. Late in 1969, the U.S. Food and Drug Administration announced a ban on general use of cyclamate because of harmful effects observed in laboratory animals given very large amounts of cyclamates. No harmful effects have been observed in humans, and cyclamate still has a restricted use in the diet of diabetics, where the advantages outweigh the possible dangers.

SACCHARIN is currently the only artificial sweetener in unrestricted use, but products containing saccharin must carry a warning statement that it is a weak carcinogen.

ASA

The abbreviation for *a*cetylsalicylic *a*cid, commonly sold in the United States as ASPIRIN.

In Canada, Aspirin is the trade name of one manufacturer, and the product is sold by other Canadian drug companies as ASA.

ASBESTOSIS

A disease of the lungs that is caused by breathing in minute particles of asbestos. The disease (pronounced as"bes·toh'sis) is often contracted by persons who work with the material.

ASCARIASIS

See ROUNDWORM. (Pronounced as·ka·rie'a·sis.)

ASCITES

An unusual buildup of fluid in the abdomen. Ascites (pronounced a·sie'teez) can appear in diseases of the heart, kidneys, liver, and other vital organs. See also EDEMA.

ASCORBIC ACID

Known also as vitamin C, it is found in citrus fruits such as oranges, grapefruits, lemons, and limes. Tomato juice (fresh or canned) is a good source, as are fresh berries such as strawberries and raspberries. The ascorbic (pronounced a·skawr'bik) acid content of fruits and vegetables is much reduced by canning or prolonged cooking. A lack of ascorbic acid in the body may lead to the disease called SCURVY. See also VITAMIN.

ASEPSIS

The absence of bacteria and other disease-producing microorganisms or germs. The care of the sick and modern surgical techniques are based in good measure on aseptic methods of avoiding infection. The meaning of asepsis (pronounced a·sep'sis) is summed up in one word: *sterile*.

In surgery, asepsis includes the sterilizing of the air in the operating room, the furnishings and equipment, the surgical instruments, and the hands and clothing of the doctors and nurses. An autoclave or other type of sterilizer is frequently used for the sheets, instruments, and other items. The dry heat of an oven, as well as ultraviolet light, may be used for special purposes.

In the sickroom, asepsis is strictly maintained. Masks and gowns are worn whenever there is a possibility of spreading disease. ANTISEPTIC methods are also used to prevent the spread of disease—that is, substances such as alcohol and carbolic acid are employed to destroy germs or to slow down their growth.

ASIAN FLU

See INFLUENZA.

ASPHYXIA

Suffocation; a condition in which breathing has been interfered with, resulting in a lack of oxygen in the blood. If the condition continues for more than about five minutes, the individual will die.

Asphyxia (pronounced as·fik′see·a) can be produced in many ways. In giving first aid, the cause of the suffocation should be eliminated or otherwise dealt with at once. Thus, if the individual is suffocating as a result of carbon-monoxide poisoning, he should be carried out into the open air. If he has suffered an electric shock and is lying on the wire or wires, remove him with the help of some nonconducting material, such as rubber or dry wood. In case of strangulation, untie the constricting object around his neck. If a person is choking on an object lodged in his throat, remove the object by using the Heimlich maneuver described in the FIRST AID section.

After eliminating the cause of suffocation, begin artificial respiration immediately (see the FIRST AID section). At the same time, ask someone to telephone the police or a hospital to ask for an ambulance. Fast action may save a life.

ASPIRATOR A medical instrument used to remove fluids from cysts or body cavities, such as the lungs, by the process of suction. (Pronounced as′pi·ray″tor.)

ASPIRIN A name for acetylsalicylic acid, a drug prescribed primarily as an ANALGESIC (pain-killer). It is also useful in reducing fever. When properly used, it is effective and relatively safe. The adult dosage is one to two 5-grain tablets every three to four hours, not to exceed 12 tablets in any 24-hour period.

Before giving aspirin or any other medicine to children, consult your doctor. The proper dosage of the standard tablets or the special children's aspirin varies with the age of the child. Flavored aspirin can be dangerously mistaken for candy or chewing gum and, like all medicines, should be kept out of the reach of children.

Aspirin is the basic ingredient of many types of pain-relieving tablets with dozens of different brand names. The only significant difference between brands is price. If the bottle is kept tightly closed, aspirin has a shelf life—that is, remains effective—for up to two years.

The precise means by which aspirin diminishes pain is still not known. It is believed to affect some part of the nervous system which, within 15 to 30 minutes, causes lessened sensitivity to pain. It has been found to be most effective in easing low-intensity pain such as headaches and muscular aches, thus accounting for its popularity as a cold remedy.

Aspirin can reduce body temperature, but it should not be taken routinely for fever without consulting your doctor.

Three to five tablets stirred vigorously in a glass of warm water and used as a gargle are an effective pain reliever for minor sore throats. Aspirin gargle reduces soreness, not infection, and must not be regarded as a cure. Aspirin's remarkable effect of reducing swelling and pain in ARTHRITIS and RHEUMATIC FEVER is not completely understood.

The side effects of aspirin taken as prescribed are minimal. When you swallow aspirin, the acetylsalicylic acid is turned into salicylic acid during digestion. Salicylic acid then passes through the intestinal wall and into the bloodstream to produce its effect. It may cause some slight stomach irritation, which can often be alleviated by taking the prescribed dosage with milk. There are various brands of buffered aspirin which contain an alkaline buffer to neutralize stomach acidity. Peptic ulcer sufferers should avoid taking aspirin without their doctor's consent.

In some cases, aspirin seems to act as a mild sedative by relieving minor pain, but "two aspirins at bedtime" will not guarantee a sound night's sleep. An allergic reaction to aspirin may occur, but this is not common.

Warning: The fact that aspirin is a medicine means that it should be taken in prescribed dosages at regular intervals. You will not get better results by taking more aspirin tablets than are recommended by the doctor; furthermore, an overdose of aspirin can cause serious stomach upset, nausea, and vomiting. In excessive doses it can even be fatal.

ASTHMA A disorder of the bronchial tubes in which the individual has difficulty in breathing. Most asthmatic attacks are mild, but the condition is a chronic one, and if it remains untreated, the consequences can be serious.

Causes: Basically, there are two major causes of asthma. The first is an infection of the nose, sinuses, bronchi, or lungs, such as BRONCHITIS. The second, and more common, type of asthma is caused by an allergic reaction that is usually hereditary in origin. In allergic asthma, the individual may be sensitive to POLLENS, house dust, animal dander, molds, insecticides, wool, certain foods or medicines, or some similar substance. When he takes them into his body or comes in contact with them, histamine forms in his system, triggering the allergic reaction. (See ALLERGY.) In either type of asthma, the bronchial passages are narrowed by swelling of the mucous membranes that line them and by the formation of mucous plugs.

A number of factors have an influence on the severity of an asthmatic attack. Of these, emotional stress is probably the most important. A nervous person is likely to suffer more frequently and more intensely. Fatigue can bring on the spasms of asthma. So, also, can changes in temperature, and, particularly, a rise in humidity.

Symptoms: In a typical attack, the individual feels a tightness in his chest; he wheezes, coughs, and has difficulty in breathing. His face may turn blue, and there may be a feeling of suffocation. The attack may last an hour, sometimes less, sometimes much longer. Toward the end of the attack, thick mucus is coughed up, and there is a feeling of relief.

Treatment: It is easy to confuse asthma with breathing difficulty caused by some other disorder, such as EMPHYSEMA or heart disease. (See HEART DISEASE—SYMPTOMS.) Only a physician is capable of making the diagnosis. Treatment of asthma consists in bringing any infection under control, usually with antibiotics. If an allergic factor seems likely, the individual should be given a series of tests to determine what allergens are involved. Then a course of injections may be prescribed to reduce sensitivity. To bring an asthmatic attack under control, such drugs as epinephrine, isoproterenol, or aminophylline may be used. During a severe attack the doctor may give the drug by injection.

Some persons who live in damp areas have obtained effective relief by moving to a warm, dry climate such as that of the American Southwest. But such a drastic measure ought not to be undertaken without a long trial visit to the region. Children with "intractable" or severe asthma of psychological origin have been helped by being removed from their homes and placed in a special institution for asthmatics. Such a step, however, should not be taken without full medical advice. In many children, the condition improves as they get older.

ASTIGMATISM An eye defect, usually in the cornea, which prevents the eye from focusing properly and results in distorted or blurred vision. Astigmatism (pronounced *a·*stig′ma·tiz″em) is common in children, and may be present if the child tilts his head to one side when reading. It can be corrected with eyeglasses or contact lenses. See also EYE.

ASTRINGENT A preparation that helps to stop bleeding and reduce body secretions by causing blood vessels and tissues to contract. The familiar witch hazel solution and styptic pencil, used to stop bleeding from small cuts, contain astringents, as do after-shave lotions and other skin preparations.

ATABRINE The trade name of quinacrine, a medicine used in the treatment of malaria. Atabrine (pronounced at′*a·*brin) was developed in the 1930's and came into wide use when it became difficult to obtain QUININE during World War II. Like quinine, however, it has been to a large extent replaced by newer and better medicines. See also MALARIA.

ATAXIA Loss of control of muscular movements. It is often due to damage to the nervous system and not to weakness in the muscles. (Pronounced *a·*tak′see·*a.*) See also LOCOMOTOR ATAXIA.

ATELECTASIS A condition in which a newborn baby's lungs fail to expand properly; also collapse of

part of an adult's lung. If it is not quickly corrected, severe atelectasis (pronounced at″*e·*lek′tah·sis) in a baby results in death. Mild atelectasis in an adult generally corrects itself (see PNEUMOTHORAX). Severe cases are corrected by treating the cause.

ATHEROSCLEROSIS A condition associated with HARDENING OF THE ARTERIES. (Pronounced ath″er·oh·skle·roh′sis.) See also CORONARY HEART DISEASE.

ATHLETE'S FOOT A contagious infection of the foot caused by a FUNGUS that thrives in wet, warm places. There are LESIONS and blisters between the toes, and scaling of the skin. Often, the sole becomes involved. Excessive perspiration aggravates the condition.

Athlete's foot is normally a minor irritation, and people may have it for some time without being particularly bothered by it. It may, however, spread to other parts of the body, where it can produce an annoying rash. The cracks or blisters may also become a site for other infections. Thus, if the condition persists, it should not go untreated.

Treatment: Good foot care is indispensable. The scaly or damp peelings should be rubbed gently away. Dry the feet. Apply water mixed with a little rubbing alcohol. Dry the feet again, and apply a dusting powder. Try to expose the feet to the air as long as possible. When you go to bed, and again in the morning, put a mild fungicidal ointment obtainable at your drugstore on the infected area. Wear cotton or wool socks, which absorb perspiration, unlike socks of synthetic materials. In summer, light shoes should be worn.

Potassium permanganate solution, in the strength your doctor advises, makes a helpful footbath if the blisters are oozing. Soak your feet in the warm bath for 10 to 15 minutes; then dry them, and apply CALAMINE LOTION. If the condition persists or becomes more troublesome, visit your physician. He can often provide quick and thorough relief.

ATHLETE'S HEART A supposed condition of heart damage due to overdevelopment of the heart muscle as a result of participation in strenuous athletic activity. In the past, it was believed that former athletes were likely to suffer from heart disease in later life because of this condition. However, surveys of thousands of high school and college graduates have revealed that there is no difference in the death rates of those who took part in school athletics and those who did not. Physiological tests have confirmed that exercise does not impair a heart that is healthy to begin with. Fear of contracting "athlete's heart" need not keep any boy or girl in good health off the athletic field.

ATROPHY A wasting away or reduction in size of an organ or tissues of the body. An example is atrophy (pronounced at′ro·fee) of the leg muscles in POLIOMYELITIS. Lack of use is one of the causes of atrophy.

ATROPINE A substance that is used in the treatment of a large number of disorders. Atropine (pronounced at′ro·peen) is extracted from BELLADONNA and other plants of the nightshade family. It is most familiar in the form of TINCTURE of belladonna.

Atropine paralyzes certain nerve endings and thus relaxes the smooth muscles. It is used chiefly internally to control spasms and contractions of the digestive system. Because it decreases the activity of the stomach, it is helpful in cases of peptic ULCER. It also dilates, or widens, the pupil of the eye, so it is employed in drops used in eye examinations. It is an antidote in some cases of mushroom poisoning and may provide relief in asthma and whooping cough.

As a side effect, atropine may slow down the activity of salivary and sweat glands.

AUDIOGRAM A tracing produced by an audiograph, a machine used to test a patient's hearing. Sound waves of various frequencies are transmitted directly to the patient's inner ear through leads from the machine, and the results are recorded on a graph. This is also a useful test to establish the type of HEARING AID a deaf or partially deaf patient needs. (Pronounced aw′dee·oh·gram″.) See also DEAFNESS.

AURA See EPILEPSY. (Pronounced awr′a.)

AUSCULTATION Listening with the ear or with a STETHOSCOPE to sounds within the body. Doctors find auscultation (pronounced aws″kul·tay′shun) a useful method in determining the general health of various parts of the body: usually, any irregular sounds will be further investigated by more precise means, such as the X ray.

In auscultation, the physician listens for sounds, such as murmurs in the heart, that may indicate an abnormal condition for an organ. These sounds are amplified by the stethoscope. When the person breathes in or out, for example, the doctor can tell from the sounds of the air in the respiratory passages whether or not they are clogged or infected. Auscultation is used to check the state of organs such as the lungs, the heart, and those in the abdomen.

AUTISM The state of being absorbed in oneself and one's fantasies in order to escape from the real world. It is found in children, and it is also one of the symptoms of SCHIZOPHRENIA, a severe psychotic disturbance that afflicts some 50 percent of the inmates of our mental institutions.

Autism (pronounced aw′tiz·em) may show itself in early childhood. The autistic child, as the victim of this condition is known, lives in a world of his own. If an object is dropped close to him, he may

not show the slightest response. He appears insensitive to pain. He does not relate to people; when they are present, he does not even seem to be aware of them. He develops a few limited patterns of behavior, and he forms an emotional attachment of a sort to some objects. He may alternate between periods of intense physical activity (hyperactivity), sometimes even causing self-injury, and periods of impenetrable calm. He resists and resents any change in his surroundings.

The mother is the center of the universe to the normal child; the autistic child, however, may not even notice her. An early sign of autism observed by parents is that the child does not answer them when they speak, although his hearing is perfectly normal. He does not smile or respond to them. They cannot get to him. He may develop a set of signals by which he imperiously lets his parents know his wishes, but that is the limit of his communication.

In an adult, autism is fairly similar. The person, unable to respond to the world in a normal way and feeling threatened by it, shuts it out altogether. There is complete withdrawal from reality; the schizophrenic becomes utterly absorbed in his inner life. There may be regression to a childlike type of behavior.

No single method for treating autism has been found effective in all cases, but research into its cause and treatment is ongoing. Parents of autistic children can obtain information about local treatment facilities by writing to the National Society for Autistic Children, 1234 Massachusetts Avenue, N.W., Washington, D.C. 20005.

AUTONOMIC NERVOUS SYSTEM The part of the nervous system that regulates the unconscious functions of the body, such as breathing, beating of the heart, digestion, rate of glandular activity, and contraction and dilation of the blood vessels.

The autonomic nervous system is made up of two systems: the *sympathetic* nervous system and the *parasympathetic* nervous system.

The sympathetic system comes into play following a fright or an emergency, preparing the body to defend itself by aggression or flight. In such a situation, various changes take place in the body. Blood is diverted from the vessels surrounding the stomach and intestines to those serving the muscles; the person concerned may have a sinking feeling in his stomach. At the same time, the rates of working of the heart and lungs speed up, thus pumping more oxygenated blood to the muscles. Small blood vessels near the surface of the skin dilate, and the person my go white in the face.

After the emergency is over, the nerves of the parasympathetic system "switch off" these changes and the person relaxes. The two systems check and balance each other, so that the body can adjust to many types of situations and function effectively in times of stress.

AUTOPSY Examination of a dead body to determine the cause of death or for purposes of study. An autopsy (pronounced aw'top·see) is also known as a postmortem ("after death") examination.

When the cause of death is unknown, or a person dies unattended by a doctor, the law generally requires an autopsy. It is also required when there are suspicious circumstances surrounding the death. If a physician is not certain why a person has died, he may ask for a postmortem; however, in these circumstances, the family of the dead person must give its consent. In many cases, an autopsy can contribute to the understanding of a disease and hence to the treatment of others suffering from it.

The postmortem examination is usually performed by a coroner, a medical examiner, or a pathologist, who makes a systematic study of the remains. Various tissues or substances may be subjected to microscopic or chemical analysis in the process. The findings are then submitted in a report to medical or legal authorities and recorded on the death certificate.

Many persons will their remains to hospitals or medical schools for examination after death. Usually, the next of kin must give permission. Both the training of future physicians and medical understanding of health and disease have been advanced by this practice.

B

BABINSKI'S REFLEX The involuntary turning upward of the toes when the sole of the foot is stroked. Babinski's (pronounced ba·bin′skeez) reflex is a sign of brain injury or disease of the spinal cord. It also occurs in normal babies, up to about the age of two.

BABY CARE The average new mother, although she may be inexperienced in handling a baby of her own, knows much more about child rearing than she may give herself credit for. She has probably helped friends or relatives in taking care of their babies. No doubt she has done some reading in preparation for her new role, and she may even have attended a class in baby care. She has every reason to feel confident in her ability to raise her baby to be a healthy, happy child. And remember—husbands are parents, too. They are usually eager to help take care of the child if they are given encouragement and guidance.

Babies may look delicate and helpless, but they are only relatively so. Actually, they are strong, vigorous little creatures with self-protecting instincts of their own. They need love and good care, of course. Given a reasonable amount of each, they will do very well indeed.

Choosing a Doctor: Often the doctor who delivers the baby is a specialist whose practice does not extend beyond childbirth. If this is the case, he will usually recommend a competent pediatrician (children's specialist). The pediatrician is a valuable ally for the new mother. She should bring her child to him regularly for examination and vaccinations and call him whenever she is confronted by a problem in child care. It does not pay for her to guess or worry when she can easily obtain this help.

Breast or Bottle-Feeding: An important decision facing the expectant mother is whether to feed her baby from her breasts or by bottle. Breast milk contains the food elements the infant needs, and the feeling of affectionate closeness to his mother that he experiences in nursing is no doubt good for him. Also, most mothers find the nursing relationship emotionally satisfying.

If the mother is unable to breast-feed her baby, there is no need for her to feel inadequate or guilty. Countless millions of babies are bottle-fed and grow up perfectly normally. The mother should just give the baby as much attention when feeding him as she would if she were nursing him, and hold and cuddle him while she gives him the bottle.

The doctor will recommend a bottle formula that is easy to make. There are also "just add water" commercial preparations available. In spite of an old tradition, it is not necessary to heat the formula before giving the baby his bottle. He will drink it as readily just as it comes from the refrigerator, unless he has become accustomed to drinking it warm.

Baby Grows and Develops: The infant grows and develops very rapidly in the first year of life. At 12 months he may weigh three times as much as he did at birth. Although all babies follow certain patterns of development, each is an individual. One baby at 15 months may be walking everywhere without support and have an impressive vocabulary; another who is the same age may still be crawling and incapable of uttering a single word. There is no reason to worry if a child seems slow in maturing. Every baby has his own rate of development. Do not try to rush the child or be impatient with him because he does not do as well as the neighbor's youngster. Just give him time and he will. But if you have any nagging questions about your baby's development, do not hesitate to discuss these with your baby's doctor.

BACILLARY DYSENTERY A form of DYSENTERY. (Pronounced bas′i·ler″ee dis′en·ter″ee.)

BACILLUS (plural, **bacilli**) Any of a large group of BACTERIA having a long, rodlike shape. Many types of bacilli (pronounced ba·sil′ie) are harmless and are present all around us in the air, water, and soil, and within living organisms, including man. Like all bacteria, a bacillus (pronounced ba·sil′us) is so tiny that it can be seen only by means of the magnifying power of a microscope. Most varieties require oxygen to exist and reproduce; some become inactive for long periods in the form of spores, when conditions are unfavorable for their growth. Some cause diseases in human beings. As its name indicates, bacillary DYSENTERY is caused by a bacillus, as are such diseases as anthrax (a disease of cattle that can be transmitted to man), botulism, diphtheria, leprosy, tuberculosis, typhoid fever, and whooping cough.

BACITRACIN An ANTIBIOTIC derived from the bacterium called *Bacillus subtilis*. Bacitracin (pronounced bas″i·tray′sin) is effective against many bacterial skin infections. It is usually applied only externally in an ointment.

BACKACHE Pain in the back, especially low-back pain, may take many forms and can result from many conditions and causes. Sometimes the cause is obvious, as when a person has had a fall or has lifted an exceptionally heavy load. Often enough, however, the backache comes on gradually, and the cause is not easy to find.

Poor posture lies at the root of many cases of chronic backache. Nervous tension may also be responsible; the muscles in the back tense up when one is under constant strain, as so many persons are, from the pressures of business or private life. If, associated with backache, there is dull or shooting pain going from the buttock and down into the leg, SCIATICA or a slipped disk (see VERTEBRAL DISK) may be suspected. ARTHRITIS in the region of the lower back may also be a cause. Many a woman has her first serious encounter with backache when she takes up her heavy duties as a housekeeper after she has borne a child.

Treatment: If the condition is a mild one, relief may be obtained by taking aspirin every four hours. (See ASPIRIN for precautions in the use of this medicine.) Application of a heating pad to the affected region is helpful, and so, frequently, is soaking in a warm bath only slightly above body temperature. You may also find that warm, moist compresses help. You should get as much bed rest as possible, and this must be on a very firm mattress. Placing a bed board under the mattress is a good idea.

If, in spite of these measures, the pain persists, or if it is acute at any time, medical attention should be sought without delay. Diagnosis of the cause of back trouble is not always a simple matter, and often it is necessary to consult an orthopedist, or specialist in bone, spine, and joint disorders. The sooner you visit your physician, the sooner you can hope to obtain relief.

Prevention: In addition to sleeping on a hard bed, it is advisable to sit in straight chairs. Soft, heavily padded chairs do not give the strained back the support that it needs.

Careful examination of your work habits is also in order, if you are to avoid recurrence of this common discomfort. Be very careful in lifting or carrying heavy loads. If you have to lift anything, use your strong leg muscles and spare the relatively weak back muscles. The correct method is to keep the back straight and bend your knees until you are low enough to grasp the object you want to lift. Then raise the object and yourself by simply straightening your legs. A housewife should see to it that she does not lean too far forward when ironing clothes and washing dishes. An office worker needs to be aware that relaxed but upright posture will help protect him against backache. If he has to spend most of the day sitting, he should shift his position or get to his feet from time to time. If a person is required to spend many hours behind the wheel of a car, he should stop at regular intervals and get out and stretch. Automobile seats may need extra support, and low-slung cars may prove troublesome.

Everyone should be aware that bad posture places a heavy strain on the spine, distorting its normal curvature. This is an open invitation to back trouble. Carry your body upright, in a natural, comfortable way. Do not slouch or slump. Keep the chest raised somewhat. Good posture will not only make you feel better, it will make you look better as well. Also, your doctor may suggest simple exercises to strengthen the abdominal and back muscles.

BACKBONE See SPINE.

BACTEREMIA A medical term for BLOOD POISONING. (Pronounced bak″te·ree′mee·a.)

BACTERIAL ENDOCARDITIS Inflammation of the thin membrane (endocardium) that covers the valves and the inner surface of the cavities of the heart. Bacterial endocarditis (pronounced bak·tir′ee·al en″doh·kahr·die′tis) may be acute or chronic. It is caused by strains of STREPTOCOCCI and STAPHYLOCOCCI bacteria. It may follow even the unnoticed, slight TOXEMIA (blood poisoning) that may result from surgery or tooth extraction. People with hearts damaged by earlier disease, such as rheumatic or congenital heart disease, are especially susceptible. If not treated with ANTIBIOTICS and bed rest, bacterial endocarditis may prove fatal.

BACTERIUM (plural, **bacteria**) A microscopic organism commonly called a microbe, or—if it causes infection or disease—a germ. Bacteria are one-celled living organisms and have various shapes: rodlike (BACILLUS), spherical (COCCUS), and spiral (SPIROCHETE). Bacteria are everywhere—in water and soil and inside other living organisms, including human beings; *anaerobic* bacteria flourish in airless environments. They are not necessarily harmful. Some types are essential for the growth and production of food by plants.

Disease-bearing bacteria produce poisons called TOXINS, against some of which medical science has developed ANTITOXINS. Among the diseases caused by bacteria are cholera, meningitis, pneumonia, tuberculosis, the venereal diseases, and STAPHYLOCOCCUS and STREPTOCOCCUS infections such as strep throat. The discovery that certain bacteria destroy others led to the development of ANTIBIOTICS.

BAD BREATH See HALITOSIS.

BAG OF WATERS See AMNION.

BAKER'S DERMATITIS A type of allergic skin irritation of the hands caused by constant handling of yeast; also called baker's itch. This type of DERMATITIS (pronounced dur″ma·tie′tis) is common among people who bake professionally.

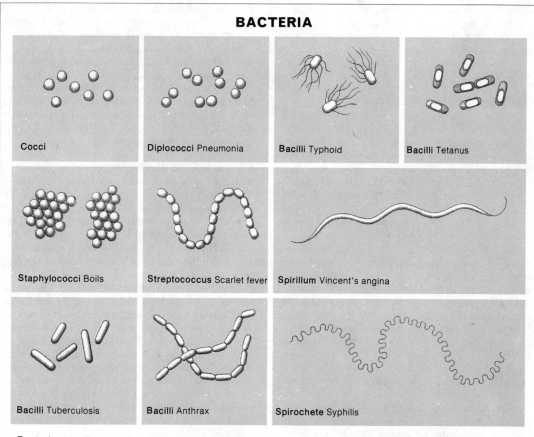

BACTERIA

Cocci

Diplococci Pneumonia

Bacilli Typhoid

Bacilli Tetanus

Staphylococci Boils

Streptococcus Scarlet fever

Spirillum Vincent's angina

Bacilli Tuberculosis

Bacilli Anthrax

Spirochete Syphilis

Bacteria are microscopic organisms, generally only a few ten-thousandths of an inch across; these are shown enlarged about a thousand times. Many bacteria are harmless or beneficial to man, and are found living in the soil as well as in the human intestines. Some, called pathogenic bacteria, cause diseases in human beings, although most of these can be combated by treatment with antibiotics.

BAKING SODA See SODIUM BICARBONATE.

BALANCE, SENSE OF Keeping our sense of balance relies upon a number of factors. When any of these is interfered with, as in certain diseases, we experience dizziness and are unable to remain in an upright position.

One factor is our vision. With the eyes open, it is easy for us to judge our position and our surroundings and balance ourselves accurately. You can easily demonstrate this to yourself by trying to stand on one leg with your eyes closed. Another important factor is our kinesthetic sensations, or sensations of movement. As a part of the body—say, an arm—moves, it sends continual messages to the brain, thus keeping the brain advised of the relative position of the arm; meanwhile the rest of the body makes adjustments to keep in balance.

But by far the most vital factor in balance is found in the inner EAR. The external and middle parts of the ear are concerned with hearing; the inner ear, however, in addition to its auditory func-tion, helps to control posture and equilibrium. It does this chiefly by means of three semicircular canals, which are at right angles to each other, like three sides of a box. These canals, each shaped like the letter U, contain fluid. As the body changes position, the fluid touches different nerve endings inside the canals. The sensation is communicated to the brain by nerve cells, and automatically muscles are called into play to keep the body in equilibrium.

When taking a trip on a ship or in a car or other moving conveyance, you may feel MOTION SICKNESS. This unpleasant sensation is caused by the fluid in the inner-ear canals making unaccustomed movements. In motion sickness and related disorders, there is often not only a feeling of dizziness, but also nausea and vomiting. These symptoms show up, too, in diseases of the inner ear.

BALDNESS See ALOPECIA.

BALNEOTHERAPY The treatment of disease by specially prepared baths. Once a popular remedy for many illnesses, balneotherapy (pronounced bal″nee·oh·ther′a·pee) is now chiefly used to relieve the discomfort of certain skin disorders. See also HYDROTHERAPY.

BANDAGING See FIRST AID section.

BARBER'S ITCH See FOLLICULITIS.

BARBITURATE A medicine that is used as a sedative, to overcome insomnia, or for general anesthesia. PHENOBARBITAL is probably the most familiar kind, but there are many others, including SECONAL and AMYTAL. A barbiturate (pronounced bahr·bich′ur·it) is often prescribed in connection with psychotherapy or to relieve tension.

Barbiturates can be purchased only with a physician's prescription, and the exact dosage that he indicates should not be exceeded. An overdose can be fatal. There are many barbiturate preparations. One kind, for example, may be prescribed for the person who has trouble falling asleep, and another kind for the person who keeps waking up during the night. However, do not suppose that you need sleeping pills if you occasionally suffer from INSOMNIA. Recent research has shown that barbiturates alter the normal pattern of SLEEP. You can often do yourself as much good—or more—by going for a long walk or taking a warm bath before retiring. Relaxed reading in bed also helps.

Barbiturates have other uses. Phenobarbital is administered to prevent or reduce epileptic seizures. Rapidly acting barbiturates such as PENTOTHAL are used for anesthesia of brief duration.

Barbiturate Dependency: If you have barbiturates in your possession, make certain that they do not fall into anyone else's hands. Do not use them any longer than your doctor advises. Barbiturates can be habit-forming. Alcoholics sometimes take them in place of liquor and become just as dependent on them. Symptoms of barbiturate dependence are sleepiness, slurred speech, confusion, slow reflexes, and other types of behavior that we associate with drunkenness. There is also a tendency to become involved in accidents. When the person stops taking barbiturates, he suffers typical withdrawal symptoms: convulsions, tremors, nervousness, and insomnia. Treatment is by reducing the dosage gradually and administering psychotherapy.

Barbiturate Poisoning: This is another of the risks of taking barbiturates to excess. Symptoms of barbiturate poisoning include slow, shallow breathing, muscle twitching, slow reflexes or none, bluish skin, and deep sleep. The police or a hospital should be called at once to send an emergency respiration unit. If the victim is not asleep, vomiting should be induced by inserting a finger in his throat. Loosen constrictive clothing around the throat; mouth-to-mouth artificial respiration should be begun if breathing is weak. (See FIRST AID section.)

BARIUM SULFATE A compound of barium that is given orally, in a pleasantly flavored liquid mixture, to patients being X-rayed for disorders of the intestinal tract. X RAYS cannot pass through barium, so the organ in question, usually the stomach or intestines, stands out on the developed X-ray film. The barium (pronounced bar′ee·um) compound is used to locate disorders such as ulcers, tumors, and colitis. A barium enema, injection of a barium-containing fluid through the anus, is given when X-raying the rectum or lower intestine (colon).

BASAL METABOLIC RATE (BMR) The rate at which a person uses energy just to remain alive—to carry on the basic vital functions of breathing, circulation, and METABOLISM. The rate of metabolism is regulated by the THYROID GLAND, and the BMR was formerly much used to diagnose disorders of that gland. In theory, the BMR can be measured by measuring the amount of heat produced by the body when completely at rest. In practice, the BMR is determined by measuring how much oxygen a person at rest uses in a short period of time. This indicates how much energy the body has generated. (The amount of oxygen used is an indirect measure of the heat produced.) The results of a BMR test can be influenced by a number of other things: pregnancy, diabetes, various medicines, the presence of food in the stomach, and even emotions such as anxiety during the test. Other tests that are easier to perform and just as reliable have largely replaced the BMR as a test of thyroid function.

BATTERED-CHILD SYNDROME Willful and serious physical injury, which is sometimes fatal, to infants and young children by their parents or guardians. Until recent years, children brought to hospitals or to doctors' offices suffering from skull fractures, broken limbs, and extensive burns, bruises, and lacerations were usually regarded as victims of "accidents." Today, however, doctors are paying increasing attention to the battered child and are reporting suspicious or recurring cases to the police.

The parents or guardians of such children are deeply disturbed people who have usually experienced neglect and maltreatment in their own early years. Parents who have the urge to injure their children should voluntarily seek help and advice from a PSYCHIATRIST.

B COMPLEX See VITAMIN.

BEDPAN A shallow enamel pan of a special, somewhat oval shape that can be used as a toilet by a person who is confined to his bed.

BED REST A good, comfortable bed is indispensable in general, but especially in illness. Too many beds have soft or sagging mattresses that do not give the back the support that it requires. So a firm, well-made mattress, resting upon a bedspring in good condition, must be provided.

A soft mattress can sometimes be helped by placing under it a strong plywood board. If you cannot purchase one of the right size, you can have one made to the measurements of your bed at your local lumberyard. In cases of sciatica, slipped disk, or lower-back pain, a bed board is essential. Often complaints about not sleeping comfortably are resolved by firming up a soft mattress with a bed board or obtaining a harder mattress.

Bedding should be chosen with the health and comfort of the individual in mind. If he is a young child or an elderly person with poor bladder control, a plastic or rubber sheet should be placed between the bed sheet and mattress. But normally this item may be dispensed with, as it makes the bed too hot. If a bedridden person is allergic to dust, it is advisable to use a mattress and pillows of foam rubber or synthetic fibers. Pillows stuffed with feathers or kapok may produce an allergic reaction in sensitive persons.

The position of the bed in the room deserves careful consideration. Do not set it too close to a window, or there may be a draft. It should also be at a comfortable distance from the heating unit. There should be adequate light for reading, and it ought to be possible to put the light out just by reaching out a hand. A table at the head of the bed, to hold the objects that the occupant needs, is a convenience.

The Bed in the Sickroom: If there is prolonged illness at home, it may be advisable to rent a bed of the adjustable kind used in hospitals. Usually, though, the sick person's own bed will do. If the patient is confined to bed constantly, the linen should be changed every day. If he is able to leave the bed for periods of time, then three changes a week are sufficient. It is important that the linen be clean, and that the bed be made very smooth.

In ordinary sickness bed linen may be washed in the usual way. In infectious disease, however, it must be made germ-free by boiling. Boiling should last five minutes or longer. Then allow the linen to soak in hot water and soapsuds. Next, remove it and follow your normal washing procedure. When practicable, hang it in the sunlight to dry.

A person may feel weak and dizzy when he tries to get up after a long period of bed rest. Here is a good way to handle this problem: Have the person sit first on the edge of the bed with his feet on the floor. If he feels all right after a few minutes, assist him in walking to a seat close by. Have him return to the bed if he complains of dizziness. If he does not, after resting a few minutes more, he may proceed farther, and gradually increase the distance he walks day by day.

BEDSORE A serious condition resulting from lying in one position in bed over a long illness.

When a person is lying in bed, most of the weight of the body bears down on just a few small areas. The pressure reduces the blood supply to the soft tissues and skin in the affected areas. A healthy person resting or sleeping will normally make many slight changes in position to relieve the pressure. In a seriously ill person, weakness or pain may prevent these movements. Under prolonged pressure, the soft tissue and skin begin to break down. The first sign of trouble is usually local skin redness, which disappears if pressure is applied with a finger. At a later stage, the area feels somewhat hard and the skin has a bluish tinge. If untreated, an ulcer finally develops. A neglected ulcer may cause so much tissue damage that the bone underneath may be exposed.

Elderly patients are most likely to suffer from bedsores, which are also called decubitus ulcers. Also highly susceptible are bedridden patients whose skin is sensitive because of a nervous or circulatory ailment and those for whom paralysis makes change of position impossible.

If the patient cannot change his own body position frequently, he should be helped to do so—*this is most important.* Assistance should be gentle and slow, and prolonged pressure on the bony parts of the body should be avoided. Continued pressure from the bed can be relieved by improvising little cushions or pads made of soft clean material or of pieces of foam rubber wrapped in a handkerchief. These pads should be placed under the back of the heels, the elbows, and the ears. A rubber air ring covered with an absorbent cloth can be placed under the buttocks if the patient is lying on his back, or under the hipbones if he is lying on his side.

Bedsores are easier to prevent than to cure. There are several procedures that should be followed by anyone caring for a patient immobilized in bed at home for a long time. The patient's skin should be kept clean and healthy by frequent bed baths and massaging. Powdering the exposed areas of skin with plain talc is also a good preventive measure, but be sure to pat off excess powder to prevent caking. Sheets should lie absolutely smooth and be kept dry and free of any crumbs or irritants.

At the first sign of any sore spots on the skin, call the doctor immediately for further instructions.

BED-WETTING See ENURESIS.

BEE STING Bee or wasp stings can be serious. The stinger and the attached poison sac are usually left in the wound and should be removed. Do not use tweezers which would squeeze the sac and inject all the poison into the wound. Beekeepers recommend using the edge of a knife or a fingernail, instead, to scrape the stinger out of the wound. Apply household AMMONIA, CALAMINE LOTION, or a paste of SODIUM BICARBONATE and water to relieve the pain. Do *not* plaster the wound with mud. This old-fashioned remedy may cause infection.

If the sting is on a very sensitive place, such as the eyelid, lip, or tongue, or if the victim complains of weakness or swelling of the body, call a doctor immediately. If you have been prescribed medicine for bee-sting allergy, take it as soon as possible. To avoid stings, keep away from hollow trees and other places where hives may be.

BELCHING The sudden release of air, gas, or stomach acid through the mouth; burping. By eating too much or too fast, one tends to swallow air along with the food. This air is then released by belching.

BELLADONNA A toxic substance obtained from the roots and leaves of the belladonna, or deadly nightshade, plant, which is native to Europe and Asia and is cultivated in North America. ATROPINE and related medicines are derived from belladonna (pronounced bel''a·don'a). Although it is poisonous in concentrated or prolonged use, in proper dosages it relieves peptic ulcer and spasms of the gastrointestinal tract. It is also used to dilate the pupil of the eye in order to facilitate examination of the retina.

BELLADONNA

The deadly nightshade plant, scientific name *Atropa belladonna*, contains the poisonous drug atropine, or belladonna, which is used to dilate the pupil in treating eye disorders.

BENADRYL The trade name for an ANTIHISTAMINE used in the treatment of allergic reaction, as well as for alleviation of the symptoms of MOTION SICKNESS and PARKINSONISM. Benadryl (pronounced ben'a·dril) is available by prescription only.

BENDS A disorder occurring in tunnel workers, divers, and others who work under increased atmospheric pressure. The bends (also called caisson disease or decompression sickness) has become a problem in space travel when men are required to move from their pressurized space cabins to the near-vacuum of outer space, as on "space walks" or on the surface of the moon. This is one reason why astronauts must wear space suits that protect them against sudden drops in pressure. Scuba diving can also lead to the bends if a person returns to the surface too rapidly after a period under water.

The bends results when the individual makes a too-rapid return from a high-pressure atmosphere to a lower pressure. Bubbles of nitrogen gas, freed from the bloodstream, block small blood vessels and collect in the tissues. The victim suffers from headache, dizziness, vomiting, and pains in the upper abdomen and limbs.

The bends can be prevented by the use of a decompression chamber in which the air pressure is gradually reduced to that of the atmosphere. Treatment for a person who has contracted the disorder consists of prompt recompression in a "lock," a medical machine built for this purpose, followed by gradual decompression. To avoid the bends, a diver may breath a mixture of helium and oxygen instead of air, because helium does not dissolve in the blood and cannot cause the disorder.

BENEMID The trade name (pronounced ben'-e·mid) for a probenecid, a medicine used to promote excretion of uric acid, as in the treatment of GOUT.

BENIGN A term used to indicate a disorder that is not likely to get worse and is essentially harmless. It is often applied to the type of growth or TUMOR that is not in itself harmful and not likely to recur after it has been removed. The opposite of benign in this sense is MALIGNANT. The term is also used for any abnormal condition that is harmless or transitory. For example, the presence of protein in the urine (ALBUMINURIA) is a symptom of serious kidney disease. However, under certain conditions, benign albuminuria may occur in a person with perfectly healthy kidneys.

BENTYL A trade name for dicyclomine, a medicine used in relieving spasms arising from functional disorders (such as COLITIS) in the large intestine, or colon.

BENZEDRINE A trade name for an AMPHETAMINE. It is a medicine that stimulates the central nervous system, increasing energy and mental alertness, and raises the blood pressure. Benzedrine (pronounced ben'ze·dreen) may be obtained only with a physician's prescription and is taken orally, in tablet or capsule form.

Doctors may prescribe Benzedrine to counteract mental depression and the effects of alcoholism. It may also be used as an appetite depressant for persons on reducing diets. After taking Benzedrine, the individual experiences a sense of well-being and feels little desire to eat.

Unpleasant side effects, such as ANXIETY, tremors, and INSOMNIA, have limited the use of Benzedrine in recent years. It is rarely prescribed for people with known CORONARY HEART DISEASE or HYPERTENSION, or for women in the early stages of pregnancy.

BENZIDINE TEST   A diagnostic test to detect blood in the feces, urine, or other substances. Benzidine (pronounced ben'zi·deen″) is a chemical that turns blue and then purplish in the presence of blood.

BENZOCAINE   A local anesthetic used in some ointments and dusting powders for relieving the pain of minor burns, sunburn, hemorrhoids, and similar conditions. Benzocaine (pronounced ben'zoh·kayn″) may cause a local inflammation in some persons who are sensitive to it. In such a case discontinue its use.

BERIBERI   A deficiency disease caused by a lack of vitamin B₁ (thiamine) in the diet. Beriberi (pronounced ber'ee·ber'ee) attacks the nervous system, causing NEURITIS, circulatory disturbances, stiffness in the legs, and sometimes paralysis. Although now rare among people who have access to adequate nutrition, beriberi is still prevalent in the Orient where polished (or white) rice forms the main part of the diet. It also occurs in prisons or during wartime when food is scarce. A more widespread use of unpolished (or brown) rice, which is rich in thiamine, could practically wipe out the disease in many parts of the world. See also VITAMIN.

BICARBONATE OF SODA   See SODIUM BICARBONATE.

BICUSPID   A tooth with two "points," or cusps. There are normally eight bicuspids (pronounced bie·kus'pidz) in the mouth, two on the top and two on the bottom of each side of the mouth. Another term for bicuspid is premolar. See also TOOTH.

BIFOCALS   A type of eyeglasses (pronounced bie·foh'kalz) that have lenses of two different strengths combined in the same pair of glasses. The upper lens is used for distance, while the lower lens is used for close work, such as sewing and reading. Also available are trifocals for distance, intermediate, and close viewing, as well as "no-line" bifocals, lenses that increase in strength gradually from top to bottom. Do not be discouraged about the time required to get used to bifocals; the convenience is worth the effort.

BILE   A bitter, greenish-yellow fluid manufactured continuously by the LIVER and stored in the gallbladder. Bile, also known as gall, enters the small intestine directly from the liver through a small tube, the common bile duct. A smaller duct, the cystic duct, connects the gallbladder to the common bile duct. Whenever fat leaves the stomach and enters the small intestine, it stimulates the flow of bile from both the liver and the gallbladder. Bile helps in the digestion and absorption of fats; it also helps to neutralize acids from the stomach. A brownish substance in bile, bilirubin, is present in small amounts in the blood and urine. In jaundice the yellow color of the skin and eyeballs results from abnormal amounts of bile pigment in the blood.

BILIARY COLIC   A form of COLIC involving the bile duct. (Pronounced bil'ee·er″ee kol'ik.)

BINET TEST   A graded series of questions developed between 1905 and 1911 by the French psychologists Alfred Binet and Théodore Simon for the purpose of comparing the mental ability of school children. The questions were designed to call upon a variety of mental functions, such as memory, reasoning, and the perception of spatial relations. By giving the test to a large number of children of different ages, Binet and Simon determined which questions were within the capacity of the average child of any given age. It was then possible for them to tell whether any particular child had more or less mental ability than the average French child of his age. (See INTELLIGENCE QUOTIENT.)

The Binet tests, also known as the Binet-Simon tests, were the models for a great number of different intelligence tests which were devised to evaluate the mental ability of both children and adults. Tests may be written or oral, given individually or to groups. One of the best-known revisions of the Binet tests is the Stanford-Binet. Other widely used tests include the U.S. Army General Classification Test, the Wechsler-Bellevue Scale, and the Cattell and Otis tests.

Intelligence tests are often criticized because they are not "culture free"—that is, they reflect not only native intelligence but also the amount of encouragement and practice the individual has previously had in performing the sort of mental tasks set by a test. Nevertheless, if it is necessary to grade people according to mental ability, the results of intelligence tests are less biased than any subjective judgment of the mental ability of another person.

To obtain a typical test, write American Mensa, Ltd., 1701 West 3rd Street, Brooklyn, New York 11223. For a small fee they will grade your test and give you the results.

BIOFLAVONOID Any of a group of compounds that are involved in maintaining the walls of small blood vessels. Certain bioflavonoids (pronounced bie"oh·flay'vo·noydz) occur along with vitamin C in citrus and other fruits. These bioflavonoids are sometimes called vitamin P, but there is no evidence that they are needed in the human diet.

BIOPSY Removal of a bit of tissue from the living body for examination, generally under the microscope, to diagnose a disease. Biopsy (pronounced bie'op·see) is one of the surest ways that medical science possesses to determine whether or not a disorder is present. Usually only a small piece of tissue is removed and sent to a laboratory, where it is analyzed by a specialist in pathology.

Biopsies are important in the investigation of cancer, skin diseases, and other conditions. If there is a small growth on the surface of the body, the entire growth may be removed by the surgeon and sent to the laboratory. Biopsy specimens may be taken within the body with the help of special instruments. If lung cancer is suspected, for example, the BRONCHOSCOPE is used not only to view the lungs but to remove a minute section for analysis. To diagnose kidney diseases, or a liver disease such as CIRRHOSIS, a bit of tissue is taken with a long needle passed through the skin and other tissues.

A biopsy may be performed either before an operation or as part of one. For example, a lump in the breast is removed in the hospital with the patient under general ANESTHESIA. Then, immediately, the lump of tissue is prepared for examination. It is quick-frozen and then cut into minute sections. After these tiny slices have been stained and mounted on glass slides, the pathologist studies them under his microscope. If no evidence of cancer is found, the surgeon sews up the incision, and the patient is released soon afterward. If the growth is MALIGNANT (cancerous), a more extensive operation proceeds at once, so that the disease may be arrested. A similar procedure is followed when the growth is inside the body.

BIRTH See CHILDBIRTH.

BIRTH CONTROL See CONTRACEPTIVE METHODS AND DEVICES; FAMILY PLANNING.

BIRTH DEFECT An abnormality present at birth; a congenital defect. Such abnormalities may be inherited from the parents or they may be the result of an illness, a toxic condition of the pregnant mother, or an abnormal condition in the uterus or the birth passage. Sometimes, more than one cause may be responsible for a birth defect.

A difficult birth may also injure a baby, resulting sometimes in a more or less permanent physical or mental handicap. This is called a BIRTH INJURY rather than a birth defect.

Exactly what is a birth defect? Just about all of us are born with minor defects such as asymmetry (for example, one eye higher than the other), BIRTHMARKS, or slight oddities of bone structure. Only about 3 percent of infants are born with a defect that imposes a handicap on them. One of the most publicized—and also one of the rarest—birth defects is SIAMESE TWINS. Others include such varied conditions as MONGOLISM, CLEFT PALATE, COLOR BLINDNESS, HEMOPHILIA, and CONGENITAL HEART DISEASE. Some of these show up at birth, but some may not become apparent until later in the child's life. A large number of defects can be corrected by surgery or other treatment, especially if detected early. *This is one good reason why infants and young children should have frequent and thorough medical, dental, and eye examinations.*

Conditions in the Mother's Body: As many as 80 percent of birth defects are attributable to conditions in the mother's body, or these same conditions working in combination with heredity. Sometimes, but by no means always, the specific cause of a birth defect is known. Exposure during pregnancy to X rays or other radiation may produce deformity. The taking of certain medicines may also lead to birth defects. A child may be born with a defective heart or nervous system or other abnormalities if the mother catches German measles (RUBELLA) during the first three months of pregnancy. A gonorrheal infection in the mother's birth canal may cause blindness in a baby (although this is not strictly speaking a birth defect, since the newborn infant's eyes are normal at birth and are blinded *after* birth by infection picked up during delivery). This can be prevented by the routine precaution of treating the eyes of a newborn baby with a solution of silver nitrate or an antibiotic.

Hereditary defects are those birth defects that are inherited and passed on in the GENES, the minute elements that transmit characteristics from generation to generation. Mental deficiency, eye defects, and tendencies to develop various types of disease are only a few of the abnormalities that may be inherited.

Most people are aware of some family traits they would rather be without. If these are serious hereditary defects, the possibility must be faced that they may be passed on to future children. The chances that this will happen in any particular case range all the way from certainty to impossibility. A new specialty in medicine called genetic counseling is concerned with predicting quite accurately what the chances are in specific cases, and thus helping people decide whether or not to have children. If you want a child but fear that you may pass on hereditary defects, talk it over with your doctor. If you live in a large population center, he may be able to refer you to a qualified genetic counselor.

Some birth defects are unavoidable, but others might be prevented by visiting your physician regularly all through pregnancy and following his instructions. Pay particular attention to his advice about food, medication, and rest. Report any illness or abnormal symptoms to him as soon as possible. *Do not take any medicines or have any injections during pregnancy without first getting your doctor's consent.*

BIRTH INJURY Injury suffered by an infant while it is being born. Thanks to the increasingly widespread practice of paying visits to the physician early in pregnancy, as well as throughout its course, it is possible to anticipate and avoid difficulties in delivery. Improvements in techniques of handling abnormal deliveries have also helped greatly to minimize birth damage.

CESAREAN (CESARIAN) SECTION is one of the techniques now frequently used when a difficult birth is anticipated. If the mother's pelvis is too narrow or if she is unwell, the baby may be brought safely into the world by surgical removal from the uterus by way of the abdomen. The same procedure may be used for subsequent babies.

Head injuries are sometimes suffered by infants during prolonged labor or because of difficulties in delivery. Injury of the nerves branching from the spinal cord may cause paralysis of the arms and hands. The brain may also be damaged during birth, resulting in some degree of MENTAL RETARDATION. Another possible result is CEREBRAL PALSY, a condition in which there is partial paralysis and defective muscular coordination. (Not all cases of cerebral palsy are caused by birth injuries, however. Techniques of helping cerebral palsy children are highly developed, and outlook is improved if treatment is begun early and continued.)

Brain damage may also result from oxygen starvation during birth. The infant receives oxygen from its mother through the PLACENTA and the UMBILICAL CORD until its own lungs take over after birth. In some instances the placenta may become detached before the baby is born or the cord may become so twisted while the infant is passing through the birth canal that oxygen is temporarily cut off and areas of the brain suffer damage.

Some especially well-equipped hospitals have electronic equipment by which, in a difficult or premature birth, a continuous check can be made of the baby's condition, including the concentration of oxygen in its blood. If the equipment signals any dangerous condition not evident to the eye, emergency measures are taken immediately. At the opposite extreme are cases where the moment of birth has been artificially delayed by attendants until the doctor can arrive on the scene. Only recently has it been shown that this procedure is extremely dangerous for the future development of the baby.

Premature infants are especially susceptible to injury because of their delicate condition. Thus, the best policy is for a mother to avoid anything that may bring the pregnancy to an early termination. The pregnant woman should go about her activities in a sensible way; if anything unusual happens, the doctor should be called immediately.

BIRTHMARK A blemish or other mark present on the skin at birth; also called a NEVUS. Usually, birthmarks develop before the baby is born. Precisely what causes them is not known. If they are annoying or disfiguring, certain types may be removed by surgery, reduced by medical treatment, or concealed by the use of cosmetics.

Blood-Vessel Birthmark: This type of birthmark is known as a HEMANGIOMA. It includes the familiar dark red strawberry or raspberry birthmark, which consists of an enlarged group of blood vessels in the skin. Often the mark subsides early in life. If it does not, and is located in a prominent place, such as on the face, it may be best to seek medical assistance in treating it. The mark may be shrunk by injections, removed by a surgeon, or treated with dry ice.

Port-wine stain, another type of blood-vessel birthmark, presents more of a problem. Dermatologists have developed various methods of treating it to make it less conspicuous. There are also cosmetic preparations available for covering it.

If a child has a large birthmark in a conspicuous place, he should not be made self-conscious about it by his parents. It is best to avoid discussions of such a disfigurement in his presence. However, if treatment is contemplated, or if a child is to visit a plastic surgeon for removal of a birthmark, he should be told about it in a simple, comforting way, in advance. A few well-timed words with a tone of reassurance can often prevent long-lasting emotional upset.

See also MOLE.

BISMUTH A silver-white metal, the salts of which are now rarely used in treating certain inflammations of the stomach and intestines. Before the discovery of PENICILLIN, bismuth (pronounced biz'-muth) preparations were employed in the treatment of syphilis.

BITE See ANIMAL BITE; DOG BITE; INSECT BITE.

BLACK-AND-BLUE MARK Bluish or purplish discoloration caused by blood that accumulates under the skin after the rupture of small blood vessels in the surrounding tissues. Black-and-blue marks usually follow a fall, blow, or pressure severe enough to be noticed when it happens, and are often accompanied by cuts or scrapes. Although unsightly, such a BRUISE is not serious and gradually fades away. Pain may be relieved by applying an ice bag, or a cold cloth.

If you find the black-and-blue mark is very painful and there is much swelling, or a hard knot persists under the skin, consult your doctor. He can help relieve the pain and discoloration. Besides, he may discover a fracture or other injury requiring treatment. If black-and-blue marks appear without external cause, they should have medical attention promptly. Such "unexplained" marks are not ordinarily painful, but they may be a symptom of one of a number of serious diseases affecting the blood. See also BLOOD DISEASE.

BLACK DEATH   See BUBONIC PLAGUE.

BLACK EYE   Discoloration of the skin and swelling of tissue in the region of the eye, usually resulting from an injury that has ruptured minute blood vessels beneath the skin. Because of the many blood vessels and the transparency of skin in this area, a minor blow near the eye often produces a darker BRUISE than it would elsewhere. Pain and swelling may be reduced by applying ice packs or cloths soaked in very cold water and wrung out. A doctor should be consulted if there is any injury to the eye itself, or if pain and swelling are severe.

BLACKHEAD   A plug of hardened fatty material in a skin pore, formed by oil secreted by small glands in the skin. If a great many form, a doctor should be questioned about the possibility of ACNE. Blackheads may be removed by gentle pressure with a special extractor you can buy in a drugstore. First wash the face gently with warm, soapy water and a clean washcloth; if the blackhead does not come out easily, leave it for a few days. Never apply such pressure that the skin is injured, and avoid pressing or touching blackheads with the fingers, which may carry and spread infection.

BLACK LUNG   See SILICOSIS.

BLADDER   A part of the URINARY TRACT, consisting of a hollow organ with muscular walls, in which URINE collects before voiding, or urination. Urine, excreted by the kidneys, drains continuously into the bladder through two long tubes, the ureters. The bladder expands and contracts as urine is collected and voided. In adults, the bladder has a capacity of about one pint. As it fills up, discomfort causes the urge to urinate. Release of urine from the bladder is controlled by a circular muscle (a SPHINCTER) surrounding the URETHRA, which leads out from the lower part of the bladder. Conscious control of this sphincter muscle develops after infancy. A number of disorders can affect the bladder, including CALCULUS (stones), benign and cancerous TUMORS, HERNIA (protrusion through an opening), and CYSTITIS (inflammation). These are dealt with in the branch of medicine called UROLOGY. If urination is painful or difficult, see your doctor.

BLAND DIET   A diet of easily digested, nonirritating foods prescribed in the treatment of peptic ULCERS of the stomach and duodenum, GASTRITIS (inflammation of the stomach lining), and other stomach and intestinal disorders. In such cases, the purpose of the diet is to neutralize the acidity of the gastric juices and to reduce irritation in the digestive tract. The doctor may recommend a bland diet for a sick person or someone convalescing from an illness.

Milk is the basic food in any bland diet. In the first stage of treating peptic ulcers, a mixture of milk and cream (called the Sippy diet) is frequently given hourly for two or three days. Other foods, added gradually as the person improves, include Cream of Wheat, cottage cheese, lean meat, eggs, poultry, custards, potatoes, rice, cooked fruits, and vegetables (such as strained squash) that do not produce gas. Spicy and fried foods are prohibited, as are raw fruits and vegetables, salads, meat broths, coffee, and tea. In a bland diet, supplements of vitamins and minerals are usually needed.

BLASTOMYCOSIS   An uncommon infection, caused by a fungus, that first appears in the skin or the lungs and may spread to other organs. Usually slow to develop, blastomycosis (pronounced blas″-toh·mie·koh′sis) produces painless areas of small, wartlike spots on the skin. If present in the lungs, the symptoms, very mild at first, may include shortness of breath, coughing, and occasionally pain. Diagnosis is certain only if the minute, yeastlike fungus is identified under the microscope. Treatment involves a stay in a hospital for careful, regulated administration of a medicine such as amphotericin B or hydroxystilbamidine isethionate.

BLEEDER'S DISEASE   See HEMOPHILIA.

BLEEDING   Most abrasions or surface injuries that produce bleeding are not serious. If a cut is washed promptly with soap and clean water, preferably under a water tap, there is little danger from infection. There is no need to apply an antiseptic if you do a good job of cleansing the wound; some antiseptics are so strong they produce considerable pain. Place a sterile dressing over the injury and fasten it in place with a bandage. A ready-made adhesive-gauze bandage may be used for a minor cut.

In a healthy person NOSEBLEED usually means only that a minor blood vessel has ruptured. The simplest way to stop a nosebleed is to pinch the nose between two fingers for about 10 minutes.

Severe wounds can cause heavy loss of blood. The quickest way to halt bleeding is to apply direct pressure to the wound with a gauze compress or clean cloth. Even a clean hand alone may be used. Continue the pressure for 15 minutes. Then bandage the cloth tightly in place. For other types of bleeding, see the FIRST AID section.

Bleeding as a Symptom: When bleeding occurs without any noticeable cause, it may be a warning that there is something wrong in the body. For example, if blood is coughed up, it should be reported to the family physician without delay. It may be a slight, relatively meaningless occurrence—but it can also be the first symptom of lung disease.

Blood may show up in the urine. This can signal the presence of urinary or other disease. In the stool, blood may be caused by HEMORRHOIDS (most commonly) or intestinal disease. Bleeding between menstrual periods calls for investigation. So does bleeding after the MENOPAUSE. The sooner such a symptom is reported to your doctor, the sooner he can reassure you—or take prompt, effective steps to bring the problem under control.

BLEMISH Any small spot or mark on the skin, as a PIMPLE, WART, or MOLE. The word is often used loosely: a well-placed mole may be considered a beauty spot rather than a blemish; and even FRECKLES may be called blemishes by someone who would rather be without them. A good attitude toward blemishes is to think twice before deciding they are unsightly, and then to consult your doctor about the advisability of their removal.

BLINDNESS Partial or total loss of vision. The ability to see consists of two parts: the ability to focus sharply (visual acuity); and the ability to see things without looking at them directly (peripheral vision). A person with very good visual acuity is said to have 20/20 vision. This figure is based on his ability to read, at a distance of 20 feet, the fine print in the lower lines of the standard chart that the doctor uses to test eyesight. If a person can read at 20 feet only as much as a person with good vision can read at 200 feet, his visual acuity is 20/200. Poor visual acuity can be corrected to some extent by EYEGLASSES. A person is generally considered to be blind if visual acuity cannot be corrected to at least 20/200 in the better eye.

A person whose visual field is very severely limited is also considered to be blind. Normally, peripheral vision takes in an area somewhat greater than would be marked off by a straight line across the face at right angles to the line of sight; in technical terms, normal vision subtends an angle greater than 180°. A person whose peripheral vision subtends an angle of 20° or less is considered to be blind, even if acuity is good within his narrow field of vision. (The special conditions called NIGHT BLINDNESS and COLOR BLINDNESS are not blindness at all in this sense.)

There are many different causes of blindness. It may result from injury to the EYE itself, or from some abnormality or lesion in the brain or the optic nerve. It is sometimes due to a disorder affecting the whole system, such as diabetes. In some cases, it is congenital. Bacterial infections in the eyes of newborn babies were once a fairly common cause of blindness, but this is now prevented by routinely treating the eyes with a solution of silver nitrate when a baby is born. Formerly, blindness in premature babies was also fairly common, until it was discovered that this was the result of putting them in an atmosphere of almost pure oxygen in the incubator. Other causes of blindness are described in CATARACT, DETACHED RETINA, GLAUCOMA, IRITIS, KERATITIS, OPHTHALMIA, and TRACHOMA.

In many cases, blindness can be prevented by taking good care of the eyes and by getting a doctor's help promptly if any abnormality develops. An OPHTHALMOLOGIST is a doctor who specializes in eye disorders.

Since we depend more on vision than on any other sense, blindness is a very serious handicap. Most blind persons learn unconsciously to depend on hearing and other clues to give them information about their surroundings, and they take pride in their ability to function despite their handicap. In helping blind persons, use tact, and avoid thrusting upon them more help than they really need.

There are a number of ways in which blindness can be made somewhat less hard to bear. Many books are published in Braille (see BRAILLE SYSTEM) or are available in recorded form. One promising new device, still in the development stage, is an instrument that scans a printed page with a photoelectric eye and translates it into patterns of pressure that the blind person can recognize by the sense of touch. Almost every community of any size has agencies to help the blind. For more information on all aspects of blindness, write the American Foundation for the Blind, 15 West 16th Street, New York, New York 10011.

BLIND SPOT A small area at the back retina of the EYE where the optic nerve fibers enter. This spot is insensitive to light and hence "blind."

BLISTER A collection of fluid in the epidermis (the outer layer of the SKIN). The fluid is usually colorless, watery SERUM. Blisters containing serum are often caused by rubbing or burning by heat or the sun's rays. A blister containing blood sometimes forms if a small area of skin is sharply pinched. Blisters can also be a symptom of a disease, such as CHICKEN POX. Exposure to certain substances, such as the poisonous element in poison ivy, may also result in blisters.

The fluid in a small blister, or bleb, is usually reabsorbed fairly rapidly. (A large blister is sometimes called a bulla.) New epidermis forms under the blister, and when healing is complete the old bit of damaged skin is sloughed off. If the epidermis covering a blister is removed before healing takes place underneath, it leaves a painful, moist surface of dermis (the lower layer of skin) exposed to infection. Blisters on the feet, caused by a shoe rubbing against the skin, are especially likely to be rubbed open accidentally. It is advisable to put a gauze dressing or adhesive bandage over a blister if it is in any danger of being damaged before it heals.

Healing normally takes place after a blister breaks and the serum is drained off. A dressing should be applied. First, wash the area with soap and water. Then put a gauze dressing or adhesive bandage over the area.

Serious burns that cause blisters require a doctor's attention. See a doctor immediately, too, if any blister shows signs of infection, such as inflammation or the formation of pus.

BLOCK Any interruption of normal function. A *nerve* block, used to prevent the sensation of pain in a specific area of the body, consists of injecting an ANESTHETIC into a NERVE at the point where it branches out to that area. A *spinal* block usually refers to an injection of anesthetic near the spinal cord, deadening pain in the entire portion of the body below the point of injection. "*Speech* block" and "*mental* block" are terms for involuntary obstacles to mental functioning. See also BLOCKING; HEART BLOCK.

BLOCKING In PSYCHIATRY, sudden stoppage in a train of thought. Blocking is one of the characteristic symptoms of SCHIZOPHRENIA, a serious and widespread type of mental illness. Typically, the person jumps repeatedly from one idea to another idea that has no connection with what he has just been thinking or talking about. Or he may suddenly stop talking (and presumably thinking) altogether, without taking up another subject. In this extreme form, blocking is called obstruction.

According to psychoanalytic theory, blocking is due to painful memories and thought associations, which the individual unconsciously recognizes and tries to avoid. However, it is not advisable to try to persuade the person to face up to painful thought associations; this does not relieve the symptom.

The word "blocking" is often used popularly to account for temporary lapses of memory, such as inability to remember a word or a name.

BLOOD The fluid that circulates in the VEINS, ARTERIES, and CAPILLARIES; it carries digested food elements and oxygen to the cells of the body and removes carbon dioxide and other waste products from them. In addition, it performs many other functions vital to health and growth.

Blood appears to be a simple red fluid; under the microscope we see that it is actually a very complex substance. Over half (55 percent) of our blood is not red at all. It is a clear liquid known as plasma that is 92 percent water. The other 8 percent includes many essential substances, among them the protein fibrinogen, which enables the blood to clot. GAMMA GLOBULIN, another protein in plasma, contains antibodies and provides protection against certain infections; it is produced by the lymph glands. Other plasma materials include hormones manufactured by the endocrine glands, vitamins, enzymes, additional proteins, and salts.

What of the other 45 percent of the blood? It is made up largely of red and white corpuscles (blood cells) and platelets suspended in the plasma.

Of these minute particles, the most numerous are the red blood cells (ERYTHROCYTES), which give the blood its color. The average person may have as many as 30 trillion red blood cells. These are con-

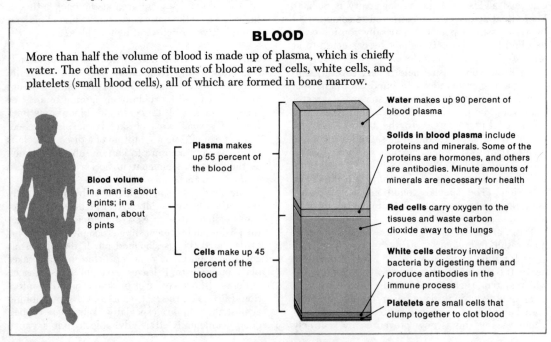

BLOOD

More than half the volume of blood is made up of plasma, which is chiefly water. The other main constituents of blood are red cells, white cells, and platelets (small blood cells), all of which are formed in bone marrow.

Blood volume in a man is about 9 pints; in a woman, about 8 pints

Plasma makes up 55 percent of the blood

Cells make up 45 percent of the blood

Water makes up 90 percent of blood plasma

Solids in blood plasma include proteins and minerals. Some of the proteins are hormones, and others are antibodies. Minute amounts of minerals are necessary for health

Red cells carry oxygen to the tissues and waste carbon dioxide away to the lungs

White cells destroy invading bacteria by digesting them and produce antibodies in the immune process

Platelets are small cells that clump together to clot blood

stantly wearing out and are replaced with new ones—at the rate of 5 million per second—produced in the marrow of the bones. The red blood cells contain HEMOGLOBIN, a protein substance. As the blood passes through the capillaries of the lungs, the red blood cells release carbon dioxide, a waste gas, and pick up oxygen, which attaches very readily to the hemoglobin.

There are a number of different types of white blood cells (LEUKOCYTES), some originating in the bone marrow and some in the lymph glands. These cells are the body's first line of defense against bacterial invaders. When bacteria enter the body, white blood cells are produced in great numbers. They travel to the infection and engulf the invaders.

The platelets (thrombocytes) are minute colorless bodies that are also manufactured in the marrow. Their main role is to help blood to clot.

"Tired Blood": Much has been said about "tired blood," especially by promoters of popular remedies. It is maintained that people feel weary and spiritless because of a deficiency of iron and other elements in the blood. This may happen in the case of ANEMIA, but the sensible approach is not to jump to conclusions but to obtain an accurate medical diagnosis. Iron-poor blood is better treated with an iron supplement and a good diet than with expensive and unnecessary tonics. In general, most complaints of fatigue are corrected by getting adequate rest and engaging in diverting activities.

BLOOD BANK A place in a hospital or other health agency where whole BLOOD and BLOOD PLASMA are kept ready for use in TRANSFUSIONS. In some banks, blood donors are given credit for blood "on deposit," and can make withdrawals from their account if they or their family should need it. Similar banks of organs for transplantation exist, such as eye banks, where corneas are kept in storage. See also ORGAN TRANSPLANT.

BLOOD CLOT A plug that normally forms whenever a BLOOD VESSEL is injured or so weakened that it begins to leak. A clot is formed by a series of chemical reactions that begin when substances in the blood come in contact with a substance released by injured tissue. Thus, any scratch or cut in the skin is quickly sealed off to prevent loss of blood. Later, when the injured tissue has healed, the clot is sloughed off. Clots also form inside the body. A clot, or thrombus, on the inner wall of a weak or injured vein or artery (THROMBOSIS) can have serious consequences. If it breaks away and floats off in the bloodstream, it may suddenly block off the flow of blood (EMBOLISM) in a vital area. New techniques are being developed to locate and remove such dangerous clots.

Clot formation can be temporarily prevented by injecting an ANTICOAGULANT. This is a precaution taken in some major operations and after serious accidents involving internal injuries. However, continued failure of blood to clot (HEMOPHILIA) is a serious condition, requiring the closest supervision of your doctor.

BLOOD CORPUSCLE Any of the minute particles that together make up about 45 percent of the volume of the BLOOD; a red blood cell (ERYTHROCYTE), white blood cell (LEUKOCYTE), or platelet (thrombocyte).

BLOOD COUNT The determination of the number of particles in a cubic millimeter (a small fraction of a drop) of blood. An actual count is made, under a microscope, of the number of particles in an exceedingly small, accurately measured volume of diluted blood, and from that the number of particles in a cubic millimeter of whole blood is calculated. The three main kinds of particles in the blood are counted separately. In a cubic millimeter of blood from an average healthy person, there are about 5 million red cells, 5,000 to 10,000 white cells, and about 200,000 to 500,000 platelets. Sometimes special stains are used on the microscope sample in order to distinguish the proportion of different kinds of white cells and platelets.

If a person's blood count differs greatly from the average, the doctor has valuable clues in making or confirming a diagnosis. A low red-cell count may indicate various kinds of ANEMIA, a serious infection, or a disorder in blood production. A high white-cell count may signify leukemia or certain infections. The platelet count is usually low in leukemia and some other blood diseases.

Some ANTIBIOTICS and other medicines also tend to upset the blood count. When these are administered, blood counts are made in order to obtain warning of possible side effects.

BLOOD DISEASE Signs of many types of disease often make their appearance in the BLOOD. The following are only a few of the more widespread disorders involving the major substances in the blood—the red blood cells, the white blood cells, the platelets, and plasma.

Anemia: This condition is caused by a deficiency in the number of red blood cells or the amount of hemoglobin in these cells. It may be the result of hemorrhage, iron deficiency, disease, or extreme overexposure to radium or X rays. The treatment varies, depending on the cause. See also the separate entry, ANEMIA.

Polycythemia: In this condition there is an excess of red blood cells. It may be a hereditary condition, or the result of a decrease in the plasma or of a disease. The symptoms include weakness, malaise, headaches, and nosebleed. Radioactive phosphorus may be used in treatment.

Agranulocytosis: A sudden decline in the number of white blood cells marks this disorder. It may be brought on by exposure to radioactivity or poisoning with drugs, antibiotics, or other substances. Symptoms include sores in the mouth and fever. See also separate entry, AGRANULOCYTOSIS.

Leukemia: Here the number of white blood cells increases, sometimes enormously. There may be an associated anemia and swelling of the LYMPH NODES. The disease may take an acute or chronic form. The cause is not fully understood. Treatment includes the use of X rays, radioactive isotopes, and chemical medicines. See also separate entry, LEUKEMIA.

Hemophilia: This hereditary disorder is caused by a deficiency in the clotting mechanism. Unlike the other blood diseases described here, hemophilia is not associated with an abnormal BLOOD COUNT. The condition varies greatly from extremely mild cases, in which there is only a slight delay in clotting time, to dangerous and uncontrolled bleeding. Plasma, whole blood, and a recently developed clot-forming protein (called the antihemophilia factor) are used in treatment. See also separate entry, HEMOPHILIA.

Thrombocytopenia: In this disorder there is a deficiency of blood platelets, whose function is to aid in clotting. The result may be purple patches—evidence of bleeding from small blood vessels—in the mucous membranes and skin, a condition known as purpura. Certain diseases and chemical poisonings or an overactive SPLEEN may be responsible.

BLOOD PLASMA The liquid portion of blood, as distinct from the BLOOD CORPUSCLES. It is a watery solution containing all the vital substances (except oxygen) that must be transported throughout the body. These vital substances include digested foodstuffs for the body cells, salts, HORMONES, ANTIBODIES, ENZYMES, and substances essential to the formation of a BLOOD CLOT; in addition, blood plasma absorbs and carries away waste products from the body cells. It also provides a medium in which corpuscles can move freely. Because plasma keeps better than whole blood and can be used for persons of any BLOOD TYPE, it is used rather than whole blood for some TRANSFUSIONS.

BLOOD POISONING The presence in the bloodstream of bacteria from a local infection, such as a boil, an abscessed tooth, or an infected scratch or cut. Blood poisoning is also a grave risk in clandestine abortion because bacteria may be introduced into the uterus by instruments that have not been properly sterilized. Many different bacteria can cause blood poisoning, but STREPTOCOCCUS and STAPHYLOCOCCUS are the most common. The body's defenses normally keep such infections localized. Physical manipulation, such as lancing a boil or CURETTAGE of the uterus, seems to increase the danger of bacteria entering the blood. If pus as well as bacteria is present in circulating blood, the condition is known as PYEMIA.

Once in the bloodstream, bacteria can produce abscesses throughout the body and in vital organs such as the lungs and the heart (see BACTERIAL ENDOCARDITIS). The condition is very serious. The symptoms vary. There is usually weakness accompanied by chills and fever. If blood poisoning is suspected, a doctor may confirm the diagnosis by growing the bacteria in the laboratory from samples of infected blood. Prompt treatment is necessary, including medication with ANTIBIOTICS and complete bed rest in a hospital. Treatment must be continued until every trace of the infection has disappeared.

Septicemia and *bacteremia* are two medical terms for blood poisoning. TOXEMIA refers to a condition in which bacterial TOXINS are present in the victim's bloodstream.

BLOOD PRESSURE Circulating blood presses against the walls of the blood vessels with a force that fluctuates with every heartbeat. The pressure is greatest during the SYSTOLE, when the heart contracts and forces blood into the arteries of the body. This maximum pressure is known as systolic pressure. During the DIASTOLE, when the heart muscle relaxes, the pressure drops to a minimum, which is called diastolic pressure.

Blood pressure varies from person to person, as well as from time to time in the same person. It is influenced by general health, heredity, age, activity, and emotional state. The blood pressure gives the doctor an indication of two important factors in a person's health: the volume of circulating blood and the elasticity of the blood vessels. For example, a rapid decline in blood pressure following severe injury warns the doctor that a person is going into SHOCK—a very serious condition associated with a decrease in the volume of circulating blood. Blood pressure increases as a person grows older and the walls of the blood vessels lose their elasticity. The rate at which the heart is beating affects blood pressure; therefore, blood-pressure measurements must be taken when a person is in a relaxed, resting condition.

Taking the Blood Pressure: The doctor uses a STETHOSCOPE and a device called a SPHYGMOMANOMETER to take the blood pressure. A rubber cuff attached to the sphygmomanometer is wrapped around the upper arm. Then air is pumped into the cuff, arresting the flow of blood in the artery of the upper arm. Listening through the stethoscope, which is placed against the artery at the bend of the elbow, the doctor cannot hear any heartbeat because the blood flow through the artery has been stopped. Now the air pressure is slowly released. Blood begins to flow into the artery when the systolic pressure from the heart's contraction exactly equals the pressure of the partly inflated cuff on the person's artery. The doctor reads and records the pressure (in millimeters of mercury) shown on the sphygmomanometer at the moment when he first hears the thumping sound of blood entering the artery at every systole. Then more air is released from the sleeve. The thumping stops when the artery is no longer obstructed by any outside pressure—blood is then flowing freely through the artery. The reading on the sphygmomanometer at the moment the thumping stops gives the diastolic pressure. Blood pressure is always recorded as two numbers; 120/80, for example, means that the systolic pressure is 120 and the diastolic pressure, 80.

What Blood Pressure Means: On the average, a woman has a systolic pressure as much as 10 millimeters lower than a man's. A normal young person's systolic pressure may range up to 140, and an older person's up to about 170.

When someone has a systolic pressure above 160 millimeters, he is usually considered to have high blood pressure, or HYPERTENSION. If the systolic pressure is below 90 millimeters, low blood pressure, or HYPOTENSION, may be suspected. A diastolic pressure of 90 or 100 should be looked into.

There is no truth to the folk tradition that the systolic pressure should be "100 plus your age." What is normal for one person may indicate high or low blood pressure in another. Moreover, people may react emotionally to having their blood pressure taken, particularly as part of a medical examination for insurance or a new job. The result may be a reading that is not truly the "normal" one. Thus, before a firm diagnosis of abnormal blood pressure can be made, the pressure must be measured on a number of different occasions and confirmation obtained by other tests, such as examination of the blood vessels of the eye.

It is important to be aware that elevated blood pressure, or hypertension, is a symptom and not a disease. In about 10 percent of all cases, it is associated with hardening of the arteries, nervous tension, kidney disease, or other disorders. In the remaining 90 percent, however, no disease is found. This condition is described as essential hypertension. Most persons with moderately high blood pressure are not handicapped by it, but are able to keep it under control with medical help.

BLOOD SERUM   See SERUM.

BLOOD TEST   A test made to measure the blood's component parts and establish whether or not disease is present. Two important kinds of blood tests are described under BLOOD COUNT and BLOOD TYPE. These are concerned especially with the blood corpuscles—the white and the red blood cells. Other tests are made on whole blood and on serum—the liquid remaining when the corpuscles are removed.

BLOOD is always circulating throughout the body. It carries oxygen, digested food, hormones, enzymes, and other elements to the cells; it removes carbon dioxide and other waste products from them; it carries antibodies that protect the body against

disease. Because of the great number of functions that the blood performs, it closely reflects the condition of the body, whether in health or sickness.

A multitude of blood tests are made to diagnose disease or other physical conditions, ranging from pregnancy (see PREGNANCY SIGNS AND TESTS) to ANEMIA and DIABETES. Some of these tests are so simple that the physician can draw a few drops of blood from a patient's finger and analyze them in a moment under his microscope. But often more elaborate chemical tests or measurements must be performed over a period of days in a laboratory by skilled technicians. Many blood tests require more than a few drops of blood—sometimes several ounces are needed. New techniques are being developed by which fairly elaborate tests can be performed on one or two drops of blood. These are being used where taking a larger sample might be dangerous—as with a tiny baby.

The findings in some blood tests are not always conclusive. Do not be surprised if your doctor is not satisfied with just one test and orders another. His only aim is to supply you with the most accurate diagnosis, and this is not always possible with a single blood test.

One very simple blood test consists of observing the color of a drop of blood absorbed on a piece of special paper. The color of the spot is matched with a series of standardized colors to give an estimate of the percentage of HEMOGLOBIN present. If great accuracy is desired, more elaborate tests are done.

In some examinations of the blood the sedimentation rate is measured. The blood sample is treated with an ANTICOAGULANT; this causes red blood cells and other elements in the blood to sink to the bottom of the container, leaving the plasma, a clear liquid, at the top. The sedimentation rate is the rate at which the cells fall to the bottom. If the rate is rapid it may be a sign of cancer, tuberculosis, or some other condition.

Other important tests include those made to measure blood sugar, cholesterol, calcium, hormones, and the acid-alkali balance of the body (pH test). Complement-fixation tests are antibody tests used for the diagnosis of syphilis (WASSERMANN TEST), as well as for various infections produced by bacteria and viruses.

BLOOD TRANSFUSION   See TRANSFUSION.

BLOOD TYPE   If you took a drop of your own blood, mixed it with the blood SERUM of another person, and examined it under the microscope, the chances are that you would see the red cells sticking together in clumps. If you gave this person some of your blood in a transfusion, the same thing would happen in his blood system. The clumps would clog the blood vessels, and the results could well be disastrous.

Fortunately, this would not be allowed to happen. Before giving a blood transfusion, a doctor always performs a test to determine the patient's blood type. Certain blood types can be mixed without clumping: they are said to be compatible.

There are four main blood types: A, B, AB, and O. These types differ in the presence or absence of two factors (A and B) in the red blood cells, and in the presence or absence of two factors (anti-A and anti-B) in serum. The table below shows which factors are present in each type of blood and which types can be mixed without clumping.

In practice, it is only the red cells in donated blood that are likely to clump and cause trouble. The serum in donated blood is so much diluted by the volume of the recipient's blood that no clumping due to donated serum occurs. Thus, if your blood is type O, you can safely give a transfusion of whole blood to anyone, because your red cells contain neither factor A nor B. You are what is called a universal donor. But you cannot receive whole blood from anyone but another type O, because your serum contains both anti-A and anti-B factors. Fortunately, type O blood is not rare. About 44 percent of the white population of the United States has type O blood. On the other hand, if your blood is type AB, you can receive a whole-blood transfusion from any donor, but you can donate blood only to another type AB. Type AB blood is found in about 4.5 percent of the white population of the United States. The same four types are found among people of all racial groups, but the frequency of each type varies. You can receive or donate blood regardless of racial group or sex or age—only the blood types must be compatible.

There are many other types of blood besides the four main types based on A and B factors. Most of these are of little significance to health. The main exception is the RH FACTOR, which must also be taken into account when a transfusion is made.

The various blood types are inherited according to a definite but complicated pattern. It is possible to tell by his blood type whether a child could or could not possibly be the offspring of given parents.

Donor's blood type	Factor in red cells	Factor in serum
A	A	anti-B
B	B	anti-A
AB	A,B	none
O	none	anti-A, anti-B

Donor's blood type	Incompatible blood types	Compatible blood types
A	O,B	A,AB
B	O,A	B,AB
AB	O,A,B	AB
O	none	A,B,AB,O

BLOOD VESSEL Any of the tubular channels through which blood circulates; an ARTERY, a VEIN, or a CAPILLARY. Capillaries, the last link between the blood and the body tissues, carry substances to and from the larger blood vessels; they are networks of tubes made of a thin tissue called ENDOTHELIUM. The arteries, through which the heart pumps blood to the capillaries, have an inner lining of endothelium surrounded by a double wall of muscular and connective tissue. The veins have a similar three-layered outer wall; in addition, they have valves at intervals that keep the rather sluggish blood in the veins moving in the right direction—toward the heart.

BLUE BABY A baby whose lips and skin have a blue tinge because of a CONGENITAL heart defect. Some of his blood bypasses the lungs and is recycled through his system without oxygen, which normally gives blood a bright red color. CYANOSIS (the bluish tinge of lips and skin) and other symptoms are not always present immediately after birth, and, in fact, more often appear when a baby is a few months old. The baby grows more slowly and tires more easily than a normal child. His fingers may show clubbing (enlargement) at the tips. The condition can very often be corrected by surgical repair of the defective heart before permanent damage is done. See also CONGENITAL HEART DISEASE.

BLUES See DEPRESSION.

BODY BRACE A device used to provide rigidity or support for a physical disability. It is worn around the part of the body involved, such as the neck, back, arm, or leg. A body brace is also called an orthopedic appliance.

Brace users include individuals who have injuries or diseases of the joints, bones, spine, tendons, or muscles. A large—and, unfortunately, growing—group is made up of persons who have suffered injuries in automobile accidents. Braces are also used to correct deformities and to control movements that are involuntary.

How Braces Are Made: Many materials are used to make body braces, including wire, metal, leather, plastic, and plaster of Paris. If made of a hard material such as metal, the brace is covered with a softer substance where it comes in contact with the body, so that it will not produce irritation. The general aim is to make the brace as light, but also as strong, as can be. Although two braces made for the same purpose look much alike, each is made to fit a particular person and to help him overcome his problem.

Braces for children are often made to allow for growth and to encourage the child to develop his muscles and general coordination. It may take quite a while to become accustomed to wearing braces, but eventually a handicapped person comes to view them as a blessing.

BODY ODOR See BROMIDROSIS.

BODY TEMPERATURE The degree of heat of the body. The average body temperature is 98.6°F, but the average does not apply to everybody. Some people have a normal temperature a little above 98.6°F, some have a temperature a little below. It is wise to take your temperature while you are in good health so that you know what is normal for you. A temperature that is higher—or lower—than your normal one can be a sign of illness.

Normal body temperature is not stable; it changes during the course of the day and night. Usually it rises approximately a degree by about 4 p.m. and goes down during sleep. Your temperature goes up during periods of activity.

Young children have a wider range of normal temperature than grownups. Sometimes sickness will show itself only by a low fever; this happens occasionally in DIPHTHERIA. It is better to judge the child's condition by the way he behaves than by a temperature reading slightly above normal. In adults, if the temperature is 100°F or higher, fever may be presumed present.

Some persons know they have a slight fever but, unwisely, ignore it. If low-grade fever persists, it requires investigation. It may be a symptom of tuberculosis or other serious infection, rheumatic heart disease, or some other disorder that is much more readily controlled when detected early.

Temperature may provide a clue to pregnancy. During ovulation (10 to 14 days after the beginning of the last menstrual period) there is normally an increase of approximately 1° in the morning. After a few days it returns to normal. However, should the temperature maintain its elevated level for 20 days, pregnancy may be suspected.

The temperature is measured by means of the clinical THERMOMETER. This comes in two types, oral and rectal. The oral thermometer has a narrow bulb, the rectal a wider one. Temperature is usually taken by mouth because it is more convenient. On the other hand, rectal temperature is less subject to error. It usually registers approximately 1° higher than mouth temperature. If you use a rectal thermometer, do not insert it without first coating the bulb end with petroleum jelly (Vaseline), cold cream, or some other lubricant.

BOECK'S SARCOID See SARCOIDOSIS. (Pronounced beks' sahr'koyd.)

BOIL A raised, tender, pus-filled area on the skin caused by bacterial infection; also known as a furuncle. The BACTERIA, usually staphylococci, may enter the outer layer of skin through a hair follicle or sweat gland or through a scratch or break in the skin. The bacteria do not generally thrive unless resistance has been lowered by poor nutrition or some illness such as ANEMIA or DIABETES. If it remains localized, a boil may be painful but not serious. However, the consequences can be grave if bacteria enter the bloodstream and cause BLOOD POISONING. For this reason, you should never try to open a boil yourself—leave this to your doctor.

Treatment: A doctor should be consulted if a boil develops on the upper lip, nose, or groin, in the ear or armpit, or anywhere on the skin of an elderly person or an infant. See a doctor also if several boils appear at once or follow each other in quick succession. For a single, small boil in an area that is not sensitive or vital, the following treatment may be safely applied to relieve discomfort and help the boil to drain: Wash the area with soap and warm water several times a day, dab it lightly with alcohol, and protect it with an antiseptic gauze pad. In addition, hot compresses may be applied for 10 minutes several times a day. The COMPRESS may be a gauze pad dipped in warm water that contains as much salt as will dissolve in it. Between treatments, protect the area with a dry gauze pad. See also CARBUNCLE; SKIN ERUPTION.

BONE A rigid structure of connective tissue interlaced with NERVES and BLOOD VESSELS and hardened by deposits of (chiefly) calcium phosphate. The entire bone is sheathed in a tough tissue called the periosteum. Babies' bones are pliable and contain a high proportion of CARTILAGE, which is gradually replaced by more rigid bone tissue. In adults, each bone has a very dense outer layer with a high content of calcium. Under this layer, the structure is spongy, with pores and cavities of various sizes.

Bones are the source of vital constituents of BLOOD. They are the storehouse from which the calcium in BLOOD PLASMA is obtained. The pores and cavities—at each knob-like end (epiphysis) of the jointed bones, in the ribs, the skull, the vertebrae, and the numerous short bones of the hands and feet—are filled with red MARROW. Red marrow consists largely of blood corpuscles in all stages of development. About 5 million mature red blood cells (ERYTHROCYTES) are produced and released into the bloodstream every second. The blood platelets, which are essential for BLOOD CLOT formation, and the white blood cells (LEUKOCYTES), which protect the body against infection, are also formed in the red marrow. The shafts (middle sections) of the long bones of the arms and legs are hollow and filled with yellow marrow. Yellow marrow is a fatty substance whose function is not known.

Bones are hinged and held together by LIGAMENTS to form the SKELETAL SYSTEM. This system provides support, mechanical leverage for movement, and protection. The flat bones (skull and ribs) protect the delicate tissues of the brain and the lungs. The long bones move on interlocking joints that are lined with cartilage. In childhood, the shafts of the long bones are separated from the epiphysis at each end by a layer of cartilage. Growth of the bone takes place at this point until adult size is reached. Then the shaft and the epiphysis fuse together. In old age, the bones become increasingly brittle. See FIRST AID section for treatment of bone fractures.

BONE, BROKEN See BROKEN BONE.

BONE DISEASE There are relatively few diseases that directly involve the bone. Arthritis, for example, is a disease of the joints rather than the bones, although a person with arthritis may complain that his bones ache. Conditions outside the bone may sometimes lead to deformed or stunted bone growth in children. For example, clubfoot and congenital hip dislocation (see below) are birth defects that can lead to bone deformity if not corrected. A limping gait or any other sign of abnormality in a child's arms or legs calls for a visit to the doctor. (See ORTHOPEDICS.)

Clubfoot: This deformity, also known as TALIPES, is present at birth. If it is not treated early it may require surgery. However, when medical attention is sought promptly, the condition may be corrected by relatively simple measures.

Congenital Hip Dislocation: At the time a child begins to walk, this condition reveals itself by a limp. This is one of many good reasons that babies should have regular checkups. The doctor will check for excessive tightness of the hips when pushing the baby's legs apart. If such tightness is found, the doctor may recommend X-raying the hip. The dislocation grows worse if neglected, and may require extensive surgery. When treatment is begun as soon as the condition becomes apparent—if possible, even before the child begins walking—there is good hope of correction without surgery.

Rickets—Osteomalacia: This disease is called by the first name when it occurs in children; by the second, in adults. The bones do not harden normally, due to lack of calcium and phosphorus, and may become deformed, as with BOWLEG. The disease is frequently relieved by means of a high-calcium diet and vitamin D. See also OSTEOMALACIA; RICKETS.

Paget's Disease: This disease, also known as osteitis deformans, usually strikes the middle-aged. Typically, the bones in the leg, skull, or spine become overgrown and deformed by deposits of calcium. The cause is not known. The condition may develop so slowly that it is hardly noticed. Pain is controlled by various types of treatment, including the use of vitamins C and D, calcium, and aspirin. Sodium fluoride may arrest the progress of the disorder. ("Paget's disease" also refers to an unrelated condition, a form of breast cancer.)

Osteoporosis: In this condition the bones become porous and brittle. The first sign is often a fracture produced by a minor jolt. Poor nutrition and inadequate blood supply to the bone are two of many possible causes; the treatment varies with the cause. In time, most old persons suffer from osteoporosis to some degree. Estrogens may be required in women after menopause to control osteoporosis.

Osteomyelitis: This disease occurs in both acute and chronic forms. It is an infection of the bone and is produced by bacteria. OSTEOMYELITIS most frequently strikes younger persons and usually involves the arms and legs. Antibiotics very often can cure acute osteomyelitis if administered soon after the onset of the disease. Methods in addition to antibiotics must be used to cure the chronic form.

Pott's Disease: Another name for this disease is tuberculosis of the spine. It is marked by inflammation or destruction (caries) of the spinal vertebrae, and is usually produced by a germ from infected cows. Pasteurization of milk has made Pott's disease relatively uncommon.

Other Diseases: There are many other disabilities of the bones and joints. Some involve the marrow, where blood cells are produced. (See BONE.) ARTHRITIS, BURSITIS, and certain types of CANCER also involve the bones.

BOOSTER SHOT An injection of a VACCINE or a TOXOID given some time after a previous injection in order to increase or renew IMMUNITY to a disease. Booster doses are usually weaker than initial doses. The time between doses varies for different diseases. It is wise to have booster shots if there is any increase in the probability that you will be exposed to a particular disease—if, for example, there is a threatened outbreak. Also, booster shots may be required if you plan to travel in countries where certain diseases such as typhoid fever commonly occur. See also IMMUNIZATION; VACCINATION.

BORAX A white powdery or crystalline substance with slightly antiseptic properties, sometimes used as a household cleanser or water softener. Because it is a compound of sodium and BORIC ACID, which is toxic, other safer cleaning compounds may be considered preferable. But if you do use borax, keep it out of children's reach.

BORIC ACID A white powder that can be dissolved in water. It is very mildly antiseptic, but toxic if swallowed or absorbed through an open wound or scratch. Therefore it should never be used as a baby powder. Although formerly used to rinse out the eyes, such application is no longer recommended.

BOTTLE-FEEDING Many mothers feed their babies with a bottle instead of at the breast. With an adequate formula and *affectionate, attentive treatment by his mother*, the bottle-fed baby should fare as well as the one who is breast-fed. *There is absolutely no cause to think you are failing your child if you are unable to breast-feed him*, or choose not to for reasons of your own. See also BABY CARE; BREAST-FEEDING.

The Formula: Your pediatrician will recommend a suitable formula for your baby. The typical formula consists of evaporated milk, water, and a sweetener, such as sugar or corn syrup. It is boiled to make certain it is germ-free. The bottle may be given to the baby directly from the refrigerator, if you want to spare yourself the bother of heating it. There are also convenient disposable plastic feeding bottles on the market. These are really plastic bags that fit into a rigid permanent container. They are presterilized, and eliminate the bother of continually washing and boiling glass bottles.

There are many types of commercial formulas available, containing vitamins or other special dietary ingredients. Milk allergies can occur among infants, and there are formulas for these babies, too.

The Feeding Schedule: Your doctor will suggest a feeding schedule for your baby. As a rule, the infant is fed about every four hours. Many physicians and parents favor demand feeding. Under this system the baby is given the bottle whenever he indicates that he is hungry. The theory is that the baby guides the parents in establishing a schedule that is suitable for him as an individual. Other parents find demand feeding unreliable and prefer to make the child accustom himself to a regular schedule.

Giving the Bottle: When you give the baby his bottle, be careful to hold it slanting downward a bit toward his mouth. That way he will not be able to swallow much air because there will be milk in the nipple until the very end. Burp him once or twice during the feeding period as well as afterward by patting him on the back. If you burp him on your shoulder, put a diaper over it first, as he is likely to regurgitate a bit.

BOTULISM   A rare type of FOOD POISONING. (Pronounced boch′*u*·liz″em.)

BOWEL   An INTESTINE, especially the relatively short large intestine. The term is used in such expressions as bowel movement (the elimination of solid waste matter from the body).

BOWLEG   Outward curvature of one or both legs, leaving space between the knees. Some bowing of the legs is normal in infants and disappears in healthy babies as the bones develop. If the bones remain pliable because of deficiencies in the baby's diet, his weight may cause further curvature when he begins to walk, and his legs may be permanently bowed, even if the diet is corrected. The same condition may appear in adults as a secondary symptom of other diseases affecting the bones. See also RICKETS; OSTEOMALACIA.

BRACE, BODY   See BODY BRACE.

BRACES, TEETH   See ORTHODONTICS.

BRADYCARDIA   Very slow pulse resulting from decreased heart action. It is sometimes caused by

HEART BLOCK or head injuries, but more often it arises during convalescence after an acute infectious disease such as DIPHTHERIA, INFLUENZA, PNEUMONIA, or TYPHOID FEVER, or when the blood carries toxic matter, as in JAUNDICE. The patient's pulse returns to normal as his general health improves, unless the cause of bradycardia is a heart block. (Pronounced brad″i·kahr′dee·*a*.)

BRAILLE SYSTEM   A kind of writing for the blind in which the letters and common words are represented by simple patterns of raised dots that are read by touch. A blind person can write in Braille (pronounced brayl) with either a portable Braille slate or a machine like a typewriter, called a Braillewriter. Books and periodicals in Braille are available for loan in the public libraries of most cities and from the National Library Service for the Blind and Physically Handicapped, Library of Congress, Washington, D.C. 20542.

BRAIN   The center of the NERVOUS SYSTEM; the soft mass of nerve tissue encased in the skull. The brain, or *encephalon,* consists of billions of cells with a total weight of about 2½ to 3 pounds in adults. The brain cells are organized in connected parts whose detailed functions are only partly understood. The main structures are the CEREBRUM, the CEREBELLUM, and the brain stem, which narrows down to connect with the SPINAL CORD. The cerebrum consists of two hemispheres controlling opposite sides of the body; it is covered with several layers of gray matter in rounded folds (the cerebral cortex), which is the center of all the activities considered distinctively human: speech, memory, logic, and imagination.

Behind and below the cerebrum is the cerebellum, the center of muscular coordination. A small

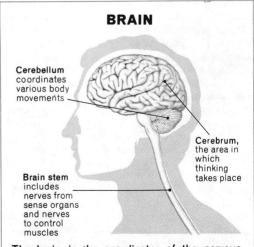

BRAIN

Cerebellum coordinates various body movements

Cerebrum, the area in which thinking takes place

Brain stem includes nerves from sense organs and nerves to control muscles

The brain is the coordinator of the nervous system, and its various areas control most of the body's conscious and unconscious actions.

structure near the center of the brain, the HYPO-THALAMUS, has to do with the regulation of body temperature and the activities of the internal organs; it is also thought to play a role in various other body responses. The entire brain is cushioned in a liquid medium (cerebrospinal fluid) contained in delicate membranes. The brain has also a tough, protective outer membrane (the dura mater). The brain has no capacity to repair injury, but the cells of the cortex are able gradually to take on new functions if a limited area is injured (see BRAIN DAMAGE). And because the two hemispheres duplicate each other to a certain extent, one can take over some of the functions of the other.

BRAIN DAMAGE The brain, with its 15 billion cells, regulates a vast number of the activities of the body. Brain cells use oxygen at a faster rate than do other cells of the body. About one-fifth of the oxygen absorbed in the lungs is used by the brain. The most serious and general kind of brain damage occurs if the oxygen supply is interrupted. This kind of brain damage sometimes occurs during birth (see BIRTH INJURY), but it may happen at any age as a result of drowning, suffocation, heart stoppage, or any condition that prevents delivery of oxygen to the brain for more than three or four minutes.

Other local brain damage may be caused by a tumor, stroke, or injury. Since the functions of some sections of the brain are well understood, medical specialists can often identify the area involved by the activity that is impaired. If, for example, a person suddenly loses the ability to speak (see APHASIA), damage to the speech center of the brain is immediately suspected. However, the functions of many portions of the brain are not definitely known, so that certain areas may suffer injury without it being possible to diagnose the exact area involved.

A number of disorders are caused by damage to the brain, or inflict damage upon it. A STROKE, for example, is produced by the blocking or rupture of a blood vessel in the brain. MENINGITIS is an inflammation of the meninges, or membranes, covering the brain and spinal cord. SYPHILIS, TETANUS, and RABIES will ultimately damage the brain unless they are treated properly and promptly. Brain injury may occur before or during birth, as in the case of CEREBRAL PALSY, which is manifested by partial paralysis and by deficient muscular coordination.

The rigid, compact casing of the skull surrounds the brain very closely. All spaces are filled with cerebrospinal fluid.

If an injury or a disorder of any sort—such as internal bleeding or a tumor (see BRAIN TUMOR)—causes even a slight increase in the contents of the skull, there is a corresponding increase in the pressure on the sensitive tissues of the brain, and this may produce a severe and lasting headache. Such a condition calls for prompt consultation with your physician. If the pressure is not relieved, it may cause vomiting, paralysis, and blindness. This does not mean that a headache is necessarily a sign of interference with normal brain function, or can lead to such consequences; but a headache that is painful and long-lasting does call for attention from a doctor.

Mild external injury to the head or brain, such as may result from a fall or a blow, can cause momentary dizziness or brief unconsciousness. The physician will often take an X ray to rule out the possibility of a fracture. There may be headaches for a while, but generally, in such cases, there is no permanent harm to the brain.

If a person suffers a severe blow and feels intense head pain, CONCUSSION must be suspected, especially if blurred sight, dizziness, and unconsciousness occur. Prompt emergency treatment and medical attention are required. However, most skull injuries are not serious. But it is wise to caution youngsters who engage in diving, hockey, football, and other potentially hazardous sports to be on their guard against the danger of head injuries.

BRAIN SURGERY See NEUROSURGERY.

BRAIN TUMOR Any growth inside the skull will cause pressure and interfere with the blood supply, producing symptoms that depend on the part of the brain affected. Headaches in a person who formerly had none, disturbance of vision, dizziness, and nausea may suggest to a doctor that a number of tests should be made. The tests, including the BRAIN WAVE pattern, seek to determine if a tumor is present, and then to find its exact location. Many different kinds of tumors are known, and they may occur at any age. Treatment is by NEUROSURGERY or IRRADIATION or both.

BRAIN WAVE An electric impulse generated in the brain. Brain waves occur continuously, whether one is awake or asleep. They are detected and recorded with a special instrument, the electroencephalograph. (See ELECTROENCEPHALOGRAM.) The recorded waves have various characteristic patterns for different areas of the brain in different states of activity. Many factors—for example, a brain injury, a tumor, epilepsy, and certain medicines—affect the pattern in special ways. Thus, brain waves give exceedingly valuable clues for diagnosis of brain disorders.

BREAKBONE FEVER See DENGUE.

BREAST One of a pair of organs situated on the chest of females and composed of milk glands, fatty tissue, and milk ducts leading to the nipple. Breasts normally develop in girls at puberty in response to hormones secreted by the OVARIES and the pituitary gland. The secretion of milk (LACTATION) is initiated by a hormone (OXYTOCIN) produced by the pituitary gland at childbirth, and is stimulated by BREAST-FEEDING. In boys and men, unusual breast development (GYNECOMASTIA) sometimes occurs because of hormone disturbances, but it can occur normally to a slight degree during adolescence or in obese, mature males.

The shape and size of the breasts is determined largely by heredity. If the breasts are overlarge because of obesity, reducing excess weight will, of course, make them smaller. Excessive development or underdevelopment may in rare cases be due to a glandular or other disorder, which should be treated medically. Extremely large and pendulous breasts can be corrected by COSMETIC SURGERY (surgery performed to improve appearance). Never submit to such an operation by anyone but a professional surgeon.

The practice of injecting a "harmless" plastic material into the breast tissue in order to enlarge the breast is foolhardy and dangerous. Normally, all that should be done to conform to fashion—and it is a great deal—is to practice good posture, do upper-arm exercises to tone up muscles in the breast area, and wear a well-fitting brassiere that is not too tight, with some padding, if desired. Adequate support and protection, as well as cleanliness, are as essential for health as for appearance.

Disorders of the breast include inflammation (MASTITIS), CYSTS, ABSCESSES, and TUMORS. They are fairly common and usually yield readily to treatment. Even the most serious, BREAST CANCER, can be treated successfully if detected at an early stage. Any lump, a change in the nipple, an injury, pain, or discharge should be referred to your doctor without delay.

Palpation: Regular monthly examination and PALPATION of the breasts is advisable, especially for women over 40. Make a regular routine of self-examination, as follows: Once a month, before you dress in the morning, stand in front of a mirror and raise your arms above your head. Look carefully for any dimple or depression. Also look closely for any change in shape or size of one breast compared with the other. Then, lower the arms and, using the hand of the opposite side, press each breast in turn gently against the chest to find if any part seems denser than the rest. Finally, feel for lumps in the armpits. If you notice anything suspicious, see your doctor. If the condition is harmless, an examination will save you needless worry. If it should be malignant (cancerous), treatment is most likely to be successful if the malignancy is detected early.

BREAST CANCER This occurs most commonly in women between 45 and 64 years of age. It is estimated that it appears in about 108,000 women every year in North America. The cause of breast cancer is unknown. The earlier breast cancer is detected, the better the chances are of successful treatment. Unfortunately, too many women delay in reporting the presence of a lump or other telltale signs to their physicians.

Some Warning Signs: The commonest symptom is a tumor, or lump. It is usually in the top outward part of the breast. The breast should be palpated, or felt, systematically after the menstrual period or once a month to make certain there is no tumor present. (See BREAST.) If a suspicious lump is found, it should be reported to the physician immediately. One out of 11 women, it is estimated, will develop breast cancer. Most lumps, fortunately, are not cancerous; they are benign TUMORS or CYSTS. But only a doctor is qualified to tell which is which.

Other symptoms to report to the doctor are:
1. A rash around the nipple.
2. Bleeding or other discharge from the nipple.
3. Sinking or rising of the nipple.
4. Dimpling of the skin of the breast.
5. A marked change in the shape of the breast.
Pain occurs only in later stages.

The physician's examination, which may include the X-ray technique known as mammography, will often rule out the presence of cancer. If it does not, a tiny sample of tissue must be removed and examined by a pathologist. The BIOPSY is taken in a hospital operating room, with the patient under anesthesia. If the finding is positive, the operation, known as a MASTECTOMY, proceeds at once. Usually, the breast and the surrounding lymph nodes are removed; skin grafts may be used to cover the incision. Later, the chest area may be treated with X rays, or anticancer drugs may be used to destroy any remaining cancer cells.

The Outlook: The majority of women who have had mastectomies continue to lead healthy, meaningful lives. There are psychological and physical adjustments to be made, of course. With the help of a breast form, it is possible to duplicate the breast contours perfectly. Certainly, with the removal of a breast, a woman does not lose her particular personality or her attractiveness.

BREAST CYST See CYST.

BREAST-FEEDING Breast milk contains almost all the nutrients the baby needs during the first six months of life. The colostrum, or first milk, includes substances that help protect the baby against disease, and the breast milk that comes later is relatively free from harmful bacteria. Feeding the infant at the breast gives him a feeling of warmth and security that is important to his well-being.

Breast nursing can be emotionally rewarding to the mother. On the strictly physical side, breast-feeding appears to stimulate contractions of the uterus, which restore this organ to the size it was before pregnancy. Breast-feeding may delay or completely prevent menstruation from reoccurring. However, breast-feeding is no insurance against becoming pregnant again, since the normal monthly cycle of ovulation can resume before the baby is weaned. On the practical side, some mothers find breast-feeding more convenient than preparing a formula. See also BABY CARE; BOTTLE-FEEDING.

The Mother's Diet: The nursing mother, like the pregnant woman, must pay special attention to her diet. She has a greater need now for calcium (the bone-building mineral), which she can obtain by drinking extra milk every day. She should have about six cups of milk (or the equivalent in milk products, such as cheese and ice cream) each day, compared with the average adult requirement of two cups. She should eat more fruits, vegetables, and meats to supply the proteins, vitamins, and other elements her baby needs for growth. In terms of calories, her recommended daily allowance is about 1,000 more than it would otherwise be. It is, however, unnecessary and undesirable to put on weight.

How to Nurse: A good diet, with plenty of water, is important in avoiding an insufficient supply of milk. (See LACTATION.) So, too, is a relaxed attitude. The mother should rest a bit before nursing. As a rule, feedings are every four hours. The baby is nursed at both breasts at each feeding, but the breast that is offered first is alternated. He is usually burped one or two times during, as well as after, nursing. Report to your doctor any soreness of the nipples or problem with your milk supply.

BREAST PUMP A small, hand-operated device for removing milk from the breast by suction. Such a pump should be used only on the advice of your doctor.

BREATHING DIFFICULTY See DYSPNEA.

BREECH DELIVERY A birth in which the baby's buttocks (or sometimes the knees or feet) are the first part of its body to come out of the mother's birth canal. About one out of 25 births are breech deliveries. In a normal delivery, the largest part of the baby, the head, is born first. When the head is born last, the baby runs a somewhat greater risk of being deprived of oxygen during the critical moments when breathing must start. In addition, a breech delivery is usually slower than a normal birth. It is sometimes necessary for the doctor to use instruments (such as FORCEPS) to help the breech baby into the world. During the last week or two before the baby is due, the doctor can learn the baby's position in the uterus by feeling with his hands.

Many breech deliveries proceed without trouble. However, if the baby cannot be delivered normally, the doctor may have to perform a CESAREAN (CESARIAN) SECTION, an operation in which the child is delivered through an incision made in the mother's abdomen. If the baby is in a transverse position—that is, lying crosswise with neither its head nor its buttocks near the birth canal—the doctor may prefer to reach in and turn the baby to a more favorable position.

BRIDGE A partial DENTURE; one or more artificial teeth set in a mounting that is attached at each end to a sound natural tooth. There are two types of dental bridges: fixed and removable. The fixed bridge is attached to the natural teeth by a crown or gold inlay. The removable type is a cast metal framework that fits into the natural teeth and can be removed whenever desired. Both types of bridges can be cleaned by regular brushing.

BRIGHT'S DISEASE See NEPHRITIS.

BROKEN BONE A break in a bone is known as a fracture. To ensure proper healing, the parts of the bone must be carefully manipulated (by a qualified physician only) so that the ends at the break are in the most favorable position for growing together. X rays are used to find the exact nature of the break and check the progress of the healing. With a young person, an uncomplicated fracture usually requires several weeks in a plaster cast. Broken bones heal more slowly in older persons.

A bone may fracture in a number of different ways. There are two main types of fracture: simple and compound. The *simple* (closed) fracture is a break in the bone that does not pierce the skin or cause severe damage to surrounding tissues. In the *compound* (open) fracture, the skin and tissues are broken through. Fractures vary considerably. A fracture may be *complete*, dividing the bone into two or more separate pieces; or it may be *incomplete*, or partial. A type common in children is the *greenstick* fracture; here the pliable bone bends like a living branch of a tree, and the break is incomplete. A *transverse* fracture is one in which the break is straight across the bone; in an *oblique* fracture, the break is diagonal. In a *comminuted* fracture, the bone is broken into little pieces at the point of fracture. There are other, less common, types of fracture in which the break may extend lengthwise in the bone in a spiral or a straight line.

How to Recognize a Fracture: There are a number of ways to recognize a fracture. The surest sign is when the individual is unable to move the limb or other part involved. The part will also not have its usual appearance. (In the case of an arm or leg, compare the injured to the uninjured one.) The skin may be discolored, with accompanying swelling. The individual may feel great pain when he attempts to move the part. If the fracture is a compound one, there is often bleeding. If you are uncertain whether or not a bone is broken, it is wise to treat it as a fracture until the doctor can examine it.

What to Do: Have someone telephone for medical assistance. It is important to avoid moving the fractured bone; if possible, get a doctor to come to the injured person, rather than rushing the person to a doctor or a hospital. If there is bleeding, apply direct pressure on the wound with sterile gauze, a clean handkerchief, or your hand in an emergency. If the victim must be moved from a dangerous area, make a simple SPLINT. An umbrella, a board, or any other stiff object may be used. Cover it with something soft, such as clothing or bed linen. Make sure the splint extends beyond joints, to restrict motion. With a fractured limb, a useful splint is a folded pillow that is loosely tied to the arm or leg. See also the FIRST AID section.

Prevention: Most accidents that result in broken bones can be avoided. Good lighting is essential— there should be ample illumination of halls and stairways. Do not allow toys or other objects to build up to a clutter. Steps and railings should be kept in good repair, and floors should be level. In winter, snow on steps and walks around the house should be shoveled promptly, and ice should be spread with ashes or sprinkled with ice dissolvers. If you must use a stepladder or a chair to reach something high up, first make sure that it is perfectly steady and strong enough to support your weight. These few, simple precautions will make your home a much safer place to live in.

BROMIDE Any of the various compounds of bromine formerly much used to soothe mental distress and in the treatment of epilepsy. Bromides are toxic, and their harmful effects build up if bromine is allowed to accumulate in the body. A single large dose or small doses taken over a period of time can produce a skin rash resembling acne, as well as nausea, vomiting, fever, and delirium. Today, bromides are rarely used, and only under the strictest medical supervision.

BROMIDROSIS This formidable looking term is derived from two Greek words meaning "ill-smelling perspiration." Bromidrosis (pronounced broh"mi·droh'sis) is the medical term for what we call body odor or B.O. To the collectors of odd words, here is an additional term: "bromidrosiphobia"—the fear of body odors. Manufacturers of soaps, deodorants, and antiperspirants have built a multimillion-dollar industry on bromidrosiphobia.

The body has about 2 million SWEAT GLANDS. These glands may produce from one pint to three quarts of PERSPIRATION in 24 hours, depending upon the individual's amount of physical exertion, the temperature to which he is subjected, his nervous tension, and so on. Fresh perspiration does not produce an offensive odor in a healthy, clean person if it is free to evaporate. However, when perspiration occurs in contact areas such as between the thighs or under the arms, or when it is absorbed by clothing, BACTERIA soon produce an offensive odor.

Body odor can be avoided if the individual takes a bath or shower every day and lathers liberally with

soap; twice a day is advisable in warm weather. A daily change of socks, stockings, and underclothing is also important. Dresses and shirts need to be changed frequently, too.

Talcum powder of the nonmedicated type can be applied under the arms. A DEODORANT or antiperspirant may also be used. The claims made for "magic" ingredients or "newly discovered formulas" in deodorants should be viewed with some suspicion. Antiperspirants suppress perspiration in areas where they are applied, which simply means that the perspiration will be excreted by sweat glands in other areas. An unfamiliar brand should be used in moderation at the start, as a sensitive person may react allergically to certain ingredients.

BRONCHITIS Strictly speaking, inflammation of the bronchial tubes (see BRONCHUS), but often much more is involved. The infection strikes the air passages of the nose, the throat, the larynx, and often the bronchioles, the small air passages in the lungs. In its mild form, it may seem like a severe chest cold; in its worst forms, it may lead to pneumonia. Bronchitis may be either acute or chronic.

Acute Bronchitis: This is frequently due to viral infections such as the COMMON COLD or INFLUENZA. But it may also be associated with whooping cough, measles, chicken pox, an allergy, or chemical irritants such as acid or ammonia fumes. Fever may be present for one or two days without other symptoms. Then there is considerable coughing, with SPUTUM containing pus. The disease lasts for a week and a half, sometimes longer. It is dangerous in elderly persons, particularly those with EMPHYSEMA or heart disease.

Chronic Bronchitis: This condition usually comes about after repeated infections of the upper respiratory tract. It may follow influenza, or it may be a reaction to excessive smoking or to breathing polluted air. It strikes city residents much more frequently than country people, and men more than women. In mild cases, the only symptom may be a persistent cough. In advanced cases, breathing may grow difficult and lung function may be impaired.

Treatment: EXPECTORANTS are taken to loosen the mucus in the air passages. The inhalation of steam from a VAPORIZER is helpful. Drink plenty of liquids. Antibiotics are prescribed only if the inflammation is due to bacteria; they have little effect if the cause is a virus, as it often is.

To avoid recurrence, try not to inhale smoke and dust. Air in bedrooms should not be too cold. If you frequently catch colds, get plenty of rest and ask your doctor how to improve your general health.

BRONCHOPNEUMONIA Inflammation of the lungs localized around the small, branched air passages (bronchioles) leading from each BRONCHUS. If mucus accumulates in the bronchioles, it forms a favorable breeding ground for bacteria. This is most likely to happen in persons confined to bed, unless preventive measures are taken, such as encouraging the patient to cough. Also, after surgery, periods of exercise out of bed are often recommended. In persons who are not bedridden, bronchopneumonia (pronounced brong''koh·noo·mohn'ya) sometimes results from infection in the upper respiratory tract (TRACHEA and bronchi). Any chest pain accompanied by a cough and breathlessness should be reported to your doctor promptly to determine if bronchopneumonia is present. He will then be able to treat the condition with ANTIBIOTICS before the lungs become further infected and bacterial TOXINS affect the system.

BRONCHOSCOPE An instrument for examining the air passages to the lungs. It consists of a long, thin tube, which is inserted through the mouth under a local ANESTHETIC. A tiny light and a system of lenses and mirrors in the tube enable the doctor to see the inside of the TRACHEA and the bronchi (see BRONCHUS).

BRONCHOTOMY The medical term for any operation that involves cutting into a BRONCHUS. (Pronounced brong·kot'oh·mee.)

BRONCHUS (plural, **bronchi**) One of the two main branches of the windpipe (TRACHEA), leading to either lung. The right bronchus (pronounced

brong'kus) extends nearly an inch from the windpipe before dividing and subdividing into many branches; the left bronchus is about twice as long and narrower. Like the windpipe, the bronchi (brong'kie) are ringed with cartilage that keeps them open for the free passage of air. They are lined with moist tissue (epithelium) whose surface is covered with microscopic, hairlike projections that push upward and help to keep particles, such as dust and pollen, from reaching the lungs. Inflammation of the bronchi is known as BRONCHITIS.

BRUCELLOSIS Infection by the bacterium *Brucella*, which primarily infects cattle and other livestock. (See BACTERIUM.) Brucellosis (pronounced broo''se·loh'sis) is also called undulant fever, Malta fever, and mountain fever. It is transmitted to man by contact with an infected animal or its carcass, or by drinking unpasteurized infected milk. Butchers and farmers are more likely to contract the disease; it is rarely passed from person to person.

The symptoms of brucellosis may develop either slowly or suddenly. They include weakness, great exhaustion at the least exertion, headache and general aches and pains, irritability, chills and fever that come and go, and night sweats. The glands in the neck and the armpits may be swollen and the SPLEEN enlarged. Without treatment, the infection may last for months or even years. It is rarely fatal. A person who recovers from the infection may continue to be irritable and have some degree of mental or emotional disorder. If a doctor suspects brucellosis, he will confirm the diagnosis by growing the bacteria in the laboratory from a sample of the person's blood. Treatment includes bed rest, high vitamin intake, and the use of ANTIBIOTICS.

BRUISE Any surface discoloration and swelling resulting from a blow or pressure; in medical language, a contusion. Usually without breaking the skin, the small blood vessels under the skin are ruptured, and internal bleeding shows through as a typical BLACK-AND-BLUE MARK. Minor bruises heal without special treatment, although cold wet compresses will speed healing and reduce pain. If a bruise is severe, it should be examined by a doctor to determine if the damage is extensive.

BUBO (plural, **buboes**) A painful swelling of a LYMPH NODE, especially in the groin or the armpit. The word bubo (pronounced byoo'boh) accounts for the name BUBONIC PLAGUE, of which one of the symptoms is a swelling of the lymph nodes. See also LEISHMANIASIS.

BUBONIC PLAGUE An acute CONTAGIOUS disease caused by a microscopic BACTERIUM that is transmitted to people by fleas from infected rats and other rodents. The severe symptoms of bubonic plague (pronounced byoo·bon'ik playg')—chills,

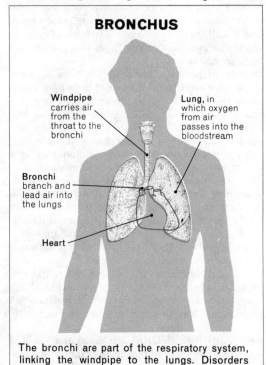

BRONCHUS

Windpipe carries air from the throat to the bronchi

Lung, in which oxygen from air passes into the bloodstream

Bronchi branch and lead air into the lungs

Heart

The bronchi are part of the respiratory system, linking the windpipe to the lungs. Disorders affecting them, such as bronchitis, interfere with breathing and generally cause a cough.

fever, vomiting, thirst, general pain, and delirium—appear suddenly. Painful swellings develop in the LYMPH NODES. (See BUBO.) In one form of the disease, known as pneumonic plague, the lungs are affected.

Bubonic plague has also been called the Black Death, because of the dark spots that develop from bleeding under the skin. Severe epidemics raged through Europe and Asia in the 14th and 17th centuries; outbreaks have occurred in recent times in Asia and Africa. Isolated cases turn up even now in all countries, since the disease is still harbored by rodents around the world. Public health agencies keep on the alert for epidemics among rodents and maintain programs of flea and rat control. A VACCINE has been developed, but it gives only short-term IMMUNITY and requires yearly BOOSTER SHOTS. When any human case is suspected and proved, bubonic plague is kept from spreading by strict QUARANTINE and treatment with STREPTOMYCIN and SULFONAMIDES, both of the victim and of everyone known to have been in contact with him.

BUFFERED ASPIRIN A kind of ASPIRIN tablet containing in addition to the aspirin a material that is intended to neutralize the acid reaction of aspirin in the stomach.

BULBAR POLIO See POLIOMYELITIS.

BUNION A painful deformity of the big toe, caused by shoes that bend this toe inward toward the smaller toes, putting pressure upon the joint connecting the big toe with the foot. First the bursa (the lubricating pouch of the joint) becomes inflamed and tender. With continued irritation a bony deposit develops, and a corn or callus at the pressure point often adds to the pain. Bunions can be avoided or corrected at an early stage by wearing properly fitting shoes. Minor pain may be relieved by heat, and foot-strengthening exercises may help. In severe cases, specially fitted shoes or surgery may be necessary; a doctor or podiatrist should be consulted. See also FOOT.

BURN Injury to the skin by heat, chemicals, electricity, or radiation. There are three types of burn. A *first-degree* burn is one in which the skin turns red, but there are no blisters. Only the epidermis, the outermost part of the SKIN, is injured. A *second-degree* burn goes somewhat deeper. There is blistering, and the skin turns very red. A *third-degree* burn penetrates the skin completely and destroys both epidermis and dermis (the part of the skin beneath the epidermis). Because nerve endings in the skin are destroyed, a third-degree burn may actually cause less pain than a more superficial first- or second-degree burn.

Any burn suspected of being severe should be seen at once by a doctor. If you cannot obtain medical help immediately, turn to the FIRST AID section.

In practice, it is not possible to determine right away how deeply a burn has penetrated. Any burn that involves one-tenth or more of the body's surface may be regarded as a potentially serious or major burn, requiring emergency attention. SHOCK is the first danger in any major burn, especially if a large area of skin is involved. The second danger is infection, which the doctor can control by administering antibiotics. Rapid and complete healing can be expected if the burn is a first-degree one, but scarring may be expected if the burn penetrates deeper. Skin grafting is necessary to repair skin destroyed by a third-degree burn.

Mild Burns: Everyone has experienced a minor burn, and most of us instinctively do the right thing in treating it. If we burn a finger on something hot, for example, we immediately put the finger in our mouth. This keeps air away from the burn and cools it off to body temperature. The same result can be achieved by immersing the burn in cold water.

If the burn is still painful after you have removed the affected part from the cold water, mix baking soda and water and apply it to the area. Or, if you have a burn-soothing ointment or petroleum jelly (Vaseline) available, apply it to the wound and cover with a sterile bandage. This treatment is recommended only for mild burns. Never put medication on a severe burn before consulting a doctor.

Major Burns: The injured person should be wrapped in clean sheets and a blanket and transferred to the hospital at once. If this is not possible, the victim may be put in a bath of water at room temperature until help arrives. This will reduce pain and delay shock resulting from fluid loss. Do not attempt to remove clothing, and do not wash, grease, powder, or medicate severe burns. Give the person fluids to drink if he is conscious.

Chemical Burns: These are burns produced by a chemical, such as an acid or alkali. Remove at once all clothing that has been in contact with the chemical. Place the injured part under running water. If a substantial area of the skin is involved, rush the victim into a shower and help him strip under the running water. See also ACID BURN.

Electric Burns: These include burns produced by lightning. Immediate attention should be given to the effects of ELECTRIC SHOCK rather than to the burn itself. If breathing has stopped, give artificial respiration. (See FIRST AID section.) In the meantime, have someone telephone for an ambulance.

Powder Burns: Powder burns are commonly caused by careless handling of cap pistols or fireworks. In addition to the burn, the skin may be cut and thus exposed to infection by germs. Remove any splinters or dirt that can be picked off easily, and wash with soap and water. A sterile dressing may be applied. If the person has not had a TETANUS inoculation recently, he should be given one as soon as possible.

Avoiding Burns: A little care will go a long way in preventing burns. If a grease fire starts on the stove or in the oven, do not make the mistake of pouring water on it; use salt or baking soda instead. Keep pot handles turned inward on the stove. Take special precautions if there are children about. Hot radiators should be shielded. Do not allow a small child to put wood in a fireplace or campfire. Keep matches where little hands cannot reach them.

BUROW'S SOLUTION A soothing, ANTISEPTIC solution used to treat minor skin disorders. Applied as a wet dressing, its ASTRINGENT action lessens the "weeping," or oozing, of poison ivy blisters and fever sores. As sold by druggists, Burow's solution should be diluted with about 15 parts of water.

BURPING See BELCHING.

BURSITIS Painful inflammation of a bursa, a pouch containing a small amount of fluid that is usually found at a spot subject to friction such as a joint or where a tendon and bone come together. Bursitis (pronounced bur·sie′tis) occurs when a bursa becomes inflamed, and there is an accumulation of fluid. The bursal sac around the joint becomes swollen. Any of the joints in the body may be affected.

Bursitis of the knee, known as HOUSEMAID'S KNEE, results from the strain and pressure of much kneeling on hard floors. Bursitis of the big toe (BUNION) is likewise associated with chronic irritation of the affected joint. In other cases, bursitis flares up suddenly with no known cause. The pain may be eased by application of hot or cold wet compresses and by taking aspirin. Avoid all strain on the affected joint. If pain or swelling is severe, call a doctor. He may find it necessary to drain off excess fluid. X ray may reveal calcium deposits, which may need surgical removal.

BUTTERFLIES IN THE STOMACH A feeling of NAUSEA due to fear or other emotional stress, especially in situations where pain or failure is anticipated. Typical sufferers are a passenger in a plane about to take off or land, a student just before an examination, a job-seeker going to an interview, or an actor about to go onstage. The reaction is not harmful to health. If it is very troublesome, a mild SEDATIVE prescribed by a doctor will help; but the effects of a sedative may be worse, from the student's or the actor's point of view, than a temporary feeling of queasiness.

BUTYN A trade name of a local ANESTHETIC used chiefly in operations on the eye. A very dilute solution of Butyn (pronounced byoo′tin) rapidly deadens feeling at the site of contact.

C

CAESAREAN (CAESARIAN) SECTION See CE-
SARIAN (CESARIAN) SECTION.

CAFFEINE A colorless, crystalline substance
found in coffee, tea, and the kola nut. It is also
present in cocoa in much smaller quantity. Caffeine
(pronounced kaf′een) is a stimulant to the nervous
system and is widely used in beverages. It is also a
diuretic—that is, it stimulates the kidneys to produce urine.

When coffee, tea, or cola drinks are consumed
moderately, they have a bracing effect and are
harmless to adults in good health. But when large
quantities are consumed, the individual may feel
nervous and restless and he may suffer from PALPI-
TATIONS. Many of us have experienced some INSOM-
NIA if we have drunk too much coffee too close to
bedtime. Individual susceptibility to caffeine is
highly variable, however; some persons may take it
immediately before bedtime and be able to fall
asleep at once.

The caffeine content differs in various beverages.
The average cup of coffee made from ground coffee
beans contains from 90 to 120 milligrams of caffeine; instant coffee contains only two-thirds of
these amounts, and decaffeinated coffee that contains as little as 3 to 4 milligrams is available. Tea
usually has about the same percentage of caffeine as
coffee, as does the typical cola drink.

Children should not be encouraged to drink too
many beverages containing caffeine, since the caffeine may overstimulate them. Caffeine has only
slight nutritional value.

Caffeine pills are available for people who want
to stay awake. They should be used very cautiously
to avoid dependence upon them. It is always better
to sleep when tired than to force oneself to stay
awake.

CAISSON DISEASE See BENDS. (Pronounced
kay′son.)

CALAMINE LOTION The familiar name for a
medicated liquid containing ZINC OXIDE. Calamine
lotion has a soothing effect when applied to a painful SUNBURN, and it helps to relieve the itch of
POISON IVY and INSECT BITES.

CALCIFICATION Hardening of tissue resulting
from the deposit of calcium salts. Calcification (pronounced kal″si·fi·kay′shun) is the normal process
by which bones are formed and kept in repair; but
abnormal calcification in the moving parts of a joint
can be very painful, and surgery may be required to
correct the condition.

CALCIUM A chemical element whose presence in
the body is essential for the maintenance of good
health. The combination of calcium and phosphorus
produces calcium phosphate, the substance that,
together with carbonate, makes up most of the
mineral part of bones and teeth.

If sufficient calcium is lacking in the body, such
diseases as RICKETS and OSTEOMALACIA may occur.
Foods that are high in calcium include whole milk
and skim milk, many cheeses, broccoli, cabbage,
molasses, and watercress.

CALCULUS (plural, **calculi**) Any abnormal, hard
mass formed in the body. A calculus (pronounced
kal′kyu·lus) is usually small and pebblelike, but
some forms of renal calculi (kidney stones) have a
branched structure that follows the shape of the
inside of the kidney. Dental calculus takes the form
of a hard deposit that coats the surfaces of teeth.
Failure to remove the deposits is the cause of PYOR-
RHEA, a common dental disease. Calculi may form in
various other parts of the body, such as the joints,
the salivary glands, and the bronchi. The most common and troublesome calculi are GALLSTONES and
URINARY TRACT stones.

Except for gallstones, which are composed of
cholesterol and bile salts, most calculi consist
largely of crystals of calcium salts that have separated out of body fluids. It is not known what causes
calculi to form. In some cases they are associated
with disorders that can be treated, such as abnormal
calcium levels in the blood. The tendency to form
stones in the urinary tract can sometimes be held in
check by a high intake of fluids. Calculi may cause
serious irritation and inflammation at the site where
they form. If they are carried into a duct leading
from a vital organ, as often happens with stones
formed in the kidney, the urinary bladder, and the
gallbladder, they can cause intense pain, irritation
of the duct wall, and blockage of the normal flow of
secretions. Once a stone has formed and begun to
cause trouble, it may be necessary to remove it
surgically. See also LITHOLAPAXY; LITHOTOMY.

CALLUS An area of the skin that has become hard
and thick. Calluses usually appear on the palms of

the hands or soles of the feet, where the skin is continously exposed to pressure and friction.

A CORN on the foot is a form of callus. Calluses may become troublesome if much hard skin has built up. They may be treated by rubbing off the callus with an emery board, or soaking the calloused area thoroughly in water and then rubbing the softened callus with a rough towel. However, if you have DIABETES or your calluses are painful, you should never attempt to treat calluses yourself, but should seek the advice of your doctor, who may recommend a visit to a PODIATRIST (foot specialist).

CALORIE A unit of measurement by means of which the amount of energy produced in the human body by different kinds of foods is calculated. A person's needs depend on his activity and such other factors as age and body build. A man doing very heavy work may need as much as 3,500 calories daily. An elderly, inactive woman may need less than 2,000 calories. If the food you eat supplies more calories than you need, the excess is stored as fat. You gain about one pound for every 3,500 calories in excess of your needs. Many people control their weight by counting up their daily calorie intake. The number of calories supplied by average servings of all kinds of foods has been determined; a boiled egg, for instance, supplies about 80 calories, and a pat of butter, about 100.

One of the many available calorie guides is *Calories and Weight,* published by the U.S. Department of Agriculture as Agricultural Bulletin #364. It is obtainable from the Superintendent of Documents, U.S. Government Printing Office, Washington, D.C. 20402.

CAMPHOR A colorless or white substance with a penetrating odor. Used as an ingredient in ointments, camphor (pronounced kam'for) stimulates the nerve endings under the skin and increases the supply of blood locally where it is applied to the skin. It relieves itching and has a soothing effect on minor sprains and muscular aches. Camphor is sometimes an ingredient of mothballs and of lacquers and varnishes.

If taken internally, camphor can cause rapid pulse, dizziness, convulsions, and coma. If a child should accidentally swallow any preparation containing camphor, call the doctor at once and try to induce vomiting.

See *Poisoning* in FIRST AID section.

CANCER All the tissues of the body normally grow and renew themselves by an orderly process of CELL division. It is not known exactly how this process is kept within limits, nor why it sometimes goes out of control. When it does go out of control, the result is cancer. Cancer is not a single disease but a large number of different diseases, all characterized by cells that repeatedly subdivide in a random, disorderly way. Through the uncontrolled growth of these MALIGNANT cells tumors are usually formed that crowd out healthy tissue and eventually interfere with the vital functioning of affected organs. Further, cells from the orginal, or primary, cancer site have a tendency to enter the lymph vessels and the bloodstream. By this route, malignant cells can be carried to a distant part of the body and give rise to secondary NEOPLASM, or tumor, which is also malignant. This process is know as METASTASIS.

Cancer can originate in practically any part of the body. A tumor is usually formed, although in some cancers involving the blood, tumors may not occur. Most cancers are classified as either CARCINOMA or SARCOMA, depending on the kind of tissue in which they originate.

How Cancer Develops: Cancer affects not only man, but animals and plants as well. Some cancers in animals have been shown to result from infection by a virus, but human cancer is not contagious.

Certain conditions and habits favor the development of cancer. Smoking is probably the most notorious. Air pollution and other environmental agents may also be involved in the incidence of lung cancer. Overexposure to the sun or to other sources of radiation definitely increases the risk of cancer of the skin. Irritation from such sources as shaving and badly fitting dentures may also be a factor.

Signs of Danger: Not all tumors are malignant; many are BENIGN. Although a benign tumor may grow very large, so that it must be removed by surgery, it lacks the worst characteristic of the malignant tumor: it does not spread into neighboring tissues or other parts of the body. The only certain way of distinguishing between a benign and a malignant tumor is by a BIOPSY. Any persistent lump or unusual growth should be regarded as suspicious. Only a physician is qualified to say whether a tumor is malignant or benign.

A lump in the breast or discharge from the nipple may or may not indicate BREAST CANCER. Unusual vaginal bleeding may be a sign of cancer of the uterus. (The PAP TEST has been of great benefit in the early detection of cervical cancer.) Unexplained loss of weight, blood in the bowel movement, persistent hoarseness, sores that refuse to heal—all call for your doctor's early attention. If only for your own peace of mind, see your family physician without delay should you have any of these symptoms.

Controlling Cancer: The outlook for a person with cancer is excellent if diagnosis is made early enough so that he receives timely treatment. Many thousands of people are alive today who have recovered from cancer. Surgery, radiation of various kinds, and chemicals are being used, either singly or in combination, to bring the disease under control.

CANINE TOOTH The single, pointed tooth on each side of the incisors (the four central teeth) in the upper and lower jaws; also called the eye tooth or cuspid. Canine teeth are so named because they resemble the corresponding fanglike teeth in dogs. See also TOOTH.

CANKER SORE   A small, ulcerated sore on the inside of the mouth that usually clears up within a week or two. The exact cause of canker sores is not known, but some contributing factors may be a VIRUS, ANEMIA, or a VITAMIN deficiency. Rinsing the mouth with a mild solution of one teaspoonful of table salt to a pint of water may help to soothe the irritation. Temporary abstinence from nuts, chocolates, and citrus fruits may help speed the healing. If canker sores persist, check with your doctor.

CAPILLARY   A minute blood vessel with very thin walls. Capillaries form a network in close contact with all the living CELLS in the body. They are the connecting links between ARTERIES and VEINS. One end of a capillary (pronounced kap'i·ler''ee) connects with an arteriole (a fine branch of an artery), and the other end connects with a venule (a very fine vein). All exchanges between blood and body cells take place through the thin capillary walls. Oxygen and other essential substances in arterial blood diffuse into the fluid between the cells and then through the cell wall into the cell. Waste material from the cell, such as carbon dioxide, diffuses out into the capillary. Then pressure (from the heart's beating) forces the blood to flow out through the venule into a vein and back to the heart.

CARBOHYDRATE   One of the three main kinds of foodstuffs needed for a healthy DIET. (The other two are protein and fat.) To the chemist, a carbohydrate (pronounced kahr''boh·hie'drayt) is a compound of carbon, hydrogen, and oxygen, put together in a particular way. All carbohydrates come originally from plants, which manufacture them out of carbon dioxide in the air and water. All the plants and plant products that we eat contain carbohydrates. Refined sugar, starch, and flour are practically pure carbohydrate. When carbohydrates are eaten, ENZYMES in the digestive system break them down into simple sugars that can be absorbed into the bloodstream. The body uses these simple sugars as fuel.

Carbohydrates are a main source of CALORIES. They supply the energy we use in moving, working, or just breathing. If we eat more carbohydrates than we use as fuel, the excess is converted to fat. Most people attempting to lose weight are advised to cut down on the amount of carbohydrates they eat. Some foods, such as candy and cake, are especially rich in sugar and starch, but poor in vitamins and other essential nutrients.

CARBOLIC ACID (phenol)   This chemical has a strong odor and a very destructive effect on living tissue. It is not a true acid. Although it is a powerful DISINFECTANT and ANTISEPTIC, it is too dangerous for household use.

CARBON-MONOXIDE POISONING   Poisoning of body tissues resulting from the breathing of carbon monoxide. If too much of this highly toxic gas is inhaled, death follows.

Carbon monoxide itself is difficult to detect, for it has no smell, color, or taste. It is found in the gas of a gas heater, in fumes from gasoline engines, and in smoke from burning coal or wood. Industrial workers may be exposed to the effects of carbon monoxide. Miners, plumbers, refinery workers, and garage mechanics must constantly be on the alert against this poison. Because carbon monoxide is present in automobile exhaust fumes, an automobile engine should not be kept running in a closed garage.

When the gas is inhaled, it combines very quickly with the HEMOGLOBIN in the red blood cells. The body cannot obtain the oxygen it requires, and suffocation begins. The symptoms include headache, giddiness, shortness of breath, reddening of the skin, faintness, and collapse.

What to Do: The first step in treating the victim of carbon monoxide is to shut off whatever is producing the gas and carry him out of the poisonous atmosphere. (Remember that covering the nostrils or mouth with a damp cloth doesn't keep the fumes out.) Mouth-to-mouth resuscitation should be given at once if breathing is poor or appears to have ceased. (See FIRST AID section.) Constricting clothing should be loosened. Keep the victim warm. While you are giving first aid, have someone call your nearest hospital, the fire department, or the police to bring a RESPIRATOR.

Proper ventilation is a most essential step in avoiding carbon-monoxide poisoning. A gas heater should be provided with a vent. Furnaces and automatic exhausts should be checked regularly to be certain they are in good working order. If you run the engine of your automobile in a garage, make sure the door is open.

CARBON TETRACHLORIDE   A colorless, dangerously toxic solvent that dissolves greases and waxes. Never use carbon tetrachloride (pronounced te''tra·klohr'ied) indoors for dry-cleaning clothes or dewaxing floors. Breathing its fumes can be fatal. Carbon tetrachloride's toxic effects are increased if a person has alcohol in his system.

CARBUNCLE   A painful skin eruption that has a hard covering and is filled with pus. It is larger than the ordinary BOIL, or furuncle, which it resembles in its tendency to spread. A carbuncle has a number of openings, and it reaches deeper than a boil into the underlying tissue.

Carbuncles are usually the result of an infection caused by the bacterium *Staphylococcus aureus*. They are most frequently found in areas subject to irritation, where there are sweat glands and hair—on the chest, neck, and face, between the thighs and on the buttocks, and under the arms. Often they are associated with poor health.

Carbuncles should receive prompt medical attention in anyone (and particularly in persons suffering from DIABETES or NEPHRITIS).

CARCINOGEN Any substance or irritant that contributes to the development of CANCER. (Pronounced kahr·sin′o·jen.)

CARCINOMA Any CANCER that originates in epithelium, which is the special kind of TISSUE that forms the skin and mucous membranes. Carcinoma (pronounced kahr″si·noh′ma) is one of the two main types of malignant tumor. (The other is SARCOMA, which is found in connective tissue and especially in muscle and bone.)

Carcinomas may spread by METASTASIS via the blood and the lymph, or they may simply invade adjacent tissues. Surgery, radioisotopes, and X rays play a major part in eradicating these malignant growths. See also CANCER.

CARDIAC Referring to the HEART.

CARDIAC ARREST Stopping of the heartbeat; also called heart stoppage. Sometimes, if the heart is not severely damaged and action can be taken immediately, the heart can be stimulated to resume its beating by medicines or special techniques of HEART MASSAGE. See also FIRST AID section.

CARDIAC CONDITION A disorder or disease of the heart. See CORONARY HEART DISEASE; HEART DISEASE—SYMPTOMS; ANGINA PECTORIS.

CARDIAC MURMUR See HEART MURMUR.

CARDIAC PACEMAKER Normally, all the chambers of the HEART function with precise timing: left and right auricles send blood into the ventricles at the same time; left and right ventricles pump blood out of the heart simultaneously. The rhythm of the heart action is established by the natural cardiac pacemaker (heart pacemaker), or sinoatrial node. This is a small piece of tissue made up of nerve cells and muscle cells in the wall of the right auricle. These cells not only cause the auricles to contract but also telegraph electric impulses through the atrioventricular node to the ventricles, thus pacing their action, too. The pacemaker keeps stimulating the parts of the heart so that they continue to work rapidly. In effect, the rhythm of the pacemaker is the rhythm of the heart.

In certain heart conditions, the natural pacemaker may not function properly. (See HEART BLOCK.) To make up for this shortcoming, an artificial pacemaker may be used to stimulate the heart

with tiny electrical impulses and restore the normal rhythm.

CARDILATE The trade name of a nitrogen compound that relaxes smooth MUSCLES and dilates BLOOD VESSELS when taken by mouth. Cardilate (pronounced kahr′di·layt) is often prescribed in the treatment of ANGINA PECTORIS.

CARDIOGRAM A graph showing the strength and rhythm of the heartbeat. A cardiogram (pronounced kahr′dee·o·gram″) is made by a special instrument, a cardiograph, which is placed over the heart. Although not strictly correct, the word is sometimes used for ELECTROCARDIOGRAM.

CARDIOLOGY The study of the HEART and the diagnosis and treatment of its diseases. A physician who specializes in this branch of medicine is known as a cardiologist.

CARDIOPULMONARY RESUSCITATION See HEART MASSAGE.

CARDIOVASCULAR Relating to the system through which blood circulates—HEART, ARTERIES, CAPILLARIES, and VEINS. (Pronounced kahr″dee·oh·vas′kyu·lar.)

CARIES A medical term (pronounced kair′eez) for decay of a tooth or a bone. See BONE DISEASE; DENTAL CARIES.

CARISOPRODOL A medicine sometimes prescribed by doctors to relax muscles and relieve pain in cases of SPRAIN or BACKACHE. A mild sedative, carisoprodol (pronounced kar″i·sop′ro·dohl) is sold under the trade names "Soma" and "Rela."

CAROTENE Any of several related orange pigments that are utilized by the body to form vitamin A. Carotene (pronounced kar′o·teen) compounds are present in all plants and are essential in the diet. Foodstuffs with a distinct orange or yellow color, such as carrots, sweet potatoes, egg yolks, and butter, are especially rich in carotene. See VITAMIN.

CAROTID ARTERIES Two major arteries in the neck which supply blood to the head. See also EMBOLISM.

CARRIER 1. A person who harbors germs of an infectious disease in his body but does not develop symptoms of the disease. Although apparently healthy himself, a carrier unwittingly infects others. Diseases such as TYPHOID FEVER and DIPHTHERIA are sometimes transmitted by carriers.

2. In HEREDITY, an apparently normal person whose chromosomes carry a gene for some abnormality which may appear in his children—or *her*

children, in the case of HEMOPHILIA. In a broader sense, anyone whose hereditary makeup includes a RECESSIVE gene paired with a DOMINANT gene is a carrier of the recessive trait.

3. A VECTOR, such as the *Anopheles* mosquito, which harbors the parasite that causes malaria in humans.

4. In biochemistry, a substance that enters into temporary combination with another substance and releases it under certain conditions. Thus, HEMOGLOBIN is a carrier that combines with oxygen in the lungs and releases oxygen in the tissues.

CAR SICKNESS See MOTION SICKNESS.

CARTILAGE Flexible white tissue or gristle around the joints and in other parts of the body. Cartilage (pronounced kahr′ti·laj) is present in the windpipe (TRACHEA), the LARYNX, the ears, and the tip of the nose. It also makes up the disks between the vertebrae of the spinal column. In general, cartilage improves flexibility, serves as padding, and prevents friction. The skeleton of the FETUS, or unborn infant, is made up of cartilage. Later the cartilage hardens into bone.

Cartilage is subject to a number of disorders. ARTHRITIS produces degeneration of the cartilage as well as the bones of the joints. A VERTEBRAL DISK may slip out of position and cause severe backache. The cartilage in the knee may be damaged by an accident; surgery is sometimes required to correct this condition.

CASCARA A mild CATHARTIC, or LAXATIVE, obtained from the bark of the cascara buckthorn. Cascara sagrada (pronounced kas·kair′a sa·grah′da), to give its full name, stimulates muscular action of the COLON. Since it needs about eight hours to reach the colon, it is best taken at bedtime.

CAST (for broken bones) A rigid dressing used to prevent movement of a fractured bone or a dislocated joint so that it can heal rapidly without being deformed.

Casts are made of bandage impregnated with plaster of Paris or other hardening material. The weight of a cast should be borne largely by a sling or other support rather than by the body's muscles and joints. The person's general circulation should be stimulated as much as possible by exercise. Wearing a cast always causes a certain amount of discomfort, but complaints should not be brushed aside; pressure on nerves and blood vessels under the cast may be causing complications. Watch for danger signals, such as odor, swelling, or any differences in temperature and skin color between affected and unaffected parts of the body. Any unusual conditions such as these should be reported to your doctor immediately.

See also BROKEN BONE in FIRST AID section.

CAST (in bodily discharges) An abnormal body discharged in the urine, the sputum, or other body fluids.

Casts are composed of a variety of tissue debris and fatty or waxy substances. They are formed by the hardening of fluids in tiny body cavities and, like a liquid that solidifies in a mold, they retain the shape of the cavity. A renal cast, for example, has a shape of the tubule (tiny tube) in the kidney in which it was formed.

CASTOR OIL A thick, colorless vegetable oil with a faint odor and an unpleasant taste. Castor oil is a powerful CATHARTIC. It irritates the intestine and should not be self-administered for CONSTIPATION. See also LAXATIVE.

CASTRATION Surgical removal of the testicles. The operation is performed in men to combat disease of the testicles and cancer of the prostate gland. If the operation is done before puberty it arrests the development of the male sexual characteristics. The voice remains high-pitched, the beard does not grow, and the figure softens in outline.

If performed after puberty, castration produces little or no change in secondary sexual characteristics. There is complete sterility (inability to father children) as soon as the seminal vesicles, which store sperm, are empty. But there is not necessarily impotence (inability to have sexual intercourse), although castration does lessen sexual desire. See also VASECTOMY.

CATALEPSY See CATATONIA.

CATARACT A clouded condition in the lens of the EYE, resulting in blurred vision. Cataracts sometimes, but very rarely, are present at birth or develop in young people. However, the condition is usually seen in elderly people. Heat, X rays, or injury, as well as diseases such as DIABETES, may cause cataracts in some cases.

The clouding of the lens increases very slowly. In its early stages, difficulty in seeing may be helped by eyeglasses. Later, vision may be aided if the clouded natural lens is removed by surgery. Special techniques have been developed that make this operation a relatively minor one. Extreme cold is sometimes applied to freeze the lens to a surgical instrument, which then removes it. (See CRYOSURGERY.) Or the lens may be liquefied by very-high-frequency sound waves and drained off through a tiny tube inserted through a small incision. Thereafter, the person must wear special eyeglasses or CONTACT LENSES. It is not necessary to wait until the cataracts become complete before an operation can be performed.

CATARRH A term that refers to the inflammation and discharge that occur with a COMMON COLD or

375

SINUSITIS. The word "catarrh" (pronounced ka·tahr') is not generally used today.

CATATONIA A medical term applied to certain kinds of abnormal behavior that are characteristic of some patients with the mental illness called SCHIZO-PHRENIA. Typical symptoms of catatonia (pronounced kat"a·ton'ee·a) include a tendency to remain motionless in one position for prolonged periods (catalepsy), phases of stupor and excitement, repetition of aimless motions or sounds, and seeming unawareness of other persons or active resistance to spoken requests. It is futile to deal with the illness by trying to persuade the catatonic person to correct his behavior. Professional psychiatric help should be sought immediately. See also EMOTIONAL AND MENTAL DISORDERS.

CATHARTIC A medicine that promotes emptying of the bowels. It is stronger than a laxative and more rapid in its action, although the terms are sometimes used interchangeably. A cathartic (pronounced ka·thahr'tik) may also be referred to as a purgative or a physic. Cathartics should only be used under the supervision of a physician.

Perhaps the most familiar of the strong cathartics is CASTOR OIL. This medicine causes irritation of the bowel, and is now not used as much as formerly.

Saline (salt-containing) cathartics produce their effect by causing the intestine to retain water that is normally absorbed into the blood. This causes fluid to accumulate in the bowel and aids in evacuation. EPSOM SALTS and sodium phosphate are familiar examples.

No cathartic (or laxative) should be taken regularly in the treatment of CONSTIPATION. Often the constipation can be overcome with a good diet and simple, healthy living.

Never take a cathartic when there is abdominal pain. This pain may be a warning signal of APPENDICITIS, and the cathartic may cause rupture of the infected appendix. See LAXATIVE for a discussion of mild cathartics.

CATHETER A thin, flexible tube designed to be introduced into a body passage or a body cavity in order to withdraw or inject some substance, or to keep the passage open. One common type of catheter (pronounced kath'e·ter) is used to draw urine from the bladder.

CAT-SCRATCH FEVER A mild disease thought to be caused by a VIRUS transmitted through scratches inflicted by apparently healthy cats. The symptoms include swelling of LYMPH NODES, headache, and fever. The disease disappears without treatment after a period that may last for a few weeks or several years. It is sometimes treated with certain ANTIBIOTICS, such as TETRACYCLINE and CHLORAMPHENICOL.

CAULIFLOWER EAR Lumpy disfigurement of the ear due to injury, such as repeated blows in boxing or fistfighting. As with any BRUISE caused by impact, there is bleeding under the skin. Instead of being absorbed, a large pool of blood may harden into a clot, and excessive repair tissue may form, causing permanent disfigurement. This can usually be prevented by having a doctor draw the blood off with a special needle before it hardens. A fully developed cauliflower ear can be repaired only by PLASTIC SURGERY.

CAUTERIZE To destroy abnormal or injured tissue by applying a hot iron, a corrosive substance such as nitric acid, an electric current, intense cold, or other means. It was once common practice to cauterize (pronounced kaw'te·riez) almost any wound in order to destroy an infection that might be present, but such cauterization is now used mainly on the bites of animals suspected of having RABIES. At the same time, cauterization has become a common technique in modern surgery, due to the development of instruments that can be applied with great precision to diseased tissue without affecting healthy tissue nearby. One such instrument is the laser, which produces an extremely intense beam of light that can be focused on a very small, definite area for as short a time as a fraction of a second.

CAVITY See DENTAL CARIES; TOOTH.

CELIAC DISEASE A relatively rare disorder of the intestines, usually occurring in children between the ages of six months and six years; the symptoms may continue into adulthood. It is characterized by an inability to digest and absorb fats, starches, and some sugars. Celiac disease is related to nontropical and tropical SPRUE, disorders occurring in adults. Its cause is not completely understood, but heredity and vitamin deficiencies may play a part.

The child with celiac disease becomes anemic, irritable, and weak. He fails to grow properly and has a poor appetite. The abdomen is distended with gas; stools contain undigested fat and are pale and frothy.

Treatment is based largely on the feeding of a high-protein diet from which fat and gluten (found in cereal flours) are eliminated. Fruit sugars and honey are substituted for ordinary sugar. VITAMIN supplements are given to treat the anemia and other vitamin deficiencies.

A child who responds well to the diet for six months is gradually introduced to new foods, one at a time. With good treatment, the chances for recovery are excellent.

CELL Any of the similar units out of which all living tissue is built. A cell consists of a membrane

CELL

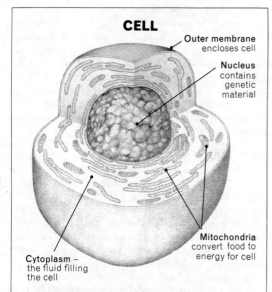

Outer membrane
encloses cell

Nucleus
contains
genetic
material

Mitochondria
convert food to
energy for cell

Cytoplasm –
the fluid filling
the cell

Nearly every tissue in the body is made up of microscopic cells, generally only a few hundred-thousandths of an inch across. Each cell has a central nucleus containing 23 pairs of chromosomes, which bear the genes that determine a person's inherited characteristics.

surrounding a mass of jellylike cytoplasm in which a variety of specialized structures are suspended. The largest of these internal bodies is the nucleus, a sort of cell within the cell, containing the material by which the cell reproduces itself. Cells vary in shape and size according to the work they do. Most cells are so small that they can be seen only with a microscope, and some of the structures inside the cell cannot be seen at all except in photographs taken by an electron microscope.

CELSIUS The temperature scale used in most parts of the world (also known as the centigrade scale). In the United States, however, the FAHRENHEIT scale is commonly used. In the Celsius system, the normal body temperature is 37°C. Any Celsius temperature can be changed to Fahrenheit by multiplying the Celsius reading by 9, dividing by 5, and then adding 32. Thus 37°C is the same temperature as 98.6°F. To change Fahrenheit to Celsius, reverse the calculation: subtract 32 from the Fahrenheit reading, multiply by 5, and divide by 9.

CEMENTUM Bonelike material forming a thin, hard covering over the roots of a TOOTH.

CEREBELLUM The second largest part of the BRAIN, located toward the back of the head under the CEREBRUM. The cerebellum (pronounced ser"e·bel'um) is the center where voluntary movements, posture, and equilibrium are coordinated.

CEREBRAL Pertaining to the CEREBRUM, the upper part of the BRAIN. (Pronounced ser'e·bral.)

CEREBRAL CORTEX The outer layer of the CEREBRUM in the BRAIN, sometimes referred to as the gray matter.

CEREBRAL HEMORRHAGE Bleeding inside the BRAIN from a ruptured BLOOD VESSEL, usually from an artery that has been weakened by HARDENING OF THE ARTERIES (arteriosclerosis). When the blood vessel ruptures, certain brain cells are deprived of blood and are permanently damaged. Blood from the ruptured vessel also irritates healthy brain tissue. A cerebral hemorrhage may be brought on by unusual exertion or emotional excitement, especially in a person who has high blood pressure (HYPERTENSION). The symptoms depend upon the severity of bleeding and the part of the brain where it occurs. Usually there is headache and nausea followed by unconsciousness that lasts for six hours or longer.

The victim of a cerebral hemorrhage should be put to bed and given medical attention immediately. Skilled nursing care is essential to help the person maintain normal body functions as long as he is unconscious or unable to move. When consciousness returns, there may be considerable paralysis and speech disturbance. It is impossible during the first few weeks to tell how much of this impairment will be permanent. Improvement takes place very gradually over a period of months. Sometimes complete recovery occurs.

CEREBELLUM

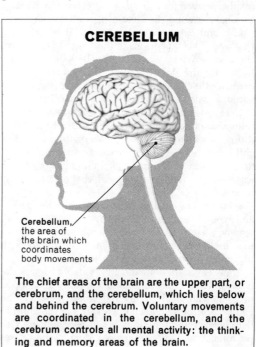

Cerebellum,
the area of
the brain which
coordinates
body movements

The chief areas of the brain are the upper part, or cerebrum, and the cerebellum, which lies below and behind the cerebrum. Voluntary movements are coordinated in the cerebellum, and the cerebrum controls all mental activity: the thinking and memory areas of the brain.

The chances of recovery are greatly improved if physical therapy is begun without delay. Parts of the body that are paralyzed should be put through a regular program of exercise, and the person should be encouraged to try to move himself. With patience, encouragement, and skillful guidance, it is often possible for a person to relearn lost functions by using other brain cells in place of cells that are damaged. See also STROKE; BRAIN DAMAGE.

CEREBRAL PALSY A nonprogressive disability caused by damage to the developing brain, which may occur before, during, or after birth. (Pronounced ser′e·bral pawl′zee.) Typical disabilities include poor muscular coordination, muscular spasms and weakness that interfere with movement, and speech disturbances. The degree of disability varies greatly. In mild cases, the condition may not be noticed until the child is found to have difficulty performing acts normal for a child his age, such as grasping objects or learning to walk. Typical signs include odd movements of the arms, legs, and head, inability to coordinate movements, tremors, and a stiff "scissors" gait. In severe cases, vision and hearing may be affected and the child may suffer convulsions.

Any of a number of different causes may be responsible for the brain damage associated with cerebral palsy. It may be due to incompatible blood types in the parents, insufficient oxygen before birth, premature birth, injury during birth, diseases such as encephalitis and scarlet fever, or other causes. In medicine, the term "cerebral palsy" is commonly reserved for the condition caused by damage to a baby around the time of its delivery.

Cerebral palsy is not uncommon; it is estimated that over 700,000 persons in the United States have the disorder. Every year about 10,000 infants are born with the disease. Their life expectancy is as great as the general average. Many persons with cerebral palsy are able to lead normal lives.

Cerebral palsy children frequently have the intelligence of normal children. Because of their condition, however, they may appear subnormal. The child may slobber and grimace or utter incomprehensible sounds. The fact that a child has trouble in expressing himself does not mean that he is mentally retarded.

Treatment: The treatment varies with the degree and type of cerebral palsy. In severe cases, surgery may be used to help some of the physical aspects of the disease. The convulsions are controlled with phenobarbital or other medications.

Many cases are mild and a reasonably normal life is possible. For the others, a carefully developed program can lead to marked improvement. The emphasis must be placed upon training the child to help himself and building his self-confidence. With persistence and encouragement, even serious cases can make remarkable progress.

Physical therapy, aimed especially at the development of the muscles, is important in any program. Speech training may also be needed. Psychological testing is used to determine whether there is any mental retardation and to point the way to a suitable educational program. Guidance in all these matters is available from the United Cerebral Palsy Associations, 66 East 34th Street, New York, New York 10016, which has branches throughout the United States. See also PALSY.

CEREBRUM The main part of the BRAIN, occupying the top part of the skull above the level of the eyes. The cerebrum (pronounced ser′e·brem) is composed of a soft, wrinkled outer layer, called the cerebral cortex, and an underlying mass of nerve fibers. It is divided from front to back into two similar halves, or hemispheres. Each hemisphere has five distinct parts, or lobes. The cerebrum is larger and more complex in man than in any other mammals except, perhaps, dolphins and whales.

All "intelligent" mental activity takes place in the cerebrum. Distinct regions of the lobes in each hemisphere are devoted to particular kinds of mental activity. These regions have been mapped by noting the effects of brain injury and of stimuli applied directly to different areas during brain surgery. One region is a memory storehouse; another controls speaking; another makes it possible to understand the sounds of speech; still another controls writing. Thus a person who cannot speak following a STROKE may be fully able to understand what is said and even to communicate by writing instead of speaking, because these functions are controlled by separate parts of the brain.

CERUMEN Another name for earwax, a secretion found within the canal leading from the outer EAR to the eardrum. Never use a hard object like a hairpin or a matchstick to remove cerumen—you may puncture the eardrum. Cerumen (pronounced se·roo′men) normally drains out of the ear very slowly, carrying with it any small particles of dust and dirt that may have drifted into the ear canal. All that is usually needed is to wash the outer part with soap and water. Sometimes a plug of stiff or hardened cerumen accumulates in the ear canal, causing pain and interfering with hearing. A doctor can soften and remove it by using a syringe.

CERVICAL CANCER Cancer of the neck of the uterus (cervix). It is one of the most common types of cancer in women, especially among middle-aged women who have had several children. It can be detected at an early stage by a cervical smear (see PAP TEST), and successfully treated. The American Cancer Society recommends that women between the ages of 20 and 65 have a Pap test every three years. A family doctor can advise a woman how she can have a test. See also CANCER; UTERUS.

CERVICAL CYTOLOGY Study under the microscope of a small bit of tissue removed from the cervix—the narrow, lower end of the UTERUS. (Pronounced sur'vi·kal sie·tol'o·jee.) See also PAP TEST.

CERVICAL EROSION A small ulcer on the neck of the womb (cervix). It may bleed or cause a vaginal discharge. It is not serious if treated promptly, usually by cauterizing (see CAUTERIZE). (Pronounced sur'vi·kal e·roh'zhun.)

CERVICAL SMEAR See PAP TEST.

CERVIX The Latin word for neck. Often, the word "cervix" (pronounced sur'viks) refers to the lower, constricted part of the UTERUS, which projects into the VAGINA.

CESAREAN (CESARIAN) SECTION Incision of the abdominal wall and the uterus to deliver a baby. This type of childbirth is practiced in cases where delivery by the birth passage presents difficulties or complications—as in placenta previa, where the placenta has attached itself directly over the cervix, or in cases of premature separation of the placenta from the uterine wall.

In cases where the mother's pelvic passage is too narrow to allow for safe delivery of the baby, for instance, subsequent births will probably also be by cesarean section. In theory, there is no limit to the number of cesareans that a woman can have; many have delivered four or five babies this way. However, much depends on individual circumstances. Some women who have had an initial cesarean section later deliver their babies vaginally.

In the cesarean (pronounced si·zair'ee·an) operation, the surgeon makes an incision in the abdomen, cuts through the fatty tissue and other layers, and incises the wall of the uterus. He lifts out the baby, the placenta, and the rest of the afterbirth. Then the uterus and abdomen are sewn up in layers. The patient experiences brief discomfort, as one inevitably does after an operation. She normally leaves the hospital only a little while later than she would have if she had had a normal delivery.

CHAGAS' DISEASE The South American form of SLEEPING SICKNESS. (Pronounced chah'gahs.)

CHALAZION (plural, **chalazia**) A swelling of a sebaceous oil gland of the eyelid. See STY. (Pronounced ka·lay'zee·on.)

CHANCRE See SYPHILIS. (Pronounced shang'ker.)

CHANCROID A small, soft sore caused by the bacterium *Hemophilus ducreyi*. A chancroid (pronounced shang'kroyd) develops rapidly at the site of infection, usually in the genital area. It should be promptly treated with ANTIBIOTICS.

CHARLEY HORSE Muscular soreness and stiffness caused by overstrain, excessive or unaccustomed exercise, or physical impact. Pain may be relieved by soaking in warm baths and taking ASPIRIN. If the pain persists more than a few days, consult your doctor about the condition.

CHEMOTHERAPY In the broadest meaning of the term, the use of chemical agents to prevent or fight disease and to promote healing, whether of mind or body. Chemicals have a whole spectrum of uses in medicine. They may be applied locally, like iodine, to a particular part of the body, or taken systemically (by mouth or injection) to combat infection throughout the body. Chemicals are also used in the treatment of EMOTIONAL AND MENTAL DISORDERS. Following the development of ANTIDEPRESSANTS and TRANQUILIZERS, chemotherapy has become at least as important as PSYCHOTHERAPY in treating the mentally ill.

The use of the word "chemotherapy" (pronounced kem"oh·ther'a·pee) is sometimes restricted to treatment of infectious diseases and cancer with chemicals that act like "magic bullets," seeking out and killing the disease-producing microorganisms or abnormal cancer cells in the body without hurting normal tissue. Paul Ehrlich (1854–1915), a German bacteriologist, was the first to develop this kind of chemical therapy. He discovered that Salvarsan, a chemical containing arsenic, had a selective lethal action on the organism that causes syphilis. Although Salvarsan is no longer used, it was the first effective treatment ever found for syphilis.

Sulfonamides: Chemotherapy has made enormous strides in the 20th century. The development of the sulfonamides, or sulfa compounds, opened a new era. They were first used in 1908 as dyes for wool, but such use was subsequently discontinued. In 1932 their medical value was recognized, and they were soon being used to treat streptococcal infection (see STREPTOCOCCUS). Large numbers of sulfonamides have been developed, but many of them proved to have undesirable side effects and have been replaced by other chemical agents discovered later. They continue to be used effectively against meningitis and certain infections of the urinary tract. See also SULFONAMIDE.

Antibiotics: PENICILLIN, discovered by Sir Alexander Fleming in 1929, is a chemical agent that is very effective in killing bacteria. It is a natural substance produced by a type of green mold, like that which may grow on stale bread. This antibiotic was first used in 1940 against infection caused by STAPHYLOCOCCUS germs, and saved numerous lives in World War II. Because some persons are allergic to penicillin, doctors are cautious in prescribing it, but it has proved effective against a wide range of diseases, including pneumonia and syphilis. Penicillin and most other antibiotics have no effect whatever on virus-caused diseases, however. More recently developed antibiotics include AUREOMYCIN, TERRA-MYCIN, and TETRACYCLINE. Although antibiotics were orginally derived from molds and bacteria, efforts have been made to produce them synthetically and to alter them to eliminate undesirable side effects. New ones are being constantly created and tested for safety and effectiveness. See also ANTIBIOTIC.

Certain highly toxic chemicals have been found useful in controlling some kinds of cancer. Cancerous cells, without exception, are cells that grow and subdivide more rapidly than normal cells. Chemotherapy in the treatment of cancer depends on the fact that rapidly growing cells are more easily damaged by chemicals than are mature, slowly growing cells.

CHEST The upper part of the body, above the abdomen and below the neck, and separated from the abdomen by the muscular wall of the diaphragm. The chest cavity contains the heart and lungs, which are protected by the bony cage of the ribs. The esophagus (gullet) passes down through the chest from the throat to the stomach.

Muscles between the ribs, called intercostal muscles, help to change the size and shape of the rib cage and allow maximum expansion of the lungs during deep breathing.

Pain in the chest may be a symptom of strain or overuse of one of the muscles, or it may be a sign of a respiratory disorder such as BRONCHITIS or PNEU-

MONIA. It may be caused by INDIGESTION. Sometimes chest pain is a symptom of HEART DISEASE.

CHEWING Breaking down food into small particles in the mouth. Chewing mixes SALIVA, which contains the enzyme ptyalin, with the food. The ENZYME begins the digestion of starches, and the chewing and the saliva make the food easier to swallow.

Chewing, or mastication, is an important part of the digestive process. Early in this century the American nutritionist Horace Fletcher advocated, in a doctrine that came to be known as Fletcherism, that food be eaten in small amounts, that it be taken only when one is hungry, and that it be chewed ("Fletcherized") very thoroughly. It is unnecessary to follow his method to the last extreme detail, but good chewing does help to prepare the food so that it can be used by the cells of the body.

Persons who have lost a good many teeth or who gulp their meals obviously cannot chew their food properly. This serves to increase the work that the stomach has to do, and contributes to indigestion.

CHICKEN BREAST See PIGEON BREAST.

CHICKEN POX An acute, infectious disease of childhood that is caused by a virus and marked by eruptions on the skin. The disease is not considered serious, and generally lasts about two weeks after the first appearance of symptoms. Chicken pox is highly CONTAGIOUS, so the patient should be isolated, that is, kept away from contact with others. The disease, also known as varicella, is among the commonest occurring in childhood. It is rare among adults simply because most people are exposed to the disease in childhood and develop immunity to it.

Symptoms: Chicken pox is spread by contact with a person who has the disease, or by breathing infectious droplets in the air. From 10 to 20 days after exposure—two weeks, on the average—the first symptoms appear. Fever and discomfort are usually mild in children but more severe in adults. The patient has little or no appetite. Small red marks appear on his back and chest and continue to spread in successive crops for several days to his face, scalp, arms, and elsewhere. After some hours the marks become blisters; these soon fill with pus, and, finally, they form crusts. In one to two weeks the crusts drop off. There is much itching during this period.

Treatment: Call your doctor for a reliable diagnosis when symptoms first appear. If he confirms a case of chicken pox, the individual should be put to bed and kept isolated until the primary crusts are gone—about 12 days. Caution the person to avoid scratching, since there is risk of infection and scarring. If the sick person is a child, cut his fingernails close and make sure that his hands are kept clean. Have him take baths or showers frequently when

CHEST

The chest cavity, protected by the rib cage and separated from the abdomen by the diaphragm, houses the lungs and the heart and its major blood vessels. The esophagus (gullet) passes through the chest, carrying food to the stomach.

the fever is gone, to keep his skin clean. The itching may be relieved by applications of CALAMINE LOTION, or by taking a cold bath containing several handfuls of starch. An ANTIHISTAMINE, prescribed by your doctor, can also be helpful. If signs of infection of the PUSTULES appear, call them to the physician's attention promptly. Change sheets, pillow cases, and the patient's clothing often.

A single attack of chicken pox generally confers immunity. Unfortunately, there is no reliable vaccine available to protect against the disease.

CHILBLAIN A local reddening, swelling, and itching caused by exposure to cold. A chilblain (pronounced chil'blayn") may occur on the fingers, toes, ears, and nose. It can be treated with drugs and by improving the circulation with hot baths or exercise.

CHILDBIRTH For the vast majority of women, bearing children is a natural and inevitable part of life. For most, it is a safe and relatively minor interruption of day-to-day living—especially so when modern medical and also anesthetic techniques are available.

Attitudes toward childbirth, or parturition, vary greatly from person to person and gradually change in groups of people over a period of time. A few generations ago, childbirth was a fearful mystery shrouded in taboos. Today, there is a healthy trend toward frankness and complete honesty. Many wives—and their husbands—look forward to childbirth eagerly. Large numbers of women bear their children with little anesthesia or none, and witness every part of the birth. Frequently, in preparation, they follow a program (known as natural childbirth) that helps them to strengthen and prepare the parts of the body most involved in childbearing. Such a program obviously appeals to some women more than others, and every woman should make her own choice. In general, every mother-to-be should get some exercise, eat well, and follow the advice given by her physician.

Labor: A normal pregnancy lasts about 40 weeks from the start of the last menstrual period, although the baby may come a few weeks earlier or a few weeks later. Its impending arrival is announced by contractions of the uterus. These may start gently and irregularly, coming about every 15 minutes; they may not last much more than 10 seconds. When they become more frequent and pronounced—at intervals of less than 10 minutes and lasting half a minute—it is time to call the doctor. Labor is more rapid in the woman who has borne children before.

It happens, rarely, that labor proceeds so rapidly that there is no time to obtain expert help when it is most needed, at the moment of birth. However, babies have been known to arrive in taxis and buses and completely unexpectedly at home. For what to do in such an emergency, see FIRST AID section.

With the first baby, a woman generally feels the first mild twinges of labor some 15 or 16 hours before delivery. With later babies, it may take half this time. These are only averages, of course, and there is considerable normal variation within them. (See OBSTETRICS.)

Labor is usually divided into three stages.

First Stage: In this stage the cervix, or mouth of the uterus, very gradually dilates from a minute opening to about four inches, making it possible for the baby's head to pass through. The contractions grow longer and more intense until each is 40 seconds or longer. The first stage varies greatly in length and is usually the longest stage of childbirth.

Second Stage: The baby is born in this stage. The process may take up to two hours for a first child, and 30 minutes or less for a later one. The infant passes through the cervix and the vagina. Sometimes a small incision (called an EPISIOTOMY) is made in the perineal tissue to prevent tearing and make passage of the infant easier.

Third Stage: In the final stage, which lasts 10 or 15 minutes, the placenta and the rest of the AFTERBIRTH are expelled.

Treatment After Birth: At birth, the baby normally begins to breathe and cry on his own. The umbilical cord is cut, the infant's eyes are treated with an antibacterial medication, and he is placed in a heated crib. The baby is thoroughly examined, weighed, and cleaned.

What of the mother? She is examined and the episiotomy is closed with stitches. Her abdomen is massaged to help the stretched tissues contract, and she may be given a sedative to make her sleep. The afterbirth is checked by the doctor to make sure that all of it has been expelled. If the mother has been awake during the delivery, her baby may be given to her to suckle, because suckling causes uterine contractions and helps the uterus to regain its tight, hard shape. Usually, the mother will be taken back to her room only after the doctor is sure that the uterus has contracted sufficiently. See also POSTPARTUM.

Delivery Problems: With regular visits to the doctor, delivery problems may be anticipated and handled in a satisfactory way. In one out of 25 births, the infant's buttocks will emerge first, rather than the head. This is called a BREECH DELIVERY. It is slower than the usual type and generally requires a more extensive episiotomy.

If the mother's pelvis is too narrow, birth by CESAREAN (CESARIAN) SECTION may be necessary. This is a surgical operation used to remove the baby from the mother's abdomen. A cesarean may be performed, too, if the mother is ill or if some other condition makes normal delivery unwise. This operation is safe under normal conditions, and may be done repeatedly for subseqent births.

Occasionally, for medical reasons, it is necessary to induce labor. This is done by rupturing the membranes enclosing the infant or by giving the mother a medicine that stimulates the uterus to contract, so that labor may begin.

CHILD PSYCHOLOGY Building emotional security in a child is a challenging task. Nowadays it is widely felt that the early years of childhood are critical in determining the kind of adult the youngster will grow up to be. The mother and father, in their behavior toward each other and the child, establish patterns that may well have a lasting influence on him. This does not minimize the roles played by brothers and sisters, school, playmates, and relatives in forming the emerging personality.

Childhood has its own special psychological or emotional problems. It is impossible to lay down precise rules for handling all these problems, but there are some general principles that can light our way in dealing with them.

Love Your Child: Never be afraid to show your children that you love them and want to understand them. Loving them will not spoil them, so long as you follow certain commonsense rules of discipline.

Discipline: Most young children look to their parents for direction. They become bewildered and confused if they are unfailingly allowed to have their own way. It is the parents' role to set the limits in important matters. Yet, although parents must be authority figures, they should not be authoritarian. Children should be encouraged to explore and to learn for themselves. Parents should learn not to expect more of a child than is justified by the child's age and development.

A family atmosphere in which you are constantly shouting, "No, you mustn't do that!" is not a wholesome one. Think things through and see if you aren't being too severe. Perhaps you can establish new ground rules and make clear to your child what you expect of him. Most children desire and have need for their parents' approval.

Sleeping Problems: Every child has a sleeping problem at some time. If your child has difficulty getting to sleep, don't just scold him. Find out what the trouble is. Bad dreams may make him afraid of the dark. Perhaps you can solve the problem by reassuring him or installing a night-light. Provide a period of relaxation at bedtime so the child is not too stimulated. Above all, never punish a child by making him go to bed early.

Feeding Problems: Just as some children are poor sleepers, others are poor eaters. Don't be disturbed if your child refuses his food. It isn't wise to force him to eat. Simply take the food away—but not as a punishment. Usually by the time the next meal comes, he will be hungry enough to eat. Try to see to it that the child is relaxed at mealtimes, and the atmosphere is restful.

Toilet Training: Many psychiatrists believe that good toilet training is important in providing the basis of a good personality. Don't try to toilet train a child before he is ready, or make him ashamed of soiling himself. You may resent the smell and the mess, but avoid letting him see your attitude. He will generally take to the toilet easily enough when his organs are sufficiently developed to make control possible for him; usually this is in the third year, but it may be later or earlier.

Sibling Rivalry: This term means the jealousy or dislike that exists between children in the same family. When a second child is born, the first one usually resents having to share the affection of the parents, whether he shows it or not. It is important to prepare the older child for the coming of the baby and to get him to help in its care, so that he feels it is his baby as well as his mother's. Above all, let the older child know without reservation that you love him as much as the baby.

For a discussion of the emotional problems of teenage children, see ADOLESCENCE.

CHILL A sensation of being cold, accompanied by shivering and pallor. In a healthy person, these symptoms are a normal defense against exposure to cold. The work done by the muscles in shivering produces heat and keeps the body's temperature from falling. However, a chill may be a sign of a serious disorder. Chills followed by fever are the first stage of several acute infections, including pneumonia, scarlet fever, malaria, and influenza. The presence of a toxic substance in the blood may cause chills. A chill is also one of the symptoms of SHOCK following injury, severe fright, or unusual exertion, as in childbirth. Any chill that is accompanied by a feeling of being unwell should be brought at once to the attention of a doctor.

CHIROPODIST Another name for a PODIATRIST. (Pronounced ke·rop′e·dist.)

CHLOASMA The medical term for the harmless, light-brown patches of irregular size and shape that are popularly, and incorrectly, called liver spots. (Pronounced kloh·az′ma.)

CHLORAMPHENICOL An ANTIBIOTIC effective against many disease-producing organisms, but especially against the BACILLUS that causes TYPHOID FEVER. Chloramphenicol (pronounced klaw″ram·fen′i·kohl″) is not generally used except where other antibiotics are ineffective. Frequent blood tests and other precautions must be taken to guard against dangerous side effects. It is sold under various trade names including Chloromycetin.

CHLOROFORM A volatile (rapidly evaporating) liquid with a strong smell. Chloroform (pronounced klawr′o·fawrm″) is a powerful ANESTHETIC, but it is toxic and therefore rarely used in modern surgery. It has a limited use as an ingredient of some LINIMENTS for relieving muscle SPASM.

CHLOROMYCETIN A trade name for CHLORAM-PHENICOL. (Pronounced klawr"oh·mie·seet'in.)

CHLOROPHYLL The green substance in plants, which enables them to absorb light energy and to manufacture plant tissues out of water and carbon dioxide. Chlorophyll has been said by some manufacturers of chlorophyll compounds to promote healing and destroy bad odors; it is used in certain nonprescription formulas for ointments and deodorants. Its effectiveness has been debated, however. Chlorophyll has no known harmful or toxic effects.

CHLOROQUINE A compound used in the treatment of amebic HEPATITIS, MALARIA, LUPUS ERYTHEMATOSUS, and, only occasionally, in rheumatoid ARTHRITIS. When chloroquine (pronounced klawr'e·kwin") is prescribed, a careful watch must be kept for possible side effects, including blurring of vision and loss of appetite.

CHLORPROMAZINE The GENERIC name of a tranquilizing medicine often prescribed to overcome anxiety and agitation in some types of mental illness. Chlorpromazine (pronounced klawr·prom'a·zeen') is sometimes prescribed to control nausea and vomiting, or to strengthen the effect of certain pain-relieving compounds. In some persons, chlorpromazine produces undesirable side effects, including rapid heartbeat, jaundice, drowsiness, and overweight. It should never be used except under careful medical supervision. Chlorpromazine is often prescribed under the trade name Thorazine.

CHOKING Obstruction of the LARYNX or TRACHEA (windpipe) so that breathing becomes difficult or impossible. Anything that cuts off the supply of oxygen to the brain for more than a few moments is dangerous. If a child has an attack of CROUP, a doctor should be contacted immediately, before blockage of breathing becomes severe. In cases where an obstruction develops suddenly, first aid measures must be taken without delay—there is no time to wait for a doctor. See the FIRST AID section.

CHOLERA An acute epidemic disease caused by a BACTERIUM found in the feces of infected persons. Cholera (pronounced kol'er·a) is spread through polluted water and contaminated food or insects. Cholera is a danger only in countries that lack modern sanitary techniques, such as frequent testing and purification of water supplies and proper disposal of human excrement. The chief symptoms of cholera are sudden onset of severe vomiting and copious diarrhea, sometimes referred to as ricewater stools. The resulting dehydration (loss of water from the system) is often fatal.

Treatment consists of combating dehydration by administering large quantities of special fluids intravenously (directly into a vein). The vaccine that has been developed against cholera is effective for only a few months and requires frequent BOOSTER SHOTS. If you visit a region where cholera occurs, use only boiled water, avoid uncooked fruits and vegetables, and see that your living quarters are well protected by screens to keep out any disease-carrying insects.

CHOLESTEROL A STEROID substance present in the blood, the brain, and all other tissues throughout the body, as well as in many foods. Pure cholesterol (pronounced ko·les'te·rohl") consists of white crystals, something like sugar, but it dissolves in fat and not in water. It is manufactured by the body, chiefly in the liver and adrenal glands, and is the principal constituent of GALLSTONES. In the brain and spinal cord, about 14 percent of the dry weight of the white matter consists of cholesterol. It is undoubtedly one of the key substances in the METABOLISM of the body, although its exact role is not well understood. Cholesterol of animal origin is used commercially to synthesize steroid hormones.

Hardening of the Arteries: Cholesterol has been implicated in HARDENING OF THE ARTERIES, or arteriosclerosis, one of the commonest disorders of middle-aged and older persons. Large numbers of deaths from STROKE, heart disease, and kidney disease are linked to arteriosclerosis.

How does cholesterol contribute to hardening of the arteries? In the disorder called atherosclerosis, the lining of the arteries is covered with fatty deposits that contain large amounts of cholesterol. In some cases, but by no means all, a significant rise in the quantity of cholesterol and related substances in the blood precedes the appearance of these deposits. The deposits attract compounds of calcium, which further thicken the walls of the arteries and make them hard and inelastic.

Low-Cholesterol Diet: Research on the relationship of cholesterol and disease is still going on. In the meantime, it makes sense to consider reducing the amounts of both cholesterol and fat in our diet. Some kinds of fats, especially fats of animal origin, are found to increase the amount of cholesterol in the blood. These *saturated* fats are found in whole milk, butter, cream, cheese, bacon, eggs, and fatty meats. *Unsaturated* fats (polyunsaturates) do not increase the cholesterol level in the body. These are found in oleomargarine, soybean products, and cottonseed and corn oils. Not all vegetable fats are unsaturated fats, however. Coconut oil, for example, is largely saturated fat. Foods low in saturated fats include nonfat fish, poultry, lean meat, skim milk, vegetables, and fruits.

CHOREA Irregular, involuntary twitching movements, which in severe cases may involve all the muscles except those that move the eyes. Chorea (pronounced ko·ree'a) is a symptom of several diseases affecting the nervous system. Sydenham's chorea, or Saint Vitus's dance, is a disorder often associated with RHEUMATIC FEVER in children. The loss of muscular control first shows up as unusual clumsiness. This type of chorea runs its course in about two months and causes no permanent damage to the brain.

It is essential that a child with signs of chorea be given special medicines and nursing care promptly in order to lessen the damage to the heart that is often a sequel of rheumatic fever. BED REST and TRANQUILIZERS are important for the chorea victim. HUNTINGTON'S DISEASE, or Huntington's chorea, a type of mental defect, is a totally different disorder.

CHROMOSOME One of a number of minute bodies present in every cell of a living thing. The chromosome (pronounced kroh′mo·sohm) is the carrier of the genes, which determine the physical characteristics of the individual that are handed down from generation to generation. Thus, chromosomes carry the "instructions" that determine the color of our eyes and hair, our height, body structure, and other characteristics.

Chromosomes are present in pairs in the nucleus of each CELL. By using special methods of dyeing, it is possible to see them under a microscope. In the human being, each ordinary body cell has 46 chromosomes, arranged in 23 pairs. The number of chromosomes varies with different SPECIES of organisms, but is fairly constant for the same species. Plants typically have 12 to 24. The fruit fly, widely used in studies of genetics, has eight chromosomes. A human sex cell, male or female, has half the ordinary number of chromosomes. Instead of 23 chromosome pairs, there are 23 single chromosomes in each sperm cell and each egg cell, or ovum. When the two sex cells unite, the number of chromosomes becomes 46 again, and the individual resulting from the union inherits genetic traits from both the father and the mother. Certain chromosomes (called X and Y) determine the sex of the new individual. (See HEREDITY.)

An abnormal condition of the chromosomes is responsible for the disorder called MONGOLISM. Other irregularities, such as duplication or absence of chromosomes, may produce individuals who possess the characteristics of both sexes. Breakage of chromosomes can be caused by a number of factors—for example, an overdose of radiation—and leads to a variety of hereditary defects.

CHRONIC Lasting for a long time, without any rapid change for the better or the worse. The opposite of chronic is ACUTE, which describes a condition or a disease that has a relatively sudden onset and runs its course in a short time. It is a mistake to think that the two words mean anything more than this. A chronic disease is not necessarily either more or less serious than an acute disease; nor it is necessarily an incurable disease. Some "chronic" conditions can be cured or greatly helped by proper treatment.

CHYME Food that has been changed in the stomach into a mushy, homogeneous mass. At this stage, chyme (pronounced kiem) has been partly digested by SALIVA and by the ENZYMES and ACID that are secreted by the stomach. The chyme is then ready to pass into the small INTESTINE, where further digestion will take place.

CIGARETTE See SMOKING.

CINEPLASTY Another spelling for KINEPLASTY.

CIRCADIAN RHYTHM The natural daily rhythm of certain bodily activities, such as eating and sleeping ("circadian" means "about a day"). Such activities are probably under the control of an internal "biological clock" and are thought to be largely independent of external influences. (Pronounced sir·kayd′ee·an.)

CIRCUMCISION Cutting off the foreskin, or prepuce, a fold of skin at the end of the PENIS. Sometimes the foreskin covers the end of the organ, causing difficulty in urination. The foreskin may also be formed in such a fashion that it is difficult to keep clean, which can open the way for infection. In these and similar instances, the physician may recommend circumcision as a hygienic measure.

Circumcision is best performed soon after the baby is born, perhaps when he is about a week old. It is often done while baby and mother are still in the hospital. The operation is a slight one, taking only a few minutes; it is completely routine and safe when performed under hospital conditions by your physician or someone he recommends. If circumcision is put off until the child is two or three years old, he may find it a frightening experience.

Circumcision is not only a sanitary measure, but it is also a religious practice of great antiquity. It is prevalent among Jews and Moslems and was practiced in ancient Egypt.

CIRRHOSIS A chronic disease of the liver, marked by destruction of liver cells and their replacement by fatty or fibrous tissue.

Cirrhosis (pronounced si·roh′sis) is often associated with alcoholism, but it also occurs in people who never drink. The precise cause is not known. Poor nutrition, particularly a deficiency of vitamin B, can play a part. So can diseases such as MALARIA or HEPATITIS. Chronic disease of the bowel appears to be a factor, and sometimes exposure to toxic chemicals, such as CARBON TETRACHLORIDE, may be the cause. The disease most often strikes men, especially those between the ages of 40 and 60.

Symptoms: Symptoms may be late in appearing and, in some cases, never bother the person at all, as long as enough healthy liver cells remain to carry on the various vital functions of the liver. But the disease, if untreated, can be profoundly serious. Typically, the circulation of blood through the liver is impaired. The liver increases in size and, as the condition progresses, fluid accumulates in the abdomen, causing it to become enlarged. The person suffers from indigestion, nausea, and vomiting. He has no appetite and loses weight. The legs may swell, and the skin eventually takes on the yellowish hue of jaundice. Eventually, the liver may become shrunken and deformed, as more fibrous tissue accumulates.

Diagnosis and Treatment: Chemical tests and a liver BIOPSY (done with a needle) are used to confirm the diagnosis of cirrhosis suggested by the symptoms described. The person is put on a salt-restricted diet rich in carbohydrates and proteins, and vitamin supplements may be given. Medicines that help the person lose the accumulated fluid may also be used. He is not allowed to take alcoholic beverages. Cortisone is used in some cases. The outcome ultimately depends on how early the disease is diagnosed and treated.

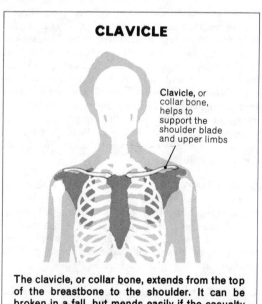

CLAVICLE

Clavicle, or collar bone, helps to support the shoulder blade and upper limbs

The clavicle, or collar bone, extends from the top of the breastbone to the shoulder. It can be broken in a fall, but mends easily if the casualty keeps his arm in a sling for a week or two.

CLAVICLE The collarbone; either of the two bones connecting the breastbone to the shoulder blades. The two bony humps at the base of the throat are the front ends of the clavicles. Fractures of the clavicle are fairly common, but they are among the easiest of all fractures to heal—usually within a month.

CLEFT LIP See HARELIP.

CLEFT PALATE A split, or cleft, in the roof of the mouth. It is a CONGENITAL condition that is due to failure of the two sides of the palate to grow together. It frequently occurs in combination with a cleft lip (HARELIP). Modern techniques of surgery and dentistry can correct the condition, assuring the child of normal appearance and speech, provided treatment is begun early.

There are numerous varieties of cleft palate. The cleft may be slight or large; it may extend through the hard palate or soft palate or both. The infant frequently has feeding difficulties, being unable to chew or swallow in a normal way. There are usually speech difficulties.

Treatment: Correction of cleft palate requires PLASTIC SURGERY. The palate may be reconstructed in one operation or more, depending on the condition. The work is usually begun when the child is about a year and a half old. Dental problems often appear that call for special attention. The child also may need the help of a speech therapist. It is most important, through it all, to encourage the youngster to lead a normal life with other children and to keep him from becoming overly self-conscious.

CLERGYMAN'S THROAT Dysphonia; HOARSENESS and other difficulty or pain in speaking, resulting from overstraining or misusing the voice. People who do much public speaking can usually avoid or lessen this kind of hoarseness by using less strenuous patterns of voice production and control. Hoarseness may, of course, arise from other causes, and it may be a symptom of a serious throat disorder. It is advisable, therefore, to see a doctor if such a condition persists.

CLIMACTERIC See MENOPAUSE. (Pronounced klie·mak′ter·ik.)

CLINIC An institution providing medical treatment for people who are not confined to a hospital. Clinics are maintained by public and private hospitals, some of which are affiliated with medical schools; by industrial and labor organizations; and by private groups of medical specialists. Many hospital clinics, including those connected with a medical school, offer treatment at little or no charge. (See OUTPATIENT DEPARTMENT.) Those operated by labor and industrial organizations provide services to organization members.

The term "clinic" may also refer to a large hospital facility such as the Mayo Clinic at Rochester, Minnesota, that specializes in diagnosis of disease, and the Menninger Clinic at Topeka, Kansas, that treats and does research in mental illness.

A clinic may be maintained by several doctors who are specialists and who cooperate in studying and treating a patient. This is called group practice, or group medicine. In such a clinic, regular fees are charged for the services provided. However, the total amount for examination and treatment is generally less than the total of corresponding separate fees charged by individual specialists.

CLITORIS A small structure located at the front of the VULVA. The clitoris (pronounced klit′ohr·is) contains erectile tissue that is stimulated by touch during COITUS (sexual intercourse) or MASTURBATION. It is the counterpart of the penis in the male but it is not connected with the URINARY TRACT. See also GENITALS.

CLOT A soft, jellylike mass formed from a liquid. See also BLOOD CLOT.

CLOVE, OIL OF A fragrant oil obtained from the dried buds of a tropical tree. Applied to an aching tooth, oil of clove affords temporary relief.

CLUBFOOT See TALIPES.

COAGULATION The process of changing from a liquid into a soft solid. The formation on a wound of a clot of solidified blood and the curdling of milk are two examples of coagulation (pronounced koh·ag″yu·lay′shun).

COCAINE A white, bitter drug, originally obtained from the leaves of the coca, a South American shrub, and later synthesized. Cocaine is an analgesic—that is, it relieves pain. It is used as a local ANESTHETIC especially in operations involving the mouth, nose, throat, or eyes. If a solution of cocaine in proper strength is applied to mucous membrane, it rapidly deadens all sensation in the area.

Most doctors are wary of prescribing cocaine-containing medicines. In some persons, even a small surface dose produces harmful side effects. An overdose may cause delirium, convulsions, respiratory failure, and death. BARBITURATES help to counteract the dangerous effects of cocaine and are often administered before cocaine is used. A number of synthetic derivatives of cocaine, such as procaine hydrochloride, have been developed. All of them are toxic, but some are considerably less so than pure cocaine.

Repeated use of cocaine leads to ADDICTION. In most countries, the use of cocaine is regulated by strict laws governing addictive narcotics.

COCCIDIOIDOMYCOSIS A disease caused by inhaling minute, airborne particles of a fungus that grows in the soil in certain dry regions of the southwestern United States, Mexico, and Central and South America. Coccidioidomycosis (pronounced kok·sid″ee·oy″doh·mie·koh′sis) is also known as San Joaquin Valley fever, or desert fever.

People vary greatly in susceptibility to the disease. Symptoms may be absent or so mild as to pass unnoticed. In other cases, symptoms of varying severity develop from 10 to 30 days after a person has inhaled the fungus. There may be mild or severe chills and fever, inflammation of the respiratory system, muscular aches, backache, headache, and pain under the ribs. Given bed rest, most such cases recover without further treatment. In a small proportion, however, the disease becomes progressively more severe. The fungus destroys lung tissue and produces lesions that can easily be mistaken in X-ray pictures for tuberculosis or lung cancer. Any or all of the organs besides the lungs may become involved.

Whatever the symptoms, a doctor cannot be sure whether or not coccidioidomycosis is present until he makes a series of laboratory tests of the person's blood serum and microscopic examinations of sputum and affected tissue. Once properly diagnosed, coccidioidomycosis can usually be cured by treatment with the ANTIBIOTIC amphotericin B. The treatment can be carried out safely only under carefully controlled hospital conditions.

COCCUS (plural, **cocci**) Any BACTERIUM that appears spherical or egg-shaped when examined under the microscope. A coccus (pronounced kok′us) has characteristic ways of growing that provide further clues in identifying it. The simple cocci, such as the bacteria that cause gonorrhea, tend to grow as separate, individual spheres. Others grow in pairs and short chains, like the bacteria responsible for a common form of pneumonia. Cocci that are paired in this way are called diplococci. STAPHYLOCOCCI are cocci that grow together in clumps, and STREPTOCOCCI grow in long chains. A number of diseases are caused by cocci, but not all cocci cause disease.

COCCYGODYNIA Severe pain in the area of the coccyx, the lowest bone of the spine. It may be due to injury, such as a blow or a fall, or to a disorder of the spinal nerve (see NEURALGIA). The cause must be found and treated, and in some cases surgical removal of the coccyx may be recommended. (Pronounced kok″see·goh·din′ee·a.)

COCCYX A bony structure at the lower end of the spine. It consists of four rudimentary vertebrae which fuse together as a person grows to adulthood. The coccyx (pronounced kok′siks) corresponds to the tail that many other animals possess. In man it serves to anchor the external SPHINCTER of the anus (the terminal opening of the digestive tract).

CODEINE A white, crystalline substance used to relieve pain and to control coughing. As an ANALGESIC (pain reliever), codeine (pronounced koh′deen) is usually prescribed in tablet form for pain more severe than can be treated with aspirin or a similar common analgesic. Dentists may prescribe codeine

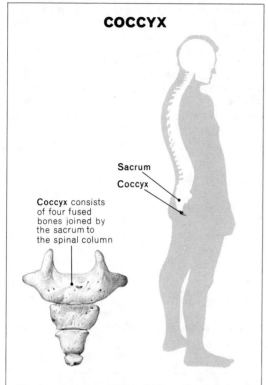

COCCYX

Sacrum
Coccyx

Coccyx consists
of four fused
bones joined by
the sacrum to
the spinal column

The four lowermost bones in the spine are fused
together to form the coccyx, or tailbone. Pain in
the coccyx, called coccygodynia, may be caused
by an injury or inflammation of a spinal nerve.

for patients who are having extensive dental work
done. Unlike aspirin, codeine is a NARCOTIC; it may
cause drowsiness and depress the central nervous
system, thus reducing REFLEX action. It is often used
in cough syrups because it lowers the cough reflex.
It also reduces PERISTALSIS (rhythmic contractions
of the intestine), and hence tends to cause CONSTI-
PATION. In some individuals, it causes nausea and
other severe symptoms. Codeine is habit-forming,
and its use can result in ADDICTION. It should therefore be used sparingly, and only under a doctor's
orders.

COD LIVER OIL A pale yellow, liquid fat with a
fishy odor and taste, obtained from the fresh liver of
cod. It is rich in VITAMINS A and D and, like all
animal fats, has a high CALORIE content. Cod liver
oil was formerly used very widely to prevent or
treat RICKETS and as a general tonic. It has been
largely replaced by purer and more concentrated
vitamin preparations.

COFFEE See CAFFEINE.

COGENTIN A trade name for a synthetic compound, benztropine mesylate. Cogentin (pro-

nounced koh·jent'in) is used in the treatment of
PARKINSONISM to relieve rigidity and tremor.

COITUS The act of sexual union, also called sexual
intercourse. Coitus (pronounced koh'i·tes) is preceded by a number of involuntary mechanisms.
Sexual stimulation results in an increased blood
supply to the sexual organs. The PENIS consists
largely of erectile tissue which becomes filled with
blood, causing the penis to become stiff and erect.
At the same time, increased mucous secretions lubricate the VAGINA and the male urethra.

Insertion of the penis into the vagina and continued stimulation is normally followed by ejaculation
of about a teaspoonful of semen, which may contain
as many as 400 million live sperm cells. Many of the
commonly used methods of contraception are devices to prevent ejaculated sperm cells from entering the Fallopian tubes and fertilizing an egg cell.
See also CONTRACEPTIVE METHODS AND DEVICES.

COLA See CAFFEINE.

COLD See COMMON COLD.

COLD COMPRESS See COMPRESS.

COLD SORE See FEVER SORE.

COLIC An attack of abdominal pain. Colic (pronounced kol'ik) is common among babies in the first
three months of life. The infant's abdomen may be
distended because of a cramp; he draws his legs up,
cries from discomfort, and releases gas.

Colic in babies is sometimes due to swallowing air
during feeding. To avoid this problem, burp the
infant occasionally to get the air out of his system.

ALLERGY may be a factor in causing colic. The
child may have a sensitivity to vitamin drops, to
cow's milk, or to some element in the formula, such
as sugar. If any of these are suspected as a cause of
the baby's colic, your doctor can recommend a
substitute.

Adult Colic: Older persons are subject to quite different types of colic than babies. As the word itself
suggests, colic is often related to some disorder in
the COLON. It may be due to constipation, appendicitis, or colitis. RENAL colic is produced by stones in
the ureter or kidney. There may be acute pain in
the loins and legs. The person urinates frequently,
and the urine may be an abnormal color. In *biliary*
colic, the cause may be inflammation of the gallbladder or a GALLSTONE in the bile duct. The chief
symptom is acute, intense pain in the upper abdomen. In women, colic may be associated with MEN-
STRUATION or with some disorder in the ovaries,
uterus, or Fallopian tubes.

Finally, pain in the face caused by a CALCULUS, or
stone, in the salivary gland is called salivary colic.
This condition has nothing to do with the abdomen.

COLITIS Inflammation of the COLON. (Pronounced ko·lie′tis.)

Mucous colitis, or SPASTIC colon, is a relatively mild ailment in which there is little or no inflammation. The condition results from spasms of the muscles in the colon wall, which interfere with the normal wavelike motion of PERISTALSIS. The symptoms (cramps and constipation with copious passage of mucus rather than normal feces) are usually associated with nervousness and worry. The condition can generally be relieved by dealing with the cause of the emotional tension—with psychiatric help (PSYCHOTHERAPY), if it is necessary.

Ulcerative colitis is a potentially serious disease whose cause is not known. It usually begins at the end of the colon near the rectum (the terminal part of the large intestine) and may extend upward. Marked redness and ULCERS (open sores) develop in the affected area, and blood is often present in the feces. There may be severe diarrhea, with as many as 15 to 20 watery bowel movements a day. In most cases, ulcerative colitis is a chronic condition interrupted by remissions (temporary improvement or disappearance of symptoms). Emotional tension is often very great, but it is not clear whether this is a contributing cause or an effect of the pain and disability that go with the disease. Psychiatric help is sometimes of value.

Treatment usually consists of BED REST and a BLAND DIET without fruits or vegetables but with plenty of vitamins and essential minerals. CORTISONE is often administered either in pills or enemas. In extreme cases, the affected part of the colon may be relieved and given a chance to heal by a surgical procedure (COLOSTOMY) in which a temporary artificial anus is made in the abdominal wall.

COLLAPSED LUNG See PNEUMOTHORAX.

COLON The lower part of the digestive tract, consisting in adults of a tube about $4\frac{1}{2}$ feet long, and about 2 inches wide when distended by material passing through it. Watery waste material enters the colon (pronounced koh′lon) from the small intestine, loses water in its passage toward the rectum, and is discharged in semisolid form from the anus. The colon is coiled in a single large loop beginning at the lower right side of the abdomen, passing upward and crossing under the liver and stomach to the left side, and then leading downward to the rectum. The colon wall contains a muscular layer and is lined with mucous tissue. The muscles in the colon wall contract in successive waves (PERISTALSIS), forcing the contents to move along toward the rectum.

For disorders affecting the colon, see COLITIS and CONSTIPATION.

COLOR BLINDNESS An eye condition that makes it impossible to distinguish one color from another. Inability to tell red from green is the commonest type. This red-green confusion affects many more men than women. Complete inability to distinguish among colors, or total color blindness, is extremely rare. Red-green blindness is also known as Daltonism, after John Dalton (1766–1844), the English scientist, who had the condition himself and studied it.

Causes: Color blindness is a deficiency, not a disease. In a limited number of cases, it is a result of alcoholic poisoning, infection, or a disorder of the optic nerve; but in an overwhelming number of instances, it is an inherited trait, and nothing can be done to correct it. Both eyes are commonly involved. In normal vision, the cones of the retina respond to various wavelengths of light and identify them as colors; in color-blind persons, certain of these cones may be missing or defective. (See EYE for location of optic nerve, retina, and cones.)

Usually, color blindness is inherited from the mother. She is not color-blind herself, but her father was. Most color-deficient persons are unaware of their problem until it is discovered in a test. Those who cannot discriminate between green and red see these two colors as shades of gray or yellow. In a typical test, mosaic patterns of colored dots are shown in which there is a symbol, such as a number

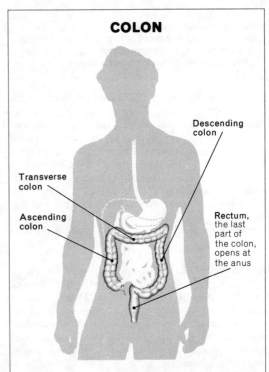

COLON

Descending colon

Transverse colon

Ascending colon

Rectum, the last part of the colon, opens at the anus

The 4½-foot-long tube of the large intestine is made up of the colon and the rectum. In it, water is absorbed from food residues, leaving the undigested material as feces.

or a letter, that is partly concealed. The color-deficient person is unable to see this symbol.

COLOSTOMY The establishment by surgical means of an artificial opening in the wall of the abdomen through which waste matter is discharged directly from the colon instead of passing out through the rectum and anus. A colostomy (pronounced ko·los′to·mee) is performed when part of the colon or the rectum is removed because of CANCER, or when it seems advisable to bypass the lower colon in order to relieve a condition such as ulcerative COLITIS.

COLOSTRUM See LACTATION; BREAST FEEDING. (Pronounced ko·los′trum.)

COMA A state of unconsciousness from which it is impossible to awaken a person. Coma may be produced by disease, poison, alcoholism, drugs, or injury. The brain stops operating in its normal way, and the individual no longer reacts intelligently to stimuli. A coma differs from a fainting spell in that it is much deeper and lasts longer. It is also much more serious, and it requires medical treatment as quickly as possible. See also UNCONSCIOUSNESS.

COMBAT FATIGUE See FATIGUE.

COMMON COLD An infectious disease of the RESPIRATORY SYSTEM, particularly its upper portion. A large number of VIRUSES are known to cause colds, and new cold-causing viruses continue to be found.
Symptoms: The common cold is the most widespread of the contagious diseases. Its symptoms usually appear 18 to 48 hours after infection. They include a stuffy or runny nose, moderate headache, and cough. There may be a feeling of chilliness, the sensations of smell and taste may become less acute, and the person may run a slight fever. He may also suffer from malaise—a general feeling of listlessness and discomfort. As the disorder develops, there may be a sore throat, varying from mild to severe. The typical cold may produce only some or all of these symptoms. It may last from a few days to a few weeks.

The average cold rarely calls for a physician's attention—unless complications arise. However, for certain individuals, even the common cold may pose a dangerous problem. These include the small infant, and persons with asthma, a heart disease, kidney disease, tuberculosis, or chronic bronchitis.
Treatment: When you feel a cold coming on, go to bed. If you can't, then get as much rest as possible. Take two aspirins every four hours if there is a fever, headache, or sore throat. A light diet and plenty of fluids are recommended in case of fever. If there is a bad cough, the doctor may prescribe a cough medicine containing codeine. Steam inhalations from a VAPORIZER may also bring relief, especially for a child. A DECONGESTANT can temporarily relieve a stuffy nose; and an allergic individual may take ANTIHISTAMINES.

There are numerous remedies on the market, all of them heavily advertised, which provide slight or illusory relief for the symptoms of the common cold. Cold laxatives, germicides, gargles, and lozenges promise much, but viruses are utterly indifferent to them. Rubbing oil of wintergreen or other preparations into the skin may distract your attention briefly from your cold, but will not cure it or shorten it. Painting a sore throat with a distasteful solution is equally ineffective, as are antibiotics.
Prevention: What can you do to avoid colds? You can keep away from people who have colds, or persuade them to cover their sneezes. The viruses travel in infective droplets, which can be propelled several feet by a single sneeze. Maintain a good diet and avoid excessive fatigue. Cold weather and getting chilled may set the stage for a cold, although they do not by themselves cause it; only a virus can.

There is no proof that colds may be prevented by drinking orange juice or taking large doses of vitamin C; however, these precautions may help to improve your general physical condition. Even vaccines are of limited usefulness against the constantly multiplying virus population.

COMMUNICABLE DISEASE A disease that is transmitted from one person to another, or from an animal to a person; an INFECTION. A communicable disease may or may not be CONTAGIOUS. It may be communicated by touching objects that an infected individual has handled, or by direct or indirect contact with him. Communicable diseases are sometimes transmitted by carriers—individuals who exhibit no signs of the disease but are carrying the organisms that produce it.

Communicable diseases are often described as caused by GERMS, although parasitic worms are sometimes responsible, as in the case of PINWORM INFECTION. What exactly are germs? They are potentially disease-causing microorganisms—organisms so small that they are visible only when viewed under a microscope.

There are a number of types of microorganisms that produce communicable disease. Of these, BACTERIA, first observed under a microscope in the 17th century, are probably the most familiar. Among the communicable diseases caused by bacteria are diphtheria, pneumonia, and gonorrhea. VIRUSES, another type of microorganism, produce a vast number of diseases, including measles, chicken pox, smallpox, influenza, poliomyelitis, and the common cold. Many of the diseases produced by viruses and bacteria are transmitted by coughs or sneezes which fill the air around the infected person with the germs. Other disease-producing organisms include types of FUNGUS, PROTOZOA, and the already mentioned parasitic worms.

Preventing Infection: IMMUNIZATION helps in avoiding communicable disease. Every child should receive inoculations against such diseases as whooping cough and measles. Tetanus, poliomyelitis, diphtheria, and smallpox are other diseases against which everyone should be immunized. Periodic booster shots ought to be obtained as required.

When someone in the household has a communicable disease, his dishes and cutlery should be kept apart from the rest and immersed in boiling water after meals. All wastes should be disposed of promptly. Persons nursing the sick individual should wash their hands thoroughly after each contact with him.

COMPAZINE A trade name for prochlorperazine. Compazine (pronounced kom′pa·zeen″) is prescribed to calm agitation in some types of mental illness. It is also sometimes used as a sedative for patients before and after surgery, and to help control nausea and vomiting. It may cause drowsiness and a slowing down of reaction time. Anyone taking Compazine should obtain his doctor's permission to drive a car or to do anything where safety depends upon mental alertness.

COMPLEMENT-FIXATION TEST See BLOOD TEST.

COMPLEX A group of ideas or feelings with significant emotional meaning to an individual. These ideas and feelings stem from the experience of the individual and have a strong influence on his personality. The term is used in PSYCHIATRY in such expressions as inferiority complex and Oedipus complex.

Inferiority Complex: Alfred Adler (1870–1937), an Austrian psychiatrist, held that a feeling of inferiority is at the root of all personality disorders. This feeling may be a reaction to a physical handicap, real or imagined, or to a conflict with society that prevents the individual from fulfilling his desires. As a result of his inferiority complex, the individual attempts to overcompensate for his failings. The undersized person who develops aggressive, domineering traits is a familiar type. Napoleon is a well-known example; the Napoleonic complex, a type of inferiority complex, has been named for him. Feelings of inferiority may lead to a PSYCHONEUROSIS or to constructive, socially valuable activity, as in the case of the puny youngster who builds himself into an extraordinarily vigorous, masculine adult—Theodore Roosevelt was an excellent example.

Oedipus Complex: Sigmund Freud (1856–1939), the founder of PSYCHOANALYSIS, introduced this term to describe what he regarded as a stage in the development of every young boy: deep love for his mother and hatred for his father. Oedipus, according to Greek mythology, was a man who unwittingly killed his father and married his mother. In a girl

there may be hatred for the mother and love for the father; this female Oedipus complex is sometimes known as an Electra complex. Freud held that people normally outgrew the Oedipus complex early in adolescence, and he sought to explain various psychiatric problems in adults as a failure to develop beyond the Oedipal stage. It is perfectly normal for a child to favor one parent over the other; but in some persons, the favoritism exists in an exaggerated, neurotic form, requiring treatment by PSYCHOTHERAPY.

The theories of Freud, Adler, and other early psychoanalysts have enjoyed an immense popular vogue, and the word "complex" is often used loosely by amateur psychologists to account for all kinds of puzzling behavior. Applying such a label, of course, explains nothing and helps nobody.

COMPRESS A pad of folded gauze or cloth for applying moisture, heat, cold, or pressure to a part of the body. A compress is usually, but not always, applied moist.

The value of a compress lies mostly in its soothing effect. A cold compress may relieve a headache or a toothache. Warm compresses are used to relieve pain in sore muscles, and also in treating surface infections, such as a BOIL or a STY. A dry compress applied with pressure is one of the most effective first aid methods of checking the flow of blood from a wound. See also FIRST AID section.

CONCEPTION The beginning of a new individual. Authorities differ in their use of the term. Some hold that conception occurs at the moment when the male sperm cell fertilizes the ovum, or egg cell. Others consider conception to take place later, when the fertilized egg, or ZYGOTE, becomes implanted in the wall of the uterus. (See also PREGNANCY entry.)

CONCUSSION Injury to the brain by severe mechanical jarring or shaking, which may or may not involve a fracture of the skull. A person who has suffered a concussion from a fall or a blow on the head may experience dizziness, impaired vision, and severe headache. If the concussion is very severe, there may be irregular breathing and total loss of consciousness.

The victim of an accident in which there is any likelihood of brain or spinal injury should be kept lying down until medical help arrives. Cover the victim with a coat or blanket to prevent him from becoming chilled, even if the weather is warm. Do not give stimulants of any kind or attempt to clean or bandage any bloody bruises he may have. If breathing begins to fail, give ARTIFICIAL RESPIRATION. (See FIRST AID section.) These precautions are necessary to protect the accident victim from further injury in case of skull fracture or damage to the backbone.

In cases of a simple concussion alone, the injured person's symptoms will gradually decrease until, within a few days or a few weeks, his recovery is complete.

CONDITIONED REFLEX See REFLEX.

CONDOM A sheath that is fitted over the penis before sexual intercourse. The condom (pronounced kon′dom) serves two purposes. As a PROPHYLACTIC, it affords considerable protection against infection if the partner has a venereal disease. It is also a contraceptive device, preventing sperm-bearing semen from entering the vagina and causing pregnancy. Condoms are commonly made of a thin film of rubber. The condom should be fitted in such a way that a loose space remains at the tip to hold ejaculated semen. Many other CONTRACEPTIVE METHODS AND DEVICES are available.

CONGENITAL Existing at birth. Any condition, good or bad, that is present at the moment of birth is a congenital (pronounced kon·jen′i·tal) condition, no matter what caused it. For example, if a healthy fetus becomes infected at the moment of birth by venereal-disease organisms in the birth canal of the mother, the infection is a congenital infection. A congenital defect may also be inherited; MONGOLISM, for instance, results from an abnormality, present before conception, in the GENETIC makeup of the ovum (egg cell) or sperm from which the baby develops.

Other congenital defects arise from the presence of various abnormal substances in the mother's blood during the early stages of fetal development in the uterus, when the heart and other organs are being formed. For example, a number of pregnant women who had taken the sedative thalidomide gave birth to deformed babies in the late 1950's. If the mother becomes infected with RUBELLA (German measles) at this time, congenital defects are very likely to result. See also BIRTH DEFECT; CONGENITAL HEART DISEASE; RH FACTOR.

CONGENITAL DEFECT See BIRTH DEFECT.

CONGENITAL HEART DISEASE Impaired circulation and heart trouble due to any of a number of possible defects in the heart at birth. One such defect is an open connection between the pulmonary artery (the artery leading to the lungs) and the aorta (the artery leading to the rest of the body). This open connection is always present in the newborn, but normally it closes off soon after birth. If it does not close, some of the blood that should go to the lungs is pumped back into the body without carrying its normal load of oxygen. As a result, the heart has to work harder to supply the oxygen needs of the body, and it is gradually damaged or enlarged by overwork. Other defects include abnormal openings in the walls that divide the four chambers of the heart, narrowness in the aorta or the pulmonary artery, and a variety of misplaced connections between the heart and the large blood vessels.

One cause of congenital heart disease in infants is RUBELLA (German measles) contracted by the mother during early pregnancy. The infant may have no heart symptoms if the defect is a minor one, or symptoms may only develop later in life as a result of prolonged overwork by the heart. In some cases, other and more obvious defects may also be present at birth, putting the doctor on the alert to watch for symptoms of heart disease. In severe cases, the condition known as BLUE BABY may be present at birth or develop shortly afterward. A highly skilled surgeon using modern surgical techniques can alleviate most congenital heart defects.

CONGESTION An accumulation of blood in the blood vessels of a tissue or an organ. Anything that interferes with the return flow of blood through the veins will cause congestion. Thus, a tight bandage around the arm will constrict the veins and produce congestion in the hand. Most commonly, however, congestion begins as a defense against local infections or to repair injured tissue. The tiny blood vessels in the affected tissue become enlarged and swollen with blood. When this happens in the mucous membranes of the nose and the sinuses, the resulting nasal congestion can be uncomfortable and interfere with breathing.

Nasal congestion is a symptom of the common cold, and may also be caused by chronic infections, allergies, nasal POLYPS, or infected adenoids. For the treatment of nasal congestion with nose drops and other medicines, see DECONGESTANT.

CONGESTIVE HEART FAILURE A condition in which the heart is not strong enough to keep blood circulating in sufficient quantity to supply the body's needs. The lungs and other vital organs become congested, due to the accumulation of blood. See also HEART FAILURE.

CONJUNCTIVITIS Inflammation of the conjunctiva, the mucous membrane covering the eyeball and the inner part of the eyelids. Conjunctivitis (pronounced kon·jungk″ti·vie′·tis) is often associated with the common cold, with hay fever, and with chemical irritation from severe air pollution. It may also be a symptom of TRACHOMA.

A fairly common eye infection is caused by bacteria. The eyes become pink from inflammation; hence the condition is also called pinkeye. It is very contagious and is commonly transmitted by fingers or towels carrying the bacteria to the eye. There may be a pus-containing discharge, and the eyelids swell and tend to stick together. Pinkeye is a bothersome but minor disease that can usually be cured by simple home treatment. The eyes should be kept free of discharge by washing them with clean, warm water, using a disposable tissue or cloth. Apply warm, moist compresses for five minutes three or four times a day. Morning and night, apply yellow oxide of mercury ophthalmic ointment on the inner lid and spread it over the eyeball by rolling the eye. If improvement is not rapid, see your doctor. He may prescribe ANTIBIOTIC or SULFONAMIDE (sulfa compound) eye drops to heal the infection.

CONNECTIVE TISSUE See TISSUE.

CONSTIPATION Difficulty in emptying the bowel. Usually the waste material has become compact and hard, making it painful to evacuate. Improper diet, nervous tension, bad toilet habits, insufficient exercise, and overuse of laxatives may contribute to the condition. It is rarely serious unless it is the result of organic disease.

After food has been digested, the waste is passed along the COLON by the action of the intestinal muscles (PERISTALSIS; see also DIGESTIVE SYSTEM). It is in the form of a thickish liquid. Water is absorbed from the waste through the wall of the colon. For various reasons, the colon muscles may become temporarily inactive and not pass the waste out of the body promptly. There may be associated discomfort in the lower intestinal tract, as well as a headache.

How often you should have a bowel movement depends on your habits and physical makeup. One movement every 24 hours is average. However, there are plenty of individuals who have a movement every 36 or 48 hours, or at even greater intervals, and do not suffer from constipation. If you have no discomfort, there is nothing to worry about. Nor is there any cause to worry about occasional minor irregularity or discomfort.

How to Avoid Constipation: If you suffer from constipation frequently, a simple program may help you to overcome it. First, examine your diet carefully. Does it include enough roughage, such as leafy green vegetables, fruit, and whole-grain cereals and bread? Add dates, raisins, figs, and prunes to your diet. Fluids and lubricants are essential; drink ample quantities of water, milk, fruit juice, and soups, and use salad dressings, oils, and butter with your food.

Nervous tension may contribute to constipation. If you are tense or constantly worried, discuss your problem with your physician. Talking it out helps; besides, he has other aids at his disposal. Poor muscular tone, especially of the abdominal muscles, should be considered as a possible cause of a sluggish colon. Try to get more exercise.

If constipation recurs, try an ENEMA preparation, which is available at a drugstore. Alternatively, but only if absolutely necessary, take a LAXATIVE, such as milk of magnesia or mineral oil; use a CATHARTIC

only as a last resort and preferably after checking with your doctor. Stop relying on these as soon as possible. It is necessary to train the colon to function regularly, and an enema or laxative does not promote this.

CONSUMPTION See TUBERCULOSIS.

CONTACT LENS A tiny lens of hard or soft plastic fitted directly over the CORNEA. Contact lenses are often worn in place of EYEGLASSES for cosmetic or occupational reasons. Hard lenses are less costly, easier to care for, and last almost indefinitely (provided your prescription does not change). But they may cause eye irritation. Soft lenses, on the other hand, are easier to get used to, but are susceptible to breaking and tearing. They are hard to keep clean and need replacing at least once every three years. In a person who has had a CATARACT removed, a contact lens replaces the diseased lens that has been taken out, and may give the wearer better vision than thick eyeglasses.

Drawbacks: Care must be taken in inserting and removing contact lenses, which is not the case with standard eyeglasses. Moreover, contact lenses are easily mislaid or lost—sometimes they fall out of the eyes and may be extremely difficult to find because of their tiny size.

Advantages: On the other hand, contact lenses have very distinct advantages. They are virtually invisible when worn, which makes them especially appealing to persons who feel that ordinary eyeglasses detract from their appearance. In occupations where eyeglasses are cumbersome, contact lenses may prove a boon—for example, athletes often wear them. For certain eye conditions they may be particularly advantageous. Consult with your OPHTHALMOLOGIST or OPTOMETRIST.

Care: The use of contact lenses calls for special care. The hands should be washed thoroughly before the lenses are inserted. Soft lenses must be cleaned with an antiseptic solution before you put them over the corneas, and after they are removed. If there is any pain, discoloration of the eye, or other problem, see an ophthalmologist or optometrist.

CONTAGIOUS Spread from person to person by direct contact or by contact with objects that have been touched by an infected person. "Contagious" and "infectious" are often used to mean the same thing, but this is not strictly correct. All contagious diseases are infectious (that is, due to infection by a microscopic organism), but not all infectious diseases are contagious. Malaria, for example, is an infectious disease that is transmitted by a mosquito. Malaria is not contagious—it cannot be caught by contact with someone who has malaria.

CONTRACEPTION See CONTRACEPTIVE METHODS AND DEVICES; FAMILY PLANNING.

CONTRACEPTIVE METHODS AND DEVICES
Techniques and contrivances used to prevent conception, or pregnancy, and an effective means of birth control and FAMILY PLANNING.

An extensive variety of contraceptive devices and techniques are available today, and new ones are under study. Before deciding on any particular type, it is wise to discuss the subject with your physician.

The Rhythm Method: One technique, known as the rhythm method, relies solely on a woman's natural OVULATION cycle. It achieves its objective by restricting intercourse to a "safe period" before and after ovulation. This method is sanctioned by the Roman Catholic Church. See also separate entry, RHYTHM METHOD.

The "Pill": Regarded as highly reliable, the "pill," an oral contraceptive, is available only with a physician's prescription. The "pill" contains sex hormones that prevent ovulation. Like any medicine containing hormones, it changes the body's metabolism. Most women experience minor or temporary side effects, such as nausea, cramps, or facial discoloration. The "pill" involves serious risks for women who have diabetes, or who have had blood clots, cancer, or disorders of the liver. See also separate entry, ORAL CONTRACEPTION.

The Vaginal Diaphragm: This is a dome-shaped rubber device inserted in the VAGINA before coitus. It is used with a spermicidal (sperm-killing) cream or jelly. The diaphragm is fitted by a physician and should be checked periodically. The woman inserts the device before intercourse and does not remove it until at least six hours afterward. For further information, see DIAPHRAGM (*birth control*).

The Condom: If used correctly, this is a highly reliable device. A thin rubber sheath, it is worn on the PENIS. See also CONDOM.

Sterilization: This is the most reliable of all methods. It should be seriously considered by couples who, for any reason, wish to have permanent insurance against the risk of pregnancy. It involves a surgical operation in which either the vas deferens (in men) or the oviducts (in women) are tied or severed. Sterilization does not interfere in any way with the production of sex hormones in the testes or the ovaries. In other words, it does not affect normal sexual activity. See also separate entry, VASECTOMY.

Other Devices: Spermicidal foams, gels, creams, jellies, suppositories, and tablets are available at drugstores. These are of varying effectiveness, and it is best to consult your doctor before placing reliance on any particular type. A vaginal DOUCHE following intercourse is a popular method with some, but it is not effective, and repeated use of certain preparations may injure the delicate membranes of the genital passage. A new device, the plastic loop, has been tried and found effective in many countries. See also INTRAUTERINE DEVICE.

Local Planned Parenthood associations maintain birth control clinics throughout the United States. Their staffs include doctors who are well informed about contraceptive devices. If your local telephone directory contains no Planned Parenthood listing, more information may be obtained from Planned Parenthood Federation of America, 810 Seventh Avenue, New York, New York 10019.

CONTRACTION See MUSCULAR CONTRACTION; CHILDBIRTH.

CONTUSION See BRUISE. (Pronounced kon·too' zhun.)

CONVALESCENCE The period during which a person gradually returns to health following an illness. People who have been gravely ill, or who cannot obtain adequate care at home, may pass the period of convalescence in a nursing home. For most, however, it is much more cheerful (not to mention economical) to convalesce at home. If there is no one in the home to take care of the sick person, it may be possible to obtain the assistance of a trained nurse from the local Visiting Nurse Service.

The Patient's Schedule: It is wise to discuss the problems of home care with your doctor and work out a schedule with him. Find out when the patient should be given his medicine, whether his temperature should be taken, and if so, when (generally it is in the morning and at night).

Keeping the Patient's Spirits Up: Bear in mind that the convalescent needs emotional as well as physical care. An elderly person who has been ill a long time can easily become despondent. Almost any patient appreciates being reminded that his condition is improving and that he looks better, especially when recovery seems to be lagging. Cheerful decorations and a bright rug or pictures in the sickroom are helpful. There should be a table close by the bed with plenty of room for the patient's medicine and water, and perhaps a bell so that he can let you know when he has special needs. A radio or a television set within easy reach can help shorten long hours; so, also, can a good supply of magazines, newspapers, and books.

Comfort in Bed: Staying in bed a long time can be wearying to the body as well as to the spirit. Encourage the patient to change his position periodically, and help him if necessary. Provide one or two large pillows and perhaps a small one or two, arranged in varying ways, to make him more comfortable. Bed linen and clothing should be changed frequently. (See also BED REST.)

See that the room is adequately ventilated. Opening windows on opposite walls a little at the top will provide cross ventilation without exposing the patient to a draft. Try to maintain a temperature of 72° to 74° F by day and lower it a few degrees at night. Do not let the room get too cold, but always consider the patient's comfort.

A patient should be encouraged to pay attention

to his appearance. Looking better often makes a convalescing person feel better. A man should shave, if possible, and a woman should be allowed to comb her hair and use cosmetics.

Some convalescences are short, others must be long. Your physician can tell you regularly about the patient's condition and when he should be ready to resume normal activities.

CONVERSION HYSTERIA A form of PSYCHO-NEUROSIS which results when an individual with a severe emotional conflict unconsciously converts it into a physical symptom, such as blindness, deafness, or paralysis. Treatment is by PSYCHOTHERAPY.

CONVULSION Powerful involuntary contractions of the muscles, producing contortions of the body or of a part of it, such as an arm or a leg. A convulsion, or seizure, may be caused by many factors: interruption of the flow of blood to the brain; brain tumors; excessive use of alcohol; drugs; an overdose of insulin in a diabetic (see DIABETES); injury to the brain; EPILEPSY; or an inflammation of the brain resulting from a disease such as ENCEPHALITIS or MENINGITIS. In an older person, convulsions may be associated with HARDENING OF THE ARTERIES of the brain.
Children: Convulsions may occur in young children who have fever or one of the childhood diseases, or they may be brought on by the violent coughing found in WHOOPING COUGH. In a small child, they may be produced by holding the breath. An unexplained convulsion or a wave of convulsions requires prompt medical attention.
What to Do: Although many convulsions end by themselves, a doctor should be called immediately.

It is essential to keep the individual from hurting himself during the seizure. There is a chance that he may bite his tongue or his lips, so place a rolled handkerchief or a hard object that is too large to swallow between his jaws. Lay him flat on his back and turn the head to one side. Loosen his collar and his belt. Don't give him alcohol to drink or throw water in his face. If the individual is a stranger, see whether he has a card identifying him as an epileptic or a diabetic. (See also FIRST AID section.) Do not be unnerved by his contortions; they look much worse than they are, and come to an end within a few minutes.

CORN A painful thickening of the skin on or between the toes. A corn is almost always the result of pressure or friction by badly fitting shoes. Even well-fitting shoes may press and rub against the feet and can cause thickening of the skin on the toes.
Treatment: First, try soaking the foot in hot water and then scraping the thickened skin away. A corn pad may relieve the pressure. Commercial corn-removing preparations should be used with great care to prevent injuring the tissue surrounding a

corn; they contain salicylic acid or stronger chemicals that can injure the skin. If corns are very troublesome and do not yield to simple care, it is advisable to consult a PODIATRIST (specialist in treatment of the feet).

CORNEA See EYE.

CORONARY From the word *corona*, meaning "crown." Blood is supplied to the heart muscle by branching ARTERIES that encircle it like a crown. The term "coronary" (pronounced kawr′*o*·ner″ee) usually refers to these heart arteries.

CORONARY HEART DISEASE Narrowing or blockage of the coronary arteries that supply blood to the HEART muscle. As a result, the muscle receives insufficient blood to meet the demands made on it. This is the commonest type of heart disease. It affects about four times as many men as women, and is most prevalent after the age of 50.

Coronary heart disease is most often due to CORONARY SCLEROSIS, in which deposits on the coronary artery walls slow down the flow of blood. One type of coronary heart disease, coronary thrombosis, occurs when a blood clot forms in the narrowed, roughened artery and obstructs the blood supply. The term coronary occlusion simply means obstruction in or blockage of coronary arteries.

It is not known exactly what produces the degeneration of the heart blood vessels that precedes coronary heart disease. A number of factors are involved. People with coronary heart disease often have a high level of CHOLESTEROL in their blood. High blood pressure (see HYPERTENSION), DIABETES, and OBESITY increase one's susceptibility to coronary heart disease. Another factor is heredity. In families that tend to have coronary heart disease, there is usually a tendency also to have large quantities of cholesterol in the blood, diabetes, or high blood pressure.

Infrequently, coronary heart disease occurs without coronary sclerosis. Other possible causes include CONGENITAL HEART DISEASE, RHEUMATIC FEVER, an EMBOLISM, and SYPHILIS.
Symptoms: Coronary heart disease does not necessarily produce any symptoms whatever. When symptoms do occur, they are symptoms of heart disease in general. (See HEART DISEASE—SYMPTOMS.) These include shortness of breath as a result of some effort, such as walking up the stairs; pain in the chest or neck, or over the heart (ANGINA PECTORIS), which may be acute or simply a feeling of constriction; PALPITATIONS and heart pounding.
Treatment: A person having a heart attack must lie down at once. Try to make him comfortable while you send someone to call the doctor. Keep everyone out of the room so that the victim is not disturbed. If the attack is a severe one, the person *must* be taken to a hospital.

Prevention: The outlook for the victim of a heart attack is more promising today than ever before. But certain precautions must be taken to avoid recurrence—precautions that are just as valid for the person who wishes to avoid coronary disease. Weight control is essential. Avoid excessive sugar and fatty foods. Get some exercise regularly, adjusted to your age and condition. Smoking is a hazard—cigarettes may seem relaxing, but they can lead to disaster, since they produce constriction of the blood vessels. Regular medical checkups should also be part of any health program.

CORONARY OCCLUSION See CORONARY HEART DISEASE. (Pronounced kawr′o·ner″ee o·kloo′zhun.)

CORONARY SCLEROSIS A local accumulation of fatty and fibrous tissue inside the arteries that supply blood to the heart muscle. This accumulation obstructs the circulation of blood to the heart. In severe cases, parts of the heart muscle itself may be damaged and replaced with scar tissue. Coronary sclerosis (pronounced kawr′o·ner″ee skli·roh′sis) is the commonest underlying cause of heart attacks and heart failure. On the other hand, some degree of arteriosclerosis, or HARDENING OF THE ARTERIES, is common in most people as they grow older, and it may not produce any symptoms.

CORONARY THROMBOSIS See CORONARY HEART DISEASE; THROMBOSIS. (Pronounced kawr′o·ner″ee throm·boh′sis.)

CORPUSCLE See BLOOD CORPUSCLE.

CORTEX (plural, **cortices**) The outer layer of an organ, especially if it is markedly different from the underlying tissue. For example, the CEREBRUM and CEREBELLUM of the brain have a cortex of gray matter covering a mass of nerve fibers.

CORTISONE One of the numerous HORMONES produced in the cortex (outer layer) of the ADRENAL GLANDS. Cortisone influences the utilization of carbohydrates (sugars and starches) and the maintenance of the body's connective tissue. The adrenal glands are stimulated to produce cortisone by another hormone, ACTH, which is made by the PITUITARY GLAND.

Cortisone for medical use is either manufactured synthetically or obtained from animals. It is used to treat ADDISON'S DISEASE, in which the patient's adrenal glands are underactive. Cortisone and a closely related hormone, hydrocortisone, have also been found effective in relieving a number of conditions that are not associated with a lack of natural cortisone. These diseases include arthritis, rheumatic fever, certain allergic conditions, and some skin ailments.

Cortisone is usually prescribed only if other treatment is ineffective. A number of side effects often occur, including mental disorder, retention of water and swelling of tissues, restlessness, insomnia, and increased growth of hair on the body.

CORYZA The medical term (pronounced ko·rie′za) for inflammation of the upper respiratory tract combined with discharge of a large volume of mucus in the nasal passages. This combination of symptoms appears in hay fever (allergic coryza) and a common cold in the head (acute coryza).

COSMETIC SURGERY Surgery undertaken to improve the appearance. It differs only in purpose from PLASTIC SURGERY. The major purpose of plastic surgery is to overcome a serious handicap through the restoration or repair of damaged, deformed, or missing parts of the body; in contrast, cosmetic surgery aims to correct healthy features that are displeasing to their owner.

Cosmetic surgery may be no more complicated than the removal of a mole or a group of moles. Fine wrinkles or the scars of acne may be removed by planing with an electric brush; this work is usually handled by a DERMATOLOGIST (skin specialist).

More pronounced wrinkles and sagging skin of the face and chain require a face-lifting by the plastic surgeon. Incisions are made at the ears or another border area of the face. Some tissue is removed, the skin is pulled tight across the underlying structure of the face, and SUTURES (stitches) are made. The results of a face-lifting operation do not last more than seven or eight years, so that persons such as actresses, to whom a youthful appearance is important, may have a series of them.

Cosmetic surgery may be used to correct a displeasing feature—to make a nose prettier or ears less prominent. However, it should be borne in mind that improving the features may not make an individual significantly more attractive; attractiveness is often a matter of personality rather than of appearance. Occasionally, PSYCHOTHERAPY may accomplish more for a person dissatisfied with himself.

COUGH A forceful, noisy expulsion of breath. A cough is an attempt to clear the air passages of anything that causes irritation, such as mucus. One cause of irritation is BRONCHITIS (inflammation of the bronchi); heavy smoking is another. Coughing is a symptom of many different conditions, from the common cold to serious diseases like whooping cough, emphysema, tuberculosis, and lung cancer. If a cough persists for more than a few weeks, or if bloody sputum is coughed up, consult a doctor. A cough in infants should have medical attention without delay.

Coughing may be relieved, but not cured, by a COUGH MEDICINE. Those that are sold without a prescription are seldom very effective. Most of the cough medicines that effectively suppress coughing can be habit-forming, and should be taken only according to your doctor's directions.

COUGH MEDICINE The COUGH, like the headache, is one of the commonest of ailments. Just because it is so common, there are scores of syrups and PALLIATIVES available that are represented as offering relief from cough due to the common cold. So, too, are cough drops in all their vast variety of flavors, pleasant and unpleasant alike. They may momentarily relieve a tickle in the throat, but they will not cure a cough, much less the underlying condition.

Cough medicines, in medical language, are known as antitussives, or cough suppressants. In the past, almost all antitussives contained NARCOTICS, CODEINE being the most widely used. Many cough medicines now contain a substance called dextromorphan instead. Dextromorphan is not a narcotic, but has an antitussive action much like codeine. These medications act on the cough center of the brain to suppress or reduce coughing. To obtain cough medicine containing a narcotic, a physician's prescription may be required.

It should be remembered that the cough serves a useful purpose. It is a reflex mechanism which helps to clear the respiratory tract when it is invaded by dust, mucus, or other substances that irritate it. For this reason, it is not wise to take a medicine that completely suppresses coughing. If you have a hacking or otherwise annoying cough, your physician will prescribe a mild medicine to bring it under control. ANTIHISTAMINES may also be prescribed to dry up the secretions.

A few simple measures often help to reduce coughing. If the nose membranes are congested, a VAPORIZER or even a steaming kettle may bring relief. A cup of hot milk or cocoa may also be helpful.

COUGH SUPPRESSANT See COUGH MEDICINE.

COUNTERIRRITANT A substance that produces a mild inflammation when applied to the skin. Counterirritants such as menthol, methyl salicylate (oil of wintergreen), and CHLOROFORM are used in liniments to produce a soothing sensation of warmth when rubbed on the skin over sore muscles or joints, or over areas of the chest and throat congested as a result of a common cold.

COWPOX See SMALLPOX.

CRAMPS A popular (nonmedical) term for painful MENSTRUATION or any sharp pain in the abdomen. For a discussion of the type of involuntary muscular contraction known as a cramp, see SPASM.

The basic cause of menstrual pain is not known. It very often occurs for only a short time at the onset of menstruation and can usually be relieved by taking aspirin. If severe pain occurs at every menstrual period, a doctor should be consulted.

Acute pain in the abdomen may be also due to some temporary disorder of the digestive tract, and is often vaguely referred to as upset stomach, although it is the intestine and not the stomach that is affected. Cramps can sometimes be traced to poor eating habits, such as rushing through meals, or to eating hard-to-digest foods (causing GAS) and highly spiced foods that irritate the food canal. Simply eating and drinking too much may cause cramps; or the pain may be due to a nervous habit (usually unconscious) of swallowing air, which distends the stomach and intestines. Mucous COLITIS, a condition that often results from nervous tension, is another possible cause of abdominal pain. However, acute pain in the abdomen can be due to a great variety of disorders, some of them serious, such as appendicitis, gallstones, and gastric or duodenal ULCER. In some cases, pain in the abdomen may be referred pain, caused by some disorder outside the abdomen, such as a heart condition.

For the mild, chronic cases, self-treatment should begin with good, commonsense eating and living habits. The effects of occasional overindulgence may be relieved by home remedies, such as a teaspoonful of sodium bicarbonate (baking soda) in a glass of water, or a few drops of peppermint oil on a sugar cube. Self-medication with LAXATIVES should be avoided, since it may aggravate the condition. If the pain is severe or tends to recur, see your doctor.

CRANIAL NERVE Any of the 12 pairs of nerves that connect directly and independently with the BRAIN, as distinguished from the system of nerves that branch out from the SPINAL CORD. For the most part, the cranial (pronounced kray′nee·al) nerves carry information to the brain from the sense organs located in the head, and they control the muscles in the head and neck.

CRANIOTOMY See NEUROSURGERY.

CRETINISM See DWARFISM.

CRISIS The turning point in a fever or a disease. The term is used especially to describe the point when the patient's condition begins to improve. With a FEVER, the crisis occurs when the individual's skin turns warm, and he starts to perspire; these are signs that the heat-discharging mechanisms of the body have gone into operation, and the temperature begins to drop.

A crisis of this kind is not encountered so frequently as it used to be. Today's ANTIBIOTICS and other medicines usually cut off the infection before a crisis occurs.

CRITICAL Sometimes a sick or injured person is described as being in a critical condition or on the critical list. Many people interpret this as meaning that the person is dangerously or hopelessly ill. Although this may indeed be the case, the more exact meaning of "critical" relates to the medical term CRISIS, a stage of a disease or condition at which a sudden change either for the better or for the worse is expected at any time.

CROSS-EYE   A condition in which one or both eyes tend to turn inward toward the nose, or outward. The eyes of most very young babies are more or less crossed. Normally, by the time a baby is three months old, his eye muscles develop enough strength to keep his eyes in focus. If the baby's eyes appear to be permanently crossed, or if at six months his eyes still tend to cross, consult a doctor.

For the various corrective measures the doctor may take, see STRABISMUS.

CROUP   An acute respiratory infection, the victims of which are generally children, although it may strike persons of any age. It is most common in winter and spring, and usually occurs first at night. The medical term for croup is laryngotracheobronchitis, which simply means inflammation of the larynx (voice box), trachea (windpipe), and bronchi (the air passages between the windpipe and the lungs).

By far the largest number of cases is the result of infection with a VIRUS or a BACTERIUM. Occasionally, the attack is associated with an allergic reaction (see ALLERGY).

Croup can be dangerous. Call your doctor without delay as soon as the symptoms appear. See also the FIRST AID section.

CRYOSURGERY   Surgery in which tissue is destroyed by extreme cold instead of being cut into. With special instruments, cold can be applied very precisely to tissue that is too delicate to be manipulated with ordinary surgical instruments. Another advantage is that cryosurgery (pronounced krie″oh·sur′je·ree) produces no bleeding. The technique is used especially in repairing a DETACHED RETINA of the eye, and in brain surgery for the treatment of PARKINSONISM. See also CATARACT.

CURARE   A drug that temporarily paralyzes the nerves that control muscles. Extracted from plants, curare (pronounced kyoo·rahr′ee) was first used as a deadly arrow poison by South American Indians. It is now produced artificially and used in carefully controlled dosages to relax muscles during surgery and to relieve muscle spasms in conditions such as TETANUS.

CURETTAGE   The scraping out of a body cavity with a special instrument called a curette. Curettage (pronounced kyoor″i·tahzh′) is usually performed to remove abnormal tissue or growths or to obtain a sample of tissue for examination. (See BIOPSY.) Curettage of the uterus is a common minor operation. See also DILATATION AND CURETTAGE.

CURVATURE OF THE SPINE   See the entry SPINAL CURVATURE.

CUSHING'S SYNDROME   A group of symptoms produced by excessive amounts of CORTISONE and other adrenal hormones in the system. The symptoms include obesity, which is confined to the face and the trunk; muscular weakness; loss of calcium from the bones; high blood pressure; retention of salt and water; and excess sugar in the blood and urine. The overproduction of adrenal hormones may be caused by a tumor growing in either the ADRENAL GLANDS or the PITUITARY GLAND. Treatment consists of surgical removal or irradiation of the tumor.

CUSPID   Having a single point, or cusp; another name for the CANINE TOOTH. See also TOOTH.

CUT   A wound caused by a sharp edge or a point penetrating the skin. See FIRST AID section for measures to take in treating a cut.

CUTANEOUS   Affecting, resembling, or relating to the SKIN. (Pronounced kyoo·tay′nee·us.)

CUTICLE   The protective outer layer of the SKIN; the epidermis. Dead cuticle cells are continuously sloughed and rubbed off the surface and are continuously replaced by the living cuticle underneath. The cuticle is thinnest in areas like the eyelids and thickest on the palms of the hands and the soles of the feet. The fingernails and toenails are specialized outgrowths of horny cuticle. CORNS and CALLUSES are abnormal thickenings of cuticle caused by excessive pressure or friction. The word "cuticle" is sometimes used to mean particularly the thin layer of dead cuticle cells that adheres to the base of the nails and may split away in strips that remain attached to the living cuticle underneath. See also HANGNAIL.

CYANOSIS   A bluish or purplish discoloration of the skin and mucous membranes due to lack of oxygen in the blood. (Pronounced sie″a·noh′sis.) See also BLUE BABY.

CYCLOPROPANE   A potent ANESTHETIC gas. Cyclopropane (pronounced sie″klo·proh′payn) can be mixed with a large proportion of pure oxygen and still produce complete anesthesia.

CYST   A sac containing gas, fluid, or a semisolid substance. Cysts may develop in any part of the body.
Breast Cysts: Cysts of the breast occur as part of a condition known as chronic cystic mastitis (see MAS-

TITIS). Breast cysts are most common at the menopause. They cause much anxiety because a lump in the breast is often one of the first signs of BREAST CANCER. A BIOPSY may be necessary to determine whether such a lump is a harmless cyst or a malignant tumor. Any lump in the breast should be brought to a doctor's attention.

Ovarian Cyst: A number of different types of cysts may occur in the ovary. Small ones may disappear without treatment. However, some grow quite large. Others produce pain that may be mistaken for the pain of appendicitis. Large or troublesome cysts have to be removed.

Parasitic Cyst: The bones, kidneys, liver, and other organs may become infested by parasites that produce cysts. The cysts may grow quite slowly. Liver cysts sometimes become calcified, or they may grow so large that they exert pressure, making it necessary to remove them. AMEBAS and TAPEWORMS are among the parasites that produce cysts.

Sebaceous Cyst: These cysts are formed when the sebaceous glands of the skin, which produce oil, become clogged. Often they develop from BLACKHEADS. Sebaceous cysts frequently occur on the face, ears, scalp, and back. It is not uncommon for them to form an ABSCESS. The abscessed sac is removed by surgery. If it is on or near the skin's surface, it may be punctured by a physician and the contents squeezed out. Sebaceous cysts are also known as wens.

CYSTIC FIBROSIS (C/F) A disease of children and adolescents in which the sweat glands and the mucus-secreting glands do not function properly, and the lungs and PANCREAS become involved. The child suffers from malnutrition and respiratory infections. Cystic fibrosis (pronounced sis'tik fie·broh'sis) is among the most serious lung problems of American children. The disease is also known as mucoviscidosis and pancreatic fibrosis.

Cause: Cystic fibrosis is a hereditary disease. Although neither the mother nor father of a C/F child is affected by the disease, both must carry a predisposing factor in their genes as a RECESSIVE trait. Cystic fibrosis was first recognized in relatively recent times, so that much still remains to be learned about it.

Symptoms: Cystic fibrosis often shows up soon after birth. Up to 10 percent of C/F babies have intestinal obstructions that require prompt surgical relief. The individual has severe coughing spells, due to the presence of a thick mucus that clogs the air passages. There is repeated infection of the lungs, and the child is especially subject to bronchitis, pneumonia, and emphysema.

In most children, the mucus prevents the enzymes of the pancreas from reaching the intestine and aiding in the digestion and absorption of food. The result is malnutrition and underweight.

Another pronounced symptom in C/F children is the loss of excessive amounts of salt in body sweat. As a result, in hot weather or in episodes of fever, they are dangerously subject to heat exhaustion. The salt loss, which may be more than three times as great as that of healthy children, provides the principal diagnostic indication of the disease.

Treatment: To overcome the problem of underweight, the child is put on a high-protein diet, with vitamin supplements. Pancreas extract is given to help digestion. Respiratory diseases are treated with ANTIBIOTICS. Extra salt must be taken. A respiration machine or a plastic mist tent is used to loosen the thick mucus clogging the air passages. Physical therapy also helps to free the lungs of mucus and ventilate them.

For further information on cystic fibrosis and the location of your nearest C/F clinic, write the Cystic Fibrosis Foundation, 6000 Executive Boulevard, Suite 309, Rockville, Maryland 20852.

CYSTITIS Infection or inflammation of the bladder. The bladder is subject to a considerable number of infections from both inside and outside the body. For example, cystitis (pronounced sis·tie'tis) may be caused by BACTERIA traveling down inside the body from the KIDNEYS by way of the ureters, the tubes that conduct the urine to the BLADDER. In infection from the outside, which is the more usual form, the bacteria enter by way of the URETHRA, the passage leading from the bladder. Prolonged bed rest, childbirth, major surgery, and untreated diabetes mellitus (see DIABETES) increase the risk of cystitis. Women, especially when pregnant or if past the menopause, are particularly subject to this type of infection; but bladder infections occur at all ages, including infancy.

Cystitis frequently occurs in combination with other disorders or as a result of them. Stones in the bladder or inflammation of the urethra (URETHRITIS) may trigger the condition. An enlarged prostate gland may interfere with normal emptying of the bladder, providing favorable conditions for the growth of bacteria.

Symptoms: Cystitis occurs in many forms. It can be acute or chronic, and the symptoms may range from extremely troublesome to mild. Generally there is a need to void urine frequently, and this act is accompanied by a burning, painful sensation. There may be fever and chills as well as backache.

Treatment: It is important to keep the sexual organs clean and reduce the possibility of further infection. The condition is combated with SULFONAMIDES and ANTIBIOTICS. Bladder sedatives and analgesics may be given. Highly seasoned foods and alcoholic beverages are eliminated from the diet, since they may irritate the bladder. The bladder may be investigated by the cystoscope (see CYSTOSCOPY), an instrument for viewing the inside of the bladder, or by the cystogram, which is an X-ray picture of the bladder.

CYSTOGRAM See CYSTITIS.

CYSTOSCOPY Examination of the inside of the urinary tract with a special instrument, the cystoscope. This instrument is a narrow tube fitted with lights and mirrors. Cystoscopy (pronounced sis·tos′ko·pee) involves inserting the lighted end of the cystoscope into the bladder through the meatus, the opening into the URETHRA. The examining doctor can then see the inside of the bladder. If CALCULI (stones) are present, they can be located and removed by the operation known as LITHOLAPAXY. If the doctor wishes to introduce a CATHETER into the upper part of the urinary tract nearer the kidneys, he will use the cystoscope to locate the openings into the bladder of the ureters that lead to the kidneys.

CYTOLOGICAL SMEAR A very small sample of body fluid or tissue mounted on a glass slide so that the individual cells may be examined under a microscope. (Pronounced sie·to·loj′i·kal.) See also BIOPSY.

CYTOLOGY The study of CELLS. (Pronounced sie·tol′o·jee.)

D

D AND C See DILATATION AND CURETTAGE.

DANDRUFF Small flakes of dead skin. It is usually confined to the SCALP, but in severe cases the skin of the eyebrows and other parts of the body may be affected. The condition is often accompanied by itching.

Dandruff is associated with some disturbance of the tiny glands in the skin that excrete SEBUM, or oil. There may be too little sebum, and the hair becomes brittle and dry. More commonly, too much sebum is excreted. Then the hair becomes oily, and the dandruff has a yellowish color.

There is no specific cure for dandruff, but a wholesome diet and rigorous cleanliness will usually help. Wash the hair often, and wash your comb and hairbrush at the same time. Massage the scalp to improve circulation and brush the hair regularly. If these measures do not help, see a doctor.

DARVON-N A trade name for propoxyphene, a powerful pain reliever. Other trade names include Algodex, Depronal-SA, Novopropoxyn, Pro-65, and 642. *Take only the dosage prescribed by your doctor.* An overdose (more than four capsules a day) or a combination of propoxyphene and alcohol can cause CARDIAC ARREST and death.

DDT The familiar name for the chemical jaw-breaker *di*chloro*di*phenyl*tri*chloroethane. In 1939 it was discovered that DDT killed insects on contact, and it was put into use as an insecticide. DDT is not easily broken down. It accumulates in soil and water and in the bodies of animals, threatening the survival of some species. At the same time, many insects have developed resistance to it. Many countries, including the United States have banned DDT for all but a very few uses.

DEAFNESS Partial or complete loss of the ability to hear. It is estimated that as many as 20 million persons in North America have some degree of hearing difficulty, but only a small percentage of these are totally deaf. Fortunately, today's electronic HEARING AIDS and medical techniques can do a great deal to help correct hearing problems.

Hearing impairment may stem from numerous causes. It can be CONGENITAL, or it can be the result of an injury. Wax in the ear (see CERUMEN), infection of the middle ear, otosclerosis (overgrowth of bone in the ear), syphilis, or certain drugs may produce hearing impairment, as can continuous exposure to loud noise.

There are two types of deafness. One is *nerve* deafness. Nerve tissue, unfortunately, cannot be repaired; however, the loss of hearing is sometimes only partial. The second type is *conduction* deafness. Here there is some impairment or blockage of the structures of the EAR, such as the tiny bones, the eardrum, or the ear canal. Many of these conditions may be relieved or cured by medical treatment or surgery. They may also be helped by a hearing aid that is carefully fitted by a medical specialist.

Warning Signals: Symptoms that may be forerunners of serious ear trouble include persistent ringing and pain in the ears and a discharge of pus or blood from the ear canal. Any of these indicates the need for a prompt medical examination. Early treatment of an ear infection or disorder lessens the chances of impaired hearing.

DEATH At one time a person was considered dead when his heart stopped beating and breathing ceased. But with modern methods of resuscitation and artificial respiration, this definition has had to be reexamined. A stopped heart may be restarted, and breathing may be maintained in an apparently dead person until he recovers and can again breathe for himself. For this reason, anyone who is apparently dead from drowning, electric shock, or suffocation should be given artificial respiration immediately, and this should be continued until medical help arrives. For emergency treatment, see FIRST AID section.

Many doctors today define death in terms of the activity of the brain. The heart and lungs can be kept working by machines, but when there has been no electrical activity of the brain for many hours (as shown by an ELECTROENCEPHALOGRAM), the person is considered medically dead.

From the moment a person is born he begins to die; most cells in the body are dying all the time. The external surface of the skin consists entirely of dead cells which are being renewed from beneath. Red blood cells have a life of only two or three months and die at a rate of 1,000 per second; new blood cells are continuously manufactured in the bone marrow, while dead cells are removed by the liver and spleen.

In most countries people are living longer. The average life expectancy of a person in the United States is about 73 years. The present annual U.S.

death rate is about 878.1 per 100,000 of the population (at the same time the birth rate is about 15 per 1,000 women each year). Apart from accidents and deaths at the time of birth or soon afterward, the chief causes of death are cancer, heart disease, stroke, pneumonia, diabetes, cirrhosis of the liver, and arteriosclerosis.

DEBRIDEMENT   The removal of foreign matter and diseased or injured tissue from the surface of an open wound, usually by excision. Contaminated wounds or those involving extensive tissue damage often require debridement (pronounced di·breed'ment). By debridement, obvious sources of possible infection are removed and any infective organisms present are deprived of the nourishment that dead tissue would provide for them.

DECALCIFICATION   Abnormal loss of calcium compounds from BONES or from teeth. (Pronounced dee·kal"si·fi·kay'shun.) See also TOOTH.

DECIDUOUS TOOTH   Another name for baby, or primary, TOOTH. (Pronounced di·sij'oo·us.)

DECONGESTANT   An agent that reduces congestion or swelling; in particular, a medicine used to relieve a stuffed or runny nose. Decongestant (pronounced dee"kon·jest'ant) medications shrink the MUCOUS MEMBRANES and thus widen the air passages. They are employed in treating the nasal symptoms of HAY FEVER and the COMMON COLD.

Decongestants are available in a number of forms, including tablets, liquids, nose drops, inhalants, and sprays. Effective decongestants include ADRENALIN (epinephrine) and EPHEDRINE. Applied to the swollen membranes of the nose, they not only cause the membranes to shrink, but they also have an antiallergic action; however, they may produce a rise in blood pressure. Oily nose drops should be avoided, as they have a tendency to drip into the lungs, where they may cause damage.

DEHYDRATION   Abnormal loss of fluid from the body. (Pronounced dee"hie·dray'shun.) Water makes up the greater part of the blood and the PROTOPLASM, the fundamental material of which the body is composed.

We normally take in between two and three quarts of fluid every day in the liquids we drink and the food we eat. Dehydration begins when we take in less fluid than we are losing in our urine, exhaled breath, perspiration, and stool.

Dehydration often accompanies excessive urination, vomiting, diarrhea, or loss of blood. Excessive use of DIURETICS (drugs taken to increase the volume of urine) may produce the condition. Heavy perspiration in hot weather is frequently responsible. Fever also causes water loss. Dehydration is sometimes a symptom of DIABETES and other diseases.

Treatment is to drink plenty of water, juice, or any healthful fluid. In severe dehydration, SALINE solutions, BLOOD PLASMA, or whole blood may be injected. The diarrhea, vomiting, or other condition producing the dehydration must also be treated.

DELIRIUM   An acute mental disturbance marked by excitement, restlessness, confusion, disordered speech, and, frequently, hallucinations. Sometimes there is a high fever. Delirium (pronounced di·lir'ee·um) may be due to any of a number of causes. These include physical or mental shock, INSULIN shock, toxins produced by certain bacteria, alcoholism, and excessive use of sedatives (especially BROMIDES).

The condition is very serious and requires medical attention without delay. Treatment depends upon the underlying cause.

DELIRIUM TREMENS (DT's)   An acute mental and physical disturbance associated with chronic ALCOHOLISM. The symptoms of delirium tremens (pronounced di·lir'ee·um tree'menz) include extreme excitement and mental confusion, anxiety, trembling, fever, and rapid and irregular pulse. The person may have terrifying hallucinations. The onset often occurs after a period of especially heavy drinking followed by several days of abstaining. It is usually preceded by sleeplessness, extreme nervousness, irritability, and restlessness.

A person with delirium tremens requires intensive hospital care. Call a doctor without delay. Until the doctor arrives, try to calm the affected person. Confine him in a room free of frightening shadows, and remove any objects with which he could harm himself or others.

DELIVERY   See CHILDBIRTH.

DELUSION   An erroneous belief which is unshaken by reasoned argument. It may arise from an exaggerated or mistaken response to something in the real world, or it may have no basis in reality. A HALLUCINATION, by contrast, is a false sense perception that has no basis in the real world. Thus, to hear a voice when there is no one speaking is a hallucination.

Delusions, like hallucinations, occur to normal persons when they are extremely tired or have been subjected to great emotional strain. Severe delusions without a rational basis are characteristic of psychosis. See also EMOTIONAL AND MENTAL DISORDERS.

Delusions of being unjustly persecuted are frequently encountered in psychotics. The individual may appear rational in many ways, but he has a fixed belief that some person or force is bent upon injuring him. Delusions of grandeur are another familiar type. In these, the psychotic is convinced that he is a great hero or ruler, such as George Washington or Napoleon.

DEMENTIA A general term for serious impairment or loss of mental capacity, usually accompanied by disturbances in emotion and behavior. The onset of dementia is a gradual process. Dementia (pronounced di·men′sha) may be associated with a number of different diseases or conditions, including SENILITY, HARDENING OF THE ARTERIES of the brain, syphilitic PARESIS, ALCOHOLISM, BRAIN TUMOR, and SCHIZOPHRENIA.

A person with dementia needs medical help. In a few cases, a complete cure is possible. In other cases, symptoms may be controlled. Medicines such as TRANQUILIZERS may be prescribed to improve the person's sense of well-being

DEMENTIA PRAECOX See SCHIZOPHRENIA. (Pronounced di·men′sha pree′koks.)

DEMEROL A trade name for meperidine, a synthetic compound that is used as an ANALGESIC (pain reliever). It is somewhat more effective than codeine, and is prescribed to relieve labor pains. Meperidine is also a NARCOTIC (causing sleep) and is sometimes used as a SEDATIVE. Repeated use can lead to addiction; hence, Demerol (pronounced dem′e·rohl″) is under federal control in the United States and Canada.

DENGUE An acute, infectious disease usually seen only in the tropics, although epidemics have occurred in the southern United States. Dengue (pronounced deng′gee) is also known as dengue fever and breakbone fever. It is caused by a virus transmitted by the same family of mosquito that carries yellow fever. The symptoms are headache, fever, weakness, and severe pain in the joints and muscles. These symptoms usually appear for two to four days, disappear for a day, and then return along with a rash.

There is no specific cure for dengue. Complete recovery usually takes place within a few weeks, and an attack gives immunity for a year or more. Treatment consists of BED REST, ANALGESICS to relieve pain, and enough fluid to counteract DEHYDRATION through sweating.

DENTAL CARIES Tooth decay. Dental caries is the most widespread of human diseases, experienced by 98 percent of the population.

How Caries Develop: It seems almost certain that caries are produced by colonies of BACTERIA of many different kinds present in the mouth. When we eat, small deposits of food accumulate between the teeth and in the grooves on the chewing surfaces. The bacteria form ENZYMES that act on the starches and sugars in the food deposits, producing a substance called LACTIC ACID. Fifteen minutes after we have eaten, this acid is already present. It starts to dissolve the enamel—the protective covering of the tooth—and then goes to work on the next layer, the dentin. (See TOOTH for illustration of tooth structure.) In this manner a *cavity* develops, a toothache being the eventual result if the decay is not checked. A dentist must drill away (see DENTAL DRILL) the decayed material and replace it with a filling.

A hereditary factor appears to be involved in the development of dental caries. However, there are a number of steps that everyone can take to keep his teeth as healthy as possible.

Prevention: Tooth brushing is indispensable, and it should be done soon after eating. The action of the bacteria begins almost at the instant the food is deposited on or between the teeth. Using dental floss or dental tape helps to remove particles the brush cannot reach.

A DENTIFRICE containing stannous fluoride is helpful in controlling tooth decay, especially when combined with the direct application to the tooth surfaces of a stannous fluoride solution at regular intervals. In communities that add a regulated amount of fluoride to their drinking water the occurrence of dental caries in children has dropped 60 percent or more. (See FLUORIDATION.)

Obviously, the more sugar and starch taken into the mouth, the greater the risk of tooth decay. You should cut down on cake, soda, candy, jams, sugary desserts—everything rich in carbohydrates. When these are taken repeatedly throughout the day, the harmful effect is multiplied.

No matter how healthy your teeth seem, or how dutiful your care, a visit to the dentist at least every six months is desirable for everyone. This is especially true for children, beginning after the age of two. Some dentists specialize in the treatment of children, or pediatric dentistry.

DENTAL DRILL Advances in *dentistry* are nowhere more conspicuous than in the high-speed drills of today.

Dental drills in use until very recently vibrated jarringly, were noisy, and soon heated the cavity so that the dentist had to pause frequently in his work. Moreover, old-fashioned drills were slow, seldom surpassing 5,000 revolutions per minute. In contrast, today's most advanced drills work at almost incredible speeds in excess of 200,000 revolutions per minute, with the result that the drilling is completed much more rapidly. New air drills cooled by water are in use, so that the tooth being operated upon does not get painfully hot.

DENTAL FILLING A good filling material must be able to stand the heavy strain of chewing. It must not change color or absorb the moisture of the mouth. It must not contract or expand.

Today it is possible to save many teeth that would formerly have been lost. Infected pulp can be removed, and even the nerve of a tooth. To fill a tooth, the dentist first removes the area of decay with a high-speed drill that operates with a minimum of friction. (See DENTAL DRILL.) Then he treats the inside of the tooth with medicine and inserts the filling.

For a gold inlay, a cast must be prepared. The dentist fills the cavity with wax; from this a mold is made which is filled with a gold alloy. Dental cement is used to fasten the gold inlay into the tooth. For a silver filling, an amalgam made of silver, mercury, and tin is packed into the cavity bit by bit. Then the dentist shapes it with his instruments. Porcelain fillings are more fragile than metal, but they can be tinted to match the rest of the tooth and are generally preferred for teeth that show at the front of the mouth.

DENTIFRICE A substance used on the toothbrush to clean the teeth. Dentifrices come in three forms: paste, powder, and liquid. Toothpaste and tooth powder usually contain a detergent and an abrasive material. To create the consistency of paste, a substance such as glycerin is added.

In recent years, much has been heard about sodium fluoride and stannous fluoride, chemicals that help to prevent DENTAL CARIES, or tooth decay. Fluoride is included in several dentifrices, and has been added to the local water supply in many communities. Strontium chloride is used in some dentifrices to relieve the sensitivity of teeth resulting from the wearing away of dentin.

As yet, there is no perfect toothpaste or powder. Those containing harsh abrasives or strong antiseptics should be avoided. Rely on the recommendation of your dentist or of such nonprofit organizations as the United States Public Health Service or the Council on Dental Therapeutics of the American Dental Association.

Brushing: More important than the type or brand of dentifrice is how you use it in brushing the teeth. Proper brushing helps prevent decay by removing food particles from the surfaces of teeth, massaging the gums, and cleaning the crevices where the teeth and gums meet. Most dentists believe that a soft brush with rounded end bristles is the best kind to use. The brush should be held at an angle of about 45 degrees to the teeth and gums, and should be moved in a short, vibrating action, with the teeth brushed in groups of three or four at a time. Use two toothbrushes so that each of them gets a chance to dry out thoroughly before being used again. Rinse the brush after using it to prevent bacteria from breeding on any remaining food particles.

DENTIN See TOOTH.

DENTISTRY See DENTAL DRILL; DENTAL FILLING; DENTURE; ORTHODONTICS.

DENTURE An appliance or BRIDGE containing an artificial tooth or teeth. Dentures may be perma-

nently fixed in place or removable; they may be partial, with just one or several teeth, or they may be complete, replacing all the teeth of the upper and lower jaws. Not only do dentures enable a person to enjoy a full range of foods, they also fill out the face and support any natural teeth that remain in the mouth.

If you have a new set of complete dentures, or plates, do not start eating foods that require a lot of chewing. Choose softer foods and eat on both sides of your mouth. As you get accustomed to the dentures, you can shift to harder foods. There may be some soreness of the gums at first. If this persists, it is important to wear the dentures the day before you go to the dentist, so he can identify the points of irritation and correct the plates, if necessary.

New dentures also present some problems in speaking. Tongue, lips, and teeth all work together in forming speech sounds, and the tongue and lips must become used to the dentures. Speak with careful precision at first, until your tongue and lips get the feel of the dentures. Read out loud from a newspaper or book. Drill yourself on the sounds that give you difficulty.

Complete dentures should be brushed after every meal. Scrub them thoroughly. Place them in water overnight and add salt or a dental-plate cleanser. You should have periodic checkups by your dentist to make certain that the dentures continue to fit correctly, since changes may take place in the bone structure of your mouth.

DEODORANT A preparation that counteracts or prevents unpleasant odors. The odor of sweat is produced by BACTERIA that normally inhabit the skin and thrive in areas that are kept moist by perspiration. The common deodorants and antiperspirants that are applied under the arms generally contain aluminum chloride, which reduces or prevents sweating by causing the pores in the skin to close. These deodorants prevent odor indirectly by depriving the bacteria of moisture and nourishment. The deodorant soaps, on the contrary, do not interfere with sweating. These soaps are effective and seem to be quite harmless.

DEPERSONALIZATION A term sometimes used in PSYCHIATRY for a state in which a person appears to have lost his sense of self. He may behave as if he were a detached observer of his own actions, without any ownership or control of the parts of his body. (Pronounced dee·pur″so·na·li·zay′shun.)

DEPILATORY A cosmetic preparation for removing unwanted hair. Ordinarily, a depilatory (pronounced di·pil′a·tawr″ee) does not permanently affect the hair roots, and the hair grows in again. Most depilatories consist basically of a caustic chemical (a sulfide) that dissolves hair so that it can be washed away in water. Perfume is usually added to disguise the unpleasant smell of the sulfide; and oily substances are added to soothe skin irritation.

Hair and nails are composed of a very tough substance called KERATIN. Anything that is caustic enough to dissolve keratin must be handled very cautiously, or it may injure the skin and more sensitive tissues. If you use a depilatory, test it first on a very small area. If there is any evidence of a skin rash after the depilatory is removed from the skin, do not use it. Be sure not to get it near the eyes.

For safer and more pleasant methods of getting rid of unwanted hair, see HAIR REMOVAL.

DEPRESSANT Any medicine that slows down some activity of the body, mental or physical. TRANQUILIZERS are depressants that calm nervous excitement by acting on the central nervous system. Medicines that reduce the rate and force of contraction of the heart are cardiac depressants. Thyroid depressants reduce the production of hormones by the thyroid gland.

DEPRESSION The state of feeling dejected or dispirited. Depression is most likely to occur at critical or unsettled times in life: in the adolescent years, during pregnancy, shortly after giving birth to a child, at menopause, or in the later years. It may be triggered by the death of a loved one or by a profound disappointment.
Symptoms: A depressed person tends to have a bleak, pessimistic outlook on his future and to be apathetic toward activities he formerly regarded as meaningful. He may complain of constant fatigue or exhibit a variety of physical complaints, usually minor in character or difficult to identify. The individual may lose all interest in sex activity. He may no longer have an appetite for food, with a resulting sharp loss in weight; or he may overeat compulsively. Sleeping difficulties and fits of weeping are common.
Help for the Depressed: Getting a depressed person to talk out his problem is often helpful. Although the listener should lend an understanding ear, it is a mistake to be oversympathetic. Encouraging the individual to feel pity for himself may do more harm than good. It might be pointed out to the depressed person that the situation is best met in a realistic, unemotional way. The individual should be assisted to recognize his own value and make the most of his resources.

A doctor can prescribe medicines to fight depression (see ANTIDEPRESSANT) and to help the depressed person sleep if he has difficulty in doing so. When the condition is very severe, a PSYCHIATRIST should be consulted.

DERMATITIS Inflammation of the SKIN. Dermatitis (pronounced dur″ma·tie′tis) is not a disease but a skin condition that may have any of a large variety of causes.

DERMATOLOGIST A specialist in the diagnosis and treatment of disorders of the SKIN. Since the skin is the largest and most exposed part of the body, the dermatologist (pronounced dur″ma·tol′o·jist) deals with a wide range of conditions of varying seriousness, from WARTS and RASHES to cancer of the skin.

DESENEX The trade name for the synthetic chemical zinc undecylenate. Desenex (pronounced des′e·neks) is effective in destroying the fungus that causes ATHLETE'S FOOT. It is available either as an ointment or a powder.

DETACHED RETINA The retina, the part of the EYE that is sensitive to light, is a delicate film covering about two-thirds of the inner surface of the eyeball. Normally, the retina is closely attached to an underlying layer, the choroid. Sometimes, a small area of the retina separates, or becomes detached, from the choroid. Separated from its support, the detached retina tears. There is no pain, but the person sees sparks and flashes of light, followed by a blank area in the field of vision. By looking into the eye with an ophthalmoscope, a doctor can easily see the location and extent of the damage. If untreated, the condition becomes steadily worse.

Treatment consists of one or more operations by a specialist skilled in the technique. Using a tiny point of intense light or extreme cold for a fraction of a second, the eye surgeon creates minute patches of scar tissue that serve to "glue" the retina back in place. Treatment is usually completely successful if it is done before the damage progresses too far.

DEVIATED SEPTUM A common defect in which the nasal septum (the wall of bone and cartilage that separates the nostrils) is situated off center, or deviated, so that one nostril is smaller than the other. (See NOSE.) A deviated septum (pronounced dee′vee·ayt″ed sep′tum) may result from injury but is usually CONGENITAL.

If the malformation is severe, it is sometimes advisable to have part of the septum removed surgically. The operation, called submucous resection, is a relatively minor one.

DEVIATION See PERVERSION.

DEXAMYL The trade name of a combination of DEXEDRINE and a BARBITURATE, sometimes prescribed to control the appetite in the treatment of obesity. Dexamyl (pronounced dek′sa·mil) is also used to improve depressed moods.

DEXEDRINE A trade name for dextroamphetamine sulfate, an AMPHETAMINE with a slightly inhibiting effect on the appetite. Dexedrine (pronounced dek′si·dreen″) is sometimes used in the treatment of PARKINSONISM. Undesirable effects include drug dependence, sleeplessness, and cumulative fatigue. Dexedrine should never be taken by persons with high blood pressure (HYPERTENSION).

DIABETES There are two types of diabetes, diabetes mellitus (pronounced die″*a*·bee′tis me·lie′t*u*s) and diabetes insipidus (in·sip′*i*·d*u*s). These diseases, although unrelated, are both characterized by the symptoms of excessive thirst and excessive secretion of urine.

Diabetes mellitus is a disease that runs in families, but its precise cause is not known. In many people, the condition arises when the PANCREAS fails to produce the hormone INSULIN in sufficient quantity (a defect known as hypoinsulinism), or when the body does not use the insulin properly. Insulin helps the body to utilize carbohydrates. In diabetes, sugar builds up in the blood; eventually, this excess sugar is passed off in the urine, a condition known as glycosuria. The disease is diagnosed by testing the urine and the blood for sugar. (See GLUCOSE TOLERANCE TEST.)

Diabetes mellitus requires continued medical attention. If the person is overweight, a program of weight reduction and exercise is immediately embarked upon. In mild cases, these measures are sufficient to bring the disease under control. If the condition is more severe, or if it starts in childhood, insulin injections or another medicine in tablet form is prescribed. The amount and kind of insulin given varies with the individual. If diabetes is not treated, the results may be extremely serious. A diabetic diet, consisting of highly nutritious foods that are low in sugar, is usually prescribed by the doctor.

The diabetic who takes insulin may undergo a dangerous drop in blood sugar (hypoglycemia), accompanied by trembling, weakness, and hunger, or even by coma or convulsions. A diabetic should carry an identification card telling that he has diabetes—it could well save his life.

Diabetes insipidus is produced by a disturbance in the secretion of the PITUITARY GLAND, which controls the use of fluid in the body. Pituitary extracts or synthetic substitutes are prescribed to regulate the disorder.

DIAGNOSIS The art and science of identifying the disease that causes any particular group of symptoms. A doctor may have to make numerous laboratory tests and X-ray examinations before he can make a correct diagnosis of a disease.

DIAPER RASH Reddening and soreness of a baby's skin in the areas usually covered by a diaper. The condition makes the baby fretful and unhappy, and may expose him to secondary skin infection.

At the first sign of diaper rash, take the following precautions. Keep the baby as dry and clean as possible by changing diapers frequently. If you launder the diapers yourself, always rinse them

thoroughly to remove all traces of soap and bleach. Keep the diapers free of bacteria by boiling them and pressing them with a hot iron. Do not use a fiberglass ironing-board cover or any washing machine that may contain lint from fiber-glass material. If the rash persists, you should consult a doctor.

DIAPHRAGM (anatomy) The flexible dome-shaped partition that lies between the chest and the abdomen. The diaphragm (pronounced die′*a*·fram) is attached to the lower ribs at each side and to the breastbone and the backbone in front and back. It bulges upward against the heart and lungs, arching over the stomach, liver, and spleen underneath. There are openings in the diaphragm through which pass large blood vessels, nerves, and the ESOPHAGUS.

The diaphragm is a muscle that contracts and relaxes rhythmically—usually about 16 times a minute. It plays an essential part in breathing. When it contracts, its dome shape becomes flatter, creating empty space in the chest cavity. Air immediately rushes into the lungs, which expand to fill the empty space. The diaphragm then pushes upwards, deflating the lungs and causing the person to breathe out. During bowel movements and childbirth, the contracted diaphragm contributes to downward pressure on the abdominal cavity.

A hernia sometimes occurs in the diaphragm as a result of a defect in one of its openings; the one for the esophagus is especially vulnerable. Part of the stomach may push up into the chest cavity, sometimes causing severe pain. Surgery can correct the defect in most cases. (See illustration on the following page.)

DIAPHRAGM (birth control) A contraceptive device that is worn by a woman to prevent sperm from entering the womb (UTERUS). It is made of a dome-shaped piece of thin rubber surrounding a flexible metal ring. When the device is properly inserted, the rubber film covers the cervix, or mouth of the womb, and the metal ring encircles the cervix and holds the film in place. A contraceptive jelly is usually spread over both sides of the diaphragm as an additional barrier against the live SPERM CELLS. The diaphragm should remain in place for at least six hours after intercourse. After it has been removed, it should be carefully rinsed and dried.

The initial fitting of the diaphragm should always be made by a physician, who will at the same time demonstrate how it should be inserted and removed. See also CONTRACEPTIVE METHODS AND DEVICES.

DIARRHEA Frequent and excessive discharge of watery material from the bowel. The chief danger is excessive loss of water (DEHYDRATION). In addition, diarrhea interferes with nourishment: PERISTALSIS is so speeded up that digested food passes through the intestine before it can be absorbed into the system.

Diarrhea may be due to many different causes.

DIAPHRAGM

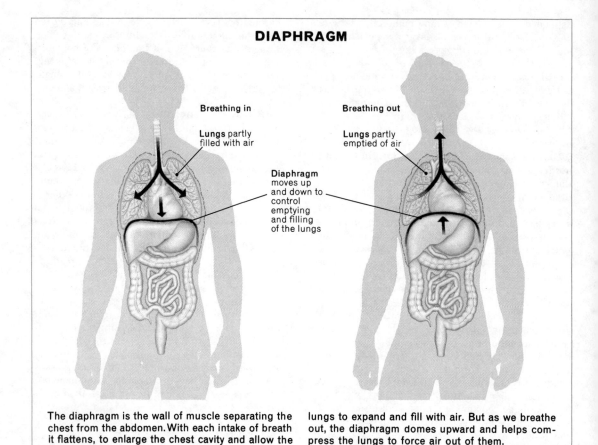

Breathing in

Lungs partly filled with air

Breathing out

Lungs partly emptied of air

Diaphragm moves up and down to control emptying and filling of the lungs

The diaphragm is the wall of muscle separating the chest from the abdomen. With each intake of breath it flattens, to enlarge the chest cavity and allow the lungs to expand and fill with air. But as we breathe out, the diaphragm domes upward and helps compress the lungs to force air out of them.

Unwise eating or drinking may bring on a mild and brief attack. Allergic reactions, and even unusual emotional stress or excitement, may cause diarrhea.

More serious causes of diarrhea include FOOD POISONING, which results from eating food that has been contaminated by bacteria. Nausea and vomiting accompany this more serious type. Accidental swallowing of chemical substances harmful to the body, such as arsenic or lead (see LEAD POISONING), will also bring on diarrhea, usually accompanied by severe cramps and vomiting.

Various infections may also cause diarrhea; among them are bacillary and viral DYSENTERY. A change in water or diet during travel may be a cause. The chance of such minor infections occurring is reduced if you are careful about the water you drink and the food you eat on your travels.

The discomfort of a mild case of diarrhea can usually be relieved by a simple remedy available at a pharmacy, such as a KAOLIN-PECTIN PREPARATION. Most important, restore fluid balance in the body by taking plenty of liquids, such as tea and light soups. If diarrhea lasts more than a day or two, a doctor should be consulted.

Diarrhea in Children: Before babies reach their second year, they usually suffer at least a few mild attacks of diarrhea. The results are likely to be more serious than in adults, because babies cannot stand much fluid loss. Any conspicuous difference in the composition of a baby's stools, particularly if they are watery or contain mucus or blood, is cause for calling your doctor at once.

If an older child has a mild attack of diarrhea, he may be given a soft drink diluted with an equal amount of water. An older child with diarrhea, however slight, should be kept away from younger members of the family, just in case he has a contagious infection.

DIASTOLE The rhythmic relaxation and dilation of the heart after each SYSTOLE, or contraction. The diastole (pronounced die·as'to·lee) coincides with the interval between pulses. See also the entry BLOOD PRESSURE.

DIATHERMY A treatment in PHYSIOTHERAPY using heat generated in the tissues by electricity passing between two metal electrodes placed on the skin. Diathermy (pronounced die'a·thur"mee), which is completely painless, may be used to relieve muscular disorders. A surgeon may use a diathermy needle to destroy diseased tissues, such as tumors on the wall of the bladder, or to stop bleeding from small blood vessels during an operation.

DICK TEST A test for IMMUNITY to SCARLET FEVER. A small amount of toxin is injected under the skin. If redness develops within 48 hours, the subject is susceptible (i.e., not immune).

DIET The nourishment that a person takes regularly. The type of diet that you follow has a direct influence on your health and emotional well-being. It is important to eat adequate amounts of the essential nutrients described below; otherwise, the body will not have the fuel it needs for energy and the building blocks used for the growth and repair of tissue.

Carbohydrates: Starch and sugar are collectively known as carbohydrates. They are the body's basic source of energy. Starch is found in potatoes and in grains, such as wheat and rice, as well as in the foods made with them—spaghetti, bread, crackers, cake, and so on. Sugar is supplied by vegetables, fruits, and honey. See also CARBOHYDRATE.

Proteins: Proteins are essential for the growth and repair of our tissues. Good sources of these building blocks include lean beef, veal, fish, poultry, milk and milk products, nuts, grains, peas, lentils, and beans. See also PROTEIN.

Fats: Fats are major sources of energy, yielding more than twice the number of calories that carbohydrates do. They are also needed in the functioning of all tissues. Fats are found in milk and milk products, nuts, oils, meat, fish, and some vegetables. See also FAT.

Minerals: Many minerals are needed for health. Calcium and phosphorus, which make up most of the human skeleton and teeth, are found in milk, meats, fish, green vegetables, and whole grains. Iron is needed for the red corpuscles of the blood. Good sources are liver, spinach, and raisins. IODINE, essential to the thyroid gland, is obtained from iodized salt and seafood. Other necessary minerals include sodium, potassium, and copper. A good diet will provide them in sufficient quantity.

Other Essentials: Water is a vital part of all living tissue, making up about two-thirds of the weight of the body. We can do without food much more readily than we can without water. VITAMINS are also essential for health at every age. Normally, all that you need are provided in a good diet.

Planning the Diet: The caloric values of foods must be considered in planning the diet. Young persons need more CALORIES and older ones fewer. If your diet supplies more calories than required, the result may be OBESITY.

The requirements of good NUTRITION are satisfied by including in the daily diet one pint of milk (a quart for a child), one serving of meat or fish, two servings of whole wheat bread or cereal, two portions of leafy green or yellow vegetables or fruit or tomato, a potato, an egg, and a small amount of fat, such as butter or margarine. The diet should be varied, since the body needs nutrients of different types.

DIGESTION The process by which food is broken down into simpler elements so that it may be absorbed into the bloodstream and used for energy, repair of tissues, and growth. Digestion takes place in the alimentary canal: the mouth, stomach, small intestine, and large intestine, or colon.

The Mouth: Digestion begins as soon as food enters the mouth. Here the food is chewed into a fine texture. Three pairs of salivary glands pour saliva into the mouth, moistening the food. Ptyalin, an enzyme in the saliva, acts on the CARBOHYDRATES (starches and sugars), and begins to break them down into more digestible form.

What Happens in the Stomach: The food makes its way into the stomach through the esophagus, moved by contractions of the muscles (PERISTALSIS). The stomach, a muscular organ that bears a rough resemblance to a football bladder, churns the food with a series of contractions. The food is mixed with the gastric juices (pepsin, lipase, and hydrochloric acid) secreted by the stomach, which help to prepare it for absorption. Pepsin and hydrochloric acid act on PROTEINS; lipase begins the breaking down of certain FATS. After several hours, what was formerly food has been churned into an acid liquid called CHYME, which is then forced out of the stomach and into the small intestine.

The Small Intestine: The small intestine is so called because of its diameter; its greatest width is less than two inches. Actually, however, it is the longest part of the alimentary canal, making up 22 feet or more of the canal's overall length of 30 feet. Digestion continues here, and it is here that absorption of the food takes place. Digestive juice from the PANCREAS empties into the duodenum, the first part of the small intestine, to work further on protein, fats, and carbohydrates; bile from the liver also helps the digestion of fats. This action continues as the food is propelled along by the contractions of the intestine. As the food is converted into chemical compounds simple enough for absorption, it passes through the intestinal wall into the bloodstream and lymph.

The Large Intestine: Next, the bulk left after absorption is forced into the COLON. Moisture is absorbed through the wall of the intestine and the residue, or feces, is condensed into semisolid form. Mixed in with it are mucus, worn-out cells from the intestinal wall, and bacteria which work on the waste, producing certain vitamins. Finally, about 20 hours after the meal was eaten, the residue is evacuated from the body by way of the rectum and anus.

DIGESTIVE SYSTEM The food canal from mouth to anus, together with accessory glands, including the liver and the pancreas.

DIGITALIS

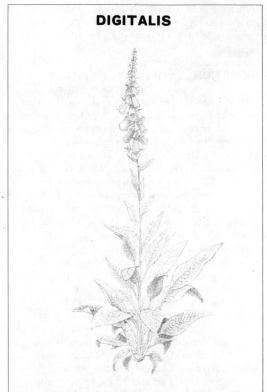

The leaves of the common foxglove contain the poisonous drug digitalis, named after the plant's scientific name, *Digitalis purpurea*. The drug is often used for treating heart complaints.

DIGITALIS Any of a number of similar compounds obtained from the leaves of the foxglove and other plants. Digitalis (pronounced dij"*i*·tal'is) is prescribed by doctors to treat disorders of the heart and circulatory system. It strengthens the heartbeat and slows down its rate.

DILANTIN A trade name for diphenylhydantoin, a synthetic preparation. Dilantin (pronounced di·lan'tin) is prescribed to prevent convulsive seizures. It slows down excessive activity in the part of the brain that controls movements, but it does not affect mental alertness or produce sleep. Dilantin is usually taken with meals in order to lessen nausea and gastric irritation.

In some persons, Dilantin produces other side effects, including swelling and inflammation of the gums, blurred vision, and a skin rash similar to acne. These toxic effects vary greatly from person to person. The doctor therefore starts treatment with very small doses and increases the amount gradually and cautiously.

DILATATION AND CURETTAGE (D and C) This is a common operation on the female organs. Dila-

tation and curettage (pronounced kyoor"i·tahzh') consists of widening, or dilating, the opening of the cervix (the narrow mouth of the UTERUS) and scraping the wall of the uterus with a curette, a surgical scoop or ring. The operation is performed while the patient is under ANESTHESIA.

A "D and C," as this operation is called by physicians, may be performed for any one of a number of medical reasons. It is a common method for early termination of a pregnancy that threatens the life of the mother. It may also be recommended after a miscarriage, when the physician has cause to believe that a portion of the membranes that surround the embryo may still be lodged in the uterus. Performed in a hospital by a qualified surgeon, it is a safe and uncomplicated operation for a woman in general good health. She can usually return home in a day or two.

When abnormal bleeding leads the doctor to suspect that there may be tumors in the cervix or uterus, this surgical procedure is used to explore the organ, to obtain a tissue sample for a BIOPSY, and to remove MALIGNANT growths. Benign cysts, polyps, and other growths are removed in the same manner.

DILATION Expansion of any opening, cavity, or passageway in the body, whether occurring naturally or induced artificially. Dilation (pronounced die·lay'sh*u*n) of the pupil of the eye, for example, occurs naturally to admit more light to the retina whenever lighting is dim. Dilation of the pupil can also be induced by the action of certain medicines, such as BELLADONNA; this permits easier examination of the retina. Except for bone, most body tissues are quite elastic and adapt to a great deal of dilation and contraction during their normal functioning.

DIPHTHERIA An acute, contagious disease caused by a BACILLUS. The diphtheria (pronounced dif·theer'ee·*a*) infection first lodges in the upper respiratory tract, producing symptoms much like the common cold, such as sore throat, fever, and generalized discomfort and weakness. A grayish membrane forms in the throat, constricting the air passages. As the bacillus multiplies, it produces a powerful toxin which circulates throughout the system. The fever gets much higher, and the person appears very weak and sick.

Treatment and Prevention: Prompt administration of ANTITOXIN and absolute bed rest are necessary for recovery.

The disease is spread by apparently healthy persons (CARRIERS) as well as by acutely ill persons. It was formerly one of the most common childhood diseases. Due to a public health program of immunization, diphtheria is now rare in North America. Your child should be immunized at an early age. A simple skin test, the SCHICK TEST, has been developed to show whether a person is susceptible or immune to infection by the diphtheria bacillus.

DIPLEGIA See PARALYSIS. (Pronounced die·plee'ja.)

DIPLOPIA The medical term for seeing double. Diplopia (pronounced di·ploh'pee·a) is usually caused by an inability to focus both eyes together (STRABISMUS).

DIPSOMANIA A form of ALCOHOLISM in which periods of excessive drinking alternate with periods of abstinence. Dipsomania (pronounced dip"so·may'nee·a) is often a reflection of underlying MANIC-DEPRESSIVE PSYCHOSIS, in which the individual attempts to relieve periods of depression by drinking to excess. Psychiatric treatment is needed.

DISINFECTANT A chemical used to destroy GERMS, especially in the surroundings rather than on the person. Solutions containing cresol or related chemicals are often used as disinfectants. These are toxic and must be kept out of children's reach.

DISK, VERTEBRAL See VERTEBRAL DISK.

DISLOCATION Displacement of a bone from its normal connections at a JOINT. Smooth working of the affected limb becomes impossible, and if the bone is moved or disturbed there is usually intense pain. When a bone is dislocated there is always injury to the connecting LIGAMENTS and to the lubricating sac surrounding the joint. In addition, there is danger that BROKEN BONES may have resulted from the same blow or fall that caused the dislocation. Every joint has its own particular way of fitting together, and it is highly advisable to have only a doctor repair a dislocation. For what to do for accidental dislocations and broken bones, see the FIRST AID section.

DIURETIC A substance that increases the output of urine by the kidneys. Normally, any increased intake of liquid results in more liquid being excreted as urine. In this sense, water, tea, beer, or any liquid is a diuretic (pronounced die"yoor·et'ik). In some abnormal conditions, the tissues accumulate excess water, and EDEMA (swelling), or dropsy, is the result. The medicines prescribed to relieve such conditions are called diuretics.

Losing only water from the body upsets the delicate balance that must be maintained in the concentration of salts in body fluid. Diuretics cause salts to be excreted along with water. A number of different substances are effective diuretics. The list of drugs includes the compounds known as xanthines and thiazides.

DIURIL A trade name for chlorothiazide. Diuril (pronounced die'ur·il) is a DIURETIC, a medicine prescribed to relieve swelling (EDEMA) due to the retention of excess fluid in the tissues.

DIVERGENT STRABISMUS See STRABISMUS.

DIVERTICULITIS A complication of DIVERTICULOSIS, in which the pouches (diverticula) in the wall of the COLON (large intestine) are filled with waste matter and become inflamed and infected. The symptoms of diverticulitis (pronounced die"ver·tik·gu·lie'tis) include muscle spasms and pains, often in the lower left side of the abdomen.
Treatment: Mild cases may be treated by bed rest, a special diet prescribed by your doctor, and medicines to reduce the infection. Severe cases are usually treated by surgery.

DIVERTICULOSIS An abnormal condition of the COLON, or large intestine. Small pouches (diverticula) form along the mucous membrane that lines the colon, and they protrude through the colon's muscular outer wall. These pouches occur usually near the rectum, and can be seen upon X-ray examination after taking BARIUM SULFATE. Diverticulosis (pronounced die"ver·tik"yu·loh'sis) is harmless unless DIVERTICULITIS develops.

DIZZINESS See BALANCE, SENSE OF; MÉNIÈRE'S DISEASE; VERTIGO.

DMSO Short for dimethylsulfoxide, a synthetic chemical. DMSO (pronounce each letter) has many poorly understood but remarkable effects on living tissue. Applied to the skin, it relieves pain and reduces inflammation. It passes through the skin readily and carries with it any medicine or other substance dissolved in it, and it enhances the usual effects of these substances. DMSO stops the growth of BACTERIA, or kills them. In carefully controlled experiments, *pure* DMSO seems to be nontoxic. Any impurities, however, could make the compound potentially dangerous. Because of this danger, and because the compound's side effects have not been sufficiently studied, DMSO has had limited medical use.

Unpurified DMSO is widely used as a solvent in industry. If this industrial DMSO is taken for unauthorized use as a pain-killer, the results can be disastrous.

DNA Short for deoxyribonucleic acid. DNA (pronounce each letter) is found in the central part, or nucleus, of every living CELL. The DNA molecule differs in structural arrangement from one person to another. It is made up of four basic building blocks, called nucleotides, which are joined together in two long, connected coils. The detailed patterns in which the DNA constituents are arranged constitute a set of instructions for reproducing other cells of the same kind. Thus DNA is the mechanism by which an organism reproduces other individuals similar to itself. See also GENE; HEREDITY. (See illustration on following page.)

DNA

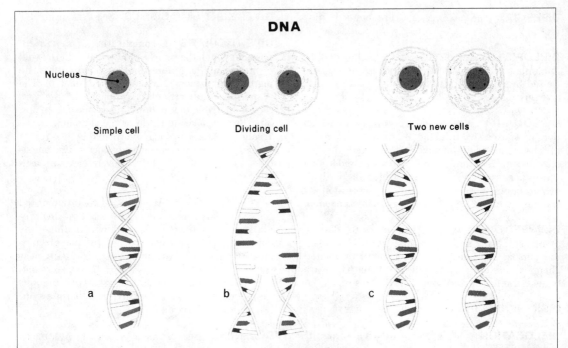

Nucleus

Simple cell

Dividing cell

Two new cells

a

b

c

The giant DNA molecule contains within its complex structure a wealth of genetic information, coded according to the order of components along its twisted coil (a). When a cell divides to form two new cells—the normal method of cell reproduction— the DNA molecules in its nucleus split down the middle (b). The two resulting half-molecules take on fragments to give two new complete DNA molecules, each an exact replica of the original (c). In this way, genetic instructions are passed on.

DOG BITE A dog bite may be very slight, or it may be a serious wound that bleeds profusely. In either case, it is important to have the bite inspected and treated by a physician as soon as you can. Until you are able to get to the doctor, first aid treatment will reduce the risk of infection. (See FIRST AID section.)

Rabies: The danger with a dog bite is that the animal may have rabies. This disease is produced by a VIRUS present in the saliva of infected animals— not only dogs, but cats, skunks, bats, and other animals as well. If there is any suspicion of rabies, the victim should be immunized at once.

Since the injections for rabies are painful, it is best to determine first whether the animal actually has the disease. The disease is fatal if it is not treated, so injections must be started if rabies cannot be definitely ruled out. See also RABIES.

DOMINANT When two or more factors compete, the one that wins out is said to be dominant. If vision is better in one eye than the other, the good eye tends to dominate.

In GENETICS, having brown eyes is known to be a dominant trait; blue eye color is a RECESSIVE trait. Thus, if a baby inherits a GENE for blue eyes from one parent and a gene for brown eyes from the other, the baby's eyes will usually be brown.

DORIDEN The trade name for glutethimide, a synthetic compound. Taken in pill form, Doriden (pronounced dawr′i·den) calms excitement or produces sleep, depending on the dosage. It is sometimes prescribed to prevent motion sickness. Repeated use can lead to addiction, and in some persons Doriden produces a skin rash.

DOUCHE A stream of water directed against some part of the body or into a body cavity. The word is often used to mean particularly the washing of the VAGINA with a stream of water or a medicated solution. Although sometimes advocated as a necessity for adequate feminine hygiene, a douche (pronounced doosh) is not essential. Ordinary bathing is usually sufficient.

DOWN'S SYNDROME The medical name for MONGOLISM.

DRAMAMINE The trade name for dimenhydrinate. Dramamine (pronounced dram′a·meen″) is prescribed in pill form to control the nausea and vomiting that occur in MOTION SICKNESS and during pregnancy.

DRESSING A protective covering applied to a wound or LESION. The simplest dressing is the familiar adhesive strip with a small, sterile gauze insert (Band-Aid), used to protect minor skin injuries from infection and physical injury. Be sure that the area is clean before applying such a strip; wash the wound gently with soap and water. It is not necessary to apply an antiseptic solution before covering a minor scratch or cut.

Wet dressings, moistened with water or a medicated solution, have a soothing action on inflamed or itchy areas. (See COMPRESS.) Splints and casts are special kinds of dressings that protect by holding a part of the body rigid.

DROOLING Dribbling of saliva out of the mouth. The salivary glands are constantly producing saliva during our waking hours. The amount is increased by the sight or even by the thought of appetizing food and by other stimuli, such as pain. Drooling is universal among babies; it often increases during teething, when pain stimulates the flow of saliva. Anyone will drool if swallowing is interfered with, as it is during dental work, for example.

DROPSY Another word for EDEMA.

DRUG The word has several meanings. Broadly, a drug is any substance that is introduced into the body or applied to the skin for the purpose of changing or reinforcing the ways the body reacts. In this sense, ANTIBIOTICS are referred to as wonder drugs, and aspirin is one of the pain-relieving, or analgesic, drugs. Such medicines have government approval and are sold in drugstores.

The word "drug" is used here to refer only to those substances that cause physical or emotional addiction. Some drugs, like morphine, codeine, and the barbiturates, are highly valuable medicines. Others, like heroin, LSD, and marihuana, are never prescribed by physicians because they tend to be habit-forming and harmful to the habitual user. (See DRUG ADDICTION.)

DRUG ADDICTION The compelling need to take a drug, often in increasing amounts. The person is dependent on the physical and emotional effects that the drug produces.

Addiction sometimes occurs in persons who are given a drug for a medical reason, such as the relief of pain, and then become so dependent upon the drug that they continue to take it after the reason has disappeared. Most cases of drug addiction are the result of a desire to escape from reality and enjoy the "high," or special type of stimulation, afforded by various kinds of drugs.

Addictive drugs are those on which the body becomes physically dependent. If the drug is withdrawn, there is a bodily reaction, often quite violent when the addiction is severe. A whole series of symptoms, known as a withdrawal syndrome, commonly appears. Addictive drugs include opiates

(NARCOTICS) such as codeine, morphine, and heroin; BARBITURATES, or sedatives, such as Seconal and phenobarbital; and certain TRANQUILIZERS. Nonaddictive drugs include peyote and MARIHUANA. Although no physical dependence on these two drugs occurs, a neurotic individual may develop an emotional need for the release they provide, and this may lead him to try more dangerous HALLUCINOGENIC DRUGS such as LSD or the opiates.

Treatment: Treatment for drug addiction may be obtained in many city hospitals, or call the Health Department in your state capital for information on their drug treatment programs. Total withdrawal of the drug, such as occurs when an individual is jailed for possession of narcotics, can produce the violent reaction already referred to; this may include vomiting, nausea, cramps, and convulsions. Gradual withdrawal is favored by many physicians. The dosage is cautiously reduced over a period of days or weeks. In narcotics cases, a medication is often substituted and then reduced gradually. PSYCHOTHERAPY is used to uncover the reasons why the person took to drugs, and to reeducate him. The help of former addicts is frequently beneficial.

For the taker of nonaddictive drugs, the corrective program is usually simpler. The person abstains from the drug, and psychotherapy is administered if there are indications that it will be helpful.

Prevention: This may be summed up in one word: avoidance. Do not be tempted to try any drug, addictive or nonaddictive. Do not take an AMPHETAMINE, SEDATIVE, or sleeping pill without first discussing the matter with your physician. If your doctor prescribes such pills, do not seek to have the prescription renewed without his recommendation.

DRUGGIST See PHARMACIST.

DRUGSTORE See PHARMACY.

DT'S See DELIRIUM TREMENS.

DUODENAL ULCER See ULCER. (Pronounced doo"o·dee'nal.)

DUODENUM See INTESTINE. (Pronounced doo"o·dee'num.)

DWARFISM A condition of seriously retarded, or stunted, growth. A dwarf's mental development may be either normal or retarded, and his body may be either well-proportioned or deformed, depending upon the cause of the dwarfism.

It has been found that a child whose DIET is deficient in any of the essential food elements will not grow to his full potential, either mentally or physically. Normal growth may also be prevented by PITUITARY GLAND disturbances. Pituitary dwarfs are usually well-proportioned and of normal intelligence. Thyroid deficiency (see THYROID GLAND) before birth and in early childhood retards physical and mental development, causing cretinism. MON-GOLISM, a congenital and sometimes hereditary disorder, is marked by similar retardation.

DYSENTERY An infection of the intestinal tract marked by repeated attacks of DIARRHEA. Dysentery (pronounced dis'en·ter"ee) may be caused by bacteria, amebas, viruses, or parasitic worms.

Amebic Dysentery: Also called amebiasis, this disease is caused by an AMEBA. It is often spread through contaminated drinking water, and occurs chiefly where human excrement is employed as a fertilizer. In severe cases an ABSCESS of the liver or HEPATITIS may develop as a complication. Medications include TETRACYCLINE and emetine hydrochloride.

Bacillary Dysentery: Also known as shigellosis, this disease is caused by BACTERIA. The disease is spread by contact with the feces of an infected person, or simply by touching an article that such a person has handled. It is also frequently spread by flies.

Bacillary dysentery is characterized by severe diarrhea with watery stools that sometimes contain blood and pus. The person has fever and cramps; nausea and vomiting are common. The disease is treated with ANTIBIOTICS and frequent consumption of liquids to avoid DEHYDRATION. It usually comes to an end in a week or 10 days.

Viral Dysentery: A virus is responsible for this form of dysentery. Fortunately, this infection runs its course in two to three days. Travelers in tropical countries are particularly exposed to one form or another of viral dysentery.

DYSLEXIA Inability to read properly because of a brain disorder that causes the victim to confuse various letters; sometimes known as "word blindness." It is different from mere slowness in learning to read and does not indicate low intelligence—some dyslexic children are of above average intelligence. Dyslexia (pronounced dis"lek'see·a) is difficult to diagnose (although special tests for children have been devised), and it may be present to some degree in one person in 20. It responds to treatment, especially if begun early, in which the child is encouraged to read as much as possible at home and at school. Parents of children with dyslexia can seek advice about education from the various dyslexia associations.

DYSMENORRHEA The medical term for painful MENSTRUATION. (Pronounced dis"men·o·ree'a.)

DYSPEPSIA See INDIGESTION. (Pronounced dis·pep'sha.)

DYSPHAGIA The medical word for difficulty in SWALLOWING. (Pronounced dis·fay'jee·a.)

DYSPHONIA Difficulty in speaking. It is usually applied to difficulty caused by disease affecting the speech organs themselves—such as inflammation (see LARYNGITIS; SORE THROAT) or a tumor in the throat. (Pronounced dis·foh'nee·a.)

DYSPNEA Difficulty in breathing. It is not a disease, but the body's attempt to increase the supply of oxygen to the tissues. Everyone experiences temporary dyspnea (pronounced disp·nee'a) after any extra physical exertion.

Dyspnea is a symptom of many diseases. ASTHMA and BRONCHITIS are associated with wheezing and labored breathing. Any condition that reduces the volume of air being pumped in and out of the lungs, such as PNEUMOTHORAX, a painful broken rib, or a tumor, can cause shortness of breath. Dyspnea accompanies diseases that interfere with oxygen absorption inside the lungs, such as emphysema, pneumonia, and lung cancer. It is a common symptom of heart disease. Some hormone disturbances, such as overproduction of thyroxine in GOITER, create greater than normal demands for oxygen. OBESITY is often accompanied by shortness of breath because any movement of a heavy body requires more than ordinary effort and hence more oxygen. In some cases, dyspnea has no physical cause, but results from ANXIETY or other emotional stress. Only a thorough medical checkup can find the cause and indicate the treatment in any individual case.

DYSTROPHY Although it strictly means faulty nutrition, the term dystrophy (pronounced dis'tro·fee) is used to describe several diseases in which there is a wasting away of tissue. An example is progressive MUSCULAR DYSTROPHY, a chronic condition in which the muscles weaken because of a breakdown in muscle fibers.

DYSURIA The medical word for any difficulty or pain in urinating. (Pronounced dis·yoor'ee·a.)

E

EAR The organ of HEARING and of equilibrium. The ear is divided into three parts: the external ear, the middle ear, and the inner ear. Sound waves enter the ear canal and cause the EARDRUM, or tympanum, to vibrate. In the middle ear, three small bones, or ossicles, transmit the vibrations to an intricate, snail-shaped organ, the cochlea, in the inner ear. Nerve endings in the cochlea pass the impulses along the auditory nerve to the brain, which interprets them as sounds.

Several other parts of the ear are of special interest. The EUSTACHIAN TUBE, leading from the throat to the middle ear, admits air and thus helps to equalize air pressure on either side of the eardrum. In the inner ear are three semicircular canals which are filled with fluid. These canals are of primary importance in enabling us to maintain our physical equilibrium. See also BALANCE, SENSE OF.

EARACHE Pain in the ear is usually caused by an infection. A boil in the ear canal is extremely painful, because the skin is fixed to the bone and cannot stretch easily. Wax in the canal can also cause earache (for treatment of earwax, see CERUMEN). Aspirin will stop minor pain, and putting a heating pad or warm cloth over the ear may relieve some of the discomfort. Consult a doctor if the ache is very painful or if the pain persists.

If the lining of the ear canal is inflamed—a condition known as otitis externa—there may be a minor earache, which becomes worse if the jaw is moved, and there may be a slight discharge from the ear. A doctor will clean out the ear passage and instruct the patient to keep his ears free from dirt by wiping them gently with the corner of a dry towel.

The most common cause of severe earache, particularly in children, is MIDDLE-EAR INFECTION (otitis media). Germs readily spread from the throat up the Eustachian tube to the middle ear, and ear infection is common after tonsillitis, measles, influenza, and a head cold. In addition to pain there may be deafness, ringing in the ears, and—if the EARDRUM perforates—a bloodstained discharge from the ear. All such infections are serious, and a doctor should be consulted if any of these symptoms occur. He will probably prescribe antibiotics to combat the infection, and other drugs to relieve the pain. Most cases of ear infection recover completely.

If infection spreads from the middle ear to the bone behind the ear, acute MASTOIDITIS may develop, although this disorder has become rare since the introduction of antibiotics.

Not all earache, however, is caused by a direct disorder of the ear. Tonsillitis, swollen neck glands, neuralgia, and even a bad tooth may cause earache. The condition should be treated by a doctor or, in the case of a diseased tooth, by a dentist.

EARDRUM A concave membrane at the end of the inch-long external ear canal; also called the tympanum. The eardrum separates the outer EAR from the middle ear. When sound enters the ear canal, it makes the eardrum vibrate. These vibrations are intensified and transmitted by the bones of the middle ear.

Sometimes the eardrum is perforated by a forceful blow on the ear, by diving, or by probing with a pointed object, such as a hairpin. This type of injury may be accompanied by bleeding and pain, and prompt medical attention is called for. Fortunately, there are usually no serious aftereffects.

EARWAX See CERUMEN.

ECG An abbreviation for ELECTROCARDIOGRAM. (Pronounce each letter.)

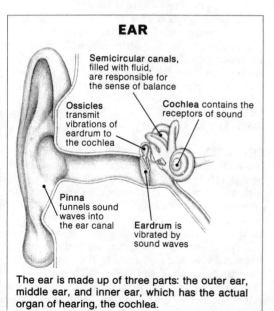

EAR

Semicircular canals, filled with fluid, are responsible for the sense of balance

Ossicles transmit vibrations of eardrum to the cochlea

Cochlea contains the receptors of sound

Pinna funnels sound waves into the ear canal

Eardrum is vibrated by sound waves

The ear is made up of three parts: the outer ear, middle ear, and inner ear, which has the actual organ of hearing, the cochlea.

ECLAMPSIA A serious condition causing convulsions and coma which may occur, although rarely, during the last three months of pregnancy or immediately after childbirth. Eclampsia (pronounced ik·lamp′see·a) is an advanced stage of what is called TOXEMIA of pregnancy, the cause of which is not known. There is retention of fluid in the system, with resultant EDEMA that may involve the brain and damage the eyes. Treatment includes complete bed rest and close medical supervision.

ECTOCARDIA See EXOCARDIA.

ECTOPIC PREGNANCY

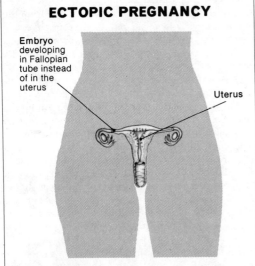

Embryo developing in Fallopian tube instead of in the uterus

Uterus

Sometimes, although very rarely, a fertilized egg lodges in the Fallopian tube instead of passing along it to develop in the uterus. The developing embryo in the tube, called an ectopic pregnancy, has to be removed by surgery.

ECTOPIC PREGNANCY A pregnancy in which the embryo begins to develop elsewhere than in its normal place, the UTERUS. The union of the sperm cell and the EGG CELL, or ovum, takes place in the FALLOPIAN TUBE. Sometimes the fertilized ovum becomes lodged there and is unable to make its way to the uterus, as it would normally.

Symptoms show up in the second or third month, as the embryo grows. These may include acute pain on one side of the abdomen, slight swelling, and vaginal bleeding. An ectopic (pronounced ek·top′ik) pregnancy is a dangerous situation, and its symptoms should be reported to the doctor without delay. It is usually necessary to remove the tube and embryo by surgery. Fortunately, the woman has a second tube, so she can become pregnant again.

ECZEMA A skin condition characterized by a red, itchy rash and blisters. In eczema (pronounced ek′se·ma), the skin often crusts and scales. These symptoms may appear on any part of the body and at any time of life, including infancy. Since there are a number of different kinds of eczema, it is often necessary to have the precise condition diagnosed and treated by a DERMATOLOGIST (skin specialist).

Eczema may occur if the skin is excessively oily or dry, or is repeatedly irritated by domestic cleansers, alkalis, or grease solvents. The condition is often an allergic reaction to such substances as pollens, dusts, or molds that are inhaled or sometimes to drugs such as barbiturates and sulfonamides. Tests will determine the substance or substances that produce allergic eczema, and the condition may be cleared up simply by avoiding the cause. See also ALLERGY.

Eczema is particularly trying for infants, and makes them restless and irritable. Often children with eczema have a family history of some type of allergy. Try to find the cause of the condition, which may be a certain soap, a powder, a woolen blanket, or a food. Each of the possible allergy-producing substances should be dispensed with for a brief period to see whether the rash disappears. If it does not, consult a doctor who may prescribe an ointment and, occasionally, a sedative.

EDEMA An abnormal accumulation of fluid in the body tissues, producing swelling. Edema (pronounced i·dee′ma) is not a disease in itself, but it may be a symptom of a disease or the result of an injury or dietary deficiency. It is sometimes known as dropsy.

Edema of the ankles and feet is quite common. People who are on their feet a lot may have puffy ankles. This is not a serious condition and may simply require rest. Severe swelling, however, should be reported at once to your physician, as it may be a symptom of heart, kidney, or other disease.

Treatment is directed at the cause. Keeping the leg raised provides relief for that limb. Restriction of fluids and the taking of DIURETICS under your doctor's direction may help reduce certain edemas.

EEG Abbreviation for ELECTROENCEPHALOGRAM. (Pronounce each letter.)

EGG CELL The female cell, or ovum, which is released monthly from the ovary during a woman's reproductive years. (See OVULATION.) When it unites with the SPERM CELL, a new individual begins to develop. See also EMBRYO.

EGO The conscious mind. The ego is a basic concept of PSYCHOANALYSIS, the method of treating emotional disorders developed by the Viennese psychiatrist Sigmund Freud (1856–1939) and others. Freud saw the human psyche, or mind, as made up of three parts: the ego, the ID, and the SUPEREGO. The id is the primitive, raw, unconscious self, which moves instinctively and immediately toward the satisfaction of desires, in accordance with what Freud called the pleasure principle. The superego is the conscience, formed by the restraints imposed by one's parents and society; it functions as a censor, keeping the id and the entire personality within bounds. The ego is, loosely, the conscious self, in touch with both id and superego.

The ego's function is to make us think, behave, and interpret things in a realistic way. It is helped in this by the superego. When the ego is strongly swayed by the unconscious or conscious drives in disagreement with the restraints imposed by the superego, tensions and feelings of guilt are aroused, according to Freud's theory.

EJACULATION Discharge of SEMEN, a whitish fluid containing SPERM CELLS, from the male penis. Ejaculation (pronounced i·jak″yu·lay′shun) is the process by which these cells are transferred to the female vagina so that fertilization and pregnancy may take place. See also COITUS.

EKG An abbreviation for ELECTROCARDIOGRAM. (Pronounce each letter.)

ELBOW The joint between the forearm and the upper arm. Like other joints, it is subject to dislocation and fracture. Any persistent pain or discomfort in the area, particularly after a wrench or fall, should be brought to the attention of a physician.

Any condition marked by pain on the outer side of the elbow is popularly labeled a tennis elbow. This pain may involve all the muscles of the forearm and is felt especially when the hand grips an object. It may be a symptom of BURSITIS. Relief is obtained by rest, application of heat, massage, or injection of local anesthetics. Carrying the arm in a sling is sometimes advisable.

ARTHRITIS may produce stiffness of the elbow, as well as pain when the joint is moved.

ELECTRA COMPLEX See COMPLEX.

ELECTRIC SHOCK A shock produced when a strong charge of electricity enters the body. (For emergency measures, see the FIRST AID section.) The electricity may paralyze the breathing centers in the brain, resulting in unconsciousness and breathing failure, and may also affect the rhythm of the heart. In cases of electric shock caused by lightning, electric BURNS are also a factor.

A few commonsense precautions help in avoiding electric shock. Electric outlets should not be exposed if there are small children in the house. Check electric cords to make certain they are not frayed, and discard or repair defective electric ap-

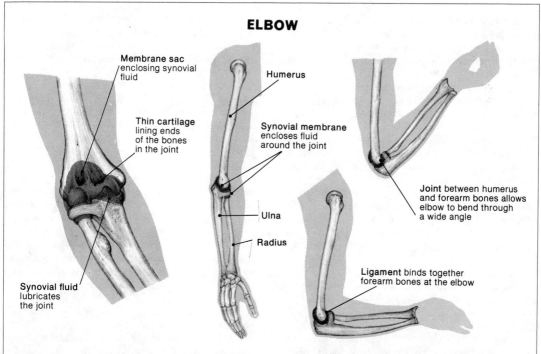

ELBOW

Membrane sac enclosing synovial fluid

Humerus

Thin cartilage lining ends of the bones in the joint

Synovial membrane encloses fluid around the joint

Synovial fluid lubricates the joint

Ulna

Radius

Joint between humerus and forearm bones allows elbow to bend through a wide angle

Ligament binds together forearm bones at the elbow

The elbow is a typical hinged joint, lubricated by a thin layer of synovial fluid. Inflammation of the synovial membrane, or synovitis, causes a painful swelling. Continual jarring of the joint produces the pain and stiffness of tennis elbow. Overflexing of the elbow can tear ligaments and cause a sprain. The general treatment for these and other common disorders of the elbow joint is rest.

pliances promptly. Stay away from high-tension wires—a necessary piece of advice, since every month failure to heed it produces fatal accidents.

For the use of electric shock in the treatment of mental disorders, see SHOCK THERAPY.

ELECTROCARDIOGRAM (ECG, EKG)

A tracing, or graph, made by amplifying the minute electric impulses generated in the HEART. The pattern produced by the impulses indicates whether the heart is in good condition or whether it is damaged, and to what degree. An electrocardiogram (pronounced i·lek″troh·kahr′dee·o·gram″) poses no danger; it is often part of a thorough medical examination.

The instrument used to record the tracing is called an electrocardiograph. Electrodes connected to this apparatus are fastened over the heart and usually on both arms and a leg. These pick up tiny electric impulses that the heart produces as it beats. The impulses are amplified by the electrocardiograph, which produces a tracing on a sheet of graph paper. The pattern that is recorded provides information on the heart's rhythm and other actions.

A specialist examines the electrocardiogram for deviations from the normal. Slight irregularities may show up if infectious diseases are present. More serious ones will appear if the individual is suffering from a cardiac condition.

ELECTROENCEPHALOGRAM (EEG)

A tracing, or graph, made by an instrument (the electroencephalograph) that records brain waves—the electric impulses in the brain. Electrodes with small metal disks are attached to the scalp. These disks pick up the minute electric waves generated in the nerve cells of the brain. Wires conduct the impulses to the electroencephalograph, where they are amplified millions of times and recorded on a strip of paper to produce the electroencephalogram (pronounced i·lek″troh·en·sef′a·lo·gram″), also called an encephalogram. The recording of an electroencephalogram is entirely painless.

The recorded brain waves are interpreted by a specialist to indicate various conditions of the brain. Different patterns of waves may indicate EPILEPSY, brain tumor, or other serious disorders involving the central nervous system.

ELECTROLYSIS

A technique used to remove unwanted hair permanently. A small electric needle is inserted into the hair follicle, which contains the root of the hair. Then an electric current is sent through the needle, destroying the root, and the hair is removed.

Electrolysis (pronounced i·lek·trol′i·sis) is used to remove hair only from small areas of the skin, usually on the face, for cosmetic reasons. It is a slow process, requiring great care, and should be performed by a skilled practitioner, preferably one recommended by your family physician. In general, it is far easier to make hair less conspicuous by bleaching it, or by removing it with tweezers, cuticle scissors, or an electric shaver. See also HAIR REMOVAL.

ELEPHANTIASIS

A disease of tropical countries, marked by swelling of part of the body, most commonly the arms, legs, or scrotum. Elephantiasis (pronounced el″e·fan·tie′a·sis) is caused by a wormlike parasite, filaria (hence the term "filariasis," another name for the disease). The larvae of these parasites are transferred from the body of one human being to that of another by the bite of numerous species of mosquitoes. The mature worms, about two inches long, live in the lymphatic system or the tissues, eventually producing inflammation, swelling, and hardening.

Elephantiasis is prevented by sanitary control aimed at eliminating the mosquitoes and parasites. Medicines are available that kill the parasites in the body, but this treatment is not always completely successful. The affected part of the body may be helped by bandaging or surgery.

EMACIATION

The condition of being or becoming extremely underweight. (Pronounced i·may″-shee·ay′shun.) Any considerable or sudden loss of weight that cannot be accounted for may be a symptom of disease. A prompt and thorough physical examination is in order. Among the disorders that may interfere with the way the body maintains its normal weight are malfunction of the endocrine glands, disturbances of the digestive tract, cancer, and diabetes.

People who do not eat enough—including alcoholics who "drink" their meals—or who do not maintain a proper balance of carbohydrates, fats, and proteins are also subject to emaciation. The condition is sometimes precipitated by an emotional state, such as DEPRESSION.

EMBOLISM

Blocking of a blood vessel by material that has originated somewhere else. (Pronounced em′bo·liz″em.) This material (called an embolus) may be a part of a blood clot that has broken off, a clump of bacteria, a globule of fat, a gas bubble, or a similar object. The embolus, carried through the circulatory system from its point of origin, may arrive at a place in a blood vessel too narrow for it to pass. There it lodges, producing the obstruction. When a BLOOD CLOT causes blockage at the site of origin, it is called a thrombus, and the condition produced is a THROMBOSIS.

Embolism is one of the causes of a stroke. Generally the obstruction is produced by a portion of a blood clot that lodges in an artery of the brain or in one of the carotid arteries, the pair of major blood vessels in the neck that lead to the brain. The blood supply to an area of the brain is cut off, and the brain cells starve and die. The victim may lose the power to speak, to move his limbs, or to coordinate his movements, depending on the cells affected and the severity of the stroke. See also the separate entry, STROKE.

Other areas may be affected by an embolism. The embolus may cause obstruction of an artery in a leg or arm, leading to GANGRENE. A dangerous clot may lodge in the lung (pulmonary embolism). Blood clots that produce blockage elsewhere frequently form in the blood vessels of the heart or the leg. Clots sometimes arise in the legs as a result of inflammation (PHLEBITIS), when there has been damage to the walls of the veins. Poor circulation can also be a cause.

Treatment: A basic treatment for embolism is administering anticoagulants—medicines that combat the tendency of the blood to clot. Drugs that dilate the blood vessels assist in increasing the flow of blood to nearby areas. Surgery may be recommended when the blockage is traced to a blood vessel within the surgeon's reach, such as the carotid artery.

EMBRYO The unborn infant, from conception to the end of the second month. (Pronounced em′bree·oh″.) After the second month, the developing baby is known medically as a FETUS.

A new life comes into existence when the sperm cell from the father enters the ovum, or egg cell, of the mother and fertilizes it. The two cells become one, which inherits qualities from both parents. (See CHROMOSOME.) About 30 hours later, the fertilized ovum divides into two cells. Cell division continues as the tiny developing mass of life makes its way from the FALLOPIAN TUBE to the uterus, or womb.

Every month, in preparation for the arrival of an embryo, the lining of the uterus grows thicker and its blood supply more abundant. If pregnancy does not occur, this blood and tissue are discharged from the vagina during MENSTRUATION.

The developing ovum attaches itself to the wall of the uterus and draws nourishment from it. As the weeks go by, membranes form around the embryo, and it is cushioned in fluid. (This is the familiar bag of waters, or AMNION.) A structure called the PLACENTA grows on the wall of the uterus, and the developing infant is connected to it by the umbilical cord. The mother's blood circulates in the placenta, and food and oxygen are passed from it into the infant's blood through the umbilical cord. (The baby will not breathe for himself until after birth.) Wastes from the infant's body, including carbon dioxide, are passed into the mother's bloodstream by the same route and excreted by her lungs and other organs.

Gradually the embryo grows, and rudimentary organs are formed. At one month it is only an eighth of an inch long. It is about an inch in length at two months. In the third month, the fetus may be 2½ to three inches long and weigh an ounce. At this stage its major organs are fairly well developed, and it is recognizably human.

EMBRYOLOGIST A specialist concerned with the development of the infant from conception to birth. (Pronounced em″bree·ol′o·jist.) See also EMBRYO.

EMESIS The process of VOMITING. See also EMETIC. (Pronounced em′e·sis.)

EMETIC A substance used to produce vomiting. An emetic (pronounced e·met′ik) is important in certain cases of poisoning when a stomach pump is not available. Before administering an emetic for poisoning, see the FIRST AID section. For some types of poisoning—swallowing kerosene, for example—emetics are life-endangering.

Perhaps the simplest method of bringing on vomiting is the insertion of a finger in the throat. Another common treatment is to swallow large quantities of warm water to which salt has been added.

Drinking water with mustard in it is also effective. IPECAC is often recommended by doctors.

EMETINE HYDROCHLORIDE A medicine that is helpful in bringing severe cases of amebic DYSENTERY under control. (Pronounced em′e·teen″ hie″dro·klawr′ied.)

EMOLLIENT A substance that produces a soothing effect, particularly on the skin and mucous membranes.

EMOTIONAL AND MENTAL DISORDERS Approximately 10 percent of the population of the United States suffers from some type of mental or emotional difficulty that is serious enough to warrant professional care. Mental and emotional illnesses include a multitude of disorders, many of which are not fully understood. Some may be associated with physical diseases or injuries which involve impairment of the brain. Others are functional disorders in which no organic brain damage is apparent.

Neurosis, or PSYCHONEUROSIS, sometimes cripples the individual's ability to function normally, although usually he manages to hold his own. The neurotic individual may be unable to relate to others emotionally. ANXIETY is a common type of neurosis—the individual feels fearful and threatened, although his anxiety is basically without foundation. Or he may suffer from a PHOBIA—a morbid fear of germs, dirt, falling, ill health, death, or almost anything else. Prolonged or intense DEPRESSION is another form a neurosis may take.

Psychosis, unlike neurosis, is a severe mental illness that requires the individual (known as a psychotic) to be confined to a mental hospital or to have regular psychiatric attention. The PSYCHOSIS may be organic—the result, for example, of alcoholism,

HARDENING OF THE ARTERIES, or brain injury. Presumably nonorganic disorders include PARANOIA, SCHIZOPHRENIA, and MANIC-DEPRESSIVE PSYCHOSIS.

Treatment: PSYCHIATRY utilizes various procedures in the treatment of emotional and mental disorders. Neuroses and certain psychoses may be treated by PSYCHOTHERAPY. The core of this method is to help the patient to overcome his difficulties by constructive discussions with a psychiatrist. PSYCHOANALYSIS is one of several types of psychotherapy; the psychoanalyst delves into the patient's unconscious mind to lay bare the origins of the disorder. Another technique is GROUP THERAPY, in which a number of individuals discuss their problems under professional supervision.

If patients are disturbed, TRANQUILIZERS may be administered to quiet them; other medicines are used to rouse patients from depression. Extremely withdrawn patients may be treated by electric SHOCK THERAPY.

EMPHYSEMA A condition in which the air sacs of the lungs are enlarged. In severe cases, there is difficulty in breathing. Emphysema (pronounced em"fi·see'ma) is generally a chronic condition and is not contagious.

Causes: The lungs contain millions of air sacs, known as alveoli. These air sacs receive carbon dioxide from the blood and exchange it for the oxygen breathed into the lungs. In emphysema, the air sacs lose their elasticity, grow larger, and can no longer function efficiently. The blood tends to become overloaded with carbon dioxide. In addition, mucus may be produced which plugs up the small air tubes (bronchioles) leading to the air sacs.

Emphysema frequently afflicts heavy smokers or people who live in industrialized areas where the air is polluted. Individuals with a long history of bronchitis or asthma also appear to be susceptible.

Symptoms: The severity of the symptoms varies. Persons who have the disease in a mild form may not even be aware of it. In severe cases, the symptoms include shortness of breath or wheezing, bluish skin, and a chronic cough that brings up sticky sputum. As the condition worsens, the individual has increasing difficulty in breathing.

Treatment: The progress of the disease may be halted, but there is no specific remedy for it. Persons subject to bronchitis or asthma should obtain help in bringing these conditions under control. If the individual lives in a smog-infested area, he may wish to consult his physician about the possibility of moving somewhere else. The smoker who gives up the habit may find this measure alone will arrest the disease. Certain drugs relieve the secretions obstructing the lungs, and breathing exercises may help to make fuller use of the lungs' decreased capacity.

EMPYEMA A condition in which pus is formed in a body cavity. Empyema (pronounced em"pee·ee'ma) is most commonly found in the chest cavity around the lungs.

The person with empyema may find it hard to breathe, and he may cough frequently and run a temperature. Treatment of the condition includes the use of antibiotics and removal of the pus through a hollow needle inserted in the chest cavity—a process known as aspiration. (See ASPIRATOR.) If the empyema persists, surgery may be required to drain the pus.

ENAMEL See TOOTH.

ENCEPHALITIS An acute inflammation of the brain. It is popularly known as sleeping sickness because of the sleepiness that is often a prominent symptom of the disease. However, encephalitis (pronounced en·sef"a·lie'tis) is quite different from the tropical disease called SLEEPING SICKNESS (trypanosomiasis).

There are a number of types of encephalitis, some of which are caused by a virus transmitted by mosquitoes or ticks. One type, equine encephalomyelitis, is basically a disease of horses and mules, but it can be transmitted to people. The patient may run a high fever and fall into convulsions followed by a coma. In later stages of encephalitis, there may be seemingly neurotic behavior and depression.

Another type of encephalitis may occur as an aftereffect of vaccination or infectious diseases such as chicken pox, mumps, and influenza. Symptoms may include headache, fever, vomiting, sore throat, and drowsiness. Prompt medical attention will provide relief and a good outlook for recovery.

ENCEPHALOGRAM See ELECTROENCEPHALOGRAM.

ENCEPHALOMA A type of BRAIN TUMOR; the term can also apply to HERNIA of the brain. (Pronounced en·sef"a·loh'ma.)

ENCEPHALON Another word for BRAIN. (Pronounced en·sef'a·lon".)

ENDEMIC A term describing a disease that persists in a particular locality. (Pronounced en·dem'ik.) See also EPIDEMIC.

ENDOCARDITIS An inflammation of the heart lining, or endocardium. Endocarditis (pronounced en'doh·kahr·die'tis) may be produced by bacteria (BACTERIAL ENDOCARDITIS) or by other causes. See also HEART; HEART DISEASE—SYMPTOMS.

ENDOCRINE GLAND A gland that produces and releases a HORMONE directly into the bloodstream. Hormones influence our height and build, sexual activity, mental sharpness, ability to respond to stress, and numerous other qualities and capacities.

There is not a single body cell whose activity is not in some way affected by these "chemical messengers" secreted by the endocrine glands.

Endocrine (pronounced en'do·krin) glands are also known as ductless glands because they do not have ducts to carry off their products as, for example, sweat glands do. The hormones find their way through the bloodstream to the area where they are needed. If there is a hormonal deficiency, serious disease may ensue. However, these deficiencies may often be remedied by administering hormones that are produced synthetically.

The PITUITARY GLAND, or hypophysis, is located at the base of the brain. Its secretions stimulate the other glands. This gland regulates sexual characteristics, growth, blood pressure, and numerous other activities. The THYROID GLAND is found in the neck. Its hormone, thyroxine, influences growth and metabolism. The four parathyroid glands are embedded in the thyroid or located near it. They influence the way the body uses calcium and phosphorus, two essential minerals.

In the PANCREAS are the islets of Langerhans. They secrete the hormone insulin, which regulates the use of sugar in the body. Many vital jobs are done by the secretions of the adrenal glands, located on the kidneys. See also ADRENALINE.

The gonads, or sex glands, consist of the OVARIES in the female and the TESTICLES in the male. The female hormones, produced chiefly in the ovaries, are called ESTROGENS; they influence menstruation, pregnancy, and female characteristics and keep the reproductive organs in condition. Testosterone, a male hormone, controls the male characteristics. (See SEX HORMONES.) The thymus, in the upper part of the chest cavity, is concerned with the production of ANTIBODIES and LYMPHOCYTES early in life and so helps the body combat infection. The function of the pineal gland, in the brain, has not been established.

ENDOCRINOLOGIST
A specialist in endocrinology—the study of the ENDOCRINE GLANDS, the HORMONES they secrete, and the effect these glands have on each other and the entire body. (Pronounced en"doh·kri·nol'o·jist.)

ENDOMETRIOSIS
A condition in women which occurs when cells like those lining the uterus grow on the surfaces of other organs inside the pelvis. Cysts may form from the blood produced by these patches of tissue. The woman has pain in the lower abdomen, particularly at the time of menstruation. Treatment may be by operation or with hormones. (Pronounced en"doh·mee·tree·oh'sis.)

ENDOTHELIUM
A membrane made up of thin, flattened cells; it lines the lymph and blood vessels, the heart, and the body cavities. (Pronounced en"doh·thee'lee·um.)

ENEMA
Injection of a liquid into the rectum and colon. An enema (pronounced en'e·ma) is generally given to clean out bodily waste, but sometimes it is administered as part of a medical examination (see BARIUM SULFATE) or for some other purpose, such as the treatment of ulcerative COLITIS.

A simple type of enema preparation is available at the drugstore. It contains an adequate amount of solution for one use and is thrown away afterward. A douche bag or an enema bag with a long rubber tube may also be used to give an enema. The bag is filled with warm water, and a teaspoonful of salt for each pint of water is added. (Soapsuds should be avoided, as they may irritate the bowel lining.) Apply a lubricant to the tube nozzle. The nozzle is best inserted by the person getting the enema, who is lying on his side on a rubber pad, with his knees pulled up. Hold the bag about a foot and a half above him. If the solution appears to be flowing too fast, pinch the tube. When the bag is empty, remove the nozzle. Urge the person to retain the liquid for five minutes, if possible. Then have him go to the bathroom or give him a bedpan.

It is unwise to rely on enemas for relief of CONSTIPATION because any artificial aid of this kind tends to undermine the normal functioning of the bowel. A person should preferably have an enema only if a doctor recommends it. Never give an enema if there is fever, nausea, abdominal pain, or any other indication of APPENDICITIS.

ENTERITIS
An inflammation of the intestine. Enteritis (pronounced en"te·rie'tis) may be due to a bacterial or virus infection, allergenic foods or medicines, or other causes. See also GASTROENTERITIS.

ENURESIS
Habitual bed-wetting; also called nycturia. Many children cannot overcome the tendency to wet their beds until their bladders have grown sufficiently to hold a night's production of urine—about 11 ounces. This is usually achieved between the ages of four and five. Enuresis (pronounced en"yu·ree'sis) should not be a source of anxiety to either parent or child.

Parents should not be overeager or anxious about training the child. When he is ready both physically and emotionally, he will learn control. For late bed-wetters, it may be helpful to restrict fluids moderately for two hours before bedtime, without making an issue of it. The child should be reminded to visit the bathroom before going to bed. Some parents have obtained good results by waking the child gently at about 11 p.m. and taking him to the bathroom. Scoldings and spankings only tend to make the difficulty worse. Time is the best trainer.

If a youngster is very slow in developing bladder control, your doctor may advise a thorough medical examination, including a urinalysis. In most cases, however, prolonged enuresis is the result of emotional insecurity. The birth of a new child in the family, sickness, or the parents' separation may be a cause of bed-wetting. These and other emotional problems are likely to cause a return of the habit in a child who has already learned bladder control.

ENZYME   A substance secreted by living cells, which breaks complex substances down into forms in which they may be used by the body.

Thousands of enzymes are present in our bodies. A number of them play a major role in DIGESTION. These digestive enzymes have been classified according to the substances upon which they act. One of the enzymes that helps to digest CARBOHYDRATES is ptyalin, which is secreted by the salivary glands. Ptyalin begins to break down starches while they are still in the mouth. Another one, lactase, reduces the sugar in milk to glucose molecules, which in this form can be absorbed into the bloodstream from the small intestine. PROTEINS are reduced to simpler forms by pepsin, secreted in the stomach. Trypsin, produced in the pancreas, flows through a duct into the small intestine, where it, too, acts upon proteins. Other enzymes in the pancreatic juice break down FATS and starches.

EPHEDRINE   A substance used in the treatment of nasal congestion, bronchial ASTHMA, and HAY FEVER. Ephedrine (pronounced i·fed′rin) is also employed to dilate the pupil of the eye in eye examinations. See also DECONGESTANT.

EPIDEMIC   An outbreak of a communicable disease that affects a large number of persons within an area at the same time. When the disease is unusually widespread in terms of geographic area or of proportion of the population contracting it, it is known as a pandemic. The influenza epidemic of 1918, which took the lives of vast numbers of persons in many countries, was a pandemic. A disease may also be endemic—that is, it may occur fairly persistently in a certain region.

EPIDERMIS   The outermost layer of the SKIN.

EPIGLOTTIS   A yellowish, leaf-shaped flap of fibrous cartilage that slants upward behind the root of the tongue. During swallowing, the epiglottis is pressed against the opening to the LARYNX and prevents solids and liquids from entering the TRACHEA (windpipe).

EPILEPSY   A chronic disorder of the nervous system in which there is periodic loss of consciousness accompanied by convulsive seizures. The convulsions are usually not harmful. With the help of medication, most seizures can be brought under control or prevented.

Causes: Epilepsy may be the result of brain injury or brain infection; occasionally a brain tumor is responsible. Often, however, it is impossible to de-

tect a specific cause, and the condition is called idiopathic epilepsy. There appears to be a slight hereditary tendency to epilepsy.

Types of Seizure: The severest and commonest type of seizure is called grand mal. It is sometimes preceded by an aura (pronounced awr′a), a sensation that recurs before each attack but differs from person to person. The epileptic may fall to the ground unconscious and have convulsions. He may salivate at the mouth; bite his lips, cheek, or tongue; and become incontinent. The seizure lasts only a few minutes.

Petit mal is the name of a lesser type of seizure. This is generally seen in children, who may outgrow it. The youngster suddenly seems to be daydreaming or absentminded. There may be slight twitching, but no falling or convulsions. The attack is over in seconds.

A third type, the PSYCHOMOTOR seizure, is marked by restlessness, loss of memory, and repeated, purposeless behavior, such as wandering around aimlessly or picking at a part of the clothing.

Epilepsy is diagnosed by the symptoms, as well as by ELECTROENCEPHALOGRAMS, skull X rays, and other tests.

Treatment: If a person has a convulsion, he should be placed on the ground, away from any obstacle on which he might injure himself. A soft, rolled-up handkerchief or similar object should be placed in one side of his mouth between the teeth to keep him from biting his tongue or lips. Turn him on his side, in case he should vomit. If one seizure follows another, call a physician or get the patient to a hospital.

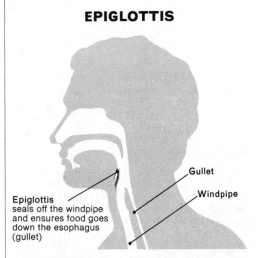

EPIGLOTTIS

Gullet

Windpipe

Epiglottis seals off the windpipe and ensures food goes down the esophagus (gullet)

To prevent swallowed food from going down the windpipe and causing choking, a flap of cartilage called the epiglottis swings across and diverts the food down the esophagus (gullet).

EPINEPHRINE Another name for ADRENALINE, a hormone secreted by the adrenal glands. (Pronounced ep"*i*·nef'rin.)

EPISIOTOMY A small incision at the edge of the vagina, running toward but at a slight angle away from the rectum. Performed during the last stage of childbirth, an episiotomy is employed to enlarge the vaginal opening so that the tissues will not tear, and the baby may pass through more easily and safely. An episiotomy (*e*·pee"zee·ot'*o*·mee) is usually performed under anesthetic. After the baby has been born, the incision is sewn up in natural layers.

EPITHELIUM A layer or layers of cells that form part of the sense organs and the glands, and produce secretions. The MUCOUS MEMBRANES and the skin are formed by the epithelium (pronounced ep"*i*·thee'lee·*um*).

EPSOM SALTS The popular name of magnesium sulfate, a bitter white crystalline salt that is used as a purgative, or CATHARTIC.

ERECTION The rigid, swollen state of the PENIS when filled with blood. Normally, this organ is soft and relatively short. However, under the influence of stimulation, either mental or physical, blood rushes into the arteries of the penis. The erectile tissue of the organ is dilated by the blood, causing the penis to grow longer and become hard and erect. In its erect state the penis is able to penetrate the female VAGINA. (See COITUS.)

Inability to have an erection is a sign of IMPOTENCE. This should not be confused with STERILITY, which is the inability to produce offspring.

ERYSIPELAS A painful, infectious disease of the skin, produced by STREPTOCOCCUS bacteria. A dark red, patchy inflammation, especially on the face, is one of the most striking symptoms of the disorder. The skin is as hot as it looks—probably the reason that the disease is sometimes called Saint Anthony's fire. The person has fever and headache, and vomits.

Erysipelas (pronounced er"*i*·sip'*e*·las) is quickly brought under control by ANTIBIOTICS. A physician should be contacted at the first appearance of the disorder.

ERYTHEMA Abnormal redness of the skin, produced by an accumulation of blood in the capillaries. Erythema (pronounced er"*i*·thee'm*a*) may be a sign of inflammation or infection.

ERYTHROBLASTOSIS FETALIS A relatively uncommon blood disease of the newborn. (Pronounced i·rith"roh·bla·stoh'sis fee·ta'lis.) It is caused by the RH FACTOR.

When an Rh-negative woman marries an Rh-positive man, their children usually inherit the father's Rh factor. This may provoke the formation of antibodies in the mother. The antibodies may pass into the baby's bloodstream through the placental membrane, producing erythroblastosis fetalis.

Only one in 25 children born to Rh-negative mothers and Rh-positive fathers has the disease. It seldom occurs in the first pregnancy and may be prevented in a later pregnancy by a special gamma globulin preparation given to the mother. If an infant with erythroblastosis fetalis is given an exchange transfusion of Rh-negative blood, the outlook for recovery is good.

ERYTHROCYTE A red blood cell. (Pronounced i·rith'ro·siet".) These cells carry oxygen and nutrients to the cells of the body and also help remove carbon dioxide from them. They owe their color to HEMOGLOBIN, an iron-rich pigment. See also BLOOD.

ERYTHROMYCIN An antibiotic that is much like PENICILLIN in its action. Erythromycin (pronounced i·rith"roh·mie'sin) is used in the control of infections by STREPTOCOCCI and other bacteria, and by some special forms of viruses.

ESOPHAGOSCOPY Examination of the ESOPHAGUS, the tube connecting the throat and the stomach. Esophagoscopy (pronounced i·sof"*a*·gos'ko·pee) is performed with an esophagoscope, a slender tube about 18 inches in length, with an electric light and a lens. The physician inserts it into the esophagus and moves it gradually downward toward the stomach while he views the interior. The esophagoscope is also used to remove objects stuck in the esophagus.

ESOPHAGUS A 10-inch-long muscular tube extending from the PHARYNX to the stomach. At the upper end of the esophagus (pronounced i·sof*'a*·gus) there is a ring of muscle—called a sphincter—that keeps the esophagus closed. When food has been chewed, it is pushed back into the pharynx. The sphincter relaxes, opening the esophagus, and the food is forced down into it by muscular contraction. In five to 10 seconds the food comes to the end of the tube. There, another sphincter, the cardiac sphincter, relaxes, allowing the food to pass into the stomach. See also DIGESTION.

ESTROGEN The general term for the female SEX HORMONES, which are produced chiefly in the OVARIES. There are a number of different kinds of estrogens (pronounced es'tro·jenz), including estrone, estriol, and estradiol. Estrogens are the substances that are responsible for the maturation of a woman's sexual organs, the development of her breasts, and her rounded form and high voice.

Estrogens are secreted in particular abundance during OVULATION. They stimulate the uterus to prepare for pregnancy, causing a thickening of the

ESOPHAGUS

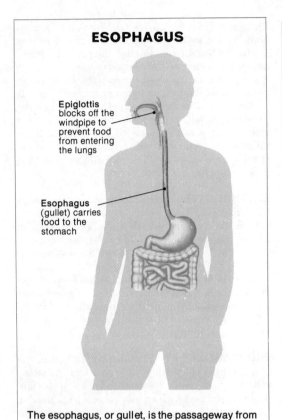

Epiglottis blocks off the windpipe to prevent food from entering the lungs

Esophagus (gullet) carries food to the stomach

The esophagus, or gullet, is the passageway from the throat that carries swallowed food to the stomach. It lies behind the windpipe in the neck.

lining and enrichment of the blood supply. If conception occurs, the estrogens also stimulate growth of the milk glands.

Estrogens are produced synthetically and sometimes used in the treatment of female disorders. They may also be used to alleviate the symptoms, both physical and emotional, of the MENOPAUSE. However, physicians prescribe estrogens with extreme care because of studies showing a link between estrogen therapy and the development of uterine cancer.

ESTRONE A female hormone, or ESTROGEN. (Pronounced es'trohn.)

ETHER An ANESTHETIC used to produce loss of sensation, so that surgery may be performed painlessly. Ether (pronounced ee'ther) is a general anesthetic that renders the patient unconscious, often for a long period of time. The patient breathes it in through a tube attached to a cone or a face mask. Generally, ether is given only after the patient has been made unconscious by an injection of a fast-acting drug, such as a BARBITURATE.

Many other anesthetics have been developed since ether was first introduced, in the mid-19th century, so that it is not as widely used as it once was. See also ANESTHETIC.

ETHYLENE A colorless gas used as an ANESTHETIC. (Pronounced eth'i·leen".)

ETIOLOGY The cause, or the study of the causes, of a disease. (Pronounced ee"tee·ol'e·jee.)

EUGENICS The science that deals with the planning of human mating and reproduction for the purpose of improving the mental and physical qualities that are passed on from generation to generation. Eugenics (pronounced yoo·jen'iks) takes into account the fact that various severe defects, such as bone and blood abnormalities, are inherited. It can predict how often defective children will be produced from mating between members of two families exhibiting certain hereditary weaknesses. However, there is much that science does not know about heredity. Many abnormalities—for instance, some types of mental deficiencies—are transmitted as RECESSIVE traits for a number of generations and only show themselves from time to time.

EUPHORIA A feeling of comfort and well-being, particularly one that does not have a basis in an individual's general circumstances and condition. Alcohol, taken in small quantities, may produce a sensation of euphoria (pronounced yoo·fawr'ee·a). A decided feeling of well-being and escape from reality may also result from taking certain drugs, such as the AMPHETAMINES.

EUSTACHIAN TUBE One of two tubes connecting the middle ear to the PHARYNX at the back of the throat. The Eustachian (pronounced yoo·stay'kee·an) tube helps to equalize air pressure on both sides of the eardrum. See also EAR.

EUTHANASIA The act of causing or enabling someone to die painlessly. Euthanasia (pronounced yoo"tha·nay'zha), also known as mercy killing, has many advocates. They maintain that incurably ill people have a right to be spared prolonged suffering. Some opponents of euthanasia have religious objections; and some emphasize its possible dangers to aged persons and the mentally disturbed. Euthanasia poses an ethical paradox for physicians; they do what they can to keep their patients alive, while doing everything in their power to relieve the discomfort of the person for whom there is no hope. Recently there has been much controversy over the increased ability of medical science to keep individuals alive even after they have suffered apparently irreversible brain damage.

EXACERBATION In medical usage, an intensification of the severity of a disease or its symptoms. (Pronounced ig·zas"er·bay'shun.)

EXCISION   The action or procedure of cutting something out (see DEBRIDEMENT); the surgical removal of a part, such as a portion of a limb or organ. (Pronounced ik·sizh′un.)

EXCORIATION   A raw, scraped area of the skin or of a mucous membrane. (Pronounced ik·skawr″ee·ay′sun.)

EXCRETION   The elimination of waste matter from the body. Sweat, carbon dioxide, urine, and feces are eliminated by the process of excretion.

EXFOLIATION   The shedding or peeling off of dead skin. (Pronounced eks·foh″lee·ay′shun.)

EXHIBITIONISM   Indecent exposure of the body for the purpose of sexual stimulation. Exhibitionism is a form of PERVERSION, or sexual deviation, requiring psychiatric help.

EXOCARDIA   Congenital displacement of the heart. The condition is also known as ectocardia. (Pronounced ek″soh·kahr′dee·a.)

EXOPHTHALMOS   A condition in which the eyeball protrudes abnormally. Sometimes exophthalmos (pronounced ek″sof·thal′mos) is the result of a tumor in back of the eyeball or of an infection. More usually, however, it is a side effect of hyperthyroidism (overactivity of the THYROID GLAND). This disease is often referred to as exophthalmic goiter. The condition can be partially relieved by administering a chemical or radioactive iodine, or by surgical removal of part of the overactive thyroid gland.

EXPECTORANT   A medicine that promotes expectoration, or the discharge of sputum from the respiratory tract. It is often helpful to take an expectorant (pronounced ik·spek′tor·ant) in disorders such as bronchitis, in which there is an accumulation of dried or sticky mucus in the air passages.

EXPLORATORY   A medical term used to describe an examination for the purpose of diagnosing a physical condition. It commonly refers to a surgical operation. If the cause of the trouble is found during the operation, it is frequently possible to correct it at that very time.

EXTREMITY   See ARM; LEG.

EXTROVERT   A person who is mainly interested in things outside himself. (Pronounced eks′tro·vurt.) By contrast, the INTROVERT is a somewhat withdrawn person who prefers to be by himself and is largely concerned with his inner life. The concept of these two basic psychological types was developed by Carl Jung (1875–1961), a Swiss psychiatrist.

Actually, it is no simple matter to classify human beings as extroverts or introverts. Each of us has certain traits of both types. However, there is usually more of one type in most of us.

EXUDATE   A fluid containing white blood cells that escapes into inflamed or injured tissue from a blood vessel. (Pronounced eks′yood·ayt″.)

EYE   The organ of sight, or *vision*. The eyeball is a sphere set in a bony socket called the orbit, and protected above by the ridge of the brow.

The outer layer of the eye, which we see as the white, is the *sclera*. The *cornea*, a transparent membrane in the middle of the white, helps to focus the rays of light entering the eye. The colored portion of the eye, the *iris*, is a muscle; in its center is the *pupil*, actually an opening in the eye that admits light. The iris dilates or contracts the pupil, just as does the iris diaphragm of a camera, thus controlling the amount of light entering the eye. In back of the iris, the crystalline *lens* receives the light rays and continually changes its shape to assist in focusing, changes known as accommodation.

The inner layer of the eye is a cup-shaped membrane called the *retina*. It is an intricate structure of

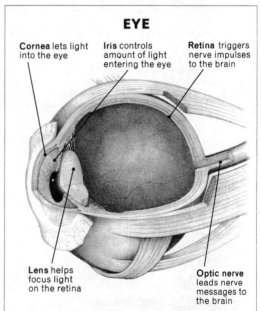

EYE

Cornea lets light into the eye

Iris controls amount of light entering the eye

Retina triggers nerve impulses to the brain

Lens helps focus light on the retina

Optic nerve leads nerve messages to the brain

Light enters the eye through the transparent cornea at the front and is then focused by the lens onto the retina, the light-sensitive surface on the inside of the eyeball. The size of the pupil, the hole in the center of the colored iris, changes automatically to control the amount of light passing through it. In the retina, light triggers nerve cells which pass nerve impulses along the optic nerve to the brain, where they give rise to the sensation of sight.

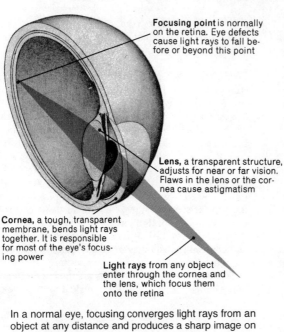

Focusing point is normally on the retina. Eye defects cause light rays to fall before or beyond this point

Lens, a transparent structure, adjusts for near or far vision. Flaws in the lens or the cornea cause astigmatism

Cornea, a tough, transparent membrane, bends light rays together. It is responsible for most of the eye's focusing power

Light rays from any object enter through the cornea and the lens, which focus them onto the retina

In a normal eye, focusing converges light rays from an object at any distance and produces a sharp image on the retina. The cornea is mainly responsible for focusing, but the lens adjusts for near and far vision. However, in a subnormal eye, poor focusing power converges light rays at points which are not on the retina, causing blurred vision. Faulty focusing may be due to irregularities in the shape of the eye, which cause far or near sight, or defects in the cornea and the lens, which cause astigmatism. Eyeglasses improve vision by compensating for the inability to focus properly.

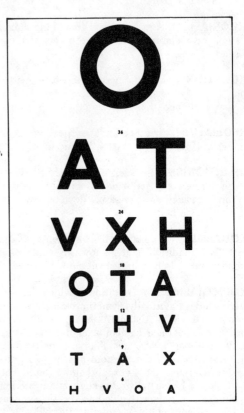

Eye-chart tests are used by optometrists to measure the ability to distinguish detail at a distance.

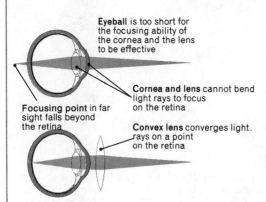

Eyeball is too short for the focusing ability of the cornea and the lens to be effective

Cornea and lens cannot bend light rays to focus on the retina

Focusing point in far sight falls beyond the retina

Convex lens converges light rays on a point on the retina

A person with far sight can see distant objects more clearly than near ones. This condition, which is known as hypermetropia, is caused by the eyeball being too short for the focusing ability of the lens and the cornea. As a result, light rays fall beyond the retina. Far sight can be corrected by eyeglasses with convex, or converging, lenses.

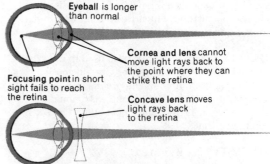

Eyeball is longer than normal

Cornea and lens cannot move light rays back to the point where they can strike the retina

Focusing point in short sight fails to reach the retina

Concave lens moves light rays back to the retina

A person with short sight can see clearly only nearby objects; distant objects appear out of focus. This condition, which is known as myopia, is caused by the eyeball being longer than normal. As a result, light rays are focused on a point that is in front of the retina. Short sight can be corrected by spectacles with concave, or diverging, lenses.

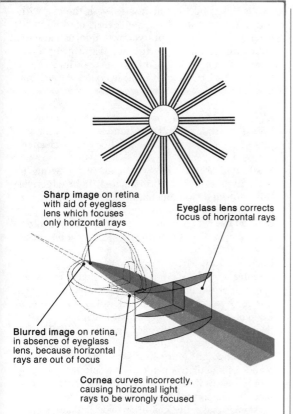

Sharp image on retina with aid of eyeglass lens which focuses only horizontal rays

Eyeglass lens corrects focus of horizontal rays

Blurred image on retina, in absence of eyeglass lens, because horizontal rays are out of focus

Cornea curves incorrectly, causing horizontal light rays to be wrongly focused

Astigmatism makes it impossible to focus simultaneously on objects that are at an angle to each other, as in the illustration of horizontal and vertical objects above. An astigmatic person looking at the spoked chart may find the horizontal lines blurred, whereas the vertical ones are in sharp focus. Eyeglasses with specially shaped lenses correct this.

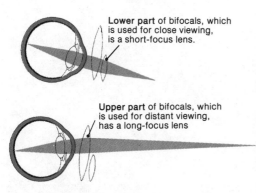

Lower part of bifocals, which is used for close viewing, is a short-focus lens.

Upper part of bifocals, which is used for distant viewing, has a long-focus lens

As people get older, their eye lenses lose elasticity and the ability to focus clearly. This condition is called presbyopia, and can be corrected by using bifocal eyeglasses, which have upper and lower parts. The upper part of the eyeglasses is used for focusing on distant objects; and the lower part for seeing clearly objects that are close at hand.

vast numbers of nerve endings in the form of rods and cones. They pick up light rays and convert them into nerve impulses. The cones are sensitive to color. Cone deficiency is the most common cause of COLOR BLINDNESS. The cones and rods lead to cells that are connected to the optic nerve, which ends in the brain. Here the impulses received from both retinas are fused into a single image.

The complex structure of the eye is only suggested here. Much of the eyeball in back of the crystalline lens is a semifluid mass, the *vitreous body* (vitreous humor). The tear glands in the upper part of the eye socket produce a liquid that cleanses the eye; it contains lysozyme, an enzyme that combats bacteria. Tears drain through a channel that leads to the nose and thence to the throat; this accounts for the runny nose associated with crying, and for the fact that you may *taste* eye drops.

Defects and Disorders: Deviations in the shape of the eye or its structures produce nearsightedness (MYOPIA), farsightedness (HYPEROPIA), and ASTIGMATISM. (See REFRACTION.) These conditions may be corrected by wearing EYEGLASSES. Like other organs, the eye may be infected and injured. (See EYE INFECTION; EYE INJURY.) Serious diseases of the eye include CATARACT, a clouding of the crystalline lens that blocks the passage of light; GLAUCOMA, a condition produced by pressure within the eyeball; and DETACHED RETINA, in which the retina becomes separated from its bed.

EYE CARE Our eyes are a priceless treasure and should be treated accordingly. It is important not to abuse them by reading or writing in a poor light. When possible, the light should be a little above and behind the shoulder. After you have been reading steadily for a while, look up from the text and into the distance; this provides relief for tired eye muscles. See also EYEGLASSES.

Foreign Bodies in the Eye: Dust, cinders, or other foreign bodies are often caught under the eyelid. Before attempting to remove such objects, wash the hands with soap and hot water. Now lift the lid by the lashes. The object will usually be visible on the inner lid and should be removed promptly with a twist of sterile cotton. Do not rub the eye. Rubbing the other eye will cause both eyes to tear and may help in removal of the object. If the difficulty persists and is painful, visit a physician. See also FIRST AID section.

EYEGLASSES Devices that correct or improve poor vision. The lenses are made of glass or plastic and are ground to a shape suitable to help overcome the defect.

Eye Examinations: The eyes should be examined at least every two years. Children's eyes should be examined early, because certain eye defects, such as AMBLYOPIA (dimness of vision), become much more difficult to correct after early childhood.

An OPHTHALMOLOGIST is a doctor of medicine, and so can not only prescribe glasses or contact lenses but can also examine the eyes for the presence of disease and treat them. In most states an OPTOMETRIST is licensed only to examine eyes in order to prescribe glasses or contact lenses.

Lenses and Glasses: Three common defects, produced by deviations in the shape or structure of the eyes (see REFRACTION), are nearsightedness (MYOPIA), farsightedness (HYPEROPIA), and ASTIGMATISM. These defects are corrected by lenses ground to different shapes—respectively, concave, convex, and cylindrical—which bring the image into sharp focus on the retina. Bifocal lenses are two different lenses combined in one frame, the top one for distance viewing, the bottom one for close work. CONTACT LENSES are tiny lenses fitted to the corneas.

EYE INFECTION If the eye is painful, persistently pink, swollen, or otherwise troublesome, an infection may be present and you should bring the condition to the attention of your family physician.

Sty: Sometimes bacteria infect the glands of the eyelid or the roots of the eyelashes. The result is often a swelling, or cyst, filled with pus. Apply a moist, warm compress to the eye for about a quarter of an hour every three hours. This helps to bring the sty to a head so that it opens and the pus escapes. If this treatment is not effective after several days, see a doctor. See also separate entry, STY.

Conjunctivitis: The conjunctiva is the membrane covering the inner eyelids and the outer surface of the eyeball. When this membrane is infected, the eyeball appears red, and the lids become sticky and swollen. A good treatment is to wash the eye with warm water, using a tissue, every morning and evening, and then apply yellow oxide of mercury ophthalmic ointment to the lid. Warm compresses should also be placed on the eye several times a day. If the infection does not clear up quickly, see your doctor. See also separate entry, CONJUNCTIVITIS.

EYE INJURY Many needless injuries occur to the eyes. If there are small children about, it is important to keep sharp objects and household cleaners out of their reach.

Black Eye: Wet a cloth with cold water, wring it out, and press it on the bruised area. To be effective, this must be done immediately after the injury. See also separate entry, BLACK EYE.

Blow on the Eye: A blow may damage the eye internally. Apply a cold compress and get to a doctor as soon as possible.

Chemical Burn: The essential measure is to wash the chemical out of the eye instantly. Hold the eye wide open under running water. Lift the upper and lower lids to be sure that water penetrates under them. Keep flushing the eye for at least five minutes. See a doctor as soon as possible. See also FIRST AID section.

Eye Wound: An injury that perforates the eye demands immediate medical attention. Nothing should be applied to the eyes before the doctor is seen. It is important to reduce eye movements, since they may make the condition worse. Place sterile gauze on each eye and run a bandage gently around the head to hold the gauzes in position over the eyes.

F

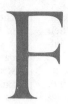

FAHRENHEIT The temperature scale commonly used in the United States. (Pronounced far'en·heit''). The term is usually shortened to "F" when a particular temperature is given. Thus, normal body temperature is about 98.6°F. More widely used in other parts of the world and in scientific work is the CELSIUS scale.

FAINTING Falling unconscious, generally for a very brief period. Fainting is usually caused by a decrease in the amount of blood—and thus in the quantity of oxygen—reaching the brain. The medical name for fainting is syncope.

Certain symptoms usually precede a fainting spell. The individual feels light-headed and weak, and the color goes out of his face; he may feel as though he is falling asleep. To increase the flow of oxygen to the brain, have the person sit down immediately, spread his legs apart, and lean over until his head is between his knees. He should keep this position for a few minutes and then straighten up. As an alternative, if there is a bed available, he should lie down.

When a person has fainted, he should be placed on his back and his legs elevated above his head. Constricting parts of his clothing should be loosened. If he is indoors, open the window to provide better air circulation. Never force an unconscious person to drink anything. If aromatic spirits of ammonia or smelling salts are available, hold them under his nose, or else apply cold water to his face. In several minutes, he should regain consciousness. When he does, keep him lying down for 10 minutes; then he should get up slowly. If he fails to revive, the condition may be more than a simple fainting spell, and a doctor should be summoned without delay. See also UNCONSCIOUSNESS.

FALLEN ARCH A foot condition produced by walking on the inside of the lengthwise arch instead of on the sole. In time, the weight of the body on the ligaments of the inside of the FOOT may cause considerable pain.

A fallen arch is quite different from a FLATFOOT. If you think you have either, consult your doctor.

Fallen arches are corrected by wearing shoes with built-in arches. These should be purchased only after a careful examination by your physician, who may prescribe them. He will also prescribe exercises; if you do these faithfully, they can help the condition considerably.

FALLOPIAN TUBE One of two tubes, each about 4½ inches long, which connect the UTERUS to an ovary situated on either side of the abdomen. Also known as oviducts, the Fallopian (pronounced fa·loh'pee·an) tubes play an important part in the fertilization of an egg cell.

About midway between two menstrual periods, an unfertilized EGG CELL, or ovum, is released from an ovary and is moved slowly toward the uterus by contractions of the muscular wall of the tube. The ovum can be fertilized only if it unites with a SPERM CELL while it is moving through the tube. PREGNANCY follows when the fertilized ovum reaches the uterus and becomes implanted in the wall of the uterus. In some instances implantation takes place within the Fallopian tube, resulting in an ECTOPIC PREGNANCY.

FALLOPIAN TUBE

Fallopian tube leads an egg from the ovary to the uterus

Ovary from which egg is released

Uterus

..A woman has two Fallopian tubes, or oviducts, one connecting each ovary to the top of the uterus. Once a month, an ovary releases an egg, which passes along one tube and into the uterus. Tying off or cutting the tubes, an operation called salpingectomy, blocks the passages for eggs and so is a method of sterilization.

FALSE LABOR PAINS Pains resembling those of labor felt by a pregnant woman (or by a woman who believes herself pregnant), but not caused by the actual start of labor in CHILDBIRTH.

FAMILY PLANNING Control by individual couples of the number and spacing of births in their family; also called birth control or planned parenthood. For most parents, family planning involves the regular practice of methods to avoid conception. (See CONTRACEPTIVE METHODS AND DEVICES.) For others, it involves measures to increase the chance that conception will occur. (See STERILITY.)

How many children should a couple have? This is largely a matter of private choice. Certainly they should not have more children than can be provided with adequate shelter, food, clothing, health care, education, and individual affection and attention. It should be remembered that the cost of these necessities is only partly borne by the parents. When many couples decide to have large families, even wealthy countries like the United States have difficulty in providing the rapidly increasing needs for public services of all kinds.

Family planning began as a movement to improve maternal and child health among the poor by helping women avoid unwanted pregnancies. A pioneer in birth control education in the United States was Margaret Sanger (1883–1966). Her efforts led to the establishment of birth control clinics throughout the country. Today their services are available for all aspects of family planning. The Planned Parenthood Federation of America, 810 Seventh Avenue, New York, New York 10019, will furnish information about planned parenthood groups, clinics, or centers in your locality.

FARSIGHTEDNESS See HYPEROPIA.

FAT One of the essential elements in the DIET. Fats supply energy in concentrated form. They serve to carry the fat-soluble VITAMINS A and D, and they are the chief source of vitamin E, all essential to nutrition. The digestion of fat is begun in the stomach and completed in the small intestine, where it is acted upon by the enzymes in bile.

Fats may be solid, like the fat in bacon, or liquid, like oil. Fats occur in all meats, in whole milk, and in milk products such as cheese. Butter is the practically pure fat removed from milk. Fats are also found in plant seeds, which are the source of vegetable oils.

Fats are composed of fatty acids and glycerin. Saturated fats contain more hydrogen than unsaturated fats. Research has shown that saturated fats are more likely to be harmful to your health because they contribute to an excess of CHOLESTEROL in the blood that may lead to atherosclerosis.

FATIGUE A feeling of tiredness. It may range from slight to severe; if severe, the condition may be referred to as exhaustion.
Causes: Usually, fatigue is the result of prolonged or excessive activity without obtaining sufficient rest. The failure to get enough sleep, poor diet, and other bad health habits may also produce a general sense of fatigue.

Chronic fatigue, however, may have more serious causes. Frequently it is produced by emotional strain. A person may be so deeply troubled that he is unable to eat or sleep regularly; eventually there is such a buildup of fatigue that he may suffer from mental exhaustion. In wartime combat conditions, the strain can be so intense that a PSYCHONEUROSIS or PSYCHOSIS develops. This is the condition called fatigue syndrome, or combat fatigue.

Serving as a warning signal, fatigue may be one of the first signs of an illness, such as influenza. Fatigue also occurs as a symptom in a large number of more serious disorders, among them anemia, diabetes, kidney disease, cardiac trouble, cancer, drug addiction, and dysfunction of the endocrine glands. A person who finds himself feeling tired much of the time would be well advised to have a medical checkup.

FAVUS A contagious disease of the hairy surfaces of the body. Favus (pronounced fay'vus) is caused by a FUNGUS. The skin, particularly that of the scalp, is covered with yellowish, cup-shaped crusts, and the hair may fall out. It is treated with antibiotics.

FDA The *F*ood and *D*rug *A*dministration of the U.S. Department of Health, Education, and Welfare. The FDA (pronounce each letter) and its Canadian counterpart, the Food and Drug Directorate, regulate the marketing of food, medicines, cosmetics, and veterinary preparations. Their primary purpose is to protect the health of the public. They also protect consumers from misleading advertising and labeling. Among their other responsibilities are limiting the kind and amount of preservatives and other substances that may be added to food; enforcing laws regarding the safety of cosmetic and household products; and policing the quality of standard medicines that are in general use. Also, before any newly developed medicine is introduced, both agencies must be satisfied that the medicine has no harmful side effects when used as prescribed and is effective for the use intended.

FECES The material discharged from the bowels; also called the stool. Feces (pronounced fee'seez) consist not only of indigestible food residues, but also of various body secretions (chiefly from the liver), mucus and worn-out cells from the intestinal lining, and bacteria that are normally present in the intestines.

FEEBLEMINDEDNESS A term used at one time by psychologists to indicate the least severe degree of MENTAL RETARDATION; feeblemindedness ranged from low normal intelligence down to an adult mental capacity that would be normal in a seven-year-old.

FELON See NAIL; PARONYCHIA. (Pronounced fel'en.)

FEMININE HYGIENE See DOUCHE.

FEMUR The thighbone. The femur (pronounced fee'mer) is the longest, largest, and strongest bone in the human body. See also LEG.

FERTILIZATION The union of the SPERM CELL and the EGG CELL, or ovum. This usually occurs in the FALLOPIAN TUBE. See also EMBRYO.

FETUS (foetus) The unborn infant, two months or more after the beginning of pregnancy. (Pronounced fee'tus.) From conception to the end of the second month, the infant is usually described as an EMBRYO. By the third month most of the unborn baby's organs are fairly well developed; by the sixth month, these organs are capable of normal functioning. The heart is already pumping blood in the third month.

By the seventh month the baby reaches half the weight it will have at birth, and by the eighth

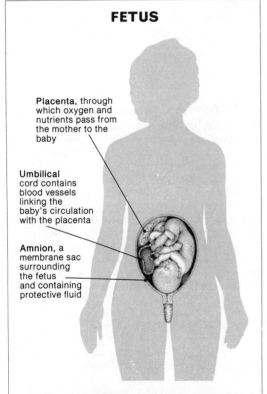

FETUS

Placenta, through which oxygen and nutrients pass from the mother to the baby

Umbilical cord contains blood vessels linking the baby's circulation with the placenta

Amnion, a membrane sac surrounding the fetus and containing protective fluid

In medical terms, a developing baby in the uterus is known as a fetus only from the ninth week until the end of pregnancy; before that time it is called an embryo. However, the term fetus is commonly used to mean any unborn baby.

month, three-quarters of that weight. An adequate diet is especially important for the mother at this time to provide the calcium, protein, vitamins, and other nutrients needed by the vigorously growing fetus.

FEVER An abnormal rise in BODY TEMPERATURE; also known as pyrexia. It is most often the result of viral or bacterial infection and is an important clue to the seriousness of the condition.

Temperature is measured with a THERMOMETER of either the oral or rectal type. When the temperature rises above 100°F on the oral thermometer, the individual is febrile, or running a fever. When the fever reaches 101°F, a doctor should be consulted.

Other Symptoms: Fever usually occurs in combination with other symptoms. While the temperature is still rising, the person's skin is often dry and he feels a chill. He may feel very weak and light-headed. Often, he has an ache in the joints. His pulse rate increases. The febrile individual loses his appetite, and he may be constipated. When he begins to perspire, it is a sign that the temperature is falling.

Treatment: For the person running a slight fever, the doctor may advise taking ASPIRIN several times a day to help bring down the temperature. Encourage the individual to drink water and juices. For the person with a high fever (104°F or more), sponging the forehead with alcohol may provide relief. The doctor may prescribe an ANTIBIOTIC or SULFONAMIDE, depending on the cause of the fever. The individual should be given something light to eat, to help maintain his strength.

FEVER BLISTER See FEVER SORE.

FEVER SORE One of the common names, along with cold sore and fever blister, for an acute viral infection known medically as herpes simplex, which is caused by a virus called Herpes Simplex Virus Type 1. The infection tends to break out repeatedly in people who carry the virus in their skin. The first symptom is a stinging, burning sensation on the skin of the face, usually about the mouth or on the lips. After a day or two, small clusters of blisters form on the face. The blisters usually dry up in less than 10 days. They should be left alone, and a doctor or dermatologist should be consulted. See also HERPES SIMPLEX.

FIBROBLAST A type of long, flat cell present in connective TISSUE. (Pronounced fie'bre·blast.)

FIBROID TUMOR (fibroid) A benign TUMOR made up mainly of fibrous tissue, especially one growing in the muscle fibers of the walls of the UTERUS. There may be only a single large tumor or a scattering of small ones. Sometimes a fibroid (pronounced fie'broyd) enlarges to the point that it causes the uterus to press on neighboring organs and to interfere with their normal functions. Fibroids may also cause menstrual disturbances such as pain, irregular menstrual periods, and profuse bleeding; they can interfere with pregnancy.

Doctors usually prefer to leave small fibroids alone if they cause no trouble. Large fibroids may have to be removed by surgery. In some cases, it may be necessary to perform a HYSTERECTOMY.

FIBULA One of the two long bones between the ankle and the kneecap. See LEG. (Pronounced fib'ye·la.)

FILARIASIS See ELEPHANTIASIS. (Pronounced fil"a·rie'a·sis.)

FINGER See HAND.

FINGERNAIL See NAIL.

FIRST AID These are major emergency first aid situations:
Bleeding—Severe
Breathing Stopped
Poisoning
Shock—How to Treat It
Other life-threatening emergencies include:
Bites—Snake
Burns
Carbon-Monoxide Poisoning
Childbirth—Emergency
Choking on an Obstruction
Convulsions
Electric Shock
Heart Attack
Heat Exhaustion and Sunstroke
Moving an Injured Person
Stomach Pain—Appendicitis
Stroke
Should any occur, see the FIRST AID section.

FISSURE A groove or deep fold in an organ, or a break in the skin or a membrane. A fissure (pronounced fish'ur) may occur in the rectum as a complication of constipation or HEMORRHOIDS. Rectal fissures are usually accompanied by a sharp, burning sensation that may be very painful during and following a bowel movement.

FISTULA An abnormal passage connecting two hollow organs or a hollow organ and the body surface. It may be CONGENITAL, or it may develop from a FISSURE, an ABSCESS, or some other abnormal condition in a tissue. Secretions, pus, or waste products are sometimes passed through the abnormal passage. The fistula (pronounced fis'choo·la) may become infected, and the infection may spread to other parts of the body. The condition may be extremely sensitive or painful. It requires prompt medical attention.

FIT A popular term for CONVULSION.

FLATFOOT A condition in which the whole sole rests flat on the ground, because the arch of the instep has flattened. A solid footprint made on soft earth by a FOOT is a sign of a flatfoot; a foot with a sound arch leaves a raised area in the print on the side with the big toe.

A flatfoot is sometimes a hereditary trait. It may also be the result of being overweight or of standing for long periods without good foot support. In the event of painful symptoms, the physician prescribes an arch support and exercise to strengthen the ligaments of the foot and help correct the condition. The feet of children, in particular, should be examined to see if they are flattening.

FLATULENCE An uncomfortable accumulation of air or GAS in the stomach or the intestines. The discomfort may usually be relieved by forcing the excess gas out through the mouth (BELCHING) or the anus. Flatulence (pronounced flach'yu·lens) in the stomach may be caused by excessive drinking of carbonated beverages. Often it is caused by a nervous habit of swallowing air. Intestinal flatulence sometimes accompanies mucous COLITIS.

Sometimes intestinal flatulence follows the eating of gas-producing foods. These include most raw fruits and vegetables, sugar in large quantities, beans, fried foods, nuts, and spices.

FLU See INFLUENZA.

FLUORIDATION The addition of a small amount of FLUORIDE to public water supplies for the purpose of preventing DENTAL CARIES in children. The amount added is about one part of fluoride per million parts of water.

Fluoridation is known to reduce the amount of tooth decay in all children in a community, including those whose parents have not the means to provide adequate dental care. In the few communities where the water supply is rich in natural fluoride, no ill-effects from fluoride are evident. However, there is evidence that, for some very specialized uses, fluoridated water may be harmful. In artificial-kidney machines, for example, the use of fluoridated water may result in a harmful concentration of fluoride in the patient's tissues.

If your water supply is fluoridated, you should not be uneasy about using water in the ordinary way. If your water supply is not fluoridated, your dentist should be consulted about other methods to prevent dental decay.

FLUORIDE A compound of the chemical element fluorine and another element, such as sodium or potassium. A compound of tin and fluorine—stannous fluoride—is used in certain toothpastes. See also FLUORIDATION.

FLAT FEET

Arch in normal foot

Arch in flat foot

Print of normal foot at rest

Print of flat foot at rest

Weak or fallen arches in the feet, often found in people who are overweight, cause flat feet. Instead of the ball of the foot and the heel carrying most of the weight, the arch of the instep makes firm contact with the shoe or the ground, as revealed by the broad shape of the footprints.

FLUOROSCOPE An instrument that permits direct X-RAY examination without taking and developing X-ray photographs. A fluoroscope (pronounced floor′o·skohp″) is simply a projection screen coated with chemicals that glow when X rays strike them. By using a fluoroscope rather than a camera in X-ray examinations, the doctor can instantly observe internal organs in motion.

FOLIC ACID See VITAMIN.

FOLLICLE A very small cavity or sac that occurs in many parts of the body. A follicle (pronounced fol′i·kel) has various forms and functions. Hair follicles are tiny cylindrical depressions in the skin, from each of which a single hair grows. In the ovary, each EGG CELL (ovum) is enclosed in a membrane; egg cell and membrane make up a Graafian follicle.

FOLLICULITIS Inflammation and the formation of PUSTULES due to bacterial infection of individual hair FOLLICLES. Folliculitis (pronounced fo·lik′yu·lie″tis) is most likely to occur on areas of the skin that are frequently shaved. Chronic cases are commonly called barber's itch—the medical term is "sycosis vulgaris." There may be considerable itching and burning, and gradual enlargement of the inflamed area. Scar tissue may form. If the infection does not clear up, see a doctor for special treatment.

FOMENTATION A warm, pulpy mass applied to the outside of the body to relieve pain and inflammation. Various substances are used. The mustard plaster is a fomentation (pronounced foh″men·tay′shun), or poultice.

FONTANEL Any of the soft areas on a baby's head where the skull bones have not yet fused. There are normally six fontanels (pronounced fon″ta·nelz′). The largest, about an inch across, is at the top of the head. Another is toward the rear, and there are two more on each side, one at the temple and one behind the ear. The fontanels usually close and harden by the time the baby is 18 months old. (See illustration on next page.)

FOOD AND NUTRITION See DIET.

FOOD POISONING Acute illness resulting from eating contaminated food. Food poisoning should always be suspected if several persons at the same time suddenly develop such symptoms as nausea, vomiting, diarrhea, and pain or tenderness in the abdomen. The symptoms may develop shortly after the food is eaten, or they may be delayed for 24 hours or more. Call the doctor at once if food poisoning is suspected.

Although most cases of food poisoning are caused by BACTERIA, there are also nonbacterial forms.

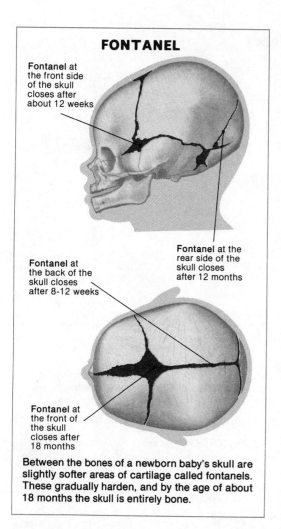

FONTANEL

Fontanel at the front side of the skull closes after about 12 weeks

Fontanel at the rear side of the skull closes after 12 months

Fontanel at the back of the skull closes after 8-12 weeks

Fontanel at the front of the skull closes after 18 months

Between the bones of a newborn baby's skull are slightly softer areas of cartilage called fontanels. These gradually harden, and by the age of about 18 months the skull is entirely bone.

Nonbacterial food poisoning can result from eating poisonous mushrooms, plants, or berries mistakenly thought to be edible. Acute or chronic poisoning can develop from eating residues of insecticide and other sprays on fruits and vegetables. Never eat anything growing wild unless you are sure it is not poisonous. Wash thoroughly any unpeeled fruits and leafy vegetables before consuming them.

Bacterial food poisoning is of two types. One type is due to food-borne bacteria infecting the system, the other to toxic substances produced by bacteria and present in the food before it is eaten.

The commonest food-borne infection is salmonellosis, caused by several kinds of bacteria belonging to the genus *Salmonella*. Shellfish growing in sewage-polluted waters or vegetables fertilized by human manure are often contaminated with such bacteria. Food may also be contaminated by human carriers during the process of handling.

A number of different bacteria cause food to spoil, and many of them produce toxic substances in the process. The commonest of these food-spoiling

bacteria are STAPHYLOCOCCI. Persons otherwise in good health usually recover from this kind of food poisoning in from one to four days.

Botulism is a serious, but fairly rare, form of food poisoning that is due to a toxin produced by the bacterium *Clostridium botulinum*. This toxin is one of the most potent poisons known; fortunately, an antitoxin has been developed. If not treated, botulism is often fatal. The organism grows slowly in food of low acid content. Home-canned food that has not been properly processed may contain dangerous amounts of the botulism toxin.

FOOT A remarkably flexible organ adapted to supporting the continually shifting weight of the body. The foot muscles work with the tendons and ligaments in momentarily holding the foot in certain positions.

The 26 bones and 33 joints in the foot are bound together by over 100 strong ligaments. The bones fall into three groups. Just below the ankle are the *tarsals*, a group of strong, compact bones that are jointed in such a way that the foot can be rotated in any direction. The tarsal bones include the strong heel bone. In front of the tarsals are the *metatarsals*, which form the framework of two flexible arches. The main arch runs lengthwise between the tarsals and the phalanges, or toe bones. The second arch runs crosswise at the ball of the foot. These arches, formed of bones, ligaments, tendons, and muscles, play an important part in walking.

The imprint of a normal foot shows that the lengthwise arch touches the ground only at the outer edge. The height of the inner part of the arch varies from person to person. The arch may be naturally rather flat (see FLATFOOT) without interfering with normal functioning. Babies generally have flatfeet, and the arch gradually becomes higher as the ligaments, tendons, and muscles strengthen with use. It is important that a child's shoes fit well so that this development is not impaired.

In adults, trouble arises when undue strain is put on the foot. Strain may be due to overweight, poor posture, fatigue, or ill-fitting shoes that prevent the foot from freely altering shape under the stresses of shifting body weight. Ill-fitting shoes are often the cause of FALLEN ARCHES and other painful conditions such as CORNS, BUNIONS, and INGROWN TOENAILS. If you have persistent foot trouble, it is advisable to consult a podiatrist, or foot doctor.

FORCEPS A hinged, two-pronged instrument used to grasp an object and then pull or compress it. Specially designed forceps (pronounced fawr'seps) are used by surgeons, obstetricians, and dentists. Obstetrical (childbirth) forceps are shaped so that they grasp a baby's head or hips firmly but without harmful pressure if the doctor finds it necessary to assist the emergence of the baby from the birth canal. See also BREECH DELIVERY. The dentist uses special short, strong forceps to grasp and extract teeth. The surgeon uses many different kinds of forceps to grasp tissue and hold it in a particular position during an operation, and also to compress blood vessels and thus control bleeding.

FORESKIN The fold of skin that covers the rounded head of the PENIS; also called the prepuce.

FORMALDEHYDE A pungent, poisonous gas that can be readily dissolved in water. The solution of water and formaldehyde (pronounced fawr·mal'de·hied") known as Formalin is a powerful DISINFECT-ANT. It should be used with great caution.

FORMULA See BOTTLE FEEDING.

FRACTURE See BROKEN BONE; also FIRST AID section.

FRECKLE A brown spot on the skin. Freckles are due to the excessive development of the pigment MELANIN by isolated clusters of skin cells when exposed to the sun. As a person grows older, the tendency to have freckles diminishes.

CHLOASMA, popularly known as liver spots, is the medical term for the light-brown patches that can occur on the skin of older persons.

FRIGIDITY In women, inability to derive pleasure from sexual relations, usually accompanied by failure to achieve an ORGASM. This may have a physical cause, such as insufficient lubrication of the genitals, or by lack of adequate stimulation of the clitoris. Rarely, it may be the result of injuries or physical abnormalities. More often, frigidity is the result of psychological factors. Failure to enjoy intercourse (COITUS) or distaste, dislike, or actual abhorrence of it can be due to fear of pregnancy or to conscious or unconscious feelings of guilt related to sex. In such cases PSYCHOTHERAPY is usually required to discover and remove the underlying cause.

FRONTAL LOBOTOMY See LOBOTOMY.

FROSTBITE Injury to the skin and the tissues under the skin by exposure to severe cold. Ears, nose, toes, and fingers are most often affected. The process of freezing is quite painless. The tissue turns numb and white and may freeze solid without the person's being aware of it. See also CHILBLAIN.
Treatment: The process of thawing out is painful, and very careful treatment is needed to avoid further damage. The person should stay in gently warm surroundings, but never near a stove or heater. Hot drinks and soup should be given if the individual feels chilly; an ANALGESIC will relieve pain.

A severe case of frostbite may lead to GANGRENE and possible loss of a limb. A doctor should be called immediately to prevent this happening. While waiting for the doctor, never massage the frozen part with the hands or with snow. Outer clothing should be removed very gently. If the toes are frostbitten, do not permit the person to walk; any pressure on frozen tissue is likely to injure it.
Prevention: Whenever you go out in freezing temperatures, take precautions against frostbite. Wear adequate, warm, dry clothing. Be sure that it is loose enough to allow free circulation of blood everywhere, including the fingers and toes. Avoid smoking when you are out in very cold weather; smoking constricts the blood vessels and increases the possibility of frostbite.

FULMINATING Occurring with great suddenness and severity. A serious condition that rapidly worsens is said to be fulminating (pronounced ful'mi·nayt"ing).

FUNCTIONAL DISEASE OR DISORDER An ailment that cannot be traced to any physical cause. When a physical cause can be found, the ailment is known as organic. See also EMOTIONAL AND MENTAL DISORDERS.

FUNGUS (plural, **fungi**) Any of a large group of organisms that includes mushrooms, molds, mildews, yeasts, and various single-celled microorganisms. Fungi occur everywhere in the soil and as tiny particles floating in the air. Most fungi are harmless, but some cause a variety of diseases in plants and animals. There are some fungi that cure disease: PENICILLIN and many other ANTIBIOTICS are obtained from fungi.
Fungal Skin Infections: Many of the disease-producing fungi affect the skin. Fungi are responsible for ATHLETE'S FOOT and different kinds of RINGWORM.

Mild cases of fungal skin infection can often be cured by good hygiene and various ointments or powders, such as DESENEX, which may be obtained from a druggist without a prescription. In stubborn or severe cases, consult a doctor.
Systemic fungus diseases (those that infect the whole system) include ACTINOMYCOSIS, BLASTOMYCOSIS, COCCIDIOIDOMYCOSIS, and MONILIASIS.

The systemic fungus diseases require medical attention. In some cases, a vaccine produced in the laboratory from the person's own body fluids is effective. The antibiotic amphotericin B, given intravenously, is effective against most systemic fungus diseases.

FURUNCLE Another name for BOIL. (Pronounced fyoor'ung·kel.)

G

GALL Another word for BILE. See GALLBLADDER.

GALLBLADDER A pear-shaped sac, 7 to 10 centimetres long, situated in the right upper part of the abdomen, under the liver. The gallbladder is a storage tank for bile produced by the liver. Fat present in the intestine stimulates the flow of bile from the gallbladder. Bile enters and leaves the gallbladder through the cystic duct, which branches off the main (common) bile duct leading from the

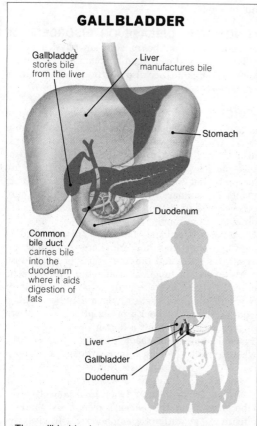

GALLBLADDER

Gallbladder stores bile from the liver

Liver manufactures bile

Stomach

Duodenum

Common bile duct carries bile into the duodenum where it aids digestion of fats

Liver

Gallbladder

Duodenum

The gallbladder is a pear-shaped sac which stores bile from the liver, and releases it into the duodenum after a meal to help with the digestion of fats. Obstruction of the bladder or its duct by gallstones prevents the flow of bile and often has to be treated by surgery. Each day the liver produces about half a litre of bile, which is stored 50 millilitres at a time in the gallbladder.

liver to the small intestine. Serious gallbladder trouble is usually treated by removing the organ surgically—it is not essential to health. The most common abnormal conditions are GALLSTONES and acute inflammation due to infection.

Acute Inflammation: Symptoms include intense pain in the upper abdomen, fever, nausea, vomiting, and extreme exhaustion. Immediate medical attention is needed. If untreated, the inflamed gallbladder may rupture or become gangrenous. Either of these complications can be fatal.

GALLSTONE A solid, pebblelike mass (CALCULUS) formed in the gallbladder, often in large numbers. The cause of the formation is not known. Autopsies show that many persons have gallstones without having had any symptoms. However, gallstones may cause chronic inflammation of the GALLBLADDER, marked by nausea and discomfort in the upper abdomen. Acute, intense pain may be experienced if a gallstone passes through the bile duct. This is especially likely to occur after a meal high in fats, which stimulate the flow of bile from the gallbladder. Sometimes a gallstone becomes lodged in the bile duct, blocking the flow of bile. If this happens, the person develops jaundice and serious inflammation of the gallbladder and the duct. Gallstones are treated by a controlled diet and medication; in some cases, surgery is required.

GAMMA GLOBULIN A protein that is found in the BLOOD PLASMA and contains many different kinds of ANTIBODIES. Antibodies are essential in combating infection; when GERMS invade the body, the antibodies go to work and help destroy them.

Gamma globulin (pronounced gam′a glob′yu·lin) serum is extensively used to produce IMMUNITY against disease. When it is extracted from a number of people and blended, it contains antibodies that can help to fight off a large number of the diseases prevalent in the region. Injections of gamma globulin are used to provide protection against some of the diseases of childhood, such as measles. The serum also has a record of effectiveness against hepatitis.

GANGLION (plural, **ganglia**) (1) In the peripheral NERVOUS SYSTEM, a ganglion (pronounced gang′glee·on) is a knotlike group of nerve cells that form a nerve center. A network of ganglia is called a plexus. Absence of ganglia in the COLON causes in young children a condition called congenital MEGACOLON. See also PARKINSONISM.

(2) A ganglion may be a cystic TUMOR containing fluid. Usually it is connected to a tendon or a membrane on a joint and forms a small, firm mass under the skin. As a rule, it causes no pain. Surgery is often recommended if a ganglion becomes troublesome.

GANGRENE Death of tissues in an area of the body, produced by infection or by loss of the blood supply and the nourishment and oxygen it provides. Gangrene (pronounced gang'green) most often affects the hands and feet as a result of frostbite. Other causes include injury, embolism, and severe burn. Common symptoms are discoloration of the skin, pain in the affected area, and fever.

Types: Gangrene occurs in three principal forms: gas, dry, and moist. Gas gangrene is caused by anaerobic BACTERIA, which produce a gas under the skin. A toxin is formed that decomposes tissue. Dry gangrene occurs gradually and is usually the result of a slow reduction in the blood flow owing to a disease such as ARTERIOSCLEROSIS. The tissue shrinks, loses its warmth, and begins to change color, until finally it is black. Moist gangrene results from the sudden stoppage of blood because of burning, freezing, or injury. It turns the skin purple and causes swelling and blistering.

Treatment and Prevention: Gangrene is treated with ANTIBIOTICS. If gas gangrene is present, an ANTITOXIN may be used. Rest is important. In severe cases, it may be necessary to remove the diseased area by surgery.

Preventive measures include close attention to the hands and feet, especially in the case of DIABETES. Wounds should be kept free from infection. Frostbitten parts of the body should be covered with gently warmed blankets or immersed in lukewarm water. See also FROSTBITE.

GANTRISIN The trade name of a SULFONAMIDE (sulfa compound). Gantrisin (pronounced gan'tri·sin) is used to combat bacterial infections in the URINARY TRACT.

GARGLING Over the decades, a great many gargles have been promoted. At best, these commercial products contain weak antibacterial agents. For a severe sore throat you need treatment by a physician. Relief for a mild sore throat may be obtained by gargling every few hours with a half glass of warm water in which two crushed aspirins have been dissolved. Or a half teaspoonful of salt in a large glass of warm water may help.

GAS Air or gas accumulated in the stomach or intestines. It may distend the abdomen and cause pain. The condition is also called FLATULENCE.

Gas is a typical symptom of INDIGESTION and may be the result of eating too fast or too much, eating spoiled food, or eating while emotionally upset. Relief is sometimes obtained by taking a teaspoon of sodium bicarbonate in a glass of water.

Infants are often troubled by gas when they gulp in air with their milk. The condition is avoided by burping the baby. See also COLIC.

GAS POISONING Poisoning by carbon monoxide from coal gas, a car exhaust, or a gas stove is the most common form of gas poisoning. But there are many other kinds, including poisoning by sewer and cesspool gases and "damp" gas in mines. Gas-poisoning victims should be taken into the fresh air and any tight clothing loosened. Give artificial respiration until a doctor arrives. See also CARBON-MONOXIDE POISONING and the FIRST AID section.

GASTRECTOMY Surgical removal of a part of the stomach (subtotal gastrectomy) or of the entire stomach. The subtotal gastrectomy (pronounced gas·trek'to·mee) is sometimes used for the removal of an ulcer; the surgeon removes the section of the stomach where most of the glands that secrete HYDROCHLORIC ACID are located. Total gastrectomy, or removal of the whole stomach, may be necessary in the case of a malignant TUMOR.

GASTRIC JUICE A number of gastric juices are secreted in the stomach.

An important secretion of the stomach is HYDROCHLORIC ACID; it helps to prevent bacteria from multiplying and promotes the action of certain enzymes. Pepsin, an ENZYME, splits protein (the main constituent of meat) into simpler molecules. Other gastric secretions also assist in the process of DIGESTION.

GASTRIC ULCER See ULCER.

GASTRITIS Inflammation of the stomach. (Pronounced gas·trie'tis.)

Acute Gastritis: It may be caused by an infection, overeating, eating food that has turned bad, taking a particular medicine or poison, or—most commonly—drinking too much alcohol. The person may have a fever and vomit. Sometimes it is necessary to empty the stomach by inducing vomiting or using a stomach pump.

Chronic Gastritis: In its chronic form, gastritis may be the result of long-term use of an irritant, or caused by ulcers, repeated emotional upsets, or a vitamin deficiency. Symptoms range from mild to severe; they may resemble those of indigestion, acute gastritis, or stomach ulcer.

Treatment for chronic gastritis is much the same as for a stomach ULCER. SEDATIVES may be helpful in reducing tension. In certain cases, vitamin injections provide relief. The person should avoid alcohol and fried and highly seasoned foods, and should eat his meals in a relaxed atmosphere.

GASTROCELE A HERNIA of the stomach. (Pronounced gas′troh·seel.)

GASTROENTERITIS An inflammation of the membrane that lines the intestines and the stomach. Gastroenteritis (pronounced gas″troh·en″te·rie′tis) may be produced by a contagious disease, an allergic reaction to certain foods, emotional disturbance, and irritation of the intestine by overindulgence in food or drink. Symptoms include fever, vomiting, and diarrhea.

GASTROENTEROLOGIST A physician who specializes in gastroenterology, the diagnosis and treatment of disorders of the intestines and stomach. (Pronounced gas″troh·en″te·rol′o·jist.)

GASTROENTEROSTOMY A surgical operation for the purpose of creating an artificial passageway between the stomach and the small intestine. (Pronounced gas″troh·en″te·ros′to·mee.)

GASTROINTESTINAL SERIES (GI series) A procedure for X-ray examination of the digestive tract. By means of a gastrointestinal (pronounced gas″troh·in·tes′ti·nal) series, the doctor can locate and diagnose an abnormality in the esophagus, stomach, or intestines. The digestive tract itself does not show up on ordinary X-ray examination. It is made visible by means of a barium meal (see BARIUM SULFATE), a harmless, chalky liquid that the person drinks on an empty stomach at the beginning of the test. As the barium preparation passes down the esophagus into the stomach and through the intestines to the rectum, the shape and movement of all these organs are outlined by X ray. Any obstructions or swellings in the tract are made visible.

GASTROSCOPY Visual inspection of the stomach. Gastroscopy (pronounced gas·tros′ko·pee) is performed to determine whether there are tumors, ulcers, or other abnormal conditions present. It enables the doctor to examine the stomach in detail and make a more specific diagnosis.

The instrument employed in viewing the interior of the stomach is known as a gastroscope. Two kinds are in use. The fiberscope is several feet long and contains a large number of glass fibers that transmit the image of the stomach's interior. The flexible gastroscope, also a long instrument, is equipped with a number of lenses. Either instrument is inserted through the esophagus and into the stomach.

GASTROSTOMY An operation by which an opening is made into the stomach through the wall of the abdomen, usually for the purpose of introducing food. (Pronounced gas·tros′to·mee.)

GASTRULA An early stage in the development of the EMBRYO. In its simplest form, a gastrula (pro-nounced gas′trool·a) is made up of only two layers of cells.

GENE A unit in the CHROMOSOME that determines a particular inherited characteristic. Each of the 46 chromosomes in the cells of human beings contains hundreds, perhaps even thousands, of genes arranged in a definite order. Each gene determines some detail (such as eye color) of the inherited makeup of the individual. See also GENETIC.

GENERIC The generic (pronounced je·ner′ik) name of a medicine is the name given to it by chemists according to certain rules of naming that are internationally agreed upon. Generic names cannot be protected by patent or registration. The generic name, based on the chemical structure and composition of a compound, is often long and difficult to remember and to pronounce. On the other hand, pharmaceutical manufacturers may register with the U.S. Patent Office short and easily recalled names for the medicines they manufacture; these are known as proprietary medicines. A medicine prescribed and sold under its generic name is usually less costly than the same medicine sold under the pharmaceutical company's trade name.

GENETIC Having to do with the GENES, the units of HEREDITY. Genetic (pronounced je·net′ik) studies, or genetics, are concerned with the structure of the CHROMOSOMES, which consist of many genes arranged in definite patterns. Chromosomes are present in every cell of the body as well as in the egg and sperm cells that unite to form a new individual. Their structures control the functioning of the body and the physical makeup of succeeding generations.

Many abnormal conditions are the result of abnormalities in the chromosomes that can be inherited; abnormalities may also arise from exposure to certain chemicals, to viruses, or to radiation. Genetic engineering may someday make it possible for scientists to alter chromosomes to produce desired characteristics or repress others, and to cure diseases caused by abnormalities in the chromosomes.

GENITALS The organs of reproduction, especially the external organs. The term does not usually include the female ovaries and uterus inside the abdominal cavity.

The male genitals consist of the TESTICLES, which produce SPERM CELLS, and the PENIS, through which SEMEN is deposited in the female vagina. The testicles develop inside the abdominal cavity and descend gradually into the SCROTUM as the fetus grows in the womb.

The testicles become active at puberty (see ADOLESCENCE), producing male sex hormones and sperm cells. A long duct, the VAS DEFERENS, leads from each testicle up toward the prostate gland, inside which the duct connects with the URETHRA. At this

GENITALS

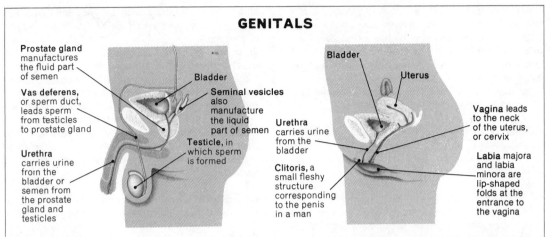

Prostate gland manufactures the fluid part of semen

Vas deferens, or sperm duct, leads sperm from testicles to prostate gland

Urethra carries urine from the bladder or semen from the prostate gland and testicles

Bladder

Seminal vesicles also manufacture the liquid part of semen

Testicle, in which sperm is formed

Bladder

Uterus

Urethra carries urine from the bladder

Clitoris, a small fleshy structure corresponding to the penis in a man

Vagina leads to the neck of the uterus, or cervix

Labia majora and labia minora are lip-shaped folds at the entrance to the vagina

The male genitals consist of the penis and the testicles, which are contained in the pouchlike scrotum. Ducts from the testicles carry sperm to the prostate gland, where they join the urethra, the tube from the bladder. The urethra extends along the center of the penis, where it serves the dual function of carrying urine or semen. Glands called seminal vesicles, below the rear of the bladder, and the prostate, produce the liquid part of semen. The female genitals, or vulva, have two pairs of lips, called the labia majora and the labia minora. The labia flank the entrance to the vagina, which may be partly blocked by a membrane called the hymen. The vagina leads, by way of the cervix, to the uterus. Below the clitoris, a fleshy structure corresponding to the penis in men, is the exit of the urethra, the tube from the bladder.

point, other fluids enter the urethra and mix with the sperm cells from the testicles to form the SEMEN. These fluids are produced by the two seminal vesicles, long pouches that lie beside each vas deferens, and by the prostate gland, which is situated just under the bladder.

The end of the penis bears a sheath called the foreskin, or prepuce. This is often removed in babyhood by the simple operation of CIRCUMCISION. If the operation is not performed, special attention should be given to keeping this area clean. The penis contains a network of tiny artery branches. When sexually stimulated, these small vessels become filled with blood and cause the penis to become stiff and erect.

The female external genitals (called the VULVA) include two pairs of folds (the labia), one pair on either side of the opening to the VAGINA; the HYMEN; and the CLITORIS.

GENITOURINARY Relating to both reproduction and urination. Although these are two distinct processes, the reproductive and urinary organs are so closely associated that it is often convenient for doctors to treat them as a single system, known as the genitourinary (pronounced jen″i·toh·yoor′i·ner″ee) system. In addition to the external and internal genital organs (see GENITALS), the genitourinary system includes the KIDNEYS and the urinary tract (URETERS, BLADDER, and URETHRA).

GERIATRICS The branch of medicine concerned with the diseases and health problems of old people.

With the constant rise in the number of persons who reach old age, the science of geriatrics (pronounced jer″ee·at′riks) is becoming increasingly important.

Old age, like every other period of life, has its special problems. The body changes with time. In the later years, HARDENING OF THE ARTERIES occurs, and changes in the bones may be associated with arthritis and bone fracture. Loss of teeth and impaired ability to see and hear are fairly common.
Secrets of Long Life: It has been said that the secret of living to a ripe old age is to choose the right parents. However, whether or not our parents lived long and healthy lives, there are a number of things we can do to help lengthen our own lives. Regular medical examinations, prompt attention to our health needs, good DIET, a sensible amount of exercise, and—above all—maintaining an involvement in living can add years to our lives.

GERM A microorganism; a tiny living thing that usually cannot be seen without the aid of a microscope. Germs include bacteria, viruses, rickettsiae, and protozoans (one-celled animals).

The word "germ" is popularly applied to a microorganism that is capable of causing disease. Disease-producing germs are also called pathogens or microbes.

GERMAN MEASLES See RUBELLA.

GERMICIDE A substance that is capable of killing disease GERMS and other microorganisms. By contrast, a fungicide will destroy only fungi, and a bactericide, only bacteria. Germicides must be used with care, since many are so strong that they may injure the skin or cause serious burns. Your doctor can advise you about them. Iodine is a familiar example of a germicide that should be used with particular care. Hydrogen peroxide is a safe general-purpose germicide for external use.

GERONTOLOGY The study of aging and of the social, medical, and psychological problems of the elderly. (Pronounced jer"on·tol'o·jee.) See also GERIATRICS.

GESTATION The period that begins with the conception of a child and ends with delivery. Gestation (pronounced jes·tay'shun) is the biologist's term for PREGNANCY.

GIANTISM (gigantism) Excessive growth of the long bones of the arms and legs during childhood and adolescence. Like ACROMEGALY in adults, giantism is caused by overproduction of growth hormone in the PITUITARY GLAND. A noncancerous pituitary tumor is often the cause. In addition to excessive growth, other symptoms may include headaches, weakness and lack of energy, a narrowing of the visual field, and absence of normal sexual development at puberty.
Treatment: If medical diagnosis shows that a pituitary tumor is present, it may be treated by irradiation or by surgery. In some cases, sex hormones are administered.

Occasionally, excessive height is associated with a GENETIC abnormality in the chromosomes.

GIARDIASIS An intestinal disorder caused by infestation with the parasite *Giardia lamblia*, contracted by eating contaminated food. Sometimes it causes diarrhea, although usually the parasite produces no symptoms, and the fact that it is present may be discovered only by chance in microscopical examination of feces for some other purpose. It can be treated with drugs such as atabrine metronidazole. (Pronounced jee"ahr·die'i·sis.)

GINGIVITIS An inflammation of the GUMS that begins around the teeth. Bleeding of the gums is a prominent symptom. If gingivitis (pronounced jin"ji·vie'tis) is not treated promptly, it may lead to PYORRHEA (formation of pus) and the eventual loss of teeth.
Causes: Failure to brush the teeth allows minute particles of food to lodge themselves between the teeth, or between the teeth and the gums; bacteria go into action at once, preparing the way for gum infection. Among the potential causes of gingivitis are TARTAR on the teeth, decaying teeth, spaces where food may lodge between the teeth, and dentures that produce gum irritation. Also, poor health

and a poor diet may lead to gum inflammation. VINCENT'S ANGINA (trench mouth) is an acute form of gingivitis.
Treatment: Good dental care is indispensable. The dentist will scale away the tartar, treat decayed teeth, and make certain that fillings and dentures fit correctly. The teeth must be brushed after every meal; the brush should also be used to massage the gums. If poor health is a contributing factor, a medical checkup is essential. A well-balanced diet that is light on sugary foods and rich in vitamins and minerals will usually help restore the gums to good condition.

GI SERIES See GASTROINTESTINAL SERIES. (Pronounced gee'ie' sur'eez.)

GLAND An organ that secretes a substance for use by the body or for elimination from it. Some glands, such as the salivary and sebaceous (oil-producing) glands, are provided with ducts that carry their secretions to the places where they perform their actions. Other glands, known as ENDOCRINE GLANDS, are ductless; they pour their hormones, or secretions, directly into the bloodstream. The PITUITARY GLAND and the ADRENAL GLANDS are examples of this type. The PANCREAS produces secretions of both types. In addition, there are the so-called lymph glands, or LYMPH NODES, which produce certain white blood cells (lymphocytes) and play an important role in the body's defense against infection.

GLANDERS A serious disease of horses, mules, dogs, and other mammals, which can be caught by human beings who come into contact with a diseased animal; also called equinia. Glanders (pronounced glan'derz) is caused by bacteria, and symptoms include ulcers in the skin and mucous membranes. It may be treated with antibiotics or prevented with a vaccine.

GLANDULAR FEVER See MONONUCLEOSIS.

GLAUCOMA A disorder of the eyes caused by increased pressure of fluid within the eyeballs. In glaucoma (pronounced glaw·koh'ma), fluid accumulating in the EYE exerts pressure on the retina and the optic nerve. If treated promptly, before the retina and the optic nerve have been damaged, there is good hope of complete recovery.
Symptoms: In *acute* glaucoma, there may be considerable pain within the eye. The vision may be blurred; the person often finds it difficult to see on the side, and he may see halos around electric lights. *Chronic* glaucoma often comes on slowly; the nerve structure of the eye may already have been damaged before glaucoma is diagnosed. This is an important reason for having the eyes examined regularly—at least every two years—especially after a person reaches 40.

Diagnosis and Treatment: Glaucoma is diagnosed with a tonometer. After making the eyeball insensitive to pain with anesthetizing drops, the eye doctor presses the tonometer painlessly upon the cornea. The pressure of the fluid in the eye makes a plunger in the tonometer rise, providing an index to the degree of pressure present. Measurement of the field of vision and examination of the optic nerve and the structure of the eye also help in diagnosis. Treatment with medicines often gives good results. If this is ineffective, surgery may be performed to open the outflow canal. If the retina and the optic nerve have been damaged, there will be partial or complete loss of sight.

GLOSSITIS Inflammation of the TONGUE. (Pronounced glos·sie′tis.)

GLUCOSE A SUGAR that is found in the blood; also known as dextrose. When sugars and starches (CARBOHYDRATES) are taken into the body, they are broken down into simpler sugars, including glucose; in this form they can be assimilated into the cells and used to produce energy. In DIABETES the body is unable to use glucose properly; the result is an excessive amount of sugar in the blood and urine.

Glucose is stored in the liver in the form of glycogen. When the blood needs sugar, the glycogen is readily converted back into glucose.

GLUCOSE TOLERANCE TEST A test used in the diagnosis of DIABETES. A person is given sugar in the form of glucose. At periodic intervals for up to six hours, the urine and blood are examined for the amount of sugar present; the results show how efficiently the body is using the sugar.

GLYCEMIA The normal presence of sugar in the bloodstream. (Pronounced glie·see′mee·a.) Too much sugar in the blood is called hyperglycemia; too little, hypoglycemia.

GLYCOSURIA The presence of an abnormally large quantity of sugar in the urine. (Pronounced glie″ko·syoor′ee·a.) See also DIABETES.

GOITER An abnormal enlargement of the THYROID GLAND, which regulates the rate of the METABOLISM of the body. The swollen thyroid shows up conspicuously in the front of the throat. Goiter is a symptom in not just one but a number of disorders of the thyroid gland.

Hyperthyroidism: In this disorder the thyroid gland produces a greatly increased amount of the hormone THYROXINE. The gland swells to two or three times its normal size. The basal metabolism rate rises steeply. The person is extremely nervous and has diarrhea, and his heartbeat speeds up. He may also lose a considerable amount of weight. In severe cases, edema or excess tissue develops behind the eyeballs, causing them to bulge. This condition is known as exophthalmic goiter. (See EXOPHTHALMOS.) Hyperthyroidism is treated by surgery or with various chemicals. An effective treatment is the administration of radioactive iodine.

Hypothyroidism: In this condition the situation is just the opposite: the thyroid gland produces too little thyroxine, often because of an insufficient amount of natural iodine in the person's diet. The rate of metabolism decreases, and the individual may put on weight and become lethargic; he may sleep much longer than normal. Constipation is a recurrent symptom. In severe cases the legs may swell, and the skin and hair are very dry. (A related condition is called myxedema. In this disorder, the underfunctioning of the thyroid gland is usually not caused by a dietary deficiency of iodine.) The thyroid, in its effort to produce enough thyroxine, enlarges enormously—as much as 15 times. Thyroxine is used in the treatment of hypothyroidism.

GONAD A sex gland; the OVARY in the female, and the TESTICLE in the male.

GONORRHEA A contagious venereal disease caused by a gonococcus, a type of BACTERIUM. Gonorrhea (pronounced gon″o·ree′a) is usually, but not always, transmitted during sexual intercourse. If detected in its early stages, gonorrhea is readily cured with ANTIBIOTICS or SULFONAMIDES (sulfa compounds).

Gonorrhea is not as serious a disease as SYPHILIS, but it is much more widespread and can do considerable damage. It may cause sterility or arthritis in adults. If a pregnant woman is infected, the disease may be transmitted to her child as the baby passes through the birth canal, and blindness may result. To avoid this, a solution of silver nitrate or a penicillin preparation is applied to the eyes of all newborn children.

Symptoms: Generally, about a week after infection, a man may experience a burning sensation when he urinates. There may also be a discharge of pus from the penis. The symptoms are often slower to appear in a woman. Pus may be discharged from the vagina; a burning sensation is sometimes felt during urination, or the abdomen may be painful. If the disease is not arrested, it may spread deep into the urinary and reproductive systems.

Prevention and Treatment: To avoid gonorrhea, sexual relations with individuals likely to carry the disease should be avoided. A CONDOM offers some protection, but a diaphragm does not.

The only person qualified to treat the disease is a physician. Do not rely on self-treatment with a prophylactic kit or even with a sulfonamide or penicillin.

GOUT A metabolic disease caused by the production of abnormally large amounts of URIC ACID.

Gout, also known as podagra, is most common in men over 30. Sometimes it occurs in women after the menopause.

Cause: The cause of gout is not well understood. Due to a metabolic defect (see METABOLISM), excess uric acid is produced. The kidneys are unable to excrete the uric acid rapidly enough, and it is deposited in the tissues, particularly the cartilages of the joints. An attack of *acute* gout may be triggered by an operation, a penicillin injection, a diet rich in fats, emotional strain, or other causes.

Symptoms: The joint of the big toe may become inflamed and extremely painful. The toe is swollen, and the skin is hot and red. Sometimes the ankle or another joint is involved. The person may have a fever. The attack usually subsides after a few days or weeks. If the condition is neglected for a long time, it may become chronic, and the joints are likely to become lumpy and stiff. Occasionally the kidneys may be affected. Overall, advanced symptoms resemble those of rheumatoid ARTHRITIS.

Treatment: For an acute attack of gout, the patient is given a medicine such as phenylbutazone or colchicine; corticosteroids may also be used. The patient should stay in bed until pain and swelling subside. Drinking large quantities of water helps the kidneys discharge the uric acid.

GRAFT The transplanting of an organ or a tissue to take the place of one that does not function adequately. Grafts may be made from one person to another, or from one part of a person's body to another part. The latter type is more successful. When a tissue or an organ is transplanted from another individual, there is considerable likelihood that the recipient's body will "reject" it. (See ORGAN TRANSPLANT.) However, marked success has been achieved with the transplantation of cartilage, bones, and corneas, which are stored in so-called banks. Skin grafts are used frequently to replace burned, diseased, or scarred tissue. The skin is generally taken from the thigh, chest, or some other relatively inconspicuous area.

GRAMICIDIN See TYROTHRICIN. (Pronounced gram″i·sied′in.)

GRAND MAL See EPILEPSY. (Pronounced grahn mahl′.)

GRANULATION The formation of patches of grainy tissue on the raw surface of a wound. Granulation is an important step in the process of healing.

GRANULOMA A tumor or nodule that frequently occurs in connection with an infection and is made up of GRANULATION tissue. Granuloma (pronounced gran″yu·loh′ma) inguinale is a disease of the anal and genital region caused by BACTERIA. It can generally be treated with antibiotics.

GRIPPE See INFLUENZA.

GRISTLE Elastic white tissue found at the joints and in other parts of the body. Another name for this tissue is CARTILAGE.

GROIN The region on the front of the body at the top of each leg; it includes the lower part of the abdomen and the upper part of the thigh. A pain in the groin is generally caused by a strained muscle or ligament. If accompanied by a lump or swelling, it may be a sign of a rupture (inguinal HERNIA) or of an inflamed lymph gland in the groin (see LYMPH NODE).

GROUP MEDICINE A group of private doctors, usually representing several different specialties, who cooperate in providing medical diagnosis and treatment; also known as group practice.

GROUP THERAPY Essentially, there are two major types of group therapy. In the first, persons with a similar problem attend a series of meetings in which members of the group unburden themselves of their difficulties and try to analyze them in open discussion. The meeting is guided by one or more leaders, and its aim is to inspire the participants and encourage them to overcome their troubles. ALCOHOLICS ANONYMOUS is an example of this type.

The second type is more accurately called group PSYCHOTHERAPY. This kind of group is led by a psychotherapist or psychiatrist. The members are persons with emotional difficulties, and the psychotherapist guides them in analyzing their own and each other's problems. From five to 10 persons usually participate. In the course of their discussions, they become more acutely aware of their problems in getting along with other people and gain a deeper insight into their inner drives. As a result, there may be an improvement in the individual's ability to cope with his emotional difficulties and to relate effectively to other people.

GROWING PAINS Many parents expect their children to suffer from "growing pains" at some time, but this is not a normal symptom of growing up. Often muscular pain in a child's legs is merely a result of excessive exercise. But any pain could be a symptom of some disorder, and leg pains in a growing child can be a sign that the child has a rheumatic infection, however slight, which could progress to affect the heart if not treated early. If a child complains of persistent pain, put him to bed and consult a doctor.

GULLET A common term for the ESOPHAGUS and PHARYNX together.

GUM The tissue that covers the portions of the jaws where the teeth grow. The gum, or gingiva, surrounds the lower portions of the teeth and gives them support. Between the enamel of each TOOTH and the gum there is a slight space, the gingival crevice, which may grow larger as the gum tissue shrinks with age. If food lodges in the gingival crevices, they may become sites of bacterial infection that can result in two troublesome disorders: GINGIVITIS and PYORRHEA alveolaris.

GUMMA See SYPHILIS.

GYNECOLOGIST A medical doctor who specializes in the diseases of women, or GYNECOLOGY. (Pronounced gie″ne·kol′o·jist.)

GYNECOLOGY The branch of medicine concerned with the treatment of female diseases, particularly those of the reproductive system. (Pronounced gie″ne·kol′o·jee.) The specialist who practices gynecology is called a gynecologist. Many qualified gynecologists are also obstetricians, taking care of women during pregnancy and childbirth.

Menstrual problems of many types are brought to the gynecologist, ranging from delayed beginning of MENSTRUATION in the adolescent girl to dysmenor-rhea (painful menstruation) and the MENOPAUSE. Improper development of the female organs, infectious diseases of the vagina and other genital organs, tumors, and disturbances of the sexual ENDOCRINE GLANDS are other problems that the gynecologist is called upon to treat. Gynecologists also treat women who have difficulty in becoming pregnant.

The Gynecological Examination: Many women, in addition to obtaining a regular medical checkup from their family physician, also visit a gynecologist periodically for an examination. In the gynecological examination, the specialist carefully investigates the organs of the pelvis as well as the breasts to determine whether there is evidence of malignancy or any other abnormality. An examination and consultation with a gynecologist is particularly desirable for the girl about to be married.

GYNECOMASTIA An overdevelopment, in a man, of one or both breasts. The breasts may produce a secretion. In gynecomastia (pronounced gie″ne·koh·mas′tee·a), along with the development of female characteristics, there is a reduction of male ones. The condition is most frequently the result of a hormone imbalance.

H

HAIR A specialized structure of dead cells filled with a tough substance called KERATIN. Each hair grows from the base of a small cavity, known as a follicle, that extends into the inner layer of the skin. Associated with every hair follicle are one or more minute oil glands and a tiny muscle that makes the hair "stand on end" when the muscle contracts. Hair follicles occur almost everywhere on the skin except on the lips and the undersurfaces of the feet and hands. They are thickest on the scalp.

The color and texture of hair are inherited characteristics. The hair of children becomes coarser as they grow up. Hair cells develop tiny air pockets as a person ages that change the color to white when the pigment disappears.

Care of the hair involves cleanliness most of all. Frequent washing does no harm. Gentle massage and frequent brushing help to stimulate the scalp and keep it in healthy condition. Chemical dyes and other cosmetic treatments should be used cautiously to avoid injuring the scalp. See also ALOPECIA (baldness); HAIR REMOVAL.

HAIR, LOSS OF See ALOPECIA.

HAIR REMOVAL The commonest and most convenient method of removing HAIR is by shaving. In general, any type of razor will do the job. Shaving or cutting the hair with scissors does not alter the hair follicle. Hair will not grow in coarser or more quickly than before, but it will grow in again.

When hair is pulled out, it takes a little longer to reappear than when it is cut. If only a few isolated hairs are to be removed, tweezers are useful. Many hairs can be pulled at the same time from insensitive areas by wax preparations that are spread on the skin. The wax grips the hairs as it solidifies, and then pulls them out when it is stripped away. Abrasives, such as pumice, are sometimes recommended for wearing away unwanted hair. This method may injure the skin and is time-consuming. A chemical DEPILATORY dissolves hair, but must be used cautiously; never use it on the face.

Instead of removing hair, it can be made almost invisible by bleaching with ordinary HYDROGEN PEROXIDE to which a drop of ammonia has been added.

The only method of removing hair permanently is by ELECTROLYSIS. This is a complicated process and must be performed by a careful, skilled operator in order to be effective and leave no disfiguring marks on the skin.

HALITOSIS The medical term for bad breath. It is not used for the temporary breath odor that follows eating foods containing garlic or onions. True halitosis (pronounced hal''i·toh'sis) can be caused by DENTAL CARIES or by infections of the gums, tonsils, nose, or sinuses. Disorders of the stomach and intestines, uremia, and many other conditions can also cause halitosis.

Treatment depends on the underlying cause. As a matter of course, the teeth should be brushed regularly and the dentist visited, whether or not the breath is bad. If halitosis persists, you should see a doctor.

HALLUCINATION A vivid perception of something that is not present in reality. The hallucinations produced by taking LSD and other such drugs have received wide attention in recent years.

Hallucinations can occur with any of the senses. The most common hallucinations involve "seeing things" or "hearing things." Amputees sometimes feel intense pain in a foot or a hand that is no longer there, an experience known as phantom limb or stump hallucination. In such a case, the pain is real, but it is mistakenly interpreted. Hallucinations are often associated with extreme fatigue, emotional stress, or some other abnormal condition. They may be brought on by toxic substances such as alcohol (see DELIRIUM TREMENS) and certain HALLUCINOGENIC DRUGS such as LSD. Severe EMOTIONAL AND MENTAL DISORDERS are often accompanied by hallucinations. Anyone who has hallucinations should have medical advice.

HALLUCINOGENIC DRUG A substance that alters ordinary mental and emotional processes, producing HALLUCINATIONS, bizarre states of consciousness, and unusual reactions to ordinary stimuli. Hallucinogenic (pronounced ha·loo''si·noh·jen'ik) drugs are sometimes called psychedelic or mind-expanding drugs.

The hallucinogenic drugs, or hallucinogens, include MESCALINE, MARIHUANA (hashish), psilocybin, and LSD. A few of them are now made synthetically, but all were originally obtained from certain plants and fungi.

It is not understood how these drugs act on the nervous system, or whether they all act essentially the same way or in different ways. The effect produced by any particular drug depends on the individual who takes it, as well as on the dosage. The emotional effects may range from feelings of intense pleasure to extreme terror. Most of these drugs produce mild physical reactions, such as a slight increase in heartbeat and blood pressure, an increase in the KNEE JERK and other reflexes, and sometimes dilation of the pupils of the eyes. Some, such as LSD, may produce severe and long-lasting mental derangement.

Some of the hallucinogens—mescaline, for example—have a long history of ritual use in certain religious cults. Today, hallucinogens have a limited application in medical research and no standard application in the treatment of disease.

The illegal use of hallucinogens is widespread, especially among young people. Repeated use is not believed to lead to true addiction (see DRUG ADDICTION), though some psychological dependence may result. In the United States and Canada, the unauthorized possession and use of any of the hallucinogens leads to severe legal penalties, including imprisonment. Some people claim that the mild hallucinogens, such as marihuana, are less harmful than tobacco and alcohol; but since the long-term effects of these drugs are not known, their use should be avoided for health reasons, as well as on account of their legal status. The use of marihuana may lead to use of more dangerous drugs.

HAMSTRING Either of the two groups of tendons at the back of the knee, which attach the muscles at the back of the thigh to the bones in the lower leg.

HAND The structure of the hand is similar to that of the FOOT, except that the shape and size of the parts are modified and adapted to handling things. The thumb is placed sideways, so that it can move in a direction opposed to the fingers. (See illustration on the following page.)

It takes nothing more than the pain of a minor injury, such as a HANGNAIL, to remind us how much we depend on our hands and how much they are exposed to rough usage.

It is surprising that normally the hands need no special care beyond trimming the nails. If the skin becomes dry and chapped, it can usually be restored by using a hand lotion or cream. Itchy, reddened areas (see ECZEMA) sometimes occur on the skin, especially on hands that are much exposed to detergents and other cleansers.

HANGNAIL A piece of partly dead skin torn away from the side or root of a fingernail, leaving a painful area not protected by epidermis (outer layer of the skin). Hangnails are apt to develop whenever the skin of the hand lacks sufficient natural oil to keep it moist. The use of a hand lotion or cream will prevent the skin from drying out.

HANGOVER The aftereffects that sometimes follow drinking too much alcohol. Alcohol is a toxic substance that affects the entire system. It takes some time for the body to recover from excessive drinking. The aftereffects include headache, dizziness, upset stomach, thirst, and feelings of depression and anxiety. The severity of the symptoms depends on the individual's tolerance for alcohol and the amount that has been drunk.

Mild symptoms may be relieved by common-sense remedies. Take aspirin for headache. Drink plenty of fluids to relieve thirst. Eat bland food to relieve stomach irritation. Severe symptoms may require a doctor's help.

On no account should another alcoholic drink be taken to relieve a "morning after" feeling. A hangover is a warning to drink less or to stop drinking altogether. See also ALCOHOLISM.

HANSEN'S DISEASE Another name for LEPROSY.

HARDENING OF THE ARTERIES In the middle and later years, the arteries tend to become less efficient in piping blood through the body. Fatty mineral deposits accumulate in the walls and on the inner surfaces of the arteries, and the walls gradually become thickened and less elastic. In many persons this condition, known medically as arteriosclerosis, does not progress so far as to be disabling. In others, fatty deposits on the inside of the artery walls may narrow the passageways so that the flow of blood is seriously curtailed. This type of arteriosclerosis, known medically as atherosclerosis, can be serious.

It is not known what causes atherosclerosis to develop. There is a tendency for the condition to run in families. This tendency may be associated with eating habits as well as with heredity. People whose diet contains much FAT, especially the saturated fats in meat and dairy products, appear to develop atherosclerosis more often than those on a lean diet. (See CHOLESTEROL.)

The symptoms and complications of atherosclerosis depend on which arteries in the body are most affected. Frequently, signs of inadequate blood supply appear first in the legs. There may be numbness and coldness in the feet and cramps and pains in the legs after even light exercise. In other cases, the coronary arteries may be chiefly affected, causing the pain characteristic of ANGINA PECTORIS. If the arteries of the kidneys are impaired, kidney disorders will develop. There may be partial loss of memory and other brain damage if the arteries of the brain are affected.

Treatment: No known treatment will restore hardened arteries to their original condition, but arteriosclerosis can be relieved and prevented from getting worse. Competent medical advice should be obtained, since the disabilities accompanying hardening of the arteries are so varied that treatment must be prescribed individually. In some cases, surgery may be performed to remove blood clots or

HAND

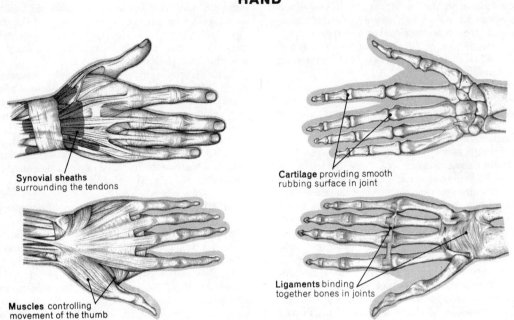

Synovial sheaths surrounding the tendons

Muscles controlling movement of the thumb

Cartilage providing smooth rubbing surface in joint

Ligaments binding together bones in joints

Man owes his unique ability to grasp and manipulate objects to the evolution of the bones, joints and ligaments in his hands. The thumb can be moved across the palm by the muscle at the base of the thumb to oppose the fingers and apply counter-pressure against one or more of them for gripping.

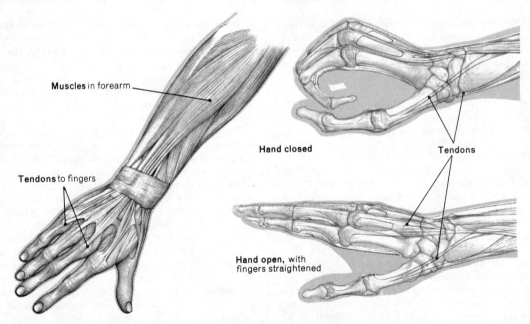

Muscles in forearm

Tendons to fingers

Hand closed

Tendons

Hand open, with fingers straightened

The movements of the fingers are controlled by tendons attached to muscles in the forearm. Rotation of the hand is made by twisting the pair of bones in the forearm, which are parallel when the palm is facing forward or upward. The fingers can spread or converge; but most movements involve opening and closing the fist, generally to wrap the fingers around an object and hold it.

widen the diameter of certain large arteries. Medication such as nitroglycerin may be prescribed to increase blood flow of the coronary arteries. The doctor may order a diet low in cholesterol and saturated fats. In any case, overweight should be avoided. Smoking, which further constricts the blood vessels, should be cut down or discontinued altogether.

HARELIP   A birth defect of the upper lip. For reasons not understood, the two sides of the face sometimes fail to unite before birth. There may be a single fissure in the fleshy tissue below the nose, or the upper lip may be missing entirely. The condition is often associated with CLEFT PALATE. Besides being disfiguring, a harelip causes difficulty in sucking and interferes with speech when the infant begins to talk. In most cases, a doctor will advise that a harelip should be corrected by surgery as soon after the baby's birth as possible.

HASHISH (HASHEESH)   See MARIHUANA.. (Pronounced hah'sheesh.)

HAY FEVER   The popular term for allergic RHINITIS, or inflammation inside the nose due to an ALLERGY. The symptoms resemble those of a common cold, except that there is no fever. The mucous membrane in the nose and eyelids becomes puffed up, there is sneezing and a watery discharge from nose and eyes.

There are many substances that are capable of causing an allergic reaction. Pollen from ragweed and other plants is often responsible. Animal dander (particles shed by skin, feathers, and fur) and household dust may also produce hay fever. In some cases, hay fever is caused by eating certain foods to which an individual has become sensitized.

Anyone with repeated "colds" should suspect hay fever. There are a number of laboratory tests by which the doctor can determine whether or not hay fever is present. By making a series of skin tests, he may also be able to determine what allergen is responsible in a particular case. Substances suspected of causing hay fever are applied in minute amounts to pricks or scratches in the skin. The responsible allergen is identified when swelling develops at any of the scratches.

Treatment: After the allergen has been identified, a person can sometimes be made immune to it by a series of injections.

ANTIHISTAMINES are available without a prescription, but may produce undesirable side effects. It is advisable to have a doctor's guidance in searching for an effective medicine. It may take a great deal of experimentation to find the right one.

It is sometimes possible to avoid the allergen responsible. You can refrain from inhaling pollen indoors by using air conditioners. Individual nose filters can be used, indoors and out. Some people find that their symptoms disappear if they use synthetic-foam pillows instead of feather ones. If you have household pets, remember that their dander can bring on hay fever.

HEADACHE   The blood vessels in the brain are interlaced with many nerves, and it is in these nerves that headache pain originates. The brain tissue itself and most of the brain covering are incapable of feeling pain; but the blood-vessel nerves are especially sensitive to changes of pressure and to abnormal pressure within the skull.

Tension headaches are the commonest kind of headaches. They occur without any other symptoms, and are due to conscious or unconscious emotional stress. They are usually temporary and disappear if one or two tablets of aspirin are taken. Stronger medication should be avoided except under a doctor's orders.

Migraine headaches, like tension headaches, cannot be traced to any general bodily disorder. They are much more severe and disabling than ordinary tension headaches. There is intense, throbbing pain in the front and top part of the head, usually on one side only. There may also be flickering vision, nausea, and vomiting. Migraine headaches occur repeatedly in some persons, and in certain families. There is a biological predisposition to migraines that, when coupled with certain psychic factors, probably produces the headaches.

Relaxation in a warm bath followed by quiet bed rest may help to relieve a migraine headache. Aspirin is not effective in soothing the pain. It is advisable to consult a doctor, who may prescribe a more potent painkiller (ANALGESIC). Some sufferers from recurring severe migraines may be helped by PSYCHOTHERAPY.

Other Types of Headaches: Sometimes the origin of a headache can be traced to other parts of the body. Almost any disease may be accompanied by a headache. Such headaches can only be treated effectively by getting at the cause. A doctor should be consulted without delay for a headache that will not go away or one accompanied by such symptoms as fever, nausea, vomiting, and disturbed vision.

HEARING   We live in an ocean of sound waves, many of which we cannot, or do not, hear. Some sounds are too high in pitch for the human ear, although dogs, bats, and other mammals can hear them. At the other end of the scale, there are sounds too low in pitch for us to hear, although we may sense them and react by a feeling of anxiety or even of dread. Children can hear sounds of much higher pitch than can adults. Keen hearing of this kind is related to the physical functioning of the EAR and nerve tissues, which tend to deteriorate with age.

The ability to pick out and attend to sounds that have meaning for us is what is sometimes meant by "hearing." This is partly a mental process that is greatly reinforced by seeing. Everyone does a certain amount of lipreading, as we realize when the sound in a motion picture is not exactly synchronized with the lip motions of the actors.

A low level of background noise, which we do not consciously hear, seems to be absolutely necessary for our emotional and physical well-being. On the other hand, a very high noise level can be a source of stress and actually injure the ears. Noise pollution is a serious problem. See also DEAFNESS; HEARING AID.

HEARING AID The simplest and oldest kind of hearing aid is a hand cupped behind the ear so that it collects sound waves and reflects them into the ear. The old-fashioned ear trumpet was a development of this natural hearing aid. Modern, battery-operated hearing aids work on a different principle. They consist of a tiny receiver, an amplifier, and either an earpiece or a vibrator. The earpiece, usually a small plastic mold that fits into the EAR, feeds the amplified sound into the ear so that it strikes the eardrum in the normal way. The vibrator is a device that is fitted behind the ear over the mastoid bone, and the sound reaches the ear by conduction through the bone. It is advisable to seek the advice of a specialist before buying a hearing aid. See also DEAFNESS.

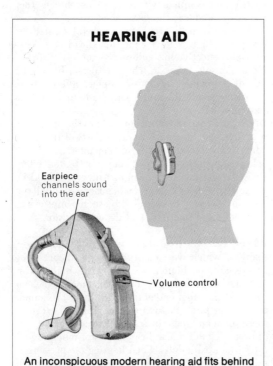

HEARING AID

Earpiece channels sound into the ear

Volume control

An inconspicuous modern hearing aid fits behind the ear—or in the hair or in special eyeglass frames—and transmits amplified sounds along a tube into the ear canal, or passes them directly through the bones at the side of the skull.

HEART A muscular organ that pumps blood to every part of the body. It lies in the middle of the chest more to the left side than the right, and is about the size of a fist. It is enclosed in a membrane called the pericardium.

The heart is divided into two major parts separated by the septum, a muscular wall. The right part receives blood from the veins and propels it to the lungs, where it discharges carbon dioxide and absorbs oxygen. The left part receives the blood from the lungs and pumps it to the rest of the body through the aorta.

Each part of the heart is divided into two chambers, an auricle (atrium), which receives the blood, and a muscular ventricle, which propels it. The two sides of the heart function in unison, contracting, relaxing, and refilling at the same time; the contraction is known as the systole, the relaxation as the diastole. See also HEART VALVE.

HEART ATTACK An ailment brought on by failure of the heart to function normally. A frequent cause is coronary thrombosis, which occurs when a blood clot blocks an artery leading to the heart. (See CORONARY HEART DISEASE.) The circulation to the heart is cut off, and the tissues may be damaged in the area affected. Older persons who have HARDENING OF THE ARTERIES are particularly likely to suffer heart attacks; but heart attacks may also strike individuals who have no record of circulatory trouble. The majority of persons survive a first heart attack. With good medical care and attention to health, the outlook for the heart patient is favorable.

Causes: A coronary thrombosis frequently has a long history. There is increasing evidence that persons with a high level of CHOLESTEROL in the blood are more subject than others to hardening of the arteries. The cholesterol is deposited in the walls of the arteries. As a result, the arteries become narrower, so that the blood flows more slowly. A piece of tissue may break off and block a narrower vessel (see EMBOLISM), or a blood clot may form on the damaged arterial tissue. The circulation is obstructed (occluded), and the heart may not be able to function normally.

Symptoms: A heart attack may occur without any pain. The victim may feel faint or lose consciousness. He turns very pale, and his pulse is weak. He may go into a state of shock. Usually, there is a feeling of suffocation or a crushing pain over the heart, which may go down the left arm (ANGINA PECTORIS). See also HEART DISEASE—SYMPTOMS.

What to Do: Call an ambulance and notify the victim's doctor. Help him into a comfortable position. If he has angina pectoris and the doctor has prescribed nitroglycerin, see that he gets it instantly.

For further information on emergency care of a heart-attack victim, see the FIRST AID section.

Prevention: Certain conditions predispose us to coronary disease. One is overweight. Do not eat too

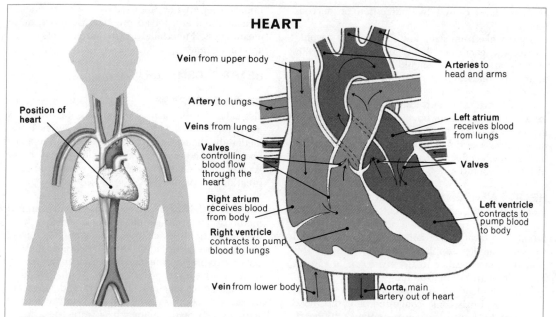

HEART

Vein from upper body

Artery to lungs

Veins from lungs

Position of heart

Valves controlling blood flow through the heart

Right atrium receives blood from body

Right ventricle contracts to pump blood to lungs

Vein from lower body

Arteries to head and arms

Left atrium receives blood from lungs

Valves

Left ventricle contracts to pump blood to body

Aorta, main artery out of heart

The heart consists basically of two pumps side by side, one receiving blood from the veins and pumping it to the lungs, and the other receiving oxygenated blood from the lungs and pumping it around the body along a network of arteries. The pumping action is achieved by the two lower chambers (ventricles) which consist of a powerful muscle that contracts to force blood out of the pulmonary artery to the lungs, and out of the aorta to the body. Blood flow from the upper chambers to the lower ones and out of the heart is controlled by various one-way valves, and the heart muscle itself is supplied with blood by means of the coronary arteries, which encircle the outside of the heart.

much; it is better to be a little under the average normal weight for your height. Avoid fat. If you smoke cigarettes, you are endangering your heart. Heart disease occurs three to five times more frequently among heavy smokers than among non-smokers. Regular exercise keeps the heart and circulation in good condition. Have a thorough medical examination at least once a year.

HEARTBEAT The cycle of contraction and relaxation of the heart muscle. The average adult heart beats approximately 72 times a minute. A child's heart beats more rapidly, averaging 90 beats a minute for ten-year-olds. The heart will beat faster or slower, depending on whether you are at rest or exerting yourself. Excitement and various medicines may speed up the heartbeat.

The rate and rhythm of the heartbeat are established by the body's natural CARDIAC PACEMAKER, located in the right auricle. It transmits its impulses to a group of fibers called the atrioventricular node, located in the lower right auricle (atrium).

HEART BLOCK A heart disorder in which the auricles (atria) and ventricles no longer beat in coordination. The blockage is actually an obstruction of the impulses from the body's natural CARDIAC PACEMAKER.

Heart block may range from minor to severe. If the damage is only slight, there will be a greater than normal delay between the beat of the auricle and the ventricle. In more serious cases, the auricle beats two, three, or four times to the ventricle's one.

Surgery may be recommended in cases of severe heart block caused by disease. A small artificial electric pacemaker may be embedded surgically in the heart to make the rhythm normal again.

HEARTBURN See PYROSIS; INDIGESTION.

HEART DISEASE—SYMPTOMS Heart disease has certain typical symptoms. One or two of these do not necessarily indicate heart trouble, for similar symptoms are found in a number of other disorders. No one but a physician, however, is qualified to determine whether the symptoms are caused by heart disease or some other condition. He will make such a diagnosis only after a thorough examination, including an ELECTROCARDIOGRAM. Sometimes a very specialized test called cardiac catheterization is necessary before an exact diagnosis can be made.

Pain in the chest, or ANGINA PECTORIS, calls for an examination. The pain may be over the heart, in the middle of the chest, or in the neck, back, or left arm. The person may feel a sensation of constriction or suffocation rather than an acute pain. (Similar pains are sometimes caused by indigestion or nervous tension.)

If you wake from sleep and find you are gasping for air, the condition should be brought to your doctor's attention. So should breathlessness that follows normal exertion that formerly placed no strain on your system.

Rapid heartbeat or fluttering of the heart may last for a few minutes or for hours. TACHYCARDIA, as the condition is known medically, may be the result of nervousness, exertion, smoking too much, or drinking too much coffee or tea, or it may be a symptom of a heart condition.

HEART FAILURE A condition in which the heart is so weakened that it is unable to pump the blood rapidly enough to maintain a normal rate of circulation. The term "heart failure" is sometimes used to mean a sudden stopping of the heartbeat, but this is more properly called HEART STOPPAGE, or cardiac arrest. In heart failure, the lungs may become congested with blood, causing breathing difficulty. The heart may also become congested, and the blood may push back into the veins supplying the heart. Fluid may escape from the blood into the tissues, causing the ankles to become puffy and swollen. Causes of heart failure include extremely high blood pressure, CORONARY HEART DISEASE, and, less commonly, congenital birth defects of the heart.

Treatment: Heart failure may be corrected by attention to the underlying condition. Usually, a low-salt diet and medication are prescribed to bring down the blood pressure. The medicine DIGITALIS is used to improve the action of the heart.

HEART-LUNG MACHINE See HEART SURGERY.

HEART MASSAGE An emergency measure, also called cardiopulmonary resuscitation, to restart a heart that has stopped beating. If it is begun promptly, skillful heart massage can temporarily keep the blood circulating, at least enough to prevent permanent brain damage through lack of oxygen. See the FIRST AID section for instructions on cardiopulmonary resuscitation.

Open-chest heart massage, in which the chest wall is opened and the heart massaged directly, is applied by medical personnel only under special circumstances, such as when the heart stops beating in a patient undergoing surgery.

HEART MURMUR A sound, other than the heartbeat, heard by the physician when he applies his STETHOSCOPE in the region of the HEART. The sound may indicate that the heart is not functioning normally, the HEART VALVES are not closing properly, or there is some structural defect, possibly present since birth.

Many cardiac murmurs, on the other hand, are described by physicians as innocent, or func-

tional—they are not produced by any heart damage or defect and are, for all practical purposes, quite meaningless. Functional heart murmurs often disappear in time.

HEART PACEMAKER See CARDIAC PACEMAKER.

HEART STOPPAGE Stopping of the heartbeat, also called cardiac arrest. Sometimes, if the heart is not severely damaged and action can be taken immediately, the heart can be stimulated to resume its beating by medicines or special techniques of HEART MASSAGE. For emergency measures when a person's breathing stops, see FIRST AID section.

HEART SURGERY Developments in surgical methods, medication, and medical devices have opened a whole new chapter in heart surgery during the past several decades. ANTIBIOTICS now make it possible to prevent the fatal infections that formerly made heart surgery so dangerous. With the aid of the heart-lung machine, the heart and lungs are bypassed: blood is drawn from the veins, recharged with oxygen, and pumped back into the arteries supplying the body. The ailing heart, relieved of the need to keep pumping the blood, may be opened up by the surgeon and repaired where necessary. Hypothermia (chilling the body) is used to slow down the body processes, thus reducing the need for oxygen-rich blood; this enables the surgeon to perform brief operations without having to use the heart-lung machine.

Heart surgery is performed to correct an increasing number of defects, some of which may have been produced by disease while others may have been congenital. Much of the damage caused by rheumatic heart disease can now be corrected. HEART VALVES damaged by RHEUMATIC FEVER can be repaired. Narrowing, or STENOSIS, of the valves can be corrected by widening the valve opening. Sometimes a valve becomes so weak that it will not close properly. The surgeon may suture the valve or substitute a valve of synthetic material.

ANEURYSM of the aorta is another circulatory difficulty that may be helped by an operation. In this condition, the wall of the aorta becomes weakened, forming a bulging sac of blood. To prevent the danger of rupture, the surgeon may remove the damaged segment and substitute a graft of human tissue or synthetic material.

Congenital heart problems corrected by surgery include septal defects—openings in the wall, or septum, between the two auricles (atria) or ventricles. The hole may be stitched up, or the surgeon may close it with a synthetic graft.

HEART VALVE The chambers of the HEART have valves that close after the blood has passed through, so that it cannot flow back. The mitral valve separates the left auricle (atrium) from the left ventricle;

the tricuspid valve controls the opening between the right auricle and right ventricle. The exits from the ventricles are also controlled by valves. The aortic valve separates the left ventricle from the aorta, and the pulmonary valve shuts the right ventricle off from the pulmonary artery.

When a sufficient amount of blood accumulates in the auricles so that the pressure is greater than in the ventricles, the valves separating the chambers are forced open and allow the blood through. As soon as it has entered the ventricles, the valves shut tight. The contractions of the heart force the exit valves to open for the blood to leave the ventricles; immediately afterward the valves shut.

If a valve is damaged so that it permits blood to escape, or if it does not function properly in some other way, it may produce a sound known as a HEART MURMUR. If there is damage to valves, HEART SURGERY may be recommended. See also MITRAL DISEASE.

HEATING PAD An electric appliance consisting of thermostatically controlled heating elements with a fabric cover. It is a very convenient method of applying dry heat, but it must be used with caution. Never use a heating pad with frayed wires or exposed connections. Keep it dry—water and moisture conduct electricity. Never use pins to keep a heating pad in place. Have your doctor's approval before using a heating pad for any acute pain in the abdomen or elsewhere, or for treating any seriously ill patient. Although heat is soothing for some conditions, it is harmful for others.

Finally, be sure that the thermostatic control works and that it is set at a comfortable temperature. An overheated pad can cause a serious burn. Do not depend on the patient to warn you if the heat is too great. It is usually best to use the lowest setting.

HEAT PROSTRATION Exhaustion and collapse caused by overexposure to heat. The temperature of the body is normally kept from rising above 98.6° F by the cooling effect of evaporation. When the temperature outside the body is high, a great deal of water is lost in perspiration. As the fluid volume in the body decreases, the circulation of the blood is affected.

Heat prostration is especially likely to occur in persons with poor circulation, but even a person in good health can suffer the same effects if the cooling system of the body is overworked. The skin becomes pale and clammy; there is weakness, dizziness, headache, and stupor.

Treatment: Call a doctor at once. In the meantime, put the person in a cool place in a reclining position. Loosen his clothing, and let him drink cool, lightly salted water.

Heat prostration can be prevented by avoiding excessive activity in hot weather, increasing the amount of salt intake, and drinking enough fluids to take care of extra losses through perspiration.

HEAT RASH See PRICKLY HEAT.

HEAT STROKE See SUNSTROKE.

HEBEPHRENIC A psychiatric term referring to a group of symptoms of SCHIZOPHRENIA that usually appear at puberty. (Pronounced hee″be·free′nik.) They include giggling without apparent cause, infantile behavior and mannerisms, delusions, and hallucinations. Persistently inappropriate behavior may indicate schizophrenia.

HEMANGIOMA The medical term for a type of BIRTHMARK, such as those popularly called strawberry marks or port-wine stains. Hemangiomas (pronounced hi·man″jee·oh′mas) may occur internally as well as on the skin. They consist of clusters of small blood vessels.

HEMATOMA A localized pool or clotted lump of blood. A hematoma (pronounced hee″ma·toh′ma) is usually the result of injury. BLACK-AND-BLUE MARKS are familiar examples, but hematomas are not limited to tissue immediately under the skin. Fractures are almost always accompanied by hematomas in the surrounding tissue.

The most serious hematomas are those that sometimes form under the skull following a head injury. By pressing on the brain, they may cause severe physical symptoms.

Surgery is usually necessary to remove the more serious kinds of hematomas. Minor hematomas are reabsorbed by the body, gradually disappearing without treatment.

HEMATURIA The presence of blood in urine, usually giving the urine a red color. In some cases, however, the blood cells can be detected only under a microscope. Hematuria (pronounced hem″a·toor′ee·a) may be caused by a minor illness or it may be a symptom of a serious disorder, such as KIDNEY DISEASE. All cases of blood in the urine should be reported to a doctor at once.

HEMIANOPIA Partial BLINDNESS in which the victim cannot see in the whole of the visual field. Each half of the retina at the back of the eye has a separate nerve supply, and damage to the brain or to the nerves behind the eye can cause blindness affecting half the field of view of one or both eyes.

HEMIPLEGIA See PARALYSIS. (Pronounced hem″i·plee′jee·a.)

HEMOGLOBIN The red pigment that gives blood its color. Hemoglobin is contained within the red blood cells (erythrocytes), which are formed in the bone marrow. Hemoglobin (pronounced hee′mo·

gloh''bin) is the vehicle by which oxygen is carried from the lungs to the tissues of the body. It also carries carbon dioxide, a waste product, from the tissues to the lungs. Hemoglobin is a complex compound of AMINO ACIDS and iron.

The exact nature of a person's hemoglobin is an inherited GENETIC characteristic. Inherited abnormalities in hemoglobin are responsible for sickle-cell ANEMIA, Mediterranean anemia, and other less serious blood conditions.

HEMOPHILIA A congenital disorder in which the blood clots very slowly. As a result, any wound or injury, no matter how minor, gives rise to prolonged bleeding. The individual with hemophilia (pronounced hee''mo·fil'ee·a) risks anemia and dangerous loss in blood volume. In addition, pools of blood (HEMATOMAS) in the tissues or joints may produce varying degrees of disability. Hemophilia is owing to a deficiency of one of the factors (the *anti*hemophilic *factor*, or AHF) in blood plasma that contribute to the process of clotting. Treatment for, or prevention of bleeding or hemorrhaging, is by transfusions of blood plasma containing the clotting factor or by injections of concentrated preparations of AHF.

Hemophilia occurs almost exclusively in males, and is due to a genetic defect that is transmitted only by women. (See HEREDITY.)

Information about hemophilia is available from the National Hemophilia Foundation, 19 West 34th Street, Room 1204, New York, New York 10001.

HEMOPTYSIS The process of spitting up blood or blood-stained sputum from the lungs or from the bronchial tubes. (Pronounced hee·mop'ti·sis.)

HEMORRHAGE Copious or abnormal loss of blood from the blood vessels. If a large volume of blood is lost in a hemorrhage (pronounced hem'or·ij), the result is SHOCK or, if the loss is very great, death. Swift action is needed in cases of accidents in which any of the large blood vessels are severed. For emergency treatment of severe bleeding, see the FIRST AID section.

Blood transfusions are required whenever much blood is lost. Internal bleeding can also be dangerous. A heavy blow or impact in a traffic accident, for example, can produce serious internal hemorrhage.

Apart from accidents, various disorders are characterized by hemorrhages. Ulcers in the stomach or intestines sometimes produce massive bleeding. Certain blood disorders, such as HEMOPHILIA and purpura (see "thrombocytopenia" in the entry BLOOD DISEASE), are characterized by abnormal bleeding. See also CEREBRAL HEMORRHAGE.

HEMORRHOID The medical term for an enlarged vein in the region of the anus (the terminal opening of the rectum). Hemorrhoids (pronounced hem'o·roydz), also known as piles, may bring discomfort or severe pain, and may be accompanied by bleeding. They are usually caused by pressure on the anal area, which can arise in several ways. Excessive straining to relieve constipation and habitual or excessive use of laxatives are frequent factors. Hemorrhoids often develop during pregnancy, when the fetus crowds against the abdominal organs. A tumor or large cyst may also cause pressure and lead to hemorrhoids.

Treatment: As an emergency measure to relieve pain, apply very cold water on tissues or a cloth for a few minutes directly to the anal area. A warm bath several times a day will help to relax muscle spasm that sometimes develops in the muscle that encircles the anus. If there is much discomfort or persistent aching, if the hemorrhoids protrude from the rectum, or if there is bleeding, see a doctor, who will prescribe treatment. He may recommend surgical removal of the hemorrhoids. This is not a serious operation and is a permanent cure for any hemorrhoids that are present.

HEMOSTAT Anything—medicine or mechanical device—that arrests the escape of blood from a blood vessel. (Pronounced hee'mo·stat''.)

HEPARIN A natural chemical compound that is administered medically as an ANTICOAGULANT to prevent blood clots from forming. Heparin (pronounced hep'a·rin) may be used to treat or prevent THROMBOSIS (formation of a blood clot in a blood vessel) or EMBOLISM (blockage of a blood vessel).

HEPATITIS Inflammation of the liver, usually due to infection by a virus. Infectious hepatitis (pronounced hep''a·tie'tis) and serum hepatitis are acute infections with similar symptoms. They are caused by two different viruses.

Infectious hepatitis is spread by food or water that has been contaminated by the feces of CARRIERS. The incubation period is from two to six weeks.

Serum hepatitis has a longer incubation period—from 6 to 26 weeks. It is spread by transfusions of blood and blood products from infected donors, and by injections given with contaminated needles.

After the incubation period has passed, the symptoms of viral hepatitis develop suddenly. They include loss of appetite, nausea, fever, and pain or tenderness in the right upper part of the abdomen. The urine may have a very dark color, due to the presence of bile pigments.

Treatment: A doctor should be called at once if the above symptoms occur, or if an individual has been knowingly exposed to infection. Bed rest is important. Injection of GAMMA GLOBULIN may help to control the disease, if given soon after exposure. Precautions must be taken to protect others.

Recovery usually follows in six to eight weeks after onset, but relapses may occur. The disease may become chronic, causing prolonged disability.

Inflammation of the liver can also be caused by certain toxic agents, such as alcohol and CARBON TETRACHLORIDE. It may also occur in infectious MONONUCLEOSIS, amebic DYSENTERY, CIRRHOSIS of the liver, and other diseases.

HEREDITY The repetition in children of their parents' characteristics. Inherited (GENETIC) characteristics are carried from parents to children by CHROMOSOMES. There are 46 chromosomes in every cell of the human body, grouped into 23 pairs. SPERM CELLS and EGG CELLS have 23 chromosomes, one from each chromosome pair. When egg and sperm unite, the baby that develops obtains half of its 46 chromosomes from the mother and half from the father. The 46 chromosomes bear innumerable GENES, each determining a distinct characteristic.

One pair of the 23 pairs of chromosomes determines sex. There are two distinct sex chromosomes, called X and Y. The X chromosome is larger than the Y chromosome; the pair are easily identified under the microscope. Sex chromosomes furnish a simple illustration of how characteristics in general are inherited. Normal men have an XY chromosome pair in each of their body cells, and normal women have an XX chromosome pair. When two sperm cells are formed by the division of the male chromosome pairs, one carries an X chromosome, the other a Y chromosome. The sex chromosome in the egg cell is always an X, since it arises from the division of an XX chromosome pair.

The sex of the offspring depends on whether an X-chromosome or a Y-chromosome sperm cell fertilizes the X-chromosome egg cell. If the X egg cell is fertilized by a Y sperm cell, the offspring is XY, or male. If the X egg cell is fertilized by an X sperm cell, the offspring is XX, or female.

The X chromosome carries genes that are not related to sexual characteristics. Such genes are said to be sex-linked. For example, it carries a gene that is essential for the normal clotting of blood. A defect in this gene is responsible for the blood disorder known as HEMOPHILIA. Like most gene defects, this defect is RECESSIVE—that is, a person usually develops normally if the defective gene is matched with a normal gene in a chromosome pair. In the XY chromosome pair of males, the tiny Y chromosome lacks any gene to mask the effect of a defect in the X chromosome. Hence hemophilia develops in males. Since females have two matching X chromosomes, the defect usually remains latent if it is present.

HERMAPHRODITE A person whose body contains tissue of both female ovaries and male testicles. The GENITALS of a hermaphrodite (pronounced hur·maf'ro·diet'') may be either male or female, or there may be some combination of the two. True hermaphroditism is a rare congenital abnormality.

Pseudohermaphroditism is a condition in which a person of one sex develops secondary sexual characteristics normally seen in the opposite sex. (Secondary sexual characteristics include such things as a beard and a deep voice in men and breast development in women.) These characteristics develop in response to sex hormones. Every normal person produces both male and female hormones in various proportions. In a pseudohermaphrodite there is some imbalance in the production of sex hormones.

HERNIA A condition in which there is weakening of the tissue surrounding an organ, and a portion of the organ bulges at the weak point. The term "hernia" (pronounced hur'nee·a) is applied especially when a loop of the intestine protrudes through the wall of the lower abdomen.

Inguinal Hernia: This is the most familiar kind of hernia. The inguinal area is the groin, the abdominal wall near where the thigh joins the trunk. Under strain, the groin sometimes weakens, and the intestine pushes out. Occasionally a hernia is strangulated—a loop of the intestine is constricted in the bulge, and the blood that normally nourishes it is cut off. Any hernia requires medical attention, but a painful one requires it immediately.

Other Types of Hernia: Another hernia is the femoral hernia, which occurs in the upper part of the thigh. In the *cystocele*, the bladder bulges into the vagina, and in the *rectocele*, the rectum protrudes at the anus or, in a woman, bulges into the vagina. In *hiatus* hernia, the stomach pushes through an opening in the muscles of the diaphragm, producing symptoms similar to those of an ulcer. A hernia of the wall of the stomach is known as a *gastrocele*. *Umbilical* hernia is marked by bulging in the area of the navel; it is especially likely to occur in children. There are numerous other kinds of hernia, including hernia of the brain.

Treatment and Prevention: Hernia is best remedied by surgery. The operation, which corrects the weakness of the muscles, is quite simple, as a rule. The wearing of a truss is generally not recommended.

HEROIN A NARCOTIC derived from opium. Because of the great danger of ADDICTION, heroin (pronounced her'oh·in) may not be used legally for any purpose in the United States and Canada. See also DRUG ADDICTION.

HERPES SIMPLEX A viral skin infection causing clusters of red, fluid-filled blisters on the skin or mucous membrane. The blisters cause burning and itching sensations for from 5 to 10 days, then dry up or form yellowish crusts that fall off easily. Herpes simplex (pronounced hur'peez sim'pleks) is a latent disease that recurs suddenly within months or sometimes years. It is triggered by exposure to sunlight, emotional upset, intestinal infection, pregnancy, or sexual intercourse—and often for no apparent reason.

There are two main types of the virus: oral and genital. The oral type, herpes simplex virus type 1, attacks the face, usually near the mouth or on the lips (see FEVER SORE), and occasionally the genital area. The genital type, herpes simplex virus type 2, infects the genital organs; in women it often infects the vagina and the cervix, and it is a possible cause of cervical cancer. The virus is spread chiefly by sexual contact.

There is no known cure for genital herpes, but a doctor can prescribe medicines to relieve pain and prevent secondary infections. The best prevention is to avoid sexual contact with a carrier of the virus.

HERPES ZOSTER The medical term for the viral nerve infection known as SHINGLES. (Pronounced hur′peez zoss′tur.)

HEXACHLOROPHENE An ANTISEPTIC substance formerly used in soaps and detergents to kill or slow up the growth of bacteria on the skin. Its general use was banned by the U.S. Food and Drug Administration when it was found to have a toxic effect on the brain. (Pronounced hek″sa · klohr′o · feen″.)

HICCUP (hiccough) An involuntary, spasmodic contraction of the DIAPHRAGM between the chest and abdomen. The characteristic clicking sound is caused by the sudden closure of the glottis (the upper opening of the LARYNX) at the moment of taking a breath. Hiccups occur from eating too fast, from disorders of the digestive tract and respiratory system, and from nervous tension. They may follow certain types of surgery and may be present in serious illnesses such as UREMIA and ENCEPHALITIS.

Ordinarily, hiccups last only a few minutes and are no cause for concern. However, if an attack is prolonged and severe, do not wait until it has caused exhaustion and anxiety. Call your doctor. He may be able to end the attack by giving one of several SEDATIVES or by washing out the stomach.

HIGH BLOOD PRESSURE See BLOOD PRESSURE; HYPERTENSION.

HIP The important, weight-bearing joint formed where the top of the femur, or thighbone, meets the pelvis. The hip is subject to a number of disorders, including dislocation, fracture, and arthritis.
Congenital Dislocation: This is a condition that a child is born with. A malformation of the bony socket allows the thighbone to slip out. If uncorrected, the child will limp when he begins to walk. Girls are much more likely than boys to have congenital dislocation of the hip. If diagnosis is made early, the condition may be corrected with a plaster cast or splints. In advanced cases, surgery may be necessary.

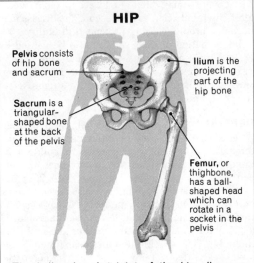

HIP

Pelvis consists of hip bone and sacrum

Ilium is the projecting part of the hip bone

Sacrum is a triangular-shaped bone at the back of the pelvis

Femur, or thighbone, has a ball-shaped head which can rotate in a socket in the pelvis

The ball-and-socket joint of the hip allows a wide range of movements for the leg. The ball on the top of the thighbone, or femur, fits into a socket on the side of the pelvis. Through the hip joints, the whole of the weight of the body is transferred to the legs.

Fracture: The top of the thighbone is the part of the hip that usually fractures. The flesh around the joint may appear swollen and livid, and there is pain when the leg is moved. Only a physician is qualified to deal with a hip fracture. For emergency treatment of broken bones, see the FIRST AID section.
Arthritis: Degenerative ARTHRITIS (osteoarthritis) of the hip is usually the result of aging. Often the symptoms are not severe, and may be relieved with aspirin, massage, and application of heat. The disorder sometimes occurs in younger people as a result of disease, injury, or congenital defects. An operation may be recommended to correct the condition; sometimes metallic devices are inserted to reconstruct parts of the damaged joint.

HIRSCHSPRUNG'S DISEASE Another name for MEGACOLON.

HIRSUTISM A condition in which a woman grows superfluous hair on the face and body, sometimes because of a hormone disorder. See HAIR REMOVAL.

HISTAMINE A substance present in all body tissues. Normally, most of the histamine (pronounced his′ta · meen) in the body remains inactive. Only small amounts are released to stimulate the stomach walls to produce gastric juices and to dilate the walls of the capillaries (tiny blood vessels).

Occasionally, however, large amounts of histamine are released with irritating, and often dangerous, effects. An excess of histamine may so dilate the small blood vessels that they leak blood into surrounding tissues and cause the redness and swelling present in INFLAMMATION. It is known that a person suffering from SHOCK has a high histamine content in his blood.

When irritating substances (allergens) enter the body or come in contact with the skin, the body reacts by releasing histamine in large amounts, causing the symptoms of ALLERGY. Compounds known as ANTIHISTAMINES are prescribed to counteract the action of histamines.

HISTOLOGY The branch of anatomy that deals with the study of the minute structure of body tissues as seen under the microscope. (Pronounced his·tol′o·jee.)

HISTOPLASMOSIS A disease caused by infection with *Histoplasma capsulatum*, a FUNGUS found in the soil and in the dried dung of bats and of various birds. Histoplasmosis (pronounced his″toh·plaz·moh′sis) occurs most often in the lungs, and is caused by inhaling the fungus's tiny, airborne spores (seeds).

The disease may show few outward symptoms and be discovered only during a routine chest X ray. The acute form of the disease usually begins with fever, malaise, and other symptoms similar to those of influenza. In most cases, the patient recovers after a period of bed rest.

HIVES An acute or chronic allergic reaction in the form of reddish, circular WHEALS that form on the skin and itch and burn. They may range from small spots to areas the size of a saucer. The medical name for the condition is urticaria.

The usual cause of hives is sensitivity to certain foods. (See ALLERGY.) Some people are sensitive to PENICILLIN, aspirin, or other medicines. Dust and pollen can also cause hives, as can emotional stress.

A more serious form of hives, known as giant hives, or angioedema, appears as large swellings on the lips, tongue, eyelids, throat, and other parts of the body. The appearance of giant hives is an emergency. Call your doctor immediately. He will prescribe an antihistamine or other drug.

There are various home remedies to help relieve the itching and burning of ordinary hives. A lukewarm bath containing two cups of old-fashioned laundry starch may be helpful. Calamine lotion or a paste of bicarbonate soda applied to the skin may be soothing. If the itching persists, you can get relief from medicine your doctor will prescribe.

HOARSENESS The quality of the voice depends on the size and shape of the LARYNX, or voice box, and the elasticity of the vocal cords. A husky voice may indicate a larynx that has been misused or overworked. However, hoarseness may accompany the common cold as well as more serious infections. A hoarse quality to a baby's cry should always be

reported to a doctor. It may be the first sign of CROUP.

Hoarseness is often accompanied by a SORE THROAT or LARYNGITIS. Persistent hoarseness may be due to a tumor of the vocal cords or other parts of the throat. A thickening of tissue on a vocal cord, known as singer's node, may result from incorrect or excessive use of the voice. Hoarseness may sometimes be an early warning of cancer of the larynx.

HODGKIN'S DISEASE A disease of unknown cause that attacks the LYMPH NODES, SPLEEN, liver, bone marrow, and sometimes other tissues. Hodgkin's disease is seen most commonly among adults between the ages of 35 and 55, and in children.

The earliest sign of the disease is the enlargement of the lymph nodes in the neck, armpits, and groin, often accompanied by excessive itching. Swelling of these nodes occurs also in many less serious disorders. However, if the swellings persist for a week or longer, a doctor should be consulted. Diagnosis is made by BIOPSY—the removal and examination under a microscope of a tiny slice of affected tissue.

As the disease progresses, the person becomes feverish and experiences sweating, weakness, anemia, loss of weight, and increasing inability to resist infection.

Treatment: The principal treatment for Hodgkin's disease is radiation therapy (see RADIOLOGY), which may be followed by chemotherapy. In many cases, under proper treatment the disease can be controlled for years. Treatment begun in the very early stages may bring about remission of all symptoms.

HOMEOPATHY A system of treating diseases that was developed by Samuel Hahnemann, a German physician (1755–1843). Homeopathy (pronounced hoh″mee·op′a·thee) is based on the principle of "like cures like." Thus, a homeopathist would prescribe in small amounts a medicine that would produce in healthy persons symptoms similar to those of the disease to be treated.

Although homeopathy is seldom practiced today, Hahnemann's investigation of the effects of medicines and drugs upon healthy persons was a significant contribution to medical science. Hahnemann discovered that large doses of cinchona bark, used to treat malaria, caused the symptoms of that disease.

HOMOSEXUALITY Preference for a member of the same sex as one's sexual partner. A homosexual relationship may exist between men or between women; in the latter case, it is called lesbianism. Some individuals may have sexual relationships with members of both sexes. Such persons are known as bisexuals.

A Complex Problem: Homosexuality usually has a psychological foundation. A boy may identify too strongly with his mother or a girl with her father and ultimately be led to assume that parent's sexual role. Children normally relate more directly to members of their own sex until puberty, when their sexual drive asserts itself and they become heterosexual, or interested in members of the opposite sex. One theory of the cause of homosexuality is that some youngsters fail to mature in this way, but for psychological reasons remain fixated on their own sex.

Many homosexuals are not happy about their condition and would prefer to be heterosexual. But if their deviation is deep-rooted, it is not easy to correct. PSYCHOTHERAPY is helpful for homosexuals who are disturbed by their sexual preference or are unable otherwise to function normally.

HONG KONG FLU See INFLUENZA.

HOOKWORM DISEASE (necatoriasis) A disease still prevalent in parts of the southern United States, Africa, and Asia. It is caused by infestation of the intestines by a parasitic worm. The hookworm derives its popular name from the hooked teeth by which the adult worm fastens itself to the lining of the small intestine, where the worms, about one half inch long, suck the victim's blood. When present in large numbers, hookworms cause anemia and malnutrition and may retard normal mental and physical development in children. The victim becomes pale, weak, and underweight.

How Hookworms Enter the Body: The life cycle of the hookworm begins when the eggs, which the female worm produces in the human intestine, are passed out in the feces. If they are deposited on warm, moist soil, they develop into the larval stage, at which time they are able to burrow into the skin and enter the bloodstream. Several weeks after the larvae have entered the skin, they reach the small intestine as adult worms.

Diagnosis and Treatment: Diagnosis is made by examination of a feces specimen, in which the eggs can be easily seen. Treatment consists primarily in improving the person's general health by means of a high-protein diet and iron supplements. The doctor may prescribe any of several medicines to eliminate the worms from the intestinal tract.

Prevention: Hookworm disease is still a serious public health problem in areas where sanitary toilet facilities are inadequate. Control of the disease depends largely upon the installation of sanitary flush toilets or, where this is not possible, privies with deeply dug pits, to prevent the hookworm larvae from infesting the soil at ground level. Children should not be permitted to go barefoot in areas where the disease is prevalent.

HORMONE A substance present in very small amounts in the circulating blood and producing specific effects in some part of the body. Most of the hormones that are essential for normal functioning are produced by the ENDOCRINE GLANDS; during pregnancy, the PLACENTA also produces important hormones.

Hormones regulate many, perhaps all, of the vital body processes. The amount of the hormone released into the blood varies according to need. ADRENALINE, for example, is released in greater than normal amounts under conditions of stress. When the temporary need has passed, any excess adrenaline in the system is broken down chemically and disposed of by the liver.

Some hormones are used in medicine to treat conditions associated with hormone deficiencies or to produce certain desired effects. For the effects and medical uses of some specific hormones, see the entries ACTH; CORTISONE; INSULIN; OXYTOCIN; THYROXINE; VASOPRESSIN.

HOT FLASH A common symptom during the menopause, in which the woman feels hot and sweats. She may also feel slightly dizzy or lightheaded. The symptoms accompany the changes that are taking place in the woman's hormone balance. See also MENOPAUSE.

HOUSEMAID'S KNEE An injury to the bursa in the front of the kneecap, caused by kneeling for long periods on hard surfaces.

The knee becomes swollen and tender and is painful to bend. Inflammation of the bursa (BURSITIS) may develop, requiring treatment or even minor surgery by a doctor. In order to avoid injuring the bursa of the knee, use a thick, soft rubber mat or other pad when working in a kneeling position.

HUMERUS (plural, **humeri**) The bone of the upper part of the arm, extending from the shoulder to the elbow. (Pronounced hyoo′mer·us.)

HUNCHBACK A familiar term for KYPHOSIS.

HUNTINGTON'S DISEASE A relatively rare hereditary disease, also called Huntington's chorea. The symptoms usually appear in the adult between the ages of 30 and 50.

The disease is marked by the group of symptoms called CHOREA: jerky, involuntary movements of the face, neck, and arms and unsteadiness in walking. Speech disturbances also occur, along with intellectual deterioration. There is no known cure for Huntington's disease, but sedatives and tranquilizers help to relieve the symptoms.

HYDROCELE A collection of watery fluid in a saclike body cavity, usually the SCROTUM. A hydrocele (pronounced hie′dro·seel″) may either be congenital or follow an injury. The fluid accumulates between the layers of tissue that cover the testicles. The swelling is painless, but may cause some discomfort due to the increase in size.

A hydrocele can sometimes be removed by drawing off the fluid through the outer layer of tissue. If the condition recurs, surgery will be required to correct the condition.

HYDROCEPHALUS A rare condition resulting in abnormal enlargement of the head and pressure on the brain tissues. Hydrocephalus (pronounced hie″dro·sef′a·lus) is usually congenital, becoming apparent during infancy; occasionally, it may occur in adults. It is caused by increased accumulation of cerebrospinal fluid in the ventricles (cavities) of the BRAIN.

A type of operation called the shunt technique has met with success in the treatment of hydrocephalus. A small tube is placed under the skin behind the ear to drain off the excess fluid from the brain into the jugular vein. In a similar operation, the fluid is shunted to the URETER and excreted through the bladder.

HYDROCHLORIC ACID A strong acid that is normally present in very dilute amounts in the GASTRIC JUICES to aid in digestion. The presence of too much hydrochloric (pronounced hie″dro·klawr′ik) acid in the stomach is called hyperchlorhydria and is an important factor in causing peptic ULCER.

HYDROGEN PEROXIDE A liquid ANTISEPTIC used in weak solution for cleansing cuts and scrapes, and also for infections of the mouth. Hydrogen peroxide (pronounced hie′dro·jen pe·rok′sied) is also used to lighten the hair.

HYDRONEPHROSIS Distension of the kidney and pelvis by accumulated urine, usually caused by a birth defect, infection, or a stone or tumor obstructing the ureter, the tube leading from the kidney to the bladder. Sometimes the ureter becomes kinked, causing an obstruction. Symptoms include pain in the loins, nausea, and vomiting (see COLIC). Hydronephrosis (pronounced hie·dro·ne·phroh′·sis) is more common in women than in men. It is treated by removing the cause of the obstruction or, in severe cases, by removing the affected kidney (the patient can live a normal life with only one kidney).

HYDROPHOBIA See RABIES. (Pronounced hie″dro·foh′bee·a.)

HYDROTHERAPY Formerly, the treatment of certain disorders or disabilities by the external application of water to the body. At one time, hydrotherapy (pronounced hie″dro·ther′a·pee) was one of the standard treatments for mental illness. Continuous baths and hot or cold packs were given to calm or stimulate disturbed patients. Tranquilizing and antidepressant drugs have now replaced this use of the treatment. Today, hydrotherapy in

orthodox medicine is restricted to the use of swimming pools in the rehabilitation of patients with arthritis or partial paralysis. See PHYSICAL THERAPY.

HYGIENE The general care of the body and its individual parts. For example, "dental hygiene" means taking good care of your teeth and keeping them clean.

HYMEN A membrane, also called the maidenhead, that in most cases partially closes the entrance of the vaginal passage in virgins. (Pronounced hie′-men.) During the first sexual intercourse, or COITUS, the rupture of the hymen may be accompanied by some pain and slight bleeding, especially if the hymen is tough and resistant to penetration. In many girls and young women, the membrane is very thin, full of perforations, or completely ruptured because of injury or participation in sports.

It is wise for young women about to be married to have a complete physical examination. If the doctor finds that the hymen is tough and inelastic, he may remove it surgically or stretch it. Either of these simple procedures is performed in his office.

HYPERACIDITY See ACID STOMACH. (Pronounced hie″per·a·sid′i·tee.)

HYPERCHLORHYDRIA See HYDROCHLORIC ACID. (Pronounced hie″per·klohr·hie′dree·a.)

HYPEREMIA Congestion of blood in a body organ or part resulting from either dilation of blood vessels or a blockage of normal blood flow. A related condition, called plethora, is an abnormal increase in the total volume of the blood in the body. (Pronounced hie″per·ee′mee·a.)

HYPERESTHESIA Unusually acute sensitivity of any of the senses, especially extreme sensitivity of the skin. (Pronounced hie″per·is·thee′zha.)

HYPERGLYCEMIA A condition in which a person has too much sugar (glucose) in his blood, generally because his pancreas is not producing enough of the hormone INSULIN. Hyperglycemia is a feature of DIABETES mellitus and may be corrected by a controlled diet, regular injections of insulin, or by taking an antidiabetic drug by mouth. (Pronounced hie″per·glie·see′ mee·a.)

HYPERINSULINISM In persons having DIABETES mellitus, a reaction from too large a dose of insulin or from failure to eat sufficient food to use up the insulin that has been injected. In hyperinsulinism (pronounced hie″per·in′su·lin·iz′em), the blood sugar falls to an abnormally low level (hypoglycemia); the person may break into cold sweats, have tremors, and feel weak (a reaction known as insulin shock). In some cases, dizziness and coma may occur. A glass of orange juice or a few pieces of sugar will relieve the symptoms. They will also respond dramatically to an injection of GLUCOSE given by a doctor.

A second type of chronic hyperinsulinism and hypoglycemia—not related to diabetes—is commonly called low blood sugar. For some reason, the PANCREAS tends to produce too much insulin, occasionally because of tumors within the pancreas, or because of a disorder of the liver. Most cases of this type are relatively mild and improve with a high-protein and low-carbohydrate diet.

HYPEROPIA The ability to see clearly only things that are relatively far away. Hyperopia (pronounced hie"per·oh'pee·a) is usually called farsightedness. (The individual with nearsightedness, or MYOPIA, sees clearly only things that are close at hand.)

The eyeball of a farsighted person is shorter from front to back than the eyeball of a person with normal vision. As a result, rays of light entering the EYE do not focus properly on the retina, the intricate network of nerve endings toward the rear of the eye. Instead, they focus behind it. EYEGLASSES with convex lenses are prescribed to correct the condition. See also PRESBYOPIA.

HYPERPLASIA Enlargement of an organ or of tissue because of an abnormal increase in the number of cells that is not due to TUMOR formation. (Pronounced hie"per·play'zha.)

HYPERTENSION High blood pressure. Hypertension (pronounced hie"per·ten'shun) is not itself a disease, but it is important as a warning signal or a symptom of a disease. In many cases it is not a serious problem and can be controlled by simple dietary measures and medication.
Symptoms: In high blood pressure, weakness or exhaustion, breathing difficulty, headache, dizziness, or faintness may be present. In malignant hypertension, a severe form of the disorder, the person may have blurred vision.
Causes: Many persons react nervously to having their BLOOD PRESSURE taken, and this often results in a high reading. The blood pressure has to be measured a number of times before a definite diagnosis can be made. It must be confirmed by a number of tests and examinations. A specific cause is found in only a small percentage of all cases. In the rest, the high blood pressure is described as primary, or essential—which simply means that the cause of the condition cannot be determined.
Treatment: In cases with a known cause, the treatment is aimed at correcting that cause or relieving it. In essential hypertension, overweight may be a predisposing factor and it may be possible to bring down the pressure by bringing down the weight. Antihypertensives, or medicines that reduce the pressure, may be given, as well as sedatives.

HYPERTHYROIDISM See GOITER; THYROID GLAND. (Pronounced hie"per·thie'roy·diz"em.)

HYPERTROPHY Excessive development, or overgrowth, of an organ or part of the body. This may occur because of increased use or activity, or it may be related to disease in that part of the body. (Pronounced hie"pur'tro·fee.)

HYPNOSIS A sleeplike state, or trance, that is induced by suggestion. In hypnosis (pronounced hip·noh'sis), an individual is often able to recall experiences that he cannot remember when awake. Hypnosis is sometimes used in PSYCHOTHERAPY. Suggestions may be made to a person's unconscious mind to help him overcome certain emotional handicaps or habits. The use of hypnosis in treating disease is called hypnotherapy.

Persons under hypnosis may respond to the suggestion that they should not feel pain, and so this technique is sometimes used by physicians in medical procedures in which it is not desirable to use ANESTHETICS.

HYPNOTIC A medicine or other agent that is used to induce sleep. The term also describes a person who is capable of being hypnotized.

PENTOTHAL is probably the most familiar of the hypnotic (pronounced hip·not'ik) medicines. In addition to its use as an anesthetic, Pentothal is used to put persons into a sleeplike state in which they can recall experiences that have been repressed from consciousness. Thus it is sometimes useful in PSYCHOTHERAPY.

HYPOACIDITY A decrease in the normal amount of acid in the GASTRIC JUICES of the stomach. Hypoacidity (pronounced hie"poh·a·sid'i·tee) is also called subacidity.

HYPOCHONDRIA Abnormal worry about one's health or a physical defect that may be minor or imaginary. Concern with one's health is normal, and occasionally anyone may become worried about it. Such normal concern is not hypochondria (pronounced hie"po·kon'dree·a). The hypochondriac, however, is in a constant state of depression about his imagined poor health, and all of his thoughts center upon it. He will take a small or meaningless symptom and exaggerate it into a warning of a fatal disease.

In its extreme form, hypochondria is a PHOBIA, a form of PSYCHONEUROSIS. It does not appear by itself, but in combination with other symptoms of EMOTIONAL AND MENTAL DISORDERS.

HYPODERMIC Beneath the skin. Describing an INJECTION of a fluid medicine or an immunizing substance under the skin by means of a syringe connected to a hollow needle. This type of syringe is also called a hypodermic (pronounced hie"po·dur'mik) or a hypodermic needle.

HYPOGLYCEMIA See DIABETES; GLYCEMIA; HYPERINSULINISM. (Pronounced hie"poh·glie·see'mee·*a*.)

HYPOINSULINISM See DIABETES. (Pronounced hie"poh·in'*su*·lĭn·iz"*e*m.)

HYPOPHYSIS Another name for the PITUITARY GLAND. (Pronounced hie·pof'ĭ·sis.)

HYPOPLASIA Defective or incomplete development of an organ or tissue, resulting in a subnormal size or a state of immaturity. (Pronounced hie"po·play'zh*a*.)

HYPOTENSION Low blood pressure. In the great majority of cases, hypotension (pronounced hie"po·ten'shun) is not a symptom of ill health. It is sometimes even a health asset. In many instances, persons with low BLOOD PRESSURE enjoy healthier, longer lives than individuals whose blood pressure is closer to the average.

In a small number of cases, low blood pressure is caused by improper functioning of one or more ENDOCRINE GLANDS, or by circulatory trouble. Hypotension is also one of the main features of shock. A person with a systolic blood pressure below 90 should have a thorough medical examination.

HYPOTHALAMUS The portion of the middle part of the BRAIN that is known to regulate body temperature and help control the functions of the internal organs. (Pronounced hie"po·thal'a·mus.)

HYPOTHERMIA Deliberate and controlled lowering of the body temperature to treat a disorder or to lessen the body's oxygen requirements during extended surgery on the brain or heart. The patient is warmed up immediately after the treatment or operation has been completed.

A patient's body temperature may be lowered by passing his blood through a cooling machine, or by surrounding him with ice packs or iced water. Normally the temperature is reduced by about 14° F., although much lower temperatures have been achieved. The same machine can be used to warm the patient's blood after the operation.

Accidental chilling of the body, caused by exposure to cold weather, is also known as hypothermia. The older a person is, the less chance he has of recovering from extreme chilling. For this reason, it is important that old people in cold climates should have the proper food, clothing, and heating in their homes to prevent accidental hypothermia.

HYPOTHYROIDISM See GOITER; THYROID GLAND. (Pronounced hie"po·thie'roy·diz"em.)

HYPOXEMIA See ALTITUDE SICKNESS. (Pronounced hie"pok·see'mee·*a*.)

HYSTERECTOMY The removal by surgery of the UTERUS, or womb—also known as a uterectomy or total or complete hysterectomy. Occasionally the CERVIX is allowed to remain, and the operation is then called a subtotal hysterectomy (pronounced his"te·rek'to·mee).

In older women approaching or past the MENOPAUSE, the ovaries usually are also removed during a hysterectomy to prevent later complications such as ovarian CANCER. (The removal of one or both ovaries is termed an OVARIECTOMY.) When operating on young women in their twenties and thirties, the surgeon leaves one or both ovaries in place (unless they are badly diseased) to avoid the onset of premature menopause.

Conditions That Require a Hysterectomy: The most common condition calling for a hysterectomy is the presence of one or more large FIBROID TUMORS. However, surgery is not always required in such cases, but depends on the size and rate of growth of the tumors and on symptoms such as hemorrhage and pain.

A second condition that may require surgery is excessive uterine bleeding which is not relieved by curettage (scraping of the lining of the uterus). Another indication is the presence of precancerous cells in a microscopic examination of tissues from the uterine lining or from the cervix. A fourth reason is cancer of the cervix or of the uterus. Radiation therapy, however, may also be used in the treatment of cervical cancer. (See RADIOLOGY for a discussion of radiation therapy.)

Period of Recovery: The hospital stay following a hysterectomy is usually from 8 to 12 days, if there are no complications. Most patients are encouraged to get out of bed 24 to 48 hours after surgery and walk a little. Light household duties or employment may be resumed, in most cases, six to eight weeks after the operation. Heavy household tasks requiring bending, lifting, or straining should generally not be undertaken for two months or more. Any woman recovering from a hysterectomy will want to follow her doctor's advice carefully.

Many women are upset and concerned about the aftereffects of a hysterectomy upon their health, femininity, and sexual activity. A diseased or enlarged uterus, or one that causes pain, discomfort, and excessive bleeding, will sap a woman's energy and dampen her good spirits. Removal of the uterus and of any of the other organs connected with it has no effect upon marital relations, which may be resumed after full recovery. After they have had a hysterectomy, many women experience improvement in their general health and renewed vitality. There may be, of course, in the case of younger women, some disappointment that pregnancy is no longer possible.

HYSTERIA A condition in which the individual shows uncontrollable emotion. During hysteria (pronounced his·teer′ee·*a*) he may laugh and cry wildly and toss his arms about. Usually the condition wears itself out in a short while. If it does not, throw some water in the hysteric's face. A few light slaps may help to bring him around. Sometimes the person may faint. (See FAINTING.) Keep him warm and put some aromatic spirits of ammonia or smelling salts under his nose.

This type of hysteria may be a defense mechanism. When a person finds himself in an unbearable situation, the hysterical spell provides a way out.

Other types of hysteria are forms of PSYCHONEUROSIS. In conversion hysteria, the individual suffers from severe anxiety over a psychological conflict and converts it into a physical problem, such as the paralysis of a limb or inability to see, hear, or speak. In dissociative hysteria, parts of the memory or personality are cut off from the consciousness so that the person is totally unaware of them. AMNESIA is an example of dissociative hysteria. Treatment is by PSYCHOTHERAPY.

HYSTEROTOMY See UTEROTOMY. (Pronounced his″te·rot′o·mee.)

I

ID In psychoanalytic theory, the instinctive, most unconscious part of the mind. It is the reservoir of our psychic energy and drives, a part of ourselves of which we are not aware. The id utilizes the pleasure principle, according to Sigmund Freud, the founder of PSYCHOANALYSIS. Many of the wishes of the id are pushed out of the mind or repressed by the EGO, or consciousness. These unconscious wishes then emerge in dreams, where they appear in disguise. If the tensions produced by repression become too severe, the result is a PSYCHONEUROSIS.

IDIOCY A term formerly used for a very severe degree of MENTAL RETARDATION. The INTELLIGENCE QUOTIENT is in the range below 20, and the mental age is less than three years.

IDIOPATHIC Denoting a disease or a disorder that arises spontaneously or from an unknown cause. (Pronounced id″ee·oh·path′ik.)

ILEITIS An inflammation of the ILEUM, the lower section of the small intestine. Ileitis (pronounced il″ee·ie′tis) may develop after abdominal surgery, after an intestinal infection such as dysentery, from an obstruction, or from irritation of the intestinal lining. The typical symptoms of ileitis are pain on the right side of the lower abdomen, attacks of diarrhea alternating with constipation, poor appetite, and loss of weight. Ileitis may respond to medication, but sometimes surgery is necessary to remove or bypass the inflamed section. See also ILEOCOLOSTOMY.

ILEOCOLOSTOMY An operation to create a new connection between the ILEUM, or lower portion of the small intestine, and the COLON, or large intestine. An ileocolostomy (pronounced il″ee·oh·ko·los′to·mee) is done in severe cases of ILEITIS to prevent the passage of food through the affected part so that it can heal.

In some cases of ulcerative COLITIS and other disorders, an operation called an ileostomy is performed. It consists of bringing out a loop of the ileum through an opening made in the abdominal wall to create an artificial anus. The contents of the small intestine are drained into a specially designed container placed over the opening.

ILEOSTOMY See ILEOCOLOSTOMY. (Pronounced il″ee·os′to·mee.)

ILEUM The lower portion of the small intestine, measuring about 12 feet in length and opening into the large intestine. (Pronounced il′ee·um.)

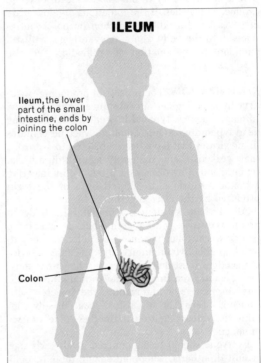

ILEUM

Ileum, the lower part of the small intestine, ends by joining the colon

Colon

In the ileum, the lower part of the small intestine, digestion of fats and carbohydrates is completed. Inflammation of the ileum, or ileitis, interferes with the digestive process and can cause diarrhea and constipation. In severe cases, a surgeon may divert the ileum to the exterior (an operation called an ileostomy) or remove a section and join the small intestine directly to the colon (an ileocolostomy).

IMBECILITY A term used at one time by psychologists for mental retardation which was more severe than that of a MORON but less severe than IDIOCY. Imbecility corresponded to the mental development of a seven-year-old.

IMMUNITY The condition of being resistant to an infectious disease. When infectious organisms, or GERMS, invade the body, they carry with them on their surfaces certain protein substances called AN-

TIGENS. Each kind of germ has its own particular antigen. The human body fights the infection by producing substances called ANTIBODIES, which counteract the germs' antigens and thereby the germs themselves. Certain antibodies are known as ANTITOXINS; the body produces them to counteract TOXINS released by the germs. These infection-fighting substances circulate in the blood plasma and contribute to recovery from the infection. After recovery from some diseases, the antibodies that remain in the blood make the person immune to being infected again by the same type of germ.

It is not necessary to have a disease in order to produce antibodies. If the infectious organisms are first weakened or killed and then purposely introduced into the body, the germs' antigens will still stimulate the production of antibodies. See also IMMUNIZATION.

IMMUNIZATION The process of producing IMMUNITY by injecting certain substances into the body. Immunity against typhoid is produced by injecting dead typhoid BACTERIA. Smallpox vaccine contains living viruses that have been subjected to a process that weakens them. Immunity against diphtheria, tetanus, and other diseases is produced by injecting a TOXOID, which is an altered form of the toxin produced by the disease germ.

All of these substances stimulate the body to produce disease-fighting antibodies. It may take several weeks following an injection for the body to build up effective immunity. In some cases a series of injections must be given, or BOOSTER SHOTS must be repeated from time to time to maintain immunity. In passive immunization, the injected substance is a serum or an antitoxin that already contains the disease-fighting antibodies. (See GAMMA GLOBULIN.)

Everyone should be immunized at an early age against diphtheria, whooping cough, tetanus, poliomyelitis, and measles. Immunizations against mumps and against rubella (German measles) are also available.

IMPACTED Packed or wedged very firmly. An impacted tooth, often a WISDOM TOOTH, is one that cannot break through the gum. Sometimes fractured bones are impacted because the jagged ends have been driven tightly together.

IMPERFORATE Describing an organ lacking the normal opening. For example, a baby may be born with an imperforate (pronounced im·pur'for·it) ear with no outer opening, or the esophagus may be closed so that it is not connected with the stomach. Fortunately, such defects can usually be corrected by surgery.

IMPETIGO. A skin infection that may occur at any age, but is most commonly seen in babies and chil-

dren. Impetigo (pronounced im"pe·tie'goh), which is caused chiefly by STAPHYLOCOCCI and sometimes by STREPTOCOCCI bacteria, begins with redness of the skin followed by blisters that break open and leave yellowish, crusty sores. Impetigo appears most often on the face, hands, and limbs. It is highly contagious and is spread by discharged matter from the sores, either by direct contact or by means of towels, clothing, and similar objects handled by other people. Prompt treatment is necessary, as the disease may spread rapidly over skin surfaces.

Treatment consists of gently removing the crusts from the sores with soap and water, and then applying any of several ointments your doctor may prescribe. Severe cases may require treatment with ANTIBIOTICS. To prevent the spread of impetigo, the skin around the sores should be cleansed frequently. The individual should wash his hands often with medicated soap and should be careful not to touch or scratch the sores.

IMPOTENCE Inability of a male to consummate the sex act. Although the term "impotence" (pronounced im'pe·tens) is sometimes given the same meaning as sterility, technically it means something quite different. A sterile man cannot produce healthy SPERM CELLS; an impotent male may produce good sperm cells but is unable to have an ERECTION and perform sexual intercourse.

Impotence may have physical or emotional causes. On the physical side, there may be a defect in the sexual organs, a deficiency of the thyroid or pituitary gland, a chronic disease such as anemia or diabetes, or addiction to alcohol or drugs. However, impotence of emotional origin is much more common. For many men, ability to achieve sexual fulfillment is impaired by feelings of insecurity, depression, or overstrict moral training. Or there may be a mother fixation, unwillingness to assume a male role, or a similar neurotic tendency. (See EMOTIONAL AND MENTAL DISORDERS.)

Physical problems are corrected by appropriate treatment of the condition, such as administering hormones or curing the underlying disease. Emotional impotence may be helped by PSYCHOTHERAPY. Any person worried about the possibility of impotence should seek medical advice.

IMPREGNATION The union of the EGG CELL, or ovum, and the SPERM CELL, which usually takes place in the FALLOPIAN TUBE. It is also called conception and fertilization.

INCISOR Any one of the eight front teeth—four in the upper jaw and four in the lower jaw—whose primary function is to bite off or cut solid food. (Pronounced in·sie'zor.) See also TOOTH.

INCONTINENCE A term meaning (1) excessive indulgence in sex, or (2) inability to control bowel movements or retain urine. The second of these meanings is explained here; sexual incontinence (pronounced in·kon'ti·nens) is discussed under NYMPHOMANIA and SATYRIASIS.

Incontinence is present in the very young because they have not acquired sufficient muscular control, and because their bladders have not grown large enough to hold the nightly production of urine. (See ENURESIS.)

In adults, inability to retain urine may be due to strong emotion or to physical causes. Any repeated lack of control over urination or bowel movements in an adult should be discussed with the doctor.

INCRUSTATION The formation of scabs, crusts, or scales on the skin. A scab is a hardened mass over a healing wound or sore. As the wound heals, the scab protects the new tissues and skin forming beneath it, and later it drops off. Crusts are found on the lesions of such skin diseases as IMPETIGO and ECZEMA. In PSORIASIS, the affected areas are covered by whitish, dry scales of horny EPITHELIUM.

INCUBATION PERIOD The time between the entry of GERMS into the body and the appearance of symptoms. Many infectious diseases have characteristic incubation periods. The period may be as short as one to four days, as with influenza, or as long as one year, as in some cases of RABIES. The incubation period determines the duration of QUARANTINE imposed as a safeguard against the spread of a disease.

INCUBATOR A transparent container in which a newborn baby can be kept under uniform, controlled conditions and isolated against possible infection. Incubators are essential in caring for babies that are born prematurely and for those born with defects that must be corrected before they can stand the stress of living in a normal atmosphere.

INDIGESTION A nonmedical term sometimes used vaguely, like stomachache and upset stomach, for almost any kind of disturbance in the digestive system, including nausea, vomiting, excessive belching, heartburn, a feeling of fullness or discomfort in the abdomen, cramps, constipation, and diarrhea. All of these are symptoms that are common to a great many diseases, some of them serious. If any of these symptoms are severe or long-lasting, or if they recur frequently, it is important to have an examination by a doctor.

Dyspepsia is the medical term for the minor digestive upsets that often occur when no other disease is present. The symptoms may include any of those listed above, usually in mild form. Dyspepsia may be due to various causes, such as eating under emotional stress, overeating, or gulping down food without chewing it properly. Some people find that there are one or two foods that just do not agree with them. Aspirin or other medicines sometimes irritate the stomach. Dyspepsia can often be avoided simply by adopting commonsense eating habits and not rushing at meals. It may usually be relieved by taking a teaspoonful of sodium bicarbonate (baking soda) in water or fruit juice.

INDOCIN A trade name for indomethacin, a medicine used to help relieve the pain and inflammation of rheumatoid ARTHRITIS and osteoarthritis. (Pronounced in'doh·sin.)

INFANTILE PARALYSIS See POLIOMYELITIS.

INFARCTION The death of tissue when the blood that supplies it with oxygen and nutrients is cut off. Infarction results from blockage of an artery, usually by a thrombus (a blood clot) or an embolus (a plug of clotted blood or foreign material). (See THROMBOSIS; EMBOLISM.) Infarction can occur in any tissue.

INFECTION A disease caused by a microscopic living organism, such as a VIRUS or BACTERIUM. The word is also used for the process by which disease organisms invade body tissue.

A secondary infection is one that occurs as a complication of some preexisting but unrelated primary infection or condition. Thus INFLUENZA, a viral infection, sometimes weakens the body's defenses and makes a person especially susceptible to certain kinds of secondary infections by bacteria, among them pneumonia. One of the most frequent types of secondary infection is the bacterial invasion during a virus cold, which leads to such infections as sinusitis, ear inflammation, bronchitis, and bacterial pneumonia.

INFERIORITY COMPLEX See COMPLEX.

INFERTILITY See STERILITY.

INFLAMMATION A reaction of the body tissues and blood circulation to injury, irritation, and INFECTION. Blows, cuts, burns, sprains, extreme cold, and invasion of certain bacteria produce inflammation. The body reacts by sending an increased flow of blood and body fluids to the affected part to promote healing. As a result, the area swells, becomes red, and is tender and hot to the touch.

INFLUENZA An acute, infectious disease, often called flu or grippe. (Intestinal flu is a popular, nonmedical term for several kinds of intestinal upsets that have no connection with influenza.) The symptoms of influenza include chills and fever, headache, loss of appetite, general aches and pains, weakness, and inflammation of the mucous membranes of the nose and throat.

The influenza virus weakens the body's defenses against bacteria. Persons with influenza risk developing pneumonia, either from the influenza virus itself or from a secondary bacterial INFECTION. In uncomplicated cases, the acute symptoms usually last for only a few days, followed by gradual recovery of normal strength and fitness.

Treatment: There are no specific medicines for influenza. A person should stay in bed while the acute symptoms last, and during convalescence should only gradually return to normal activity. Your doctor will prescribe medication to relieve the symptoms, as well as appropriate antibiotics if bacterial infection threatens or has developed.

Epidemics: Since influenza is exceedingly infectious and has an incubation period of only from one to four days, the disease spreads rapidly. Infection enters the body by way of the nose and mouth, and is transmitted partly by sneezing and coughing. EPIDEMICS of influenza occur every few years, but the virus that causes an epidemic may not be exactly the same as that which brought on the previous one.

The name of the place where any particular epidemic starts is often used in referring to that epidemic. Thus, the serious and often fatal pandemic of 1918 was known as Spanish influenza. In 1957, Asian flu swept across North America. Hong Kong flu, which proved to be relatively mild, was first identified in Hong Kong in 1968 and reached North America several months later.

Temporary immunity to a particular variety of flu virus can be acquired by injection of virus vaccine. After injection, it takes about two weeks for a person to develop immunity. It is useless to have flu shots once symptoms have developed.

INGROWN TOENAIL A toenail, often the one on the big toe, that has a tendency on the sides to curve into the flesh instead of to grow straight out. An ingrown toenail is not only painful, but if left untreated, can cause an inflamed sore and even infection. Ingrown toenails can be prevented by cutting the nails short, preferably with the sides a little longer than the middle. See that your shoes are roomy so that they do not press on the top or sides of the toes. *This is most important.*

If a badly ingrown nail continues to hurt or becomes infected, it should be treated by a doctor or by a PODIATRIST (also called a chiropodist), who specializes in foot troubles.

INH The abbreviation for *isonicotinic acid hydrazide,* a medicine used in treating certain types of tuberculosis. It is also called isoniazid.

INHIBITION The blocking or restraint of an action or a process. Inhibition may be physiological—for example, the function of an organ of the body may be inhibited or interfered with.

In popular use, the term generally has a psychological meaning. Often, it describes the restraint of a normal, instinctual reaction as a result of fear, psychological conflict, or social conditioning.

INJECTION The insertion of a fluid substance into the body, usually by means of a syringe connected to a hollow needle (popularly called a HYPODERMIC needle).

Injections may be administered in any of four main ways. An injection between the layers of the skin (intracutaneous, or intradermal) is used for diagnostic purposes, for local ANESTHESIA, and to test allergic reactions to substances. (See ALLERGY.) An injection under the skin (SUBCUTANEOUS) is generally employed for injecting pain-relieving medicines, such as morphine, or giving INSULIN to diabetics. Certain medicines, such as ANTIBIOTICS, are injected into a muscle (intramuscular) in the upper arm, upper thigh, and frequently in the buttock. When a substance must be absorbed rapidly, the injection is made into a vein, usually at the inside of the elbow, and is called an intravenous injection. See also INTRAVENOUS FEEDING.

INKBLOT TEST See PERSONALITY TEST.

INOCULATION The introduction into the body of a SERUM or VACCINE in order to produce immunity against certain infectious diseases. Inoculation is usually given by INJECTION, although certain poliomyelitis vaccines are given by mouth. See also IMMUNIZATION; VACCINATION.

INSANITY A term used to describe severe mental illness. In the legal sense, an insane individual is considered incapable of moral judgment and of managing his property and affairs. The word, while still used in law, has been largely abandoned by psychiatrists.

INSECT BITE Very few insects bite, in the ordinary sense of gouging out a piece of skin. Most insects that attack people simply puncture the skin. The damage they do results from substances they leave in the wound. Mosquitoes, lice, and other bloodsucking insects inject a substance that temporarily prevents the blood from clotting. A local allergic (see ALLERGY) reaction usually occurs at the site of the bite, with inflammation and itching. The discomfort usually disappears in a few hours, and the bite in itself has no serious consequences. However, many bloodsucking insects are carriers of serious diseases, such as malaria, typhus, and yellow fever.

There is always a temptation to scratch an itching bite, thus exposing the damaged skin to secondary infection. The itch can usually be relieved by covering the bite with a paste of bicarbonate of soda (baking soda) and a few drops of water, or by applying calamine lotion. Bites can often be prevented by using any of the numerous insect repellents.

Painful and sometimes very serious bites or stings are inflicted by many insects that do not feed on blood. They bite or sting only when someone unintentionally disturbs and annoys them. Bees, wasps, hornets, and some kinds of spiders and ants inject a venom that not only produces a local reaction but may affect the entire body. Some of the insects leave a venom-filled stinger at the site of the sting. You should try to remove this immediately—and completely—with tweezers or your fingernails.

Anyone who reacts strongly to a bite or sting should have himself desensitized by a series of venom doses carefully administered by a doctor. Such a person should always carry with him medicine to be used in case he should be bitten or stung.

If a person who has been stung or bitten shows any signs of physical distress such as swelling of the face or body, a doctor should be called at once, or the person should be taken to a hospital. See also the FIRST AID section.

INSEMINATION   The depositing of semen in the vagina during sexual intercourse (COITUS). (Pronounced in·sem"i·nay'shun.) See also ARTIFICIAL INSEMINATION.

INSOMNIA   Inability to fall asleep or to sleep restfully. Insomnia is a problem to everyone at one time or another. However, if insomnia is recurrent, it is important to track down its causes and correct them, with the help of a physician, if necessary.
Causes: Any of a large number of simple factors may make it difficult for a person to fall asleep or remain asleep. His mattress may be too soft or too hard. If there are too many blankets, he may be too warm; if the bedclothes are too light, he may feel cold during the night. The bedroom itself may be chilly or overheated. If it is not dark enough, he may have difficulty in sleeping.

Eating shortly before retiring may be responsible for insomnia. Stimulating beverages, such as coffee or tea, can also cause sleeping problems. If you share your bedroom with a loud snorer or a restless sleeper, you may also have trouble.

Inability to fall asleep is most often caused by nervous tension, but it may also be a symptom of some EMOTIONAL AND MENTAL DISORDER or of a physical disease.
Treatment: If you can determine the cause of your insomnia, it may be easy to correct. Check the mattress, bedclothes, and bedroom temperature, and make necessary adjustments. A dark eye mask will keep light out, and ear plugs will shut out sound.

If you have trouble getting to sleep, relax for an hour or two before bedtime: read a diverting book, watch television, or take a warm bath. If you wake up during the night, turn on the light and resume reading for a while. Taking warm milk and a cookie or two may be helpful.

If necessary, you may ask your physician for a tranquilizer or sleeping pills. Take only the dosage that he prescribes. An overdose is dangerous.

INSULIN   The hormone produced by the PANCREAS, specifically by the cell groups in the pancreas known as the ISLETS OF LANGERHANS. Insulin is used by the body to help burn the sugar (GLUCOSE) in the blood and convert it into energy. When the pancreas produces too little insulin, it causes diabetes mellitus. In some types of DIABETES, there is an adequate supply of insulin, but the body does not react to it normally.

INSULIN SHOCK   See HYPERINSULINISM.

INTEGUMENT   A medical word for the SKIN. (Pronounced in·teg'yu·ment.)

INTELLIGENCE QUOTIENT   A score obtained on the BINET TEST or other intelligence tests. The IQ, as it is popularly called, is defined as 100 times the mental age divided by the actual age in years of the child tested. Mental age is based on the results of testing many children of different ages. If it is found that a particular child of ten can solve problems in an intelligence test that are beyond the ability of most ten-year-olds but can be solved by approximately 75 percent of 13-year-olds, the child is said to have a mental age of 13. This child's IQ would be 130. An IQ of 100 indicates average, or normal, performance on intelligence tests.

INTERCOSTAL   Situated or occurring between the ribs. (Pronounced in"ter·kos'tal.)

INTERMISSION   A symptom-free interval between two occurrences of the manifestations of a disorder. A REMISSION differs from an intermission in that it is a temporary lessening of the symptoms of a disease.

INTERN (interne)   A recent graduate from a medical school who is being trained in a hospital before being licensed to practice medicine. In the United States, all doctors must serve an internship of at least one year.

INTERNIST   Not to be confused with INTERN, an internist (pronounced in·tur'nist) is a physician who specializes in treating diseases of the heart, lungs, stomach, intestines, and other internal organs. He does not perform obstetrical work or any type of surgery. When necessary, an internist will refer the patient to other specialists for further treatment or for surgery.

INTERTRIGO   Chafing that takes place when two layers of skin rub against each other—for example, in the armpit or between the thighs. When intertrigo (pronounced in"ter·tree'go) is severe, small blisters develop and they may burst and become infected. The treatment is by regular washing, and the doctor may also·prescribe an ointment or an antibiotic cream. Once the condition is better, a recurrence may be prevented by careful washing and drying of the areas, followed by the use of talcum powder or cornstarch.

INTESTINAL FLU   See INFLUENZA.

INTESTINAL OBSTRUCTION   Any condition that blocks up or seriously interferes with passage of the contents of the intestine. It requires immediate medical attention. The symptoms include intense, cramplike pain; vomiting; constipation; rumbling or gurgling in the bowels; weakness; copious perspiration; and shock. The condition is made worse by laxatives or food. The cause is usually a mechanical obstruction, such as INTUSSUSCEPTION; constriction of a loop of the intestine resulting from HERNIA or from an abnormal twisting; pressure from an adjacent tumor; pressure from adhesions; or an impacted foreign body or FECES.

The method of treatment depends on the exact cause of the blockage. The obstruction may need to be removed by surgery.

INTESTINE   The long, coiled tube of the digestive system, extending from the stomach to the anus. There are two main parts, the small intestine and the large intestine, or COLON. The small intestine is about 22 feet long. It is widest where it joins the stomach. This fairly wide section, called the duodenum, has one duct leading into it from the pancreas and another, the common bile duct, from the liver and gallbladder. Digestive juices from these organs mix with the partly digested food, or CHYME, from the stomach, and digestion continues as the contents are pushed forward through the intestine by muscular contractions of the intestine wall.

The wall of the small intestine is lined with countless tiny projections, called villi. The villi contain capillary blood vessels into which nutrients are absorbed. From the villi, the nutrient-rich blood is transported to the liver. By the time the intestinal contents reach the colon, most of the nutrients have been absorbed.

The intestine has extensive nerve connections, so that fear, anger, and other nervous upsets can set off attacks of nausea, cramps, diarrhea, and other symptoms. Diseases such as ulcer and cancer can occur in the intestines; contagious diseases such as typhoid fever and various virus infections can affect them, as well as such conditions as food poisoning, constipation, dyspepsia, and allergies. See also COLITIS; INTESTINAL OBSTRUCTION.

INTRAUTERINE DEVICE (IUD)   A simple, effective contraceptive device. The most common types of IUD are spirals or loops of flexible plastic that can sometimes be inserted without dilation of the cervix. A small extension of thread is left protruding into the VAGINA, so that it is easy to remove the device or check to see that it has not been expelled accidentally. After the device has been inserted, it may cause some discomfort for a short time, but this normally disappears. IUD's have been used extensively and with great success in India and some other developing countries.

INTRAVENOUS FEEDING   When a patient is too ill or too weak to take food or liquid by mouth, he is often given intravenous (pronounced in·tra·vee'nus) nourishment temporarily through a hollow needle, usually inserted into a vein in the lower arm and held in place with strips of adhesive tape. A glass bottle containing sterile water and GLUCOSE is hung upside down a few feet above the patient. It is connected to the needle by plastic tubing, through which the flow is regulated as required by the doctor. Sometimes solutions of AMINO ACIDS are given to chronically ill patients, to help build proteins in their systems.

INTRAVENOUS PYELOGRAM   An X-ray photograph of the kidneys and urinary system; known also as an IVP. The soft tissues of the kidneys and ureters (the tubes leading from the kidneys to the bladder) do not show up well on an ordinary X-ray photograph. To make them visible, the radiologist injects the person being examined with a liquid containing a substance (such as a compound of iodine) which is opaque to X rays. The injection is generally made into a vein in the arm; the substance then travels through the bloodstream and eventually reaches the kidneys. There it is removed from the blood by the normal filtering action of the kidneys, and it enters the urine. Eventually the substance, which is harmless, passes out of the body in the urine.

On a pyelogram, the radiologist can see the sizes of the kidneys and ureters, whether their shapes are normal, and the position of any calculus (stone) in the kidneys or ureters. A specialist can use the photographs in planning treatment. A pyelogram is also a good test of how the kidneys are working. For instance, if there is a stone blocking one of the ureters, only the kidney and ureter above the obstruction shows.

Other special X-ray tests on the urinary system include arteriography, in which the blood vessels are shown up by a radio-opaque dye injected through a fine tube passed into the artery supplying blood to a kidney. In a retrograde pyelogram, dye is introduced through a tube passed into the bladder and up a ureter into the kidney's drainage system. See also KIDNEY STONE; CYSTOSCOPY.

INTROVERT   A person who is mainly concerned with his own thoughts, or inner life. The opposite type is the EXTROVERT, the outgoing individual whose chief interest is in the world around him.

The terms "introversion" and "extroversion" were popularized by the work of Carl Gustav Jung, a Swiss psychiatrist. Jung held that, as a rule, people belong to one type or the other, but that we all have something of both types in our character.

INTUSSUSCEPTION The telescoping of a section of the small intestine into the adjoining part, resulting in a serious obstruction. Although intussusception (pronounced in"*tus·su·*sep'sh*u*n) can occur at any age, it is more common among small children, especially boys. The first signs are severe pain in the abdomen, fever, vomiting, and diarrhea. Later, bloody mucus is passed by the rectum.

Early diagnosis and treatment of intussusception are important. A barium enema (see BARIUM SULFATE) given to help diagnose the condition may often correct it. Otherwise, surgery is necessary.

INVOLUTIONAL MELANCHOLIA A mental disorder that is also known as involutional (pronounced in"*vo·*loo'sh*u·*n*al*) psychosis. It is found in older persons and is marked by a deep depression. See also MELANCHOLIA; EMOTIONAL AND MENTAL DISORDERS.

IODINE A chemical element that is essential to health, though only in very minute amounts. The thyroid gland needs iodine in order to produce the hormone THYROXINE. Lack of iodine before birth and in early childhood produces severe physical and mental retardation. Adults who lack iodine may develop GOITER.

Radioactive iodine compounds are sometimes given to help in the diagnosis of thyroid disease and to treat overactive goiters or some forms of cancer in the thyroid gland.

A weak solution of iodine in alcohol (tincture of iodine) was formerly much used as a household antiseptic to apply to minor wounds.

IODOFORM A yellow powder with a strong, penetrating odor, used as a local antiseptic. (Pronounced ie·oh'do·fawrm".)

IPECAC A substance obtained from the dried root of a Brazilian shrub. Ipecac (pronounced ip'*e·*kak") is often used as an EMETIC to induce vomiting in cases of poisoning. In some cases of chest congestion, a cough medicine containing a small amount of ipecac may be prescribed to help dilute the mucus and make it easier to cough up.

IRIS See EYE.

IRITIS An acute or chronic inflammation of the iris, or colored part of the EYE. Iritis (pronounced ie·rie'tis) may arise from other infections in the body or from an injury. The disease causes severe pain in the eyeball that then spreads into the forehead and temples.

Iritis is treated by regular use of ATROPINE, to keep the pupils dilated and prevent adhesions. Drops or ointments containing CORTISONE help clear up the inflammation quickly. It is most important, however, to find and treat the underlying causes.

IRON See ANEMIA; DIET.

IRON LUNG An old type of RESPIRATOR, or "breathing machine," in the form of a long, airtight cylinder. A person with paralyzed chest muscles, usually resulting from POLIOMYELITIS, was encased in the machine, except for his head. Automatically operated bellows forced the lungs to expand and contract and thus to inhale and exhale air.

IRRADIATION The use of X RAYS, radioactive material, ultraviolet rays, or infrared rays in the treatment of disease. (See RADIATION THERAPY.) Irradiation (pronounced i·ray"dee·ay'shun) is also used to kill bacteria in foods in order to prevent spoilage.

ISLETS OF LANGERHANS Clusters of cells scattered through the tissues of the PANCREAS. Also known as islands of Langerhans (pronounced lahng'-er·hahnz), they produce the hormone INSULIN. They also secrete another hormone, glucagon, that counteracts the effect of insulin by raising (instead of lowering) the level of the blood sugar.

ISODINE A trade name for povidone-iodine, an ANTISEPTIC that contains IODINE and is used locally, usually in the form of an ointment. (Pronounced ies'o·dien".)

ISONIAZID A drug, full chemical name isonicotinic acid hydrazide (INH), used for treating certain types of tuberculosis.

ITCHING A mild irritation of the many tiny nerve endings in the skin. The medical name for itching is pruritus. Moderate itching may be due to insect bites or allergic reactions. More severe and lasting itching occurs in scabies (see MITE) and in infectious diseases, such as chicken pox, in which a rash occurs. Sometimes itching is the only early symptom of such serious disorders as DIABETES, liver disease, and HODGKIN'S DISEASE.

The urge to scratch is instinctive in anyone who itches, but it may injure the skin and admit infection. The best way to cure persistent itching is to have your doctor find and treat the cause. Temporary relief may be obtained by applying cold compresses, witch hazel, or calamine lotion. See also HIVES.

IUD Abbreviation for INTRAUTERINE DEVICE. (Pronounce each letter.)

J

JAUNDICE A yellowish color of the skin and the whites of the eyes caused by the presence of too much bile in the blood. In many cases of jaundice, the stools become light and the urine dark. Jaundice is not in itself a disease, but rather a symptom of other diseases and disorders.

Sometimes a GALLSTONE is responsible. Infectious HEPATITIS, CIRRHOSIS, and hemolytic ANEMIA are usually characterized by jaundice. It may be an unfortunate side effect of some medications.

Consult your doctor immediately when the condition is noticed, so that he can diagnose the cause and start proper treatment.

JAW The bones that frame the mouth. There are upper and lower jawbones, known medically as the maxilla (a part of the skull) and the mandible. They include the alveoli, the sockets holding the roots of the teeth. See also TOOTH.

JOCKSTRAP ITCH An infection in the area of the scrotum and upper thighs, caused by RINGWORM, a type of FUNGUS.

JOGGING Running at a slow, regular trot. Jogging, like swimming and bicycling, is considered an excellent form of exercise. If practiced regularly over a long period of time, it can have a beneficial effect on the heart, the lungs, and the vast network of veins and arteries that make up the circulatory system.

Jogging has reached the proportions of a national hobby, enjoyed by men and women alike. Before engaging in jogging, it is important to see your physician and have a complete medical checkup.

If you are in average condition, do not undertake too much at once. Set aside a quarter of an hour or half an hour every day, or as often as you can, for jogging; you must do it regularly to derive any substantial benefit. It is helpful to do warm-up exercises for a few minutes. Then begin to walk slowly and rhythmically, arms swinging at your sides. Your head should be high, your body straight. Speed up your pace, touching the ground lightly with your feet. Now go faster in an easy, slow trot. Do not run—that is not jogging. Bend your arms at the elbows, clench your fists lightly, and swing your arms. If you get winded, slow down to a walk. When you feel rested, jog again, but do not overdo it. Over a period of weeks or months, try to increase the distance that you jog.

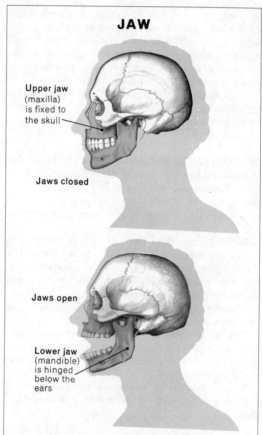

JAW

Upper jaw (maxilla) is fixed to the skull

Jaws closed

Jaws open

Lower jaw (mandible) is hinged below the ears

The upper jaw, or maxilla, is part of the skull. Hinged to it is the lower jaw, or mandible, which is controlled by the powerful masseter muscles in the sides of the face. The jaws carry the alveoli, the tooth-supporting bones.

JOINT The point where two bones come into contact. Joints may be immovable, as in the skull, or movable, as in the limbs; it is the second type that we usually think of as joints. Joints are covered with an elastic white tissue called CARTILAGE. To avoid friction, the joint is lubricated by the synovial membrane, which surrounds the joint. Ligaments attached to the bones keep the joint in position.

Movable joints are of various types. The *hinge* joint allows movement forward and backward; the joints of the finger, elbow, and knee are examples. The *pivot* joint permits rotary motion, as in the

JOINTS

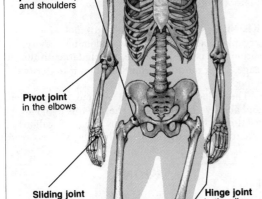

Pivot joint in the neck at the base of the skull

Ball-and-socket joint at the hip and shoulders

Pivot joint in the elbows

Sliding joint at the ankles and wrists

Hinge joint in the elbow and knees

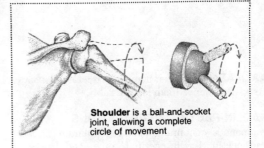

Shoulder is a ball-and-socket joint, allowing a complete circle of movement

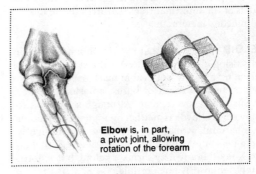

Elbow is, in part, a pivot joint, allowing rotation of the forearm

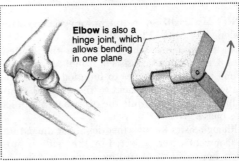

Elbow is also a hinge joint, which allows bending in one plane

There are four basic kinds of movable joints in the body: hinge joints, such as those in the fingers, elbows and knees; ball-and-socket joints, such as those at the hips and shoulders; sliding joints, like those at the wrists; and pivot joints, such as that at the top of the neck. There are also immovable joints, such as those between the bony plates of the skull. A joint of cartilage between the bones at the front of the pelvis softens and stretches to enlarge the pelvic cavity in a woman at childbirth.

neck. *Ball-and-socket* joints such as the shoulder and the hip allow for maximum movement. The *sliding* joints of wrists and ankles permit delicate movements like those used in balancing or knitting.

Joints are subject to sprains, fractures, and dislocations, as well as disorders such as BURSITIS and ARTHRITIS.

JUGULAR VEIN One of the four veins that return blood from the head to the chest. There are two, called the external and internal jugular veins, on each side of the neck. See also VEIN.

JUNGLE ROT A condition, marked by ulcers or sores on the skin, that occurs in the tropics. The disorder may be caused by various fungi, and is particularly likely to occur in individuals whose diet is inadequate. ANTIBIOTICS are of great help in controlling the sores and preventing the development of complications.

K

KALA AZAR Another name for visceral LEISHMAN-IASIS. (Pronounced kah'lah ah·zahr'.)

KAOLIN-PECTIN PREPARATIONS Various compounds containing kaolin (aluminum silicate) and pectin. Kaolin-pectin (pronounced kay'o·lin pek'tin) preparations are used to treat various disorders of the intestinal tract that irritate the intestinal mucous membrane.

KELOID Scar tissue that remains as a hard, fibrous mass rising above the surface of the skin, instead of becoming a barely noticeable mark or line. Keloids may occur as a result of burns, abrasions, surgical incisions, and severe acne. Although a keloid (pronounced kee'loyd) is neither malignant nor otherwise harmful, it may be very large and unsightly, and a person may wish to have it removed. Radium and X-ray therapy may shrink a keloid, but unfortunately removal is not possible.

KENNY METHOD A treatment for POLIOMYELITIS developed by Sister Elizabeth Kenny (1886–1952), an Australian nurse who worked in the United States. The treatment consists in stimulating and retraining paralyzed muscles to function by the application of hot, moist packs to the affected areas and by exercise, even while the disease is still in its acute phase.

Although Sister Kenny's theories about the nature of poliomyelitis were rejected by the medical profession, her methods of treatment were widely accepted and put into practice. There is no real cure for poliomyelitis, but the Kenny method and other rehabilitative treatments have been successful in lessening, or even preventing, permanent paralysis in many cases. With the development of effective vaccines, the need for rehabilitative measures has greatly diminished.

KERATIN The substance making up the horny tissues, such as the nails of the fingers and toes. Keratin (pronounced ker'a·tin) is also present to some extent in the hair and skin. In medicine, keratin is used to coat pills intended to be dissolved only in the intestine, because keratin is not affected by the gastric juices of the stomach.

KERATITIS Inflammation of the cornea, the transparent membrane that covers the front of the eyeball. Keratitis (pronounced ker''a·tie'tis) may be caused by infection, injury, or lack of vitamin A. The symptoms are usually severe pain in the EYE and sensitivity to light. The eye may water a great deal. Any inflammation of the eye demands immediate attention by your doctor.

KIDNEY One of a pair of extremely important organs located behind the abdominal cavity, on either side of the backbone, just underneath the rib cage. Their most important function is to purify the blood.

The kidneys regulate the volume, composition, and acidity of body fluids. They do this by means of a filtering system that handles about 15 gallons of blood every hour. Blood reaches the kidneys from

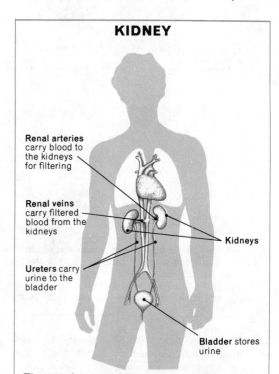

KIDNEY

Renal arteries carry blood to the kidneys for filtering

Renal veins carry filtered blood from the kidneys

Kidneys

Ureters carry urine to the bladder

Bladder stores urine

The main function of the kidneys is to filter waste products out of the blood passing through them. Blood enters along the renal arteries, and passes back to the circulation through the renal veins. The wastes, such as urea and excess water, are secreted from the kidneys as urine and pass down the ureters to be stored in and periodically released from the bladder.

the heart through the renal artery. Fluids and dissolved salts from the blood are collected in microscopic filtering units called nephrons. Then most of the water and the required salts are reabsorbed into capillaries and returned to the heart by way of the renal vein. Excess water and other waste materials are left behind as urine. This is collected into small chambers opening into the central part of the kidney, and drains away to the bladder through the ureter.

In healthy people thirst usually regulates fluid intake so that about a quart of urine is produced every day. A great deal of water is also lost by evaporation from the lungs and the skin. Usually the amount of urine increases markedly when there is a sudden change in the weather from hot to cold, because then the kidneys have to dispose of excess water that is no longer lost by perspiration.

Congenital abnormalities of the kidneys are fairly common. These abnormalities are not necessarily serious threats to health. The kidneys have a great deal of reserve capacity, and it is possible to get along quite well with only one kidney. However, it is not possible to survive without adequate kidney function. See also KIDNEY DISEASE.

KIDNEY DISEASE Any disease or injury that interferes with KIDNEY function is potentially very serious. Sometimes a heart condition prevents blood from being adequately cycled through the kidneys. In most cases, however, the condition is due to some infection or other cause that affects the kidneys directly.

Chronic kidney disease may build up very slowly over several years before it becomes serious enough to cause obvious symptoms. An annual medical checkup, including URINALYSIS and blood tests, is good insurance against such chronic conditions.

Acute kidney disease also affects the urine, often in more obvious ways. If there is blood in the urine, you should see a doctor. Other symptoms of acute kidney disease may include a marked decrease in the amount of urine voided. Elimination of urine may be frequent, or accompanied by a burning sensation. There may be puffiness in the face and limbs, and back pain just under the ribs. See also NEPHRITIS; NEPHROSIS; PYELITIS; UREMIA.

KIDNEY STONES and abnormalities in the structure of the kidney are other possible sources of kidney trouble.

Treatment: In treating severe kidney disease, an artificial-kidney machine may be used, which takes over some of the functions of temporarily or permanently damaged kidneys in a process called dialysis. See also ARTIFICIAL ORGAN.

Kidney machines are usually very expensive,

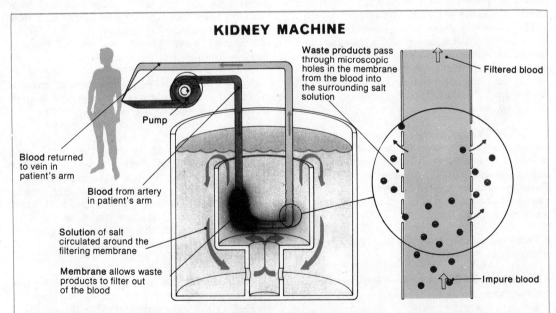

KIDNEY MACHINE

Waste products pass through microscopic holes in the membrane from the blood into the surrounding salt solution

Filtered blood

Pump

Blood returned to vein in patient's arm

Blood from artery in patient's arm

Solution of salt circulated around the filtering membrane

Membrane allows waste products to filter out of the blood

Impure blood

A patient whose kidneys have failed can be kept alive by the regular use of a kidney machine, which cleanses his blood of waste products by copying the action of a natural kidney. Blood pumped from an artery in the arm of the patient passes over a thin plastic membrane in a bath of circulating saline solution. Water and waste products such as urea pass through microscopic holes in the membrane into the surrounding solution, leaving the much larger blood cells behind. The purified blood is then warmed to blood heat and pumped back into a vein in the patient's arm. Using this machine, patients with chronic kidney failure have survived for more than 12 years. However, they are usually advised to have kidney transplant operations, if suitable donors are available.

quite large pieces of apparatus requiring expert attention while in use. Such machines are usually limited to large hospitals and a few special centers, but progress has been made in building units that can be used in the home. For more information, write the National Kidney Foundation, Inc., 2 Park Avenue, New York, New York 10016.

KIDNEY STONE A small mass of solid matter that has separated out of the urine to form a stone in the kidney. Kidney stones are fairly common in the URINARY TRACT. The stones vary in size and shape from tiny particles like grains of sand to large, branched formations filling much of the space in the kidney. Very small particles may be voided without a person's knowing it. Larger stones may cause intense pain and damage if they leave the kidney and pass through the urinary tract. They may also block the ureter and prevent urine from leaving the kidney. Stones too large to enter the ureters may cause serious mechanical damage to the delicate tissues surrounding them.

Any kidney stone that causes trouble may lead to serious complications. It must be removed as soon as possible, usually by surgery. Some persons have a tendency to form stones repeatedly. By making a thorough medical examination—including, if possible, a chemical analysis of a stone that has been voided or removed—the doctor can sometimes identify the cause in a particular case.

The doctor may prescribe a special diet or medicine to help prevent stone formation, once the cause has been determined. Frequently, treatment includes drinking larger amounts of water than usual, so that the urine is kept dilute enough to hold all dissolved salts in solution and keep them from forming a hard mass.

KINEPLASTY (cineplasty) A method used after the amputation of a hand which enables the amputee's arm and chest muscles to operate an attached artificial part. (Pronounced kin′e·plas″tee.) These muscles are treated surgically so that they can be attached to pegs which can then be made to move the artificial hand.

KINESIA Another word for MOTION SICKNESS. (Pronounced ki·nee′zha.)

KISSING DISEASE A term sometimes used for MONONUCLEOSIS.

KLEPTOMANIA An irresistible impulse to steal. Kleptomania (pronounced klep″to·may′nee·a) is found in certain persons who may appear to be otherwise normal. Often the objects stolen do not have any special value or usefulness to the individual, but seem to possess a symbolic meaning. Anyone who feels an uncontrollable impulse to steal should seek psychiatric help.

Very young children who steal are not kleptomaniacs. As a rule, they lack an understanding of what personal property is. With guidance, they usually outgrow the habit. In older children, stealing is often a sign of neurotic maladjustment.

KLINEFELTER'S SYNDROME A congenital disorder in which an apparently male person has an extra X CHROMOSOME in each cell (giving the combination XXY instead of XY as in a normal male). The testes fail to develop and some secondary male characteristics, such as facial and body hair, are lacking. The syndrome was first described by an American, Harry Klinefelter. See also CHROMOSOME; HEREDITY.

KNEE An important hinge joint, formed by the lower end of the femur (thighbone), the patella (kneecap), and the top of the tibia (shinbone). Another bone, the fibula, is connected to the tibia. A tendon extends from the muscles on the front of the thigh, runs over the kneecap, and attaches to the upper tibia. When this tendon is tapped below the joint, the leg kicks involuntarily. This is the familiar KNEE JERK.

Trick Knee: This disorder is often encountered in young athletes. It means a knee that is easily strained because the cartilage or ligaments have been weakened by a previous injury. A trick knee may be helped by wearing a bandage, or it may need to be corrected by surgery.

Dislocation of the Kneecap: A dislocated kneecap may be the result of an injury, or the dislocation may be a congenital one. The kneecap slips to the side when the knee is bent, and may be very painful. Exercises prescribed by a physician may be helpful. Sometimes an operation is needed.

See also HOUSEMAID'S KNEE; KNOCK-KNEE.

KNEE JERK A REFLEX in which the lower part of the leg kicks forward involuntarily after a tap or blow on the tendon below the kneecap. When the tendon is struck, it stimulates the big muscle (quadriceps) on the front of the thigh to stretch and then immediately to contract. Often, as part of a medical examination, the doctor taps the patient's tendon with a small rubber hammer in order to check the reflex. See also KNEE.

KNOCK-KNEE An inward curvature of the legs that causes the knees to knock or rub together during walking. The ankles are thus thrust farther apart than normal, and the feet may be flat. A person with knock-knees walks and runs clumsily, and tires easily. The condition starts in early childhood and may be caused by weak ligaments, injury to the soft bone ends of the knees, or by RICKETS.

Many children are somewhat knock-kneed at some time in their early years. They generally outgrow the condition as their bones and muscles grow

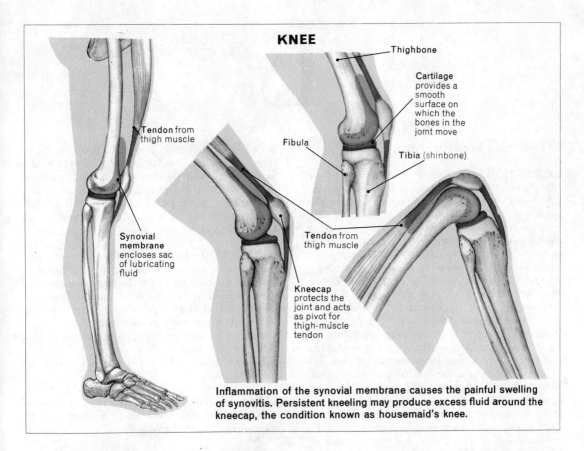

KNEE

Thighbone

Cartilage provides a smooth surface on which the bones in the joint move

Fibula

Tibia (shinbone)

Tendon from thigh muscle

Synovial membrane encloses sac of lubricating fluid

Tendon from thigh muscle

Kneecap protects the joint and acts as pivot for thigh-muscle tendon

Inflammation of the synovial membrane causes the painful swelling of synovitis. Persistent kneeling may produce excess fluid around the kneecap, the condition known as housemaid's knee.

and become stronger. Serious cases are helped by exercises to strengthen the ligaments and by manipulation of the knee joints. Occasionally, braces are needed to support and straighten the legs during growth. In some cases, surgery may be necessary to correct the condition.

KYPHOSIS Backward curvature of the spine, resulting in a hump on the upper back. The common terms for both the condition and the person who has it are hunchback and humpback. Kyphosis (pronounced kie·foh'sis) is usually caused by TUBERCULOSIS of the spine and occurs mostly in young children between the ages of 2 and 10. Treatment and prevention of deformity consist in curing the tuberculosis with medicines and in keeping the child flat on his back in a special frame until the spine heals and the vertebrae fuse properly.

471

L

LABOR See CHILDBIRTH.

LACERATION A jagged wound in the flesh or other tissues of the body made by tearing. A laceration (pronounced las″er·ay′shun) may be on the outside of the body or within.

External lacerations often contain dirt and other foreign matter. You can care for a small laceration by washing it with soap and water and bandaging it with sterile gauze. When the wound is large, deep, and full of dirt, do not try to treat it yourself. If there is much bleeding, apply pressure over the area with a gauze pad. You should see your doctor or report to a hospital emergency room as soon as possible. In addition to cleaning the laceration, the doctor may have to close the wound with stitches and administer an inoculation against tetanus.

Internal lacerations are usually more serious than external ones. The spleen or the liver may be damaged by a hard blow on the abdomen, such as from a steering wheel at the time of an automobile accident. In childbirth, there may be lacerations of the cervix (mouth of the uterus) and vaginal passage. Blows on the head in which there is no bone fracture sometimes produce lacerations of the brain tissue.

LACTASE DEFICIENCY A condition, more common among Africans and Asians than among North Americans, caused by a deficiency of lactase, a digestive ENZYME in the intestines. People with lactase deficiency, or alactasia, cannot digest lactose (milk sugar) and, if their diets include a lot of milk, they develop diarrhea and abdominal pain. Babies with inherited alactasia may suffer from malnutrition as well as diarrhea, since about 40 percent of the calories in milk, which forms their diet, are derived from lactose. Once diagnosed, the treatment for the deficiency is simple: the patient is put on a diet low in milk, so that there is a low lactose content.

LACTATION The production of milk by glands in the breast. Lactation (pronounced lak·tay′shun) does not normally begin until about three days after the birth of a baby. A fluid called colostrum nourishes the baby until the milk is formed. See also BREAST-FEEDING.

If the mother has decided to bottle-feed the newborn baby, lactation may be prevented by administering certain hormones. This must be done immediately after delivery. Lactation can usually be terminated at any time by applying a tight binder for 72 hours, and then wearing a snug brassiere. When nursing is stopped, the breasts swell at first and become tender. Pain subsides and milk production ceases in 48 to 72 hours, and the breasts return to normal in about one month.

LACTIC ACID An organic acid substance occurring in cells and muscle tissue. It is formed as a result of the burning up by the body of sugars and starches (CARBOHYDRATES). After strenuous exercise, the amount of lactic acid in the body is greatly increased. Foods such as sour cream and yogurt contain lactic acid, produced by the action of BACTERIA on carbohydrates.

For the role of lactic acid in tooth decay, see DENTAL CARIES.

LANCE To pierce or cut open a BOIL, ABSCESS, or VEIN with a surgical knife called a lancet, or with some similar sharp implement.

LANOLIN A fatty substance obtained from the wool of sheep just after shearing. Refined lanolin (pronounced lan′o·lin) is present in skin creams, shampoos, and ointments. It is readily absorbed by the skin surface and is used to soften and moisturize dry, chapped, or aging skin.

LANOXIN A trade name for digoxin, a DIGITALIS compound used in the treatment of certain heart disorders. (Pronounced lan·ok′sin.)

LAPAROTOMY Surgical opening of the abdominal cavity, either to examine the organs in the cavity or as a prelude to surgery. (Pronounced lap″a·rot′o·mee.)

LARYNGECTOMY Surgical removal of part or all of the LARYNX (voice box), usually because CANCER is present. Cancer of the larynx tends to occur most often in males over 40 years of age. The early symptoms, which are similar to the symptoms of some other respiratory diseases, are hoarseness, difficulty in swallowing, and coughing.

After a complete laryngectomy (pronounced lar″in·jek′to·mee), the TRACHEA (windpipe) is furnished with a permanent opening at the front of the neck, through which the person breathes. With patient practice and the help of a trained speech

472

therapist, persons who have undergone a laryngectomy can develop a new voice and learn to speak again.

LARYNGITIS Inflammation of the voice box, or LARYNX. Laryngitis (pronounced lar"in·jie'tis) is always accompanied by HOARSENESS. There may be coughing and a tickling feeling or soreness in the throat. If there is much swelling, breathing may be wheezy and difficult. Repeated acute attacks of laryngitis may lead to a chronic condition.

Laryngitis has a great variety of possible causes, including misuse of the voice, allergy, inhaling polluted air, and throat tumor. See also SORE THROAT.
Treatment: Give your voice a rest; if you smoke, decrease the smoking or stop it altogether. Steam inhalations may help. If the condition persists, see your doctor.

LARYNX The organ in the upper part of the throat that produces sound; also called the voice box. The larynx (pronounced lar'ingks) is part of the RESPIRATORY SYSTEM; air going to and from the lungs passes through the larynx. To keep foods and fluids from getting into the larynx, the EPIGLOTTIS, behind the tongue, closes during the act of swallowing.

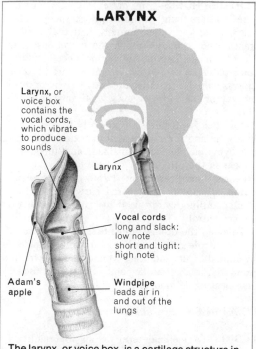

LARYNX

Larynx, or voice box contains the vocal cords, which vibrate to produce sounds

Larynx

Vocal cords
long and slack:
low note
short and tight:
high note

Adam's apple

Windpipe
leads air in and out of the lungs

The larynx, or voice box, is a cartilage structure in the windpipe. It sticks out slightly at the front of the neck to form the Adam's apple, and contains the vocal cords. Muscles control the length and tension of the cords which, aided by the tongue and lips, can be vibrated by air passing between them to give speech.

The larynx consists of cartilage, muscles, and ligaments. The largest cartilage is rather prominent—especially in men—and forms the so-called Adam's apple. The most important ligaments are the two vocal cords, reaching from the front to the back. When the air is forced through them as a person speaks, they vibrate and produce sound.

LAUGHING GAS See NITROUS OXIDE.

LAXATIVE A medicine that loosens the bowels—a mild CATHARTIC. Common laxatives include agar, milk of magnesia, cascara sagrada, vegetable mucilages such as psyllium seed, and MINERAL OIL. A glass of hot water taken half an hour before breakfast has a very mild laxative action, as does a glass of fruit juice.

Laxative medicines should be used only temporarily, and they should never be taken if CONSTIPATION is accompanied by fever, nausea, and abdominal pain. If used habitually, laxatives contribute to, rather than relieve, constipation. They may cause excessive loss of fluid from the body.

L-DOPA Another name for levodopa, a drug used to treat PARKINSONISM. (Pronounced el·doh'pa.)

LEAD POISONING Poisoning caused by the absorption of lead or lead salts by the body; the medical term is *plumbism*. Children may suffer from lead poisoning after chewing on articles painted with a lead-based paint. Workers in industries that manufacture products containing lead may breathe in lead dust from the air or eat food that has been contaminated by this dust.
Symptoms and Treatment: The symptoms of lead poisoning include anemia, severe cramps in the stomach, loss of weight, constipation, and a bluish line in the gums. In severe cases, there may even be paralysis of muscles. In children, lead poisoning may lead to convulsions and coma.

The first step in treating lead poisoning is to remove the source of contamination. Hospitalization is usually necessary for children who have enough lead in their bodies to show symptoms. Treatment consists of the administration of medicines such as EDTA (calcium disodium edetate) to help the body rid itself of the lead.
Prevention: The danger of lead poisoning to industrial workers has been lessened in recent years by more adequate ventilation systems and safer methods of handling lead-containing materials. In the home, you should be alert to the potential hazards of paints with a lead base, and see that children are not exposed to them in any way.

LEFT-HANDEDNESS Whether left-handedness is an inherited or an acquired trait is still open to dispute. It is not uncommon to find that one of the parents or a close relative of a left-handed child is also left-handed. Often a child will do certain things, such as writing, with the left hand, while he does other things quite proficiently with the right hand. Fewer girls are left-handed than boys.

In the first two years, a child does not use one hand more than the other. Later, he may favor one hand, or he may shift his preference periodically. By the time he reaches school age, the predominant use of one hand is generally well established. A person who is left-handed will often favor his left foot as well.

Most people are right-handed, and society is accordingly set up to accommodate the right-handed individual. It used to be the custom to attempt to retrain left-handed children to use their right hands. Sometimes these youngsters developed emotional problems or speech defects. Today the point of view prevails that a child should be allowed to use whichever hand he prefers.

LEG Either of the lower limbs, sometimes referred to as the lower extremities.

The leg is well adapted to its functions of supporting the body and moving it from place to place. The thighbone, or femur, is the longest and strongest bone in the body. It is set into the hip socket in such a way that it can pivot in any direction within the socket. The KNEE joint is less flexible, and can move freely in one direction only. There are two bones in the lower leg, the shinbone, or tibia, and the fibula.

The soft tissue of the leg consists largely of muscle interlaced with nerves and blood vessels. The main leg nerve, the SCIATIC NERVE, is the longest and widest nerve in the body. The femoral artery and its many branches supply most of the blood to the legs. Blood returns to the heart through two sets of veins, one set deep inside the leg near the bone, and the other near the surface. See also VARICOSE VEIN.

LEISHMANIASIS An infection caused by *Leishmania*, a genus of PROTOZOA. These tiny organisms are transmitted from rodents or dogs to man by certain species of sand flies that are found mainly in the tropics. The three forms of leishmaniasis (pronounced leesh″man·ie′a·sis) are visceral leishmaniasis, or kala azar, and cutaneous leishmaniasis, occurring in parts of Asia, Africa, Central and South America, and the Mediterranean region; and American leishmaniasis, or forest yaws, found in Mexico and Central and South America.

LENS See EYE; CONTACT LENS; EYEGLASSES.

LEPROSY An infectious disease of the skin and nerves that is found mainly in subtropical and tropical areas. Leprosy (pronounced lep′ro·see) is most common in areas where poor nutrition, overcrowding, and lack of hygienic facilities are prevalent. It occurs in the United States in Florida, Texas, Louisi-

ana, and other southern states. The disease results from infection by the germ *Mycobacterium leprae*, a bacterium of the same group that causes TUBERCULOSIS. If not treated, leprosy may result in considerable disfigurement. It is also known as Hansen's disease.

Exactly how leprosy spreads is not fully understood. It frequently does not appear until years after exposure, and it may come on almost imperceptibly. Apparently it is the result of close contact with an infected person over a long period of time. Ordinary brief contact will not transmit the disease.

Symptoms: Insensitive patches form on the skin; they may be yellow, red, or purple. The mucous membranes of the nose, throat, and eyes may also be invaded. Numbness develops in the hands and feet as the infection damages the nerves. Paralysis follows and the muscles waste away. Deformity can occur.

Treatment: Treatment is best undertaken in the National Leprosarium at Carville, Louisiana. Usually the specific treatment will vary with the character of the infection. It may be necessary to continue treatment for several years before the disease can be arrested. In some cases, however, the disorder subsides by itself.

LEPTOSPIROSIS Any of several infectious diseases that are found in rodents, dogs, sheep, cattle, goats, pigs, and other animals, and that may be transmitted to man through the excretions of infected animals. Leptospirosis (pronounced lep″toh·spie·roh′sis) is caused by several species of SPIROCHETES, which may enter the body in food or drink, by way of the lungs or eyes, or through a cut or abrasion.

Symptoms: Leptospirosis frequently begins with a headache and fever. The skin may turn yellowish, the eyes may become inflamed, and blood may appear in the urine.

Treatment and Prevention: Leptospirosis can be a serious disease if not treated early. Penicillin or similar antibiotics are used to bring the infection under control.

To avoid the disease, rodents should be exterminated. People should not bathe in ponds frequented by animals. Cuts and other wounds must be treated promptly, as they are a point of entry for the disease-bearing spirochetes.

LESBIANISM See HOMOSEXUALITY.

LESION A medical term for an abnormality in tissue, such as a wound or sore. (Pronounced lee′zhun.)

LEUKEMIA A disease characterized by abnormally large numbers and forms of LEUKOCYTES (white blood cells) in the blood or the blood-forming tissues. Leukemia (pronounced loo·kee′mee·a) is usually regarded as a type of CANCER affecting bone marrow and other blood-forming tissues.

Leukemia may be classified as either acute or chronic. *Acute* leukemia, which is more common in children than in adults, is an extremely serious disease. Some of the *chronic* forms of leukemia appear only in elderly persons and may progress very slowly for years without producing great disability; others affect persons in their middle years.

Another way to classify leukemia is according to the type of leukocyte involved. The most common form, in this classification, is *lymphocytic* leukemia, which affects the LYMPHOCYTES. The symptoms may include swelling of the lymph nodes, the spleen, and the liver. The lymphocytes invade the bone marrow and interfere with the formation of ERYTHROCYTES (red blood cells) and blood platelets, resulting in anemia and abnormal bleeding. However, chronic lymphocytic leukemia is not necessarily disabling.

The acute form of lymphocytic leukemia rarely occurs in adults. Usually the disease appears suddenly in a child, with symptoms resembling an acute infection, such as fever and loss of appetite.

Lymphocytes may rapidly invade any organ of the body, producing a great variety of symptoms. If the liver is affected, JAUNDICE may appear. If the kidneys are involved, typical symptoms of NEPHRITIS (kidney disease) may occur. Untreated, the disease may progress rapidly, but in rare cases there is spontaneous improvement. In other cases, the administration of certain chemical compounds may arrest the disease for several years.

The various leukocytes that are formed in bone marrow are associated with chronic and acute forms of *myelocytic* leukemia. The chronic form may suddenly become acute. There may or may not be enlargement of lymph nodes and spleen. ANEMIA and abnormal bleeding may occur. As the disease progresses, any of the organs of the body may be affected.

Treatment: Leukemia has long been in the category of an incurable disease, but a great deal of research is being done, and it is possible that some discovery may suddenly lead to a cure. The disease can be arrested so that symptoms are relieved or may even disappear for varying periods of time.

Radiation is often used to treat chronic and acute leukemia. Radiation may be applied either externally, with X rays or gamma rays, or internally, with medicine containing radioactive phosphorus. Certain chemical agents are sometimes effective in arresting acute cases.

LEUKOCYTE A white blood cell. A leukocyte (pronounced loo′ko·siet) is not really white, but colorless. Leukocytes are found in the circulating blood, in lymph, and in certain tissues. They are manufactured mainly in bone marrow and in lymph nodes.

There are a number of different kinds and sizes of leukocytes. One of their functions is to surround any foreign particles in the blood, thus helping the body to fight infections.

Leukocytes are larger than red blood cells (ERYTHROCYTES), but much less numerous. Normally, there is only about one leukocyte in the blood for every 1,000 erythrocytes. The number of leukocytes increases rapidly when infection and some other abnormal conditions occur in the body. The number and proportions of different kinds of leukocytes are often valuable clues in diagnosing a disease.

See also LEUKEMIA.

LEUKOCYTOSIS The presence of more than the normal number of LEUKOCYTES (white blood cells) in the body. (Pronounced loo″ko·sie·toh′sis.) See also LEUKOPENIA.

LEUKOPENIA The presence of fewer than normal LEUKOCYTES (white blood cells) in the blood. Blood normally has from 5,000 to 10,000 leukocytes per cubic millimeter. Anything over or under this range is considered to be abnormal. In severe cases, leukopenia (pronounced loo″koh·pee′nee·a) may involve increased risk of bacterial infection.

The opposite condition to leukopenia is called LEUKOCYTOSIS. Neither of these conditions is a disease in itself. They are symptoms of other disorders and help the doctor to make a diagnosis.

LEUKOPLAKIA Thickened white patches on membranes, particularly those in the tongue or lining the cheeks, caused by an overgrowth of the tissues. Leukoplakia (pronounced loo″ko·play′-kee·a) usually occurs in middle-aged men. Causes include bacterial infection in the mouth, syphilis, excessive smoking, and too much alcohol. The condition may precede cancer of the tongue; it needs treatment by a specialist.

LEUKORRHEA Discharge from the VAGINA of a white or yellowish mucous fluid; also called *whites*. Leukorrhea (pronounced loo″ko·ree′a) is not a disease but a symptom. A small amount of clear mucous discharge from the vagina is normal. The amount often increases at the time of ovulation.

An abundant vaginal discharge, especially if it is accompanied by itching and an objectionable odor, may be a symptom of infection. A doctor should be consulted about any abnormal discharge.

LIBIDO The sexual energy or drive that makes us love and create. According to Sigmund Freud, the Austrian psychiatrist who developed the concept, libido (pronounced li·bee′doh) is present in the infant. The child first directs his sexual instinct toward his own body, then toward his parents. In adulthood the libido finds a normal sexual outlet, unless it is blocked or repressed. Freud held that a good measure of the drive in adults is directed into socially constructive or creative activity of a non-sexual nature—a process referred to as sublimation. See also PSYCHOANALYSIS.

LIBRIUM A trade name for the tranquilizing drug chlordiazepoxide hydrochloride. Librium (pronounced li′bree·im) is prescribed mostly for alcoholic, nervous, or mentally ill persons to help control tension, fear, and anxiety.

LIGAMENT A band of tough tissue that helps to keep an organ of the body in place or that connects the ends of bones where they form joints. When a ligament (pronounced lig′a·ment) is injured, the damage often consists of a SPRAIN—the tearing of a ligament attached to the bones of a joint. Pain may be quite severe, and the skin around the injury may turn blue and swell up.

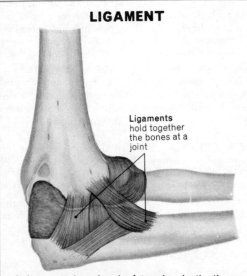

LIGAMENT

Ligaments hold together the bones at a joint

A ligament is a band of tough, elastic tissue which binds together the bones at a joint. A major joint, such as the elbow, has a set of overlapping ligaments to support the three bones that meet there. Forcing a joint beyond its normal range of movement overstretches or tears the ligaments and causes a sprain; this generally heals if the joint is rested.

LIGATION A surgical procedure employed to tie up a blood vessel or other structure in order to constrict it. (Pronounced lie·gay′shen.) See also LIGATURE.

LIGATURE A wire, thread, or other material that is used by a surgeon to tie off a blood vessel or to constrict some other part of the body. Ligature (pronounced lig′a·chur) may also refer to the device used to attach a tooth to an appliance or to another tooth in ORTHODONTIC treatment.

LINIMENT A liquid preparation applied to the skin to relieve pain or stiffness. Although liniments may relieve such symptoms, they do not cure specific conditions.

LIPS The lips have such a good blood supply that most injuries to them heal quickly and perfectly. Cracks and fissures (apart from those accompanying a head cold) may be associated with VITAMIN deficiency or anemia. A doctor should be consulted about split lips. The common FEVER SORE is an infection by a herpes virus. Treatment with CALAMINE LOTION accelerates healing.

LISPING See SPEECH DEFECTS AND DISORDERS.

LITHIUM CARBONATE A chemical compound used to treat both the manic and depressive phases of MANIC-DEPRESSIVE PSYCHOSIS. It should be taken with care under a doctor's supervision because of the possibility of dangerous side effects.

LITHOLAPAXY A common method of removing a stone, or CALCULUS, from the urinary bladder. In a litholapaxy (pronounced lith·ol′a·pak″see), the exact position of the stone is found by the method described under CYSTOSCOPY. Then a special instrument is inserted into the bladder through the urethra, the stone is crushed, and the fragments are washed out of the bladder through a CATHETER.

LITHOTOMY A surgical operation to remove a stone, or CALCULUS, from the urinary bladder. Lithotomy (pronounced li thot′o·mee) is not usually performed unless a very large stone is present. Smaller stones are usually removed by a LITHOLAPAXY.

LIVER A large, four-lobed organ situated on the right side of the abdominal cavity just under the diaphragm. The liver is the main factory and storehouse of the body. It receives about one fourth of the arterial blood pumped out by the heart at every beat. It also receives all the blood from the veins in the intestinal area; this blood contains the digested foodstuffs absorbed through the intestinal wall.

The liver stores vitamins and foodstuffs and releases them to the body as required, after converting them into usable form. For example, it stores GLUCOSE in the form of glycogen, and restores it to the bloodstream as glucose when the level of blood sugar falls. The liver purifies the blood by removing toxic substances, various waste products, and worn-out red blood cells. It helps to maintain the HORMONE balance in the body by destroying or inactivating hormones that are not needed. The liver also manufactures BILE, which is essential in digestion. At the same time, hundreds of lesser functions are performed by the liver.

The liver has remarkable powers of recovery from minor damage. Normally, no special attention is

LIVER

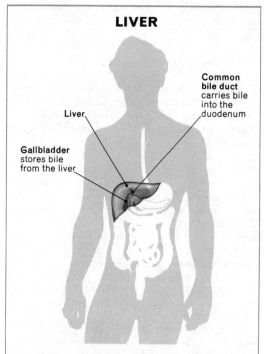

Common bile duct carries bile into the duodenum

Liver

Gallbladder stores bile from the liver

The liver is the largest gland in the body. One of its functions is to secrete bile, an alkaline liquid which passes via the gallbladder into the duodenum, where it acts on fats in food and prepares them for digestion. The liver is also a store for glycogen, a starchy substance which can be converted to sugars when the body makes demands for extra energy. Other chemical processes taking place in the liver include the building up of simple amino acids (the products of the digestion of proteins) into the various protein substances needed by the body to build tissues such as skin, bone, hair and nails.

needed to keep it in good working order. However, there are a number of abnormal conditions that affect the liver. JAUNDICE is often a symptom of liver trouble. The viruses that cause HEPATITIS and YELLOW FEVER affect the liver directly. BRUCELLOSIS and certain other bacterial infections sometimes involve the liver. The parasites that cause amebiasis (see DYSENTERY) may cause liver damage. A number of toxic substances, particularly carbon tetrachloride and chloroform, may bring about CIRRHOSIS of the liver. Certain medications may cause abnormalities of the liver. The liver is sometimes the primary site of cancer and is often invaded by METASTASIS when cancer occurs in other parts of the body. Finally, both malnutrition and obesity tend to put an excessive burden on the liver and should be avoided.

LOBOTOMY An operation in which an incision is made into a lobe of the brain, and nerve fibers are severed. When performed on the frontal lobe, the procedure is known as a *frontal lobotomy* or a leukotomy. It was formerly performed on mentally ill persons who were severely disturbed. The operation made the patient docile and gentle.

A lobotomy (pronounced loh·bot'o·mee) is seldom performed today. TRANQUILIZERS are now preferred to calm the violent patient, so that he may be receptive to PSYCHOTHERAPY.

LOCHIA A discharge from the VAGINA that occurs for a few weeks after CHILDBIRTH. After delivery, there is some bleeding; this gives way to the lochia (pronounced loh'kee·a), which is red at first but then becomes whitish.

LOCKJAW See TETANUS.

LOCOMOTOR ATAXIA A disease of the central nervous system marked by pain, loss of reflexes, inability to coordinate movements, and other symptoms. Locomotor ataxia (pronounced loh"ko·moh'tor a·tak'see·a) is also known as tabes dorsalis. It is a complication of advanced SYPHILIS.

LORDOSIS A back condition in which the inward curvature of the spine is excessive. Lordosis (pronounced lawr·doh'sis) is often the result of incorrect posture and may lead to backache. A physician or an orthopedist should be consulted.

LOUSE (plural, **lice**) A wingless insect that lives on the blood of animals and people. Two species of lice are parasitic on humans. The commonest kind has two distinct varieties. One of them, the body louse, lives and lays its eggs in the seams and wrinkles of clothing. The other, the smaller head louse, lives in the shelter of the hair on the scalp and glues its tiny white eggs, called nits, to the hair shafts. Another species, the crab louse, shelters in the hair around the genitals and sometimes in the armpits or eyebrows.

Lice obtain their nourishment by sucking blood from their host. They make a tiny puncture in the person's skin, inject a small amount of a substance that prevents the blood from clotting, and then suck blood until they are full. The substance they inject produces local inflammation and itching.

The medical term for the condition of being ·infested with lice is PEDICULOSIS. Lice are most likely to thrive wherever people live in crowded and unsanitary conditions, where the lice can easily move from one person to another and are not too often disturbed by exposure to soap and water. A few thorough shampooings with tincture of green soap and combing with a fine-tooth comb will usually remove both lice and nits from the hair. Insecticides should not be used. Many of the common insecticides are poisonous to humans as well as to insects. Several effective preparations are obtainable in drugstores. These should be used strictly as directed on the package. If you cannot easily get rid of lice, it is advisable to see a doctor about a safe and effective treatment.

Body lice are the means by which epidemic TYPHUS is spread from person to person. The crab louse is not known to spread any disease.

LOW BLOOD PRESSURE See BLOOD PRESSURE; HYPOTENSION.

LOW BLOOD SUGAR See HYPERINSULINISM.

LSD This very potent HALLUCINOGENIC DRUG derives its name from three letters of its chemical name, *l*ysergic acid *d*iethylamide. A slang term for it is "acid." LSD was originally obtained from ergot, a fungus that grows on some cereal grasses. It can now be made synthetically.

When a very minute dose of LSD is swallowed, it alters normal emotion, perception, and judgment rapidly and profoundly. The effect varies with different persons and depends also on the circumstances in which the drug is taken. The senses are confused: colors may be heard as sounds, and sounds seen as visual patterns. Emotional reactions are bizarre, and have been reported to be either extremely agreeable or terrifying. An experience with LSD is called, in slang, a trip.

The possession or use of LSD is forbidden by law and subject to severe penalties, including imprisonment. Its use for the sole purpose of "enlarging" experience is very dangerous. LSD has produced long-lasting PSYCHOSIS in some users; it may cause permanent damage to the GENETIC material in reproductive and body cells, raising the possibility of giving birth to deformed babies. Judgment is so altered that fatal accidents may occur while a person is under its influence.

LUES Another name for SYPHILIS. (Pronounced loo′eez.)

LUMBAGO Pain in the lumbar region, the lower part of the back. (Pronounced lum·bay′goh.) It may come abruptly, particularly after a sudden twisting of the spine, or it may begin gradually. Sometimes the difficulty may be due to ARTHRITIS. X rays and a careful examination by an orthopedist (specialist in disorders of the bones and joints) are first steps in diagnosing the precise cause of any persistent pain in the lower back.

Bed rest and the application of heat are often effective in treating an ordinary BACKACHE.

LUMBAR PUNCTURE A medical technique in which a hollow needle is inserted between the third and fourth vertebrae in the lumbar region (small of the back) to remove cerebrospinal fluid from the spinal canal, generally as an aid to diagnosis. For instance, the presence of blood in the fluid may be evidence of a brain hemorrhage. See also SPINAL CORD.

LUMPY JAW See ACTINOMYCOSIS.

LUNATIC A person who has a serious mental illness. (See EMOTIONAL AND MENTAL DISORDERS.) The term, although still found in legal statutes, is no longer in use among medical practitioners. See also INSANITY.

LUNG One of a pair of organs through which the blood receives oxygen from the air and gives up carbon dioxide. The lungs are two masses of porous, elastic tissue completely filling the chest cavity on either side of the heart. Each lung is partially separated into lobes, the right lung having three lobes and the left, two. Each lung is enclosed in a thin, slippery, double-layered membrane called the pleura. The outer layer of the pleura lines the chest cavity. The two layers slide against each other easily and are normally held together by suction. See also PLEURISY.

Air reaches each lobe of the lungs through branches of the BRONCHI. Inside the lungs, these branches, or bronchioles, divide and repeatedly subdivide. The smallest bronchioles end in tiny sacs, called alveoli. The lungs contain millions of these alveoli. They fill up like balloons whenever the chest cavity is enlarged by the downward motion of the diaphragm, and then collapse partially when the diaphragm pushes upward and the breath is exhaled. They are never completely emptied. The alveoli are surrounded by minute blood vessels. Exchanges of oxygen and carbon dioxide take place through the very thin walls of the alveoli and blood vessels.

The lungs are exposed to everything that a person breathes in along with air—smoke, minute particles, and a variety of toxic substances. See also AIR POLLUTION AND HEALTH; LUNG CANCER.

LUNG CANCER Malignant tumors of the lung are most common in men over 40 years of age who are heavy cigarette smokers, and rarest in people who have never smoked. The best insurance against lung cancer is to refrain from smoking.

Lung cancer readily gives rise to cancer in other parts of the body by METASTASIS, and the first noticeable symptoms may be associated with other areas. Symptoms directly involving the lungs include coughing, wheezing, pink or blood-streaked sputum, and shortness of breath. Although these symptoms do not always indicate cancer, they may signify some very serious condition that requires immediate medical attention.

In some cases, if diagnosed early, lung cancer may be cured or arrested by surgical removal of the tumor. In advanced cases, the disease may sometimes be slowed by radiation or CHEMOTHERAPY. The American Cancer Society no longer recommends an annual chest X-ray.

LUPUS ERYTHEMATOSUS A disease that is often characterized by scaly red patches on the skin. (Pronounced loo'pus er"i·thee"ma·toh'sus.)

The disease exists in two forms. The *discoid*, or mild, type manifests itself as round or butterfly-shaped lesions on the face. Usually no treatment is necessary, but the individual should avoid the sun's rays.

The *systemic*, or more serious, type affects the connective tissue. It may involve the joints, lungs, heart, kidneys, or skin. Symptoms include pain in the joints, muscles, and abdomen. CORTISONE and related medications are used to control the disease.

LUPUS VULGARIS Tuberculosis of the skin. In lupus vulgaris (pronounced loo'pus vul·gair'is), brownish lesions or nodules may form on the face or mucous membranes; the lesions then become ulcerous and form scars. There may be a tuberculous infection elsewhere in the body, which must be identified and treated.

Antibiotics are used to control lupus vulgaris. Fortunately, the disease has become fairly rare with modern methods for control of TUBERCULOSIS.

LYMPH A colorless fluid that occurs in the lymphatic vessels. Lymph (pronounced limf) contains certain white blood cells known as LYMPHOCYTES, which are manufactured by the LYMPH NODES. Lymph resembles BLOOD PLASMA, although it varies somewhat in composition throughout the body.

Lymph is pushed through the lymphatic system by contractions of the vessel walls, by differences in pressure, and by the movements of muscles in surrounding parts of the body. At the base of the neck, the two main branches of the lymphatic system merge with two veins, and the lymph becomes part of the bloodstream.

LYMPH NODE The lymphatic system forms a network of vessels in the body. It collects fluids from the various tissues and returns them to the circulating blood by way of two veins in the region of the neck. (See LYMPH.) At intervals throughout the lymphatic system, there are small masses of spongy tissue. These are the lymph nodes, or lymph glands. They are especially numerous in the neck, the armpits, and the groin. The lymph nodes have three functions: (1) they manufacture LYMPHOCYTES; (2) they act as filters, removing bacteria and other particles; and (3) they manufacture ANTIBODIES against specific infections.

The lymph nodes are stimulated to increased activity by infection, and sometimes they become swollen and painful. A cold with inflamed throat, for example, is often accompanied by painful swellings

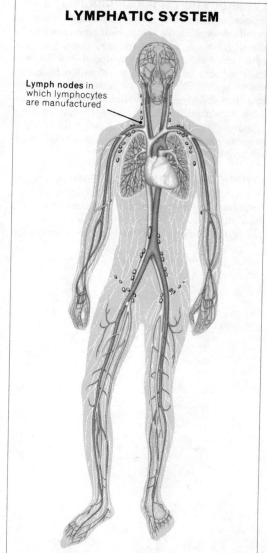

LYMPHATIC SYSTEM

Lymph nodes in which lymphocytes are manufactured

The watery fluid which makes up lymph contains various substances which the body uses to fight invading disease germs. Major glands, or nodes, which produce lymph are found in the armpits and groins, and swelling of these can be a sign that the body is mobilizing its defenses against a disease. The lymphatic ducts lead toward the neck, where they feed into veins.

in the neck which are really swollen lymph nodes. Any swelling of lymph nodes may be a sign of trouble and should be reported to your doctor.

LYMPHOCYTE A type of LEUKOCYTE (white blood cell) formed in the lymph nodes and other lymphoid tissue, as well as in bone marrow. About a quarter of the white blood cells in the circulating blood are lymphocytes (pronounced lim'fo·siets").

LYMPHOCYTIC CHORIOMENINGITIS A virus disease of mice that is sometimes transmitted to people through food or house dust contaminated by the secretions or feces of infected mice. Lymphocytic choriomeningitis (pronounced lim″fo·sit′ik kawr″ee·oh·men″in·jie′tis) is not passed from person to person. The symptoms may at first resemble influenza, followed by drowsiness, nausea, and vomiting. Lymphocytic choriomeningitis can be diagnosed by laboratory tests on spinal fluid. Beyond relieving the symptoms, there is no specific treatment. Recovery is usually complete.

LYMPHOGRANULOMA VENEREUM A venereal disease affecting the LYMPH NODES in the groin. Lymphogranuloma venereum (pronounced lim″fo· gran″yu·loh′ma ve·neer′ee·um) is due to a virus. The first reaction to infection is a sore resembling a cold sore. The virus then invades the lymph nodes, causing painful swelling.

Lymphogranuloma venereum can be cured by treatment with certain antibiotics, including TET-RACYCLINE. Early treatment is essential in order to prevent complications that may require extensive surgery.

LYMPHOID Pertaining to or resembling LYMPH or LYMPH NODES. (Pronounced lim′foyd.)

LYSIN An ANTIBODY or other substance that destroys a specific microorganism or a red blood cell. (Pronounced lie′sin.)

LYTIC Pertaining to the destruction of cells by a LYSIN. Lytic (pronounced liet′ik) may also refer to diminishing symptoms of an acute illness.

M

MACULA (plural, **maculae**) The Latin word for spot. The term "macula" (pronounced mak'yu·la) is used in anatomy for any small spot different in color from surrounding tissue. When referring to freckles or the red spots on the skin characteristic of some diseases, the form "macule" is generally used.

MADURA FOOT See MYCETOMA.

MAGNESIA Magnesium hydroxide, often used in a creamy mixture with water (milk of magnesia) as an ANTACID or a mild LAXATIVE.

MALAISE A generalized feeling of being physically unwell. With malaise (pronounced mal·ayz'), there is often a sense of being weak and run-down. Malaise is a symptom that may precede an illness or accompany it. Or, in a woman, it may occur during menstruation. Fatigue may bring on malaise in either sex.

MALARIA A disease marked by acute attacks of chills and high fever. Malaria is caused by various species of a microscopic parasite of the genus *Plasmodium*, which are transmitted to man by the bites of the mosquito of the genus *Anopheles*. The disease can also be accidentally transmitted through transfusions of blood from infected donors.

Acute attacks occur when the parasites in the blood invade red blood cells and multiply, eventually causing the red blood cells to burst. After repeated attacks, anemia develops, and the liver and spleen become enlarged. Usually, general ill health, headaches, and muscular pains follow. The intervals between acute attacks and the severity of the disease depend upon the particular kind of plasmodium parasite that has invaded the body. Some are more virulent than others.

Malaria has been brought partially under control by the use of insecticides and by draining swamps where the mosquito breeds. The cases of malaria that occur in the United States and Canada are usually contracted in countries where the disease is still common, such as in Southeast Asia and parts of Africa and South America.

Treatment: Several synthetic medicines have been developed that either cure or suppress different forms of malaria. These include CHLOROQUINE and PRIMAQUINE. QUININE was formerly the only medicine that had any effect on malaria, but the drug is rarely used today.

MALIGNANT Tending to grow progressively worse if uncorrected. A malignant tumor, or cancer, invades other tissues, produces METASTASIS, and must be removed surgically or treated by RADIOLOGY at an early stage.

MALNUTRITION A condition in which the body is poorly nourished because the individual is not getting one or more of the important nutritional elements in his diet. We must have FATS and CARBOHYDRATES (sugars and starches) to provide us with energy. PROTEINS, water, and minerals are essential to repair and maintain our body tissues. Water and minerals—as well as VITAMINS—also keep the nutritional processes of the tissues working smoothly. (See DIET.) When these nutrients are lacking, we become subject to deficiency diseases and other disorders.

Malnutrition is often the result of poverty or of inadequate knowledge of the body's dietary needs. Many persons tend to spend their money on foods high in fat, sugar, and starch, but neglect fresh vegetables, fruit, milk, and meat, which supply the all-important vitamins, minerals, and proteins. As a rule, the closer a food is to its natural state, the more it retains its original nutrients.

Severe underweight occurs when the individual has an insufficient intake of CALORIES. Underweight may also be the result of a disorder such as an overactive thyroid, cancer, or an emotional disturbance. If there is disease of the pancreas, liver, or any of the other organs of the DIGESTIVE SYSTEM, the body may be unable to absorb or use the nutrients in the diet. During pregnancy or while nursing the baby, a woman's system needs additional nutrients to avoid malnutrition.

Vitamin deficiencies produce a variety of nutritional disorders, including SCURVY, RICKETS, and BERIBERI.

MALOCCLUSION A condition in which the teeth of the upper and lower jaws do not meet correctly, due to heredity or to neglect of the first set of teeth. A poor diet or, very rarely, thumb-sucking may also be responsible for defective or badly aligned teeth. As a consequence of malocclusion (pronounced mal"o·kloo'zhun), a person may not be able to chew his food thoroughly, and the teeth are therefore more susceptible to decay, or DENTAL CARIES. Poorly aligned teeth may also cause embarrassment and self-consciousness. Crooked teeth in both children

481

and adults can be corrected with the aid of bands or braces. This work is handled by dentists who specialize in ORTHODONTICS.

MALTA FEVER See BRUCELLOSIS.

MANIA A mental disorder marked by extremely excited, overconfident behavior. It is the hyperactive phase of MANIC-DEPRESSIVE PSYCHOSIS.

The term "mania" is used more frequently in combination with other words or as a suffix to describe various kinds of violent or abnormal behavior. For example, pyromania is an uncontrollable urge to set fires, and megalomania is an abnormally exaggerated notion of one's own importance and power.

MANIC-DEPRESSIVE PSYCHOSIS A serious mental disorder, or PSYCHOSIS, in which the person is alternately extremely excited or profoundly depressed. He swings from one extreme to the other, often with great abruptness and for no apparent reason, although he may remain in one phase for long periods. In the manic phase, the person is very talkative and confident; he has wild flights of ideas and hallucinations. When he enters the depressive phase, he becomes melancholy and withdrawn.

Manic-depressive psychosis is treated by PSYCHOTHERAPY and by tranquilizing and antidepressant medicines. SHOCK THERAPY has been found effective in the acute phases. A new medicine, LITHIUM CARBONATE, has shown promising results.

MARIHUANA (marijuana) The most widely used, or abused, of the HALLUCINOGENIC DRUGS. Tea, pot, or grass, as marihuana (pronounced mar"i·whon'a) is often called, is usually smoked in cigarettes, which are prepared from the leaves, stems, and flowering tops of hemp (*Cannabis sativa*). Marihuana cigarettes vary greatly in potency, depending on the part of the hemp plant used and the conditions under which the plant was grown. The effect produced also varies from person to person.

The extracted resin of the hemp plant is called hashish. It is either smoked or eaten.

In the United States and Canada, there are legal penalties for possession or use of marihuana. It has been argued that the drug is simply a mild intoxicant with less harmful side effects than tobacco or alcohol. Some authorities disagree. Marihuana does not produce physical dependence on the drug, but users may come to rely upon it psychologically, and its long-term effects are unknown. See also DRUG ADDICTION.

MARROW The soft, gelatinous substance that fills the numerous cavities that exist in bones. The marrow consists of a network of blood vessels and fibers holding together a varying mixture of blood-producing cells, fats, and red and white corpuscles in all stages of development.

MASOCHISM An abnormal tendency to derive sexual pleasure from being abused. Masochism (pronounced mas'o·kiz"em), in terms of PSYCHOANALYSIS, is an expression of feelings of guilt or worthlessness and an unconscious wish to be punished.

Masochism derives its name from an Austrian writer, Leopold von Sacher-Masoch (1835–95). In popular usage, the term is often applied loosely to any conduct that involves discomfort or inconvenience. It is the opposite of SADISM.

MASSAGE PHYSICAL THERAPY of the muscles or other body parts by rubbing, kneading, or tapping. Massage stimulates the skin and circulation and helps prevent the deterioration that results from being in bed for long periods. Also, it has a beneficial emotional effect on chronically ill patients. To be effective, massage must be vigorous and yet not hurt the person. *The correct technique must be learned and practiced.*

Mechanical devices to provide massage include rocking beds, vibrators, and whirlpool baths.

For people in good health, massage is effective to relieve muscle strain, muscle cramps, and nervous tension. Massage is sometimes advertised as a way to remove deposits of fat from areas of the body. There is no evidence that it has any such effect.

MASTECTOMY Removal of the breast by surgery. (Pronounced mas·tek'to·mee.) The usual reason for the operation is to remove a malignant, or cancerous, tumor. In the mid-1970's there were some 89,000 new cases of breast CANCER discovered annually. No fact could underline more starkly the urgent need for early detection and treatment of such cancer.

In some cases, when the tumors are benign, a partial mastectomy is performed to remove only the area of the tissue that is diseased. However, if cancer is present, the entire breast must be removed. Since the disease can spread very rapidly, it is usually considered necessary to perform a radical mastectomy, including removal of the muscle underneath the breast and the tissue of the neighboring armpit area. Afterward, X-ray treatment is given to the area around the breast to eliminate any remaining traces of cancerous tissue.

Artificial breasts are available with astonishingly lifelike appearance. Within a relatively short time, the woman can resume all her normal activities, including sports.

MASTITIS Inflammation of the breast. The breast becomes red and feels exceptionally sensitive or painful. There are several types of mastitis (pronounced mas·tie'tis).

Chronic cystic mastitis occurs usually in women in their thirties or forties. It is the commonest type of mastitis and is the result of hormone imbalance. Cysts or lumps appear on the breast, and fluid may drip from the nipple. With these symptoms, it is natural to worry about cancer. Your doctor will make a diagnosis of the condition and recommend proper treatment.

Puerperal mastitis is an acute infection that may occur after childbirth in nursing mothers. It is caused by bacteria. Usually, the mother has to stop nursing the baby. The condition is treated with ANTIBIOTICS or SULFONAMIDES.

MASTOID PROCESS

Mastoid process, sticking out from the skull behind the ear, contains cells which can become infected

The prominent bone behind the ear, called the mastoid process, can become infected and inflamed, giving the condition mastoiditis. This can usually be treated with antibiotics or sulfonamide drugs, but in severe cases part of the bone may have to be removed by surgery.

MASTOIDECTOMY An operation on the bone behind the ear to cure an infection called MASTOIDITIS. The surgeon makes an incision and scrapes out a portion of the bone. It is usually possible to avoid a mastoidectomy (pronounced mas"toyd·ek'to·mee) by controlling the infection with SULFONAMIDES or ANTIBIOTICS.

MASTOIDITIS An inflammation of the mastoid process, the bone behind the ear. Mastoiditis (pronounced mas"toyd·ie'tis) is particularly likely to develop as a complication of MIDDLE EAR INFECTION. Symptoms include fever, pain, and swelling. The infection can usually be controlled with ANTIBIOTICS or SULFONAMIDES. See also MASTOIDECTOMY.

MASTURBATION Manipulation or rubbing of the GENITALS to obtain pleasurable sensations or an ORGASM. It was formerly believed that masturbation caused insanity, impotence, frigidity, weakness, and nervousness, not to mention pimples. Actually, it is well established that masturbation causes none of these things. The practice is almost universal among infants and very young children, and common in adolescence. Normally, the worst result of masturbation is the feeling of fear and guilt that it engenders because of generations of miseducation.

McBURNEY'S POINT A position on the right side of the abdomen, about midway between the navel and the front point of the hip, which is often extremely tender if pressed when APPENDICITIS is suspected. It was first described by the American surgeon Charles McBurney.

MEASLES A common name for two distinct diseases known medically as rubeola and rubella. Each disease is caused by a distinct virus. The disease often called German measles is discussed under RUBELLA.

Rubeola, sometimes called seven-day measles, can affect people of any age, but most people have had the disease in childhood and have thereby become immune. Babies of mothers who have ever had rubeola inherit a temporary immunity that lasts for about a year after birth.

The first symptoms resemble those of a cold: teary eyes, sneezing, cough, and nasal discharge. The body temperature becomes quite high, sometimes reaching 106° F by the fourth day. The characteristic rash appears from three to five days after the onset of other symptoms, and lasts for four to seven days. The fever subsides when the rash appears.

Complete recovery from rubeola usually occurs within a few weeks, unless complications arise. Rubeola patients should be kept in isolation not only to prevent spreading the disease but to protect them against secondary infections.

A vaccine against rubeola became available in 1963, and measles has declined dramatically since then. Babies should be vaccinated at about one year of age. But any child who has not had a measles vaccine should be given one. A single injection produces immunity, probably for life.

MECONIUM The dark-green, pasty bowel movements passed by the newborn baby during the first days of life. Meconium (pronounced me·koh'nee·um) consists of waste products accumulated in the unborn child in the last months of fetal life.

MEDICAID In the United States, a government-financed welfare program offering medical aid to the needy. See also MEDICARE.

Medicaid is financed partly by the federal government and partly by the states. Each participating state has its own program. Only the minimum services that must be provided are specified by federal legislation. Every state program must include all persons who receive federal welfare assistance, such as low-income families with dependent children and the needy blind. It must make available to them at least five services: inpatient and outpatient hospital care, doctors' services, laboratory and X-ray services, and professional nursing-home care. States may add other services and also include in their programs their own welfare clients.

MEDICARE A broad program of health insurance for persons aged 65 or older, established by the federal government in 1965. The program includes two kinds of insurance: hospital insurance and medical insurance. The hospital program is financed by payments made by individuals and their employers under the Social Security program. The medical insurance is voluntary; participants pay a set amount each month (deducted from Social Security benefits) and the federal government contributes an equal amount.

Hospital Insurance: This program helps pay the bills when the individual is hospitalized and for nursing and therapy after he leaves the hospital. It covers up to 90 days of hospital care during a period of illness. A deductible amount must be paid at the start, and the first 60 days are then fully covered, but there is a fixed charge for the remaining 30 days. After at least three days in a hospital, most of the cost for up to 100 days' care in a skilled nursing home is paid for in each benefit period. Physicians' services are not included. Hospital insurance also pays for 100 home visits by nurses and physical therapists (but not physicians) in the 365 days after the individual has been released from a hospital or nursing home.

Medical Insurance: After a deductible amount payable once in the calendar year, the program pays 80 percent of reasonable charges for physicians' and surgeons' services, no matter where received; health services in the home without a previous stay in the hospital; physical therapy services; medical equipment, surgical dressings, diagnostic tests, and similar medical and health services; and outpatient services at a participating hospital.

MEDICINES See DRUG; PHARMACIST; PHARMACOLOGY; PHARMACY; PILLS; PRESCRIPTION.

MEGACOLON A congenital condition of the colon, usually produced by absence of nerve cells in a lower portion of the intestine, or bowel. The stimulus needed for a normal bowel movement is missing, and the abdomen becomes greatly distended with fecal matter. In most such cases, surgery is necessary to correct megacolon (pronounced me″ga·koh′lon). The condition is also known as Hirschsprung's disease.

MEGALOBLAST A large abnormal blood cell found in the bone marrow of patients with perni-

cious ANEMIA and in those with a deficiency of the VITAMIN folic acid. (Pronounced meg′a·loh·blast″.)

MEGALOMANIA Delusions of grandeur or great power. Megalomania (pronounced meg″a·loh·may′nee·a) may be a symptom of PSYCHOSIS, or severe mental disturbance.

MEIOSIS See MIOSIS (3).

MELANCHOLIA A state of profound depression. Melancholia (pronounced mel″an·koh′lee·a) occurs, for example, in the depressed phase of MANIC-DEPRESSIVE PSYCHOSIS and in INVOLUTIONAL MELANCHOLIA, a mental illness of older people.

MELANIN The natural brownish or blackish PIGMENT that gives color to the skin, hair, and eyes. (Pronounced mel′a·nin.) See also MELANOMA.

MELANOMA A dark-colored TUMOR of the skin arising from cells that produce the pigment MELANIN. Some melanomas are MALIGNANT, and early diagnosis and surgical treatment are essential to prevent spread of the cancerous cells. Any new dark swelling, or any existing MOLE that gets larger or darker should be shown to the doctor without delay. (Pronounced mel″a·noh′ma.)

MELENA Black stools, caused by the presence of partly digested blood in the feces. Swallowed blood from a nosebleed; bleeding from a stomach ulcer, a ruptured vein, or a tumor; or inflammation of the intestine all give rise to melena (pronounced mel′e·na) if the blood remains some hours in the intestines. Red blood is passed with the stools when the source of bleeding is close to the anus (as in HEMORRHOIDS) or when the blood from higher up passes quickly through the digestive system.

MEMBRANE A thin, pliable layer of tissue serving to cover or line an organ or body part or to divide an organ or cavity. MUCOUS MEMBRANES line the body cavities that open to the outside. The membranes that cover certain internal organs such as the heart, stomach, and lungs are called serous membranes. The synovial membranes line the moving parts of the joints and cover the tendons.

MEMORY The ability to recall something that has been learned or experienced. The BRAIN, with its vast number of nerve cells, is the organ of memory. Very little is known about how and exactly where the brain stores away experience and later recalls certain selected parts of it. It is probable that "memory" is merely a convenient word for a number of different processes that are really distinct. For example, riding a bicycle and recognizing an old friend are acts of memory, but they involve very different mental processes.

Memory is best in early life. It is easier to learn in youth, and the retention of such learning is better. Photographic memory is much more common among children than adults. At any age it is easier to learn and recall things that are meaningful to us or that have pleasant associations for us.

Memories often become confused. We tend to weave our wishes, emotions, or dreams into our memories, and then believe that things actually happened in this way. Or we may add part of one memory to another, creating something entirely new. See also AMNESIA.

MENARCHE The first occurrence of MENSTRUATION in a young girl. (Pronounced me·nahr′kee.)

MÉNIÈRE'S DISEASE A disease of the inner ear; also called Ménière's syndrome. Ménière's (pronounced may·nyairz′) disease usually involves a single ear and is commonest among men who have passed the age of 40.

Ménière's disease may follow a blow on the ear or an infection; or it may be due to an allergic reaction, a congenital condition, or some other unknown cause.
Symptoms: An attack may come on quite abruptly. The person feels extremely dizzy and nauseated, and may vomit. There is a ringing in the ear, accompanied by a headache. The sense of balance is disturbed. Attacks may be mild or severe and long-lasting, and the hearing may become impaired.
Treatment: Medicines such as antihistamines are used to control the symptoms and a special diet is prescribed. The doctor may also recommend other medicines for acute attacks and between attacks.

MENINGITIS Inflammation of the meninges, the thin membranes covering the brain and the spinal cord. Meningitis (pronounced men″in·jie′tis) can attack people of all ages but is more common in children. It is caused by any of a number of GERMS, such as the meningococcus and pneumococcus bacteria, the influenza virus, and the tubercle bacillus. Most epidemics of meningitis are caused by the meningococcus bacterium.

Before the days of ANTIBIOTICS and SULFONAMIDES (sulfa compounds), meningitis was a dreaded disease. It could cause permanent damage to vision, hearing, and the brain. Today, if the disease is diagnosed and treated early, it can usually be cured.
Symptoms: Meningitis begins with a severe headache, high fever, vomiting, and often stiffness of the neck and back muscles. The person may become delirious or have convulsions. When such symptoms appear, you should call the doctor at once or take the sick person to a hospital.

MENOPAUSE The period during which menstruation becomes irregular and finally ceases; also called change of life or the climacteric. In most women, the menopause (pronounced men′o·pawz) begins sometime between the ages of 45 and 55 (the average in the United States is 48), and lasts for a period that may vary from six months to three years.

Menstruation may also stop prematurely—as early as the age of 30, or even before—usually, as a result of hormone abnormalities. At any age, surgical removal or irradiation of the ovaries results in an artificial menopause. The whole train of events described under MENSTRUATION comes to a halt when menstruation ceases. Egg cells are no longer released from the ovary, and pregnancy can no longer occur. The ovaries drastically curtail their production of ESTROGENS.

Because of the hormone imbalance created during menopause, many women have at least minor physical and psychological disturbances during this period. The most common complaint is HOT FLASHES, in which there is a temporary dilation of the skin blood vessels and a feeling of warmth. Other symptoms may include irritability, insomnia, bladder disturbances and frequent urination, dizziness, increased blood pressure, and backache.

It is important to consult your doctor if you have any troublesome symptoms during the menopause. If the symptoms are severe, he may prescribe estrogens to take the place of the hormones no longer produced by the ovaries. It is also possible that your symptoms may be due not to the menopause but to some other disorder.

For most women, the menopause is not a period of unusually great stress. Sexual feeling does not cease. However, some women may experience emotional problems at the menopause. Such problems should be discussed with the family doctor or a PSYCHIATRIST.

Any vaginal bleeding after menopause has been established (when there has been no menstruation for about a year) should be reported to your doctor.

MENORRHAGIA Excessively heavy bleeding during MENSTRUATION. It may be due to one of many causes, including anemia; high blood pressure (hypertension); infection, a cyst, or a tumor in the ovary, Fallopian tube, or uterus; a hormone disorder; too much alcohol; or nervous tension. Heavy periods are also common at and around the MENOPAUSE. A doctor will seek the underlying cause and treat it.

There is a wide variation in the amount of blood lost by women during menstruation, but any marked change in the pattern of bleeding should be reported to a doctor. Menorrhagia (pronounced men″o·rah′jee·a) is commonly associated with ANEMIA in women.

MENSTRUATION Periodic bleeding from the uterus in women of child-bearing age—that is, from the age of 12 or 14 to about 50. The first onset of menstruation is called the menarche, and its final

485

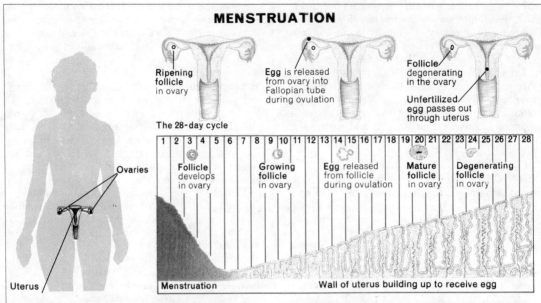

MENSTRUATION

Ripening follicle in ovary

Egg is released from ovary into Fallopian tube during ovulation

Follicle degenerating in the ovary

Unfertilized egg passes out through uterus

The 28-day cycle

| 1 | 2 | 3 | 4 | 5 | 6 | 7 | 8 | 9 | 10 | 11 | 12 | 13 | 14 | 15 | 16 | 17 | 18 | 19 | 20 | 21 | 22 | 23 | 24 | 25 | 26 | 27 | 28 |

Follicle develops in ovary

Growing follicle in ovary

Egg released from follicle during ovulation

Mature follicle in ovary

Degenerating follicle in ovary

Ovaries

Uterus

Menstruation

Wall of uterus building up to receive egg

The cycle of changes which takes place in the tissue lining a woman's uterus culminates about every 28 days when the blood-enriched lining comes away as the menstrual flow. The changes in the uterus parallel developments in an ovary, where an egg ripens and is released at ovulation, about halfway through the cycle. The egg travels along a Fallopian tube toward the uterus. If it is fertilized, it becomes implanted in the lining of the uterus, and menstruation ceases for the duration of pregnancy.

cessation is called the MENOPAUSE. The interval between menstrual periods varies considerably for different individuals. The average interval from the beginning of one period to the beginning of the next is 28 days, but any interval from 23 to 40 days may be considered normal.

Menstruation is one stage of a constantly repeated cycle in which a mucous-membrane lining (the endometrium) forms in the uterus and becomes swollen with blood and tissue in readiness to receive a fertilized egg, or ovum.

At the beginning of the cycle, on the first day of menstruation, a rudimentary egg cell in the OVARY begins to grow and continues to develop for 14 days. Then the membrane, or follicle, surrounding the egg bursts, and the egg is discharged from the ovary and enters the FALLOPIAN TUBE.

If the egg is not fertilized by a SPERM CELL during its several days' journey through the Fallopian tube, the unfertilized egg is discharged from the vagina in the menstrual flow, which consists of the sloughed-off endometrium. Then the whole process begins again. If the egg has been fertilized by the time it reaches the uterus, no menstruation occurs again until after the pregnancy is terminated.

If a girl fails to begin to menstruate at the age of puberty (a condition known as primary amenorrhea), a doctor should be consulted. Amenorrhea, both primary and secondary, may be due to a hormonal disturbance, which the doctor may correct with a hormone or a combination of hormones.

Some discomfort and minor pain may accompany menstruation and can be relieved by aspirin. There may be depression, emotional tension, headache, puffiness of the abdomen, skin, and other parts of the body, and a temporary gain of a pound or two in weight. Other menstrual disorders include excessive and prolonged menstruation (MENORRHAGIA), painful menstruation (dysmenorrhea), irregular menstruation, and bleeding between periods. If symptoms are severe, consult a doctor, especially if there is bleeding between periods or after the menopause.

MENTAL HOSPITAL A facility that provides care and therapy for the mentally ill. (See EMOTIONAL AND MENTAL DISORDERS.) Most of the hospitalized mentally ill are accommodated in state and county mental hospitals. Those whose stay will be relatively brief may be admitted to general hospitals, many of which have psychiatric wards.

MENTAL ILLNESS See EMOTIONAL AND MENTAL DISORDERS.

MENTAL RETARDATION Subnormal intelligence that is the result of defective brain development. The consequence is that the individual has trouble learning and has difficulty in taking his place in society. At one time, the terms FEEBLEMINDEDNESS, MORON, IDIOCY, and IMBECILITY were used for different degrees of mental retardation. Today, it is classified as mild, moderate, severe, or profound.

Causes: Mental retardation takes many forms and may be due to any of a large number of causes.

Disease in a pregnant woman may cause her child to be born retarded. German measles (RUBELLA) during the early months of pregnancy and syphilis can be responsible for defective brain development in a baby. Brain damage may also result from BIRTH INJURY. If the baby's RH FACTOR does not match the mother's, mental retardation may be one of the complications. A type of metabolic disorder (PHENYLKETONURIA) in the infant, a hormone deficiency such as cretinism (see DWARFISM), and malnutrition are other conditions that may produce mental deficiency. A small percentage of mentally retarded children have physical defects such as MICROCEPHALY (abnormally small head) or the features characteristic of MONGOLISM.

Treatment: Once the brain has been damaged, the condition is irreversible. Fortunately, most mentally retarded children are only moderately handicapped. As the term implies, retarded children are slow to learn, but many can learn a great deal if the teacher is patient and skilled. In many localities, special classes are available where the mentally retarded are taught useful skills.

Those of very low intelligence may be better off in an institution. However, the ultimate decision as to whether this is necessary and where to place such a child should be arrived at only after consultation with doctors, psychologists, and professionally trained people who specialize in dealing with such problems.

MEPROBAMATE A chemical substance used as a mild muscle relaxant in certain disorders and to relieve anxiety and tension. (See TRANQUILIZER.) Meprobamate (pronounced me·proh′ba·mayt″) is sold under many trade names, among the most common being Miltown and Equanil.

MERCUROCHROME A trade name for a solution of merbromin, a bright red, mildly effective, local ANTISEPTIC containing mercury.

MERCURY POISONING A serious disorder that sometimes affects people who work with mercury, corrosive sublimate, calomel, and other mercury salts. The fumes of mercury are poisonous, causing a burning pain in the mouth and stomach, diarrhea, vomiting, and ultimately collapse. Mercury poisoning may also result from POLLUTION, such as that which has occurred in Japan (see MINAMATA DISEASE). Kidney damage can occur and may lead to death.

In chronic mercury poisoning the mouth becomes inflamed, the gums bleed, and the tongue swells. The teeth sometimes fall out and the jaw bone may become diseased. There may also be tremor, paralysis, and severe anemia. Treatment consists of removing mercury from the body by a drug such as dimercaprol.

MERTHIOLATE A trade name for a skin ANTISEPTIC containing mercury. Merthiolate (pronounced mer·thie′o·layt″) usually has a reddish color.

MESCALINE A mildly HALLUCINOGENIC DRUG obtained from peyote, or mescal, a cactus that grows in the southwestern United States and Mexico. Mescal buttons (the small tubers that grow on the cactus) have a legalized, ritual use in the religious ceremonies of some American Indians. Mescaline (pronounced mes′ka·leen″) may also be used legally when authorized for psychological research. Otherwise, the possession and use of mescaline is illegal.

METABOLISM The sum total of all the complex processes by which a person converts raw material—food, water, and oxygen—into living tissue, energy, and waste. Metabolism is a continuous process that begins in the digestive tract and the lungs and goes on in every cell of the body. It consists of breaking down complex substances into simpler parts that are then recombined into countless new substances that compose the body. Every one of these chemical changes either uses up or releases energy. The following is a greatly simplified example of CARBOHYDRATE metabolism:

The carbohydrates (sugars and starches) that we eat are converted by enzymes and acids in the digestive tract into a simple sugar, called GLUCOSE. (The enzymes and acids are themselves products of metabolism.) Glucose is carried by the blood to the body's cells, where it is either combined with oxygen to release energy and waste products—carbon dioxide and water in this case—or converted into another substance, called glycogen. When needed, glycogen is changed back to glucose to supply energy. Excess glycogen is converted into fat and stored until it is needed. Carbohydrate metabolism is regulated by the hormone insulin, a protein. In this and other ways, the metabolism of carbohydrates is inseparably related to the metabolism of both proteins and fats.

The role of insulin in carbohydrate metabolism illustrates one way in which disease is sometimes associated with metabolic disorders. If the pancreas produces insufficient insulin, normal carbohydrate metabolism cannot take place. The result is DIABETES mellitus, in which abnormal amounts of glucose accumulate in the blood. Diabetes can be controlled by supplying the body with insulin from outside sources. Many metabolic processes are regulated by hormones, but the relationship between hormone deficiency and metabolic disorders is not often as clear-cut as in the case of insulin.

The term "basal metabolism" refers to the energy that the body uses when at rest. (See BASAL METABOLIC RATE.)

METASTASIS The spread of a disease from one part of the body to another by GERMS or by abnormal cells transported in the blood or the lymph. The term is usually applied to the spread of CANCER cells, which break away from the primary tumor and are carried to other parts of the body, where they grow into secondary tumors. (Pronounced me·tas′ta·sis.)

METATARSAL See FOOT. (Pronounced met″a·tahr′sal.)

METHADONE A synthetic chemical compound first developed as a pain killer and to suppress coughing. The chief interest in methadone (pronounced meth′a·dohn) lies in its use in programs to treat HEROIN addiction. Methadone does not produce the same "high" as heroin, but it may relieve the addict of the craving for heroin and so permit him to lead a normal life. Its use is under strict federal control in the United States.

METHEDRINE One of many trade names for methamphetamine hydrochloride. Methedrine (pronounced meth′e·dreen) is a stimulant very similar to AMPHETAMINE. It can be obtained legally only by prescription. However, the illegal use of Methedrine ("speed") is widespread and highly dangerous.

METHEMOGLOBIN Abnormal HEMOGLOBIN (the red pigment in blood) which has been changed chemically so that it has a dark brown color. Methemoglobin (pronounced met″hee′mo·gloh″bin) may be present in the bloodstream during an illness.

MICROBE See GERM.

MICROCEPHALY The condition of having an abnormally small head, associated with a failure of the brain to develop properly in an unborn baby. Microcephaly (pronounced mie″kro·sef′a·lee) may be caused by RUBELLA (German measles) contracted by the mother during pregnancy. The condition causes MENTAL RETARDATION.

MICTURITION Another word for URINATION. (Pronounced mik″chu·rish′un.)

MIDDLE EAR INFECTION Any infection of the part of the ear just inside the eardrum almost always arrives there by way of the EUSTACHIAN TUBE, which connects the middle ear with the back of the mouth. Because the Eustachian tubes are shorter and straighter in children than in adults, children are especially susceptible to middle ear infections. Otitis media (the medical term for a middle ear infection) may result from a common cold, infected adenoids or tonsils, influenza, measles, mumps, scarlet fever, or a STREP THROAT. Pain in the ear is usually severe with ear infection, and there may be fever, vomiting, headache, and drowsiness.

Prompt medical treatment is essential. The doc-

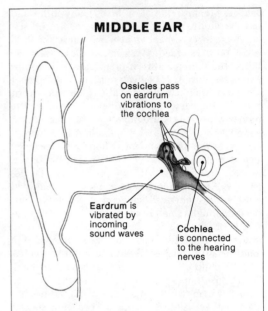

MIDDLE EAR

Ossicles pass on eardrum vibrations to the cochlea

Eardrum is vibrated by incoming sound waves

Cochlea is connected to the hearing nerves

The middle ear contains the eardrum and the three small sound-conducting bones, or ossicles. The Eustachian tube links the middle ear with the back of the throat so that air pressure is always the same on both sides of the eardrum. Infection of the middle ear, called otitis media, is generally caused by germs traveling up the Eustachian tube from the throat.

tor will administer appropriate SULFONAMIDES or ANTIBIOTICS to destroy the germs responsible for the infection in the particular case. If untreated, very serious complications may follow, including impairment of hearing, MASTOIDITIS, and MENINGITIS.

MIGRAINE See HEADACHE.

MILK LEG See POSTPARTUM.

MILTOWN A trade name for the tranquilizer MEPROBAMATE.

MINAMATA DISEASE A type of MERCURY POISONING which was first recognized in the 1950's among people living in villages bordering Minamata Bay, Japan. The disease was caused by POLLUTION. Organic mercury compounds, such as methyl mercury, were discharged into the waters of the bay and absorbed into the bodies of fish. When the local people ate the fish (their principal food), many developed symptoms of mercury poisoning—tremors, paralysis, severe anemia, and bone deformities—and nearly 50 died. (Pronounced min″a·mah′ta.)

MINERAL OIL A clear, relatively thin oil obtained from petroleum and used as a LAXATIVE.

MIOSIS (1) Contraction of the pupil of the eye. (2) The stage of a disease in which the symptoms become less severe. (3) (Usually spelled **meiosis**) The final stage in the development of a SPERM CELL or an EGG CELL, during which the number of CHROMOSOMES in the nucleus is halved. (Pronounced mie·oh'sis.)

MISCARRIAGE The expulsion of a FETUS, usually between the fourth and seventh month after conception, before the fetus is viable (able to live outside the uterus). If the expulsion occurs earlier, it is called spontaneous ABORTION.
Causes: The cause cannot be determined in many cases of miscarriage. However, when a miscarriage occurs spontaneously, the fetus is frequently defective. Sometimes, instead of being implanted in the uterus, the fetus stays in the FALLOPIAN TUBE and develops there. By the eighth to the tenth week there is no longer room for growth, and the tube ruptures. (See ECTOPIC PREGNANCY.)

A disorder may be responsible for the miscarriage. Venereal disease, poorly functioning endocrine glands, influenza, and kidney trouble are among the conditions that are sometimes to blame. Accidents, including falls, rarely cause miscarriages.
Symptoms: Vaginal bleeding is the most prominent symptom of threatened miscarriage. If the bleeding continues and there are severe cramps, the miscarriage is frequently inevitable.
Treatment: At the first sign of bleeding, the woman should get into bed and stay there. The doctor should be notified without delay. If the miscarriage takes place, sometimes the uterus must be cleaned out afterward by a simple surgical procedure known as a DILATATION AND CURETTAGE. Women who have had a number of miscarriages may still look forward to successful pregnancies. It is essential to follow the doctor's advice in every detail.

MITE Any of a large group of tiny, insectlike creatures related to ticks. Many of the mites are parasites of animals and plants. The so-called itch mite causes scabies in humans.

Other species of mites, commonly called chiggers, feed on the blood of humans and animals.
Scabies: The itch mite lays its eggs in a tunnel that it burrows in the outer layer of skin. The mites' secretions lead to sensitization (see SENSITIZED) and intense itching; PUSTULES develop on the skin. Scratching may bring secondary infections.

A doctor should be consulted about any persistent itching. If mites are responsible, the condition is treated with an ointment containing the chemical gamma benzene hexachloride. Treatment for the entire family is often necessary, as well as sterilization of bedding and clothing.

MITRAL DISEASE A rheumatic disease of the mitral valve of the heart, which separates the upper left chamber (atrium) from the lower left chamber (ventricle). Sometimes the valve fails to close completely, so that some blood flows back into the atrium instead of being pumped into the aorta. This condition is known as mitral (pronounced mie'tral) incompetence. More common is mitral stenosis, in which the two flaps of the valve stick partly together, narrowing the hole through which blood flows.

Mitral valve disease may be treated with drugs, but in severe cases surgery is needed. The surgeon may repair the valve or, in stenosis, separate the two flaps. Sometimes the complete valve is replaced by an artificial one made of plastic. See also HEART SURGERY.

MOLAR One of the 12 grinding teeth of the adult. There is a set of molars, three upper and three lower, at the rear of each side of the mouth. In some individuals, however, the third molars, or wisdom teeth, never appear. See also TOOTH.

MOLD A type of FUNGUS.

MOLE A dark spot of pigment in the skin. Moles are generally brown. They may be raised, and hairs may grow from them. If moles are small or on a part of the body covered by clothing, they are usually left untreated. Fortunately, unattractive or conspicuous moles can usually be removed by a skin specialist.

Moles should not be picked at or cut off. If moles bleed or become larger or darker, they require immediate medical scrutiny to eliminate the possibility of cancer.

MONGOLISM A congenital condition in which a child has a short, broad face, a fold of skin at the inner corners of the eyes, short fingers, and weak muscles. The child also exhibits a marked degree of MENTAL RETARDATION.

Mongolism (pronounced mong'gol·iz"em), the popular name for Down's syndrome, came into use because of the somewhat Oriental features of certain babies that were studied by Dr. John Langdon-Downs. Usually such babies are born to older mothers. The cause of the condition is an abnormality in the early development of the fertilized egg cells: the mongoloid child has an odd number of CHROMOSOMES in every cell in his body. These children usually have gentle, affectionate natures, and often can be taught to perform routine work.

MONILIASIS An infection caused by a yeastlike fungus (usually *Candida albicans*). Moniliasis (pronounced mon·i·lie'a·sis) is widespread and takes a number of different forms. Thrush is moniliasis affecting the mucous membranes of the mouth. In other cases, the infection may be confined to the skin, the nails, the vagina, the bronchi, or the lungs.

489

Sometimes the fungus enters the bloodstream and involves the heart. Moniliasis on the skin produces an oozing skin eruption, especially on areas of the body where there is friction, such as under the arms.

The antibiotic nystatin is usually effective in killing the fungus. For severe cases the antibiotic amphotericin B is used, but because it has undesirable side effects, it is administered only when absolutely necessary.

MONONUCLEOSIS A disease in which there is an abnormally large number of monocytes (a type of white corpuscle) in the blood. Mononucleosis (pronounced mon″o·noo″klee·oh′sis) is also known as glandular fever, infectious mononucleosis, or the kissing disease—it is popularly believed to be spread by kissing. The symptoms are fever, headache, scratchy throat, fatigue, and enlargement of the lymph glands.

Mononucleosis is diagnosed by means of a blood test. It is common among young people. It is believed to be a virus disease. It is usually mild, but may last for many weeks. Sometimes the spleen becomes enlarged, and the liver may be affected by a form of HEPATITIS.

There is no specific treatment for mononucleosis except bed rest and a well-rounded diet.

MONOPLEGIA A form of PARALYSIS affecting only one limb (or one side of the face). (Pronounced mon″o·plee′jee·a.)

MORNING SICKNESS The nausea and vomiting that often occur upon rising in the morning during the early months of pregnancy. Eating a dry cracker or two and sipping some weak tea or other liquid before getting out of bed will help prevent nausea. Frequent small meals may be advisable instead of three large meals a day. Greasy foods should be avoided.

MORON A term formerly used for a person with a mild degree of MENTAL RETARDATION.

MORPHINE A substance derived from opium. Morphine is a very effective pain reliever. As it is an addictive NARCOTIC, its use in the United States is under federal control.

MOTION SICKNESS A feeling of nausea, sometimes followed by vomiting, experienced by some persons when they travel on a boat, train, or airplane, or even in an automobile. It may also be felt in a swing or an elevator. The disorder is also known as kinesia, car sickness, seasickness, and airsickness.
Causes: Inside the labyrinth of the EAR, there are three semicircular canals which are sensitive to motion and assist us in maintaining our equilibrium as we move about under our own power. (See BALANCE, SENSE OF.) When we ride in an airplane or in a

rapidly accelerating elevator, the effect of the motion on the canals of the ear may result in motion sickness. Lack of fresh air or unpleasant fumes can heighten the reaction. Visual effects are also important. Many people are disturbed by watching the wake of a boat or the ground sinking from them when they are in an airplane that is climbing.
Treatment and Prevention: DRAMAMINE and BENADRYL are often effective in preventing motion sickness. Eating lightly before and during the trip also helps. If possible, adjust the ventilation so that you get plenty of fresh air.

MOTOR Having to do with, or causing, motion. Motor nerves carry messages from the central NERVOUS SYSTEM to the muscles to excite activity.

MOUNTAIN FEVER Another name for TICK FEVER; the term is also used for BRUCELLOSIS.

MOUTH Normally, the only measures that need to be taken to maintain good oral hygiene are keeping your teeth clean and visiting your dentist regularly. Even when we are not eating, the mouth is continually being washed by a faintly germicidal (germ-killing) mixture of saliva, mucus, and secretions from the tonsils and other lymphoid tissue in the mouth.

Conditions such as FEVER SORES or CANKER SORES usually disappear fairly quickly. As a rule, a coated tongue is no cause for alarm. Small growths, painless whitish patches, or any abnormal condition that lasts for more than a few days should be brought to your doctor's attention promptly.

A sore on the lips or the inside of the mouth can have any of a great variety of causes, from VITAMIN deficiency to serious infectious disease. Sore and bleeding gums may be a sign of developing pyorrhea alveolaris. (See PYORRHEA.) Sores caused by constant irritation of the mucous lining of the mouth can lead to serious trouble. See also STOMATITIS and VINCENT'S ANGINA.

MUCOUS COLITIS See COLITIS.

MUCOUS MEMBRANE The soft, smooth, moist tissue that lines most of the inner cavities and passages of the body. Mucous membrane lines the entire digestive tract (see DIGESTION) from mouth to anus, the RESPIRATORY SYSTEM from nostrils to the tiny air cells in the lungs, the URINARY TRACT, and the reproductive tracts of both sexes.

Scattered throughout the mucous membrane are mucous cells that secrete mucin. The mucin combines with water and other substances to form MUCUS.

Mucous membrane contains a great variety of special structures. In the stomach, it has the numerous tiny glands that secrete digestive enzymes. In the respiratory tract, tiny projections (called cilia) continuously sweep out microscopic foreign matter inhaled along with air. In the intestine, the projections (here called villi) form a relatively vast surface through which absorption of nutrients takes place. Inside the uterus, the mucous membrane (known as the endometrium) goes through cyclic changes that occur with MENSTRUATION.

MUCUS The thick, slippery liquid that protects and lubricates MUCOUS MEMBRANE.

MULTIPLE PREGNANCY The condition in which an expectant mother has more than one developing fetus in her uterus at once. About one in 80 pregnancies results in twins, and about one in 6,400 in triplets. Multiple pregnancies tend to run in families (the tendency being passed on from mother to daughter), and they occur more commonly in women who have been given hormones to increase their fertility. See also TWINS.

MULTIPLE SCLEROSIS (MS) A disease of the nervous system that usually begins in early adulthood. Hard, gray patches called scleroses (pronounced skle·roh′seez) form on the nerve sheaths of the brain and spinal cord. These patches make it impossible for the nerves to respond in a normal way. Multiple sclerosis (pronounced skle·roh′sis) is chronic and develops slowly, but tends to become increasingly disabling. Periods of remission or seeming improvement occur quite often, sometimes lasting for many years. The cause is unknown.
Symptoms: The symptoms of MS are variable, but one of the most obvious symptoms is an erratic, stiff walk, sometimes with a staggering gait. The hands and fingers may tremble in performing simple actions. The eyesight can also be affected: sometimes the person has a narrowed visual field and may see double; the eyeballs may move involuntarily (NYSTAGMUS). Speech may be slow or slurred. In later stages, bowel and bladder control may be affected. Paralysis, partial or almost complete, may eventually occur.
Treatment: There is at present no specific treatment, but a program of physical therapy is often advisable for muscles weakened or paralyzed by the disease.

More detailed information is available from the National Multiple Sclerosis Society, 205 East 42nd Street, New York, New York 10017.

MUMPS An acute, contagious disease that sometimes affects children between the ages of five and 15; it is also known as parotitis. It is caused by a virus that is transmitted in the saliva of an infected person. The symptoms appear from two to three weeks after exposure. One attack usually, but not always, gives immunity for life.
Symptoms: Painful swelling of the face and neck on one or both sides is the most typical symptom. This is produced by swelling of the parotid glands, saliva-secreting glands located below each ear. The person has a headache, and fever may run as high as 104° F.

In males who have passed puberty, mumps sometimes involves the TESTICLES in addition to the salivary glands. The infection is called ORCHITIS and produces a painful inflammation and swelling of one or both testicles. Mumps may also involve the pancreas, or it may attack the brain, producing ENCEPHALITIS. Complete recovery can be expected.
Treatment: Other diseases may duplicate the symptoms of mumps, so it is important to call your doctor for a diagnosis. If a child has fever, he should stay in bed. If there is no fever, the child should simply stay at home until the swelling goes down.

A vaccine is now available which provides immunity, probably life-long, against the disease. All males past puberty who have not had mumps should receive the vaccine.

MUSCLE Tissue made up of elastic cells and fibers that can repeatedly contract and relax. All the movement that takes place inside the body, as well as the motion of the body as a whole, is brought about by muscle.
Voluntary muscle is so called because it responds to our conscious control. It can also act by involuntary, reflex action. (See KNEE JERK.) Voluntary muscle is in continuous imperceptible motion; this keeps the muscle in a state of tension known as muscle tone.

Under the microscope, voluntary muscle appears as parallel bundles of long fibers, some as long as four inches or more. The fibers are striated, or marked with crosswise stripes. At each end of a muscle, the elastic muscle tissue merges into a tough, inelastic substance, called TENDON, by which muscle is attached to bone. Most of the voluntary muscles are attached to different bones of the skeleton in such a way that their contractions set in motion the complicated system of levers that is the skeletal framework.
Cardiac muscle forms the heart. Like voluntary muscle, it is striated. Of course, the heart's beating is not under voluntary control. Its rhythmic contractions are maintained by a so-called CARDIAC PACEMAKER.
Smooth muscle, also called involuntary or visceral muscle, functions entirely without our conscious control. It is arranged in flat sheets or layers. Smooth muscle forms part of the wall of all the tubes and ducts in the body, including the blood vessels, digestive tract, and genitourinary system. It moves with a slow, wavelike motion. Its contractions help to keep the contents of any duct moving forward. (See PERISTALSIS.)

As a muscle is used, it continues to grow bigger and stronger. If unused, a muscle shrivels away. For this reason, exercise is important not only to maintain health but also to prevent deterioration in persons whose activity is restricted by illness.

491

MUSCLE CONTRACTION Whenever we move, we do so by contracting some particular set of muscles attached to the skeleton. The muscles act in opposing groups. For example, when we tense the biceps muscle in the upper arm, the elbow tends to bend. It will not bend, however, unless the triceps at the back of the arm relaxes at the same time. When we want to straighten out the arm again, the triceps must contract and the biceps must relax. Even at rest, some of the muscles must be kept in a contracted state in order to maintain our balance.

MUSCULAR DYSTROPHY The name applied to a number of diseases in which the muscles shrivel away. The condition often begins in childhood.

What causes muscular dystrophy (pronounced dis′tro·fee) is not yet known, although the disorder is being actively investigated. Heredity is an important factor in most types of the disease. In affected muscles, the normal fibers of protein change, and after a while fat takes the place of the protein, swelling the fibers. Gradually, the muscles waste away. The condition may not be noticed until the child is a few years old. He does not walk normally but waddles. He has difficulty getting up from the floor or climbing stairs. The muscles become weaker and weaker, until the child may have to use a wheelchair. There is an increased susceptibility to pneumonia and other respiratory diseases.
Treatment: Massage and physical therapy are helpful in maintaining the tone of the muscles. Activity is valuable for the same reason, and also helps the person's morale. Orthopedic appliances, such as braces, aid him in getting around. He should be encouraged to do as much for himself as he is physically able to.

For further information about rehabilitation centers throughout the country, as well as the latest developments in treatment and research, contact the national headquarters of the Muscular Dystrophy Association, 810 7th Avenue, New York, New York 10019.

MYALGIA Pain in a muscle or muscles. (Pronounced mie·al′jee·a.) Since there are more than 600 muscles in the body, they will occasionally be a source of strain and pain to everyone. If you have not used certain muscles for a long time and then subject them to heavy exertion, as in prolonged walking, playing tennis, or shoveling snow, they will be sore and stiff afterward. (See CHARLEY HORSE.)

Myalgia, or diffuse muscle aches and pains, is often present when a person has a viral infection, such as the common cold. Some types of LUMBAGO and STIFF NECK are forms of myalgia.

MYASTHENIA GRAVIS A chronic disease in which the muscles are weak and tire easily. (Pronounced mie″as·thee′ni·a gra′vis.) The basic cause is not understood, but nerve impulses are not trans-mitted normally to the muscles because of a chemical abnormality. The disorder is usually found in young persons, especially women between 20 and 40.
Symptoms: The muscles of the face, tongue, larynx, throat, and chest wall, among others, may be affected. The person has difficulty in chewing, swallowing, and talking. His eyelids droop, and his smile is abnormal. Eye problems such as DIPLOPIA (double vision) may occur.
Treatment: A good, well-balanced diet is important. Complete rest is necessary during periods of crisis. A doctor can prescribe medicines that are helpful in reducing the symptoms. Sometimes the disease becomes progressively more serious, and a respirator has to be kept available. Removal of the thymus gland may be recommended (see ENDOCRINE GLAND).

MYCETOMA An infection that is caused by many varieties of FUNGI and by certain BACTERIA that are present in soil. It occurs chiefly in tropical climates. Mycetoma (pronounced mie″se·toh′ma) is also called maduromycosis, or, when caused by bacteria, actinomycotic mycetoma. Most often, it affects the feet of people who go barefoot (Madura foot), but it may involve the hands and other areas of the body.

The fungi or bacteria usually enter the body through a cut or a wound. An abscess forms, then a number of abscesses develop over a period of time.

Actinomycotic mycetoma responds favorably to the administration of SULFONAMIDES (sulfa compounds). Other types of drugs may be used to treat mycetoma caused by a fungus, but if none is effective, surgical removal of the lesion or amputation of part of a limb may be necessary.

MYCOSIS Any disease caused by a FUNGUS. Mycosis (pronounced mie·koh′sis) of the skin is common; examples include RINGWORM and ATHLETE'S FOOT. ACTINOMYCOSIS is a chronic infection that may occur in the mouth, throat, lungs, or intestines or on the skin. Other diseases caused by fungi include BLASTOMYCOSIS, COCCIDIOIDOMYCOSIS, HISTOPLASMOSIS, and MONILIASIS.

MYELITIS A medical term for an inflammation of the spinal cord or of the bone marrow. (Pronounced mie″e·lie′tis.)

MYELOMA A malignant (cancerous) disease involving the blood-making cells in the bone MARROW. (Pronounced mie″e·loh′ma.)

MYOMA A TUMOR of smooth muscle tissue, such as that in the wall of the stomach and intestines. A myoma is usually benign (noncancerous), although it can become malignant (cancerous). (Pronounced mie·oh′ma.)

MYOPATHY A term that refers to a group of diseases in which muscle weakness occurs. The cause may be poisoning, sometimes from drugs such as cortisone; or the myopathy may be part of a general disease such as DIABETES. Cancer, even in its early stages, may also cause myopathy. MUSCULAR DYSTROPHY is a hereditary form of myopathy (pronounced mie·op′a·thee).

MYOPIA The ability to see distinctly only things that are close at hand. (Pronounced mie·oh′pee·a.) The popular name of the condition is nearsightedness. (The opposite condition is HYPEROPIA.)

In a nearsighted, or myopic, person, the EYE is usually too long from the front to the back. The image of an object some distance away is not focused on the retina at the back of the eye, as it should be, but at a point in front of it. Consequently, the object cannot be seen distinctly. By squinting, the nearsighted person may obtain a clearer image. To solve his problem properly, however, he needs to have a pair of EYEGLASSES with concave lenses that focus the image correctly on the retina.

MYOSITIS Inflammation of a muscle. Sometimes the muscle loses its power and becomes rigid. If the inflammation is severe and prolonged, the muscle fibers may be replaced by scar tissue, leading to permanent weakness and stiffness. (Pronounced mie″o·sie′tis.)

MYXADENOMA A benign TUMOR made up of the same type of tissue as that of a mucous gland. (Pronounced miks″ad·e·noh′ma.)

MYXEDEMA A disease caused by the inability of the THYROID GLAND to secrete its hormone, thyroxine, in adequate quantity. (Pronounced mik″se·dee′ma.) See also GOITER.

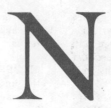

N

NAIL The nails are lifeless outgrowths of specialized skin cells. The visible, horny parts of fingernails and toenails are composed largely of the protein KERATIN. The half-moon, or lunula, appears white because it is not firmly attached to the tissue under it. The lunula is partly covered by a thin fold of cuticle, which extends up around the sides of the nail. **Injury and Inflammation:** Partial separation of the nail from the nail bed (onycholysis) can be caused by excessive exposure to water, soap, detergents, or other irritating substances. More serious disorders that affect the nails are RINGWORM and other fungal and bacterial infections. Inflammation and pus formation under and around the nail (known as felon, or whitlow) are due to BACTERIA, which may enter by way of a break in the cuticle. Such infections should be seen by a doctor. The nails may be affected in PSORIASIS. See also HANGNAIL; INGROWN TOENAIL.

NAIL-BITING Habitual biting of the fingernails. It is usually due to nervous tension.

NARCOLEPSY A tendency to fall asleep at any time, anywhere without normal tiredness. The cause may be damage to the brain in the region of the HYPOTHALAMUS—the area near the front of the brain that controls the functioning of the internal organs. This may result from an infection such as ENCEPHALITIS, from a brain TUMOR, or from a head injury. The cause should be treated, but if the condition persists a doctor may prescribe drugs to relieve the symptom and keep the person awake. (Pronounced nahr′ko·lep′see.)

NARCOTIC A medical term for any substance that produces stupor and sleep or relieves pain. Some examples are opium and substances derived from opium, or *opiates*, such as MORPHINE and CODEINE. DEMEROL and METHADONE are synthetically produced narcotics. Many narcotics induce DRUG ADDICTION if used repeatedly, because of the temporary feeling of well-being that they produce. Narcotic medicines are, therefore, under strict federal control and can be obtained legally only with a doctor's prescription.

NASAL CONGESTION See CONGESTION.

NASAL FEEDING The method of feeding a sick person who cannot swallow but whose digestive system is functioning. A thin tube is inserted into a nostril and gently pushed until it reaches the stomach. The food, usually a liquid, is then poured slowly into a funnel or other device connected to the tube, and it flows into the stomach by gravity. Nasal feeding is used after surgery of, or severe injury to, the mouth and throat regions.

NAUSEA A feeling of discomfort or queasiness in the region of the stomach which may be followed by vomiting. Nausea is associated with many disorders or conditions. It often occurs during the early months of pregnancy. (See MORNING SICKNESS.) It is also a common symptom of MOTION SICKNESS. INDIGESTION is frequently a cause of nausea. TENSION may be responsible for the nausea and vomiting produced by a so-called nervous stomach.

Persistent nausea, particularly when it occurs in combination with fever, pain, or cramps, should be brought immediately to your doctor's attention. It may be a symptom of a serious condition such as appendicitis, ulcer, or food poisoning.

NEARSIGHTEDNESS See MYOPIA.

NECROSIS The death of cells or tissues or a portion of an organ in the living body. Necrosis (pronounced ne·kroh′sis) may occur after severe burns or other injuries or in conditions where the blood supply is cut off for too long a period, as in GANGRENE. Some diseases cause necrosis in internal organs.

NEMBUTAL The trade name of a BARBITURATE medicine used as a sedative and to cause sleep. Nembutal (pronounced nem′byu·tawl″) is available only with a doctor's prescription.

NEOMYCIN An ANTIBIOTIC obtained from a soil mold. Because neomycin (pronounced nee″o·mie′sin) may have a damaging effect on the kidneys, it is usually applied only externally in ointments to combat skin infections.

NEOPLASM A new and abnormal growth in the body; a TUMOR. A neoplasm (pronounced nee′o·plaz″em) often resembles the tissue from which it arises, and may be BENIGN or MALIGNANT.

NEO-SYNEPHRINE The trade name for a medication sold, without prescription, in drops or sprays. It reduces the swelling of nasal congestion. (Pronounced nee"oh·si·nef'rin.)

NEPHRECTOMY Surgical removal of a KIDNEY. A nephrectomy (pronounced ni frek'to·mee) is usually performed if one kidney is seriously damaged by injury or disease.

NEPHRITIS Inflammation of the KIDNEYS, commonly called Bright's disease. The medical name is glomerulonephritis. There are acute and chronic forms of nephritis (pronounced ni·frie'tis). The acute form attacks children more often than adults. Nephritis is usually preceded by a STREPTOCOCCUS infection elsewhere in the body. Many cases of nephritis could be prevented if every streptococcal infection were treated promptly with penicillin or other antibiotics.

The symptoms of nephritis may be very mild or severe. They include headache, loss of appetite, nausea, and fever. The eyes and face may look puffy, and the ankles and other parts of the body may be swollen with accumulated fluid. The urine often has a dark or cloudy appearance.

See also KIDNEY DISEASE; NEPHROSIS; PYELONE-PHRITIS.

NEPHROSIS Kidney malfunction accompanied by pronounced EDEMA (swelling) due to accumulated fluid. The kidneys seem to lose the ability to regulate the fluid content of the body. In addition, abnormal protein, fats, and other substances are excreted in the urine. Nephrosis (pronounced ni·froh'sis), or nephrotic syndrome, is not a single, distinct disease. It may occur as a stage in NEPHRITIS. It may be associated with other diseases or with certain toxic substances. There is no specific cure for nephrosis except treatment of the underlying cause.

NERVE A specialized tissue through which impulses pass back and forth between the brain and SPINAL CORD and the other parts of the body. Nerve tissue consists mainly of cells called neurons. A typical neuron comprises a central body, a long threadlike extension called an axon, and a number of shorter extensions called dendrites.

Nerves are made up of long, ropelike bundles of axons whose central bodies are located in the brain or spinal cord or in clusters elsewhere in the body. The gray matter in the brain consists mostly of central bodies and dendrites. The axons are covered with a layer of white, fatty material called myelin. Impulses are received in each central body through the dendrites and leave by way of the axon. The free end of the axon is somewhat spread out, like a frayed end of string. This end comes close to the dendrites of other neurons but does not quite touch them. A nerve impulse must jump across this tiny gap, which is called a synapse.

There are two kinds of neurons, sensory and motor. Sensory, or afferent, neurons carry impulses inward to the spinal column and brain, where they are interpreted as information about the outer world. Motor, or efferent, neurons carry impulses from the central nervous system to the various parts of the body, where they are translated into action. At the outer end of a motor neuron, the frayed end of an axon spreads out to form a so-called end plate, which connects with muscle fibers. Similar structures at the ends of sensory nerves are concentrated in the sense organs and irregularly dispersed in the skin.

Impulses travel along a nerve by a series of reactions that are partly chemical, partly electrical. The impulses travel at varying speeds—up to about 200 miles an hour. See also NERVOUS SYSTEM.

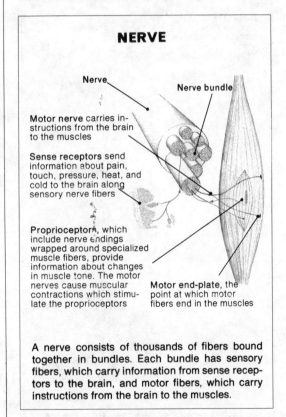

NERVE

Nerve

Nerve bundle

Motor nerve carries instructions from the brain to the muscles

Sense receptors send information about pain, touch, pressure, heat, and cold to the brain along sensory nerve fibers

Proprioceptors, which include nerve endings wrapped around specialized muscle fibers, provide information about changes in muscle tone. The motor nerves cause muscular contractions which stimulate the proprioceptors

Motor end-plate, the point at which motor fibers end in the muscles

A nerve consists of thousands of fibers bound together in bundles. Each bundle has sensory fibers, which carry information from sense receptors to the brain, and motor fibers, which carry instructions from the brain to the muscles.

NERVOUS BREAKDOWN A vague, nonmedical term for an emotional illness, or a critical point in one, that comes on suddenly.

Symptoms may include depression, profound feelings of inadequacy, fatigue, and lack of appetite. See also EMOTIONAL AND MENTAL DISORDERS.

NERVOUS SYSTEM The entire apparatus of NERVE cells that controls activities inside the body and the body's responses to the outside world. The billions of nerve cells in the body are organized into

NERVOUS SYSTEM

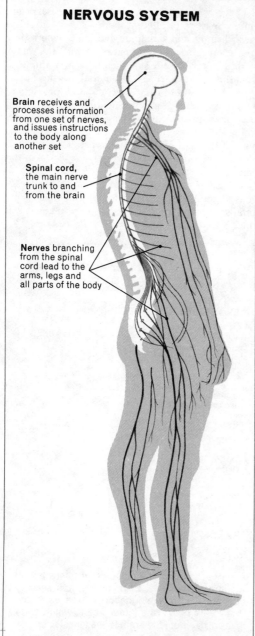

Brain receives and processes information from one set of nerves, and issues instructions to the body along another set

Spinal cord, the main nerve trunk to and from the brain

Nerves branching from the spinal cord lead to the arms, legs and all parts of the body

The central nervous system consists of the brain and the spinal cord. Major nerves branching from the cord serve every organ and part of the body. By sending and receiving impulses along nerves, the brain exercises voluntary control over muscular movements. In addition, it exercises automatic control by means of the autonomic nervous system; through these nerves, the brain can alter the pace of the heart, influence the rate of breathing, and control the processes of digestion and excretion. The activity of the autonomic system is influenced by the emotions.

a single, integrated system, but we usually consider the system as being made up of distinct parts.

The central nervous system comprises the BRAIN and the SPINAL CORD. All the nerves that branch out from the central nervous system and penetrate every part of the body make up the peripheral nervous system. The peripheral system includes the 12 pairs of cranial nerves that connect directly with the brain and the 31 pairs of spinal nerves that branch out from the spinal cord. The peripheral system also contains numerous clusters of nerve cell bodies which are known as ganglia.

The AUTONOMIC NERVOUS SYSTEM governs automatic activities such as heart action, breathing, glandular secretion, and peristalsis. The somatic nervous system serves the sense organs and the voluntary muscles.

The autonomic system consists of two subsystems, the sympathetic nervous system and the parasympathetic nervous system. These two subsystems work in opposition to each other. For example, the heart is speeded up by sympathetic impulses and slowed down by impulses from the parasympathetic system. The involuntary, automatic activity of all the internal organs is similarly regulated. The control center of the autonomic system lies largely in the HYPOTHALAMUS of the brain.

NEURALGIA Severe pain along the course of a peripheral nerve or nerves, that is, nerves outside of the central NERVOUS SYSTEM. By contrast, NEURITIS is an inflammation of a nerve, and may or may not be painful. Neuralgia (pronounced nyoor·al′jee·a) may be caused by an injury to the nerves or by an irritation, but often the cause is not easy to find. Two of the commonest types are facial neuralgia (also known as TIC DOULOUREUX and trigeminal neuralgia) and SCIATICA.

NEURASTHENIA A condition that is classified medically as a neurosis or a neurotic maladjustment. (Pronounced nyoor″as·thee′nee·a.) See also EMOTIONAL AND MENTAL DISORDERS.

NEURITIS An inflammation of a nerve or nerves. The peripheral NERVOUS SYSTEM, extending from the spinal cord and brain to the eyes, skin, muscles, and other parts of the body, is involved in neuritis (pronounced nyoor·ie′tis). Neuritis is sometimes painful: it may be accompanied by NEURALGIA.
Polyneuritis: General neuritis of the peripheral nervous system may be caused by chemical poisoning, alcoholism, diabetes, a virus infection, an allergy, or malnutrition. Removing the cause is the first step in providing relief.
Shingles: Herpes zoster, the medical term for shingles, is an inflammation of a ganglion, or mass of nerves, by a specific virus. The face, chest, or eyes are frequently the sites of the trouble, and itchy, painful blisters appear. See also SHINGLES.

Bell's Palsy: This is a temporary paralysis of the muscles on one side of the face. It is due to inflammation of a facial nerve and may be brought on by a draft, a chill, or an injury. The eye may close and the mouth droop. Warmth and massage provide relief.

Sciatica: The sciatic nerve is the largest nerve in the entire body, extending from the spinal column down through each leg. Inflammation of this nerve is sometimes responsible for the painful condition known as sciatica. See also SCIATICA.

NEUROFIBROMA A TUMOR composed of portions of nerve fibers and connective tissue. A neurofibroma (pronounced nyoor"oh·fie·broh'mₐ) is caused by the overgrowth of the cells surrounding the nerves. These tumors are BENIGN and are most common under the skin, where they form small NODES covered with brownish spots. The presence of many neurofibromas is a condition known as neurofibromatosis.

NEUROLOGY The branch of medicine concerned with the study of the NERVOUS SYSTEM and the treatment of its diseases and abnormalities. (Pronounced nyoor·ol'o·jee.)

NEUROSIS See EMOTIONAL AND MENTAL DISORDERS; PSYCHONEUROSIS.

NEUROSURGERY Surgery of the NERVOUS SYSTEM: the brain, the spinal cord, and the nerves.

In brain surgery, it is of the utmost importance to avoid injuring any sound brain tissue. By using magnifying lenses and minute instruments, neurosurgeons are able to operate on very small areas. For example, a blood clot can be removed from a tiny blood vessel.

The location of the brain operation is determined in advance by X ray and other techniques. To make an opening in the skull, it is often sufficient to drill a single small hole. In more extensive operations, a number of holes are drilled at key points. A saw is then used to cut the bone between the holes, and the piece of bone is lifted out. This preliminary operation is called a craniotomy. The same piece of bone may be replaced after the operation is completed, or a metal or plastic plate may be put over the opening.

Brain surgery may be performed for the following reasons: to remove damaged brain tissue and bone splinters in cases of severe head injury; to remove a tumor; to remove fluid, as in HYDROCEPHALUS; to remove a blood clot and seal off damaged blood vessels; and to relieve certain cases of PARKINSONISM.

Operations on the spinal cord likewise are performed to remove tumors and repair injuries.

Neurosurgery is also used to relieve severe and persistent pain when all other methods fail. If the sensory nerve that supplies the painful area is severed, the brain will no longer receive pain impulses from that area. However, once a nerve is cut, the effect is permanent. See also BLOCK.

NEUROTIC See EMOTIONAL AND MENTAL DISORDERS; PSYCHONEUROSIS.

NEUTROPENIA A condition in which there are fewer than the normal number of white cells called neutrophil leukocytes in the blood. This may happen in diseases such as influenza, measles, and typhoid fever. It can also result from taking any of a large number of drugs, such as sulfonamides, phenylbutazone, and antithyroid agents. See also LEUKOPENIA. (Pronounced noo"troh·pee'nee·ₐ.)

NEVUS The medical name for a congenital MOLE or BIRTHMARK. (Pronounced nee'vₐs.)

NIACIN See VITAMIN. (Pronounced nie'ₐ·sin.)

NICTATION (nictitation) Winking or blinking of the eye, a REFLEX of the lids that gives protection to the eye from dust, injury, and sudden bright light. The word "nictation" (pronounced nik·tay'shₐn) is also used to describe a nervous twitching of the eyelid.

NIGHT BLINDNESS Impaired ability to see in dim light. The medical term is nyctalopia. It is caused by a deficiency of vitamin A (see VITAMIN) in the diet. The condition causes no obvious changes in the eye tissues. Treatment consists of doses of vitamin A as prescribed by the doctor.

NIGHTMARE See SLEEP.

NITROGEN MUSTARD Any of a group of special chemical substances that kill or slow down the growth of rapidly dividing cells. Nitrogen mustards are used to treat cancerous conditions such as chronic LEUKEMIA and HODGKIN'S DISEASE.

NITROGLYCERIN An oily chemical liquid used in medicines and in explosives.

Nitroglycerin (pronounced nie"troh·glis'er·in) is employed medically most frequently for the relief of ANGINA PECTORIS. It is dispensed in tablet form. When there is a painful spasm, the person puts a pill under his tongue, and the chemical goes to work almost at once. It may prevent an attack if a pill is taken before one is likely to occur.

The tablets should be taken exactly as prescribed; too large a dose may cause headache or fainting.

NITROUS OXIDE A colorless gas used as an ANESTHETIC, particularly by dentists. Nitrous oxide (pronounced nie'trₐs ok'sied) is popularly known as laughing gas.

NOCTURIA Excessive urination during the night. It is often a symptom of CONGESTIVE HEART FAILURE, but can also occur in healthy persons for various reasons. (Pronounced nok·too'ree·a.)

NODE A knoblike thickening, which may be normal or abnormal. LYMPH NODES are examples of normal nodes.

NOSE The organ of smell and the entrance to the respiratory system. The part of the nose that is sensitive to smell is a small patch of olfactory bulbs. They are located at the topmost part of the nasal passage. Tiny nerve fibers lead directly from the olfactory bulbs into the central part of the brain. The sense of smell contributes a great deal to what we usually think of as taste.

NOSE

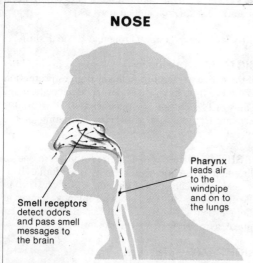

Smell receptors detect odors and pass smell messages to the brain

Pharynx leads air to the windpipe and on to the lungs

Air entering the lungs through the nasal passages passes over a series of convoluted cartilages and bones, which act as an air-conditioning system. Hairs filter out particles of dirt, sticky mucus traps dust and germs and moistens the incoming air, and the warm surfaces heat the air before it reaches the lungs. Brush-shaped receptors in the top of the nasal cavity detect molecules of scented substances in the air and provide us with a sense of smell.

The basic structure of the nose is made up of bones and cartilage. The skull behind the nose is pitted with a number of paranasal sinuses that open into the nasal cavity. These sinuses are lined with mucous membrane, as are the nasal passages. Inflammation of the lining of the nose, or RHINITIS, is the commonest nasal disorder. In most people, the two sides of the nose and the sinuses are not perfectly symmetrical. See also DEVIATED SEPTUM.

NOSEBLEED Bleeding from the nose is usually due to local injury, but in some cases it may be a symptom of any of a number of serious conditions elsewhere in the body. The commonest cause is rupture of a small blood vessel inside the nose. If heavy nosebleeds occur frequently or without obvious cause, the doctor should be consulted. For methods used to stop nosebleed, see FIRST AID section.

NOVOCAIN A local ANESTHETIC that is used in dentistry and surgery. Novocain (pronounced noh'vo·kayn) is a trade name for PROCAINE HYDROCHLORIDE.

NUMBNESS Loss of sensation, generally in the limbs. It usually results when sensory nerves are damaged or inflamed (NEURITIS), or when the arteries are diseased (RAYNAUD'S DISEASE). See also PARALYSIS.

The sensation known as PINS AND NEEDLES is caused by pressure on a nerve where it runs close to the surface of the body.

NUPERCAINE A trade name for a powerful, but toxic, local ANESTHETIC. Its chemical name is dibucaine hydrochloride. Nupercaine is used to relieve external pain in the final stages of childbirth, in eye surgery, and sometimes in spinal anesthesia.

NURSE Anyone who has ever been seriously ill knows how much a good nurse contributes to his recovery. The nurse is the one who provides continuous care and administers the treatment ordered by the doctor. Two types of nurses are legally recognized: the professional, registered nurse (RN) and the licensed practical, or vocational, nurse. Both types must successfully complete prescribed courses of study and then pass examinations set by the state authority. The professional nurse may pursue a career in hospitals, in private homes, in the armed forces (where a nurse is a commissioned officer), with the Red Cross, with public health agencies, in schools, in private industry, or as an educator in a nursing school or college.

A person who wants to become a registered nurse must be a high school graduate and pass an examination for admission to the nursing school that she (or he) chooses. She may choose one of three types of schools, which offer three different levels of professional training. A two-year course leading to an associate-in-arts degree is offered by many junior or community colleges in affiliation with local hospitals. A three-year program leading to a nursing diploma is offered by many hospitals. Four- or five-year courses leading to a bachelor's degree in nursing are offered by most universities that have a medical school and affiliated hospital.

The curriculum in all accredited nursing schools includes courses in anatomy, physiology, disease and its treatment, obstetrics, pediatrics, nutrition, pharmacology (drugs and medicines), and surgical and nursing techniques. Intensive practical training is given in the hospital wards.

Courses for licensed practical nurses are offered by a number of high schools and vocational schools, hospitals, and organizations such as the Red Cross. Most such courses take one year and emphasize techniques of tending the sick. Upon graduation, practical nurses are qualified to care for the ill in a hospital, home, or nursing home, under supervision of a doctor or professional nurse.

The graduate of an accredited nursing school is sometimes referred to as a graduate nurse. A public health nurse is a graduate nurse who works for a local board of health, assists in the prevention of disease, and educates the community in nutrition and proper health practices. A visiting nurse is a graduate nurse who works for a private community agency and cares for sick people in their homes.

Details about accredited nursing schools and training programs can be obtained from the National League for Nursing, 10 Columbus Circle, New York, New York 10019.

NURSING THE BABY See BOTTLE-FEEDING; BREAST-FEEDING.

NUTRITION The various processes involved in supplying nourishment to the tissues, especially the processes of digestion, absorption, and assimilation; also, food itself. See also DIET.

NYCTALOPIA The medical name for NIGHT BLINDNESS. (Pronounced nik″ta·loh′pee·a.)

NYMPHOMANIA Abnormally increased sexual desire in a woman. (The equivalent disorder in a male is known as SATYRIASIS.) Nymphomania (pronounced nim″fo·may′nee·a) is believed to be caused by an individual's emotional problems rather than by biological factors, such as excessive secretion of hormones. Sexual relations may serve as a temporary escape from anxiety or from a feeling of inadequacy. Such persons may obtain less satisfaction from the sex act than normal women.

NYSTAGMUS Rhythmic and involuntary movements of the eyeball, usually affecting both eyes. (Pronounced nis·tag′mus.) The condition is often caused by a congenital weakness of the EYE muscles, but it may also be the result of certain diseases, such as MULTIPLE SCLEROSIS and MÉNIÈRE'S DISEASE.

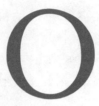

OBESITY Overweight, or excessive accumulation of fat in the body. Obesity (pronounced oh·bee′si·tee) usually results from overeating, especially of fats and carbohydrates, and from underexercise. Besides being unattractive, obesity makes the person more susceptible to DIABETES, mellitus, HEART DISEASE, atherosclerosis (see HARDENING OF THE ARTERIES), and other illnesses that can shorten life. Statistics prove that the healthiest and longest-lived people in the general population are those who avoid obesity. For information on losing weight, see REDUCING.

OBSTETRICS The branch of medicine that deals with PREGNANCY, CHILDBIRTH, and the period after birth (the PUERPERIUM). An obstetrician (pronounced ob″ste·trish′en) is a doctor who specializes in obstetrics (pronounced ob·stet′riks). See also GYNECOLOGY.

OCCIPITAL Pertaining to the back of the head. (Pronounced ok·sip′i·tal.)

OCCLUSION A blockage in the body. In coronary occlusion (pronounced o·kloo′zhun) an artery supplying blood to the heart is blocked by a blood clot or similar obstruction. See also CORONARY HEART DISEASE.

OCCUPATIONAL THERAPY AND VOCATIONAL REHABILITATION Occupational therapy is the use of selected activities to help restore health to the physically or mentally ill and retrain the handicapped or disabled. If the person is seriously handicapped, the activity will be a simple one, such as elementary needlework. Others may occupy themselves with painting, ceramics, sculpture, carpentry, weaving, leatherwork, typing, or almost anything that interests them. Being occupied tends to give the individual a positive, forward-looking point of view, and he suffers fewer of the psychological effects of protracted ill health or other impairment.
Vocational rehabilitation is concerned more specifically with restoring earning capacity. Aptitude testing, job training, and job placement are all part of vocational rehabilitation. Such programs are often conducted by a government agency.

OCULIST An OPHTHALMOLOGIST or an OPTOMETRIST. (Pronounced ok′yu·list.)

ODONTITIS Inflammation in the pulp cavity of a TOOTH. (Pronounced oh″don·tie′tis.) It may result from DENTAL CARIES (tooth decay) or injury.

ODONTOSCOPE A small mirror used by dentists to view the teeth. (Pronounced oh·don′to·skohp.)

ODYNOPHAGIA Pain in swallowing food. There may be a sensation of food sticking in the ESOPHAGUS (the tube leading from the throat to the stomach). Odynophagia (pronounced oh″din·o·fay′jee·a) may be due to temporary local irritation, or it may indicate a serious condition. A doctor should be consulted if the pain recurs or continues. See also SWALLOWING.

OINTMENT A medicine prepared in a fatty or oily base (as PETROLATUM or LANOLIN) and used to soothe, protect, or heal the skin.

OLFACTORY Having to do with the sense of smell. (Pronounced ol·fak′tor·ee.) See also NOSE.

OLIGURIA Urination that is abnormally scanty. (Pronounced ol″i·gyoor′ee·a.)

OMPHALITIS Inflammation of the navel and surrounding parts, especially in the first few days of life after the stump of the umbilical cord has dropped off. (Pronounced om″fa·lie′tis.)

ONCOLOGY The branch of medical study dealing with the origin, cause, and growth of TUMORS. (Pronounced on·kol′o·jee.)

ONYCHOLYSIS Loosening of a NAIL, usually a fingernail, at the top and sides. Onycholysis (pronounced on″i·kol′i·sis) is caused by excessive exposure of the hands to water containing strong detergents or other harsh compounds.

OPERATION See SURGERY.

OPHTHALMIA Any inflammation of the EYE or the membrane lining the eyelid. It is sometimes called ophthalmitis. Ophthalmia (pronounced of·thal′mee·a) results from such varied causes as a foreign body in the eye, overexposure to strong light, infections of various kinds, and GLAUCOMA. For some distinct forms of ophthalmia, see CONJUNCTIVITIS; IRITIS; and TRACHOMA.

OPHTHALMOLOGIST A physician who specializes in the diagnosis and treatment of eye diseases and abnormalities. The ophthalmologist (pronounced of"thal·mol′o·jist) examines the eyes and prescribes EYEGLASSES. Being a medical specialist, he is qualified to perform eye surgery and to diagnose disorders in other parts of the body that may be responsible for eye problems.

OPHTHALMOPLEGIA Paralysis or weakness of the muscles that control eye movements, caused by a disorder of the nerves from the brain. The ability of the pupil to dilate and contract may also be impaired.

Transient ophthalmoplegia (pronounced of·thal"-mo·plee′jee·a) is common after some childhood diseases such as measles. In adult life it may be an early sign of a disorder of the brain or nervous system, such as encephalitis, meningitis, multiple sclerosis, or a brain tumor.

Ophthalmoplegia affecting all the eye muscles occurs in MYASTHENIA GRAVIS and in some forms of thyroid disease. Treatment is directed at the disorder causing the ophthalmoplegia.

OPHTHALMOSCOPE An instrument used by doctors to examine the inside of the eye. (Pronounced of·thal′mo·skohp.)

OPIATE See NARCOTIC. (Pronounced oh′pee·it.)

OPTICIAN A person who makes eyeglasses to prescription.

OPTOMETRIST A professional person who is licensed to examine the eyes and prescribe lenses or exercises to improve vision. If an optometrist (pronounced op·tom′e·trist) detects eye disease, he refers the person to an OPHTHALMOLOGIST.

ORAL Pertaining to the MOUTH.

ORAL CONTRACEPTION A method of birth control in which OVULATION (the release of an egg cell from an ovary) is prevented by taking pills containing various SEX HORMONES. The pills in most common use contain some form of progesterone and ESTROGEN hormones. These must be taken on a regular schedule, usually for three weeks; for the fourth week either no pills are taken, or pills without hormones are prescribed. Menstruation then sets in, and the cycle is repeated monthly. If the schedule is followed exactly, without missing a single day, oral contraception is the most reliable of all contraceptive methods in use.

Oral contraceptives should not be taken except under the supervision of a doctor. Various minor side effects and a few serious ones have been observed in some women. Common side effects include nausea, headache, sore breasts, and a gain in weight due to fluid retention. A more serious side effect of pills containing estrogen has been seen in a very small number of women. This involves a disturbance in the mechanism of blood clotting. The "pill" is especially dangerous for women with DIABETES, liver disorders, PHLEBITIS, and certain other conditions.

Millions of women have used estrogen pills with complete satisfaction and no serious side effects since they were first introduced about 1960. Various modifications of the original pill have been developed and used in large-scale testing programs. Medical research is continuing to investigate whether long-term use of oral contraceptives is harmful. So far, it appears that, for most of a woman's childbearing years, the risks involved are less than those of pregnancy. See also CONTRACEPTIVE METHODS AND DEVICES.

ORCHIECTOMY (orchectomy) Surgical removal of one or both TESTICLES. (Pronounced awr"kee·ek′to·mee.)

ORCHIOPEXY (orchiorrhaphy) Surgical correction of a congenital abnormality in which one or both testicles remains in the abdominal cavity instead of descending into the scrotum. (Pronounced awr"kee·o·pek′see.)

ORCHITIS Inflammation of the TESTICLES. Most cases of orchitis (pronounced awr·kie′tis) occur as a complication of mumps but the inflammation may accompany syphilis or any acute infection. Orchitis may also be caused by injury.

ORGAN A distinct part of the body that performs one or more specific functions. The hand and the eye are examples of external organs. Important internal organs include the heart, the lungs, the stomach, the liver, and the kidneys.

ORGAN TRANSPLANT Replacement of a damaged organ with a sound one obtained from the body of another person.

The transplantation of organs is still a new science. A functioning eye cannot be transplanted because of the complex nerve connections required, but in cases of severe corneal damage, corneas may be transplanted from newly deceased persons to help restore sight. Kidneys have been transplanted successfully between identical twins or other close relatives, and even between unrelated persons. Other organs, notably hearts, have also been transplanted, enabling surgeons to extend life.

Rejection: In all cases, the possibility of rejection must be faced. Disease-resisting mechanisms go into action whenever any genetically foreign tissue—that is, tissue from any other person except an identical twin—is introduced into the body. The severity of the reaction can be lessened somewhat by matching donor and recipient beforehand—the technique is similar to the matching of blood types for a TRANSFUSION. Various medications are also used to bring the rejection process under control without depriving the body of its ability to resist disease.

ORGASM The climax of the sexual act. In the woman it can be produced by stimulation of the CLITORIS and may involve rhythmic contractions of the uterus. In the man it is brought on by stimulating the PENIS; the testicles and genital ducts contract, resulting in ejaculation of semen.

ORTHODONTICS The branch of dentistry concerned with the prevention and correction of irregularities in the position of the teeth. (Pronounced awr"tho·don'tiks.)

Many children have teeth with wide spaces between them or teeth that are crowded together. Premature loss of the first set of teeth, heredity, improper diet, disease, or, rarely, thumb-sucking may be responsible for a child's poorly aligned teeth. When the teeth in the upper and lower jaws do not meet properly, the condition is known as MALOCCLUSION.

To correct the irregular positioning of the teeth, they are very gradually moved to better positions by such appliances as metal *braces,* wires, or elastic bands. The appliances often have to be worn for a year or two. Orthodontic treatment is easiest if undertaken in childhood, when the bones are still growing. But many persons in middle life have had their teeth straightened successfully.

ORTHOPEDICS The branch of medicine that deals with the treatment of disorders of the bones, joints, spine, muscles, and other parts of the body used in movement. (Pronounced awr"tho·pee'diks.) Arthritis, backache, bursitis, slipped disk, dislocations and fractures, bone tumors, and bone grafts are some of the problems handled by the orthopedist or orthopedic surgeon.

ORTHOPNEA Shortness of breath (DYSPNEA) which is relieved when a person stands or sits erect. (Pronounced awr·thop'nee·a.)

ORTHOSTATIC Having to do with, or caused by, standing up. For example, orthostatic (pronounced awr"tho·stat'ik) hypotension—a momentary drop in blood pressure—occurs in some people when they stand up suddenly after a period of lying down.

ORTHOTONUS A severe muscle SPASM in which the neck, limbs, and body are held rigid in a straight line. (Pronounced or·thot'o·nus.)

OSCHEITIS Inflammation of the scrotum, the sac containing the testicles. (Pronounced os"kee·ie'tis.)

OSSICLE A tiny bone; specifically, any of the three very small bones of the middle EAR: the malleus (hammer), incus (anvil), and stapes (stirrup). (Pronounced os'i·kel.)

OSTEITIS Inflammation of bone. Osteitis (pronounced os"tee·ie'tis) is a symptom or complication in a number of diseases. See also BONE DISEASE.

OSTEOARTHRITIS See ARTHRITIS. (Pronounced os"tee·oh·ahr·thrie'tis.)

OSTEOARTHROSIS Pain and stiffness in the joints that differs from true ARTHRITIS in that there is no inflammation. However, osteoarthrosis (pronounced os"tee·oh·ahr·throh'sis) is often also called arthritis or osteoarthritis.

Osteoarthrosis usually appears in the middle years and in old age, but it can appear earlier. Overweight people often develop the condition in the joints of the knees and hips, which take the greatest strain in bearing weight. In some people the finger joints may be affected, either for no known reason or sometimes because of overuse in such activities as household chores, typing, or piano playing. The disease is believed to run in families and affects more women than men. It results from the "wear and tear" of cartilage and bone ends in the joints, and there tends to be an overgrowth of bone tissue.

Osteoarthrosis benefits from gently and continually exercising the joints, as long as they are not inflamed. The patient should keep his weight down. Aspirin and the application of heat usually help to relieve pain. Although uncomfortable, osteoarthrosis is not a progressive disease—it does not steadily worsen.

OSTEOCLASIA (osteoclasis) Destruction of bone, whether by surgery or by BONE DISEASE. (Pronounced os"tee·oh·klay'zhee·a.)

OSTEOMA A benign (noncancerous) TUMOR made up of bone tissue. Osteomas (pronounced os"tee·oh'maz) usually originate in the bones of the skull or the lower jaw.

OSTEOMALACIA An abnormal bone condition in adults, similar to RICKETS in children. The bones gradually soften owing to deficiency of calcium and phosphorus. In severe cases, the bones tend to become bowed. Osteomalacia (pronounced os"tee·oh·ma·lay'shee·a) may not be caused simply by a deficiency of calcium and vitamin D in the diet, but by some abnormality in the way the body utilizes these substances. In some cases, osteomalacia is associated with disorders of the pancreas or the kidneys.

Most forms of osteomalacia are curable if treated promptly, so it is important to see a doctor about any persistent ache in the bones.

OSTEOMYELITIS Infection of the bone marrow by pus-forming bacteria; also, any infection of bone. The bacteria usually come from a primary infection elsewhere in the body, such as a boil or pneumonia. Children are more often affected than adults. Any bone may be involved. An injury to a healthy bone may make it especially susceptible to infection. If untreated, the infection often results in disfigurement and disability due to bone destruction.

The onset of osteomyelitis (pronounced os"tee·oh·mie"*e*·lie'tis) is usually sudden, with high fever and severe pain in the area of the affected bone. Prompt medical attention is essential. Acute osteomyelitis is usually cured with antibiotics such as penicillin.

OSTEOPATHY (1) Any disease of bone.
(2) A system of treating disease mainly by massage and manipulation. The system of osteopathy (pronounced os"tee·op'*a*·thee) is based on a theory, developed in the 19th century by the American Andrew Taylor Still, that the chief obstacle to good health is faulty alignment of the bones, especially in the spine. Treatment of disease was directed to finding and correcting so-called structural derangements. Environment and diet were also taken into account, but surgery and the administration of medicines originally had no place in osteopathic treatment. Special schools were founded for the purpose of teaching osteopathic medicine. Some are still functioning but have modified both theory and practice. Accredited schools of osteopathy now have essentially the same courses of study as conventional medical schools, and their graduates take the same state licensing examinations.

OSTEOPOROSIS Loss of part of the protein framework (matrix) of the bones, leading to increased brittleness. It may be due to lack of use, as in a paralyzed limb or after severe burning, or be associated with a reduction in the amount of sex hormones in women after the menopause. In many cases, however, the cause is unknown. (Pronounced os"tee·oh·po·roh'sis.)

OTITIS Inflammation of any part of the EAR, external or internal. A serious form of otitis (pronounced oh·tie'tis) is otitis media, or MIDDLE EAR INFECTION.

OTOMYCOSIS A FUNGUS infection of the external ear and of the ear canal. Otomycosis (pronounced oh"toh·mie·koh'sis) sometimes results from swimming in fresh water containing fungus spores. It causes annoying itching. Treatment consists of applying fungus-killing ointments and antibiotic medicines prescribed by your doctor.

OTOSCOPE An instrument for examining the ear canal and eardrum. (Pronounced oh'*to*·skohp.)

OUTPATIENT DEPARTMENT A hospital department that offers treatment to patients not requiring in-hospital care. Through its outpatient department, or CLINIC, the hospital is able to provide medical services efficiently and economically to the community at large. Besides diagnosing and treating illnesses and dispensing medicines, outpatient departments also provide immunization and conduct health education programs.

OVARIAN CYST See CYST. (Pronounced oh·vair'ee·*a*n sist'.)

OVARIECTOMY The surgical removal of one or both ovaries. (Pronounced oh·vair"ee·ek'to·mee.) For further information, see HYSTERECTOMY.

OVARIOSTOMY A surgical operation to drain the fluid from a CYST of the OVARY. (Pronounced oh·vair"ee·os'to·mee.)

OVARITIS (oophoritis, oothecitis) Inflammation of one or both OVARIES. Ovaritis (pronounced oh·va·rie'tis) is usually a complication of MUMPS, but there may be other causes, such as GONORRHEA. Ovaritis produces considerable lower abdominal pain or low-back pain.

OVARY Either of the pair of female sex glands that produce egg cells (ova) and secrete SEX HORMONES. The ovaries (pronounced oh'*va*·reez) are oval-shaped glands, about one and a half inches long, located in the lower abdomen on either side of the

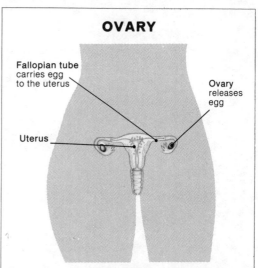

OVARY

Fallopian tube carries egg to the uterus

Ovary releases egg

Uterus

The ovaries are linked by the Fallopian tubes to the upper part of the uterus. Once a month, an ovary releases an egg, which passes along the Fallopian tube. Female sex hormones released by the ovaries bring about the changes of puberty in girls and control the menstrual cycle.

uterus. They contain thousands of tiny structures called Graafian follicles, where ova develop. From the time of puberty until MENSTRUATION ceases in middle age (see MENOPAUSE), the ovaries release one or more ova each month and secrete hormones in large amounts.

OVULATION The process by which a matured egg cell, or ovum, is released from an ovary. Ovulation (pronounced oh″vyu·lay′shun) occurs at the midpoint of the menstrual cycle. Usually only one ovum is released at a time, but occasionally there may be two or three. There is always a small rise in body temperature, and some women experience slight twinges of pain when ovulation occurs.

OVUM The medical name for EGG CELL. (Pronounced oh′vum.)

OXYGEN THERAPY The administration of oxygen to a sick person in greater concentration than exists in the ordinary atmosphere. The treatment is used to ease breathing and to raise the oxygen level of the blood.

Oxygen therapy is helpful in serious respiratory diseases, such as pneumonia and bronchitis. It eases the symptoms of congestive heart failure and coronary occlusion. (See CORONARY HEART DISEASE.) Anoxia (too little oxygen in the blood) resulting from shock, carbon monoxide poisoning, or other disorders is treated with oxygen. Occasionally, when a newborn infant fails to breathe immediately after birth, oxygen is given for a few minutes until normal respiration is established.

Oxygen is kept in a large metal cylinder under pressure. It may be administered through a mask fitted over the nose and mouth, or through a tube inserted into a nostril and passed into the throat. A transparent canopy (oxygen tent) covering the bed or the upper half of the bed is used for patients who find a mask or nasal tube irritating or who must be given oxygen for several days. Since pure oxygen represents an extreme fire hazard, any open flame, cigarette, or spark must be kept far away from the apparatus.

OXYTOCIC A drug used to hasten childbirth, usually by causing the muscles of the uterus to contract. The same drug may also be prescribed after delivery to help to shrink the uterus and lessen any bleeding. (Pronounced ok″si·toh′sik.)

OXYTOCIN A HORMONE produced by the PITUITARY GLAND. Oxytocin (pronounced ok″si·toh′sin) causes the uterus to contract during childbirth and stimulates the release of milk during lactation. Synthetic oxytocin or oxytocin obtained from animals is sometimes used to induce labor.

P

PACEMAKER See CARDIAC PACEMAKER.

PACHYCEPHALY Abnormal thickness of the skull. (Pronounced pak″i·sef′a·lee.)

PACHYDERMIA An abnormal thickening of tissue. Pachydermia (pronounced pak″i·dur′mee·a) may occur in the skin or the mucous membranes of the bladder or larynx.

PAGET'S DISEASE Either of two unrelated diseases: (1) A chronic bone disease, osteitis deformans, which is discussed under BONE DISEASE.

(2) An uncommon kind of breast cancer, characterized at first by itching and a rash resembling eczema in the region of the nipple. There may be ulceration in the nipple area. Unlike other cancers of the breast, the first signs of Paget's (pronounced paj′its) disease are plainly visible. Unfortunately, these first signs may be mistaken for a relatively harmless skin disease, and so precious time may be lost before the doctor is consulted.

PAIN Pain is a warning signal about possible injury or illness. The special nerve endings that send pain messages to the brain are distributed all over the surface of the body and the internal organs.

Some parts of the body have fewer pain receptors (nerve endings for pain) than others. Pain receptors are very plentiful on the cornea of the eye, for example, but they are absent from the surfaces of the brain. Further, different pain receptors respond to different kinds of stimuli. A prick on the finger can cause pain, but the intestine can be cut or torn without causing any sensation. Intense pain can arise in the intestine from other kinds of stimuli, such as spasms in its muscular wall.

People differ in their sensitivity to pain, much as they differ in keenness of sight and hearing. They also differ in their reaction to pain. One person might complain very loudly about a degree of pain that another would try to bear like a stoic. It is not wise to ignore pain until you have done something about its cause.

Pain may be extremely variable, ranging from slight to severe, dull to acute, spasmodic to constant. When pain originates on the surface of the body, it is easy to locate. But deep pain (that is, pain inside the body) is often deceptive because it may be felt in an area different from the place where the trouble is. With kidney disorders, localized pain is usually felt in the region of the kidneys. But pain originating in the heart in ANGINA PECTORIS may be felt in the arm. Inflammation of the GALLBLADDER may show itself by pain in the back. Such a pain is said to be referred. Both referred and localized deep pain, if severe, tend to spread beyond the area immediately affected.

Once pain has served its warning function, it is simply a nuisance to be got rid of, if possible. Some types of pain are relieved by the application of heat or cold. An ANALGESIC will also bring relief. However, for a persistent or intense pain, the treatment must be prescribed by a physician. Self-medication to kill the pain may only obscure a sign of serious illness. Methods of controlling pain in surgery are discussed under ANESTHESIA. See also ABDOMINAL PAIN; BACKACHE; EARACHE; TOOTHACHE.

PALATE The partition between the mouth and the nasal cavity that forms the roof of the mouth. The bony front part of the palate is called the hard palate, and the fleshy part toward the throat is the soft palate. During early development before birth, the right and left sides of the palate are separated by a gap that normally closes before the baby is born. The result of the two sides' failing to unite is discussed under CLEFT PALATE. (See illustration on following page.)

PALPATION An examination made by feeling with the hand. Doctors employ palpation (pronounced pal·pay′shun) as part of any thorough medical examination, since it may reveal conditions that are not readily diagnosed by other methods. Certain disorders produce changes in tissue or in the shape or the hardness or softness of an organ; by feeling or pressing various parts of the body, the physician is able to detect these changes and interpret them. Abnormalities of the PROSTATE, for example, are diagnosed by palpation of that organ by a finger inserted in the patient's rectum. Palpation of the BREAST is performed to make certain that the tissue is free of lumps.

PALPITATION Exceptionally rapid beating of a person's heart, which is perceptible to him. Palpitation (pronounced pal″pi·tay′shun) may be produced by emotional excitement, exertion, drinking too much coffee, or smoking to excess. It may also be a symptom of heart disease or of GOITER. See also CORONARY HEART DISEASE; TACHYCARDIA.

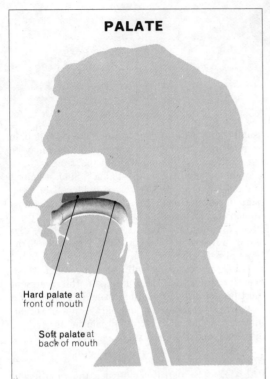

PALATE

Hard palate at front of mouth

Soft palate at back of mouth

The palate forms the roof of the mouth and separates it from the nasal cavity. It consists of the bony hard palate toward the front, and the fleshy soft palate at the back. The soft palate tapers backward to form the uvula, a small fleshy body, which hangs downward into the pharynx. An abnormally elongated uvula is called a falling palate.

PALSY A term applied to certain types of paralysis as well as to various disorders marked by constant trembling or quivering of some part or parts of the body. In palsy (pronounced pawl'zee), the ability to control the voluntary muscles is lost or impaired as a result of an injury or disorder of the brain, the spinal cord, or the nerves.

Cerebral Palsy: This may be due to abnormal conditions before birth, to birth injury, or other factors. The brain tissue is damaged and there is poor control of the muscles; there may be tremors, muscle spasms or weakness, and poor balance. Physical therapy and speech training are among the measures used to control the effects of cerebral palsy. See also separate entry, CEREBRAL PALSY.

Facial Palsy: A condition marked by paralysis of the muscles on one side of the face. Facial palsy is a type of NEURITIS. It may be caused by a draft, an infection, a tumor, or an injury. Palsy produced by the first two factors clears up in a matter of days or weeks, but more serious kinds require treatment of the underlying cause. The condition is also known as Bell's palsy.

Shaking Palsy: Palsy is one of the symptoms of parkinsonism. A brain disease, parkinsonism may be the result of hardening of the arteries, a stroke, an injury, certain infections, or other conditions. The face is immobile except for to-and-fro tremors of the head; there is trembling of the limbs, and rigidity of the muscles is pronounced. Massage, medication, and other treatments are prescribed. See also separate entry, PARKINSONISM.

Chorea: In this disorder the body jerks involuntarily. One special type is HUNTINGTON'S DISEASE, a serious hereditary condition in which the brain deteriorates. Another kind of chorea is Saint Vitus's dance. It is sometimes associated with RHEUMATIC FEVER in young children. The condition generally subsides in a few weeks. See also CHOREA.

Other Types: There are numerous other types of palsy. *Lead* palsy sometimes occurs among persons who work with lead; it is marked by paralysis of the wrist muscles. *Birth* palsy is caused by an injury suffered during a difficult delivery; in one type, *brachial* palsy, the arm may be paralyzed. A crutch pressing into the armpit may be responsible for *crutch* palsy, or paralysis of the arm.

PANCREAS A dual-purpose gland, about six inches long, lying across and behind the stomach. The pancreas produces a watery fluid called pancreatic juice, which helps to digest the proteins, fats, and carbohydrates in food. Pancreatic juice reaches the upper part of the small intestine through the pancreatic duct. In special areas, called ISLETS OF LANGERHANS, the pancreas produces INSULIN and glucagon, which are involved in the body's utilization of sugar. DIABETES results if the pancreas produces too little insulin. Too much insulin causes the condition known as HYPERINSULINISM.

PANCREATIN A whitish powder containing digestive enzymes obtained from the pancreas of the hog or ox. Pancreatin (pronounced pan'kree·*a*·tin) is used in treating digestive disorders associated with inability of a person's own pancreas to produce pancreatic enzymes.

PANCREATITIS Inflammation of the PANCREAS. (Pronounced pan''kree·*a*·tie'tis.) The cause is not known. ALCOHOLISM and GALLSTONES may be contributing factors. Attacks are sometimes brought on by excessive drinking or by eating a heavy meal. There is sudden, agonizing pain in the upper part of the abdomen, sometimes extending to the back. There may be nausea, abdominal tenderness, muscle spasm, and prostration. A doctor should be called at once so that emergency measures may be taken against the possiblity of shock. No fluid or solid food should be swallowed.

Repeated attacks may lead to chronic inflammation and permanent damage to the pancreas. Insulin may then be required, since the damaged pancreas cannot produce enough on its own. There is no specific treatment for pancreatitis. Alcohol and other factors known to aggravate the condition must be avoided. Your doctor may prescribe a special low-fat diet to help prevent recurrent attacks. Surgical operation on the pancreas is occasionally resorted to in severe, chronic cases.

PANDEMIC An EPIDEMIC affecting many countries at the same time. (Pronounced pan·dem′ik.)

PAPILLOMA A TUMOR resulting from the overgrowth of a papilla (a normal, nipple-shaped elevation) of the skin and mucous membranes. Papillomas include various types of WARTS and POLYPS. A papilloma (pronounced pap″i·loh′ma) may be caused by a virus, irritation by chemicals, or other, unknown factors. It is usually benign (noncancerous) and, when on the surface of the body, is easily removed.

PAP TEST A rapid and simple method of detecting some kinds of cancer before symptoms develop. This test is generally performed in a routine medical checkup on a woman because it detects the pres-

PANCREAS

Duodenum
in which
pancreatic
juice aids
digestion
of fats,
carbohydrates
and proteins

Pancreas
releases
digestive
juices to the
duodenum

Digestive juices produced by the pancreas flow into the duodenum, where they help to digest fats and carbohydrates in food. Within the pancreas, groups of cells called the islets of Langerhans secrete the hormone insulin, which controls the way the body uses sugars.

ence of cancer of the cervix (the mouth of the uterus). Cervical cancer is one of the commonest kinds of cancer in women. The chances of complete cure are very good—if the cancer is detected at an early stage.

To perform the test, the doctor scrapes a very small specimen of mucous tissue and secretion from the cervix. The specimen is then smeared on a small glass slide, preserved and stained by a special technique, and examined under the microscope. If cancer is present, some cells in the cervical smear will have a characteristic abnormal appearance.

"Pap" is short for George N. Papanicolaou, the name of the American physician who developed the test. A similar technique can also be used to detect MALIGNANT cells in secretions from the digestive and respiratory systems.

PAPULE Another word for PIMPLE.

PARALDEHYDE A liquid medicine with an unpleasant taste, used as a fast-acting SEDATIVE and HYPNOTIC in cases of DELIRIUM TREMENS and other disorders of the central nervous system. Paraldehyde (pronounced pa·ral′de·hied) is helpful in EPILEPSY when severe attacks occur in rapid succession, and it relieves the muscle spasms in TETANUS.

PARALYSIS Partial or complete loss of sensation or the power to move the muscles in some part or parts of the body. It is usually caused by disease or injury of some portion of the nervous system—the brain, the spinal cord, or the nerves. Sometimes a disorder of the muscles may be responsible.

Various types of paralysis may occur, depending on where and how extensive the damage is. When the whole body is paralyzed, a person is said to have general paralysis. If one entire side of the body is paralyzed, particularly by a stroke, the condition is known as hemiplegia. In paraplegia, the legs and the lower part of the body are paralyzed. Diplegia is paralysis of corresponding parts on both sides of the body. Paralysis may also be limited to the nerves or muscles in a small area of the body. See also PALSY.

Mechanical Injury: Although the backbone normally provides adequate protection for the spinal cord, it cannot withstand violent impact. Paralysis in victims of automobile accidents and casualties of war is commonly due to injury to the spinal cord.

Stroke: A paralytic stroke (APOPLEXY) may result from rupture of an artery in the brain or blocking of an artery by a BLOOD CLOT, or thrombus. This cuts off the blood supply to a portion of the brain, and the part of the body controlled by that portion is paralyzed. The ability to move an arm, a leg, or an entire side or more of the body may be lost. See also separate entry, STROKE.

Multiple Sclerosis: This disease may strike the nerves of the brain or spinal cord. Hard patches form on the nerve coverings, hampering the action of the nerves. Paralysis may come on suddenly or gradually in a leg or other part of the body. See also separate entry, MULTIPLE SCLEROSIS.

Tumors: The brain or spinal cord may be the site of tumors that sometimes bring on paralysis due to pressure on sensitive nerve tissue. Surgery to remove the tumor is usually suggested. X-ray treatment is helpful in slowing the growth of certain tumors. See also separate entry, TUMOR.

Infections of the Nervous System: POLIOMYELITIS (infantile paralysis) is an infection of the spinal cord. It may cause paralysis ranging from severe to slight. Fortunately, today this disease is on the wane, since vaccines have been developed to prevent it.

SYPHILIS is another infectious disease that may, in its advanced stage, attack the nervous system, resulting in paralysis as well as insanity.

PARANOIA A chronic mental disorder that is characterized by delusions of persecution. Different psychiatrists give slightly different meanings to the term. Usually, paranoia (pronounced par"*a*·noy'*a*) is considered to be a specific PSYCHOSIS. A person who has such a psychosis is called a paranoiac. The term "paranoid" may refer to any condition that resembles paranoia. For example, more or less systematic delusions of persecution are present in paranoid SCHIZOPHRENIA, and may also occur in less serious kinds of EMOTIONAL AND MENTAL DISORDERS. In popular usage, "paranoid" is often applied to someone judged to be unduly sensitive or suspicious.

Individuals suffering from severe paranoia must usually be admitted to a mental institution. TRANQUILIZERS and PSYCHOTHERAPY are among the methods of treatment.

PARAPLEGIA See PARALYSIS. (Pronounced par"*a*·plee'jee·*a*.)

PARASITE Any animal or plant that lives in or on another organism, the host, at whose expense the parasite obtains nourishment. Some of the parasites that afflict man, such as the LOUSE and the TAPEWORM, are large enough to be easily seen. Many parasites, however, are microscopic in size and do not resemble what we usually recognize as being either plants or animals. Parasites are responsible for a great variety of diseases in man, including malaria, amebic dysentery, scabies, hookworm disease, elephantiasis, trichinosis, and ringworm (not a worm but a fungus).

PARASITIC CYST See CYST.

PARASYMPATHETIC NERVOUS SYSTEM See NERVOUS SYSTEM; AUTONOMIC NERVOUS SYSTEM. (Pronounced par"*a*·sim"p*a*·thet'ik.)

PARATHYROID GLAND A small gland embedded in the thyroid gland or located near it. There are two pairs of parathyroid (pronounced par"*a*·thie'royd) glands. The hormones they secrete regulate the use in the body of calcium and phosphorus. See also ENDOCRINE GLAND.

PARATYPHOID FEVER An infectious disease, paratyphoid (pronounced par"*a*·tie'foyd) fever, like TYPHOID FEVER, is usually transmitted by contaminated water, food, or milk. The *Salmonella* bacterium is responsible for the disease; it is spread in the feces of infected persons and animals. The disease may be passed on by CARRIERS who show no obvious signs of the disorder.

The symptoms resemble those of typhoid fever. The INCUBATION PERIOD lasts from one to 10 days. A pink rash appears on the chest. The patient runs a fever, vomiting and diarrhea occur, and there is pain in the abdomen. Medicines such as CHLORAMPHENICOL and the TETRACYCLINES are used in treatment. Cramps and diarrhea are controlled with paregoric. Immunity may be obtained with paratyphoid vaccine.

PAREGORIC A medicine obtained from opium. Paregoric (pronounced par"*e*·gawr'ik) is useful in soothing cramps and spasms of the stomach and intestines and is helpful in cases of severe diarrhea. Taken in large and frequent doses, the medicine can be poisonous and habit-forming. See also NARCOTIC.

PARESIS Weakness or partial paralysis. A brain disease that occurs in an advanced stage of SYPHILIS is called paresis (pronounced p*a*·ree'sis) or, more correctly, general paresis.

Syphilis is relatively easy to cure with penicillin therapy if the disease is detected early enough. If it is not treated, it goes into a latent stage. Ten to 15 years later, lesions may develop in the brain or the spinal cord, causing either general paresis or LOCOMOTOR ATAXIA, or both.

The symptoms of general paresis come on quite gradually. There is a tendency to be overly lighthearted or even silly, and to have delusions of grandeur. The individual loses the ability to concentrate, and he has trouble remembering. He develops headaches; tremors of the fingers and lips occur. In time, as more and more brain tissue is damaged, the brain loses control of bodily functions and the person's condition worsens rapidly. It is possible to halt the progress of the disease with penicillin, but damaged brain tissue cannot be restored.

PARKINSONISM The medical term (pronounced pahrk'in·son·izm) for a chronic, slowly progressive disorder that affects the part of the brain that controls voluntary movement. The disorder is also known as Parkinson's disease, paralysis agitans, and shaking palsy.

Parkinsonism does not often set in before a person reaches his fifties or sixties. The onset is very gradual, usually beginning as a slight tremor in the hands when at rest and involuntary nodding of the head. The facial muscles react slowly, so that the expression tends to become masklike and the eyes fixed and unblinking. As the disease advances, muscular tremors may affect the whole body. There may be some speech impairment and involuntary rolling of the eyes. The gait becomes slow and shuffling. The afflicted person has a tendency to bend forward and to break into a run or trot in an attempt to maintain balance. Fatigue and emotional stress tend to make the symptoms worse.

There is no known single cause of parkinsonism. It may in some cases be an immediate or long-delayed sequel of ENCEPHALITIS. It may also result from CARBON-MONOXIDE POISONING, head injury, or HARDENING OF THE ARTERIES in the brain. In some cases (called idiopathic parkinsonism), no cause can be found. The symptoms are owing to a dysfunction of nerve cells in the basal ganglia, apparently related to the absence of the neurotransmitter, dopamine. The reduction of dopamine in the brain seems to be related to the aging process.

Treatment: In most cases, the symptoms are relieved by chemical substances which replace the insufficiency of dopamine in the basal ganglia: L-DOPA and anticholinergic drugs such as ARTANE and COGENTIN. Daily systematic exercise and massage of the muscles most severely affected are of value. It is advisable to have periodic consultations with a medical specialist (usually a neurologist) to discuss the treatment to be carried out by the family doctor over the many years the disease tends to last.

PARKINSON'S DISEASE See PARKINSONISM.

PARONYCHIA Inflammation of the skin and tissues around a toenail or fingernail, commonly called a whitlow, felon, or runaround. Paronychia (pronounced par″o·nik′ee·a) is usually caused by a STAPHYLOCOCCUS or a STREPTOCOCCUS, but it may be a complication of skin diseases such as PSORIASIS and FUNGUS infections. The skin around the NAIL becomes red and swollen. If not treated, the infection may spread to the tissues under the nail (nail bed), resulting in an abscess, a more serious condition.

PAROTITIS Another name for MUMPS. (Pronounced par″o·tie′tis.)

PAROXYSM A term used to mean (1) a spasm or convulsion; (2) an abrupt reappearance of symptoms; or (3) a sudden intensification of symptoms that are already present. (Pronounced par′ok·siz″em.)

PARROT FEVER See PSITTACOSIS.

PARTURITION The medical term for CHILDBIRTH. (Pronounced pahr″tyoor·ish′un.)

PAS Short for the synthetic compound para-aminosalicylic acid. PAS (pronounce each letter) is used in pill form in the treatment of certain types of TUBERCULOSIS, usually in combination with other medicines, such as isoniazid and streptomycin. PAS alone is not as effective against the tubercle bacillus as these other medicines, but it enhances their effect. It sometimes produces side effects such as loss of appetite, nausea, and diarrhea.

PASTEURIZATION A method of destroying disease-producing bacteria and delaying spoilage in milk, wine, fruit juices, and other beverages without appreciably changing their flavor. The method was devised by Louis Pasteur (1822–95), the founder of modern bacteriology. It consists of heating the liquid for about 30 minutes at a temperature about midway between normal body temperature and the temperature of boiling water, and then cooling it immediately. Pasteurizing milk destroys the bacteria that cause bovine TUBERCULOSIS and BRUCELLOSIS (undulant fever), two of several diseases that people can contract from infected cattle.

PASTEUR TREATMENT A method of preventing RABIES from developing in a person who has been bitten by a rabid animal. Daily injections of rabies virus, obtained from infected rabbits and then weakened, are given in gradually stronger doses over a period of about two weeks.

PATCH TEST A method of detecting abnormal sensitivity to a given substance. A small patch of linen or blotting paper is impregnated with the substance in question and applied to the skin. If the skin is inflamed when the patch is removed, it indicates an ALLERGY, or sensitivity, to the substance. A patch test may also be used to diagnose tuberculosis.

PATHOGEN The scientific name for any microorganism or substance that causes disease. (Pronounced path′o·jen.)

PATHOLOGICAL Caused by or related to disease. (Pronounced path″o·loj′i·kal.)

PATHOLOGIST A specialist in PATHOLOGY. A pathologist (pronounced pa·thol′o·jist) is a physician who seldom sees patients, but works in a laboratory, either private or belonging to a hospital. Among the pathologist's tools and techniques are the microscope and chemical analysis. The pathologist examines samples of blood, urine, feces, and minute sections of tissue obtained by surgery or BIOPSY; the latter is especially important in the diagnosis of CANCER.

When he acts as a public official, the pathologist is known as a medical examiner, or, in some areas, as a coroner. He performs postmortem (that is, after-death) examinations, or autopsies, to determine the cause of death.

PATHOLOGY   The branch of medicine that studies the changes causing or caused by disease in the structure and function of the body tissues.

PEDIATRICS   The branch of medicine concerned with the care of children and the treatment and prevention of the diseases of childhood. The specialist in pediatrics (pronounced pee"dee·at'riks) is known as a pediatrician (the term simply means "baby doctor"). The pediatrician is concerned not only with illness and its prevention but with every aspect of the child's growth and development from birth to the early teens.

PEDICULOSIS   The condition of being infested with lice anywhere on the body. (Pronounced pe·dik"yu·loh'sis.) See also LOUSE.

PELLAGRA   A VITAMIN deficiency disease caused by a serious lack of NIACIN (nicotinic acid), a member of the vitamin B complex. Although on the decline in North America, pellagra (pronounced pe·lay'gra) still occurs in areas where corn and corn products form the major part of the diet. Pellagra can also afflict alcoholics and drug addicts, who often suffer from MALNUTRITION.
Symptoms: Pellagra affects the skin, the mucous membranes, the gastrointestinal tract, and the nervous system. Parts of the skin that are exposed to sunlight or irritated by clothing may break out in blisters and become red and thickened. The mucous membranes of the mouth are red and tender, and the tongue may become red and swollen. Around the outside of the mouth, there are sores and cracks in the skin. Loss of appetite, nausea, vomiting, and diarrhea are the principal gastrointestinal symptoms. Emotional symptoms include sleeplessness (INSOMNIA), anxiety, depression, and irritability.
Treatment: The most important treatment is providing a well-rounded diet. Vegetables, whole-grain cereals, eggs, meat (especially liver), and peanuts are excellent sources of niacin. In addition, the doctor may prescribe tablets containing niacin and other vitamins.

PELVIS   The bony structure that connects the legs with the spine. It consists of the hip bones on each side and the sacrum and coccyx, or tailbone, behind. In front of the pelvis is the pubis, which has a normally immovable joint at the front called a symphysis. In women at the end of pregnancy, the pubic symphysis softens and stretches, widening the pelvis for the passage of the baby through the birth canal in CHILDBIRTH.

There are openings in the pelvis for the urinary and genital organs. The bladder and rectum lie inside the pelvis, which in men also houses the seminal vesicles and the prostate gland. In women, the pelvis contains the ovaries and the uterus.

PELVIS

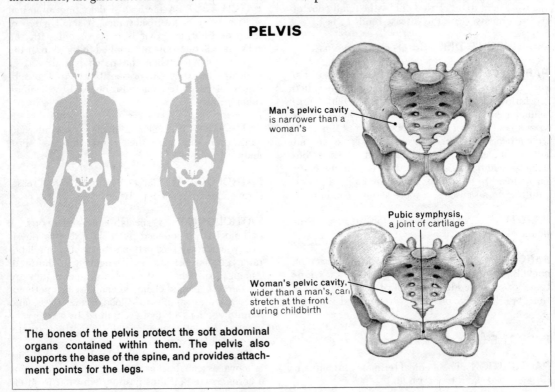

Man's pelvic cavity is narrower than a woman's

Pubic symphysis, a joint of cartilage

Woman's pelvic cavity, wider than a man's, can stretch at the front during childbirth

The bones of the pelvis protect the soft abdominal organs contained within them. The pelvis also supports the base of the spine, and provides attachment points for the legs.

PEMPHIGUS A rare but serious disease characterized by spreading clusters of large watery blisters (bullae) on the skin and on mucous membranes, especially those in the mouth. The cause of pemphigus (pronounced pem'fi·gus) is not known. Treatment involves rest, proper diet, the use of STEROID hormones, and ANTIBIOTICS to combat infection of the blisters.

PENICILLIN An ANTIBIOTIC obtained from greenish molds of the genus *Penicillium*. It interferes with the growth of the STAPHYLOCOCCUS and STREPTOCOCCUS bacteria and of those that cause pneumonia, meningitis, gonorrhea, and syphilis. It has no effect on viruses.

Penicillin is often given in very large doses, usually by INJECTION. It produces almost no ill effects except upon a few people who are allergic to it (see ALLERGY), in which case it can cause HIVES or a rash, and occasionally anaphylactic SHOCK.

PENIS The external male organ of sexual intercourse and urination. It consists of three elongated masses of spongy tissue covered with loosely fitting skin. A common duct for urine and semen, the urethra, runs through the length of the penis. At the end, a cone-shaped body, the glans penis, is partially covered by a fold of skin called the foreskin, or prepuce. Under the influence of sexual stimulation, an involuntary reflex causes blood to flow into the spongy tissue, with the result that the penis becomes swollen and erect. See also CIRCUMCISION; ERECTION.

PENTOTHAL A trade name for thiopental sodium, a type of BARBITURATE used as an ANESTHETIC before surgery. It is injected into a vein and produces unconsciousness pleasantly in less than half a minute. Because Pentothal (pronounced pen'to·thawl) keeps the patient unconscious for only a short time, it is followed up with longer-acting anesthetics in most surgical operations.

PEP PILL See AMPHETAMINE.

PEPTIC ULCER See ULCER.

PERCUSSION Tapping the body with quick, sharp blows of the fingers to cause certain sounds and vibrations of the internal organs, especially the HEART and the LUNGS. For example, if the doctor wants to find the size and exact location of the heart, he will tap the chest over the lungs in the region of the heart. Since the lungs are made up of hollow air sacs, they are resonant, but the heart is not. Therefore the sound will change in pitch when the area over the heart is tapped. In the same way, when the doctor taps the area over the lungs, any unusual sounds may indicate a need for further examination by X ray or other methods. Percussion

is a customary procedure in any general medical examination.

PERIODONTITIS (parodontitis) See PYORRHEA. (Pronounced per"ee·oh·don·tie'tis.)

PERIPHERAL NERVOUS SYSTEM The part of the NERVOUS SYSTEM that connects all the various parts of the body with the spinal cord and brain.

PERISTALSIS The slow, wavelike motion of various tubular organs and ducts in the body, such as the esophagus, the intestines, the Fallopian tubes, and the bile duct. The motion of peristalsis (pronounced per"i·stawl'sis) forces the contents of the tube to move forward. It is caused by involuntary contractions of the smooth MUSCLE that forms part of the walls of these organs. Peristalsis is controlled by the autonomic part of the NERVOUS SYSTEM.

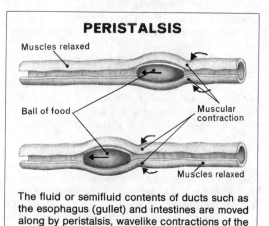

PERISTALSIS

Muscles relaxed

Ball of food

Muscular contraction

Muscles relaxed

The fluid or semifluid contents of ducts such as the esophagus (gullet) and intestines are moved along by peristalsis, wavelike contractions of the muscles in the walls of the ducts.

PERITONITIS Inflammation of the peritoneum, the membrane that forms the lining of the abdominal cavity and covers the intestine, the stomach, and other organs in the abdomen. Peritonitis (pronounced per"i·to·nie'tis) is a serious complication that can occur in many acute disorders of the abdomen. It can result from infection or from irritation by substances not normally in contact with the peritoneum, such as bile or other digestive juices. A ruptured appendix is a common cause of peritonitis, as are ulcers that have perforated any part of the stomach or the intestines. The condition may also result from infection of the uterus or Fallopian tubes following childbirth.

The symptoms include severe abdominal pain, fever, nausea, and vomiting—symptoms that should be reported to your doctor immediately. The abdominal muscles become rigid and normal PERISTALSIS is interrupted. Nothing whatever should be swallowed, since nothing will pass through the digestive tract in the absence of peristalsis. Peritonitis is a very serious condition requiring skilled hospital care. Both antibiotics and surgery are usually required to control the infection and remove its source.

PERITONSILLAR ABSCESS A severe inflammation of the throat; also called QUINSY. (Pronounced per"i·ton'sil·ar ab'ses.)

PERLÈCHE A children's disease manifested by an inflammation of the corners of the mouth. Blisters or white patches may form. Eventually the tissue in the corners become thickened, and painful cracks occur. Perlèche (pronounced per·lesh') may be caused by a deficiency of riboflavin (vitamin B₂) in the diet or infection by a fungus. The condition is treated by administering riboflavin.

PERNICIOUS Causing extreme harm or likely to result in death. Pernicious (pronounced per·nish'us) anemia, for example, is a type of ANEMIA that can have serious consequences if not properly treated.

PERSONALITY TEST Any test planned to reveal behavioral characteristics and emotional makeup. Such tests are widely used in industry, educational institutions, and mental health clinics. They must be administered and the results evaluated by professionally trained persons if they are to have any validity.

The Rorschach Test (also called the Inkblot Test) is one of the oldest personality tests. The individual is shown 10 standard cards with inkblots of varying shapes and asked to say what they suggest to him. This is a projective test—the person projects his own feelings onto the blots in interpreting them. The answers provide a clue to the person's emotional makeup, his intellectual development, and his approach to life in general.

The Minnesota Multiphasic Personality Inventory comprises hundreds of statements about feelings and attitudes an individual might have, and the subject indicates his reaction to each statement by marking it "true" or "false." His answers are then compared with those of known personality types, such as aggressive, impulsive, nervous, or depressed.

Personality tests have limitations. At best, the tests give no more than a partial insight into the character and emotional difficulties of the person taking them. However, in many instances they are helpful diagnostic tools.

PERSPIRATION The moisture secreted by the sweat glands of the skin; also, the process of sweating. Perspiration is over 99 percent water. Cooling occurs when this water evaporates. Perspiration is the mechanism by which the body temperature is kept from rising above the normal level.

Body temperature is controlled by the HYPO-THALAMUS in the brain and the sympathetic NERV-OUS SYSTEM. The amount of sweat produced does not depend wholly on body temperature, however. Some perspiring goes on constantly, even when the body is cool and the skin is dry. In some areas of the body—for example, the palms of the hands and the soles of the feet—sweating is increased by exercise, anxiety, or mental stress.

Perspiration contains very small amounts of salts, urea, and other substances. During hot weather, or under any conditions that cause much sweating, it is usually advisable to increase the intake of common salt to make up for salt lost in perspiration.

Fresh perspiration is practically odorless. Body odor (BROMIDROSIS) is due to bacteria that grow readily on the skin when it is warm and moist. See also DEODORANT.

Some persons tend to perspire to excess. This may lead to scaling of the skin, dermatitis, or other disorders. In some cases there may be an emotional cause; in others, the condition may be hereditary. Excessive perspiration is a symptom in diabetes, anemia, and hyperthyroidism.

PERTHES' DISEASE Degeneration of the upper growing end of the thighbone. It occurs most commonly in boys of about four years old, who develop pain in the knee and a limp. Treatment involves rest in bed, possibly followed by use of a splint to take the weight off the affected leg. The disease is named after the German surgeon Georg Perthes (1869–1927). (Pronounced per'teez.)

PERVERSION Broadly, any departure from what is regarded as morally right or socially acceptable. As often used, the term "perversion" refers to sexual gratification obtained in other ways than by COITUS. The various kinds of sexual perversion include HOMOSEXUALITY, EXHIBITIONISM, VOYEURISM, TRANSVESTISM, SADISM, and MASOCHISM. Many sexual perversions are punishable by law. However, many psychiatrists believe that perversion is an emotional illness and should be treated as such.

PESSARY Any device worn inside the VAGINA. A number of different forms of pessary (pronounced pes'a·ree) are made for various purposes. Some are designed to correct PROLAPSE of the uterus or to support the rectum. Another form of pessary is the DIAPHRAGM used as a contraceptive device. The term "pessary" is sometimes used for a vaginal SUPPOSITORY.

PETROLATUM A greasy, semisolid substance obtained from petroleum. Petrolatum (pronounced pet"ro·lay'tum) is used as a base for Vaseline and other OINTMENTS used to treat minor burns and skin irritations.

PHACOMALACIA Abnormal softening and whiteness of the lens of the EYE. Phacomalacia (pronounced fak"oh·ma·lay'shee·a) is also called soft CATARACT.

PHAGOCYTE Any cell that is able to engulf other cells, such as bacteria. Two of the various kinds of LEUKOCYTES, or white blood cells, are types of phagocytes (pronounced fag'oh·sietz). They digest what they engulf, defending the body against infection by "mopping up" germs and clearing the bloodstream of the remains of the cells that are constantly dying as part of the normal wear and tear that takes place in the body.

PHALANX (plural, **phalanges**) Any of the bones in the fingers and toes. (Pronounced fay'langks.) See also FOOT.

PHALLITIS Inflammation of the PENIS. (Pronounced fal·ie'tis.)

PHARMACIST A person trained in compounding medicines and filling prescriptions. A pharmacist must obtain a degree in pharmacy at a college of pharmacy (generally affiliated with a medical school) and then pass an examination and be licensed by the state where he plans to work. Professional pharmacists are employed in hospitals as well as in retail outlets for medicines.

The retail pharmacist (often called a druggist) compounds and dispenses medications. He is required to follow the physician's PRESCRIPTION with scrupulous accuracy and to keep it on file. On the container he places a label that includes the date, the name of the medicine, the number of the prescription, the person's name, the doctor's name, and instructions for the use of the medicine. He is not permitted to diagnose disease.

PHARMACOLOGY The study of medicines and other substances and the effects they produce on the living body. It includes a group of closely related sciences. One of these is therapeutics, the study of how drugs and medicines are used to cure disease. Toxicology is the study of poisons and their antidotes. Materia medica is concerned with the sources, composition, properties, and preparation of substances used in medicines.

PHARMACY The art of preparing, compounding, and dispensing drugs and medicines for use in the treatment of illness. The term is also used for the premises, whether in a hospital or a retail outlet, or drugstore, where this work is done. The practitioner of pharmacy is known as a PHARMACIST.

The preparation and marketing of drugs and medicines are supervised by agencies of the states and the Federal Government. The *United States Pharmacopeia* (see USP) and the *National Formulary* give standards for medicines and average or safe doses. The American Medical Association reviews new medications and available preparations in its annual publication, *AMA Drug Evaluation* (formerly titled *New Drugs*).

PHARYNGECTOMY Surgical removal of part of the PHARYNX. The operation usually involves some PLASTIC SURGERY to reconstruct the throat and special training afterward to relearn how to swallow. Pharyngectomy (pronounced far"in·jek'to·mee) is used mainly to treat cancer of the pharynx.

PHARYNGITIS Inflammation and soreness in the PHARYNX. Acute pharyngitis (pronounced far"in·jie'tis) is usually due to infection.

Chronic pharyngitis may follow repeated acute attacks, or it may be connected with prolonged irritation of the throat by smoke, dust, or other irritants. See also SORE THROAT; TONSILLITIS.

PHARYNX The tract between the mouth and the esophagus, serving as a passage for both food and air. The narrow entrance to the pharynx (pronounced far'ingks), called the fauces, can be seen if you look at the inside of your mouth in a mirror.

Above and extending forward from the pharynx lies the nasopharynx, which connects with the nos-

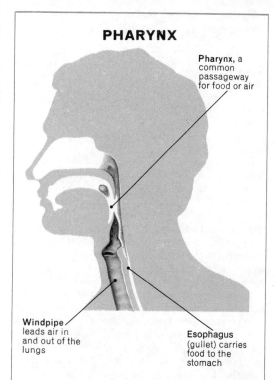

PHARYNX

Pharynx, a common passageway for food or air

Windpipe leads air in and out of the lungs

Esophagus (gullet) carries food to the stomach

The pharynx extends from the back of the throat to the top of the esophagus (gullet). Inflammation of the pharynx, or pharyngitis, is a common cause of a sore throat. It may be caused by an infection, or by irritation.

trils and the Eustachian tubes of the ears. The pharynx extends downward past the opening to the larynx and windpipe and then merges with the esophagus. The overall length of the pharynx is about 4½ inches. See also THROAT.

PHENACETIN (acetophenetidin) A medicine used to lower the temperature in fever and provide relief from pain. It is combined with aspirin and caffeine in proprietary medicines such as Empirin and APC tablets. Habitual use of phenacetin (pronounced fe·nas′e·tin) may damage the kidneys.

PHENOBARBITAL A BARBITURATE sometimes prescribed as a mild sedative to relieve nervous tension, anxiety, and insomnia. Phenobarbital (pronounced fee″noh·bahr′bi·tal) is considered to be one of the safest ANTICONVULSANTS for controlling seizures in EPILEPSY, and it is often combined with other medicines, such as DILANTIN, for this purpose. Like all barbiturates, phenobarbital can be addicting and can be obtained only with a prescription from a doctor.

PHENOLPHTHALEIN A colorless substance that turns red in alkali. Used as a CATHARTIC, it has a harsh effect. In milder dosages, phenolphthalein (pronounced fee″nohl·thal′een) is the active ingredient in many candy and chewing gum LAXATIVES.

PHENYLKETONURIA An inherited abnormality in the metabolism of the AMINO ACID phenylalanine, which is a constituent of protein food. The abnormality is a RECESSIVE trait—it does not show up unless a defective gene has been inherited from both parents.

A baby with phenylketonuria (pronounced fen″el·keet″en·yoor′ee·a) appears quite normal at birth. However, toxic products from the abnormal metabolism of phenylalanine soon accumulate in the baby's blood and urine. These toxic substances cause harm to the nervous system, especially the brain. They can be prevented from forming by giving the infant a special diet containing proteins from which most of the phenylalanine has been removed. If this diet is not followed in infancy, severe mental retardation results. At a later stage, the special diet can be discontinued without ill effects. A very simple laboratory test of a baby's blood or urine shows whether or not phenylketonuria is present. Most hospitals test every baby, and in some places, testing is required by law.

Persons with phenylketonuria are usually fair-haired and blue-eyed, since the condition also affects the production of the pigment MELANIN.

PHLEBITIS Inflammation of a vein. Phlebitis (pronounced fli·bie′tis) is often associated with THROMBOSIS, or the presence of a blood clot in the vein. It is particularly common in the legs and may

occur in persons who are overweight, who have circulatory problems such as VARICOSE VEINS, or who have suffered injury to the veins. Sometimes phlebitis follows surgery. In some cases the cause cannot be found.

In phlebitis, the area around the vein becomes red and painful. In severe cases, there may be fever and danger of GANGRENE. ANTIBIOTICS, anticoagulants, and bed rest may be prescribed. In mild cases, the condition may correct itself in a short while.

PHLEGMASIA A form of phlebitis involving inflammation and swelling of small veins in the leg, which some women suffer from after having a baby. The leg becomes swollen and very painful. A doctor should be consulted immediately because phlegmasia (pronounced fleg·may′see·a) poses a danger that a blood clot may form, break away, and move to another part of the body. See also PHLEBITIS; EMBOLISM; THROMBOSIS.

PHOBIA An extreme fear, particularly one so overpowering that the individual cannot function in a normal way. He may be unable to account for his fear, and it may appear to be completely without basis. Phobias (pronounced foh′bee·az) may be related to repressed aggressive impulses, or may symbolize fear of something else in the person's unconscious life.

Fear normally helps us to avoid real danger. A phobia, however, is distinctly abnormal and may be a symptom of PSYCHONEUROSIS or PSYCHOSIS. A person seriously troubled by an unreasonable fear should discuss it at length with his family physician or a psychiatrist.

There are a vast number of phobias: *acrophobia* is an abnormal fear of high places; *agoraphobia*, of open areas; *ailurophobia*, of cats; *algophobia*, of pain; *bacteriophobia*, of germs; *cardiophobia*, of heart disease; *claustrophobia*, of being in closed places; *cynophobia*, of dogs; *hemophobia*, of blood.

PHOTOPHOBIA A condition in which light is avoided because it produces pain in the eyes. (Pronounced foh″to·foh′bee·a.)

pH TEST See BLOOD TEST.

PHTHISIS Any gradual wasting away of tissues. The term "phthisis" (pronounced thie′sis) was formerly used especially to refer to TUBERCULOSIS of the lungs.

PHYSIC Another word for LAXATIVE or CATHARTIC; also, an old-fashioned name for any medicine given internally.

PHYSICAL EXERCISE Most Americans, especially after the age of 30, do not get enough exercise. We rely too much on machines to move us from place to place and do our work for us. Many of us work at jobs that involve little physical effort.

Muscular activity is essential to health. People confined to bed or astronauts in a space capsule rapidly deteriorate unless they are given some exercise. The muscles waste away, the circulation becomes sluggish, the kidneys cease to function well, and the bones lose calcium. Few of us, of course, suffer to such an extreme degree from lack of exercise. But our flabbiness, overweight, and lack of vitality are often due to insufficient exercise.

A moderate amount of exercise benefits everyone, young and old. Competitive sports are fine in youth, but sports that can be engaged in alone or with one or two companions may be enjoyed all through life. Bicycling, swimming, hiking, and JOGGING afford exercise that is healthful and enjoyable at any age. A daily program of simple calisthenics also helps to keep the entire body in good shape.

Before starting a program of exercise and weight reduction, let your physician advise you how much and what types of activity to undertake. The YMCA or YWCA can assist you in developing a suitable program for yourself; usually, too, they have excellent facilities for exercising singly or in groups.

PHYSICAL THERAPY The treatment of an injury, disability, or physical defect by massage, heat, exercise, and other external means. It is also called physiotherapy. Persons confined to bed or a wheelchair for long periods need physical therapy to prevent the ill effects of lack of PHYSICAL EXERCISE.

Exercise of the affected parts is one type of physical therapy. It is often combined with MASSAGE. Both may be started while the person is still in bed, as with poliomyelitis and strokes. The muscles and joints are first moved by the therapist (passive exercise) to prevent or lessen paralysis and stiffness of the joints. Later, the person is encouraged to participate (active exercise). He may be given hydrotherapy, which involves exercising in a special tub or swimming pool, where the buoyancy of the water lessens the work the muscles must do.

Heat treatments are especially useful in lessening pain and stiffness in arthritis. The method of heat application may be warm packs, soaking the affected parts in warm water, applying warm melted paraffin, or diathermy (infrared rays). In the KENNY METHOD, warm packs are used in the acute stage of poliomyelitis to help ward off paralysis.

Physical therapy is usually given in a hospital setting by a specially trained person, called a physiotherapist. The physiotherapist is often supervised by a physiatrist, a doctor who is a specialist in physical medicine and rehabilitation. Other persons, or the patient himself, may be taught to perform special exercises and treatments at home.

PHYSIOTHERAPY Another name for PHYSICAL THERAPY.

PICA A craving for eating things other than food—such as coal, dirt, and plaster—found mainly in infants, young children, and pregnant women. When the unnatural "food" is paint chippings or putty, there is a risk of LEAD POISONING (plumbism). Pica (pronounced pie′ka) gets its name from the Latin for magpie, a bird that collects, and was thought to eat, unusual objects. Pica is thought to be a sign of iron deficiency, and can be treated with drugs containing iron.

PIGEON BREAST A deformity of the chest (also called chicken breast) in which the sternum, or breastbone, is abnormally prominent. It may be CONGENITAL, or it may be due to calcium or vitamin D deficiency during infancy and childhood. See also RICKETS.

In severe instances of this deformity an operation is sometimes recommended. If the chest protrudes only slightly and the condition creates no physical problems, it is best to disregard it.

PIGEON TOES A condition in which the feet turn inward. It results from weakness of certain muscles of the legs or the bone structure of the arches. The tendency usually appears in early childhood and often is a source of serious concern to parents. The child's feet should be examined by the family physician. If the problem is so severe as to impede walking, the doctor may refer the case to an orthopedist (specialist in bone disorders). Fortunately in most cases the condition corrects itself with time.

PIGMENT Any of numerous highly colored substances manufactured by animals and plants. Pigments have very important functions. The red HEMOGLOBIN in the blood carries oxygen from the lungs to all parts of the body. The dark-colored MELANIN in the skin and the iris of the eye affords protection from harmful exposure to the sun's rays. The retina of the eye contains visual purple and other pigments that change color in the light and are essential to vision. Bilirubin and other pigments in BILE are produced by the liver. Their function is not well understood. Traces are normally present in the blood, and they give the characteristic yellow color to urine and to the skin and eyeballs in jaundice. See also CAROTENE; CHLOROPHYLL.

PILES See HEMORRHOID.

"PILL," The See ORAL CONTRACEPTION; CONTRACEPTIVE METHODS AND DEVICES.

PILLS Any medicines in small, solid form, easily swallowed whole by most people.

Pills contain a measured amount of medicine, usually mixed with some neutral material that holds the mass together. Pills are often coated with a substance that prevents them from dissolving in the mouth, so that the person taking the pill is spared the bitter or unpleasant taste that many medicines have. In the so-called time-release capsules, small pellets of medicine are coated with a variety of substances that dissolve at different rates, so that the medicine is released gradually into the system.

PIMPLE   A small, inflamed lump on the skin, containing pus. It is caused by infection of a pore that has been clogged with fatty matter secreted by the sebaceous glands of the skin. Pimples are common in adolescence. When they occur in large numbers on the face, back, and chest, they are usually referred to as ACNE. Although the temptation is great, you should not squeeze a pimple. That can spread the infection and even cause a permanent scar. Cover it with a Band-Aid and let it drain naturally.

PINEAL GLAND   See ENDOCRINE GLAND. (Pronounced pin'ee·al.)

PINKEYE   See CONJUNCTIVITIS.

PINS AND NEEDLES   A term for the uncomfortable sensation caused by the irritation of a nerve. A common cause is the buildup of pressure on a nerve, resulting from a limb being in an awkward position or having its circulation temporarily restricted. If pins and needles become frequent, it may be a sign of a nervous disorder and a doctor should be consulted.

PINWORM INFECTION   A condition caused by a small, parasitic worm, about a quarter of an inch long, that infests the large intestine. The infection is especially common among children, but also affects adults. Pinworms (sometimes called seatworms) come out into the anal region at night to lay their eggs. Intense itching around the rectum is the principal symptom of their presence; there is sometimes mild abdominal pain, nausea, and diarrhea.

The victim's sleep may be disturbed by the itching. Since he tends to scratch the area, the eggs are apt to lodge under the fingernails and cling to the hands. Unless the hands are thoroughly scrubbed, the eggs will stick to anything the infected person touches. They will be passed on to other people through the air and inhaled, or swallowed in food and drink, or acquired from bed linens. The eggs are not affected by household disinfectants or by drying. They can remain alive in dust for long periods.

Treatment: Do not attempt to treat pinworm infection yourself with a "worm medicine." The doctor will diagnose the condition by examining the stool for adult worms or by finding eggs on the anal region. He will prescribe a medicine to kill the worms. In order to prevent reinfection or infection of others, the towels, bedclothes, pajamas, and underwear of the infected person should be boiled for 20 minutes or so at least twice a week. The toilet

seat should be scrubbed with soap and water every day. Try to keep the child from scratching and putting his fingers in his mouth. Often doctors recommend that all the children in a family be treated at the same time.

PITUITARY GLAND   A very important ENDOCRINE GLAND in the body; also called the hypophysis. The pituitary (pronounced pi·too'i·ter"ee) is a tiny mass of tissue attached by a thin stalk to the HYPOTHALAMUS at the base of the brain.

The gland consists of two distinct lobes. The frontal lobe produces at least six important hormones: (1) a growth-stimulating hormone; (2) ACTH, which stimulates the adrenal gland; (3) a THYROID-stimulating hormone; (4) gonadotrophic hormones, which stimulate the production of sex hormones in the ovaries and testicles; (5) a hormone that stimulates the production of milk in nursing mothers; and (6) a hormone that stimulates production of the pigment MELANIN.

The posterior lobe receives and stores a number of different hormones that play important parts in various vital processes. These hormones are pro-

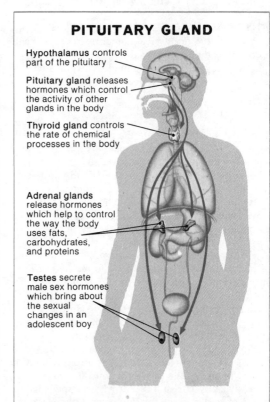

PITUITARY GLAND

Hypothalamus controls part of the pituitary

Pituitary gland releases hormones which control the activity of other glands in the body

Thyroid gland controls the rate of chemical processes in the body

Adrenal glands release hormones which help to control the way the body uses fats, carbohydrates, and proteins

Testes secrete male sex hormones which bring about the sexual changes in an adolescent boy

The pituitary gland at the base of the brain produces two chief types of hormones: those which act directly on parts of the body and those which act indirectly by stimulating other endocrine glands to secrete hormones.

duced by the hypothalamus, and one, OXYTOCIN, induces contractions of the uterus in childbirth. Another, VASOPRESSIN, acts on the kidneys and regulates the balance between water and salts in body fluids; it also makes blood vessels contract and hence raises blood pressure.

PITUITRIN A trade name for a substance containing the hormones OXYTOCIN and VASOPRESSIN obtained from the posterior pituitary glands of animals. Alternative synthetic drugs are also available. Pituitrin (pronounced pi·too′i·trin), administered by injection under the skin, is used to hasten childbirth and in the treatment of DIABETES insipidus.

PITYRIASIS ROSEA An inflammatory skin disease of unknown cause, characterized by scaly, pinkish eruptions, mostly on the trunk of the body. Pityriasis rosea (pronounced pit″i·rie′a·sis roh·zee′a) occurs more commonly in the spring and fall and is seen most often in young adults. One to two weeks before the onset of the disease, a single patch, called a herald patch, appears. There is no specific treatment for pityriasis rosea except lotions to ease the itching and medicines to combat any secondary infection. The disease is self-limiting—it runs its course in about six weeks, and then disappears.

PLACEBO A preparation containing nothing that can either help or harm the person who takes it. A placebo (pronounced pla·see′boh) is sometimes prescribed because the act of taking it can in fact relieve symptoms if the person believes it will help him.

In testing a new medicine or drug, one group of persons is given the medicine and a control group is given a placebo that looks and tastes the same. Both placebo and medicine are usually identified only by code, so that the researcher who gives them out cannot unwittingly give clues about what effect is expected.

PLACENTA A disk-shaped structure that develops in the UTERUS during pregnancy. One surface of the placenta (pronounced pla·sen′ta) is closely attached to the uterus. The opposite surface is connected to the UMBILICAL CORD, through which the developing baby (fetus) obtains nourishment and oxygen, and discharges waste products and carbon dioxide. The circulatory systems of mother and fetus are separated by a very thin barrier in the placenta, so that there is no actual mixing of blood. The placenta also functions as an ENDOCRINE GLAND for the mother, producing SEX HORMONES that regulate the course of pregnancy.

The placenta develops at the location where the fertilized egg cell has implanted itself—normally in the upper part of the uterus. The placenta remains undisturbed during the baby's birth, and continues to supply vital oxygen to the baby's system until the

PLACENTA

Placenta allows exchange of oxygen, nutrients, and waste products between the bloodstreams of mother and baby

Umbilical cord contains vessels leading blood in and out of the placenta

One side of the placenta is attached to the wall of the uterus and the other is joined to the umbilical cord of a developing fetus. Within the placenta, oxygen and waste products are exchanged between the mother's blood and the circulation of the baby.

baby takes its first breath of air. The placenta then becomes separated from the uterus and is expelled as the AFTERBIRTH.

In the abnormal condition known as placenta previa, implantation takes place in the lower part of the uterus. The fully developed placenta is in danger of being prematurely detached during birth, and CESAREAN (CESARIAN) SECTION is usually necessary to prevent the brain damage that results from interruption in the baby's supply of oxygen.

PLAGUE Any epidemic disease that causes a large number of deaths. The term is applied particularly to BUBONIC PLAGUE.

PLANNED PARENTHOOD See FAMILY PLANNING.

PLASMA See BLOOD PLASMA.

PLASTIC SURGERY The branch of medicine that deals with the reconstruction of deformed or maimed parts of the body and with the restoration of parts that have been lost. By the use of prosthetic devices (see PROSTHESIS) and tissue grafts, plastic surgeons are able today to repair disfigurements so effectively that even the trained eye has difficulty detecting them.

Plastic surgery generally has a cosmetic effect—that is, it improves the appearance. When it is performed solely for this purpose, it is called COSMETIC SURGERY.

Plastic surgery is used to correct congenital defects such as HARELIP and CLEFT PALATE.

Various materials are used to make prosthetic devices. Plastic can be molded into the shape of a missing part, such as an ear or a nose. An eye of plastic or glass can be connected to eye muscles so that it moves in a natural way.

Skin grafts are used to replace skin that has been burned or otherwise destroyed. Skin is taken usually from another part of the person's body and is left partially attached to the original site until a blood supply is established at the new site. Cartilage removed from the ribs is frequently used in restructuring the nose or a similar part. Cartilage and bone may also be obtained from a bank maintained to supply such needs. See also SKIN GRAFT.

PLEURISY Inflammation of the pleura, the double membrane that covers each lung and lines the chest cavity. The symptoms of pleurisy (pronounced ploor'i· see) are fever, coughing, shallow breathing, and pain in the chest. There are basically two types of pleurisy—dry and wet.

In *dry* pleurisy, the two layers of the pleura become swollen and chafe against each other with every intake of breath. This causes an intense stabbing pain which can be relieved by ANALGESICS and by strapping the ribs to limit the motions of the chest. This type of pleurisy is usually a complication of PNEUMONIA.

Wet pleurisy (also called pleurisy with effusion) is usually less painful than dry pleurisy but more serious. Fluid builds up between the layers of the pleura so that the lung may become compressed and breathing difficult. It also places a great strain upon the heart. Wet pleurisy may occur as a complication of tuberculosis, pneumonia, lung cancer, kidney disease, heart disease, and other diseases. Usually, the fluid must be drained off through a tube. Sometimes the fluid is infected with pus-forming bacteria, a condition known as EMPYEMA. When the pleura that covers the muscular wall of the DIAPHRAGM becomes inflamed, the condition is called diaphragmatic pleurisy. Pain, often in the shoulder blade, is the main symptom. Analgesics and strapping of the chest are the usual treatments.

PLUMBISM Another name for LEAD POISONING. (Pronounced plum'biz·em.)

PNEUMONIA Acute inflammation of the LUNGS, in which the tiny air sacs (alveoli) become so filled with fluid that breathing is affected.

Types of Pneumonia: One type of pneumonia familiar to most people is *bacterial* pneumonia, most often caused by the pneumococcus BACTERIUM. This germ is usually present in healthy mouths and throats, and when the body's resistance is lowered by colds, influenza, or general poor health, pneumonia may develop.

Bacterial pneumonia was dangerous and often fatal before antibiotics such as PENICILLIN and the sulfa compounds (SULFONAMIDES) came into use. Nowadays, if treatment is started early, the chances for full recovery are excellent.

Bacterial pneumonia may affect one or more of the lobes of the lung and is thus called lobar pneumonia. If both lungs are involved, the popular term is "double pneumonia"; the medical term is "bilateral pneumonia." In BRONCHOPNEUMONIA, the infection is not confined to one or more lobes of the lung but tends to be patchy, occurring in the alveoli surrounding the bronchial tubes.

A type of pneumonia more common in young adults than the bacterial type is called primary atypical pneumonia, or *virus* pneumonia. It is believed to be caused by VIRUSES, but other microor-

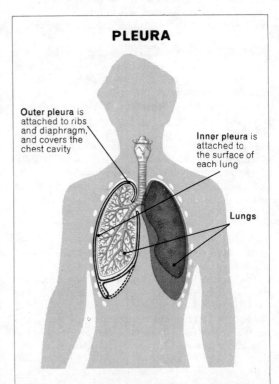

PLEURA

Outer pleura is attached to ribs and diaphragm, and covers the chest cavity

Inner pleura is attached to the surface of each lung

Lungs

The pleura is a double membrane which lines the outside of the lungs and the inside of the chest cavity. Inflammation of the pleura, or pleurisy, may cause fluid to form, and an excess of fluid is called a pleural effusion. Either condition may be associated with pneumonia.

ganisms may also be responsible. The disease usually runs its course in about 10 days, but the person may feel weak and tired for a long time afterward. Treatment with an antibiotic such as TETRACYCLINE is sometimes found to be effective.

Pneumonia may also be caused by a collection of fluid in the lungs, foreign matter such as bits of food, or irritating chemicals. In persons undergoing surgery, care must be taken to remove mouth and nose secretions by suction so that they will not get into the lungs. After consciousness returns, the postoperative patient is instructed to cough and perform breathing exercises. *Hypostatic* pneumonia may occur in bedridden older people. Frequent changes of position will help to prevent the accumulation of fluids in the lungs. Oily nose drops and some household chemicals that have been accidentally inhaled can also bring on pneumonia.

Symptoms: Pneumonia often strikes without much warning, and may be a complication of colds or influenza. The victim has a harsh, dry cough, sharp pains in the chest, fever, and often a chill. He finds it difficult to breathe and brings up rust-colored sputum containing blood or pus. When the doctor taps the chest of a patient with lobar pneumonia, he hears dull thuds instead of the hollow sounds given off by healthy lungs. In bronchopneumonia the features may be much less severe. X-ray examination of the lungs helps the diagnosis.

Treatment: Many cases can be treated at home. Severe cases are treated in a hospital where there are facilities for X rays, laboratory tests, and OXYGEN THERAPY. A patient may also need special nursing.

PNEUMORESECTION The surgical removal of part of a lung. Pneumoresection (pronounced noo″moh·ree·sek′shun) is sometimes performed in cases of chronic lung abscess, malignant TUMORS, and TUBERCULOSIS.

PNEUMOTHORAX The presence of air or gas between the two layers of the membrane (pleura) that lines the chest wall and surrounds the lung. Pneumothorax (pronounced noo″moh·thawr′aks) prevents the lung from expanding with each inhaled breath and is therefore also known as collapsed lung.

Artificial pneumothorax was formerly a common treatment for tuberculosis. By deliberately introducing air into the pleural cavity (the space between the two layers of the pleura), doctors could put an affected lung out of action and give it a chance to rest and heal. This procedure is rarely used today.

Traumatic (accidental) pneumothorax occurs when air enters the pleural cavity through injuries such as stab and bullet wounds, rupture of the pleura, fractured ribs, or accidents in which the chest is crushed.

Tuberculosis, emphysema, or other serious lung diseases sometimes perforate the pleura, resulting in *spontaneous* pneumothorax. This may also occur for unknown reasons in healthy young people. Usually the condition clears up by itself if the person rests.

Tension pneumothorax is a serious condition that occurs if an accidental or spontaneous hole in the pleura happens to be covered by a loose flap of tissue that acts as a valve, letting air into the pleural cavity but preventing its escape. Pressure builds up with each inhaled breath. The heart is forced out of place, and both lungs may collapse. Obviously, this type of pneumothorax is a medical emergency requiring immediate treatment by a doctor.

POCK A PUSTULE, or the scar left by one, especially in such diseases as CHICKEN POX and SMALLPOX.

PODAGRA Another name for GOUT. (Pronounced poh·dag′ra.)

PODIATRIST A specialist in the treatment of foot ailments; also called a chiropodist. The podiatrist (pronounced po·die′a·trist) treats disorders such as ATHLETE'S FOOT and INGROWN TOENAIL, removes corns and calluses, prescribes corrective shoes, and performs minor surgery.

Podiatrists are required by all the states to undergo prescribed training before they are licensed to practice.

POISON IVY A plant producing an oil sap that causes an itching rash on the skin. Poison ivy grows wild in most parts of North America. It may grow as a shrub, a climbing vine, or a trailing ground vine. The leaves may be notched or smooth-edged. It can always be identified by the fact that *the leaves grow in clusters of three.*

Most cases of poison-ivy rash are caused by directly touching the plant. But it is possible to get the rash by handling anything contaminated with the sap—tools, clothing, or the fur of pets. The smoke from burning poison ivy can produce a skin rash and, if inhaled, serious inflammation of the air passages. A dead, dry poison-ivy plant may be just as dangerous as a green one.

Exactly the same toxic reaction is produced by poison oak and poison sumac. The leaves of poison oak also grow in clusters of three, and somewhat resemble oak leaves. Poison sumac is a tall shrub with compound leaves of seven or more smooth-edged leaflets on a bright red stem.

Symptoms and Treatment: Ivy poisoning affects some people more than others. Sensitivity can develop after years of apparent immunity. The rash starts with burning and itching of the skin at the site of contact, followed by watery blisters.

Avoid scratching, so that the rash will not become infected. Relief can be obtained by applying Burow's solution, calamine lotion, or compresses of cool tap water. Severe cases, in which there may be large blisters, extensive inflammation, and even fever, require treatment by a doctor. It is particularly important to consult your doctor if inflammation appears on such sensitive areas as the face and the genital organs.

Prevention: Learn to identify poison ivy and its relatives. If you have accidentally touched any of them, scrub the exposed skin thoroughly with soap and water. Launder or dry-clean any clothing that has been contaminated with the sap.

POISONING See FIRST AID section.

POLIOENCEPHALITIS Inflammation of the brain due to the POLIOMYELITIS virus. It may occur alone or with paralytic poliomyelitis. Polioencephalitis (pronounced pol″ee·oh·en·sef″a·lie′tis) begins with high fever and headache followed by convulsions and sometimes coma. There is great anxiety and mental confusion. The face, hands, and feet quiver or jerk. There may be some brain damage. Treatment is the same as for polio.

POLIOMYELITIS (polio) An acute infection of the central nervous system, sometimes resulting in paralysis. Poliomyelitis (pronounced pol″ee·oh·mie″e·lie′tis) was once known as infantile paralysis. The disease is caused by a virus which enters the system through the nose or mouth and, in most cases of *paralytic* polio, attacks the nerves controlling muscles. In *bulbar* polio, breathing and swallowing are affected. Polio may attack persons of any age.

Symptoms: There is a mild form (*abortive* polio) that is often mistaken for flu or an upset stomach and does not cause paralysis. The paralytic form begins with fever, headache, vomiting, drowsiness, and stiffness in the neck and back. Since other serious childhood diseases often start in the same way, *it is important to contact a doctor immediately if your child shows these symptoms.* As polio progresses, the affected muscles weaken, develop spasms, and may become paralyzed in one to seven days. Hoarseness and difficulty in swallowing usually indicate bulbar polio.

Treatment: There is no known cure for polio. The person should be treated in a hospital where special equipment such as a RESPIRATOR is available. During the acute phase of the disease, when there is still active infection with fever and pain, the application of hot, moist packs helps to relieve the muscle spasms and may lessen or even prevent permanent paralysis. (See KENNY METHOD.)

Immunization and Prevention: The Salk vaccine, the first polio vaccine to be developed, consists of killed polio viruses that are injected into the body. Its use has largely been supplanted by the Sabin vaccine, which is given by mouth and consists of live but weakened viruses.

Every infant, child, and young adult, especially pregnant women, should be immunized against polio.

The Sister Kenny Institute at the Abbot–Northwestern Hospital in Minneapolis will give information about rehabilitation.

POLLEN See HAY FEVER.

POLYCYTHEMIA See BLOOD DISEASE. (Pronounced pol″ee·sie·thee′mee·a.)

POLYDACTYLISM A CONGENITAL abnormality consisting of having more than the usual number of fingers or toes. (Pronounced pol″i·dak′til·iz·em.)

POLYMYXIN Any of a number of ANTIBIOTIC substances obtained from the polymyxa BACILLUS, which grows in the soil. Polymyxin (pronounced pol″ee·mik′sin) must be used under careful medical supervision to prevent damage to the kidneys and the central nervous system. Effective in treating a variety of infections, polymyxins are used mainly in preparations such as ointments where large amounts will not be absorbed into the body.

POLYP A TUMOR projecting from mucous membrane, usually in the nose, bladder, intestine, or uterus. Although usually not MALIGNANT, a polyp (pronounced pol′ip) may cause obstruction.

POLYURIA The condition in which a person passes large amounts of urine. It can be the normal result of drinking a lot or taking a DIURETIC (which stimulates the kidneys), but it may also be a symptom of DIABETES or a kidney disease.

PORPHYRIA A group of uncommon inherited metabolic disorders of the blood pigments. In the usual type, the patient may suffer recurrent attacks of abdominal pain and disturbances of the nervous system. Urine passed during an attack may turn dark brown after an hour or so.

There is no specific treatment, but patients should be warned to avoid certain drugs which bring on an attack. These include some anesthetics, barbiturates, chloroquine, the contraceptive pill, and sulfonamides.

POSTMORTEM See AUTOPSY.

POSTNASAL DRIP See SINUSITIS.

POSTPARTUM Postnatal, or occurring after delivery of a child. (Pronounced pohst′pahr′tum.)

The PLACENTA is usually expelled shortly after the child is born. If it is not, the doctor removes it manually. He also makes any surgical repairs needed, such as stiching a cut or tear at the margin of the vagina. (See EPISIOTOMY.) Then the abdominal wall may be massaged gently for a short time in order to help the uterus contract. It usually takes four or five weeks for the uterus to return to its prepregnant size.

The doctor may order insertion of a CATHETER to relieve the urinary bladder, since women frequently have difficulty in urinating after childbirth. Constipation is also a common complaint. If it persists for more than a day or two, the doctor will usually order a mild cathartic or, in more stubborn cases, an enema. Bleeding from the vagina usually continues for a time. This discharge, called LOCHIA, gradually fades from blood red to a yellowish white, and normally disappears in three or four weeks.

If the baby is to be breast-fed (see BREAST-FEEDING), nursing should begin about 12 hours after delivery. Nursing stimulates the production of milk, and the clear colostrum first secreted by the breasts contains factors that help the baby resist infection. If breast feeding is not intended, hormones are administered to prevent LACTATION.

Unnecessary confinement in bed should be avoided after a normal delivery. Mild exercise aids the circulation and helps the bowels and bladder to function normally. The mother can usually leave bed for short periods the day after the baby is born. The average stay in the hospital is about three to five days.

Complications: There is always some loss of blood in childbirth. Excessive and dangerous loss of blood is called postpartum hemorrhage. If it occurs, there are a number of emergency measures that the doctor can take. In hospital deliveries, it is routine practice to have the mother's blood typed and cross-matched beforehand, so that a transfusion can be given without delay.

During childbirth, the bleeding wall of the uterus and any other bruised or torn areas are exposed to germs. Even bacteria that are normally harmless may cause serious infections. Such infections, especially puerperal sepsis, or childbed fever, were once a frequent cause of maternal death. Nowadays, such infections are controlled by using sterile techniques during delivery and with ANTIBIOTICS.

Inflammation of the breast, or MASTITIS, sometimes occurs after breast-feeding has been started. Puerperal (postpartum) mastitis is caused by bacteria that enter the milk ducts by way of the nipple. Swelling, redness, and pain in the breast are usually accompanied by chills, fever, and general malaise. Treatment includes stopping breast feeding and administering antibiotics.

Milk leg is a postpartum form of PHLEBITIS. One or both legs may become swollen and abnormally pale. If milk leg develops, it is treated by bed rest and, sometimes, medication to prevent the formation of clots in the veins.

Postpartum depression is an emotional disturbance that is experienced by some women after delivery. Some temporary tiredness and depression following the physical and emotional stress of childbirth is normal and usually disappears in a few days or weeks. In a small number of cases, however, the mother becomes profoundly depressed and is unable to carry on with the care of the baby and ordinary household chores. This should be brought promptly to the doctor's attention. Medication and, in some cases, psychiatric counseling are helpful. See also PUERPERIUM.

POULTICE   See   FOMENTATION.   (Pronounced pohl'tis.)

PPD   An abbreviation for *purified protein derivative* of TUBERCULIN. (Pronounce each letter.)

PREGNANCY   The condition of having a baby developing inside the body. Normally, pregnancy begins with the implantation of a fertilized EGG CELL on the inside wall of the uterus and ends with the birth of the infant 40 weeks, or 280 days, from the first day of the last menses.

Given special care, survival is possible if the baby is born anytime after about 28 weeks of pregnancy. A multiple pregnancy (the presence of more than one FETUS in the womb) is especially likely to end in premature birth. Other causes of premature birth include stress, infection, rupture of the membranes surrounding the fetus, and abnormalities of either the fetus or the uterus. Occasionally, pregnancy continues beyond the normal term. Healthy babies have been born following pregnancies of 300 or more days.

During the first three months, or first trimester, there is no obvious outward sign of pregnancy. However, hormones and other substances released into the mother's bloodstream from the PLACENTA will have detectable effects. (See PREGNANCY SIGNS AND TESTS.)

Following implantation, the fertilized egg cell divides and redivides, repeatedly doubling in size. First a thin, disk-shaped mass of cells is formed. Then the disk folds over on itself, enclosing a central cavity. By the end of the second week, a rudimentary spinal column has been formed, and the tiny piece of growing tissue takes on the typical curled-up shape of an embryo. At the end of four weeks, small buds appear, which will develop into arms and legs. At eight weeks, the EMBRYO is about an inch long, but different areas can be identified as future organs such as the heart, ears, lungs, eyes, and kidneys. By the end of the first trimester, the fetus begins to look recognizably human.

The first trimester is the most critical period. If the mother has German measles (RUBELLA) or certain other viral infections during this time, or if harmful substances are present in her blood, the baby may have BIRTH DEFECTS. It is a good rule to use no medicines during the first trimester unless the doctor orders them.

By the end of the fourth month, movements can

be felt by the mother, and the doctor can hear heart sounds with a stethoscope. The fetus begins to crowd the mother's internal organs and may cause various kinds of discomfort, such as shortness of breath, hemorrhoids, constipation, muscle cramps, and back pain.

No two women are alike in their physical and emotional reactions to pregnancy. Most women go through pregnancy comfortably, without complications. For a small minority, pregnancy is difficult and risky. Preexisting conditions such as chronic hypertension, heart disease, kidney disease, tuberculosis, or other serious illnesses are likely to cause complications. Another potentially serious complication is toxemia of pregnancy, which, if untreated, may lead to ECLAMPSIA.

Prenatal care, under skilled medical supervision, has made it possible to prevent or treat more of the discomforts and complications of pregnancy. Some family doctors deliver babies; others prefer to have the expectant mother cared for by an obstetrician. It is very important for any pregnant woman to see her doctor regularly, beginning when pregnancy is first suspected. See also ECTOPIC PREGNANCY.

PREGNANCY SIGNS AND TESTS Early signs and symptoms include missed menstrual periods (amenorrhea), tenderness and tingling in the breasts, and frequent urination. Some women experience nausea and vomiting and sometimes have an unusual appetite for some particular kind of food.

At about the 10th week, a slight enlargement of the uterus can be detected. The tissues at the entrance to the vagina take on a bluish hue, and the cervix (the mouth of the uterus) becomes relaxed and feels soft.

Any of these signs can be due to other conditions. Pregnancy cannot be diagnosed with certainty during the first few weeks on the basis of a physical examination alone.

A laboratory test of an early-morning sample of the woman's urine will provide early diagnosis of pregnancy. Such tests are based on changes in body chemistry that begin almost at the moment of conception. Many different kinds of tests are used. One is a type of AGGLUTINATION TEST which uses serum and preparations of red blood cells from laboratory animals that have been specially treated with human sex hormones. When the two preparations are mixed, the serum normally causes the red blood cells to come together. They will not come together if a small amount of a pregnant woman's urine is added.

PREMENSTRUAL TENSION Mental and physical distress before the onset of MENSTRUATION. Nervousness, irritability, depression, frequent headaches, general EDEMA (puffiness), and pain in the breasts may occur. These symptoms are related to retention of fluid in the tissues.

In mild cases, aspirin may relieve the symptoms. Limiting salt intake for about a week before menstruation is sometimes an effective preventive. For severe cases, consult a doctor, who may prescribe a DIURETIC.

PREMOLAR   A BICUSPID tooth.

PREPUCE   See FORESKIN; PENIS. (Pronounced pree'pyoos.)

PRESBYOPIA   A condition in which the lens of the EYE becomes less elastic with age. As a result, it is difficult to obtain a clear, sharp view of things that are close up. Presbyopia (pronounced prez''bee·oh'pee·a) necessitates the wearing of glasses for reading or close work.

PRESCRIPTION   A physician's order for medicine to be prepared by a PHARMACIST. It is written partly in symbols that stand for Latin words. It specifies the ingredients, the dosage, and directions for taking the medicine. The pharmacist is required by law to fill the order exactly as written, and to keep a record of it.

PRESSOR   Tending to raise blood pressure. ADRENALINE, for example, is a pressor (pronounced pres'or) hormone, since it causes constriction of the small blood vessels and thus brings about an increase in blood pressure. Various pressor agents are used in medicine to treat such conditions as HYPOTENSION (low blood pressure) and SHOCK.

PRICKLY HEAT   An itchy rash of minute, reddish pimples. The condition is also known as miliaria rubra, or heat RASH. Overweight people and infants are especially susceptible. The condition is most common in hot, humid weather. Perspiration and chafing are frequently contributing factors.

The rash usually disappears after the body cools off. Baths (without soap) are soothing; a light powder should be applied afterward. Keep the patient as cool and dry as possible. If the rash persists, consult a doctor.

PRIMAQUINE   A medicine effective in curing MALARIA. (Pronounced prie'ma·kween.)

PRO-BANTHINE   A trade name for propantheline bromide, a medicine used to reduce gastric acidity and relieve the spasms of stomach ULCERS and COLITIS. (Pronounced proh''ban'theen.)

PROCAINE HYDROCHLORIDE   A white substance related to COCAINE. Procaine hydrochloride (pronounced proh·kayn' hie''dro·klawr'ied) is a local anesthetic much used by dentists. It is also used in surgery. When injected into tissue near a nerve, it produces nerve BLOCK.

PROCTITIS Inflammation of the rectum. Proctitis (pronounced prok·tie′tis) may occur with colitis, dysentery, diabetes, and allergy, but often the cause cannot be found. Application of moist heat, medications, and avoidance of difficult bowel movements (see CONSTIPATION) will usually help to relieve the symptoms.

PROCTOLOGIST A specialist in proctology, the branch of medicine concerned with the diagnosis and treatment of diseases of the lower COLON, rectum, and anus. (Pronounced prok·tol′o·jist.)

PROCTOSCOPE An instrument used to examine the rectum and lower colon. It is basically a tube with an electric light and a magnifying viewer. A proctoscope (pronounced prok′ta·skohp) examination is done in any complete medical checkup.

PROGESTERONE See SEX HORMONE. (Pronounced proh·jes′te·rohn.)

PROGNOSIS A prediction of the probable future course of a disorder. A prognosis (pronounced prog·noh′sis) is based on the history of similar cases and the age, sex, and general condition of the patient. See also DIAGNOSIS.

PROJECTION Ascribing to other persons or things the feelings or motives that one has oneself. In normal PSYCHOLOGY, projection is recognized as a universal source of bias in people's judgments of events and things. Such projection is the basis for a certain kind of PERSONALITY TEST, called a projective test. In PSYCHIATRY, projection is often seen as a defense mechanism. For example an emotionally disturbed person may be able to remain comfortably unconscious of feelings he finds painful by attributing these feelings to others.

PROLAPSE Downward displacement of an organ from its usual place. The rectum and the uterus are especially subject to prolapse (pronounced proh·laps). In severe cases, they may protrude from the body. Rectal prolapse is often associated with hemorrhoids and chronic constipation. Prolapse of the uterus is usually a delayed result of injury in childbirth. It may not become troublesome until advancing age weakens the abdominal muscles and ligaments.

Prolapse is a serious condition usually requiring surgical repair.

PROPHYLACTIC Pertaining to PROPHYLAXIS. Any agent or procedure that helps to prevent disease can be described as a prophylactic agent or procedure, or simply as a prophylactic (pronounced proh″fa·lak′tik). Thus, the Sabin vaccine is a prophylactic against poliomyelitis. The CONDOM is a prophylactic against venereal disease.

PROPHYLAXIS Any procedure that is carried out for the purpose of preventing disease. To dentists, prophylaxis (pronounced proh″fa·lak′sis) means the thorough cleaning of the teeth to remove hard deposits which, if allowed to accumulate, may lead to loosening of teeth and infection of the gums. See also PROPHYLACTIC.

PROPRIETARY MEDICINE See GENERIC.

PROPYLTHIOURACIL A synthetic substance that interferes with the production of thyroid hormone. Propylthiouracil (pronounced pro″pil·thie″oh·yoor′a·sil) is prescribed to relieve the symptoms of hyperthyroidism (see THYROID GLAND).

PROSTATECTOMY Surgical removal of a portion or all of the PROSTATE GLAND. A prostatectomy (pronounced pros″ta·tek′to·mee) is usually done to relieve an enlarged prostate, which interferes with emptying the bladder. Complete removal may be recommended in the case of cancer.

A transurethral prostatectomy is done without an incision. Sections of tissue are removed through a narrow, tubular instrument called a cystoscope, which is passed up the urethra and into the bladder. In other types of prostatectomy, an incision is made between the legs or in the lower abdomen.

PROSTATE GLAND An auxiliary male gland that surrounds the urethra where it joins the bladder. Ducts from the prostate lead into the urethra, where fluid from the prostate mixes with SPERM CELLS to form SEMEN.

Enlarged Prostate Gland: In many men, there is a gradual enlargement of the prostate with age. The cause is not understood. As the gland increases in size, it presses on the neck of the bladder, interfering with the discharge of urine. Urine tends to build up in the bladder, straining and weakening it; some urine may be forced back, eventually causing kidney infection (see UREMIA).

The person with an enlarged prostate feels a need to urinate frequently. At the same time, the flow is slight, since the bladder is obstructed. Diagnosis is made by an examination in which the physician feels the prostate through the rectum. Severe enlargement usually requires surgery (see PROSTATECTOMY). If the condition is neglected, the man may find that he cannot empty his bladder at all. This is an emergency for which you should consult a doctor at once.

Cancer of the Prostate: If malignancy is suspected in an enlarged prostate, the diagnosis must be confirmed by BIOPSY. There is a good record of recovery when the condition is detected early and is treated by surgery and radiation. Older men especially should have rectal examinations regularly; otherwise a cancer may be well developed before it is recognized.

PROSTATE GLAND

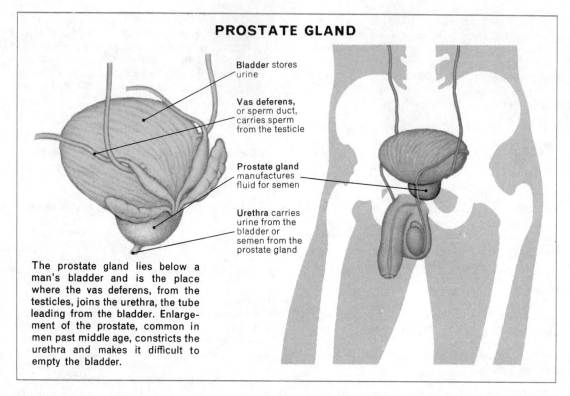

Bladder stores urine

Vas deferens, or sperm duct, carries sperm from the testicle

Prostate gland manufactures fluid for semen

Urethra carries urine from the bladder or semen from the prostate gland

The prostate gland lies below a man's bladder and is the place where the vas deferens, from the testicles, joins the urethra, the tube leading from the bladder. Enlargement of the prostate, common in men past middle age, constricts the urethra and makes it difficult to empty the bladder.

PROSTATITIS Inflammation of the PROSTATE GLAND. Prostatitis (pronounced pros″ta·tie′tis) is fairly common and may occur as a result of an infection in the urinary tract or in a remote part of the body. It can be caused by venereal disease.

In acute prostatitis, the person has fever, low-back pain, and a frequent need to urinate. Urination is difficult, and there may be a discharge of pus. In chronic prostatitis, fever is usually absent. Prostatitis responds well to treatment with ANTIBIOTICS.

PROSTHESIS Any artificial substitute for a part of the body. (Pronounced pros′the·sis.) Prosthetic devices range from dentures to artificial eyes, noses, arms, and legs.

Prostheses and Amputations: It is no longer necessary for people to be handicapped if they lose a limb. Prosthetic hands enable a person to perform both delicate and heavy tasks (see KINEPLASTY); with prosthetic legs, one can remain standing through the workday.

Before an amputation is made, the surgeon decides on the precise type of device that will replace the limb. Sometimes the muscles are rearranged or the bones given a particular form so that the prosthesis will be easier to operate.

Plastic Surgery: Prosthetic devices may be attached to the skin or inserted under the skin. Prosthetic ears and noses are molded and colored to fit perfectly with the face. See also separate entry, PLASTIC SURGERY.

PROSTHETIC DEVICE See PROSTHESIS.

PROSTRATION Extreme exhaustion. It may be physical or mental. See NERVOUS BREAKDOWN; HEAT PROSTRATION.

PROTEIN A special kind of complex chemical compound that forms an essential part of every living cell.

Proteins contain nitrogen, carbon, hydrogen, and oxygen, and sometimes other elements. All proteins are built up on smaller units, the AMINO ACIDS. Millions of different proteins are formed by different arrangements and combinations of only 20 or so amino acids. When we eat foods rich in protein (such as meat, fish, eggs, and milk), enzymes in the stomach and intestines break down the proteins into their constituent amino acids; then the amino acids are absorbed into the blood and sent to the tissues of the body; there they are built up into our own kinds of proteins.

Our bodies can manufacture some of the amino acids we need to form our own proteins, but there are eight amino acids that we cannot manufacture. These so-called essential amino acids must be supplied in the protein foods we eat. If the diet is deficient in proteins containing these essential amino acids, normal physical and mental development cannot take place during the period of growth in infancy and childhood. Anyone whose diet lacks proteins becomes weak and loses resistance to disease. In severe cases of protein deficiency, excessive fluid accumulates in the tissues and general swelling, or EDEMA, results. See also DIET.

PROTHROMBIN A protein substance in the blood that plays a vital part in the formation of BLOOD CLOTS, which help to stop bleeding. (Pronounced proh·throm'bin.)

PROTOZOA A subdivision of the animal kingdom. Like bacteria, protozoans are very tiny organisms that are found in countless billions everywhere on earth. Most protozoans are harmless, but a few are parasites and cause such diseases as amebic DYSENTERY, LEISHMANIASIS, MALARIA, and African SLEEPING SICKNESS.

PRURIGO A chronic skin condition of unknown cause, usually starting in childhood. Small, pale papules (pimples) develop deep in the skin and cause intense itching. One kind of prurigo (pronounced proor·ie'goh) occurs in people who have asthma and hay fever; another comes with warm weather.
Treatment: Prurigo is difficult to treat. Ointments and other medicines applied to the skin have little effect. STEROID hormones may help, but relapses are frequent.

PRURITUS The medical name for ITCHING. (Pronounced proor·ie'tus.)

PSITTACOSIS A lung infection caused by a VIRUS and transmitted to humans from certain birds in which it appears as an intestinal infection. Also called parrot fever and ornithosis, psittacosis (pronounced sit"a·koh'sis) affects ducks, chickens, and pigeons as well as parrots and parakeets. The disease is caught by breathing in the dust from feathers or dried droppings of sick birds. Symptoms vary from those of PNEUMONIA to those of a mild respiratory infection.
Psittacosis requires prompt treatment with TETRACYCLINES or other antibiotics to prevent complications. Infected birds must be destroyed, and their carcasses and cages, or coops burned.

PSORIASIS A skin disease characterized by itchy, red patches that become covered with loose, silvery scales. Psoriasis (pronounced so·rie'a·sis) may be acute, but in most cases it is chronic and mild.
The eruptions appear most often on the scalp, forearms, elbows, knees, and legs, but may also occur on the chest, abdomen, back, and soles of the feet. Psoriasis is sometimes associated with arthritis. The cause is unknown, but it seems to run in families. It is not communicable.
Treatment: There is no known cure, but relief from the itching and clearing of the skin lesions may be obtained from ointments and lotions prescribed by

the doctor. Sunlight is helpful, but sunburn should be avoided.

PSYCHE The mind, with its emotions, perceptions, and ideas. (Pronounced sie'kee.)

PSYCHEDELIC DRUG See HALLUCINOGENIC DRUG. (Pronounced sie"ki·del'ik.)

PSYCHIATRIST A physician specializing in PSYCHIATRY. (Pronounced sie·kie'a·trist.)

PSYCHIATRY The branch of medicine concerned with the study, diagnosis, and treatment of EMOTIONAL AND MENTAL DISORDERS. (Pronounced sie·kie'a·tree.)

PSYCHOANALYSIS A method of studying and treating EMOTIONAL AND MENTAL DISORDERS that was developed by Sigmund Freud, an Austrian psychiatrist, at the turn of the twentieth century. It is one of a number of forms of PSYCHOTHERAPY.
Psychoanalysis (pronounced sie"koh·a·nal'i·sis) holds that we are born with basic instinctive drives which, when they come in conflict with the demands of parents and others, are forced back into the unconscious mind by a process known as REPRESSION. These repressed drives then find a disguised outlet in various kinds of irrational behavior. In psychoanalysis, various methods are used to bring repressed memories and unconscious impulses into consciousness. Then the patient can learn to understand and cope with his problems.
Psychoanalysis has undergone considerable development since it was first introduced by Freud. He laid great emphasis on sexuality, or LIBIDO. Others have shifted the focus to social forces, environment, and relationships between people.

PSYCHOLOGIST A specialist in PSYCHOLOGY, the study of mental processes and their relation to behavior. Some psychologists practice PSYCHOTHERAPY. (Pronounced sie·kol'o·jist.)

PSYCHOLOGY The science dealing with the study of the mind, with special reference to behavior. (Pronounced sie·kol'o·jee.)
The field of psychology is a large one. Psychologists are interested in emotion and feeling, how we think and learn, and how we react to our environment. At one extreme, psychology is concerned with the structure and physiology of the nervous system. At the other extreme, it is involved with social relations and merges with sociology. Psychology includes many specialties, two of which are mentioned here.
Clinical Psychology: This branch is closest to psychiatry; the clinical psychologist often works with the psychiatrist in a mental health clinic or mental hospital. With the aid of such methods as intelli-

gence tests (see INTELLIGENCE QUOTIENT) and PERSONALITY TESTS, he evaluates the individual's mental and emotional problems. He gives his findings to the psychiatrist or may himself help the person through counseling.

Abnormal Psychology: The mentally ill and others who cannot function normally in society are the concern of this branch of psychology.

See also CHILD PSYCHOLOGY.

PSYCHOMOTOR Relating to muscular (motor) activity that results from mental, or psychic, activity. Stammering and tics are examples of psychomotor (pronounced sie″koh·moh′tor) disturbance.

PSYCHONEUROSIS A mild or moderately severe emotional disorder. (Pronounced sie″koh·noor·oh′sis.) Psychoneurosis (sometimes called simply neurosis) is not nearly as severe a disorder as PSYCHOSIS. The individual is able to lead a fairly normal life; however, he often suffers from feelings of depression, anxiety, or inadequacy. Everyone experiences some symptoms of neurosis, particularly when under a strain. The neurotic person experiences them frequently when there is no apparent cause; he is the victim of feelings that he cannot control. See also EMOTIONAL AND MENTAL DISORDERS; ANXIETY; DEPRESSION; HYPOCHONDRIA; PHOBIA.

Treatment: Psychoneurosis is best treated by PSYCHOTHERAPY, in which a psychiatrist or other professionally trained person explores with the individual the sources of his difficulty and guides him toward adjustment to his life situation.

PSYCHOSIS A serious form of EMOTIONAL AND MENTAL DISORDER that makes the individual unable to function in society. A person with a psychosis (pronounced sie·koh′sis) may need to be placed in a MENTAL HOSPITAL to obtain proper care.

Psychoses are fundamentally of two types, organic and functional. Organic psychosis has an obvious physical cause. Damage to the brain from alcoholism or from syphilis (PARESIS), hardening of the arteries of the brain, brain injury, tumors of the brain, and drug addiction are some of the conditions that may produce organic psychosis.

The specific causes of so-called functional psychoses are not known, although research into them is constantly going on. Heredity, physical constitution, and environment may play roles. Anxieties and conflicts that begin in childhood may become worsened as the individual encounters additional strains or frustrations with the passing years, until he retreats from an unbearable reality into a world of his own making. Some major functional psychoses are INVOLUTIONAL MELANCHOLIA, MANIC-DEPRESSIVE PSYCHOSIS, PARANOIA, and SCHIZOPHRENIA.

PSYCHOSOMATIC Having both mental and physical elements. Certain disorders, such as stomach ulcer, ulcerative colitis, heart palpitation or heart pain, infertility, arthritis, high blood pressure, and menstrual irregularities may have, wholly or in part, an emotional cause that results in physiological changes. Psychosomatic (pronounced sie″koh·soh·mat′ik) medicine is concerned with these emotionally instigated disorders.

People tend to use the term "psychosomatic" loosely and to apply it to a large number of disorders. A given disease, such as an allergy, an endocrine disturbance, or heart trouble, may or may not include a psychosomatic factor. Only a doctor is qualified to judge, and some cases are so complex that even he cannot do so with certainty.

Treatment: In psychosomatic medicine, the treatment of both body and emotions is emphasized. If, for example, the person is suffering from a peptic ulcer of largely emotional origin, he is put on a special diet and given medication to reduce the physical symptoms. He should also seek psychiatric counseling to try to resolve his emotional problems which are the basic cause of the disorder.

PSYCHOTHERAPY The treatment of EMOTIONAL AND MENTAL DISORDERS—through largely verbal means. Psychotherapy (pronounced sie″koh·ther′a·pee) may be said to have started with the system of psychoanalysis developed by Sigmund Freud (1856–1939), but many new approaches have been introduced since his day.

Methods of psychotherapy range from brief counseling to extensive individual PSYCHOANALYSIS. Group sessions under the leadership of a psychiatrist or psychologist have been effective not only with the moderately neurotic but also with the inmates of mental hospitals. (See GROUP THERAPY.)

Play therapy is often used in treating emotionally disturbed children. The psychiatrist is able to identify the child's problems by the way the child acts out his conflicts with various toys and games.

PTOMAINE Any of a group of substances produced by decaying animal or vegetable protein. Foods containing ptomaine (pronounced toh′mayn) usually look spoiled and have a disagreeable odor and taste, so that people generally avoid eating them. Contrary to widespread belief, most ptomaines are not injurious to the digestive system, where they are converted into harmless substances. They may, however, be accompanied by noxious bacteria. (See FOOD POISONING.)

PTOSIS Drooping of the upper eyelid caused by a muscle weakness or paralysis. It may be due to disease of the cranial nerve or sympathetic nerve leading to the muscle or, rarely, be of unknown cause in children who are born with it. The treatment depends on the cause.

PUBERTY See ADOLESCENCE.

PUERPERIUM The period after CHILDBIRTH, about six weeks in duration, during which the UTERUS and genital tract return to normal size and function. (Pronounced pyoo"*er*·peer'ee·*um*.) After delivery, there is a normal discharge from the uterus—called LOCHIA—which lasts for three or four weeks. Many new mothers are disappointed at not regaining a slim figure immediately. The muscles and skin of the abdomen have been greatly stretched; exercises prescribed by the doctor will help get them back into shape.

After she comes home from the hospital, the mother gradually resumes her usual household tasks in addition to caring for the new baby. She will still need rest and an afternoon nap. The help of an understanding female relative or nurse is very desirable at this time, if only for a week or two. Often, in facing her added responsibilities, a new mother becomes depressed and easily fatigued. This is not unusual or abnormal unless it persists for some time; in such a case, the doctor should be told so that a more severe mental disturbance can be prevented. (See POSTPARTUM.)

At the end of the puerperium, the mother should see her doctor for a thorough checkup.

PULMONARY Pertaining to or affecting the LUNGS. (Pronounced pul'*mo*·ner"ee.)

PULMOTOR A machine sometimes used to pump air into the lungs in cases of drowning or asphyxiation by poisonous gases. (Pronounced pul'moh"tor.) For other emergency measures when a person's breathing has stopped, see the FIRST AID section.

PULSE The alternating contraction and expansion of the arteries due to the pumping action of the HEART.

In the wrist, the pulse is felt approximately one tenth of a second after the heartbeat occurs and indicates the rate at which the heart is beating. The pulse rate of an adult at rest is about 65 to 80 per minute, women being in the upper part of this range. In children the rate is higher; a 10-year-old child's may be 90 per minute, an infant's as high as 140. As with the heartbeat, the strength, regularity, and rate of the pulse are indexes of health or disease.

Taking the Pulse: The pulse is usually taken immediately below the base of the thumb, on the inside of the wrist. Place the tips of two or three fingers over this point and apply light pressure in order to feel the pulse. Do not use your thumb; it has a pulse of its own that can be confusing. The person whose pulse you are taking should be relaxed—if he is excited or has just been active, you will obtain a high rate. Count the pulse for one minute, using a timepiece with a second hand. Make a note of your count, with the time. If you are aware of any irregularity or weakness of the pulse, note that, too.

PUPIL See EYE.

PURGATIVE See CATHARTIC.

PURGE To cause the bowels to empty by means of a strong medicine. The term is also used for a CATHARTIC or LAXATIVE that thoroughly empties the bowels.

PURPURA See the discussion of thrombocytopenia in the entry BLOOD DISEASE. (Pronounced pur'pyoor·*a*.)

PURULENT Containing or forming PUS. (Pronounced pyoor'*u*·lent.)

PUS A thick, yellow fluid produced by the body's defensive reaction against bacterial infection. It consists of serum and the remains of PHAGOCYTES (germ-destroying cells), BACTERIA, and damaged tissue. It may also contain live bacteria that are still capable of causing infection.

Pus is present in boils, pimples, and other kinds of skin lesions. However, pyogenic (pus-forming) bacteria are not confined to the skin. A pus-filled ABSCESS can form in any part of the body, including bone. See also EMPYEMA and PYEMIA.

PUSTULE A small, PUS-filled elevation on the skin.

PYELITIS Inflammation of the central part of the KIDNEY, where urine collects and drains through the ureter into the bladder. Pyelitis (pronounced pie"*e*·lie'tis) results from infection, which often reaches the kidney from lower parts of the urinary tract. In some cases, the infection originates in a different part of the body and is carried to the kidney through the bloodstream or lymph system.

Pyelitis is especially likely to occur in persons with diabetes and in women during pregnancy. The symptoms include pain in one or both sides of the lower back, chills and fever, and a burning sensation on urination. There is a frequent urge to urinate, but the total amount of urine is scanty. The urine may be bloody or cloudy with pus.

Sulfa compounds (SULFONAMIDES) and PENICILLIN or other antibiotics are very effective in clearing up the infection, but a doctor should be seen at once. If not treated promptly, pyelitis is likely to spread and involve the whole kidney, perhaps damaging it permanently. See also PYELONEPHRITIS.

PYELOGRAM An X-ray photograph of the kidneys and urinary system; known also as an intravenous pyelogram (pronounced pie'*e*·loh·gram), or IVP. The soft tissues of the kidneys and ureters (the tubes leading from the kidneys to the bladder) do not show up well on an ordinary X-ray photograph. To make them visible, the radiologist injects the person being examined with a liquid containing a substance (such as a compound of iodine) which is opaque to X rays. The injection is generally made into a vein in the arm; the substance then travels through the bloodstream and eventually reaches the kidneys. There it is removed from the blood by the normal filtering action of the kidneys, and it enters the urine. Eventually the substance, which is harmless, passes out of the body in the urine.

On a pyelogram the radiologist can see the sizes of the kidneys and ureters, whether their shapes are normal, and the position of any calculus (stone) in the kidneys or ureters. A specialist can use the photographs in planning treatment. A pyelogram is also a good test of how the kidneys are working. For instance, if there is a stone blocking one of the ureters, only the kidney and ureter above the obstruction shows.

Other special X-ray tests on the urinary system include the ARTERIOGRAM, in which the blood vessels are shown up by a radio-opaque dye injected through a fine tube passed into the artery supplying blood to a kidney. In a retrograde pyelogram, dye is introduced through a tube passed into the bladder and up a ureter into the kidney's drainage system. See also KIDNEY STONE; CYSTOSCOPY.

PYELONEPHRITIS The word is sometimes used to mean any form of PYELITIS, acute or chronic. As used here, pyelonephritis (pronounced pie"e·loh·ne·frie'tis) applies only to a serious, chronic form of pyelitis in which the initial bacterial infection has spread from the urine-collecting part of the kidney into adjacent portions. The condition may persist over many years, with continuous damage. There may be repeated attacks of fever, pain in the back, and pain on urination. The urine appears cloudy from discharged pus. Pyelonephritis is diagnosed by making laboratory tests on the urine. X rays of the kidneys may aid in diagnosis.

Treatment: Further damage to the kidneys can be prevented by getting rid of the infection by treatment with sulfa compounds and antibiotics. In addition, it is often necessary to locate and correct any condition that may be interfering with the normal flow of urine, such as a kidney stone (see CALCULUS) or a congenital defect.

PYEMIA A condition in which the blood is invaded by pus-forming microorganisms that have spread from a point of infection somewhere in the body. Pyemia (pronounced pie·ee'mee·a) is a kind of septicemia, or BLOOD POISONING.

PYORRHEA A discharge of pus. The term usually refers to pyorrhea alveolaris, a disease in which pus forms at the roots of the teeth. The tissue of the gums shrinks away, and the teeth become loose. The word "alveolaris" refers to the sockets of the teeth. Pyorrhea alveolaris (pronounced pie"o·ree'a al·vee"oh·lair'is), or periodontitis, is the commonest cause of loss of teeth in adults.

Cause: Pyorrhea is a complication of GINGIVITIS, or inflammation of the gums. Contributing factors include poor mouth hygiene, tartar around the teeth, MALOCCLUSION, worn-down old fillings, and poorly fitting dentures. The gums begin to swell and change color, and bleed easily. If gingivitis is not treated promptly, pyorrhea may develop.

Symptoms: As gingivitis worsens, the tissue begins to draw away from the teeth. Bacteria and food particles collect in the deepening spaces around the teeth, aggravating the condition. Pockets of pus form in these spaces. Gradually the teeth work loose in their sockets and eventually fall out. Wobbly or shifting teeth are always a sign that dental attention is necessary. If the disease is not checked, the bacteria may enter the bloodstream and start infections elsewhere in the body.

Treatment: Treatment may not be simple in a neglected case of pyorrhea. Removal of the tartar, which irritates the gums, is an important step. The pockets of pus must be dealt with; this may require antibiotics and, occasionally, minor surgery on the gum or removal of several teeth. Poor occlusion should be corrected. The person with pyorrhea should brush the teeth regularly and massage the gums to restore normal circulation and firmness.

PYREXIA Another name for FEVER. (Pronounced pie·rek'see·a.)

PYROSIS The medical term for heartburn. Pyrosis (pronounced pie·roh'sis) is marked by a burning sensation in the stomach and esophagus. The esophagus is distended by material forced back from the stomach. Heartburn may be due to tension and excitement. If it occurs repeatedly, it may be a symptom of organic disease and should be investigated. An occasional attack of heartburn may be relieved by taking a teaspoonful of bicarbonate of soda in half a glass of water.

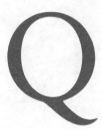

Q FEVER A usually mild disease to which dairy farmers and slaughterhouse workers are especially subject. It is caused by a RICKETTSIA microorganism. Infection often occurs following contact with infected cows, sheep, or goats, or from inhaling dust contaminated with these animals' feces and urine. The symptoms include chills and fever, headache, and persistent cough.

Like other rickettsial diseases, Q fever can be cured by treatment with CHLORAMPHENICOL or TETRACYCLINE. If untreated, repeated acute attacks may occur and recovery may be slow.

QUADRANTIOPIA Blindness or distorted vision in a quarter of the visual field. See BLINDNESS; EYE DISORDERS.

QUADRICEPS The set of four muscles on the front of the thigh, which contract to straighten the leg at the knee. See also LEG.

QUARANTINE Isolation of a person who has a communicable disease or has been exposed to one. The time an exposed person is kept in quarantine depends upon the incubation period of the particular disease. The purpose of quarantine is to protect others against infection.

QUARTAN FEVER A type of MALARIA, which causes bouts of fever every three days.

QUASSIA A type of tropical tree. A bitter extract of the wood was once used for treating fever and infection by threadworms.

QUICKENING The first signs of independent life and movement by the fetus felt by a pregnant woman. See also PREGNANCY.

QUICK TEST A test, devised by the American physician Armand Quick, used to identify clotting factors in the blood and to help determine the appropriate ANTICOAGULANT drug for the treatment of disorders such as ARTERIOSCLEROSIS (hardening of the arteries) and THROMBOSIS (blockage of an artery by a blood clot).

QUINALBARBITONE A BARBITURATE drug, used to induce sleep or anesthesia (see HYPNOTIC).

QUINIDINE An alkaloid drug, related chemically to quinine, obtained from the bark of the cinchona tree. This drug is used to treat heart disorders, such as auricular fibrillation.

QUININE A bitter substance obtained from the bark of the cinchona tree. Taken by mouth, quinine suppresses the symptoms of MALARIA, but does not cure the disease. It was once the only treatment for malaria, but other medicines have now largely replaced it.

QUINSY An acute throat infection, or sore throat. Fever and MALAISE (general discomfort) are common symptoms. An abscess forms in the tissue around the TONSIL—hence the medical name, peritonsillar abscess. The side of the throat affected is extremely swollen and tender. The swelling may extend as far up as the soft palate. The condition often occurs as a complication of TONSILLITIS, and pus-causing bacteria are usually present.
Treatment: Antibiotics are given to reduce the fever; if administered early enough, they can cure the disorder. If the case is a severe one, the doctor may make an incision in the abscess and drain the pus. After the infection has cleared up, a TONSILLECTOMY is sometimes recommended to avoid a recurrence.

R

RABBIT FEVER See TULAREMIA.

RABIES A viral disease transmitted to humans when an infected animal's saliva enters an open wound, usually inflicted by the animal's bite. Not only dogs but almost any warm-blooded animal can be infected with the disease. The virus travels along nerve fibers from the bite to the brain. Symptoms, which appear when the virus reaches the brain, include muscle spasms, convulsions, and extreme excitement and rage interrupted by periods of calm.

Hydrophobia, or fear of water, is another name for rabies, since any attempt to drink brings on extremely painful spasms of the larynx. Once symptoms appear, death follows in two or three days. The incubation period ranges from a few days to several months or longer.

Rabies can be prevented by giving an infected person a series of injections that provide immunity to the virus. Immunization should be started without delay if the bite is on the face or the neck. If the bite is farther from the brain, there is time to determine whether the animal was rabid. Rabies should be considered a possibility after a person has been bitten by any animal, especially if the bite is inflicted without provocation.

Every effort should be made to capture the animal, so that it can be confined for observation, or to kill it, so that its brain can be examined for signs of rabies.

RADIATION SICKNESS The harmful effects to the body following exposure to large amounts of radiation. The effects may be sudden and acute, or they may be delayed for days or even weeks, depending upon the rate and type of dosage.

Radiation sickness may occur as a side effect of radiation therapy (see RADIOLOGY), used in the treatment of cancer and other diseases. However, the doctor can control the symptoms by stopping the treatment temporarily or by lowering its intensity. Sometimes people who work in factories and power plants that use nuclear materials acquire radiation sickness. Safeguards against radiation hazards must be strictly maintained in such plants.

Most of the persons who survived the atomic bombings in Japan suffered from radiation sickness. Many of them died as a result, and many of those who lived bore lifelong damage from radiation.

Symptoms: The usual symptoms of radiation sickness are vomiting, diarrhea, and a feeling of weakness. There may be damage to internal organs, fever, soreness of the mouth and throat, and loss of hair. As a rule, the more severe the symptoms, the less chance the victim has of surviving. Recovery from mild radiation sickness may be fairly rapid, but sometimes the symptoms recur. Even after apparent recovery, there is always the possibility of damage to the GENES (the units that carry hereditary characteristics from parent to child). Offspring may be stillborn or defective, and both males and females may become sterile. Susceptibility to cancer may also have been increased.

RADIATION THERAPY See RADIOLOGY.

RADIOLOGY The branch of medicine in which X RAYS, radioactive substances, and other forms of radiant energy are used to diagnose and treat certain diseases. A physician who specializes in this field is called a radiologist.

Radiology in Diagnosis: X-ray photography shows up abnormalities in bones, internal organs, and teeth. Soft organs such as the digestive tract and the kidneys cannot be readily seen in an X-ray photograph unless substances are introduced into them which prevent the X rays from passing through. (See BARIUM SULFATE.) By using a FLUOROSCOPE, which projects a continuous picture on a screen, the doctor can watch internal organs in motion.

A second diagnostic procedure is the use of radioisotopes, or radioactive forms of certain elements. Since iodine salts introduced into the body concentrate in the thyroid gland, radioactive iodine is used to diagnose disorders of that gland. Radioactive iron is used in diagnosing various blood disorders, including anemia. Many abnormalities of the brain, liver, bone, and lung can be diagnosed by using radioactive materials.

Radiation Therapy: Uranium, radium, and other radioactive substances are used in radiation therapy. Radiation damages any living tissue, but it is especially destructive of cells that are multiplying rapidly. An overactive thyroid gland may be treated with radioactive iodine, which destroys the unwanted tissue. Radioactive phosphorus is useful in destroying red blood cells in a condition called polycythemia vera, in which too many red blood cells are manufactured by the bone marrow and other blood-making organs. Radioactive phosphorus is also used in the treatment of chronic leukemia. X-ray treatments may help to clear up stubborn cases of acne and certain fungal and bacterial skin infections.

In cancer therapy, there are several ways of using radium and radon, a gas that radium produces. Tiny pellets or gold needles containing radium are embedded directly into the diseased tissue, where they remain until the rays destroy the tissue. Radon is sealed into very small containers and used in the same way. For deep-seated cancers, radioactive cobalt (cobalt 60) is placed in a large device that focuses the rays on the affected part of the body. Or it can be encapsulated in minute doses in gold or silver needles and embedded in tissue.

RADIOTHERAPY See RADIOLOGY.

RADIUS (plural, **radii**) The shorter bone of the forearm. See ARM.

RANULA A small CYST or fluid-filled swelling that occurs under the tongue. It is caused by a blockage in a salivary duct. If troublesome, it may be removed by minor surgery. (Pronounced ran'yu·la.)

RASH A temporary SKIN ERUPTION. A familiar example is the itchy, raised patches that are characteristic of HIVES. Two other examples are PRICKLY HEAT and DIAPER RASH. A rash may be a local reaction or an outward sign of some abnormal condition affecting the entire body, such as an ALLERGY or a reaction to some toxic substance. Characteristic rashes accompany some infectious diseases, such as measles and scarlet fever.

Since rashes have such a variety of possible causes, there is no general treatment. If itching is bothersome, try putting a cupful of baking soda in your bath water, or use CALAMINE LOTION on the affected area. Consult a doctor if the rash persists, or if it is accompanied by other symptoms, such as fever or MALAISE.

RAT-BITE FEVER A bacterial infection transmitted to people by the bites of infected rats and, occasionally, other small animals.

The type occurring most often in the United States and Canada is also called Haverhill fever. About ten days after the bite, the wound becomes a sore filled with fluid. There is sudden high fever, a spotty rash, and swelling of the large joints and LYMPH NODES. Periods of fever lasting 24 to 48 hours alternate with periods of normal temperature, and the cycle may go on for weeks.

A related disease called sodoku occurs in Japan and the East. In sodoku, the joints are not affected and the rash erupts in the form of patches rather than spots. Both types of rat-bite fever respond to treatment with antibiotics.

RAUWOLFIA An extract of the snakeroot plant, native to India. Rauwolfia (pronounced row·

wool'fee·a) is employed as a TRANQUILIZER in the treatment of mental illness, to lower the blood pressure, and to relieve the withdrawal symptoms of narcotics addicts.

RESERPINE, a derivative of rauwolfia, is sold under various trade names.

RAYNAUD'S DISEASE A disease of the arteries in the feet, hands, and occasionally nose and ears; also called dead fingers. The blood supply to these extremities is temporarily cut off, leading to numbness, followed by severe pain when the circulation is restored. Some cases result in GANGRENE.

Treatment is by drugs or, in severe cases, by cutting the nerves controlling the blood vessels (SYMPATHECTOMY). The disease is named after the French physician Maurice Raynaud (1834–81), who first studied it. (Pronounced ray·nohz'.)

RECESSIVE In heredity, the opposite of DOMINANT. Every inherited trait is determined by a pair of GENES, one from each parent. If the two genes in a pair are contradictory, the dominant gene takes control and masks the effect of the other gene, which is said to be recessive. For example, the gene for blue eyes is recessive. In order to have blue eyes, a person must inherit a gene for blue eyes from both his father and his mother.

RECRUDESCENCE Worsening of a disease or any abnormal condition after a period of improvement. (Pronounced ree"kroo·des'enz.) The word is similar in meaning to RELAPSE.

RECTAL FISSURE See FISSURE.

RED BLOOD CELL See BLOOD; ERYTHROCYTE.

REDUCING The only way to take off excess fat and keep it off is to adjust your daily CALORIE intake to barely meet your daily energy requirements. No diet fads and reducing aids can change this fact. The best reducing DIET supplies all the essentials in an appetizing form. Then, when the desired weight is reached, it can be maintained by adding or subtracting a few extras as needed.

Take pills as weight-reducing aids only under your doctor's supervision. If you are more than a few pounds overweight, see your doctor for a checkup before you undertake a reducing diet or strenuous exercise.

REFLEX An automatic, involuntary reaction to a stimulus. A familiar example is the KNEE JERK. Another example is the contraction and dilation of the pupil of the eye according to the amount of light available. When conducting a medical examination, a doctor may test the patient's reflexes to check for possible disorders of the NERVOUS SYSTEM. (See illustration on following page.)

REFLEX

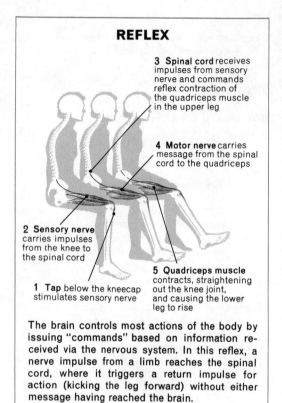

3 Spinal cord receives impulses from sensory nerve and commands reflex contraction of the quadriceps muscle in the upper leg

4 Motor nerve carries message from the spinal cord to the quadriceps

2 Sensory nerve carries impulses from the knee to the spinal cord

1 Tap below the kneecap stimulates sensory nerve

5 Quadriceps muscle contracts, straightening out the knee joint, and causing the lower leg to rise

The brain controls most actions of the body by issuing "commands" based on information received via the nervous system. In this reflex, a nerve impulse from a limb reaches the spinal cord, where it triggers a return impulse for action (kicking the leg forward) without either message having reached the brain.

REFRACTION The bending of light rays within the eye. Such conditions as nearsightedness (MYOPIA), farsightedness (HYPEROPIA), and ASTIGMATISM are due to errors in refraction that prevent proper focusing of light rays on the retina. EYEGLASSES with corrective lenses can remedy these errors.

REFRACTORY Resistant to treatment. (Pronounced ri·frak'toh·ree.)

REGRESSIVE Subsiding, or on the mend. In psychiatry, the term describes a reversion to behavior or attitudes typical of an earlier stage of life.

REGURGITATION The process of surging back. (Pronounced ri·gur''ji·tay'shun.) Examples are the vomiting up of partially digested food and the backward flow of blood through a poorly functioning heart valve.

REITER'S DISEASE A disease, usually affecting men, which causes diarrhea, URETHRITIS (inflammation of the tube leading out from the bladder), and CONJUNCTIVITIS (inflammation of the membrane lining the eyelids). It may also lead to ARTHRITIS, inflammation of the joints. Reiter's (pronounced rie'terz) disease is treated with anti-inflammatory drugs. It was named after the German physician Hans Reiter, who studied the disorder.

RELAPSE A return of symptoms that had seemingly or partly disappeared. The expression "rebound relapse" refers to a reappearance of symptoms after medication is withdrawn. See also RECRUDESCENCE.

RELAPSING FEVER An infectious disease characterized by periods of high fever that alternate with periods of normal temperature. It is caused by various spirochetes (bacteria) that are transmitted by lice or ticks, and occurs chiefly in the tropics. **Symptoms and Treatment:** The fever strikes suddenly and is accompanied by headache, muscular and joint pain, chills, and nausea. After a few days the symptoms subside, but recur several days later. In time, the symptoms grow milder and ultimately disappear.

Relapsing fever is treated with antibiotics, such as the TETRACYCLINES.

REMISSION A temporary decrease or abatement of the symptoms of a disease.

RENAL Pertaining to the KIDNEYS. (Pronounced ree'nal.)

REPRESSION In PSYCHOANALYSIS, a defense mechanism by which impulses or desires are forced out of the conscious mind because they are charged with feelings of guilt or anxiety. They remain in the UNCONSCIOUS, from which they may emerge in a disguised form.

RESECTION Surgical removal of part of an organ or bone, as, for example, a segment of intestine.

RESERPINE A tranquilizing drug obtained from the RAUWOLFIA plant. Reserpine (pronounced re'ser·peen) is also used for treating severe hypertension (high blood pressure).

RESORCINOL An ANTISEPTIC used in an ointment to treat certain skin diseases. (Pronounced ri·zawr'sin·ohl.)

RESPIRATION The process of taking in oxygen and giving off carbon-dioxide wastes. The exchange of oxygen for carbon dioxide that takes place in the lungs is called external respiration. The same exchange occurring between the circulating blood and the cells is known as internal respiration.

RESPIRATOR (1) A machine for administering ARTIFICIAL RESPIRATION. The most commonly used type of respirator (pronounced res'pi·ray''tor) is a special machine that is connected to a tube in the patient's trachea (windpipe). It alternately pushes air into the person's lungs and then releases the pressure so that the lungs relax and air is pushed out. Another type is the IRON LUNG.

(2) A mask equipped with a filter to protect the lungs from dust, harmful fumes, and smoke.

RESPIRATORY SYSTEM The complete set of structures that contribute to RESPIRATION. The central respiratory organs are the LUNGS. The respiratory system includes also the passageway between the nose and the lungs—made up of the PHARYNX, LARYNX, EPIGLOTTIS, TRACHEA, and BRONCHI—as well as the ribs that protect the lungs, the DIAPHRAGM and rib muscles that pump air in and out, and the nerves that activate these muscles.

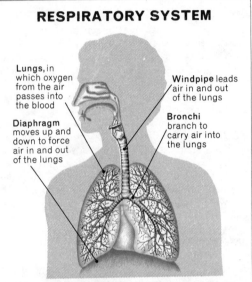

RESPIRATORY SYSTEM

Lungs, in which oxygen from the air passes into the blood

Windpipe leads air in and out of the lungs

Diaphragm moves up and down to force air in and out of the lungs

Bronchi branch to carry air into the lungs

Air enters the respiratory system through the nose and mouth, passes down the trachea (windpipe) and along the bronchi to the lungs. In the capillary blood vessels surrounding tiny air sacs in the lungs, oxygen from the air breathed in is exchanged for carbon dioxide in the blood.

RESUSCITATION Emergency measures to restore breathing and circulation in a person who is unconscious from asphyxiation, choking, electric shock, or a heart attack. (Pronounced ri·sus″i·tay′shun.) See FIRST AID section.

RETENTION A condition in which a person cannot pass urine. It may be a symptom of a disorder requiring urgent treatment. Possible causes are paralysis of the bladder muscle from injury to the brain or spinal cord; a stone in the urethra (the tube leading from the bladder to the exterior); stricture, a contraction of the urethra; or, in men, enlargement of the PROSTATE GLAND.

RETINA See EYE. (Pronounced ret′i·na.)

RETINA, DETACHED See DETACHED RETINA.

RHEUMATIC FEVER A disease of children and young adults, usually marked by fever and swollen joints. The average case is mild. In a small number of cases, heart damage occurs.

In rheumatic (pronounced roo·mat′ik) fever, the inner lining of the heart and the HEART VALVES become inflamed. As the valves heal, they may thicken with scar tissue. When the doctor listens to such a heart through a stethoscope, he can hear a HEART MURMUR as the blood passes through the damaged valves.

Cause: Rheumatic fever only occurs following untreated streptococcus infections such as strep throat, tonsillitis, and scarlet fever.

Symptoms: Fever may range as high as 104° F and last two weeks or longer. The joints of the wrists, elbows, knees, and ankles become red, swollen, and painful. Nosebleed and rashes are not uncommon. Shortness of breath and a weak pulse indicate heart damage. Saint Vitus's dance (Sydenham's CHOREA) may also occur.

Symptoms vary considerably. The disease is often so mild that it is not identified.

Treatment: Aspirin relieves the swollen, tender joints. Other drugs may be prescribed to combat the inflammation. It is essential that the person remain in bed until he has completely recovered.

Attacks of rheumatic fever tend to recur. Antibiotics or sulfa compounds (SULFONAMIDES) must be taken regularly for many years after an attack to prevent streptococcal infections, which can lead to another attack. With adequate medical supervision, even a child with some heart damage may lead a reasonably active, normal life.

RHEUMATISM A painful disorder involving the joints and bones and the tissues supporting them. (Pronounced roo′ma·tiz″em.) See also ARTHRITIS.

RHEUMATOID ARTHRITIS See ARTHRITIS.

RH FACTOR A substance present in the red blood cells (ERYTHROCYTES) of most people, who are therefore said to be Rh-positive. People who lack the Rh (pronounce both letters) factor are Rh-negative. The presence of the Rh factor is a genetic characteristic, determined by heredity.

An Rh-negative person who receives a transfusion of Rh-positive blood will form antibodies in his blood serum. It will then be dangerous for him to receive another Rh-positive transfusion. To guard against this happening, tests for the Rh factor must be made before a transfusion. See also BLOOD TYPE.

The Rh factor is important in pregnancy. If a woman with Rh-negative blood becomes pregnant with a child that has inherited Rh-positive blood from the father, antibodies against the Rh factor are formed in the mother's blood. In repeated pregnancies, more and more anti-Rh antibodies accumulate in the mother's blood. Eventually, these antibodies may enter the bloodstream of the fetus and destroy its red blood cells. The baby may be born dead or may have the serious condition known as ERYTHRO-BLASTOSIS FETALIS. Prenatal care is especially important for Rh-negative women, since the doctor can perform tests and take precautions to prevent antibodies from developing.

RHINITIS Inflammation of the mucous membranes of the nose. Rhinitis (pronounced rie·nie′tis) may be caused by HAY FEVER or a COMMON COLD.

RHINOPHYMA Swelling and redness of the nose; it is sometimes unjustly called whiskey nose. (Pronounced rie″noh·fie′ma.) Mild cases may be successfully treated by applications of cold water, ice, or a mild ASTRINGENT such as witch hazel. Advanced cases are corrected by PLASTIC SURGERY.

RHYTHM METHOD The so-called natural method of birth control, which is based on abstinence from sexual intercourse during about 10 days of each menstrual cycle. As explained under MENSTRUATION, conception can take place only if the SPERM CELL is present in the oviduct during a period of several days immediately following OVULATION. Since sperm cells can survive in the female reproductive tract for 48 hours and perhaps longer, the period of abstinence must begin at least two days before ovulation.

Ovulation occurs about midway in the menstrual cycle. It is accompanied by a slight rise in body temperature; by keeping a careful daily record of temperature (taken orally or rectally each morning before rising) for several months, a woman whose menstrual cycles are regular can predict roughly when the next ovulation will occur. The recommended period of abstinence usually includes Day 10 to Day 20 after the onset of menstruation, *provided that menstruation occurs regularly.*

See also CONTRACEPTIVE METHODS AND DEVICES.

RIBOFLAVIN See VITAMIN. (Pronounced rie′boh·flay″vin.)

RICKETS A children's disease in which the bones do not harden properly, and excessive growth of cartilage occurs at the ends of bones. It is due to lack of VITAMIN D, which is essential for CALCIFICATION of the bones. (A similar disorder in adults is known as OSTEOMALACIA.) KNOCK-KNEE, BOWLEG, PIGEON BREAST, and other deformities may develop.
Treatment and Prevention: Vitamin D is prescribed in concentrated form to overcome the deficiency. To avoid rickets, foods rich in this vitamin are recommended: egg yolk, butter, cream, and vitamin D-enriched milk. Foods such as cheese, cabbage, fish, and nuts, which contain abundant quantities of calcium, should also be eaten. Since vitamin D is formed in the skin when exposed to sunlight, sensible outdoor exposure is recommended.

RICKETTSIA (plural, **rickettsiae**) A bacterialike organism of the genus *Rickettsia* (pronounced rik·et′see·a). Various species live in ticks and mites, and in fleas, lice, and other insects that infest rodents and other animals. Introduced into a person's system by a bite or by dust containing insect feces, rickettsiae produce various illnesses.
Rickettsial Diseases: Severe headache, rash, and fever are common symptoms of rickettsial diseases. Among these are a number of disorders known as TYPHUS, as well as TSUTSUGAMUSHI DISEASE, ROCKY MOUNTAIN SPOTTED FEVER, Q FEVER, and RICKETT-SIALPOX.

RICKETTSIALPOX A disease caused by a RICK-ETTSIA microorganism that infects house mice. It is transmitted to people by mites. A small red sore forms at the site of the infection and then turns black. There may be chills and fever, muscular pain, headache, and a general rash like that of chicken pox. The disease is relatively mild and usually runs its course in several weeks.

RIGOR MORTIS Temporary stiffening of the muscles that takes place within a few hours after death and disappears after about a day. It is caused by a breakdown in the muscles of a chemical called adenosine triphosphate (ATP), a process similar to that which takes place in normal muscle contraction.

RINGWORM The popular name for tinea, a fungus infection of the skin. It causes an itchy skin eruption that spreads out ringlike from the site of infection.

Ringworm is very contagious and can be spread by direct contact or by handling infected bed linens, towels, combs, and other objects. Scratching must be avoided to prevent spreading the ringworm from one part of the body to another and also to prevent secondary bacterial infections.
Treatment: Ringworm is a stubborn disease, and used to be difficult to clear up. But now the antibiotic drug griseofulvin usually eradicates ringworm in a few weeks. In cases of ringworm of the scalp, the hair should be kept as short as possible.
Prevention: Daily washing of the entire body with soap is the best method of preventing fungus infections. Dry the skin thoroughly, especially in body folds and creases, and use a bland talcum powder, since warm, damp places encourage fungus growth.

RN Abbreviation for *registered nurse* (Pronounce each letter.) See NURSE.

RNA Short for *ribonucleic acid*. RNA (pronounce each letter) is found in all living cells. It controls many of the chemical processes that take place in the cell, such as building up proteins out of AMINO ACIDS.

ROCKY MOUNTAIN SPOTTED FEVER A disease caused by a RICKETTSIA microorganism and transmitted to humans from rats, mice, and other rodents by infected ticks. The disease is most common in the Rocky Mountain regions and in the southeastern United States.

Three days to a week after a tick bite, the person has flulike symptoms: fever, headache, joint and muscle pains, and great sensitivity to light. As the illness progresses, there is nausea, vomiting, and abdominal pain. Some persons become delirious; others are stuporous or go into a coma. From three to five days after the onset of the disease, a rash appears on the wrists and ankles, then spreads over the body.

If untreated, Rocky Mountain spotted fever can be a serious, sometimes fatal, illness. It can be treated successfully with CHLORAMPHENICOL and TETRACYCLINE antibiotics.

RORSCHACH TEST See PERSONALITY TEST.

ROSACEA A skin condition of the face, especially of the nose. The cause is unknown, but it may be associated with eating or drinking irritant foods (including strong tea) or overindulgence in alcohol. Known medically as acne rosacea (pronounced ro·za′shee·a), it involves enlarged blood vessels, giving the nose and cheeks a red, flushed appearance. The nose may become greatly enlarged, the condition known as RHINOPHYMA. Rosacea is also caused by exposure to cold winds and sometimes occurs during the menopause. A doctor will recommend a special diet that may clear up the skin.

ROSE FEVER An old name for HAY FEVER occurring in spring or early summer.

ROSEOLA A mild disease, also called roseola infantum, that occurs in young children under the age of three. Roseola (pronounced roh·zee′o·la) is probably due to a virus infection. Its principal symptoms are drowsiness and fever, sometimes as high as 104° F. Temperature returns to normal in three or four days. A pinkish rash, lasting a few days, breaks out as the fever goes down. Complete recovery is the rule, and there is no specific treatment.

ROUNDWORM A group of cylindrical worms called nematodes, some of which are parasitic in the human body. Roundworms cause ELEPHANTIASIS, HOOKWORM DISEASE, PINWORM INFECTION, and TRICHINOSIS.

The giant intestinal roundworm is a fairly common parasite, especially in children. This type of roundworm infection is called ascariasis. The feces of an infected person contain many worm eggs. Infection is spread through contaminated food. Adult worms are pearly white in color and 8 to 16 inches long. If many are present, they may obstruct the intestine or the bile duct. Occasionally, a worm may be vomited or coughed up, or it may appear in a bowel movement or emerge from the rectum at night and be found in bed.

Ascariasis requires medical attention. Home remedies or preparations from the drugstore may be useless or even harmful.

RUBELLA German measles, or three-day measles. Like seven-day MEASLES, or rubeola, rubella (pronounced roo·bel′a) is a contagious viral disease characterized by a pink rash on the face, neck, and body.

The symptoms of rubella are mild. There may be fever and tenderness in the LYMPH NODES. The person may not know he has any illness until a rash appears, two to three weeks after exposure to the disease. The rash disappears after one to three days. Recovery occurs without any specific treatment, and one attack gives protection for life.

If rubella is contracted by a woman during the first three months of pregnancy, the chances are quite high that the infant will have serious birth defects.

An effective vaccine against rubella became available in 1969.

RUBEOLA The medical name for MEASLES. (Pronounced roo·bee′o·la.)

RUPTURE (1) A break or tear. A rupture of the spleen sometimes occurs as a result of injury, causing bleeding inside the abdomen. In APPENDICITIS, the infected appendix may rupture and cause serious abdominal infection.

(2) A HERNIA. There may be no actual tear but only a weakening of the muscular wall. The most usual type is the inguinal hernia, in which a portion of the intestine pushes into a weakened area of the groin, sometimes causing a protrusion.

S

SACCHARIN A white crystalline compound, derived from coal tar and petroleum, and used as a substitute for sugar. Saccharin, (pronounced sak'*ar*·in), has been under attack since 1977 as a potential CARCINOGEN, but studies published in early 1980 indicated that moderate use of saccharin is probably safe. (See also ARTIFICIAL SWEETENER.)

SADISM Finding pleasure, especially sexual pleasure, in making others suffer pain. Sadism (pronounced say'diz·*em*) is named for the Marquis de Sade (1740–1814), who described it in his literary works. The sadist, in extreme cases, becomes sexually aroused only by beating or otherwise mistreating his sexual partner.

SAINT ANTHONY'S FIRE A common name for ERYSIPELAS, an inflamed skin condition. It is also the name given to ergotism, a chronic poisoning by ergot, a fungus disease of rye. Ergotism may result from an overdose of drugs containing ergot, which may be used after childbirth to contract the muscles of the uterus.

SAINT VITUS'S DANCE See CHOREA.

SALINE Salty. A solution in pure water of sodium chloride (common salt) in the same concentration as exists in blood is sometimes called saline (pronounced say'leen).

SALIVA A mixture of mucus and fluid secreted by the salivary glands. These glands are located in the cheeks, under the tongue, and in the lower jaw. Saliva (pronounced *sa*·lie'*va*) keeps the mouth moist and softens and lubricates food so that it can be swallowed easily. A person normally secretes about three pints of saliva a day. The flow of saliva is controlled by the autonomic part of the NERVOUS SYSTEM. The sight or smell of food, or sometimes even the thought of food, starts a REFLEX action that causes the mouth to water.

Without the stimulus of food, the salivary glands continuously produce saliva at a slow rate. If the flow is insufficient to keep the mouth comfortably moist, the cause may simply be thirst or dehydration. Anxiety, certain medicines, and deficiency of the vitamin B complex are other possible causes of dry mouth. An excessive flow of saliva can likewise result from a variety of conditions, including nervous tension, irritation from dental appliances, di-

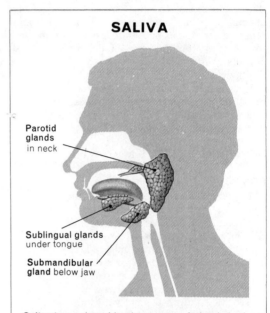

SALIVA

Parotid glands in neck

Sublingual glands under tongue

Submandibular gland below jaw

Saliva is produced by three pairs of glands in the face and neck. In the mouth, saliva mixes with food so that it can be tasted (taste buds cannot detect dry food), and enzymes in the saliva begin the digestion of starchy foods. Inflammation and enlargement of the parotid salivary gland below the ear is known medically as parotitis; the common name for the condition is mumps.

gestive disturbances, and certain toxic substances. Excessive salivation is also a symptom of certain infectious diseases, such as rabies and smallpox.

Saliva contains a digestive enzyme called ptyalin, which acts on starches. It also contains leukocytes (white blood cells) and elements of blood plasma, which help to prevent infection. When infection does occur anywhere in the upper part of the respiratory tract, the saliva is very likely to be contaminated. The tiny drops of saliva and sputum that are dispersed in the air when a person coughs are one way in which infection is spread from one person to others.

SALMONELLOSIS A type of FOOD POISONING caused by contamination with salmonella bacteria.

SALPINGECTOMY Surgical removal or cutting of one or both FALLOPIAN TUBES. (Pronounced sal″pin·jek′to·mee.) Because the egg cells cannot be fertilized by the sperm cells if both tubes are cut or removed, the operation is a completely effective and permanent method of contraception. Removal of a tube may be necessary in a tubal pregnancy (see ECTOPIC PREGNANCY).

SANATORIUM (sanitarium) An institution for the treatment of chronic disorders, such as a mental illness, tuberculosis, or alcoholism; also, a convalescent or nursing home. Sometimes, too, the term is applied to institutions that provide various types of therapy, exercise, and diet.

Sanatoriums are frequently run on a private-profit basis. If you need the type of care a sanatorium can provide, ask your physician's help in selecting an appropriate one with an adequate staff of doctors, nurses, and other personnel.

SARCOIDOSIS A chronic disease characterized by the development of small, fleshy lumps, or nodules, in the tissues. The lungs, the skin, and the LYMPH NODES are most often affected, but the nodules may appear anywhere in the body. Sarcoidosis (pronounced sahr″koy·doh′sis) in the lungs may be mistaken for tuberculosis, since both diseases show similar lesions in chest X rays. Symptoms may be absent or very mild. In more severe cases, there is low fever, weakness, lack of appetite, and loss of weight.

Sarcoidosis is also known as Boeck's sarcoid. It is not communicable, and the cause is not known. Cases occur in all parts of the world and in all races, but the disease is more prevalent among Negroes in the southern United States.

There is no specific treatment for sarcoidosis. The administration of CORTISONE and ACTH usually produces relief of symptoms. Sometimes the disease disappears without treatment. It is rarely fatal.

SARCOMA Any malignant tumor, or CANCER, that originates in connective TISSUE. (Pronounced sahr·koh′ma.)

SATYRIASIS A psychological abnormality in men, characterized by excessive desire for sexual relations. (Pronounced sat″i·rie′a·sis.)

SCABIES A skin infection caused by a MITE. (Pronounced skay′beez.)

SCALP The tough coating of skin and muscle that covers and protects the skull. The skin of the scalp is thicker than that of any other part of the body. It is covered with HAIR, which affords additional protection against accidental injury. Under the skin is a system of broad, flat muscles, some of which are continuations of facial muscles. For various disorders that may affect the skin of the scalp, see ALOPECIA (baldness), DANDRUFF, and RINGWORM.

SCAR The mark left on the skin or other tissue after a wound or sore has healed. Scars are made up of fibrous material. Most small scars fade as time goes by. Large scars can often be reduced in size and made less noticeable by means of PLASTIC SURGERY and skin grafting. The type of scar known as a KELOID, however, may be quite difficult to treat.

Scars on the inside of the body rarely give trouble. Occasionally ADHESIONS occur when scar tissue sticks to neighboring tissues and organs, sometimes interfering with normal function.

SCARIFICATION Tiny scratches or cuts in the outer layer of skin made for medical purposes. Scarification (pronounced skar″i·fi·kay′shun) is often used in VACCINATION instead of injection under the skin by a hypodermic needle.

SCARLET FEVER An infectious disease marked by fever, sore throat, and a widespread, bright red rash. It is also called scarlatina. It is caused by the same type of STREPTOCOCCUS bacterium that causes STREP THROAT. Scarlet fever develops only in people who are susceptible to the TOXIN, or poison, produced by the streptococci. (See DICK TEST.) Typically a disease of childhood, it may also occur in adults. Once a dreaded illness, it has become much milder in the last 50 years, and can now be easily treated with penicillin or other antibiotics.
Symptoms: Scarlet fever begins usually with nausea, vomiting, and headache. There is fever and sore throat, and the skin is hot and dry. In a day or so, the rash breaks out. The tongue is coated and turns a brilliant red (strawberry tongue). After about a week the rash fades, and the skin starts to peel. By this time, the disease is no longer contagious to others. The urine should be examined to ensure that NEPHRITIS (kidney disease) has not developed.

SCHICK TEST A test to show whether or not a person is immune to DIPHTHERIA. In the Schick (pronounced shik) test, a small amount of diphtheria toxin is injected just under the skin. The appearance within 48 hours of a red spot where the injection was made indicates that the person is susceptible to diphtheria and requires vaccination to produce immunity to the disease.

SCHIZOID Having some of the characteristics associated with SCHIZOPHRENIA. A schizoid (pronounced skit′soyd) person does not behave in a normal way, but has various quirks of personality that make life difficult for himself and those about him. PSYCHOTHERAPY may be useful in helping such an individual. The schizoid personality does not usually develop the extreme mental and emotional disruption characteristic of schizophrenia.

SCHIZOPHRENIA A serious mental disorder marked by irrational thinking, disturbed emotions,

537

and a breakdown in communicating with others. Schizophrenia (pronounced skit"soh·free'nee·a) is the commonest type of PSYCHOSIS. The cause is not known, although the possibility of a biochemical defect has been suggested. Environment also has an influence. Persons who develop schizophrenia often have a history of unhappiness and emotional stress in early childhood. Later, frustration and disappointment may contribute to its development. The disorder used to be known as dementia praecox.

Four different types of schizophrenia have been defined, although an individual case may change from one type to another or may have characteristics of several types at the same time. In *simple* schizophrenia, there is gradual mental deterioration and little tendency to have delusions and hallucinations. *Paranoid* schizophrenia is marked by suspiciousness and delusions of persecution. (See PARANOIA.) The CATATONIA type tends to fluctuate between extreme apathy and hyperactivity. In the hyperactive phase, erratic and confused behavior are often combined with delusions of grandeur. The HEBEPHRENIC type is marked by incoherent speech, laughing and crying without cause, and generally bizarre behavior.

PSYCHOTHERAPY has sometimes proved effective in the treatment of schizophrenia. TRANQUILIZERS and other special medicines are now replacing SHOCK THERAPY in attempting to make schizophrenics accessible to psychotherapy. With today's new approaches, the prospect for recovery is considerably better than in the past.

SCIATICA Severe pain in the SCIATIC NERVE (the large nerve that passes from the lower back into the leg), often associated with inflammation of the nerve, or NEURITIS. (Pronounced sie·at'i·ka.)

A slipped VERTEBRAL DISK may press on the sciatic nerve, causing excruciating pain in the lower back, thigh, and leg. Strain or injury of the lower back is a common cause. Frequently, no cause can be found.

Bed rest is often helpful in relieving sciatic pain. The leg is kept still, and heat is applied. Sedatives are prescribed. PHYSICAL THERAPY is useful. It is most important that the cause be identified and treated by a doctor.

SCIATIC NERVE The largest nerve in the body. There are two sciatic (pronounced sie·at'ik) nerves, one running down each leg. Each sciatic nerve begins at the lower spine and goes down the thigh to the knee, where it divides into two main branches that give rise to a complex network of nerves supplying the lower leg and the foot.

Like other nerves, the sciatic nerve is subject to inflammation. See also SCIATICA.

SCIRRHUS A hard cancerous tumor, generally rich in connective tissue. The breast is a common site of scirrhus.

SCLERA See EYE. (Pronounced sklir'a.)

SCLEROSIS Hardening of tissues. Sclerosis (pronounced skle·roh'sis) is found in a number of disorders. MULTIPLE SCLEROSIS is characterized by the development of hard areas on the nerves of the brain and spinal cord. HARDENING OF THE ARTERIES, also known as arteriosclerosis, is the most familiar type of sclerosis.

SCOLIOSIS Sideways curvature of the spine.

Scoliosis (pronounced skoh"lee·oh'sis) may be the result of habitually poor posture. In some cases, it may indicate a serious condition requiring prompt diagnosis and treatment. Scoliosis is often seen in children with rickets. Bone disease affecting either the hip or the vertebrae, weakness of spinal muscles, paralysis, sciatica, and lung disease are a few of the conditions that may produce scoliosis.

SCOPOLAMINE A substance obtained from various plants or produced synthetically. It is also called hyoscine. Scopolamine (pronounced skoh·pol'a·meen) slows down the nervous system, produces drowsiness, and interferes with the formation of memories. It has been used in combination with morphine in childbirth to produce the partial anesthesia known as TWILIGHT SLEEP. It is sometimes effective in preventing MOTION SICKNESS. It is used to relieve dizziness in MÉNIÈRE'S DISEASE and is one of many medicines used in treating PARKINSONISM. It causes dilation of the pupils and is sometimes used in eyedrops prior to eye examinations.

SCROFULA An old-fashioned name for a type of TUBERCULOSIS of the LYMPH NODES, usually those of the neck. For many hundreds of years, scrofula (pronounced skrof'yu·la) was also known as the king's evil, because it was believed that only the touch of a king's hand could cure it.

The disease usually affects children between the ages of three and seven. The germs may enter the body through the tonsils. As the disease progresses, the nodes swell and cluster together, forming abscesses that break through the skin and cause large, running sores. If left untreated, the sores eventually heal and leave unsightly scars. Once widespread, scrofula is rarer today because of the pasteurization of milk, which destroys any harmful bacteria in it, and because there are new medicines for treating tuberculosis.

SCROTUM The pouchlike structure that contains the TESTICLES.

SCURVY A disease caused by a severe lack of vitamin C (ASCORBIC ACID) in the diet. The medical name is scorbutus. Bottle-fed infants who receive no other foods may show signs of infantile scurvy between 6 and 12 months of age. (Those who are breast-fed usually obtain sufficient vitamin C from the mother's milk.) For this reason bottle-fed babies are given orange juice, which is rich in Vitamin C, or vitamin supplements.

Scurvy makes a child pale and irritable. He fails to gain weight. He may cry when he is moved, because of painful swellings in his limbs. The adult who is affected feels weak and short of breath. His skin may have many blue marks like bruises. The gums become spongy and bleed easily, and eventually the teeth begin to loosen.

Scurvy is easy to cure. A diet high in fruits and leafy green vegetables, supplemented by vitamin C tablets, can often remove all traces of the disease in less than a week.

SEASICKNESS   See MOTION SICKNESS.

SEBACEOUS CYST   See CYST. (Pronounced se·bay'shus sist'.)

SEBORRHEA   Excessive secretion of SEBUM by the oil glands in the skin. (Pronounced seb″o·ree'a.) Abnormally oily skin is often associated with certain skin disorders, such as acne, psoriasis, and eczema. In seborrhea, there is usually a tendency for the outermost layer of dead cells on the skin to come off in scales or flakes. See also DANDRUFF.

SEBUM   The oily substance secreted by the sebaceous glands in the skin. (Pronounced see'bum.)

SECONAL   Trade name for a BARBITURATE medicine used as a SEDATIVE. (Pronounced sek'o·nawl″.)

SECTION   In surgery, the act of cutting into tissue. The term is also used for a very thin slice of tissue prepared to be studied under the microscope (see BIOPSY). See also RESECTION.

SEDATION   The act of calming the emotions and relieving anxiety, especially by the administration of a SEDATIVE.

SEDATIVE   A substance that reduces irritability, excitement, and activity. Sedatives affect the nervous system. In moderate doses, they relieve emotional stress; in larger doses, they bring on sleep and also reduce sensibility to pain. Common sedatives include BARBITURATES and BROMIDES.

SEDIMENTATION RATE   See BLOOD TEST.

SEIZURE   See CONVULSION.

SEMEN   A thick, whitish fluid containing SPERM CELLS (male sex cells) as well as secretions from the PROSTATE GLAND, the seminal vesicles (two small pouches at the back of the bladder), and other glands. It is discharged during EJACULATION.

SEMICIRCULAR CANAL   See EAR.

SENILITY   Physical or mental deterioration that occurs in some persons in their later years. The term "senility" is often applied to the mental and emotional difficulties that sometimes appear in old age. These include extreme irritability, anxiety, loss of memory, depression, and a loss of ability to maintain proper feeding and dressing habits. In its most extreme form, senility is sometimes referred to as senile dementia or psychosis; the person may need constant supervision and treatment.

In many cases of senility, no sign can be found of significant changes in the brain. The elderly person may begin by feeling useless because, with advancing age, he is denied any meaningful role in society. Frustration builds upon frustration, until there is a withdrawal from life and a regression to infantile behavior. This kind of senility can be prevented, or its effects can be minimized, by involving older people in interesting and rewarding activities that give them a sense of worth. See also GERIATRICS.

SENNA   A LAXATIVE made of the dried leaves of various plants of the pea family. (Pronounced sen'a.)

SENSITIZED   The state of a person who reacts abnormally to some particular substance. A person who develops an ALLERGY to any substance is said to be sensitized to that substance. Sensitization involves the production of an ANTIBODY in the blood or tissues.

SEPSIS   The presence in the blood and tissues of disease germs or their toxins.

SEPTICEMIA   A medical term for BLOOD POISONING. (Pronounced sep″ti·see'mee·a.)

SERUM   The clear, yellowish, watery part of BLOOD. It is what remains after the blood's solid constituents have been removed by coagulation, or clotting. The process of clotting separates certain dissolved clotting factors as well. BLOOD PLASMA contains these factors, but blood serum does not. Blood serum does contain numerous substances in solution, such as digested nutrients, various salts, and a large variety of proteins, including GAMMA GLOBULIN proteins, which contain antibodies to combat infection.

Blood serum from animals that have been inoculated with bacteria or their toxins may be injected into humans to provide passive immunity against disease. See also IMMUNIZATION.

SERUM SICKNESS   A delayed reaction to foreign SERUM, such as an antitoxin injection. Certain widely used medicines, especially penicillin and other antibiotics, can also cause serum sickness. The symptoms may occur from one to three weeks after the injection is given or the medicine taken. Fever, hives, swollen lymph nodes, aches and pains in the muscles and joints, and nausea and vomiting may develop. Serum sickness usually lasts only two or three days. The doctor may prescribe ANTIHISTAMINES or other medicines.

Although serum sickness itself is not usually serious, it may sensitize a person so that a more dangerous reaction, known as anaphylactic SHOCK, may occur if the same injection or medicine is used again.

SEX ACT See COITUS.

SEX HORMONE Any of the numerous substances that normally regulate sexual development and reproduction. Like other hormones, the sex hormones are secreted under the influence of master hormones produced by the pituitary gland. At puberty, the pituitary gland normally begins to release certain substances which act on the gonads (the TESTICLES and the OVARIES). The master sex hormones released by the pituitary are FSH (*follicle-stimulating hormone*) and ICSH (*interstitial cell-stimulating hormone*). These master hormones stimulate the testicles to produce sperm cells and ANDROGENS (male sex hormones). They stimulate the ovaries to produce egg cells and ESTROGENS (female sex hormones). Normally, estrogens are secreted in insignificant amounts in men, and androgens in very small amounts in women. Irregularities in the proportions of estrogens and androgens may produce abnormal sexual characteristics, such as breast development in men or growth of facial hair in women.

The principal androgen is called *testosterone*. It stimulates the changes that take place in boys at puberty, such as increase in size of the genitals, deepening of the voice, growth of hair on the face, muscular strength, and heavy bone development. Testosterone is produced fairly steadily in the testicles throughout the adult life of a man, although there is some decline with age.

A number of estrogens are produced by the ovaries, as well as a substance called progesterone. The secretion of estrogens and progesterone regulates the changes that take place during the menstrual cycle. (See MENSTRUATION.) Estrogens also influence such secondary female characteristics as breast development and the typical distribution of fat that gives women more rounded contours than men have. These hormones are produced abundantly only during the period from puberty until the MENOPAUSE. Such hormones are the active ingredient in contraceptive pills. (See ORAL CONTRACEPTION.)

SEXUAL INTERCOURSE See COITUS.

SHINGLES Inflammation along the course of a sensory nerve leading out from the spine, characterized by great pain and crops of small blisters. The medical term is herpes zoster. It has been shown that shingles is caused by the same virus that causes chicken pox.

The nerves affected are usually those on the abdomen and chest, on one side of the body only. Sometimes the inflammation affects the nerves of the face and can result in serious damage to the sight.

Treatment: Shingles is a very painful and distressing disease. There are some medicines that the doctor can prescribe to relieve the pain and ward off eye damage. Most people recover in two or three weeks, but the pain along the nerve may, especially in the elderly, persist for many months after the rash has disappeared.

SHIVERING Uncontrollable shaking, usually caused by cold or a chill. Shivering generates heat in the muscles, and so it is a normal reaction to cold and helps to make one warmer. But when a person who is not cold shivers, it may be a symptom of a disease.

Shivering, especially when accompanied by fever, generally occurs in patients with influenza, pneumonia, or tonsillitis; it may even be an early symptom of blood poisoning or poliomyelitis. Glandular fever and malaria often give rise to bouts of shivering. Violent shivering may be a form of CONVULSION. See also CHOREA; EPILEPSY; PARKINSONISM.

SHOCK A medical term for a set of signs and symptoms (the shock SYNDROME) associated with failure or collapse of the circulatory system. The signs of shock include weakness, extreme pallor, cold and moist skin, weak and rapid pulse, irregular and shallow breathing, thirst, nausea, scanty secretion of urine, and HYPOTENSION (low blood pressure).

The shock syndrome indicates an extreme medical emergency. It may develop suddenly and become rapidly worse unless preventive measures are taken without delay. Anyone who has had a serious injury or burn should be watched very closely for signs of delayed shock, which may not develop until several hours after the injury. If signs of shock appear, call a doctor at once. Follow the directions in the FIRST AID section until the doctor arrives. If a doctor cannot be located immediately, transport the person in shock to the nearest hospital, preferably by ambulance.

Shock can be caused by many factors. *Anaphylactic* shock is a violent and sometimes fatal reaction to injection of a substance to which the body has been sensitized by a previous injection. (See ALLERGY.) The sting of a bee or a wasp may induce anaphylactic shock in a person sensitized by previous stings. *Cardiac* shock is due to a sudden decrease in the heart's pumping capacity, as in serious heart disease. Internal or external bleeding, as well as loss of fluid through burns, vomiting, or diarrhea, may cause *low-volume* shock. Severe toxic states and injury to the brain can cause blood vessels to dilate and induce shock.

The term "shock" is often used for conditions that do not resemble the shock syndrome, although they may be very serious and require emergency treatment. *Psychic* shock refers to the dazed or distraught condition seen in people who have experienced some disaster or great personal loss. *Shell* shock is a general term for a serious emotional disorder occurring among soldiers at war; it is now more commonly called combat fatigue. See also ELECTRIC SHOCK.

SHOCK THERAPY A method of treating mental patients. It consists of producing convulsions and unconsciousness by electric current or sometimes by insulin or other substances. The treatments (a series is usually required) are followed up with PSYCHOTHERAPY to treat the underlying condition. In recent years, tranquilizers and antidepressants have been used more and more in place of shock therapy.

SIAMESE TWIN Either one of twins who are joined together at birth, usually at the head, the chest, or the hip. Siamese twins are always identical twins—that is, they have developed from a single fertilized egg cell and hence have the same sex and the same genetic makeup. The condition is a rare kind of BIRTH DEFECT. The first such twins to receive wide publicity were born in Siam (now Thailand), but conjoined twins are just as rare there as anywhere else. Siamese twins can usually be separated surgically, unless a single heart or some other vital organ is shared by both twins.

SICKLE-CELL ANEMIA See ANEMIA.

SIDEROSIS Inflammation of the lungs caused by long periods of inhaling smoke and dust containing minute particles of iron. Miners of iron ore, welders, and workers who cut and grind iron and steel often develop siderosis (pronounced sid″*e*·roh′sis). Siderosis is mild, does not interfere with breathing, and requires no treatment other than measures to avoid inhaling the substances that are responsible for the inflammation. See also SILICOSIS.

SILICOSIS A disease of the lungs caused by breathing silica dust over a period of years. Hard-rock miners, stonecutters, and workers engaged in sandblasting are frequently affected. Silicosis (pronounced sil″*i*·koh′sis) develops gradually and often unnoticed. The person becomes short of breath and has a constant dry cough. The silica dust scars and thickens the lung tissue so that the person may develop bronchitis, emphysema, and tuberculosis.

In a related lung disease of coal miners—called anthracosis or anthrasilicosis—the lungs become black, thus the popular name "black lung."

Prevention: Silicosis and black lung are serious diseases. Workers exposed to silica dust or coal dust should wear breathing masks, unless there is special ventilation equipment to carry off the dust. Periodic chest X rays help detect early signs of both diseases so that they can be treated and arrested.

See also ASBESTOSIS; SIDEROSIS.

SILVER NITRATE A colorless salt that slowly decomposes and turns dark on exposure to light. A solution of silver nitrate is sometimes used as an ANTISEPTIC and germicide, especially to treat small areas of mucous membrane. Dressings soaked in dilute silver nitrate solution may be used on burns to prevent infection. It or an antibiotic is also used on a newborn baby to prevent eye infection. Solid silver nitrate crystals, or lunar caustic molded into pencils or cones, are a convenient means of applying silver nitrate locally.

SINUS, PARANASAL Any of the four sets of hollows in the skull near the nose. The paranasal (pronounced par″*a*·nay′zal) sinuses include the frontal sinuses in the forehead; the maxillary sinuses in the cheekbones; the sphenoidal sinuses at the back of the nasal passages; and the ethmoidal sinuses, behind and below the frontal sinuses. All of the paranasal sinuses have passages leading into the nose.

The function of the sinuses is not completely understood. It is known that they lighten the weight of the skull and help to warm and moisten the air as it is breathed in. See also SINUSITIS.

SINUSITIS Inflammation of the mucous membranes of one or more of the air-filled cavities in the bones of the head that connect with the nose. (See SINUS, PARANASAL.) Sinusitis (pronounced sie″nu·sie′tis) often occurs during a head cold, when the infection from the nose spreads into the sinuses. When the membranes lining the sinuses become swollen and inflamed, the tiny passages leading to the nose may become completely stopped up. Sinusitis is also caused by allergies; infected teeth and tonsils; and irritation by cigarette smoke and dry or dusty air.

Symptoms: The frontal and maxillary sinuses are the ones most often affected. There is headache if the frontal sinuses are involved, and pain in the cheekbones if the maxillary sinuses are inflamed. A thick, unpleasant discharge comes from the nose, and there may be fever. When the symptoms persist for a long period, postnasal drip may develop. Mucus from the sinuses, instead of draining through the nose, drips down the back of the throat. The mucus may infect the bronchial tubes, causing chronic BRONCHITIS.

Treatment: In severe cases of acute sinusitis, the treatment consists of bed rest and medicines to help the sinuses drain. Because the infection can spread to the ears, the neighboring bones, and, in rare cases, to the brain, the doctor may also prescribe ANTIBIOTICS. Aspirin every two or three hours and a heating pad or hot water bottle applied to the face or forehead may relieve pain.

Sufferers from chronic sinusitis should avoid smoking. A VAPORIZER in the bedroom or work space may prove helpful. Sometimes a minor surgical operation may improve drainage from the sinuses.

SKELETAL SYSTEM The jointed framework of rigid BONES that supports the soft tissues of the body. There are 206 bones in the adult skeletal system. As a system, the bones give the body its shape; they form cages and boxes that protect fragile organs; and they form a complicated lever system that permits body movements.

There are two main parts to the skeletal system: the axial skeleton and the appendicular skeleton. **The axial skeleton** consists of the skull, the spine, and the rib cage. All of these axial bones provide protection for vital parts of the body. The skull encloses the brain and supports and protects the sense organs in the head (eyes, nose, and ears). The spine, or backbone, is made up of separate bones, called vertebrae, which are joined together to form a hollow, somewhat flexible tube that protects the spinal cord. The 12 pairs of ribs are attached to the vertebrae and curve around to the front, forming a cage that protects lungs and heart.

The appendicular skeleton consists of the shoulder (pectoral) and hip (pelvic) girdles and the arm and leg bones. The pelvic girdle protects the internal organs of the reproductive and urinary systems; but the main function of the appendicular skeleton is movement. For the most part, each MUSCLE is attached by TENDONS at either end to two different bones, so that when the muscle contracts, the JOINT between the bones is forced to bend. Most movements are performed by two distinct sets of muscles acting in opposition to each other. One set pulls in one direction to bend a joint, and an opposing set pulls in the other direction to straighten it out again. Many of the muscles that move the arms and legs have one end attached to a bone of the axial system. Thus the axial skeleton as well as the appendicular skeleton is essential in movement.

At the joints, the ends of the bones are shaped to fit into each other, and the joints are strengthened and held together by bands of tough tissue called LIGAMENTS. The joints are lined with CARTILAGE, which lessens friction and acts as a shock absorber. There are separate pads, or disks, of cartilage between the vertebrae of the spine.

Some movable joints can move freely in any direction, such as the joints at the shoulder and the hip, which are constructed like a ball fitted into a socket. Other joints, such as knee and elbow joints, can move in only one direction, like the hinge on a door. Some bones, such as the skull bones, are joined together rigidly. In infancy these junctures have some flexibility to allow for growth, but in adulthood they become fused together.

SKIN The outer covering of the body, also called the integument. The skin has several functions. It is a barrier against germs. It is a tough, resilient cushion that protects the tissues underneath. It helps regulate body temperature. When it is hot, glands in the skin secrete perspiration, the evaporation of which causes cooling. Or, when it is cold, constriction of the blood vessels in the skin cuts down the flow of blood near the body's surface and so reduces heat loss.

The skin is also a sense organ whose nerve endings respond to pain, heat, cold, touch, and pressure. The skin supplies much of the body's vitamin D requirements by producing a substance that changes into vitamin D when it is exposed to the ultraviolet radiation in sunlight. Finally, the skin gives rise to special structures: the hair and the nails.

The skin is built up of two distinct layers, the epidermis, or outer covering, and the dermis, or true skin. The outermost part of the epidermis consists of flat, dead cells that are constantly being shed, or sloughed off. The underlying part of the epidermis is made up of rapidly dividing cells. These are continually pushing upward and replacing the dead cells above them. HAIRS and NAILS, which are also composed of dead cells, are produced by specialized epidermis that extends downward into the dermis.

Tiny blood vessels and nerve endings are densely woven into the flexible connective tissue that makes up the dermis, and sweat glands and oil glands are embedded in it.

Skin owes its color partly to the blood, whose tinge shows through translucent tissues, and partly to various PIGMENTS in the epidermis. The chief pigment in skin is MELANIN.

SKIN ERUPTION Any irregularity or lesion that develops suddenly on the skin. Skin eruptions take various forms, including inflammation, swelling, blistering, redness, spots, PUSTULES, and hard lumps. Some kinds of skin eruptions are accompanied by itching or pain. A special branch of medicine (dermatology) is devoted to skin eruptions. Some of the principal skin eruptions are listed below. For more detailed descriptions of these, consult the separate entries.

ACNE, LUPUS VULGARIS, and PSORIASIS are among the skin eruptions for which no definite cause is known.

Exterior injury of various kinds, including friction, extreme heat and cold, pressure, and exposure to toxic chemicals and radiation may produce skin reactions. (See ACID BURN, BEDSORE, BURN, CHILBLAIN, FROSTBITE, PRICKLY HEAT, and SUNBURN.)

Bacteria are responsible for BOILS, ERYSIPELAS, FOLLICULITIS, and IMPETIGO. FEVER SORES, SHINGLES, and WARTS are caused by viruses. ATHLETE'S FOOT, RINGWORM, and MONILIASIS are fungal infections.

HIVES is a usually minor skin eruption due to ALLERGY. Related to allergies are local reactions caused by INSECT BITES, POISON IVY, and other toxic substances. MITES, which are very like insects, are responsible for the highly contagious skin eruption known as scabies.

Skin eruptions are sometimes signs of disease affecting the whole body. SYPHILIS produces typical skin eruptions, first at the site of infection and later in other parts of the body. CHICKEN POX, MEASLES, ROSEOLA, RUBELLA, and SCARLET FEVER have characteristic skin eruptions.

SKIN GRAFT A method used to repair badly damaged areas of skin, such as a severe burn or a place where the original skin has been removed by surgery. Skin grafting is an important technique in PLASTIC SURGERY. Skin grafts are the oldest and most successful types of tissue transplants because, since the new skin is taken from another part of the patient's own body, there can be no rejection problems such as are encountered in ORGAN TRANSPLANTS. Skin grafting also works between identical twins, whose tissue types are sufficiently similar for no rejection to take place.

Skin for grafting is generally taken from the thigh, back, or abdomen. Small areas may be covered using a *pinch* graft consisting of a thin layer of surface skin about one quarter of an inch across. Larger areas need thicker grafts, containing the whole of the epidermis layer (*split-thickness* grafts) or the epidermis and dermis layers (*full-thickness* grafts). Some full-thickness grafts are left partly attached to the original site, to preserve their supply of nerves and blood vessels while they are growing. New skin grows over the area from which the graft is taken.

SLEEP During sleep, the body and nervous system become almost inactive. The conscious mind ceases to function, but processes such as breathing and digestion (controlled by the AUTONOMIC NERVOUS SYSTEM) continue. Sleep is essential to mental and physical health, but the amount varies according to age and individual needs. The need for sleep is greatest in infancy; a newborn infant sleeps most of the day. Young children should have 11 to 12 hours of sleep a night; for older children, 10 hours is usually sufficient. Adults generally require six to eight hours of sleep.

Dreaming: At intervals during sleep, the eyes of the sleeper move under his eyelids as if they were wide open and looking at moving objects. If the person is awakened at this stage, he can usually recall a vivid dream. If he is allowed to continue sleeping, he may later recall nothing. Four other distinct stages occur in normal sleep, marked by changes in electric

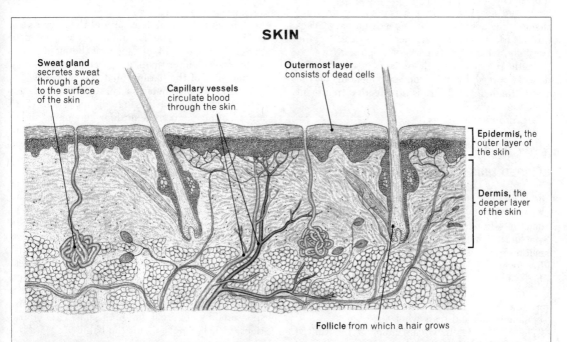

SKIN

Sweat gland secretes sweat through a pore to the surface of the skin

Capillary vessels circulate blood through the skin

Outermost layer consists of dead cells

Epidermis, the outer layer of the skin

Dermis, the deeper layer of the skin

Follicle from which a hair grows

The two main layers of the skin are the epidermis (which includes the thin outermost layer of dead cuticle cells) and the dermis beneath it. Buried beneath the skin are the various kinds of receptors of the sense of touch, and passing through the dermis are hair follicles and ducts from sweat glands. An important function of the skin is to act as a barrier against invasion by germs.

activity in the brain, in breathing, and other vital signs.

The dreaming stage seems to be very important to our well-being. The subject matter of the few dreams we remember is often so strange and puzzling that we are tempted to try to find a meaning in them. According to PSYCHOANALYSIS, dreaming is a safety valve for repressed fears and desires.

Nightmares: Dreams are usually pleasant or neutral, but sometimes we waken in terror. Nightmares are particularly frightening to children, who may cry out or wake up crying. If the parent goes into the child's room and comforts him, he will usually relax and go back to sleep. Sometimes it is helpful to have a small night-light in the child's room. When nightmares persist, and there are symptoms of emotional disturbance in the child's waking life, the problem should be brought to the attention of the family physician.

SLEEPING PILL See SOPORIFIC.

SLEEPING SICKNESS Also called African sleeping sickness. A disease caused by the presence in the bloodstream of infectious protozoans (microscopic, one-celled animals) called trypanosomes. The disease is known medically as trypanosomiasis. Characteristic symptoms are fever, skin eruptions, painful local swelling (EDEMA), and nervous disorders. The final stage of the disease is marked by prolonged sleeping. Drugs are available for treating sleeping sickness, but cure depends on early diagnosis. African sleeping sickness is spread by the tsetse fly, which infests parts of tropical Africa.

South American trypanosomiasis, or Chagas' disease, is spread by the blood-sucking bug of the family *Reduviidae*. There is no effective treatment for Chagas' disease.

See also ENCEPHALITIS.

SLEEPWALKING See SOMNAMBULISM.

SLIPPED DISK See VERTEBRAL DISK.

SMALLPOX A highly contagious viral disease characterized by a rash that leaves pitted scars. Sometimes blindness results.

Symptoms: Smallpox has an average INCUBATION PERIOD of from 10 to 14 days. About the third day after fever, headache, and nausea have developed, pinkish-red spots appear on the face, then spread over most of the body; later they become large and pustular. The lesions are deep in the skin, and leave permanent pits and scars when they heal.

The World Health Organization of the United Nations and various national health agencies have kept constant watch to prevent travel by anyone who may have contracted the disease. This vigilance, together with a worldwide program of VACCINATION and public health measures, has wiped out the disease in nearly every country. Therefore, in the United States smallpox vaccination is neither required nor recommended by the U.S. Public Health Service. Inoculation is recommended only for persons traveling to those few parts of the world where the disease may yet occur.

SMEGMA A mixture of dead skin cells and SEBUM (oil from the skin). Smegma (pronounced smeg'ma) tends to collect in the folds of the CLITORIS and the foreskin of the PENIS; hence, special attention should be given to keeping the genitals clean.

SMELLING SALTS Any of several preparations containing crystals or solutions of ammonium compounds. Held under the nose of someone who feels faint or dizzy, the ammonia from smelling salts acts as a stimulant, increasing the rate of breathing and helping the person to recover.

SMOKING In recent years, an increasing number of scientific studies have shown that cigarette smokers have significantly poorer health than nonsmokers, and that they die at an earlier average age. A heavy smoker (two or more packs a day) is 20 times more likely than a nonsmoker to have LUNG CANCER. The degree of risk is related to how much a person smokes. Emphysema, bronchitis, heart disease, hardening of the arteries, and a long list of other disabling conditions occur with increased frequency among cigarette smokers.

Pipes and cigars are less harmful than cigarettes, but not altogether safe. Even if no smoke is inhaled, there is increased risk of cancer of the mouth, lips, and tongue. A filter tip on a cigarette removes only a small part of the harmful material in smoke.

Tobacco smoke contains a substantial list of cancer-producing and noxious ingredients. Among these are nicotine, carbon monoxide, ammonia, and a variety of harmful substances called tars. Many of these substances are present in chewing tobacco and snuff as well as in smoke.

Giving Up Smoking: Many people have succeeded in stopping smoking. It may be difficult, but it is not at all impossible. The first and most essential step is to decide that you really want to stop. Then avoid temporarily any habits or activities that you associate with smoking, and just stop—either abruptly or cutting down gradually at first. The first few days are the hardest. There may be a tendency to overeat when you first give up smoking, but moderate overweight is much less harmful than smoking, and it can be corrected by diet. There are many programs, sponsored by nonprofit and profit-making organizations, to help smokers quit the habit.

SNAKEBITE The venom of snakes is produced by a special gland inside the mouth. It contains substances that act on the nervous system, as well as some digestive enzymes. Venom serves mainly to paralyze the snake's prey, which is swallowed live and whole, and aids the digestive process. Only a few kinds of snakes produce venom poisonous enough to kill the snake's enemies.

Dangerous snakes found in large areas of North America are the rattlesnake, the copperhead, and the water moccasin, or cottonmouth. These snakes all inject poison through special fangs that leave characteristic double puncture marks on the skin. There is immediate pain and swelling at the site of the bite. The small but very poisonous coral snakes, which occur only in the southern United States, leave two rows of fine tooth marks, and there is little pain and swelling. An effective antidote, or antivenin, has been developed for each of the dangerous snake venoms. For instructions on emergency treatment, see the FIRST AID section.

SODIUM BICARBONATE
A white powder, also known as bicarbonate of soda or baking soda. A teaspoonful dissolved in a glass of water is a popular and effective remedy for INDIGESTION. Sodium bicarbonate should not be taken by anyone with heart disease or on a salt-restricted diet.

A cupful dissolved in bath water along with two cupfuls of starch helps relieve the itching of allergic reactions. A paste of sodium bicarbonate and water or cold cream relieves the discomfort of insect bites.

SODIUM CITRATE
A soluble white substance with a salty taste. Sodium citrate (pronounced soh'dee·um sit'rayt) is sometimes prescribed to overcome excessive acidity in the urine, thus preventing the formation of certain kinds of urinary tract stones. This medication is always taken by mouth, since sodium citrate prevents normal clotting if it is injected into the bloodstream.

SODIUM PENTOTHAL
See PENTOTHAL.

SODIUM SALICYLATE
A substance related chemically to ASPIRIN and having similar effects in reducing fever and relieving pain. (Pronounced soh'dee·um sal'i·sil"ayt.)

SODIUM THIOSULFATE
A substance sometimes used in swimming pools and baths to prevent RINGWORM infection. Sodium thiosulfate (pronounced soh'dee·um thie"oh·sul'fayt) is also used, along with sodium nitrite, as an antidote for cyanide poisoning. Another name for this compound is sodium hyposulfite.

SOMNAMBULISM
Moving about and performing various actions while asleep; sleepwalking. Somnambulism (pronounced som·nam'byu·liz"em) is most likely to occur in children and during the first third of the night. On waking, the sleepwalker can remember nothing of what occurred. Children who sleepwalk usually lose the habit as they grow older.

SOPORIFIC
A substance used to induce sleep. A soporific (pronounced soh"po·rif'ik) is also known medically as a HYPNOTIC; in popular usage, it is a sleeping pill.

BARBITURATES are the most familiar of the soporifics. They may be obtained only with a physician's prescription and should be used exactly as directed. Phenobarbital, Amytal, Nembutal, and Seconal are some of those that are widely used. Continued taking of barbiturates may lead to dependency on them.

SORDES
Brown crusts which appear on the lips and gums of a patient with fever. They should be gently removed with a piece of bandage or lint soaked in a weak antiseptic solution. (Pronounced sor'deez.)

SORE THROAT
Inflammation and soreness may affect any part of the pharynx (PHARYNGITIS) or the tonsils (TONSILLITIS), or may extend through the entire THROAT. Throat infections may spread below the epiglottis and into the larynx (LARYNGITIS); the windpipe, or trachea (TRACHEITIS); or the esophagus (esophagitis).

Sore throat is often one of the first symptoms of an acute infection, such as the common cold, diphtheria, influenza, STREP THROAT, infectious mononucleosis, measles, rheumatic fever, scarlet fever, and VINCENT'S ANGINA. If you have a very sore throat, be sure to consult a doctor immediately, especially if you have a fever as well.

Sore throat may also be due to air pollution, smoking, and misusing the voice (see CLERGYMAN'S THROAT).

SPANISH FLY
See APHRODISIAC.

SPANSULE
A type of capsule designed to release a medicine gradually over a period of several hours within the body. (Pronounced span'sul.)

SPARE-PART SURGERY
Surgery that involves replacing or repairing parts of the body with artificial devices. Man-made spare parts include chins, tracheas (windpipes), hip joints, heart valves, arteries, and veins.

The devices are made from stainless-steel alloys, plastics, or silicones. These materials are inert and do not provoke a rejection by the body's system; the body tolerates their presence and does not form antibodies against them. These materials are also used because they do not corrode, irritate neighboring tissues, destroy red blood cells, or cause blood clots, and because they function well over a long period.

In many ways, devices made of inert materials are simpler to introduce than organs taken from other human beings. When an organ from another person is transplanted, the problem of rejection arises and

SPARE-PART SURGERY

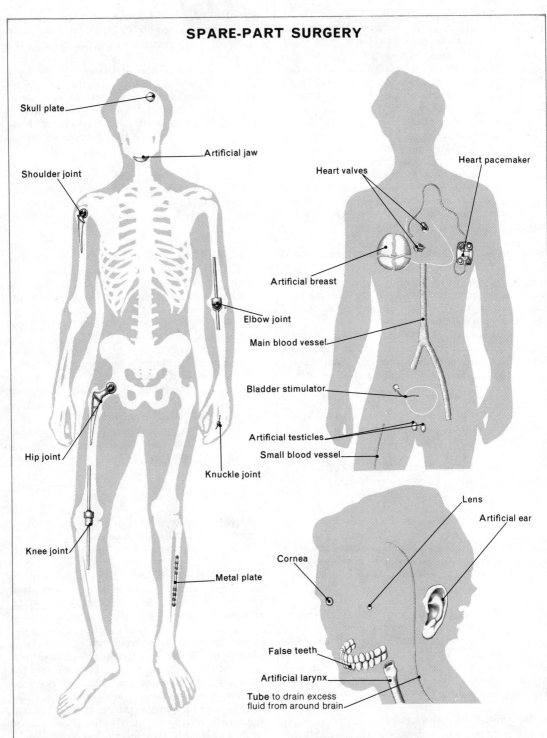

Devices of metal and plastic are used to replace organs of the body in spare-part surgery. These materials are not rejected by the body. They are also useful because they do not irritate the tissues, and they continue to function over a long period. Metal alloys are used in repairing joints, such as the knee and the elbow, or as plates and supports; plastic tubes replace arteries and veins. Other spare parts include heart valves and pacemakers, artificial larynx, and bladder stimulator.

drugs must be given to control the immune reaction (see ORGAN TRANSPLANT).

Spare-part replacements for joints are made of steel alloy. This metal is used to make the top portion (head and neck) of the thighbone, and polyethylene for the acetabulum (the socket of the hipbone into which the ball of the femur fits). The friction between the ball and socket is minimized by polishing the bearing surfaces, although the result only approximates the smoothness of movement that is found in the natural joint.

Metal can also be used to replace the humerus (the bone of the upper arm) and the elbow and knee joints. There are also metal femur supports and knee and shin plates.

Plastics are more widely used than metals in spare-part surgery. For example, tubes of Dacron can replace diseased parts of major blood vessels, such as the aorta and arteries in the legs and abdomen. The tube itself is corrugated or plaited to allow it to follow the contours of surrounding organs. Tubes of polytetrafluorethylene (PTFE, or Teflon) are used to replace smaller arteries. A plastic lens may be substituted for a diseased eye lens.

Silicones are the most promising materials from which spare parts are made. These materials produce hardly any bodily reaction, and they do not cause bacterial growth. However, injections of liquid silicones used to build up and enlarge a woman's breasts can produce adverse reactions; silicone rubber, implanted under the breasts, is safer.

Silicones are also used in the reconstruction of external features, such as the ear, or to repair damaged internal parts, such as the chin bone or a testicle. Silicone rubber rods can be implanted as temporary replacements for finger tendons.

Artificial heart valves contain a silicone-coated rubber ball enclosed in a stainless steel cage; the ring at the base of the valve is made of PTFE. These artificial valves do not have ideal flow characteristics, but they are a great improvement on defective natural valves that they are designed to replace.

Small battery-run CARDIAC PACEMAKERS are also coated with silicone. These spare parts stimulate a defective heart with tiny electrical impulses and restore normal rhythm.

SPASM A sudden, involuntary contraction involving a muscle or muscles and usually accompanied by pain. The contraction may be caused by a disturbance of the circulation, by a disease, or by some irregularity in the chemical processes of the body. There are numerous types of spasms, ranging from slight twitchings, or tics, to convulsions.

Tic: A tic is a spasmodic movement that is without pain. Often it is seen as a twitching in an area of the face, but it may be a shrugging of the shoulder, a jerking of the leg, a blinking of the eyes, or some other sudden movement that is repeated again and again. Tics occurring in CHOREA (Saint Vitus's dance) are irregular and tend to skip about from one group of muscles to another.

Cramp: A cramp is also a type of spasm—a tonic spasm, or one in which the muscles stay rigid for a long while. Cramps often occur in the legs during sleep or while swimming, and they can be extremely painful. The cause is frequently strain, cold, or impaired circulation. Massaging the leg and walking about help to relieve the cramp.

Convulsion: A convulsion is a particularly violent involuntary contraction of the muscles. Sometimes the person loses consciousness. Convulsions occur in certain childhood diseases, often in association with a high temperature; they may also be found with diabetes, alkalosis, low blood sugar, and in certain types of EPILEPSY. See also the separate entry, CONVULSION.

SPASTIC Characterized by, or resembling, spasms. The term is most frequently applied to spastic paralysis, a type of CEREBRAL PALSY. In spastic paralysis, the person suffers spasms of the muscles. The legs are generally more seriously affected than the arms, and the individual moves about with considerable stiffness in what is described as a scissors gait.

Spastic hemiplegia is a type of spastic paralysis affecting one side of the body. The most common cause of this condition is STROKE. When an attempt is made to move muscles on the paralyzed side, spasms are produced.

In spastic paraplegia, the legs are paralyzed; when the person tries to move them, he experiences spasms in the leg muscles.

Spastic COLITIS is a disorder of the gastrointestinal tract that is usually caused by nervous tension and poor eating habits.

SPECIES (plural, **species**) A group of individual organisms (plants, animals, or germs) that have some characteristic or combination of characteristics that distinguishes them from all other groups.

A special branch of biology, called taxonomy, is devoted solely to classifying and naming all the different kinds of living things. The species is usually the smallest subdivision in this scientific classification. (In certain cases, a species may be divided into a number of different races, varieties, or strains.) The next largest subdivision above species is the genus.

The names of the genus and the species to which a living organism belongs usually have a Latin form. An example of a scientific name is *Mycobacterium tuberculosis,* which a scientist of almost any country would understand to refer to the germ that causes tuberculosis. In this case, the genus is *Mycobacterium* and the species is *tuberculosis.*

SPECULUM (plural, **specula**) A medical instrument for stretching a body passageway or opening in order to examine the interior. (Pronounced spek'yu·lum.)

SPEECH DEFECTS AND DISORDERS A person may be unable to speak correctly or clearly because of physical abnormalities, emotional problems, or damage to the speech center of the brain or to the nerves involved in speech. Missing teeth may make proper articulation difficult. Malformation of the nose and tongue or abnormalities of the lungs or LARYNX may interfere with the production of normal sounds and speech. Two other causes of speech problems are HARELIP and CLEFT PALATE.

Stuttering and *stammering* are two related speech problems of psychological origin. In stuttering, the individual repeats a sound spasmodically, such as the first letter of a word. In stammering, he keeps repeating a syllable or a word involuntarily.

Stuttering is linked by many authorities to a disturbed home, an emotional shock, or, very often, to a family predisposition. Sometimes the child may have a parent who is overeager to get him to talk correctly at an early age. Good results can be obtained by speech therapy, either in individual sessions or in classes. Psychological counseling may be needed to treat underlying emotional disorders.

In *lisping*, the letters *s* and *z* are pronounced like *th* because the tongue is against the bottom of the teeth or because the jaw or teeth are malformed. If the mouth is normal, the child may outgrow the habit, or he may be trained in a corrective class to form the proper sound.

A child suffering from congenital or early DEAFNESS needs special training in speaking, since he can not hear others' voices or his own.

Other Causes of Speech Disorders: Various other speech disorders are caused by damage to the speech center of the brain or to the nerves that send impulses to the muscles involved in speech. The speech center may be damaged by a stroke, a brain tumor, syphilis, or multiple sclerosis, so that the person speaks in a slurred, singsong, or staccato manner. See also APHASIA.

SPERMATOCYSTITIS Inflammation of the seminal vesicles in the male genitourinary system. Spermatocystitis (pronounced sper"ma·toh·sis·tie'tis) is often associated with inflammation of the urinary bladder, or CYSTITIS. See also GENITALS.

SPERM CELL The male cell, or spermatozoon, which is produced in great numbers in the TESTICLES. It unites with the female egg cell, or ovum, to produce a new individual. See also EMBRYO.

SPHINCTER A circular band of muscular fibers at the exit or entrance of an organ or in some other part of the body. By contracting, the sphincter (pronounced sfingk'ter) narrows the passageway or closes it completely.

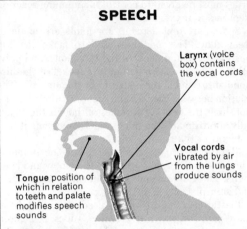

SPEECH

Larynx (voice box) contains the vocal cords

Vocal cords vibrated by air from the lungs produce sounds

Tongue position of which in relation to teeth and palate modifies speech sounds

The sounds of the human voice are produced by air vibrating the vocal cords in the larynx, or voice box. The pitch of the basic sounds depends on the length and tension of the cords – the shorter or tighter the cord, the higher the note.

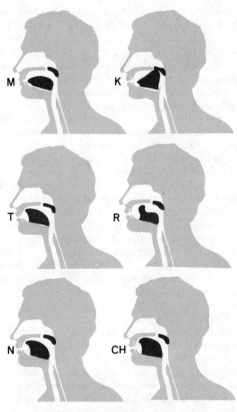

M   K

T   R

N   CH

The actual speech sounds are formed by the shape of the mouth and nasal cavities, and depend on the positions of the tongue, palate, lips and teeth. The diagrams show the positions of these in pronouncing various sounds in English.

There are numerous sphincters in the body. Typical in its action is the sphincter of the BLADDER, which is controlled by the will, as are those of the anus. The pyloric sphincter separates the stomach from the duodenum. It is relaxed automatically when the food in the stomach is ready to pass onward. (See DIGESTION.)

SPHYGMOMANOMETER An instrument used to measure BLOOD PRESSURE. (Pronounced sfig"moh·ma·nom'e·ter.)

SPIDER BITE In the United States there are two types of poisonous spiders: the black widow and the brown house spider. Tarantula bites are usually not serious.

The black widow is coal black in color and has a reddish-orange mark, shaped like an hourglass, on its belly. Only the female bites. It is found in woods, fields, and outdoor sheds and privies. The bite produces a sharp pain that may soon go away. In about half an hour the venom, which attacks the nerves, causes the abdominal muscles to become rigid. Later, there may be difficulty in breathing, tremor, and pain in the limbs. The victim should be taken immediately to a hospital for a serum injection.

The brown house spider is also known as the brown recluse because it hides in closets, dresser drawers, beds, and other dark areas of the home. It is most commonly found in the Far West and Middle West. Its venom contains a substance that is destructive to tissue and causes the site of the bite to become a large, spreading sore. The victim should call his doctor as soon as possible. ANTIHISTAMINES and CORTISONE medicines keep the sore from growing larger and help to promote healing.

SPINA BIFIDA A birth defect of the central nervous system caused by a failure of the vertebrae to close fully around the SPINAL CORD. HYDROCEPHALUS and reduced control of the BOWEL, the BLADDER, and the muscles below the waist are often caused by this condition. (Pronounced speih'na bi'fi·da.)

SPINAL CORD A thick, soft, long cord of nervous tissue that extends from the brain and the bottom of the skull to the first lumbar vertebra. It is 17 or 18 inches long and is enclosed within the spinal canal. (See SPINE.) With the brain it makes up the central NERVOUS SYSTEM.

The spinal cord is composed of white and gray matter formed by an elaborate assembly of nerves—rather like a telephone cable made up of innumerable wires—that carry messages (nervous impulses) to and from the brain. Pairs of nerves (31 in all) extending from the spinal cord to different parts of the body pick up and transmit the impulses to the brain.

Spinal Fluid: The spinal cord is surrounded by protective membranes (meninges) and the fluid of the spinal canal. This fluid undergoes changes in its chemical composition in the presence of certain diseases of the nervous system. In cases of suspected multiple sclerosis, stroke, poliomyelitis, meningitis, tumor, and similar disorders, a sample of the spinal fluid may be taken and analyzed as a help in diagnosing the disease. The sample is extracted by means of a hollow needle inserted between the vertebrae of the lower back. This procedure is known as a spinal puncture or a spinal tap.

Spinal ANESTHESIA is used to deaden pain in certain areas of the body. The anesthetic is injected into the spinal canal. The person remains awake, but is not aware of pain anywhere below the point of injection. See NEUROSURGERY.

SPINAL CURVATURE An abnormal curving of the spine that may result from poor posture, disease, or a congenital condition. See KYPHOSIS; LORDOSIS; SCOLIOSIS.

SPINAL PUNCTURE See SPINAL CORD.

SPINAL TAP See SPINAL CORD.

SPINE The flexible, bony column that gives support to the trunk of the body. It is made up of 33 small bones called vertebrae. The top seven of these, in the neck, are called cervical vertebrae. The first of these, the atlas, supports the skull. Below are 12 thoracic (chest) vertebrae, to which the ribs are attached, and the five lumbar vertebrae. All of these are mobile. The remaining nine vertebrae are fused together, forming a large bone, the sacrum, and the small coccyx, or tailbone. Bony projections at the rear of the vertebrae can be felt in the back.

Each vertebra has a hollow area inside it within which is the spinal canal or, in the sacrum, the sacral canal.

SPIROCHETE Any of a large group of spiral-shaped bacteria. (Pronounced spie'ro·keet.) LEPTOSPIROSIS, RELAPSING FEVER, SYPHILIS, and YAWS are among the diseases caused by specific spirochetes.

SPLEEN An organ lying in the upper left part of the abdominal cavity, between the stomach and the diaphragm, against the lowest ribs. The spleen is a pulpy, blood-filled mass weighing about half a pound. It stores red blood cells (ERYTHROCYTES) and removes old or damaged red blood cells and other particles from the blood. It also plays a part in fighting infection.

An enlarged spleen is a typical symptom of a number of infectious diseases: mononucleosis, typhoid fever, malaria, and syphilis. Cirrhosis of the liver and rheumatoid arthritis are often accompanied by enlargement of the spleen, as are leukemia and certain anemias. The spleen can be removed without apparent harm if injury or disease makes its removal necessary.

SPLINT Any device for supporting or preventing movement of some part of the body. A plaster cast for broken bones is one kind of splint. Lighter and more comfortable splints have been designed for various specific conditions. They permit free movement of other parts of the body so that the wearer can carry on normal activities during healing.

SPONDYLITIS Inflammation of one or more of the vertebrae of the SPINE. Spondylitis (pronounced spon"di·lie'tis) may be due to injury or to some disease, such as arthritis or tuberculosis. Spondylitis is often a chronic, crippling condition leading to some degree of stiffening (spondylosis) of the spinal joints and deformation (KYPHOSIS). Spondylitis may be treated by X ray, postural exercises, and drug therapy.

SPONDYLOSIS See SPONDYLITIS.

SPOTTED FEVER A popular name for three distinct infectious diseases characterized by spots on the skin. They are ROCKY MOUNTAIN SPOTTED FEVER, TYPHUS, and the type of MENINGITIS that is caused by the meningococcus bacterium.

SPRAIN A severe wrenching of a JOINT, causing a tearing of the supporting ligaments. It is a more serious injury than a strain. The pain is apt to be intense, and the joint swells because there is also damage to surrounding tissues and blood vessels. Most sprains are caused by falls or athletic accidents and commonly occur in the ankle, knee, wrist, or shoulder. For emergency treatment of sprains, see the FIRST AID section.

SPRUE A chronic disease of the small intestine in which certain food elements, especially fats and some vitamins, are not absorbed properly by the body. Sprue (pronounced sproo) is also known as nontropical sprue, adult celiac disease, or gluten enteropathy. It is also the name for a related tropical form of the disease.

The main symptom of nontropical sprue is diarrhea, at first watery and later consisting of foul-smelling, pale-colored stools containing undigested fat. A person with sprue loses weight rapidly and has a poor appetite. Anemia is likely to be present. If the vitamin B complex cannot be absorbed, the tongue becomes sore and shiny red in color.

Treatment is by a diet high in calories and proteins, but low in fats and gluten, the protein found in wheat and other cereal flours. Ripe bananas and skim milk are also beneficial. To treat the anemia and vitamin deficiencies, iron preparations, folic acid, and vitamin B_{12} are prescribed.

SPUTUM Fluid, principally mucus, which originates in the air passages and is discharged through the mouth. (Pronounced spyoo'tum.)

SQUINT See CROSS-EYE; STRABISMUS.

STAMMERING See SPEECH DEFECTS AND DISORDERS.

STANFORD-BINET TEST See BINET TEST. (Pronounced stan'ford bi·nay'.)

STAPHYLOCOCCUS (plural, **staphylococci**) A member of a group of BACTERIA that causes boils, pus-forming infections, and a type of FOOD POISONING. (Pronounced staf"i·loh·kok'us.)

STENOSIS The narrowing of an opening, duct, or passageway in the body. Stenosis (pronounced sti·noh'sis) occurs often in HEART VALVES that have become constricted by disease. For instance, narrowing of the mitral valve between the two chambers on the left side of the heart is known as mitral stenosis, or MITRAL DISEASE.

STERILITY Partial or complete inability to reproduce; infertility. The cause may be a defect, either organic or functional, in the man or the woman. Sometimes, difficulty in conceiving is due to a couple's not knowing that there is an optimum time for conception. This is the period midway in the menstrual cycle, beginning about two days before OVULATION, and lasting for about five days after it. People who want to have a baby should concentrate on having sexual intercourse (COITUS) during this period.

The Medical Examination: Couples experiencing difficulty in having a baby should obtain a thorough medical examination for signs of abnormality, glandular disturbance, poor nutrition, or disease—any of which may be responsible for sterility. When a specimen of the man's SEMEN is examined under the microscope, it can quickly be determined whether the sperm cells are sufficient in number and in a healthy condition.

The first consideration with the woman is whether she ovulates. If she does, it must be ascertained that her FALLOPIAN TUBES are open to receive the egg cell from the ovary. Sometimes the mucus of the CERVIX is inhospitable to the sperm.

Treatment: If no sperm cells are present in the man, little can be done to help the condition. However, if they are weak or few in number, a variety of treatments may be tried to overcome these handicaps. Failure of the woman to ovulate may be corrected by hormone treatment. In some cases an emotional difficulty is the source of the problem, and psychiatric counseling may offer a solution. If the Fallopian tubes are obstructed, surgery may be recommended. Sometimes the cause is hard to find and treat. However, GYNECOLOGISTS, fertility clinics, and the Planned Parenthood Federation can offer helpful assistance. (Information about infertility treatment can be obtained from the Planned Parenthood Federation of America, Inc., 810 Seventh Avenue, New York, New York 10019.) In numerous cases, infertility has been corrected after a period of treatment.

When the wife is apparently fertile but the husband is sterile or for emotional or physiological reasons is unable to perform the sex act (see IMPOTENCE), the couple may want to consider ARTIFICIAL INSEMINATION.

STEROID A general term (pronounced ster'oyd) for any of a large group of naturally occurring substances with a similar kind of chemical structure, many of which play important roles in the body. The SEX HORMONES (androgens and estrogens) and the hormones produced by the cortex of the ADRENAL GLAND are steroids.

DIGITALIS owes its great effectiveness to a steroid that has a specific action on the heart. CHOLESTEROL is also a steroid.

STETHOSCOPE An apparatus for listening to the sounds made by the heart, lungs, large blood vessels, and other internal organs. The modern stethoscope (pronounced steth'o·skohp) consists of two earpieces attached to flexible rubber tubes that, in most types, lead into a sort of bell, or cone, which is applied to the outside of the body.

By means of the stethoscope, the doctor listens for any sounds that may indicate the presence of a disease or abnormality. This type of examination is called AUSCULTATION.

STIFF NECK Soreness and stiffness of the neck muscles that may be either mild or severe. The common "cold in the neck" may be caused by nervous tension, exposure to drafts, or certain sitting and lying positions. Aspirin and application of heat will usually relieve it.

However, if the stiff neck is very painful, it may indicate the onset of a serious infectious disease, especially in children. You should call your doctor immediately if stiff neck is accompanied by fever, headache, and nausea. Stiff neck may also result from an injury, such as WHIPLASH.

Wryneck, or torticollis, is sometimes congenital and may be caused by a birth injury. The muscles on one side of the neck pull the head to one side and down toward the shoulder. The condition is treated by massage and careful stretching of the affected muscles. Severe cases may require surgery. Early treatment is essential. Wryneck in adults may be the result of chronic RHEUMATISM.

STILL'S DISEASE A type of ARTHRITIS (inflammation of a joint) which affects children. It was first described by the British physician George Still (1868–1941). The disease is similar to rheumatoid arthritis in adults. Treatment includes rest, drugs such as aspirin, physiotherapy, and surgery to alter any deformity.

STIMULANT Any substance that increases the rate or intensity of some mental or physical activity. A variety of stimulants are used in medicine. DIGITALIS is a stimulant that affects weakened heart muscle. The hormone OXYTOCIN is a stimulant that induces contractions of the uterus during childbirth. Some stimulants, such as AMPHETAMINE preparations, act on the central nervous system, temporarily increasing mental alertness. Amphetamines produce a temporary feeling of well-being, but they have a number of harmful side effects and should be used only under a doctor's supervision. One of their chief medical uses is to relieve apathy and depression.

Coffee and tea contain very small amounts of a stimulant (CAFFEINE), as do many popular soft drinks. However, alcoholic drinks are actually depressants—they slow down rather than stimulate mental activity.

STOMACH The curved, saclike enlargement of the ALIMENTARY CANAL between the esophagus and the small intestine, located just under the diaphragm. The mucous membrane that lines the stomach contains many small glands. These produce hydrochloric acid, digestive enzymes, and mucus. The wall of the stomach consists of smooth muscle.

When food enters the stomach, the muscle contracts rhythmically, mixing the food thoroughly with the digestive juices to produce a thick, soupy mixture called chyme. The stomach contents then pass through the pylorus at the small end of the stomach into the small intestine. The walls of the stomach stretch when food presses against them.

The stomach is subject to disturbances such as NAUSEA and INDIGESTION. The stomach lining is very sensitive to irritating and toxic substances. If certain types of toxic substances are swallowed, it may be necessary to induce VOMITING or to pump out the stomach contents. (See STOMACH PUMP; also FIRST AID section.) The most serious diseases of the stomach are ULCER and CANCER.

Wise eating habits can do much to prevent stomach disorders. Any persistent stomach distress should have prompt medical attention. See also ACID STOMACH. (See illustration on the following page.)

STOMACH PUMP A device consisting of a flexible tube to which a small suction pump is attached. The tube is inserted into the mouth or nose and passed down through the esophagus to the stomach, from which it withdraws some, or all, of the contents. Stomach pumps may be used in certain cases of poisoning.

STOMATITIS An inflammation of the inside of the mouth, stemming from a variety of causes. Thrush (see MONILIASIS), trench mouth (VINCENT'S ANGINA), GINGIVITIS, glossitis (inflammation of the tongue), and other local infections of the gums and mucous membranes are all forms of stomatitis (pronounced stoh"ma·tie'tis). Irritating substances such as tobacco and spices, certain medicines, and inadequate oral hygiene can cause mouth inflammation. Jagged teeth and poorly fitting dentures can irritate the gums or result in accidental biting of the tongue and of the inside surfaces of the cheeks. Infants can acquire mouth infections from unsanitary nursing bottles or from an infected breast nipple.

Stomatitis is one of the secondary symptoms of several diseases. Swollen tongue and bleeding gums are signs of pellagra and scurvy; white spots (Koplik's spots), of measles; and strawberry tongue, of scarlet fever.

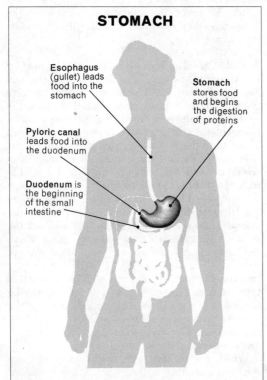

STOMACH

Esophagus (gullet) leads food into the stomach

Stomach stores food and begins the digestion of proteins

Pyloric canal leads food into the duodenum

Duodenum is the beginning of the small intestine

The stomach is a reservoir for food and the part of the alimentary canal where the major processes of digestion begin. Food reaches the stomach from the mouth along the esophagus, mixed with saliva which starts the digestion of some starchy foods. Acid gastric juices, secreted by glands in the stomach wall, begin the breakdown of proteins and milk. After two to four hours of being churned in the stomach, the food is forced along the pyloric canal and into the duodenum, the first part of the small intestine, where digestion is completed.

STOOL See FECES.

STRABISMUS A condition in which both eyes cannot be focused on the same spot at the same time. Strabismus (pronounced stra·biz'mus) is also called squint. When one or both eyes are turned in toward the nose, the disorder is called convergent strabismus, or CROSS-EYE. When one or both eyes turn outward toward the temples, the condition is known as divergent strabismus, or walleye.

Treatment by a skilled eye specialist (OPHTHAL-MOLOGIST) should begin as early as possible. Corrective glasses, eye exercises, special eyedrops, and surgery to restore muscle balance can do much to help straighten the eyes.

STRAIN Overstretching or tearing of muscle fibers causes a strain (not to be confused with a SPRAIN, which involves tearing of the ligaments of a joint). A strain generally causes swelling and pain in the affected muscle, and sometimes bruising. The pain increases if the muscle is used.

Treatment involves rest and a cold compress to reduce swelling. Aspirin or other analgesics will relieve the pain. A severe strain may need bandaging for support. For a week or so, as the muscle heals, gentle exercise lessens stiffness and hastens recovery. See also MYALGIA; RHEUMATISM.

STREP THROAT A popular term for a throat infection caused by a STREPTOCOCCUS bacterium. Strep throat is always accompanied by fever. It is very serious because the infection may involve the whole system. Acute NEPHRITIS and RHEUMATIC FEVER can follow neglected cases of strep throat.

Prompt treatment by your doctor with penicillin or another ANTIBIOTIC can prevent serious damage to the kidneys and the heart.

STREPTOCOCCUS (plural, **streptococci**) Any of a large group of spherical bacteria (pronounced strep"to·kok'us) that grow together in long chains. SCARLET FEVER and STREP THROAT are caused by streptococci, but many streptococci are harmless or even beneficial.

STREPTOMYCIN A powerful ANTIBIOTIC obtained from a mold. Streptomycin (pronounced strep"to·mie'sin) is effective against tuberculosis and some other infections.

STRESS A condition or factor that produces an intense strain on a person. The cause may be emotional, such as worry; biochemical, such as histamine produced by an ALLERGY; or physical, such as illness, injury, or overexertion.

STROKE Damage to a portion of the brain as a result of blockage of an artery or hemorrhage from a ruptured artery in the brain. A stroke is also called a cerebrovascular accident, or apoplexy. A stroke usually causes a sudden loss of consciousness and paralysis on one side of the body. The paralysis occurs because a portion of the brain that controls body movements is affected. The underlying conditions that are chiefly responsible for strokes are HYPERTENSION, or high blood pressure, HARDENING OF THE ARTERIES, and valvular heart disease which may be a complication. See also MITRAL DISEASE; RHEUMATIC FEVER.

Causes: One of the three main causes of a stroke is cerebral THROMBOSIS, in which a thrombus, or BLOOD CLOT, forms within a brain artery and gradually cuts off the blood supply to a portion of the brain. A thrombus forms because of damage to the vessel walls from hardening of the arteries. A second cause of stroke is cerebral EMBOLISM. An embolus may be a plug of fat or a mass of bacteria, but more often it is a fragment of a detached blood clot or other material from a diseased heart wall or valve. The embolus gets into the bloodstream and may block off an artery in the brain or one of the main arteries in the neck leading to the brain. The third cause of stroke, often the most serious, is CEREBRAL HEMORRHAGE, which is the rupture of a weakened blood vessel in the brain.

Symptoms: Stroke caused by cerebral embolism comes on suddenly and without warning. The person may be unable to talk, lose consciousness, and become paralyzed on one side.

Cerebral hemorrhage often causes headache, nausea, and ringing in the ears just before the onset of the stroke.

First strokes caused by cerebral thrombosis and cerebral embolism are rarely fatal unless followed later by such complications as pneumonia. Eventual, and even full, recovery is fairly certain in any stroke if only a small blood vessel is involved.

Treatment: If you suspect that a person is having a stroke, call the doctor immediately. While you are waiting for medical help, place the victim in a half-sitting position and follow the instructions for emergency treatment of stroke in the FIRST AID section. The person should be taken to a hospital, if possible, so that certain tests can be made to determine the extent of brain damage and the cause of the stroke. Careful nursing care is needed, especially for the first few critical days.

Early treatment consists in keeping the person comfortable by changing his position frequently and in preventing paralyzed limbs from assuming unnatural, cramped positions. If a blood clot has caused the stroke, an ANTICOAGULANT may be prescribed to help prevent the clot from spreading.

Rehabilitation: Depending upon the severity of the stroke, PHYSICAL THERAPY should be started as soon as possible so that the person can start regaining the use of his muscles.

Although many people recover completely from a stroke, some are left with some paralysis of an arm or leg or with a speech defect.

STUTTERING   See SPEECH DEFECTS AND DISORDERS.

STY (stye)   An inflammation of the eyelid caused by infection of one or more of the sebaceous (oil) glands of the eyelids. It is usually caused by staphlococci. A small, red area appears at the edge of the lid, and soon begins to swell. Several days after the sty's appearance, pus starts to form at the center. The pus-filled sty will usually erupt and drain of its own accord within a few days.

Warm compresses will help bring a sty to a head and relieve the pain. Do not rub or touch the eyelid. Your doctor can provide antibiotic drops or ointments that will help to keep the infection from spreading.

If the sty does not rupture after several days, a visit to a physician is advisable. He may make an incision in the sty and remove the pus.

Chalazion (plural, **chalazia**): This is a small cyst on the eyelid formed by the swelling of a sebaceous gland. It is also known as a meibomian sty. A chalazion is painless, building up gradually in the lid.

Some chalazia disappear without treatment. Application of a hot compress for 10 or 15 minutes three or four times a day may hasten the disappearance of the cyst. If not, it is wise to see a doctor.

STYPTIC   See ASTRINGENT.

SUBACIDITY   See HYPOACIDITY.

SUBCONSCIOUS   The part of mental activity that is below the level of consciousness. The word is often used to mean the UNCONSCIOUS.

SUBCUTANEOUS   Beneath the skin. A subcutaneous (pronounced sub″kyoo·tay′nee·us) injection is introduced under the skin rather than into a muscle or vein. Subcutaneous tissues lie immediately under the skin.

SUFFOCATION   See ASPHYXIA.

SUGAR   Any of a group of CARBOHYDRATES that can be dissolved in water and have a more or less sweet taste. When used alone, the term "sugar" refers to ordinary table sugar, which is processed from sucrose, present in the green leaves of all plants. Some plants, such as sugarcane and sugar beets, store large amounts of sucrose in their stems and roots and are used as commercial sources of table sugar.

Sucrose is the sweetest sugar, but others also play a part in nutrition. About 5 percent of cow's milk is lactose, or milk sugar. Fruit sugar, or fructose, is a sugar found in oranges and other fruits. Glucose is the principal sugar in the blood and is called blood sugar.

As a food, ordinary sugar is a concentrated and relatively cheap source of energy. A tablespoonful of sugar (one half ounce) represents about 60 calories. Except for people with DIABETES, the system digests and utilizes sugar very easily and rapidly. It also tends to satisfy hunger, as artificial sweeteners do not. Some reducing diets, therefore, actually specify moderate amounts of sugar.

SULFA COMPOUND See SULFONAMIDE.

SULFONAMIDE One of a group of chemical compounds used in the treatment of various diseases and infections caused by BACTERIA. A sulfonamide (pronounced sul·fon′a·mied) is commonly called a sulfa compound. Some of them kill bacteria, while others stop the growth and reproduction of certain bacteria. In recent years, sulfa compounds have to a large extent been replaced by ANTIBIOTICS, such as penicillin. But sulfa compounds are still the best weapon against certain diseases, such as those of the urinary tract, and some sulfonamides are particularly useful in treating intestinal tract infections.

Sulfanilamide was once the most widely used sulfa compound. Sulfa compounds used most often today include sulfadiazine, sulfamerazine, sulfasuxidine, and sulfisoxazole.

SULFONE One of a group of medicines related to the SULFONAMIDES, or sulfa compounds. Some of them are helpful in treating LEPROSY. (Pronounced sul′fohn.)

SUNBURN A sunburn damages the skin and may even cause a second-degree BURN. In severe sunburn, the skin becomes covered with large, watery blisters and is extremely painful to the touch. If the burn is over a large part of the body, the person may become feverish or go into SHOCK. The danger of infection of the blisters is always present. When the skin starts to heal, the burned layer sloughs off and may leave scars or unsightly patches. Constant tanning will wrinkle and dry the skin and may result in epitheliomas (skin cancers).

To avoid a sunburn and acquire a tan sensibly, limit your first sunbath of the season to about 15 minutes. Thereafter, increase the time of exposure each day by another 10 or 15 minutes. It is best not to sunbathe during the middle of the day, when the sun's rays are the hottest. Also, remember that the effect of the ultraviolet rays is intensified by reflections from water, sand, and snow. Various lotions and creams may help to prevent sunburn, but they tend to wash off and should be replaced frequently.
Treatment: While the burn is sensitive, the person should stay out of the sun. Compresses dipped in cool water or mineral oil will help relieve the pain. Mild creams, such as unscented cold cream, will help restore oil and moisture to the skin.

SUNSTROKE A serious upset of the body's cooling system, caused by excessive exposure to the hot sun or to very hot air in places having poor ventilation. The early symptoms are like those of HEAT PROSTRATION, a less serious condition. The person has a headache and feels weak and dizzy. But sunstroke differs from heat prostration in that the victim soon runs a very high fever, often 106° F or more. The skin is hot and dry and *there is no perspiration.* In severe cases there may be violent vomiting, convulsions, and coma.
Treatment: Call a doctor promptly or get the person to a hospital. Sunstroke calls for immediate emergency measures. (See the FIRST AID section.) The doctor may prescribe ice bags, cold baths, and other methods to bring down the temperature. He may need to give intravenous injections of fluids containing salt and sedatives if convulsions occur. After the temperature is brought down, the person should spend several days in bed.
Prevention: Sunstroke is prevented by avoiding strenuous activity in hot weather, especially in the sun or in overheated places. Those who must work under such conditions should drink plenty of water and take salt tablets (or salt in a glass of water) to make up for the moisture and salt lost in perspiration. A hat or scarf will protect the head from the sun. Anyone who has ever had a sunstroke must be especially cautious.

SUPEREGO One of the three major parts of the mind, or psyche, with the ID and the EGO. According to psychoanalytic theory, the superego (pronounced soo″per·ee′goh) is, in a sense, the conscience. When we go against the dictates of the superego, we have feelings of guilt. See also PSYCHOANALYSIS.

SUPPOSITORY A small, sometimes medicated cone or cylinder made of glycerin or cocoa butter, to be inserted into the rectum (the terminal part of the bowel) or the VAGINA. A plain rectal suppository (pronounced su·poz′i·tawr″ee) can provide temporary relief for constipation.

Anal pruritis (itching) and the pain and discomfort of HEMORRHOIDS (piles) may be relieved by medicated suppositories. Medicated vaginal suppositories are prescribed for treating some types of VAGINITIS (inflammation of the vagina).

SUPPURATION The formation of pus. (Pronounced sup″yu·ray′shun.)

SURGERY Every day, tens of thousands of people undergo surgery in hospitals and doctors' offices in North America. A considerable amount of surgery is *elective,* so the operation may be performed when it is convenient for both patient and doctor. By contrast, an *immediate operation of necessity* cannot be postponed.
Preparing for an Operation: Usually the patient enters a hospital with which his surgeon is associated. As a rule, he checks in the day before the operation. A laboratory technician collects samples of the patient's blood and urine and analyzes them. Other

tests and X rays may also be made at the doctor's request.

The Operation: The persons taking part form a skilled professional team. In charge is the surgeon, who may have one or two other surgeons as assistants. Two nurses are present, with other nurses and assistants as required. A key person is the anesthetist, who is usually a physician. He administers the ANESTHETIC so that the patient will feel no pain. He also watches the patient's respiration, blood pressure, and heartbeat. If oxygen is needed, he administers it.

After the Operation: When the operation is over, the patient is transferred to the recovery room. He remains there until he regains consciousness. Generally this takes an hour or longer. A nurse keeps close check on the patient's condition. Afterward, the patient is returned to his own room or ward.

The doctor will advise the patient when he can get out of bed and move about. Activity has a beneficial effect on the circulation and other body processes, and doctors tend to get the patient up as early as practicable.

See also COSMETIC SURGERY; HEART SURGERY; NEUROSURGERY; ORGAN TRANSPLANTS; PLASTIC SURGERY; SPARE-PART SURGERY.

SUTURE The drawing together of two sides of a wound by means of stitches or clamps. (Pronounced soo'chur.) The process is used to close surgical incisions and accidental cuts and gashes too large to heal easily by themselves. Suturing promotes more rapid healing and helps to prevent disfiguring scars and loss of function. The sterile materials used—silk or nylon thread, catgut, wire, and metal clamps—are also called sutures.

Some sutures, especially those placed in internal organs and deeper tissues, are made of material that is gradually absorbed into the body, so that they do not have to be removed by the doctor after the sides of the wound have grown together.

SWAB A small stick with a wad of cotton or gauze wrapped about one or both ends. Swabs are used to clean out or apply medicines to cavities of the body (such as the ears, nose, and mouth), to cleanse wounds, and to obtain samples of secretions for examination. If you use a swab yourself, be careful to avoid injuring sensitive tissues.

SWALLOWING The THROAT, a passageway to both the lungs and the stomach, is constructed so that it is generally impossible to breathe and swallow at the same time. In the act of swallowing, the breathing passages are sealed off, thus preventing solids and liquids from entering the windpipe. Involuntary contractions of the PHARYNX and the esophagus force the mouthful of food or drink to move downward toward the stomach. CHOKING results if we have food or drink at the back of our mouths and we try to talk or breathe instead of swallowing.

Congenital defects of the palate, such as CLEFT PALATE, or of the esophagus will interfere with a baby's swallowing. Any such defects should be corrected by surgery as soon as possible. At any age, difficulty in swallowing (dysphagia) or pain in swallowing (ODYNOPHAGIA) requires medical attention.

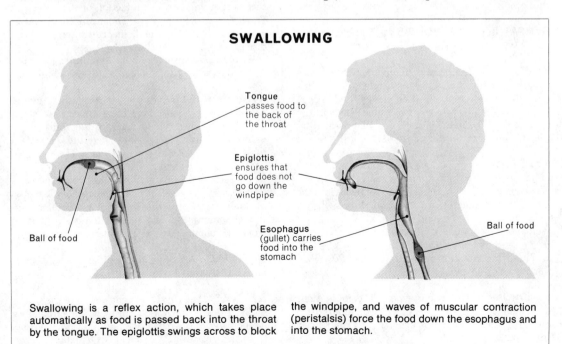

SWALLOWING

Tongue
passes food to the back of the throat

Epiglottis
ensures that food does not go down the windpipe

Esophagus
(gullet) carries food into the stomach

Ball of food

Ball of food

Swallowing is a reflex action, which takes place automatically as food is passed back into the throat by the tongue. The epiglottis swings across to block the windpipe, and waves of muscular contraction (peristalsis) force the food down the esophagus and into the stomach.

SWEAT GLAND A tiny, coil-shaped tube extending from the deepest layer of the skin to its surface. The sweat glands (there are approximately 2 million all over the skin) help regulate the body's temperature and contribute to the excretion of water and salt from the body. See also PERSPIRATION.

SWELLING The accumulation of fluid in the tissues, resulting from disease or injury, causes swelling. For this type, see EDEMA.

Other possible causes of swelling are enlargement of an organ or gland due to infection. For instance, swollen salivary glands in the neck accompany MONONUCLEOSIS and MUMPS. GOITER causes swelling of the thyroid gland at the front of the neck. Swollen lymph nodes may cause lumps, particularly in the armpit or groin (see BUBO). Other localized swelling may be due to a CYST, HERNIA, or TUMOR. Any swelling that does not clear up in a few days should be reported to a doctor.

SYCOSIS An infectious inflammation of the hair follicles caused by bacteria. Commonly known as barber's itch or rash, it is a form of folliculitis. It usually affects skin beneath the beard and sideburns of men and is treated with antibiotics. See also FOLLICULITIS. (Pronounced sie·koh'sis.)

SYMPATHECTOMY Surgical removal of a part of the sympathetic NERVOUS SYSTEM, which controls automatic movements of internal organs. (Pronounced sim"pa·thek'to·mee.) For example, one treatment for serious HYPERTENSION (high blood pressure) consists of interfering with the sympathetic nerves that normally constrict the arteries.

SYMPATHETIC NERVOUS SYSTEM See NERVOUS SYSTEM; AUTONOMIC NERVOUS SYSTEM.

SYMPHYSIS The point of union where two bones have grown together. One important joint of this type, the pubic symphysis (pronounced sim'fi·sis), is formed by the union of the two pubic bones in the front part of the pelvis. Another is that formed by the two bones of the lower jaw (the chin).

SYMPTOM Any noticeable change in a body organ or function indicating a disease or disorder. The term is also applied to changes in behavior that may point to emotional or mental illness. Fever, pain, unusual fatigue, and abnormal bleeding are well-known symptoms of a number of disorders.

SYNCOPE Another name for FAINTING. (Pronounced sing'ko·pee.)

SYNDROME The occurrence, in combination, of a number of SYMPTOMS that are characteristic of a particular ailment or condition. (Pronounced sin'drohm.)

SYNERGY A cooperative action, as when two or more muscles or nerves work together. The term "synergy" (pronounced sin'er·jee) is also applied to the joint action of medicines that together are more effective than when used individually.

SYPHILIS A VENEREAL DISEASE caused by a spirochete (spiral-shaped bacterium), *Treponema pallidum*. The germ is usually transmitted by sexual contact. Syphilis (pronounced sif'i·lis) is the most dangerous of the venereal diseases, but it can be cured with the help of penicillin.

Symptoms: There are three stages in syphilis. In the first (primary) stage, only one symptom occurs: a chancre—a hard sore—appears at the point where the germs entered the body, usually on the genitals. In the second stage, a general skin rash is seen, seven to 10 weeks after the initial exposure to the disease. Sores are frequently present in the mouth and on the genitals. The central nervous system and the eyes may be involved. The disease is highly infectious at this stage.

The symptoms of early syphilis disappear even if the disease is not treated. But the disorder remains latent, and severe complications occur with the third stage, sometimes after many years. Skin lesions and tumors (gummas) make their appearance. There may be syphilitic heart disease and PARESIS, a brain disease. Blindness and LOCOMOTOR ATAXIA (tabes dorsalis) may occur.

In congenital syphilis, the unborn baby contracts the disease from an infected mother. Many such babies are born dead; others are born blind, deaf, or otherwise handicapped. Early prenatal treatment of the mother will prevent infection of the baby.

Treatment and Prevention: The main treatment is with penicillin. This medicine can often cure the disease completely in the early stages.

Anyone who suspects he has syphilis should consult a doctor or visit a venereal disease clinic.

SYRINGOMYELIA A progressive disease of the nervous system caused by the formation of small fluid-filled cavities in the back of the spinal cord. Symptoms begin to appear when the patient is between the ages of 10 and 30 years. There is pain or weakness in a hand or arm and at the same time a loss of sensation to external sources of pain such as a burn. Later the legs may become spastic. There is no known cause of the disease, or treatment, although sometimes it may spontaneously stop getting worse. (Pronounced si·ring"goh·mie·ee'l·ee·a.)

SYSTEMIC Affecting the body as a whole. (Pronounced sis·tem'ik.)

SYSTOLE The rhythmic contraction of the HEART which propels the blood through the circulatory system. In the DIASTOLE, which follows the systole, the heart relaxes. (Pronounced sis'to·lee.)

T

TABES A wasting away of tissue during the course of a chronic disease. The term "tabes" (pronounced tay'beez) is also used to describe tabes dorsalis, or LOCOMOTOR ATAXIA.

TACHYCARDIA An abnormally rapid beating or fluttering of the heart. Tachycardia (pronounced tak"i·kahr'dee·a) may be the result of exercise, emotion, a thyroid disorder, or heart disease. In one type of tachycardia, paroxysmal tachycardia, the heart may suddenly start to beat with great rapidity—perhaps two or three times the normal rate—and then return to its normal beat just as suddenly. It is not uncommon in highstrung persons who are otherwise healthy. When it occurs in heart disease, it is rarely the only symptom.

Quinidine and certain other medicines are used to prevent spells of paroxysmal tachycardia.

TALIPES A congenital deformity (clubfoot) of one or both feet. In talipes (pronounced tal'i·peez), the foot is twisted out of normal position. The bones of the foot may be crooked, and the tendons and muscles stretched or shortened abnormally.
Treatment: If treatment is started very early in childhood, the condition can often be completely cured. In mild cases, a foot may be manipulated into the correct position and then strapped or placed in a cast. Later, the foot is exercised to strengthen the muscles and tendons. Special shoes may be needed for a while. More serious cases may require orthopedic surgery (see ORTHOPEDICS).

TAMPON A plug of absorbent material, such as cotton wool or gauze, for insertion in a body cavity. Some women prefer to use tampons rather than external pads during their menstrual periods.

TAPEWORM Any of a number of varieties of long flatworms that live as parasites in the intestines of man and animals; the scientific name is *Taenia*. Tapeworms grow up to 30 feet in length.

Tapeworm disease (teniasis) can be acquired from eating infected beef, pork, and fish containing tapeworm larvae (immature worms). Infection from fish tapeworms, which causes severe anemia, is sometimes found in the Great Lakes area.
Symptoms: A person infected with a beef or pork tapeworm may gradually lose weight, since the tapeworm continually absorbs food, and there may be mild abdominal discomfort. The flat, whitish tapeworm segments often appear in the bowel movements.

The symptoms may be more serious if the eggs of the pork tapeworm happen to hatch in the intestine. The larvae may invade the bloodstream and travel to any part of the body.
Treatment: Tapeworm infestation must be treated by a doctor and, frequently, in a hospital, to obtain a complete cure. ATABRINE, a medicine used in malaria, is one of the medicines (called teniafuges) found effective in killing tapeworms.

TARSAL See FOOT.

TARTAR A substance that builds up on the teeth, especially along the gum line. (See TOOTH.) Tartar (pronounced tahr'tar) is made up of calcium and other mineral salts found in saliva, as well as other material such as particles of food. The dentist or dental assistant scales tartar from the teeth as part of a regular dental-cleaning session.

Tartar that collects between the teeth and along the gums is an important factor in causing GINGIVITIS, which may eventually lead to pyorrhea alveolaris (see PYORRHEA).

TATTOOING Pricking indelible pigments into the skin to form images, letters, or words. An electric needle is used in Western countries.

Tattooing is prohibited in some places unless performed by licensed practitioners under strictly hygienic conditions. Many persons have been seriously infected by tattooing instruments that were not sterile. The obliteration of tattoos is a slow and painful process.

TELANGIOMA A tumor made up of clusters of dilated small blood vessels, such as CAPILLARIES or arterioles. (Pronounced tel·an"jee·oh'ma.)

TEMPERATURE See BODY TEMPERATURE; FEVER; THERMOMETER.

TENDINITIS An inflammation of a tendon; also called tenonitis and tenontitis. Tendinitis (pronounced ten"di·nie'tis) is commonly found around deposits of calcium associated with a shoulder, or other, tendon. It frequently occurs in combination with BURSITIS, an inflammation of a fluid-containing sac in the joint.

Tendinitis often announces itself with pains so

acute that the person is unwilling to move his arm or other part of his body that is affected. To relieve the condition, a local anesthetic or cortisone is injected into the site of the discomfort. Physical therapy is helpful in restoring the function of the area after the acute inflammation has subsided.

TENDON   A strong, tough band of connective tissue. Tendons connect muscle to bone, and by means of them the pull of the muscle moves the bone. The tendons attached to the bones are so strong that even when a bone is broken, they may not be harmed.

TENDONS

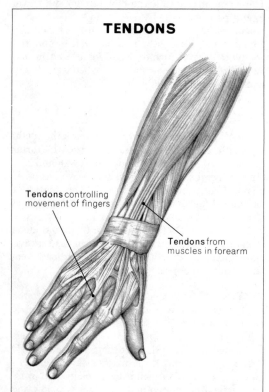

Tendons controlling movement of fingers

Tendons from muscles in forearm

Tendon is the strong elastic tissue which connects muscles to bones. Tendons may be thick and short, such as those which attach the twin ends of the biceps arm muscle to the shoulder. Or they may be long and slender, like the tendons that run from muscles in the forearm across the back of the wrist and hand to the ends of the fingers. Inflammation of a tendon or the membrane sheathing it causes the painful condition tendinitis.

TENNIS ELBOW   See ELBOW.

TENSION   A word commonly used to refer to nervous strain. People are tense in various ways. Some express their reaction to strain in repeated outbursts of anger or constant irritability. Others repress their feelings but brood or worry endlessly about their problems. In some persons, repressed tensions may produce physical effects such as backache, cramps, diarrhea, excruciating headaches, peptic ULCER, and other disorders.

Why We Are Tense: We are born into a world in which it is difficult not to experience repeated frustration and tension. As infants, we have needs and desires. When these are not satisfied promptly by our parents, we experience our first tensions.

In adulthood, the pressures become more severe. We must compete for friends, love, jobs, advancement, and social standing. Often we have to work in a less than ideal environment full of noise and distraction.

Inevitably, everyone is exposed to tension in one form or another. Some are fortunate enough to have learned in childhood how to tolerate it successfully. However, there are ways that will help virtually anyone to ease the stresses of day-to-day life.

Living with Tension: Physical activity is an excellent outlet for tension. Swimming, bicycling, or other vigorous activities are helpful, but even walking provides relief.

The person who is bored or frustrated by his job should find a different type of activity for his spare time; he may enjoy playing a musical instrument or taking up photography. Weekend trips help us get away from our daily routines.

The person who is withdrawn and broods about his tensions should find someone with whom he can discuss his problems. Normally, a husband or wife is a natural counselor. However, an old friend or a clergyman may be able to offer helpful advice.

If one's problems are too severe to be handled in this way, it is worth looking into the possibility of obtaining the assistance of a PSYCHIATRIST, PSYCHOLOGIST, or other counselor. In this case, the first step should be a frank discussion with the family physician.

TEPANIL   The trade name for a medicine that decreases the appetite. (Pronounced tep′ah·nil.) The product is also sold under other trade names, including Naterexic, Regenon, and Tenuate.

TERRAMYCIN   The trade name for an ANTIBIOTIC of the TETRACYCLINE group. Terramycin (pronounced ter″a·mie′sin) is active against many types of disease-causing germs.

TESTES (singular, **testis**)   See TESTICLE. (Pronounced tes′teez.)

TESTICLE   One of the two male sex glands, or gonads, located in an external, pouchlike structure, the scrotum. The testicles (also called testes) produce SPERM CELLS and SEX HORMONES. The sperm cells are produced in minute tubes, or tubules, which come together in a single duct leading to the

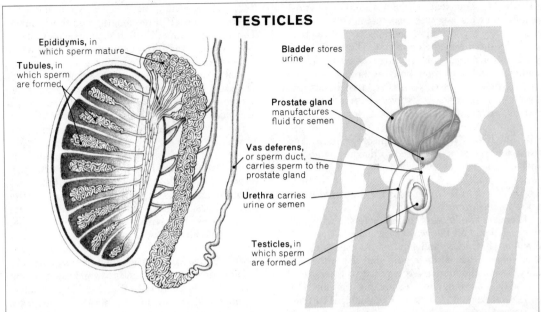

TESTICLES

Epididymis, in which sperm mature

Tubules, in which sperm are formed

Bladder stores urine

Prostate gland manufactures fluid for semen

Vas deferens, or sperm duct, carries sperm to the prostate gland

Urethra carries urine or semen

Testicles, in which sperm are formed

The testicles, or testes, are the male sex glands, located in the pouch of the scrotum. Male sex hormones produced by these glands bring about the changes in a boy at puberty. Removal of the testicles (castration) in a young boy stops him developing a man's secondary sexual characteristics, such as a deep voice and facial hair. In a man, the testicles produce sperm; castration or severing of the sperm duct (vasectomy) is an effective method of sterilization, but physical characteristics remain unchanged. In many men approaching middle age, continued production of male sex hormones results in baldness.

urethra. Production of both sperm cells and sex hormones begins at the time of puberty, under the influence of hormones from the PITUITARY GLAND.

TESTOSTERONE   See SEX HORMONE. (Pronounced tes·tos′te·rohn.)

TETANUS   A serious infectious disease caused by a type of *Clostridium* bacterium. Tetanus (pronounced tet′a·nus) is characterized by spasms of the voluntary muscles, usually beginning with a clamping together of the jaws, whence comes the name *lockjaw*. The bacteria invade the body through puncture wounds, such as those made by nails, splinters, or bullets. Such injuries should be treated by a doctor. IMMUNIZATION has helped to reduce the number of cases of tetanus. If the disease does strike, there is an ANTITOXIN to counteract the toxin produced by the bacteria, and penicillin is given to kill the germs. However, once the disease has fully developed, successful treatment is extremely difficult.

TETANY   A disorder in which a deficiency of calcium in the blood irritates the nerve tissue, causing cramps, muscular spasms, and even convulsions. Tetany (pronounced tet′a·nee) develops for any of several reasons. During pregnancy or after childbirth, a woman may have the condition because too much of the calcium in her body has gone into the

bones of the unborn baby or into the breast milk.

It is a function of the PARATHYROID GLANDS to maintain the proper calcium level of the blood. Tetany may occur because these glands are underactive. Excessive and prolonged diarrhea tends to drain the body of calcium. In children, a lack of vitamin D in the diet may be a factor in causing tetany.

The doctor may prescribe calcium, vitamin D, or injections of the parathyroid hormone.

TETRACAINE HYDROCHLORIDE   An ANESTHETIC used locally during surgery of the eyes, ears, nose, and throat. Tetracaine hydrochloride (pronounced te′tra·kayn″ hie″dro·klawr′ied) is also suitable for spinal anesthesia.

TETRACYCLINE   Any of a group of ANTIBIOTICS active against a wide variety of BACTERIA, some VIRUSES, and the RICKETTSIA microorganisms. (Pronounced tet″ra·sie′klien.) The trade names include AUREOMYCIN and TERRAMYCIN.

THALIDOMIDE   A sedative drug, introduced in West Germany and Britain in the early 1960's. If given to a woman at the beginning of pregnancy, thalidomide (pronounced tha·lid′oh·mied) can, as a side effect, result in deformities to her baby. The drug is now banned in most countries.

THERAPY The treatment of a mental or physical condition or disease with remedial agents or techniques. A very common therapy is the doctor's prescription of a medicine or rest. The term is also used as a synonym for PSYCHOTHERAPY, the treatment of mental and emotional disorders. See also CHEMOTHERAPY; GROUP THERAPY; HYDROTHERAPY; OCCUPATIONAL THERAPY AND VOCATIONAL REHABILITATION; PHYSICAL THERAPY; SHOCK THERAPY.

THERMOGRAPH A photograph of the body taken using infrared rays. It is used in diagnosing abnormal tissues such as cysts or tumors.

THERMOMETER An instrument used to indicate BODY TEMPERATURE.

There are two types of thermometers in wide use, the *oral* type and the *rectal* type. The rectal thermometer is thicker and blunter. At one end, the thermometer has a silver bulb that contains mercury. When the mercury is exposed to the heat of the body, it expands and travels along the tube. The tube is marked off in degrees Fahrenheit. The temperature is indicated by the degree mark at which the mercury stops.

Rectal temperature is one half to one degree higher than oral temperature. The rectal thermometer is less breakable than the oral type and is always used with babies. Shake the thermometer down by holding it tight at the glass end and giving your wrist a strong, sharp twist. Bring the reading down to below 97°F before taking a temperature with either the oral or rectal thermometer.

The bulb of the rectal thermometer should be covered with cold cream or petroleum jelly (Vaseline) before use. Place the child on his side with hips and knees bent or, in the case of an infant, place him on his stomach across your lap; then expose the anal opening. Insert the thermometer gently until about half its length is inserted. Hold the thermometer in place for three minutes.

THIAMINE See VITAMIN. (Pronounced thie′a·meen.)

THORAX The chest; also called the thoracic cavity. Inside this cavity, which extends from the bottom of the neck to the abdomen, are the esophagus, the heart, and the lungs. The diaphragm, a muscular wall, divides the thorax (pronounced thawr′aks) from the abdominal cavity and plays an important part in breathing.

THORAZINE A trade name for CHLORPROMAZINE, a tranquilizer. (Pronounced thohr′a·zeen″.)

THROAT As usually defined, the upper part of the muscular tube that forms a passageway from the mouth and the nose to the stomach and the lungs. It includes the TONSILS, just visible behind the uvula (the small projection that hangs down from the soft palate at the back of the mouth), and the PHARYNX. The throat branches into the upper part of the ESOPHAGUS and into the LARYNX (voice box), which leads to the TRACHEA (windpipe). Thus the throat is part of both the digestive and the respiratory tracts. They are kept separate by the EPIGLOTTIS, a flap over the larynx that closes during swallowing so that food does not enter the windpipe.

For throat infections and irritations, see SORE THROAT.

THROMBOPHLEBITIS Inflammation of a vein (generally in the leg) associated with a thrombosis, or blocking, of the vein by a blood clot. It often accompanies VARICOSE VEIN and is treated in the same way as other types of PHLEBITIS. (Pronounced throm″boh·fli·bie′tis.)

THROMBOSIS The occluding, or blocking, of a blood vessel by a BLOOD CLOT (thrombus) which has formed in the vessel. If thrombosis (pronounced throm·boh′sis) occurs in an artery leading to an arm or a leg, GANGRENE may be the result. Thrombosis in an artery of the brain or a neck artery leading to the brain causes a STROKE. If the thrombosis takes place in an artery supplying the heart, it is called coronary thrombosis, and results in a heart attack.

Thrombosis of the veins takes place most often in the legs and the pelvis, but it may also occur in the portal vein that collects blood from the liver.
Treatment: Medicines called ANTICOAGULANTS are given to restrain the normal tendency of the blood to form clots. VASODILATORS, which cause the blood vessels to enlarge so that the blood may flow freely, may also be used. Bed rest or elevation of an affected limb is necessary until the clot has dissolved.

THROMBUS The medical name for a BLOOD CLOT in a blood vessel or heart cavity. See THROMBOSIS.

THRUSH See MONILIASIS.

THUMB-SUCKING A widespread habit among children, thumb-sucking generally need not be a source of concern to parents. It rarely results in disturbance of the normal arrangement of the teeth until the second set has begun to appear, at the age of six or seven. Most children outgrow the habit by their fourth year.

Sucking is an instinctive action that we associate with the reassurance of feeding in infancy. When a child feels insecure or worried, he is likely to suck his thumb.

THYMUS See ENDOCRINE GLAND.

THYROIDECTOMY Removal of a part or all of the THYROID GLAND. A thyroidectomy (pronounced thie″royd·ek′to·mee) is performed in cases where

THYROID GLAND

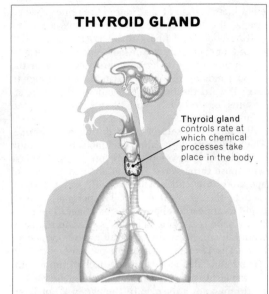

Thyroid gland controls rate at which chemical processes take place in the body

The thyroid is a shield-shaped gland in the neck. It secretes the hormone thyroxine, which controls the rate of chemical processes in the body. Thyroxine contains iodine, and for this reason iodine is an essential mineral which must be supplied in the diet. Too little iodine causes the gland to enlarge, causing a goiter.

the gland has been seriously enlarged by GOITER, and when hard lumps or cancer are detected; it is also sometimes performed when the gland is over-active, as in hyperthyroidism.

THYROID GLAND An ENDOCRINE GLAND located at the base of the neck on both sides of the windpipe below the larynx, or voice box. The thyroid gland produces the hormone THYROXINE, which regulates the speed of chemical reactions and influences the rate of growth and the development of sexual characteristics. The activity of the thyroid gland itself is regulated by a hormone secreted by the PITUITARY GLAND.

Thyroxine contains iodine, and the thyroid gland cannot produce thyroxine unless the diet contains a small amount of iodine.

If the thyroid gland produces either too much or too little thyroxine, serious disorders may result. (See GOITER; DWARFISM.) The term hypothyroidism refers to inadequate production of thyroxine; hyperthyroidism refers to excessive production.

The most widely used test to determine thyroid function is the PBI (*protein-bound iodine*) test. This is a laboratory test for which a small sample of a person's blood is required. Another test involves measuring the rate at which the body uses oxygen. (See BASAL METABOLIC RATE.) In another test, the amount of iodine taken up by the thyroid gland is measured by administering radioactive iodine.

THYROXINE A HORMONE secreted by the THYROID GLAND. A doctor may prescribe thyroxine (pronounced thie·rok'seen) if for any reason he wishes to speed up a person's METABOLISM.

TIBIA The shinbone. (Pronounced tib'ee·a.) See LEG.

TIC See SPASM.

TIC DOULOUREUX A painful nerve condition, or NEURALGIA, of the face. (Pronounced tik' doo"loo·rer'.) This disorder involves the trigeminal nerve, which branches out through the face. Irritation of this nerve can cause paroxysms of severe pain that may last only a fraction of a moment but sometimes keep coming back many times a day.

In some cases, facial neuralgia may be due to dentures that fit poorly, MALOCCLUSION, or other dental problems. There are a variety of medicines that may be prescribed. NEUROSURGERY may be proposed in extremely severe cases.

TICK FEVER A general, popular name for a number of diseases carried from rodents to human beings through bites of infected ticks.

The hard tick, which has a stiff cover over its back, burrows into the skin with its head and must be removed with care. It transmits TULAREMIA (also called rabbit fever), Colorado tick fever, and ROCKY MOUNTAIN SPOTTED FEVER. (The last two are sometimes called mountain fever.)

The soft tick, which carries RELAPSING FEVER, has no hard shell and does not burrow into the skin.

TINCTURE A medication, such as iodine, that is dissolved in alcohol.

TINEA See RINGWORM. (Pronounced tin'ee·a.)

TISSUE A collection of cells of the same general type, together with the material between the cells. The body is made up of four basic kinds of tissue.

EPITHELIUM is comprised of cells that tend to be flattened and closely packed. Skin and mucous membrane are examples of epithelium. Nerve tissue is able to conduct impulses rapidly. Muscle tissue has a unique ability to contract. In connective tissue, the cells are separated by relatively large amounts of material outside the cell walls. Bone, tendon, and cartilage are connective tissue.

TOILET TRAINING See CHILD PSYCHOLOGY.

TONGUE The movable, muscular organ in the mouth used in chewing, tasting, swallowing, and speaking. On the tongue's upper surface are scattered clusters of nerve endings called taste buds that can register only four different kinds of stimuli—sweet, sour, salty, and bitter.

Inflammation of the tongue, or glossitis, can be caused by most general infections, by anemia, and by deficiencies in the diet. In a number of disorders, the tongue may become coated, or furry. However, this condition is not in itself a sign of illness.

CANCER sometimes begins on the tongue. Irritation by tobacco smoke or by jagged teeth sometimes causes lesions that may become malignant.

TONSIL One of a pair of flat, oval masses of tissue on each side of the entrance to the THROAT. Through them circulates LYMPH, which assists in removing bacteria and impurities from the bloodstream.

The tonsils themselves, like the nearby ADENOIDS, are subject to infection (TONSILLITIS) and enlargement, especially in childhood. It is not considered advisable to remove the tonsils unless they become inflamed repeatedly or are seriously enlarged.

TONSILLECTOMY Surgical removal of the TONSILS. A tonsillectomy (pronounced ton″si·lek′to·mee) is a potentially serious operation because of the possibility of severe bleeding and should be performed in a hospital. A general anesthetic is administered. The throat may be uncomfortable for several days afterward.

If the patient is a child, the procedure and why it is necessary should be explained to him by the physician. It is also helpful if one or both parents can be with the child before and after the operation. Tonsils are generally not removed until a child is at least three years old.

TONSILLITIS Inflammation of the TONSILS. Tonsillitis (pronounced ton″si·lie′tis) is not a single specific disease but a symptom of a number of infectious diseases, including STREP THROAT and DIPHTHERIA. Any sore throat should have medical attention, especially if it is accompanied by fever. Germs that cause tonsillitis can also affect other parts of the body.

TOOTH Four different kinds of material make up the body of a tooth: dentin, pulp, cementum, and enamel.

Dentin is a substance similar to bone. Buried within the dentin body of each tooth is a central cavity, or chamber, filled with *pulp*, a soft tissue containing nerves and blood vessels.

The root of the tooth, the part below the gum, is covered by a thin layer of *cementum*. The cementum is living tissue that is capable of growth and repair. It holds the tooth firmly in its socket in the jawbone. The crown of the tooth, the part protruding from the gums, is covered with a layer of *enamel*. Tooth enamel is the hardest substance in the body, but if it is chipped or broken, or attacked by DENTAL CARIES, it cannot renew itself.

Types of Teeth: The teeth have various shapes adapted in special ways to biting and chewing. The eight incisors, four at the front of the upper jaw and four at the front of the lower jaw, have a narrow cutting edge. The four CANINE TEETH (also called cuspids or eyeteeth), one on each side of the incisors in the upper and lower jaws, are stouter than the incisors and are adapted to tearing food too tough to bite. Toward the back of the mouth, the eight BICUSPIDS, or premolars, and 12 MOLARS have broad grinding surfaces.

We have two sets of teeth during our lifetime. The baby teeth (also called deciduous teeth or milk teeth) begin to develop long before birth. The first teeth push through the gums at about six months of age, and most children have a full set of 20 milk teeth by the age of 30 months. The permanent teeth begin to appear at about six years of age. The roots of the baby teeth gradually disappear and the baby teeth fall out. Normally, an adult has 32 permanent teeth. The 12 extra teeth are all grinding teeth. The second and third molars, at the back of the mouth, are the last to appear. The third molars (the wisdom teeth) may not appear until the age of 20 or later, and sometimes they never erupt. A tooth that erupts only partially is said to be impacted. It is often painful, and must usually be extracted.

Care of the Teeth: The main enemies of teeth are DENTAL CARIES and pyorrhea alveolaris. (See PYORRHEA.) The teeth must be kept clean, but brushing too vigorously can harm the teeth and the gums. Brushing should be done in an up-and-down direction, gently removing particles of food that may be lodged in the crevices between the teeth. See also DENTIFRICE.

Regular visits twice a year to the dentist should begin early in childhood. Teeth that are lost should be replaced, in part because the diet is likely to be deficient if one has no teeth to chew with; and also because the remaining teeth tend to drift, causing MALOCCLUSION. If baby teeth are lost early because of decay or accident, the permanent teeth are deprived of the support they need. If a child's permanent teeth are out of alignment, they can be straightened by bands or braces (see ORTHODONTICS).

TOOTHACHE An ache or pain in a tooth. The most frequent cause is decay, which has penetrated the enamel and the dentin, the two outer layers of the tooth. Other causes of toothache may be an abscess, abnormal pressure from an incorrect bite, an impacted WISDOM TOOTH, or pain referred from somewhere else.

TOOTH BRUSHING See DENTIFRICE.

TOOTH DECAY See DENTAL CARIES.

TOOTHPASTE See DENTIFRICE.

TOPICAL Intended to be applied locally, as, for example, a topical medicine or anesthetic.

TOXEMIA The medical term for the presence of a poisonous substance in the circulating blood. A localized infection, such as DIPHTHERIA, may give rise to toxins which circulate in the blood and affect the whole body. In some kinds of FOOD POISONING, toxemia (pronounced tok·see′mee·a) results from eating toxic substances in spoiled food.

In toxemia of pregnancy, no bacterial infection is involved. (See ECLAMPSIA.)

TOXIN A poisonous substance that can be produced in the human body by GERMS, certain chemicals (CARBON TETRACHLORIDE, for example), and some plants and animals. See also FOOD POISONING; VENOM; ANTITOXIN.

TOXIN-ANTITOXIN One of several preparations once used for vaccination against DIPHTHERIA. In toxin-antitoxin, the poisonous quality of the diphtheria TOXIN is almost, but not quite, neutralized by the addition of diphtheria ANTITOXIN. In another kind of diphtheria TOXOID, the toxin is rendered harmless by treatment with FORMALDEHYDE. The latter is more generally used today.

TOXOID A TOXIN that has been treated in such a way that it is no longer poisonous but is still capable of stimulating the body to produce antibodies for immunization against disease. Toxoids are used in preparing vaccines against diphtheria, tetanus, and other bacterial infections. (Pronounced tok′soyd.)

TRACHEA The windpipe, the central trunk of the air passage between throat and lungs. The trachea (pronounced tray′kee·a) is a tube which extends downward from the LARYNX until it divides into the right and left BRONCHI. The passage is kept open by stiff rings of cartilage in the trachea wall.

TRACHEITIS Inflammation of the TRACHEA. The usual causes of tracheitis (pronounced tray″kee· ie′tis) are infections and allergic reactions. Inflammation is not usually confined to the trachea but affects the throat and BRONCHI as well. See also CROUP.

TRACHEOTOMY A surgical operation to make an artificial opening through the skin and neck tissue into the TRACHEA. A tracheotomy (pronounced tray″kee·ot′o·mee) is an emergency measure to bypass some obstruction in the air passage to the lungs. A rigid tube is inserted into the opening to allow the free passage of air.

TRACHOMA A highly contagious disease of the eyelids. If not treated it can lead to BLINDNESS. Trachoma (pronounced tra·koh′ma) is now rare in the United States and Canada, but is widespread in tropical countries.

The disease causes the eyelids to become very swollen and inflamed, and there is a discharge. Trachoma is treated with antibiotics of the TETRACYCLINE type.

TRACTION The application of a pulling force on a fractured bone, dislocated joint, or diseased bone to immobilize the parts in proper position during healing. The pull must be great enough to offset that of the muscles.

A system of weights suspended on pulleys above the patient's bed is used most often for fractures of the femur (thighbone) and of the pelvis. Such weights may be attached to the leg by means of a bandage (called skin traction), or by pins or wires inserted surgically into the bone (skeletal traction).

Devices made of elastic may also be used to exert pull in an injured area. Surgical collars, or neck braces, may be applied as a form of traction after fractures of the neck bones or after WHIPLASH injury. See also BROKEN BONE.

TRANQUILIZER Any of a number of different medicines that, when taken in prescribed dosages,

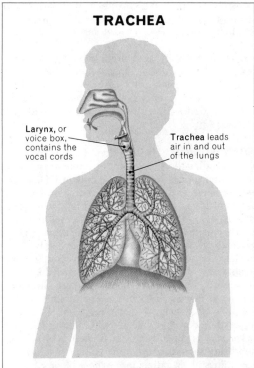

TRACHEA

Larynx, or voice box, contains the vocal cords

Trachea leads air in and out of the lungs

The trachea, or windpipe, extends from the larynx to the point where it branches into the bronchi that lead to the lungs. In patients with severe diphtheria or a throat obstruction which could cause choking, a doctor may relieve breathing by an operation called a tracheotomy; a small incision is made in the trachea, and a tube inserted to bypass the obstruction.

calm mental agitation without undue drowsiness or interference with the ability to respond to stimuli. Following their introduction in the 1950's, the tranquilizers have brought about a great improvement in the management of severe EMOTIONAL AND MENTAL DISORDERS.

Major Strong Tranquilizers: One of the first widely used tranquilizers, RAUWOLFIA, was obtained from a plant which has been known and used in India for centuries. Most of the tranquilizers now in use are synthetic substances. The strongest of them belong to a class of compounds known to chemists by the general name "phenothiazine." One of these that is widely used is CHLORPROMAZINE, sometimes sold under the trade name "Thorazine."

Mild Tranquilizers: MEPROBAMATE (Equanil and Miltown), chlordiazepoxide (Librium), and diazepam (VALIUM) are among the best known of the mild tranquilizers. They are sometimes combined with other medicines and used in the treatment of spasms of the intestinal tract, muscular spasms, and menopausal symptoms. In some alcoholics, the desire to drink may be reduced by the use of Librium.

Tranquilizers may be habit-forming and are more or less toxic, producing side effects that vary widely from person to person. Therefore, they should be used only under close medical supervision.

TRANSFERENCE When undergoing PSYCHOANALYSIS, the patient may unconsciously identify the analyst with an authority figure out of his childhood—usually a parent—and project onto him thoughts, desires, and attitudes associated with that figure.

TRANSFUSION The injection of BLOOD from one person (called the donor) into the circulatory system of another person (called the recipient). There are two general reasons why blood transfusions are required. They are given either to restore a loss in volume of circulating blood or to improve the composition of the blood in some way. The volume of circulating blood can be seriously reduced by hemorrhage, burns, and shock. In such cases, prompt restoration of volume may mean the difference between life and death. In cases where the blood volume is normal, transfusions are administered to supply vital elements that the recipient lacks, such as erythrocytes (red blood cells), ANTIBODIES, or other factors. BLOOD PLASMA or SERUM or a blood substitute such as a SALINE or ALBUMIN solution is sometimes given rather than whole blood.

Usually the transfusion fluid has been obtained in advance from various donors and preserved in a BLOOD BANK until needed. In a direct transfusion, however, blood is transferred straight from the donor to the recipient. In an exchange transfusion, the total blood supply is withdrawn and simultaneously replaced by other blood. Exchange transfusions may be performed in some cases of ERYTH-

ROBLASTOSIS FETALIS, poisoning, and liver disease.

It is essential that the BLOOD TYPES of donor and of recipient be carefully matched, or the blood cells will be destroyed after being transfused. It is also essential that the donor or donors be in good health, since diseases such as hepatitis, malaria, and syphilis can be transmitted by transfusion.

TRANSVESTISM The practice of wearing the clothing of the opposite sex. (Pronounced tranz· ves'tiz· em.)

TRAUMA A wound or injury. There are two types of trauma (pronounced traw'ma): physical and emotional. A bruise, a fracture, or a sprain is a physical trauma. An emotional, or psychic, trauma is an experience or shock that makes a profound impression on the conscious or unconscious mind and may produce symptoms of emotional disturbance, such as PSYCHONEUROSIS.

TRENCH MOUTH See VINCENT'S ANGINA.

TRICHIASIS A disorder of the eyelids in which the lashes grow inward and irritate the eyeball. It may be associated with the infection TRACHOMA. (Pronounced trik· ie'a· sis.)

TRICHINOSIS A disease caused by an infestation of a parasitic roundworm called *Trichinella spiralis*, or trichina. Trichinosis (pronounced trik"i·noh'sis) is a disease of pigs and is transmitted to human beings from infected pork eaten raw or undercooked.

The larvae get into the bloodstream and travel to all the body organs and tissues. In most tissues, they cause inflammation and are destroyed and rejected by the body's defenses. However, in the form of cysts they can survive in muscle fibers for years. **Symptoms:** During the first week, an infected person may have fever, nausea, vomiting, diarrhea, and abdominal pain. In the two-week period during which the larvae migrate in the body, there may be pain in the muscles and swelling of the upper eyelids and other affected areas. Chills and profuse sweating are common. Gradually, the symptoms subside and disappear as the larvae lodge as cysts in the muscles. At present, the usual treatment is bed rest and a nourishing diet during the acute stage. **Prevention:** Thorough cooking of all pork and pork products, such as sausages and frankfurters, will kill any trichinae that may be in the meat.

TRIGLYCERIDES A fatty substance, like CHOLESTEROL, which, if present in the blood in excessive amounts, can be a contributing factor to coronary artery disease. A diet low in saturated fats can help prevent the build-up of triglycerides, and is also the usual treatment prescribed for the condition.

TROPICAL DISEASE A disease that occurs mostly in tropical and semitropical countries. Tropical diseases are generally caused by specific micro-organisms and are communicable. Any trip to the tropics necessitates certain precautions against contracting such diseases.

Before the trip, you should have inoculations against diseases that are prevalent in the regions you intend to visit. You no longer need a smallpox vaccination within three years in order to reenter the United States or Canada from most parts of the world. Typhoid, paratyphoid, tetanus, and poliomyelitis vaccinations may be advisable. Some Asiatic countries require immunization against cholera. Your doctor will probably have all the necessary information about required immunizations. Otherwise, you can obtain it from a local passport office or from a regional office of the Public Health Service of the U.S. Department of Health, Education, and Welfare.

Insect carriers of disease germs present a problem in the tropics. Lice, fleas, ticks, mosquitoes, flies, and mites must be kept off the body. It is often wise to use mosquito netting over your bed and special insecticides that are safe to rub on the skin or on clothing.

Some Tropical Diseases: MALARIA is one of the most widespread tropical diseases, although it is no longer prevalent in the United States. There is no available immunization against malaria, but medicines can be taken to prevent the development of the disease as well as to cure it. SMALLPOX still occurs in some parts of the world. YELLOW FEVER is a virus infection spread by mosquitoes and is found in central Africa and Latin America. Immunization against yellow fever is available. TYPHUS comprises a group of rickettsial diseases and is usually spread by body lice, fleas, and mites. Epidemic (louse) typhus can be prevented by immunization. DYSENTERY, which is not wholly confined to the tropics, is spread by contaminated food and water. The bacillary type may be mild, but amebic dysentery requires treatment by a doctor.

There are a number of other diseases encountered in the tropics, such as YAWS, ELEPHANTIASIS, TRACHOMA, and JUNGLE ROT. They seldom affect the traveler who takes precautions.

See also CHOLERA, DENGUE, LEISHMANIASIS, and SLEEPING SICKNESS.

TRUSS A support worn to keep an inguinal HERNIA in place.

A truss cannot cure the condition, but for a patient whose health and medical history make a remedial operation for hernia inadvisable, a properly fitted truss may be helpful.

TRYPSIN An ENZYME, a substance that initiates and controls chemical reactions in the body, produced in the pancreas and released in the digestive juices to the duodenum. Trypsin (pronounced trip'sin) aids the digestion of proteins.

TSETSE FLY Bloodsucking insect found in tropical Africa. It can carry trypanosomes and infect people and animals by biting them, causing SLEEPING SICKNESS in human beings and wasting diseases of cattle, horses, and other domestic animals. (Pronounced tset'see.)

TSUTSUGAMUSHI DISEASE A disease, caused by a RICKETTSIA microorganism, prevalent in Japan and the Pacific area of Asia. It is also called Japanese river fever and scrub typhus. Tsutsugamushi (pronounced tsoo·tsoo'gah·moo"shee; meaning "dangerous bug") disease is spread by mice and rats through the bites of infected MITES.

TUBERCULIN A substance extracted from cultures of tubercle bacilli and used in tests as a means of diagnosing TUBERCULOSIS. (Pronounced too· bur'kyu·lin.) See also TUBERCULIN TEST.

TUBERCULIN TEST A skin test to determine the presence of TUBERCULOSIS. A small amount of PPD (purified protein derivative of TUBERCULIN) is injected into the skin. If the person has no inflammation around the site of the injection after two days, he is considered to be free of tuberculosis. Inflammation of the site always indicates some evidence of infection, but X rays and other tests may be needed to establish whether the tuberculous lesion is active.

TUBERCULOSIS An infectious, communicable disease caused by *Mycobacterium tuberculosis*. It most frequently affects the lungs, but may also involve the larynx, the bones and joints, the skin (see LUPUS VULGARIS), the lymph nodes (see SCROFULA), the intestines, the kidneys, and the nervous system. The disease is usually contracted by the inhalation of the bacilli into the lungs or by swallowing contaminated food. Droplets of sputum sprayed by an infected person during sneezing and coughing spread the germs directly to others and into the air. The germs are also able to survive for long periods in dried sputum and in dust. Because of eradication of tuberculosis in cattle and widespread pasteurization of milk, transmission of the disease from infected cows is now rare in the United States and Canada.

Types of Tuberculosis: The tuberculosis bacillus can infect almost any body tissue. *Pulmonary* tuberculosis (tuberculosis of the lungs) is the most familiar and widespread form of the disease. In its early stages, pulmonary tuberculosis may exhibit no symptoms. That is why regular chest X rays are important for everyone. If the disease is found in its early stages, it is more easily cured. The symptoms of active pulmonary tuberculosis are loss of weight, weakness, coughing, blood-streaked sputum, and fever that tends to rise gradually during the day.

Miliary tuberculosis is a condition caused by the spread of large numbers of the bacilli to many parts of the body. This type of tuberculosis can affect the meninges (the membranes covering the brain and spinal cord), causing a serious infection called tuberculous meningitis.

Pott's disease is tuberculosis of the spine and results in hunchback (KYPHOSIS). It is now rare.

Treatment: Many persons with tuberculosis can be treated at home, although a rest cure in a sanatorium may be recommended in some cases. There are several medicines used to control and cure the disease, the three chief ones being STREPTOMYCIN, isoniazid (INH), and PAS (para-aminosalicylic acid).

Prevention: The best prevention is to maintain good health and to keep away from people who have tuberculosis. If you have a cough that persists for more than two or three weeks or if you feel tired all of the time and keep losing weight, get medical advice as soon as possible. Never drink unpasteurized milk even if it is certified, because even healthy-looking cattle can transmit tuberculosis germs.

Yearly X-ray tests of the chest are no longer recommended by many physicians because of the fear that the rays may cause cancer. However, everyone should have a TUBERCULIN TEST.

TULAREMIA An acute, infectious disease that can be transmitted to human beings from infected wild animals, chiefly rabbits and squirrels. Tularemia (pronounced too″la·ree′mee·a) is also called rabbit fever.

Tularemia begins suddenly with headache, chills, nausea, and fever accompanied by extreme weakness and profuse sweating. The lymph nodes enlarge, and in some cases there is a red rash. Untreated, the disease may last for weeks and can be fatal.

Treatment and Prevention: Tularemia is treated with antibiotics, especially STREPTOMYCIN, CHLORAMPHENICOL, or one of the TETRACYCLINES.

TUMOR A swelling on or in the body resulting either from abnormal growth of tissue or, as in a CYST, a collection of body fluid or semifluid in a membranous sac. Tumors may be benign or malignant.

Benign tumors and cysts, which are usually harmless, are enclosed by walls of tissue without an opening. They may become quite large and exert pressure on neighboring organs or nerves. Under certain conditions, they may become malignant.

Malignant tumors, or CANCER, differ from benign tumors in that the multiplying cells can rapidly spread into neighboring tissues or can be carried to distant parts of the body in the bloodstream and lymphatic system by METASTASIS. See also CARCINOMA; FIBROID TUMOR; SARCOMA.

TURNER'S SYNDROME A congenital disorder in the female in which growth and sexual development are retarded and the arms and neck are slightly deformed. A person with Turner's syndrome appears to be female but has only a single sex chromosome in each cell (one X CHROMOSOME instead of two as in a normal female), and as a result no ovaries develop. The disorder is named after the American physician Henry Turner.

TWILIGHT SLEEP A type of anesthesia that was once in popular use chiefly for women in labor. The anesthetics used, MORPHINE and SCOPOLAMINE, induce a state in which all sensation of pain is blunted. Moreover, scopolamine tends to produce forgetfulness of the entire process afterward.

TWIN Either of two children born at one birth to the same mother. Twins occur about once in every 86 births. Multiple births of three or more children are much less common. A tendency to produce twins seems to be passed down from mother to daughter. Hormones play a part, and in recent years a number of multiple births have followed the administration of female sex hormones to promote conception.

About two out of three sets of twins are *fraternal* twins. They develop from two different egg cells that happen to be fertilized at the same time. Fraternal twins may be of the same or opposite sex, and they may be as different from each other as any other two siblings.

Identical twins develop from a single fertilized egg cell. At a very early stage of development, the embryo divides in an irregular way and gives rise to two individuals that are identical in hereditary make-up. Identical twins are always of the same sex, the same blood type, and the same eye color. In a very small number of cases, identical twins are not completely separated. They are called conjoined twins, or SIAMESE TWINS.

TWITCHING Involuntary movements, especially in the muscles of the face, may be merely a habit or they may be a symptom of a disorder. A habit spasm, or tic, such as blinking or sniffing, is common in children and generally passes in a few months if ignored. In middle-aged people, such habits are extremely difficult to break.

A few older people get a form of neuralgia called TIC DOULOUREUX. The condition may be treated with painkillers or, in serious cases, surgery, to cut the affected nerve.

TYMPANUM The medical name for EARDRUM. (Pronounced tim′pa·num.)

TYPHOID FEVER An infectious disease caused by a type of salmonella bacillus. The organism may be transmitted by contaminated water, milk, and other foods. The source of the disease is the urine and feces of infected people and of CARRIERS.

The typhoid bacillus gets into the body through the digestive tract. Diagnosis of the disease may be confirmed by the Widal test, in which blood serum from the sick person is mixed with a culture of the salmonella bacillus.

Symptoms and Treatment: Typhoid fever begins with headache and a fever. The temperature continues to rise (often to 105° F or more) each day for about a week. Red spots appear on the chest and abdomen, and there are periods of chills and sweating. CHLORAMPHENICOL and ampicillin are antibiotics effective in shortening the course of typhoid fever to about six days.

Prevention: Food handlers should be examined as potential carriers. Vaccination is available.

TYPHUS A group of infectious diseases caused by various RICKETTSIA microorganisms and spread by lice, fleas, ticks, and mites. Typhus should not be confused with TYPHOID FEVER.

Epidemic typhus fever (also called louse fever and European typhus) is found in cool climates throughout the world. It occurs in persons who are crowded together in unsanitary conditions. The disease is spread from person to person by infected body lice that leave their feces on a break in the skin. The disease is marked by severe headache, fever, nervous and mental disturbances, and a rash that may bleed and become gangrenous. Prevention is by vaccination.

Endemic typhus fever (also called murine typhus) is widely distributed in warm climates. Endemic typhus is a disease of rats and other small rodents, and is transmitted to man through the feces of infected fleas.

All types of typhus are treated with antibiotics. See also TSUTSUGAMUSHI DISEASE (scrub typhus).

TYROTHRICIN An antibiotic that is highly effective when applied to skin infections and wounds. Tyrothricin (pronounced tie″roh·thrie′sin) is not taken internally.

U

ULCER An inflamed open sore on the skin or on the mucous membrane lining a body cavity. There are many different kinds of ulcers.

Peptic ulcers occur in the stomach (*gastric ulcer*) and the duodenum (*duodenal ulcer*), the part of the digestive tract adjoining the lower end of the stomach. Peptic ulcers are most likely to develop in people who are habitually tense and anxious.

Pain is the most common symptom of peptic ulcer. The pain worsens when the stomach is empty, and it can often be relieved by eating, drinking milk, or taking sodium bicarbonate or other antacids. Nausea and vomiting may occur. If untreated, there may be serious complications that require emergency treatment in a hospital.

Recurring pain in the region of the stomach does not necessarily indicate an ulcer, but it should be taken as a signal to see a doctor. He may make a number of tests, including a GASTROINTESTINAL SERIES of X rays.

Treatment: There is no quick and easy cure for peptic ulcer. Treatment includes careful control of the diet, with frequent snacks of milk or other bland foods. Alcohol, tobacco, tea, coffee, and spicy foods should be avoided. The doctor may also prescribe medicine to neutralize the acidity of the gastric juices. At the same time, every effort should be made to relax and avoid worry and tension. Barbiturates and other sedatives are sometimes prescribed for this purpose. Psychiatric counseling (see PSYCHOTHERAPY) may also help.

Other Types of Ulcers: Ulcerative colitis is a condition that occurs in the lower part of the digestive tract. (See COLITIS.)

Mouth ulcers are often found in diseases such as diphtheria, leukemia, and VINCENT'S ANGINA. Syphilis may show its presence by ulcers on the genitals. Poor circulation associated with conditions such as varicose veins, diabetes, and hardening of the arteries may give rise to ulcers, especially on the lower limbs. BEDSORES, or decubitus ulcers, are due to a combination of continuous pressure and sluggish circulation. Skin cancer and a form of breast cancer (called PAGET'S DISEASE) are characterized by ulcers.

ULNA The larger of the two bones of the forearm. (Pronounced ul'na.) See ARM.

UMBILICAL CORD The structure connecting the FETUS, or unborn child, to the PLACENTA. The umbilical (pronounced um·bil'i·kal) cord encloses two arteries and a vein, through which the fetus obtains nourishment and discharges waste products. The cord reaches a length of 20 inches or so at full term.

Immediately after the baby is born, the doctor ties off and cuts the cord, leaving a stump about two inches long. The rest of the cord is expelled from the uterus with the placenta; this is the AFTERBIRTH. The stump is bandaged, and after a few days, it falls off naturally. The navel, or umbilicus, marks permanently the place where the cord was formerly attached.

UNCONSCIOUS (1) Insensible, or lacking consciousness. (See UNCONSCIOUSNESS.)

(2) The unconscious mind. According to psychoanalytic theory (see PSYCHOANALYSIS), it is a storehouse of repressed feelings, fears, and desires that the conscious mind usually cannot call up at will. Frequently, the contents of the unconscious are revealed in dreams, unconscious actions and words (as in SOMNAMBULISM and HYPNOSIS), and slips of the tongue. Repressed emotions—especially those of guilt and hatred—in the unconscious are influential in the development of PSYCHONEUROSIS.

UNCONSCIOUSNESS A loss of consciousness from which it is difficult to arouse a person.

Among the various causes of unconsciousness are concussion, electric shock, poisoning, drowning, sunstroke, convulsions, diabetes, stroke, heart attack, and excess consumption of alcohol or narcotics. It is important to find the exact cause in each case, so that the proper treatment can be given.

What to Do: If the cause of the unconsciousness is known, then the first aid treatment appropriate for the condition should be given at once before calling a doctor. (See "Concussion," "Diabetes," "Electric Shock," etc., in the FIRST AID section.) If the cause is not known, medical help should be summoned immediately. It is unwise to try to move the unconscious person, since he may be suffering from a skull fracture or other serious injury. Do not attempt to give him whiskey or water. If the person has stopped breathing or is breathing feebly, start giving him artificial respiration (see the FIRST AID section) immediately, and continue to do so until his breathing improves. See also COMA; FAINTING.

UNDULANT FEVER See BRUCELLOSIS. (Pronounced un'dyu·lant.)

UPSET STOMACH See ABDOMINAL PAIN; ACID STOMACH; INDIGESTION.

UREMIA A toxic condition of the blood due to the presence of waste products that are normally removed by the kidneys and excreted in urine. In chronic uremia (pronounced yoor·ee′mee·a), an abnormally large volume of urine (but deficient in waste materials) may be produced at one stage; acute uremia is often marked by a decrease in the volume of urine. As the level of toxic substances increases, further symptoms appear. These include anxiety, restlessness, headache, nausea, vomiting, generalized itching, muscular cramps, shortness of breath, and drowsiness. The breath may smell like urine.

Uremia is not always caused by KIDNEY DISEASE. Anything that interferes temporarily with kidney function can cause acute uremia. The long list of possible causes includes burns, a blow on the kidney, kidney stones, adverse reactions to sulfonamide drugs, and congestive heart failure.

In treating acute uremia, the first step is to give the standard treatment for the cause. For example, if the cause is SHOCK, measures are taken to restore normal circulation. The uremia itself can be relieved by circulating the patient's blood through an artificial-kidney machine, which purifies the blood and returns it to the system.

Another method of relieving uremia is called peritoneal dialysis. Special fluid is injected into the peritoneal (abdominal) cavity and allowed to remain there for a time. It is then removed, taking with it some of the body's toxic materials.

URETER One of the two tubes that convey urine from the kidneys to the bladder. The ureter (pronounced yoor·ee′ter) is about a foot long and has a very small inner diameter.

URETHRA The passageway through which urine leaves the bladder and is discharged from the body. The external opening of the urethra (pronounced yoor·ee′thra) is called the meatus. The male meatus is situated at the tip of the penis. The male urethra also serves as a passageway for the discharge of semen. The female urethra serves solely for the discharge of urine.

URETHRITIS Inflammation of the URETHRA. Urethritis (pronounced yoor″e·thrie′tis) is commonly associated with CYSTITIS (inflammation of the bladder). It is generally caused by irritant substances in the urine or by an infection, such as GONORRHEA. The symptoms include burning pain on urination and a discharge that frequently contains blood or pus. The infection may progress through the urethra to the bladder. Treatment is to remove the cause of the problem and to combat the infection with antibiotics.

URIC ACID A colorless and odorless chemical compound that is found in the blood and in the urine. Uric (pronounced yoor′ik) acid is also present in kidney stones and in the joints of a person who has gout.

URINALYSIS The detailed analysis of URINE, done with a microscope, chemical tests, and other means. Urinalysis (pronounced yoor″i·nal′i·sis) helps in the diagnosis of diabetes, diseases of the bladder and kidneys, jaundice, and other disorders.

URINARY TRACT The passageway through which urine produced by the KIDNEYS is expelled from the body. In addition to the kidneys, it includes the two URETERS (the tubes leading from the kidney to the bladder), the BLADDER, and the URETHRA (the tube leading from the bladder and opening to the outside of the body). Two different kinds of disorder may affect the urinary tract: infection and obstruction. Both can lead to damage of the

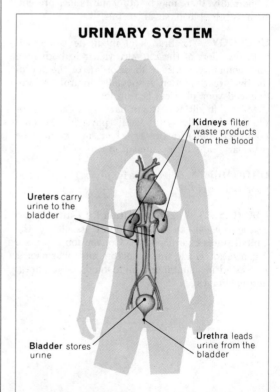

URINARY SYSTEM

Kidneys filter waste products from the blood

Ureters carry urine to the bladder

Bladder stores urine

Urethra leads urine from the bladder

The urinary system consists of the kidneys, ureters, bladder and urethra. Blood filters through the kidneys, which release excess water and waste products as urine. This travels down the ureters to be stored in the bladder, and is discharged from the body through the urethra. In a man, the urethra passes through the prostate gland, where it is joined by sperm ducts from the testicles.

kidneys if left untreated. Obstruction may be caused by a renal calculus (see KIDNEY STONE) or, in a man, by an enlarged PROSTATE GLAND. Infections of various kinds may originate at the opening of the urethra and travel up the urinary tract.

URINATION The process by which the body discharges excess fluid, salts, and other waste products. It is also known as micturition.

The kidneys normally secrete about a quart of urine a day. The amount will vary with the amount of fluid consumed, the temperature, and other factors. Normally, urination occurs about every two to four hours during the day and once at night.

URINE A liquid, normally yellowish in color, that is produced in the kidneys, carried to the bladder by the ureters, and out of the body by the urethra. (See URINARY TRACT.) Urine is mostly water, but it also contains certain waste products from the blood, such as uric acid, urea, ammonia, and creatine. Abnormally, there may be other substances present, such as bile, blood, sugar, or pus.

UROLOGY The branch of medicine concerned with disorders of the URINARY TRACT in both men and women, and also with disorders of the reproductive organs in men. A specialist in urology (pronounced yoor·ol'o·jee) is a urologist.

Many difficulties of the urinary tract can be handled satisfactorily by the family physician. When a complex problem arises or when surgery may be necessary, he will recommend a urologist.

URTICARIA Another name for HIVES. (Pronounced yoor"ti·kair'ee·a.)

USP (U.S.P.) The abbreviation for *United States Pharmacopoeia,* an official report issued by the United States Pharmacopoeia Convention, a private organization made up of doctors and pharmacists interested in maintaining high standards for drugs and medicines.

UTEROTOMY A cutting into the uterus with a surgical instrument, as in CESAREAN (CESARIAN) SECTION. Uterotomy (pronounced yoo"ter·ot'o·mee) is also called hysterotomy and should not be confused with HYSTERECTOMY, the partial or total removal of the uterus.

UTERUS The hollow, muscular organ in the pelvis of the female in which the growing fetus is protected and nourished until birth; the womb. When not carrying a fetus, the uterus (pronounced yoo'ter·us) is about the size and shape of a pear and weighs only a few ounces. The upper part of the organ is broad and branches out on either side into the FALLOPIAN TUBES. At its lower end, the uterus narrows down into the cervix, which leads into the VAGINA. The uterine walls consist of strong, elastic muscle tissue lined with mucous membrane.

From puberty to the menopause, MENSTRUATION occurs approximately every 28 days, except during pregnancy. Each month the lining of the uterus prepares itself for a fertilized egg. (See PREGNANCY.) When conception does not occur, the lining is sloughed off and passes out of the body in the menstrual flow.

Disorders and Diseases: Among the commonest uterine disorders are painful menstruation and excessive flow.

FIBROID TUMORS are benign growths in the muscular walls of the uterus. As a rule they cause little trouble, but may become large enough to interfere with pregnancy or to displace nearby organs.

Sometimes the ligaments holding the uterus in place become stretched after childbirth or other strain. The uterus may be displaced so that it sags too far backward or too far forward. Or it may drop into the upper part of the vagina, a condition known as PROLAPSE. Displacement of the uterus may be corrected by the insertion of a PESSARY to support the organ or, in some cases, by surgery.

Cancer of the uterus—if detected early—is relatively easy to cure. Every woman should have regular pelvic examinations.

VACCINATION A method of making an individual immune to disease by injecting a VACCINE or introducing it into the bloodstream in some other way. The vaccine stimulates the system to produce ANTIBODIES that neutralize the infectious agents or the toxins of the disease. Vaccination is employed to provide immunity against influenza, diphtheria, poliomyelitis, measles, mumps, tetanus, typhoid fever, and yellow fever. See also IMMUNIZATION; INOCULATION.

VACCINE A preparation containing germs that are dead, attenuated (weakened), or still virulent, or else contain modified TOXINS (poisonous material produced by these germs). The vaccine is introduced into the body to produce IMMUNITY.

Vaccines are prepared in a variety of ways. The germs may be killed by exposure to extremely high temperatures or sound waves, or treatment with chemicals. Toxins may be made harmless by chemical treatment. Sometimes a living germ is used, as in the Sabin polio vaccine. Then the virus is attenuated so that the body is immunized against the disease without being harmed. Thanks to polio vaccine, the disease has been largely eradicated. Everyone should still be immunized, however. Smallpox vaccine has also all but wiped out that ancient killer, but in this instance, vaccination is no longer required in most countries.

VACCINIA The medical name for the modified cowpox virus used to vaccinate people against SMALLPOX. It gave its name to the technique called VACCINATION. (Pronounced vak·sin′ee·a.)

VAGINA The passageway between the cervix (neck) of the UTERUS and the female external genital organs, or VULVA. The term "vagina" (pronounced va·jie′na) is also used for many other kinds of sheaths, such as those surrounding tendons and nerves and that enclosing the eyeball.

In sexual intercourse, or COITUS, the vagina becomes a sheath surrounding the erect male penis. SPERM CELLS are discharged into the vagina, and conception occurs when some of the sperm cells encounter a female egg cell, or ovum, after making their way up through the cervix and uterus and entering a FALLOPIAN TUBE.

The vagina is normally about three inches long. The vagina's walls are composed of fibrous and muscular tissue lined with a mucous membrane. In CHILDBIRTH, it becomes part of the birth canal and is stretched to many times its normal size.

Several types of infection can invade the vagina, sometimes producing inflammation (VAGINITIS) and other symptoms. Occasionally, a cyst or a cancer may form in the vagina. An abnormal passage, or fistula, may develop between the vagina and the bladder or the rectum. It is advisable for a woman to have a vaginal examination and a PAP TEST periodically, even if everything seems normal.

VAGINISMUS Painful, spasmodic contraction of the vagina, preventing satisfactory coitus, or sexual intercourse. (Pronounced vaj″i·niz′mus.) Frequently the cause is psychological.

VAGINITIS Inflammation of the VAGINA. Infections of the vagina are fairly common. Besides inflammation, they often cause itching, burning, and increased vaginal discharge, which may have an offensive odor. A number of different organisms may

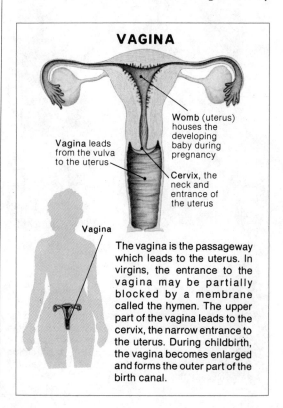

VAGINA

Vagina leads from the vulva to the uterus

Womb (uterus) houses the developing baby during pregnancy

Cervix, the neck and entrance of the uterus

Vagina

The vagina is the passageway which leads to the uterus. In virgins, the entrance to the vagina may be partially blocked by a membrane called the hymen. The upper part of the vagina leads to the cervix, the narrow entrance to the uterus. During childbirth, the vagina becomes enlarged and forms the outer part of the birth canal.

be responsible for vaginitis (pronounced vaj"'i· nie'tis). The VENEREAL DISEASES are often accompanied by vaginitis.

Other possible causes of vaginitis include polyps, cancer, lacerations during childbirth, or irritation from an ill-fitting PESSARY.

VALIUM A trade name for diazepam, one of the most commonly prescribed tranquilizers. Valium (pronounced val'ee·u·m) relieves ANXIETY, DELIRIUM TREMENS, SPASM, and TENSION. The drug has serious side effects and should be taken only under strict medical supervision. Valium may cause birth defects if taken shortly before or during pregnancy. It impairs driving ability (especially if administered in combination with other drugs or alcohol) and can lead to ADDICTION after prolonged or heavy use.

VALVE A flaplike fold of the membrane lining a blood vessel, duct, or other hollow organ, the function of which is to keep a liquid or a semiliquid flowing in one direction only.

VAPORIZER A device that produces steam to be inhaled in the treatment of respiratory disorders. Often liquid medications are added to the water.

VARICELLA The medical name for CHICKEN POX.

VARICOSE VEIN An abnormally dilated, knotted blood vessel, fairly close to the surface of the skin, and located chiefly in the leg and thigh. Varicose (pronounced var'e·kohs) veins are especially common in persons whose occupations involve long periods of standing on their feet. It is believed that the weakness is hereditary.

Varicose veins often appear first in women during pregnancy. Then they require particular attention, as there is a risk of PHLEBITIS.

There may be a crampy sensation, itching, or a feeling of heaviness in the legs. If they are neglected, the skin covering them may become inflamed, and ulcers or other complications may develop.

Treatment: The most effective treatment for severe cases is surgery. The major affected vein is stripped, or removed, from the leg. Weak veins that connect with it are tied off by a process known as ligation. After the operation, the blood makes its way to the heart through other veins.

In mild cases, a chemical solution may be injected into the troublesome veins. The veins eventually are closed off and their function is taken over by other blood vessels.

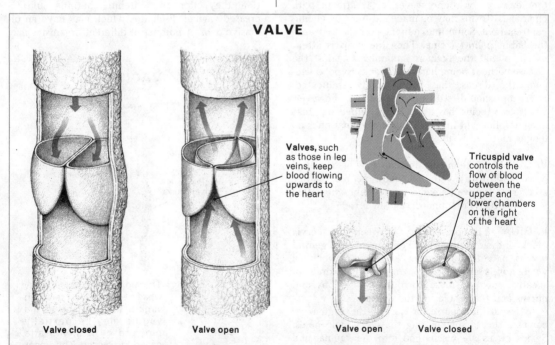

VALVE

Valve closed

Valve open

Valves, such as those in leg veins, keep blood flowing upwards to the heart

Tricuspid valve controls the flow of blood between the upper and lower chambers on the right of the heart

Valve open

Valve closed

There are various types of valves in the body, most of which serve to maintain a one-way flow of fluid through a vessel. Heart valves, for example, make sure that blood flows in only the right direction through the heart. The largest of these, at the entrances of the pulmonary artery and aorta, consist of triangular flaps which open one way under the fluid pressure of blood, then spring closed to prevent any blood flowing back. The large veins in the lower part of the body also have valves which prevent blood flowing back under the influence of gravity and tending to accumulate in the legs.

Slight cases can be controlled by avoiding extensive standing and by resting frequently with the legs in a moderately elevated position. Elastic stockings help to prevent swelling. Walking is valuable in stimulating the circulation in the legs.

VARIOLA The medical name for SMALLPOX. (Pronounced va·rie′o·la.)

VAS DEFERENS The tube through which sperm cells pass from the TESTICLES to the male PENIS. (Pronounced vas′ def′er·enz.)

VASECTOMY A surgical operation in which the VAS DEFERENS is cut, so that sperm cells cannot pass from the testicles to the penis. A vasectomy (pronounced va·sek′to·mee) is simple and virtually painless. It is a completely effective and permanent method of contraception. Vasectomy does not produce any change in virility or sexual desire.

VASOCONSTRICTOR A chemical agent that causes constriction of the blood vessels; also, a nerve fiber that, when stimulated, causes the blood vessels to constrict. (Pronounced vas″oh·kon·strik′tor.)

VASODEPRESSOR A substance that produces a drop in the blood pressure. (Pronounced vas″oh·de·pres′or.)

VASODILATOR A chemical agent that causes the blood vessels to dilate; also, a nerve fiber that, when

stimulated, causes the blood vessels to dilate. (Pronounced vas″oh·die·lay′tor.)

VASOMOTOR Influencing the contraction and dilation of the blood vessels. (Pronounced vas″oh·moh′tor.)

VASOPRESSIN A hormone secreted by the PITUITARY GLAND. Vasopressin (pronounced vas″oh·pres′in) stimulates the blood vessels to contract and thus raises the blood pressure. Its chief medical use is in controlling the excessive urination of diabetes insipidus and stimulating PERISTALSIS (muscular contraction of the alimentary canal).

VECTOR A term applied to any living CARRIER of an infectious disease, but usually limited to insects and animals that transmit such diseases in various ways to human beings. TYPHOID FEVER bacilli on the feet of house flies may be carried from the source of contamination to food, for example.

VEIN A blood vessel that carries blood back to the HEART from all parts of the body. Veins are distinguished from ARTERIES, which serve to carry blood away from the heart. *Venous* blood contains carbon dioxide and waste products picked up from the CAPILLARIES in the tissues. The blood reaches the right side of the heart and is pumped through the lungs where the carbon dioxide is removed, and the blood is replenished with a fresh supply of oxygen. The blood then returns to the left side of the heart

VAS DEFERENS

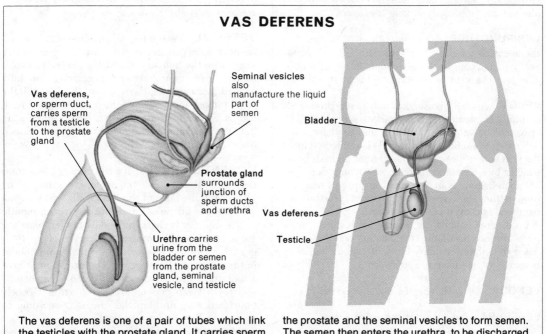

Vas deferens, or sperm duct, carries sperm from a testicle to the prostate gland

Seminal vesicles also manufacture the liquid part of semen

Bladder

Prostate gland surrounds junction of sperm ducts and urethra

Vas deferens

Testicle

Urethra carries urine from the bladder or semen from the prostate gland, seminal vesicle, and testicle

The vas deferens is one of a pair of tubes which link the testicles with the prostate gland. It carries sperm to the prostate, where they mix with secretions from the prostate and the seminal vesicles to form semen. The semen then enters the urethra, to be discharged from the body along the penis.

and is pumped out again through the arteries to all tissues of the body.

Veins contain VALVES that keep the blood flowing toward the heart and prevent it from pooling and flowing backward, especially in the lower part of the body and the legs. See also PHLEBITIS; VARICOSE VEIN.

VENEREAL DISEASE An infection transmitted chiefly through sexual contact. SYPHILIS, GONOR-RHEA, and HERPES SIMPLEX are the major venereal (pronounced ve·neer′ee·al) diseases; others include CHANCROID and LYMPHOGRANULOMA VENEREUM.
Prevention: Good hygiene is imperative in avoiding venereal disease. A CONDOM, or prophylactic rubber sheath, should be worn by the male during the entire period of exposure to the possibility of infection, not just during the sexual act. The sheath offers the best protection for male and female alike, as well as preventing conception. But it by no means eliminates all risk. After contact, the genital area should be washed thoroughly with soap and water.
Symptoms: Typical symptoms of venereal disease are pain, inflammation of the genital area, sores, and a discharge of pus. The primary chancre, or sore, of syphilis is not painful, however. Any symptoms resembling these should immediately be brought to a doctor's attention.

With the advent of such medicines as penicillin and the sulfonamides, and with the publicity given to the dangers, prevention, and treatment of venereal disease, there was a drop in its occurrence. However, in recent years there has been a noticeable increase, especially among teenagers.

VENIPUNCTURE The puncturing of a vein for therapeutic reasons. Venipuncture (pronounced ven″i·pungk′chur) is usually done to inject medicine into the vein or to obtain a blood sample.

VENOM A toxic (poisonous) substance produced naturally by various insects, spiders, scorpions, lizards, snakes, and other animals, and used for self-defense or the subduing of prey. When injected into the skin and tissues of man and larger animals by a sting or bite, venom (pronounced ven′om), depending upon its source, may produce symptoms ranging from itching and swelling to serious prostration, paralysis, and even coma and death.

Fortunately, there are various antivenins (antitoxic serums) available that counteract or slow down the effects of many types of venom. See also INSECT BITE; SNAKEBITE; SPIDER BITE.

VENOUS Of or having to do with VEINS.

VERTEBRA (plural, **vertebrae**) See SPINE.

VERTEBRAL DISK A plate, or disk, of cartilage and fiber, that contains the nucleus pulposus, a mass of white elastic fibers, in its center. The vertebral (pronounced vur′te·bral) disks are situated between the vertebrae, or bones, of the spinal column (see SPINE).
Slipped Disk: The vertebral disks tend to deteriorate with age. This deterioration or an injury or a strain may bring on the painful disorder known variously as slipped disk, herniated disk, or ruptured disk. In this condition, the nucleus pulposus in the middle of the disk bulges through the surrounding cartilage and protrudes. If it presses on the SCIATIC NERVE in the spine, the pain may be acute. (See SCIATICA.)
Treatment: For an accurate diagnosis, a medical examination by an orthopedist and X rays are necessary. The usual treatment includes strict bed rest—on a hard mattress placed over a bed board—until the symptoms have subsided. Later, the person may need to be fitted with a surgical corset or, in the case of a slipped disk in the neck, a special collar.

VERTIGO Extreme dizziness. In true vertigo (pronounced vur′ti·goh), the individual feels that he is being whirled about in space, or that things are whirling about him.

The condition is a symptom of a disturbance of the sense of balance (see BALANCE, SENSE OF) caused by infection in the middle ear or by a disease such as MÉNIÈRE'S DISEASE.

VESICOTOMY Surgery of the urinary bladder, performed to remove bladder stones and tumors, or to repair a FISTULA. Vesicotomy (pronounced ves″i·kot′o·mee) is also known as cystotomy.

VESTIGIAL Pertaining to an unessential or underdeveloped organ or structure in present-day man, or in the human embryo, that in man's evolutionary past may have been essential or fully formed. For example, the so-called third eyelid, the small pinkish membrane at the inner corner of each eye, is vestigial (pronounced ves·tij′ee·al) in man, but in some animals the membrane can be drawn over the entire eyeball.

VINCENT'S ANGINA An infection of the gums that may also involve the membranes lining the cheeks and the back of the throat. Vincent's angina (pronounced an·jie′na) is also called trench mouth.

The disorder is characterized by tender, bleeding gums and later by sores and ulcers covered by a grayish membrane. Fever and swollen lymph nodes in the neck sometimes occur. The breath may have a foul odor. People who do not keep their mouths and teeth clean or who are run-down and poorly nourished may develop the disease. According to recent studies, it is not contagious.
Treatment: In its early stages, Vincent's angina responds well to treatment with ANTIBIOTICS. Usually the dentist treats the disease, since an important

part of the treatment consists of cleaning the teeth to remove tartar and food particles lodged between the teeth or under the edges of the gums. Left untreated, Vincent's angina can lead to pyorrhea alveolaris (see PYORRHEA).

VIOSTEROL A preparation of vitamin D obtained by irradiating ergosterol, a substance present in yeast and other fungi. (Pronounced vie·os'ter·ohl.)

VIRAL DYSENTERY See DYSENTERY.

VIRILISM The presence in a woman of male characteristics, such as hair on the face and chest, a deep voice, and lack of menstruation. A woman's body hair grows in response to the balance of hormones produced by the ovaries and adrenal glands. Wide variations in sexual characteristics are found in any group of healthy women. But a marked change in the amount of hair on the face and body may be caused by treatment with steroid drugs, by oral contraceptives, or by overproduction of certain hormones by the ADRENAL GLANDS generally because they are enlarged or have a TUMOR. The condition is corrected by changing the drugs or by treating the disorder of the adrenals. (Pronounced vir'il·iz·em.)

VIRULENT Descriptive of a disease that is severe, dangerous, and rapid in its course. (Pronounced vir'yu·lent.)

VIRUS Any of a large variety of exceedingly small particles that cause many different diseases. They are sometimes called filterable viruses because, unlike BACTERIA, they easily pass through ordinary laboratory filters.

Viruses occupy the borderline between living and nonliving things. They seem to be complex molecules of protein and nucleic acid, resembling GENES. They show no lifelike activity unless they are introduced into a living cell. They cannot be grown in the laboratory on simple nutrient substances as bacteria can.

Once inside a cell, a virus can control the processes that occur within the cell, including the process of making copies of itself, or reproducing. By changing the cell's chemistry, viruses cause the cell to produce TOXINS. Viruses also act as ANTIGENS—that is, they stimulate the cell to form ANTIBODIES. This is the defense the body musters against viral disease.

Specific viruses are responsible for a host of diseases. These include the common cold, fever sores, shingles, influenza, mumps, measles, chicken pox, smallpox, rabies, poliomyelitis, and many others. Certain viruses have been proved to cause cancer in laboratory animals. There is suggestive evidence that certain types of cancer, such as leukemia, may be caused by viruses. This does not mean, however, that cancer is contagious.

Antibiotics and most other medicines have no effect on the viral diseases. In general, the control of viral diseases depends on the development of vaccines. A few diseases, such as poliomyelitis and rubella (German measles), have now been brought under control in this way.

VISCERA The internal organs of the body, particularly those in the chest and abdominal cavities. (Pronounced vis'er·a.)

VISION See BLINDNESS; EYE.

VITAMIN Any of a group of substances found in very small amounts in most foods. A well-balanced, varied diet contains all the vitamins normally needed for health. Vitamins in excess of what the body needs do not increase health or well-being, and may actually produce illness. A poor diet cannot be corrected simply by taking vitamins in concentrated form.

Vitamin A plays a part in the chemical reactions that take place in the retina of the eye when it is stimulated by light. In other words, vitamin A is essential to vision. Lack of vitamin A can lead to XEROPHTHALMIA and to poor vision in dim light (night blindness). Vitamin A is found in all animal tissues, but it is especially abundant in fish-liver oil. An indirect source of vitamin A is a substance called CAROTENE, which the body can convert into vitamin A. Carrots and orange-colored fruits and vegetables contain plentiful amounts of carotene. If pure vitamin A concentrate is taken daily in very large amounts, it can lead to severe disorders of the nervous system, bones, and other tissues.

Vitamin B (vitamin B group) contains a number of vitamins that are usually known by their chemical names. They include thiamine, riboflavin, niacin, pantothenic acid, folic acid, and vitamin B_{12}, described below, as well as other substances.

Thiamine, or vitamin B_1, is found in many foods. Yeast, wheat germ, pork, and liver are especially good sources. BERIBERI is due to thiamine deficiency as are some of the symptoms that accompany chronic alcoholism.

Riboflavin, or vitamin B_2, occurs chiefly in milk, egg white, liver, and leafy vegetables. Skin disorders, inflammation of the tongue, and cracking at the corners of the mouth may result from lack of sufficient riboflavin.

Niacin, or nicotinic acid, is abundant in yeast, wheat germ, and organ meats (liver, kidney, heart, and brain). Milk contains large amounts of a substance that the body readily converts to niacin. PELLAGRA is due to severe niacin deficiency.

Pantothenic acid is plentiful in liver, kidney, egg yolk, and fresh green vegetables. No abnormal conditions are known to result from lack of this vitamin.

Folic acid, also known as PGA (*p*teroyl*g*lutamic *a*cid), is plentiful in liver, yeast, mushrooms, and green leafy vegetables. This vitamin is essential to a number of chemical reactions that take place in the nucleus of every cell in the body. Alcohol and several other substances, including some antibiotics, interfere with the utilization of folic acid. Some kinds of anemia, sprue, and chronic alcoholism are associated with folic acid deficiency.

Vitamin B$_{12}$ is abundant in liver and other organ meats. It plays a part in the formation of red blood cells, or erythrocytes. In normal, healthy people, most of the vitamin B$_{12}$ needed is absorbed in the digestive system. People with pernicious anemia are unable to absorb this vitamin properly, and the disease is controlled by vitamin B$_{12}$ concentrate.

Vitamin C, or ASCORBIC ACID, is abundant in many fruits and vegetables, especially in oranges, lemons, and tomatoes. It is often added to canned fruit juices and fruit drinks. Lack of vitamin C causes SCURVY. Since the body cannot store vitamin C, foods containing it should be eaten daily to maintain good health.

Vitamin D is sometimes called the sunshine vitamin because it is produced in the skin when a person is outdoors in the sun. It plays a part in bone formation and the utilization of calcium. RICKETS in children is associated with lack of sufficient vitamin D. Commercially prepared foods, such as milk and bread, are often enriched with vitamin D. If pure vitamin D concentrate is prescribed by your doctor, do not take more than he orders. Deposits of calcium in the kidneys, heart, and other soft tissues can result from taking massive does of vitamin D.

Vitamin E is present in most foods and very abundant in vegetable oils. Very little is known about the role of this vitamin in human diets.

Vitamin K is very abundant in green leafy vegetables. It is also formed by bacteria normally present in the intestine. It has an essential role in the clotting of blood.

VITREOUS BODY (vitreous humor) See EYE. (Pronounced vit′ree·us.)

VITAMINS

The body requires small quantities of various vitamins to remain healthy. It cannot make enough or all of these for itself, and so they have to be provided in food. A well-balanced diet containing meat, fish, dairy products and fresh fruit and vegetables contains enough vitamins for the body's needs. A poor diet can give rise to various deficiency diseases. These charts show foods rich in the common vitamins: vitamins A and C, and thiamine, niacin and riboflavin from the B-group vitamins.

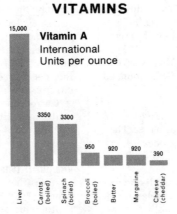

Vitamin A International Units per ounce

Daily requirement is 5000 i.u. for an adult, half this for a child.

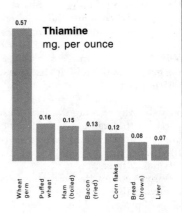

Thiamine mg. per ounce

Daily requirement is 1.5 mg. for an adult, 0.7 mg. for a child.

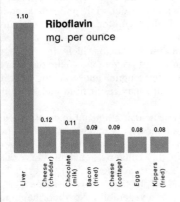

Riboflavin mg. per ounce

Daily requirement is 1.7 mg. for an adult, 0.8 mg. for a child.

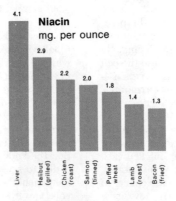

Niacin mg. per ounce

Daily requirement is 20 mg. for an adult, 9.0 mg. for a child.

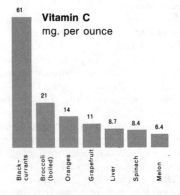

Vitamin C mg. per ounce

Daily requirement is 60 mg. for an adult, slightly less for a child.

VOCATIONAL REHABILITATION See OCCUPA-
TIONAL THERAPY AND VOCATIONAL REHABILITATION.

VOICE BOX See LARYNX.

VOLVULUS A twisting of the intestine into a loop,
causing blockage and a shutdown of the blood supply to the area. A volvulus (pronounced vol′vyu·l*u*s)
occurs most often in the COLON, or large intestine,
and is more common in middle-aged and elderly
people. The symptoms are severe pain and disten-
tion of the abdomen from gas and feces trapped in
the colon. Immediate surgery is necessary.

VOMITING Throwing up; emesis; discharging the
contents of the stomach by way of the mouth. Eating contaminated food and eating and drinking to
excess are among the commonest causes; so, too, are
disorders of the digestive tract, such as GASTRITIS.
MOTION SICKNESS frequently causes severe vomiting.
It may occur in association with an attack of migraine (see HEADACHE) and with infections and fevers. Early in pregnancy, women may have spells of
vomiting.

VOYEURISM An abnormal condition in which the
individual obtains sexual fulfillment by looking at
the sexual acts or organs of others.

VULVA The external female GENITALS, which surround the opening of the VAGINA. (Pronounced
vul′v*a*.) A thin membrane, the HYMEN, usually partly
covers the opening to the vagina before women
have had sexual relations. The vaginal opening is
surrounded by two folds of flesh. The inner folds
meet in front at the CLITORIS, a small projection of
sensitive, erectile tissue. The opening of the URE-
THRA is situated just behind the clitoris.

Disorders that produce vulvitis, or inflammation
of the vulva, are fairly common. Causes include
tight-fitting underclothes, contamination by urine or
feces, and local allergic reactions to detergents and
medicines. In many cases, the cause is more serious.
A number of infections, including gonorrhea and
syphilis, can affect both the vulva and the vagina.

Intense itching and burning pain are very common symptoms in vulvitis. Swelling and reddening
may be severe or hardly noticeable. In any case, a
doctor should be consulted about the condition.

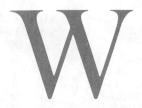

WALLEYE See STRABISMUS.

WART A small, usually hard, BENIGN growth formed on and rooted in the skin; also called verruca. It is caused by a virus. Ordinary warts tend to occur most often on the hands, fingers, elbows, and face and are most common in young people.

Plantar warts always occur on the bottom of the foot, often on the metatarsal region (see FOOT). Because of pressure from standing and walking, these warts are painful and become covered with a thick callus. Moist warts occur on the genitals and the anus, causing itching and discomfort.

Warts must be treated by a doctor. Never attempt to remove a wart yourself.

WASP STING See INSECT BITE; BEE STING.

WASSERMANN TEST The most widely known of the tests used to determine the presence of SYPHILIS. It was developed in 1906 by August von Wassermann (pronounced wos'er·man), a German bacteriologist. The test consists in taking a small quantity of blood from a vein and testing it in the laboratory to see if there is an antibody reaction to syphilis germs. Positive results do not always mean that the person tested has syphilis, and further tests and examinations should be made.

WAX IN THE EAR See CERUMEN.

WEIGHT WATCHERS An organization of persons whose aim is to lose weight. Members of Weight Watchers are supplied with recipes and information that they are expected to use faithfully to overcome their obesity. Regular meetings are held at which the individuals are weighed and their progress (or lack of progress) is ascertained. The members also discuss as a group their problems in weight control to strengthen their resolve to go on losing weight.

For further information, you can write to Weight Watchers International Inc., 800 Community Drive, Manhasset, New York 11030.

WEN Another name for sebaceous cyst. See CYST.

WHEAL A temporarily swollen spot on the skin, as in HIVES. (Pronounced weel.)

WHEEZING The whistling or grating sound made during difficult breathing, or DYSPNEA. During an attack of ASTHMA, the bronchial tubes go into spasm and are sometimes clogged with thick mucus. The airway to the lungs becomes very narrow, and the effort to breathe causes the wheezing. A bad cold, PNEUMONIA, and CONGESTIVE HEART FAILURE will cause wheezing because fluid collected in the lungs and in the pleural (lung) cavity inhibits free breathing. It is important that prolonged wheezing be reported to your doctor so that he may determine the cause and treat it.

WHIPLASH An injury that may be suffered in an automobile collision. The term is not a scientific one, but in general it describes a sudden strain or tearing of ligaments or muscles in the neck; it is usually caused by a violent jerking of the head and neck as a result of a severe jolt. The neck of a person who has suffered a whiplash injury should be supported by a special collar for several weeks until the injury heals. Analgesics such as aspirin help to relieve the pain; local application of heat also proves beneficial.

Occasionally, whiplash may involve more serious injury. Any person involved in an accident should consult his doctor, since sometimes injuries occur that are not immediately evident.

WHISKEY NOSE See RHINOPHYMA.

WHITE BLOOD CELL See BLOOD; LEUKOCYTE.

WHITES See LEUKORRHEA.

WHO Abbreviation for WORLD HEALTH ORGANIZATION. (Pronounce each letter.)

WHOOPING COUGH An acute, very contagious disease of the bronchial tubes and the upper respiratory passages. The medical name is pertussis. It is primarily a childhood disease that attacks children under 10 years of age. It is especially dangerous in early infancy. At its height, whooping cough is marked by severe bouts of coughing ending in a whooping sound, because the person must take a deep breath.

Symptoms and Course: The incubation period of whooping cough is from 7 to 14 days. The early stage, which lasts for a week or two, is much like a heavy cold, with some fever and a persistent cough. At this time, the disease may escape diagnosis. Then the cough grows worse, and the person begins to whoop. This stage lasts up to four weeks from the start of the illness, and then gradually subsides. During this period, the disease is still contagious. **Treatment:** The sick person should be kept in bed while the fever lasts. He should have plenty of fresh air, as it seems to lessen the severity of the coughing. A well-rounded, plentiful diet is important during whooping cough to prevent undue loss of weight. If vomiting occurs often after coughing spells, try serving small amounts of food at frequent intervals. Keep the sick person away from anyone with a cold. Antibiotics such as CHLORAMPHENICOL and the TETRACYCLINES help to shorten the duration of the disease.

Prevention: A vaccine against whooping cough is usually given to infants as young as six weeks, followed by two more injections at monthly intervals. It is commonly combined with tetanus and diphtheria vaccines (DPT).

WINDPIPE See TRACHEA.

WINTERGREEN OIL An aromatic oil used as a flavoring and in medicines; it is also called oil of wintergreen. The oil may be made synthetically or extracted from the leaves of wintergreen plant or the sweet birch.

WISDOM TOOTH The last tooth at each end of the upper and lower jaws. See TOOTH.

WOMB Another word for UTERUS.

WORLD HEALTH ORGANIZATION (WHO) An agency of the United Nations concerned with maintaining and achieving good health of people all over the world. The organization has its headquarters in Geneva, Switzerland.

WHO gives assistance to developing countries in training doctors, improving sanitation and water supplies, and providing medical research on diseases peculiar to certain regions. It is active in helping to control malaria, leprosy, yaws, elephantiasis, syphilis, trachoma, tuberculosis, and less well-known diseases. It also offers services to safeguard the health of mothers and children.

Through WHO, international quarantine regulations and standards for medicines and vaccines have been established. The organization also broadcasts news and information regarding epidemics in all parts of the world.

WORM Worm infections and diseases are caused by parasites that live and multiply in the bodies of human beings and some animals. The worms often infect the intestine, but some types are found in other organs, in the blood, and in muscle tissue. Worm infection is relatively infrequent in temperate regions such as the United States and Canada; in the Orient and in tropical countries, it poses a serious health problem. Most worm infections are passed from person to person through water, food, and soil contaminated with human feces that contain worm eggs. The meat of some infected animals and fish, if insufficiently cooked, is another source of infection. For further discussion, see ELEPHANTIASIS, HOOKWORM DISEASE, PINWORM INFECTION, TAPEWORM, and TRICHINOSIS.

WOUND A break in the skin and often underlying tissues. It may be a cut, puncture, contusion (caused by a blow), abrasion (graze), or laceration (tear). All wounds should be washed with soap and water or a mild antiseptic solution, and covered with a clean dry dressing and bandage, or an adhesive-plaster dressing. For emergency treatment of a bleeding wound, see FIRST AID section.

Cuts tend to bleed and may need stitching to assist healing and minimize scarring. When in doubt whether or not a cut needs stitching, consult a doctor or hospital emergency room.

The main danger from a puncture or stab wound is damage to internal organs with subsequent internal bleeding; a doctor's diagnosis is needed.

A contusion is accompanied by bruising and is slow to heal; there may also be crush injury to bones or internal organs.

Severe lacerations give rise to shock and, more than any other type of wound, are liable to infection. Antitetanus serum is generally given, and any infection is treated with antibiotics (see TETANUS).

See also BLEEDING.

WRITER'S CRAMP A muscular spasm in the hand and arm, occurring in people, such as tailors, typists, musicians, metal workers, and writers, who do much repetitive work with their hands. Although bad posture may contribute to the condition, it has no organic cause, and the hand is still able to do similar, but different tasks. For instance, a typist with writer's cramp is still able to use the same muscles to knit, indicating that the cramp may be largely psychological in origin.

XYZ

XANTHOMA A yellowish, benign, fatty tumor appearing on the eyelids, around joints, and over certain tendons. A xanthoma (pronounced zan·thoh'm*a*) is caused by faulty metabolism of fats and localized deposits of CHOLESTEROL.

X CHROMOSOME In genetics, the sex chromosome associated with femaleness (chromosomes are bodies in the cell nucleus that carry the GENES, which determine one's inherited characteristics). Every normal person has two sex chromosomes in each cell, and a person with two X chromosomes (XX) is female. There is also a Y CHROMOSOME, and a person with the combination XY is male. Certain congenital defects are associated with abnormal sex chromosomes. For instance, a person with one X chromosome only (XO) has TURNER'S SYNDROME. A person with an extra X chromosome (XXY) has KLINEFELTER'S SYNDROME. Each of these conditions involves abnormal sexual characteristics and may cause sterility (see HERMAPHRODITE).

XEROPHTHALMIA A condition of the EYE in which the cornea is dry and may become inflamed and ulcerated. Xerophthalmia (pronounced zir"of·thal'mee·*a*) is caused by a lack of vitamin A in the diet (see VITAMIN). The condition also dries out the conjunctivas (the membranes lining the eyelids and the front of the eyeball) and slows down the production of tears by the tear glands. Often an individual with xerophthalmia also suffers from NIGHT BLINDNESS.

Treatment includes taking doses of vitamin A as prescribed by a doctor and using special ointments to combat infection.

XEROSIS Abnormal dryness of the skin, the eyes, or the mucous membranes. Xerosis (pronounced zi·roh'sis) may result from a disease or other disorder, or it may be simply a normal drying of tissues associated with advancing age.

X RAY A form of electromagnetic radiation with extremely short wavelengths and great penetrating power. It is used in medicine to help diagnose certain diseases, to find the extent and location of injuries, and to treat disease. X ray is valuable in treating many types of cancer. (See RADIOLOGY.)

By means of X-ray pictures of internal organs, doctors are able to detect many conditions, including pulmonary tuberculosis, pneumonia, broken and diseased bones, stomach ulcers, and intestinal obstructions (see GASTROINTESTINAL SERIES). Dentists use X ray to photograph teeth suspected of having DENTAL CARIES or other abnormalities.

The use of X ray must always be under medical supervision, since overexposure may cause sterility, skin disorders, cancer, and RADIATION SICKNESS.

(See illustration on following page.)

YAWS A tropical disease due to infection by a SPIROCHETE bacterium. Although this organism is closely related to the spirochete that causes syphilis, yaws (also called frambesia) is not a venereal disease. It is spread by nonsexual contact with persons who have the disease. The symptoms include fever, rheumatic pain, and a skin eruption of clusters of small sores covered with a crust. The disease can be readily controlled with penicillin.

Y CHROMOSOME In genetics, the sex chromosome associated with maleness (chromosomes are bodies in the cell nucleus that carry the GENES, which determine one's inherited characteristics). Every normal person has two sex chromosomes in each cell, and at least one of them is an X CHROMOSOME. If the other is a Y chromosome, the person is male (XY); the combination XX results in a female. There are various disorders associated with an abnormal arrangement of sex chromosomes. For example, a person with the abnormal chromosome combination XXY has KLINEFELTER'S SYNDROME.

YELLOW FEVER An acute, infectious disease once common in southern coastal cities of the United States and still widespread in parts of Central and South America as well as Africa. It is caused by a virus transmitted by the female *Aedes aegypti* mosquito, as well as by other species. Yellow fever is also known as yellow jack.

Symptoms: After an incubation period of three to six days, symptoms begin to appear suddenly. The person runs a moderately high fever. But the most conspicuous symptom is jaundice, a yellowing of the skin and eyes caused by the presence of an excess of bile in the blood and tissues.

Treatment: There are no specific medications for curing the disease. For the mild form of the disease, there is a good rate of recovery, with temperature returning to normal after a week or so. In an epidemic, however, the death rate is sometimes extremely high.

X RAYS

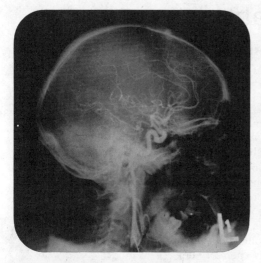

An angiogram, an X ray of blood vessels, can detect a fault in the brain's blood supply, such as a blood clot, which may cause a stroke.

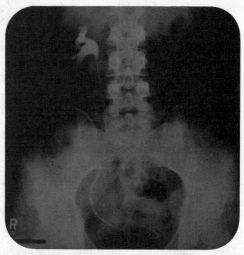

The kidney stands out on this pyelogram because it contains a substance, injected into it along the urethra, which is opaque to X rays.

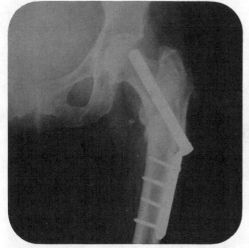

Mending of a fracture is being checked in this X ray, which shows a metal plate on the thighbone and the pinned head of the femur.

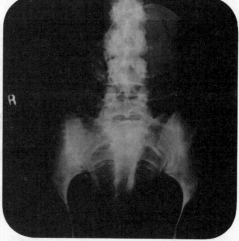

The position of a breech baby is revealed in this X ray, which shows that the baby is lying head upward in the mother's womb.

Anyone entering an area of the world where there is likelihood of yellow fever should obtain a vaccination.

ZINC OXIDE A yellowish-white, soft powder soothing to irritated skin. When combined with PETROLATUM, it is called zinc ointment, and is used for minor burns, insect bites, chafing, and other skin irritations.

ZOONOSIS A disease or infection transmitted to human beings from an infected animal. (Pronounced zoh·on'o·sis.) An example is RABIES, which is transmitted from dogs, cats, bats, and other animals.

ZYGOTE The cell formed from the union of an EGG CELL (ovum) and a SPERM CELL; a fertilized egg, which is the first stage in the development of an EMBRYO. (Pronounced zie'goht.)

Pronunciation Key

In order to assist the reader in pronouncing unfamiliar medical terms, a simplified pronunciation system has been worked out by the editors, using the ordinary letters of the alphabet. Unstressed vowels are in *italics*, as, for example, the *a* in alone (*a* • lohn′) and the *e* in happen (hap′*en*). Silent letters are dropped from the phonetic form of the word. A primary stress mark, or accent (′), and a secondary stress mark (″) are used. The primary mark follows the syllable that has the heaviest stress; the secondary mark follows a syllable, in a word of three or more syllables, on which a somewhat lighter stress should fall (book′kee″p*er*). A dot (•) indicates the division of syllables (dis • pen′s*er* • ee).

Symbol	Sample Word	Transcription	Symbol	Sample Word	Transcription
a	map	map	m	move	moov
a	alone	*a* • lohn′	n	nice	nies
ai	care; air	kair; air	o	odd	od
ah	father	fah′th*er*	*o*	melon	mel′*on*
aw	jaw; order	jaw; awr′d*er*	oh	open	oh′p*en*
ay	rate	rayt	oo	pool; took	pool; took
b	bat	bat	ow	out; now	owt; now
ch	check	chek	oy	boy; oil	boy; oyl
d	dog	dawg	p	pit	pit
e	end	end	r	run	run
e	happen	hap′*en*	s	see; acid	see; as′id
ee	tree	tree	sh	sure; attention	shoor; *a* • ten′sh*un*
f	fine; photo	fien; foh′toh	t	sit	sit
g	go	goh	th	thin; this	thin; this
h	hope	hohp	u	up; done	up; dun
i	give	giv	*u*	circus	sur′k*us*
i	easily	ee′*zi* • lee	ur	urn; term	urn; turm
ie	wine	wien	v	vim	vim
ing	sing	sing	w	win	win
j	joy; gypsy	joy; jip′see	y	yet	yet
k	take; care	tayk; kair	yoo	use; few	yoos; fyoo
ks	ox	oks	z	zoo; please	zoo; pleez
kw	quick	kwik	zh	pleasure; vision	plezh′*ur*; vizh′*en*
l	look	look			

FAMILY
HEALTH
RECORD

Family Health Record

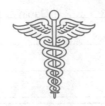

Many physicians assisted in the preparation of the *Reader's Digest Family Health Guide and Medical Encyclopedia.* All of them were agreed that, if a patient could give even some of the information that you will record in the following pages, the doctor's job—and the patient's health—would be far more trouble-free.

Keep your family's medical records complete and up to date. Most parents, of course, keep some form of record of their children's health problems and doctor's visits. But it is just as important for parents—and all adults—to keep their own "medical history."

This section has been designed as a convenient, easy-to-use method of organizing information on the health of every member of your family. *Make sure it is up to date.*

NAME

Birth Information: Date _____ Weight _____ Height _____

Place _____ Blood Type _____ RH Factor _____

Immunization Dates (including booster shots)

Diphtheria/Whooping Cough/Tetanus (OPT) _____

Tetanus/Diphtheria (TO) _____

Polio: Salk _____ Sabin _____

Smallpox _____

Other _____

_____

Allergic Reactions to medicines and other substances

_____

_____

_____

Special Conditions requiring continuing medication

_____

_____

_____

_____

_____

X-Rays, including dental (date, place, purpose)

_____

_____

_____

_____

_____

_____

_____

_____

_____

Transfusions (date, place, description)

_____

_____

_____

Insurance Policies, health and accident

_____

_____

_____

Regular Doctor (address and telephone)

Specialists _____

Dentist _____

Alternate Dentist _____

Illness, Disease, or Injury (date, description, doctor(s), hospital, or clinic)

_____

_____

_____

_____

_____

_____

_____

_____

Surgical Operations (date, description, surgeon, hospital)

_____

_____

_____

_____

_____

Continued on next page

Continued from previous page.

Routine Checkups (date, doctor, and remarks)

General Physical _____

_____

_____

_____

_____

_____

_____

_____

_____

_____

Dental _____

_____

_____

_____

_____

_____

_____

Eyes _____

_____

_____

_____

_____

_____

Notes: A record of minor illnesses, such as colds; injuries, such as slight sprains; recurrent pains; periods of constipation; etc. This information may be important to your doctor when you have your routine checkup.

Date	Description	Medication (if any)

NAME

Birth Information: Date_____ Weight_____Height_____

Place_____ Blood Type_____RH Factor_____

Immunization Dates (including booster shots)

Diphtheria/Whooping Cough/Tetanus (OPT)_____

Tetanus/Diphtheria (TO)_____

Polio: Salk_____ Sabin_____

Smallpox_____

Other_____

_____

Allergic Reactions to medicines and other substances

_____

_____

_____

Special Conditions requiring continuing medication

_____

_____

_____

_____

_____

X-Rays, including dental (date, place, purpose)

_____

_____

_____

_____

_____

_____

_____

_____

Transfusions (date, place, description)

_____

_____

Insurance Policies, health and accident

_____

_____

Regular Doctor (address and telephone)

Specialists _____

Dentist _____

Alternate Dentist _____

Illness, Disease, or Injury (date, description, doctor(s), hospital, or clinic)

_____

_____

_____

_____

_____

_____

_____

_____

Surgical Operations (date, description, surgeon, hospital)

_____

_____

_____

_____

_____

Continued on next page

Continued from previous page .

Routine Checkups (date, doctor, and remarks)

General Physical _____

_____

_____

_____

_____

_____

_____

_____

_____

_____

_____

_____

Dental _____

_____

_____

_____

_____

_____

_____

_____

_____

Eyes _____

_____

_____

_____

_____

_____

_____

Notes: A record of minor illnesses, such as colds; injuries, such as slight sprains; recurrent pains; periods of constipation; etc. This information may be important to your doctor when you have your routine checkup.

Date	Description	Medication (if any)

NAME

Birth Information: Date _____ Weight _____ Height _____

Place _____ Blood Type _____ RH Factor _____

Immunization Dates (including booster shots)

Diphtheria/Whooping Cough/Tetanus (OPT) _____

Tetanus/Diphtheria (TO) _____

Polio: Salk _____ Sabin _____

Smallpox _____

Other _____

_____

Allergic Reactions to medicines and other substances

_____

_____

_____

Special Conditions requiring continuing medication

_____

_____

_____

_____

_____

X-Rays, including dental (date, place, purpose)

_____

_____

_____

_____

_____

_____

_____

_____

Transfusions (date, place, description)

_____

_____

_____

Insurance Policies, health and accident

_____

_____

_____

Regular Doctor (address and telephone)

Specialists _____

Dentist _____

Alternate Dentist _____

Illness, Disease, or Injury (date, description, doctor(s), hospital, or clinic)

_____

_____

_____

_____

_____

_____

_____

_____

Surgical Operations (date, description, surgeon, hospital)

_____

_____

_____

_____

_____

Continued on next page

Continued from previous page.

Routine Checkups (date, doctor, and remarks)

General Physical _____

_____

_____

_____

_____

_____

_____

_____

_____

_____

_____

Dental _____

_____

_____

_____

_____

_____

_____

_____

Eyes _____

_____

_____

_____

_____

_____

Notes: A record of minor illnesses, such as colds; injuries, such as slight sprains; recurrent pains; periods of constipation; etc. This information may be important to your doctor when you have your routine checkup.

Date	Description	Medication (if any)

NAME

Birth Information: Date_____ Weight_____ Height_____

Place_____ Blood Type_____ RH Factor_____

Immunization Dates (including booster shots)

Diphtheria/Whooping Cough/Tetanus (OPT)_____

Tetanus/Diphtheria (TO)_____

Polio: Salk_____ Sabin_____

Smallpox_____

Other_____

_____

Allergic Reactions to medicines and other substances

_____

_____

_____

Special Conditions requiring continuing medication

_____

_____

_____

_____

_____

X-Rays, including dental (date, place, purpose)

_____

_____

_____

_____

_____

_____

_____

_____

_____

Transfusions (date, place, description)

_____

_____

_____

Insurance Policies, health and accident

_____

_____

_____

Regular Doctor (address and telephone)

Specialists _____

Dentist _____

Alternate Dentist _____

Illness, Disease, or Injury (date, description, doctor(s), hospital, or clinic)

_____

_____

_____

_____

_____

_____

_____

_____

Surgical Operations (date, description, surgeon, hospital)

_____

_____

_____

_____

_____

Continued on next page

Continued from previous page .

Routine Checkups (date, doctor, and remarks)

General Physical _____

_____

_____

_____

_____

_____

_____

_____

_____

_____

_____

Dental _____

_____

_____

_____

_____

_____

_____

_____

Eyes _____

_____

_____

_____

_____

_____

Notes: A record of minor illnesses, such as colds; injuries, such as slight sprains; recurrent pains; periods of constipation; etc. This information may be important to your doctor when you have your routine checkup.

Date	Description	Medication (if any)

NAME

Birth Information: Date _____ Weight _____ Height _____

Place _____ Blood Type _____ RH Factor _____

Immunization Dates (including booster shots)

Diphtheria/Whooping Cough/Tetanus (OPT) _____

Tetanus/Diphtheria (TO) _____

Polio: Salk _____ Sabin _____

Smallpox _____

Other _____

_____

Allergic Reactions to medicines and other substances

_____

_____

_____

_____

Special Conditions requiring continuing medication

_____

_____

_____

_____

_____

X-Rays, including dental (date, place, purpose)

_____

_____

_____

_____

_____

_____

_____

_____

Transfusions (date, place, description)

_____
_____
_____

Insurance Policies, health and accident

_____
_____
_____

Regular Doctor (address and telephone)

Specialists _____

Dentist _____

Alternate Dentist _____

Illness, Disease, or Injury (date, description, doctor(s), hospital, or clinic)

_____
_____
_____
_____
_____
_____
_____
_____
_____

Surgical Operations (date, description, surgeon, hospital)

_____
_____
_____
_____
_____

Continued on next page

Continued from previous page .

Routine Checkups (date, doctor, and remarks)

General Physical _____

_____

_____

_____

_____

_____

_____

_____

_____

_____

Dental _____

_____

_____

_____

_____

_____

_____

Eyes _____

_____

_____

_____

_____

_____

Notes: A record of minor illnesses, such as colds; injuries, such as slight sprains; recurrent pains; periods of constipation; etc. This information may be important to your doctor when you have your routine checkup.

Date	Description	Medication (if any)

INDEX

How to Use This Index

This index is designed to help the reader locate all the significant information throughout the book about the subject in which he is interested, while at the same time highlighting the encyclopedia article devoted to that subject. For example, under the entry "Adenoids," the boldface figure (**322**) shows the page on which the encyclopedia article about adenoids appears, while the lightface figures (73, 201, 562) refer to the other pages where adenoids are discussed. The pages on which illustrations appear are indicated by italic figures (*107, 201, 322*).

In order that first aid instructions may be found as quickly as possible, references to first aid are in boldface: **first aid for,** 301.

Circulatory system, 12, 31, 37, 49, 237
Circumcision, 64, 181, **384**, 437
Circumvallate papilla, *76-77*
Cirrhosis of the liver, 61, 264, 352, **384–385**
Clavicle, **385**, *385*
Cleaning fluid:
   first aid if swallowed, 311
Cleanliness, 11, 64, 78, 80–81, 83, 86, 112, 367
   for bed-ridden patient, 246–247, 251
   for chicken pox, 380–381
   See also Bath; Hygiene.
Cleft lip. *See* Harelip.
Cleft palate, **385**, 445, 555
Clergyman's throat, **385**
Climacteric. *See* Menopause.
Climate, elderly and, 239–240
Clinic, **385–386**
Clinical psychologist, 132, 525–526
Clitoris, 64, 148 149, 150, **386**, 577
Closed-chest heart massage:
   first aid methods of, 300–301, *301*
Clostridium bacterium, 559
Clot, **386**
   See also Blood clot; Thrombosis; Thrombus.
Clothing, 11–12, 83, 116, 120, 123, 212
   for baby, 178
   of injured person, 296, 303
   maternity, 164, 168
Clove, oil of, 313, **386**
Clubfoot, 268, 362, 557
Clumping, 324
Coagulation, **386**
Coal dust, 119
Cobalt 60, 531
Cocaine, **386**
Coccidioidomycosis, **386**
Coccus, 346, *347*, **386**
Coccygeal nerve, *44*
Coccygodynia, **386**
Coccyx, *19, 266,* 291, **386**, *387*
Cochlea, *71,* 73, *413, 488*
Codeine, 26, 321, 327, 331, **386–387**, 396
Cod liver oil, **387**
Coffee, 25, 28, 35, 45, 50, 60, 62–63, 271, 282, 371
Cogentin, **387**, 509
Coitus, **387**
   See also Sexual intercourse.
Coitus interruptus, 155
Cola drinks, 25, 282, 371
Cold (overexposure), 433
   first aid treatment of, 305
Cold, application of, 254, 297, 298, 303, 308, *308*, 311,
   312, 331
Cold, common, 106, 122, 236, 281, 375, **389**, 395
   body's fight against, *112–113*
   in child, 199, 200–201, 202
   effects of, 53, 75, 83, 111
   prevention and treatment of, 283–284, 389
Cold sore. *See* Fever sore.
Colic, 181, 185, 351, **387**
Colitis, 350, **388**, 396, 419, 430, 459
Collapsed lung. *See* Pneumothorax.
Collarbone, **385**, *385*
Colon (large intestine), *38–39,* 60, 134, 213, 276–277, 317,
   375, **388**, *388,* 407, 409, 464, 577
Colon-rectum cancer, 262
Colorado tick fever, 561
Color blindness, **388–389**, 425
Colostomy, **388**, **389**
Colostrum, 365, 472
Coma, 286, 326, **389**
Combat fatigue, 428, 541
Comminuted fsacture, 366
Common cold. *See* Cold, common.
Common headache, 282

See also Headache.
Communicable disease, **389–390**
   childhood, 210–211, 254
Compazine, **390**
Complement-fixation test, 359
Complete fracture, 366
Complex, **390**
Compound fracture, 366
Compress, 254, 281, 299, 311, 312, 331, 339, 361, **390**
Compulsion, 128
Conception, **390**
Concussion, 213, 364, **390–391**
   first aid for, 307
Condom, 151–152, 278, **391**, 393, 439, 523
Conduction deafness, 400
Cone, in color blindness, 388, 425
Conflict, in neurosis, 127, 128
Congener, 326
Congenital, **391**
Congenital bone disorder, 268
Congenital (birth) defect, 352–353, 360
Congenital heart disease, **391**
Congenital hip dislocation, 268, 362, 452
Congenital syphilis, 278
Congestion, **391**
Congestive heart failure, 257, 258–259, **391**, 578
Conjunctiva, *65, 66,* 275, 391
Conjunctivitis, 68, 212, **391–392**, 426, 532
Connective tissue, 56–58, 134, 429, 537
Consent form, hospital, 138–139
Constipation, 61, 168, 186, 209, 237, 246, 247, 277,
   286–288, 376, 387, **392**, 521
   diet for, 41, 42, 60, 287, 392
   prevention and cure of, 287–288
Consumption. *See* Tuberculosis.
Contact dermatitis, 328
Contact lens, 69–70, 342, 375, **392**, 426
Contagious, 380, 389, **392**
Contraceptive methods and devices, 56, 82, 104, 148,
   151–156, 391, **393**, 501
Contusion, 579
Convalescence, **393–394**
Conversion hysteria, 127, 131, **394**, 458
Convulsion, 48, 120, 127, 198–199, 212, 213, **394**, 420, 547
   anticonvulsant for, **335**
   first aid for, 305, 310, 311
Convulsive therapy (electroshock therapy), 131, 132
Cooley's anemia, 276
Copperhead bite:
   first aid for, 297–298
Coral snake bite:
   first aid for, 297–298
Corn (on skin), 78–79, 372, **394**, 397
Cornaro, Luigi, 239
Cornea, 65, *65, 66,* 70, 423, *423,* 468
Coronary, **394**
Coronary artery, 49, *50,* 394
Coronary artery disease, 257–258, 260
Coronary care unit (CCU), 142, 258
Coronary heart disease, **394–395**, 448
Coronary occlusion, 257, 258
   See also Coronary heart disease.
Coronary sclerosis, 394, **395**
Coronary thrombosis, *50,* 257, 258, 446
Corpuscle, blood, **357**
Corpus luteum, 103–104, *161,* 229
Corrosive substance, 327, 376
   first aid if swallowed, 311
Cortex, **395**
Corticosteroid, 288
Cortisone, 277, 280, 320, 322, 339, 385, **395**, 397
Coryza, **395**
Cosmetics, 68, 75, 81, 82, 85
Cosmetic surgery, 81, 85, 134, 237, 353, 365, 376, 385, **395**,
   543

first aid for chemical burn of, 302, 307
first aid for removing object in, 307, *307*
focusing of, *69*
movements of, *68*
See also Vision.
Eyeball, structure of, 65
Eye care, **67-71, 425**
Eyeglasses, 69-70, 71, 134, 342, 351, 355, 373, 392, *424,* **425-426,** *425*
Eye infection, 212, **426,** 500
See also Conjunctivitis.
Eye injury, **426**
See also Eye; Eye care.
Eyelid, 526
first aid for removing object from, 307, *307*
Eye muscle, 65, *65-68*
Eyestrain, 68-69
Eye tooth, 373, 562

Face, 57, 81, 83, 123, 217, 237, 270, 273, 274
Face-lifting, 81, 395
Facial nerve, *46*
Facial palsy (Bell's palsy), 269, 497, 506
Facio-scapulo-humeral type muscular dystrophy, 273
Fahrenheit, 197, 198, *252,* 377, **427**
Fainting, 46, 257, 275, **427**
first aid for, 307
Fallen arch, 78, **427**
Fallopian tube, 101, 103, 155, 157, *160-161, 162,* 169-170, 228, 229, 230, 414, **427,** *427,* 536-537, 550, 570, 571
Falls, prevention of, 242-243, 367
False labor pain, 170, **427**
Familial periodic paralysis, 273
Family planning, 151-157, **428**
Family practitioner, 133, 134, 135
Family Service Association of America, 150
Farm work, health hazards in, 117, 120-121
Farsightedness, 213, *424,* 425, 456, 532
Fat, 28-30, *38-39,* 50, 60, 61, 98, 99, 104, 166, 351, 407, **428**
cholesterol as, 31-33, 383
Fat, body, 322
Father's role, 182
Fatigue, 13, 41, 51, 60, 99, 117, 119, 120, 200, 208, 257, 264, 275, 277, 280, 357, **428**
in neurasthenics, 128
Favus, **428**
FDA, **428**
Febrile convulsion, 198-199
Feces, *39, 40,* 112, 287, 313, 338, **428,** 464
of baby, 182, 185-186
blood in, 61, 262, 264, 268, 280, 351, 355, 388, 484
Feeblemindedness, **428**
Feet. *See* Foot.
Felon, 494, 509
Female sex hormone. *See* Estrogen.
Femoral artery, *54, 55*
Femoral hernia, 277, 451
Femur (thighbone), 22, 56, *58, 192,* 338, **429,** *452,* 512, 563
Fertility, 157
Fertilization, 103, *160-161,* **429,** 570
Fetishism, 129
Fetus, 127, 160-161, *165, 166-167,* 167, 168, 170, 375, 417, **429,** *429,* 521
Fever, 48, 61, 64, 77, 78, 83, 108, 123, 170, 186, 263, 273, 276, 277, 279, 280, **429**
of child, 198-199, 200, 201, 202, 203, 208, 211, 212, 213
sordes from, *545*
Fever sore (herpes simplex), 75, 83, 84, 212, **429,** 476
of genitals, 278-279, 452, 574
Fibroblast, **429**
Fibroid tumor, 159, 231, **429-430,** 457, 570
Fibula, *22,* **430**

Fight or flight reaction, 127
Filariasis, 416
Filiform papilla, 77
Finger, *58, 165,* 169, *193,* 360
Fingernail, 87, 182, 212, 275, 443, 468, 494, 500
Fire:
first aid for person on, 303
Fire hazard, 243
First aid, 294-314
emergencies in, **430**
first steps in, 296
where to find, 295
First-aid kit, 122, 314
for automobile, 296-297
First-degree burn, 369
Fish, disease from, 113, 124
Fissure, **430**
Fistula, **430**
Fit, **430**
Flammable liquid, 243
Flare, for auto kit, 297
Flashlight, for auto kit, 297
Flatfoot, 78, **430,** *431*
Flatulence, 280, **430,** 435
Fleming, Sir Alexander, 379
Fletcher, Horace, 380
Flu. *See* Influenza.
Fluid, body processing of, *40*
Fluke, 106
Fluoridation, 91, 185, 402, **430**
Fluoride, 91, 185, 402, 403, **430**
Fluoroscope, **431,** 530
Folic acid, 42, 575-576
Follicle, **431**
Follicle, hair. *See* Hair follicle.
Follicle, ovarian. *See* Graafian follicle.
Follicle-stimulating hormone (FSH), 102, *229,* 540
Folliculitis, **431,** 556
Fomentation, **431**
Fontanel, 181, **431,** *432*
Food, 27-42
fattening, list of, 33
hospital, 140
illness from, 111-114, 124, 156, 213, 320, 328, 431-432, 438
nutrients in, 28-30, 524
See also Diet; Digestion.
Food additives, 168
Food and Drug Administration, U.S., 26, 340, **428,** 452
Food poisoning, 124, 406, **431-432,** 526, 563
first aid for, 310
See also Botulism.
Foot, 78-79, *79,* 213, 234, 237, 369, **432**
athlete's, 79, 106, **342,** 404
bones of, *57, 79*
diabetes and, 99, 101, 372
swollen, 169, 170, 414
Foot defect. *See* Clubfoot; Fallen arch; Flatfoot.
Footrest, for bed-ridden patient, *250*
Forceps, 366, **432-433**
Forearm bone, *20, 58, 59*
Foreign object, 202, 208
in eye, 425
in eye, first aid for, 307
in nose, 75
in nose, first aid for, 309
swallowed, first aid for, 313
in windpipe, 77-78
in windpipe, first aid for, 304-305
Foreskin, 64, 181, 384, **433**
Forest yaws, 474
Formaldehyde, **433,** 563
Formula, baby, 184, 362-363
Fracture, 58-59, 236, 242, 268, 366-367, 385, 563
cast for, **375**

Moccasin (snake) bite:
  first aid for, 297-298
Moist gangrene, 435
Moist wart, 578
Molar, *90*, **489**, 562
Mold, **489**
Mole, 81, 84-85, 262, 355, 484, **489**, 497
Mongolism, 156, 384, 391, 410, 412, **489**
Moniliasis, 106, 231, **489-490**, 551
Monoamine oxidase inhibitors, 335
Monocyte, *108*
Mononucleosis, 211, 277-278, 451, 470, **490**
Monoplegia, **490**
Morning sickness, 158, 168, **490**
Moron, **490**
Morphine, 26, 327, **490**, 566
Morula, *161*
Mosquito, 11, 105, 114, 121, 242, 280, 375, 402, 481, 580
Mosquito bite:
  first aid for, 297
Mother, 30, *110*
  new, 175-178
  unmarried, 158-159
  See also Childbirth; Pregnancy.
Motion sickness, 290, 347, 350, 410, **490**, 577
Motor, **490**
Motor area of brain, *46, 67*
Motor fiber, *48*
Motor neuron, 495
Mountain fever, **490**
Mountain sickness, 329
Mouth, *38*, 75-76, 83, 150, **490**
  cancer of, 23, 53, 76
  digestion in, 407
  infections of, 212
Mouth-to-mouth resuscitation, 53, 123, 258, 340
  in cardiopulmonary resuscitation, 300-301
  as first aid technique, 299-300
Mouthwash, 76
Movement sensation, 347
Mucous colitis, 276, 388, 396, 430
Mucous membrane, *107, 112-113*, 116, 200, 285, 401, 421,
  484, **490-491**, 561, 568
Mucous plug, of cervix, *161, 166*
Mucoviscidosis, 398
Mucus, *74, 107, 112*, 170, 263, 270, 284, 285, **491**
  in childbirth emergency, 304
  in child's illnesses, 201, 202, 203, 208, 212
Multiple personality, 127-128
Multiple pregnancy, **491**
Multiple sclerosis, 272, **491**, 538
  paralysis from, 507-508
Mumps, 106, 110, 115, 168, 186, 202, 210, **491**
Munroe, Ruth, 220
Muscle, *19-20, 22, 47, 48*, 49, *55, 57*, 59-60, *59*, 65, *65, 66, 79*,
  97, 100, 142, 178, 258, 260, 272, **491**, 542
  as cause of low back pain, 291-292
Muscle contraction, **492**
Muscle disease, 273
Muscle relaxant, 267, 319, 374
Muscular dystrophy, 273, 412, **492**, 493
Muscular Dystrophy Association, 273, 492
Muscular tension, 266, 281-282, 283, 292
Mushroom poisoning:
  first aid for, 310
Mustard plaster, 431
Myalgia, **492**
Myasthenia gravis, 273, **492**, 501
Mycetoma, **492**
Mycoplasmal pneumonia, 263
Mycosis, **492**
Myelitis, **492**
Myelocytic leukemia, 475
Myeloma, **492**
Myocardial infarction, 257, 258

Myoma, **492**
Myopathy, **492-493**
Myopia, 425, **493**, 532
Myositis, **493**
Myotonia dystrophica, 273
Myxadenoma, **493**
Myxedema, 95, 102, 276, 439, **493**

Nail, **494**, 509, 542

  See also Fingernail.
Nail-biting, 193, **494**
Napoleonic complex, 390
Narcolepsy, **494**
Narcotics, 25-26, 43-44, 387, 396, 411, 451, 490, **494**
Nasal cavity, *112*
Nasal discharge, 200, 263, 395
Nasal feeding, **494**
Nasal polyp, 285, 391
National Mental Health Association, 132
National Council of Senior Citizens, 240
National Council on Alcoholism, 23
National Genetics Foundation, Inc., 156
National Hemophilia Foundation, 450
National Institute for Occupational Safety and Health, 118
National Kidney Foundation, 470
National League for Nursing, 499
National Leprosarium, 474
National Multiple Sclerosis Society, 491
National Retired Teachers Association, 240
National Safety Council, 117, 242
National Society for Autistic Children, 343
National Sudden Infant Death Syndrome Foundation, 214
Natural childbirth, 163, 381
Nausea, 78, 152, 158, 169, 200, 209, 230, 264, 268, 282, 287,
  290, 370, **494**
Nearsightedness, 213, **424**, 425, 493, 532
Necatoriasis. *See* Hookworm disease.
Neck, *57, 58, 58*, 77-78, 97, *165*, 265, 270, 291
  stiff, 78, 200, 212, 273, **551**
  tension of, 281
Neck, of tooth, *90*
Neck brace, 563
Neck injury, 296, 298, 308, 309
  first aid for, 302
  See also Whiplash.
Necrosis, **494**
Neisseria gonorrhoeae, 278
Nematode, 535
Nembutal, **494**
Neomycin, **494**
Neoplasm, 372, **494**
Neo-synephrine, **494-495**
Nephrectomy, **495**
Nephritis (Bright's disease), 53, 122, 201, 264, 284, **495**
Nephron, *62-63*, 469
Nephrosis, 264, **495**
Nerve, *18, 20, 44*, 48-49, *48*, 73, *74*, 77, *80*, 84, 87, 91, 97, 103,
  273, 276, 291, **495**, *495*
  ailments of, 269-270, 272
Nerve block, 356
Nerve deafness, 400
Nervous breakdown, **495**
Nervous habits, of child, 193
Nervous system, *44-45, 47*, 48-49, 127, 134, *164, 165*, 272,
  278, 351, 363, 383, 387, 434, 490, **495-496**, *496*, 531, 556
  autonomic, *47*, **343**, 496, 511, 536, 540
  central, *44-45*, 272, 387, 490, 496, *496*, 556
Nervous system infection, paralysis from, 508
Neuralgia, 269, **496**, 561
Neurasthenia, 128, **496**
Neuritis, 269, 351, **496-497**, 538
Neurofibroma, **497**
Neurological surgery, 134

Rabbit fever, 561, 566
Rabies, 106, 110, 111, 114, 115, 120, 297, 334, 364, 376, 410, **530**, 581
Radiation, 120, 261, 357, 358, 384, 530
Radiation sickness, **530**
Radiation treatment, 262, 272, 357, 358, 365, 372, 374, 453, 475, 530–531
Radioisotope, 374, 530–531
Radiology, 134, 138, 481, **530–531**
   See also X ray.
Radium, 531
Radius, *20*, *58*, *59*, 338, **531**
Radon, 531
Ranula, **531**
Rape, 129
Rash, 80, 82, 123, 197, 210, 211, *211*, 277, 286, 342, 367, **531**, 556
   diaper, 182, **405**
Rat-bite fever, **531**
Rattlesnake bite:
   first aid for, 297–298
Rauwolfia, **531**, 532, 564
Raynaud, Maurice, 531
Raynaud's disease, 498, **531**
Reaching, *18*
Rebound engorgement of sinus, 285
Recessive, 375, 398, 410, 422, 451, 514, **531**
Reconstruction work, dental, 88
Recovery room, hospital, 142
Recrudescence, **531**
Rectal bleeding, 262, 288
Rectal examination, 136, 277
Rectal fissure, 287, 288, 289, 430
Rectal suppository, 247, 288, 554
Rectal thermometer, 197, *198*, 252, 314, 361, 560
Rectocele, 231, 451
Rectum, *38–39*, *47*, 60, 134, 231, 236, 276, 287, 288–289, 388, *388*, 516
Rectus femoris muscle, *22*
Rectus muscle, *68*
Red blood cell. *See* Erythrocyte.
Reducing, **531**
Reflex, 387, 497, **531**, *532*
Refraction, **532**
Refractory, **532**
Refrigerating food, 114
Registered nurse (RN), 498–499, 534
Regressive, **532**
Regurgitation, **532**
Reimplantation, tooth, 89
Reiter, Hans, 532
Reiter's disease, **532**
Relapse, **532**
Relapsing fever, **532**, 561
Relaxin, 103
Remission, 463, **532**
REM sleep, *14–15*
Renal, **532**
Renal artery, *62–63*, *468*, 469
Renal colic, 387
Renal vein, *62*, *468*
Renin, 103
Repression, 127, 459, 475, **532**
Research, AMA and, 330
Resection, **532**
Reserpine, 531, **532**
Resorcinol, **532**
Respiration, **532**
Respiration rate, *252*, *253*
Respirator, 373, 465, **532–533**
Respiratory infection, 198, 199, 200–208, 283
Respiratory system, **533**, *533*
Respiratory therapist, 142
Rest, 13–14, 59, 68, 117, 169, 265, 275, 277
   for elderly, 239

   See also Sleep.
Resuscitation, **533**
Retention, **533**
Reticular activating system, *24*
Retina, *44*, 65, *65*, *66–67*, *69*, *165*, *224*, 270, 423–425, *423*, 515
   detached, 397, **404**, 425
Retirement, 240–241
Reyes syndrome, **533**
Rheumatic fever, 53, 98, 201, 223, 259, 265, 284, 321, 339, 341, 384, **533**
Rheumatic heart disease, 223, 259, 284, 346, 489
Rheumatism, 236, 237, 339, **533**, 551
Rheumatoid arthritis, 225, 265, 321, 334, 339
Rheumatology, 134
Rh (rhesus) factor in blood, 53, 160, 332, 360, 421, 487, **533–534**
Rhinitis, 445, 498, **534**
Rhinophyma, **534**, 535
Rhubarb and soda, 61
Rhythm method, 153–155, *154*, 393, **534**
   reverse, for conception, 157
Rib, 56, 270, 301, 380, 463
Riboflavin (vitamin B2), 28–29, 575, 576
Ribonucleic acid, 534
Rice, white vs. brown, 351
Rickets, 362, 371, 387, 515, **534**
Rickettsia, 106, 115, **534**, 535
Rickettsialpox, **534**
Rigor mortis, **534**
Ringworm, 106, 115, 120, 213, 466, 494, **534**, 545
Ritualized behavior, 128
RN (registered nurse), 498–499, **534**
RNA, **534**
Rocky Mountain spotted fever, 106, 111, 114, 211, **535**, 550, 561
Room:
   hazards in, 243–244
   patient's, 245–246
Roosevelt, Franklin D., 14
Roosevelt, Theodore, 390
Root, tooth, *90*, 91
Root canal, 91
Rorschach test, 512
Rosacea, **535**
Rose fever, **535**
Roseola infantum, 82, 198, 210–211, **535**
Rotating joint, *467*
Roughage, 60, 287
Roundworm, 106, 213, **535**
Rubbing alcohol, 325, 327
Rubella (German measles), 82, 110, 111, 115, 156, 168, 186, 210, *211*, 352, 391, 488, **535**
Rubeola, 483, **535**
Rupture, **535**
Ruptured spleen, 209

Sabin polio immunization, 109–110, 111, 272–273, 520
Saccharin, 340, **536**
Sacher-Masoch, Leopold von, 482
Sacral nerve, *44*
Sacroiliac strain, 266
Sacrum, *19*, *266*, 291, *452*
Sade, Marquis de, 536
Sadism, 129, **536**
Safety, 117–124, 183, 199
   at home, 242–244, 367
   on job, 117–121
   on vacation, 121–124
   See also Accident.
Saint Anthony's fire, 421, **536**
Saint Vitus's dance (Sydenham's chorea), 383–384, 506, 533, 547
Salicylate compound, 339

Sinusitis, 202, 213, 284–285, 336, 376, **541–542**
Sippy diet, 354
Sister Kenny Institute, 520
Skeletal muscle, 59, *59*
Skeletal system, 56, *57, 165,* 361, **542**
  See also Bone; Spine; Vertebra.
Skin, 27, 40, *48,* 79–86, *84–85, 107,* 111, 237, 254, 281,
  397, 463, **542,** *543*
  in adolescence, 217, 320, 323
  of albino, 325
Skin allergy, 286, 328
Skin cancer, 82, 86, 122, 261, 262, 372, 484
Skin disease, 41, 83–86, 120, 122, 233, 234, 288, 348, 352,
  479
  of child, 212–213
  fungal, 433
Skin eruption, 531, **542–543**
  See also Rash.
Skin graft, 440, 537, **543**
Skin test, 286, 328, 445, 509
Skin traction, 563
Skull, 43, 56, *192*
  of baby, 431, *432*
Sleep, 13–15, *31,* 44–45, 81, 182, 187–188, 282–283, **543–544**
  for elderly, 239
  methods of getting to, 283, 348
  stages of, *14–15*
  See also Insomnia.
Sleeping pill, 26, 45, 71, 140
Sleeping sickness, 105, 115, 279, 379, 418, **544,** 565
Sleepwalking, 545
Sliding joint, *467*
Slipped disk, 266, 267, *267,* 291, 346, 538, 574
Smallpox, 106, 109, *109,* 115, 186, 210, 235, **544,** 565
Smegma, **544**
Smell, sense of, 44, *76,* 77, 500
  brain and, *74*
  threshold of, *75*
Smelling salts, 330, **544**
Smoker's cough, 285
Smoking, 50, 53, 75, 76, 111, 167–168, 219, 239, 243, 256,
  258, 260, 261, 263, 285, 372, 418, **544**
  how to stop, 24–25, 131, 544
Smooth muscle, 491
Snake, snakebite, 23, 124, **544–545**
  first aid for, *297, 297*
Sneezing, 275, 277, 283, 285
Social maturity, adolescence and, 220–221
Social service department of hospital, 144
Sodium, 30, 42, 290
Sodium bicarbonate (baking soda, bicarbonate of soda),
  26, 61, 168, 268, 297, 303, 312, 314, 319, 320, 327, **545**
Sodium citrate, **545**
Sodium pentothal. *See* Pentothal.
Sodium phosphate, 376
Sodium salicylate, **545**
Sodium thiosulfate, **545**
Sodoku, 531
Soft palate, 505, *506*
Somite, *164*
Somnambulism, **545,** 568
Sonograph, 158
Soporific, **545**
Sordes, **545**
Sore throat, 76–77, 201–202, 211, 273, 275, 277, 284, 285,
  435, 453, **545**
  See also Strep throat.
Sound location, *73*
Space travel, bends and, 350
Spanish fly, 337
Spanish influenza, 462
Spansule, **545**
Spare-part surgery, **545–547,** *546*
Spasm, 502, **547**
Spastic, 272, **547,** 556

Spastic colon, 388
Specialties, medical, 133–134
Species, 384, **547**
Speculum, **547–548**
Speech, *548*
  defects and disorders of, 260, 270, 272, 336–337, 364,
  385, 412, **548**
  dentures and, 403
Speech block, 356
Speed (methedrine), 488
  See also Amphetamine.
Spermatocystitis, **548**
Sperm cell, 101, 103, 151–152, 155, 157, *160,* 322, 339, 384,
  387, 390, 436–437, 451, 539, **548,** 558, 571, 581
Spermicidal preparation, 152, 153
Sphenoidal sinus, *285,* 541
Sphincter, *47,* 63, 319, 354, 386, 421, **548–549**
Sphygmomanometer, 358–359, **549**
Spider bite, **549**
  first aid for, 312
Spinal accessory nerve, *46*
Spinal anesthesia, 549, 559
Spinal block, 333, 356
Spinal cord, *44, 48,* 134, 212, *266,* 267, 272, 273, 276, 302,
  363, **549**
Spinal curvature, 471, 477, 538, **549**
Spinal fluid, 549
Spinal injury, 297
Spinal meningitis, 212
Spinal nerve, *266,* 267, *267,* 269–270, 291, 386
Spinal tap, 141, 212
Spine, *18–19,* 56, *57,* 134, 246, 265–266, 269, 291–292, 362,
  549
  tuberculosis of, 362, 471, 566
Spirochete, 346, *347,* **549,** 580
Spleen, *50, 107,* 209, *317,* 358, 368, **549**
Splint, 296, 367, **550**
  in first aid, 302, *302*
Splinter:
  first aid for, 311
Split-thickness graft, 543
Spina bifida, **549**
Spondylitis, **550**
Spontaneous abortion, 318, 489
Sports, 15–16, 34, 43, 56, 64, 164
Spotted fever, **550**
Sprain, 56, 242, 331, 334, 374, **550**
  first aid for, 311
Sprue, 276, 376, **550**
Sputum, 367, **550**
Squint, 329, 552
Stammering, 193, 548
Standing, *22,* 78, 79, 502
Stanford-Binet test, 351
Staphylococcus, 212, 268, 346, *347,* 358, 361, 373,
  386, **550**
Steel alloy, in spare-part surgery, 545, 547
Stenosis, 448, **550**
Sterility, 421, 460, **550–551**
Sterilization, 155, 393
Sternocleidomastoid muscle, *19*
Steroid, 321, 383, **551**
Stethoscope, 343, 358, 448, **551**
Stiff neck, 78, 200, 212, 273, **551**
Still, George, 551
Still's disease, **551**
Stimulant, **551**
Sting, 328, 349–350, 463
  first aid for, 312
Stoma, 299
Stomach, *38–39,* 41, *47, 50,* 60, 61, 93, *95,* 103, 104, *107,* 268,
  269, *317,* **551,** *552*
  digestion in, 384, 407, 551
  mild discomfort of, 320
  poison in, first aid for, 310–311

Tension, 494, **558**
Tension headache, 281–282, 445
Tepanil, **558**
Terramycin, 380, **558**
Test:
 agglutination, **324**
 for allergy, 286, 328, 445, 509
 basal metabolic rate, **348**
 benzidine, **351**
 blood, 33, 136, 139, 146, 156, 158, 159–160, 275, 278, 324, **359**, 405
 for color blindness, 388–389
 glucose tolerance, **439**
 intelligence, 126, 351, 463
 personality, **512**, 523
 pregnancy, 158, 324, 522
 Schick, 408, **537**
 tuberculin, 186, 208, 263, **565**
 urine, 139, 158, 159, 160, 271, 324, 405, 569
 Wassermann, 146, 359, **578**
 Widal, 567
Testes, *See* Testicle.
Testicle, *95*, 101, 103, 277, 375, 436, 491, 501, *516*, 538, **558–559**, 559, 573
Testosterone, 101, 103, 331, 419, 540
Tetanus (lockjaw), 105, 110, 111, 114, 115, 120, 121, 186, 210, 297, 305, 311, 335, 336, *347*, 364, **559**
Tetany, 97, 102, **559**
Tetracaine hydrochloride, 333, **559**
Tetracycline, 335, 376, 380, 480, 558, **559**, 579
Thalamus, *24*, *44–45*
Thalassemia, 156, 276
Thalidomide, 25–26, 391, **559**
Therapy, **560**
Thermograph, **560**
Thermometer, 197, *198*, *252*, 361, **560**
Thiamine (vitamin B₁), 28–29, 351, 575, 576
Thighbone. *See* Femur.
Thigh muscle, *22*
Third-degree burn, 369
Thoracic nerve, *44*
Thoracic surgery, 134
Thoracic vertebra, *19*, *266*, 291
Thorax, 53, **560**
Thorazine, 383, **560**, 564
Throat, 13, 73, 76–77, 111, 112, 134, 270, 555, **560**
 first aid for object caught in, 313
 See also Sore throat.
Throat drops, 78
Thrombocyte. *See* Platelet.
Thrombocytopenia, 358
Thrombophlebitis, 260, **560**
Thrombosis, 152, 335, 357, 416, 450, 553, **560**
Thrombus (blood clot), 225, 260, 276, 335, 357, 416, 553, **560**
Thrush, 489, 551
Thumb-sucking, 186, 193, **560**
Thymus, *95*, 102, 236, 419
Thyroid depressant, 404
Thyroidectomy, **560–561**
Thyroid gland, 78, 86, 94–97, *95*, *96*, 102, 274, 348, 419, *516*, 530, **561**, *561*
 goiter of, **439**
Thyroid hormone, 87, 94–97, *96*, 102
Thyrotrophin, 102
Thyroxine, 94, 102, 439, 465, **561**
Tibia (shinbone), *22*, 58, *192*, **561**
Tic, 547
Tic douloureux, 270, 496, **561**, 566
Tick bite, 535
 first aid for, 298
Tick fever, 490, **561**
Tincture, **561**
Tinea, 534
Tinnitus, 290
Tired blood, 357

Tissue, 374, **561**
Titian, 239
Toadstool poisoning:
 first aid for, 310
Tobacco, 24, 239, 327
 See also Smoking.
Toe, turning-in of, 78, 369
Toenail, ingrown, 79, 101, 292, **462**
Toilet training, 181, 192–193, 382
Tongue, 75, 76, *76–77*, 276, 439, *548*, 555, **561–562**
Tonometer, 439
Tonsil, 73, 76–77, 93, *107*, *112*, 201, *201*, 236, 263, 322, **562**
Tonsillectomy, 201–202, *201*, 322, **562**
Tonsillitis, 201, 545, **562**
Tooth, 27, 29, 76, 88–93, 237, 281, 377, 528, 557, **562**
 care of, 89–93, 562
 types of, *90*, 562
Toothache, 88, 91, 213, **562**
 first aid for, 313
Toothbrush, 89, 92, 403
Tooth decay, 38, 41, 88, 91–92, 402
Tooth grinding (bruxism), 92
Toothpaste, 91, 92, 403, 430
Topical, **562**
TOPV (trivalent oral polio virus vaccine), 186
Torso wound, 298
Torticollis, 551
Touch sensation, *80*
Tourniquet, 286, 314
 first aid use of, 298–299, *299*
Toxemia, 170, 346, 358, 414, 522, **563**
Toxicology, 513
Toxin, 336, 346, 358, **563**, 575
Toxin-antitoxin, **563**
Toxoid, 362, **563**
Toxoplasmosis, 156
Trachea (windpipe), *47*, *52*, 77–78, *112*, 203, 263, 270, 296, 368, *368*, 375, 383, *513*, **563**, *563*
 first aid for obstruction of, 304–305, *304*
Tracheitis, 208, **563**
Tracheotomy, **563**
Trachoma, 391, **563**, 565
Traction, **563**
Trancelike state, 127
Tranquilizer, 88–89, 219, 286, 292, 326, 379, 383, 402, 404, 411, 418, 531, 538, **563–564**
Transference, **564**
Transfusion, blood, 53, 61, 159, 275, 332, 357, 359–360, 533, **564**
Transplanted organ, rejection of, 501–502
Transsexual, 129
Transverse colon, *388*
Transverse fracture, 366
Transverse presentation, 172, 366
Transvestism, 129, **564**
Trapezius muscle, *19*
Trauma, **564**
Trench mouth (Vincent's angina), 75, *347*, 438, 568, 574–575
Treponema pallidum, 278, 556
Triceps, *20*, *59*
Trichiasis, **564**
Trichinella spiralis, 564
Trichinosis, 106, 113, **564**
Trichomonas vaginalis, 231
Trick knee, 470
Tricuspid valve, *51*, 449
Tricyclic antidepressant, 335
Trigeminal nerve, *46*, 270
Trigeminal neuralgia (tic douloureux), 270, 496, 561, 566
Triglycerides, **564**
Triplet, 491
Trophoblast, *162*
Tropical disease, 279–280, 402, 416, 467, 532, **564–565**
Troposphere, *12*
Truss, 277, **565**

Trypanosome, 565
Trypanosomiasis. *See* Sleeping sickness.
Trypsin, 420, **565**
Tsetse fly, **565**
Tsutsugamushi diease, **565**
Tubal ligation, 155
Tubal pregnancy, 159, 169–170, 414, *414*, 427, 537
Tuberculin, **565**
Tuberculin test, 186, 208, 263, **565**
Tuberculosis, 77, 115, 119, 121, 122, 156, 208, 236, 256,
    262, 263, 280, 284, 289, 345, 346, *347*, **565–566**
  of lymph node, 538
  of skin, 479
  of spine, 362, 471, 566
  types of, 565–566
Tubule, in testicle, *559*
Tubule, kidney, *62–63*
Tularemia, 111, 121, 561, **566**
Tumor, 46, 77, 85, 86, 94, 231, 232, 237, 261, 267, 269,
    270, 271, 286, 288, 365, 494, **566**
  benign, 322, 372, 429–430, 493, 502, 566
  brain, **364**, 418
  malignant, 372, 374, 481, 566
  paralysis from, 508
  uterine, 159, 232
Turner's syndrome, **566**, 580
Turpentine:
  first aid if swallowed, 311
Twilight sleep, 538, **566**
Twin, *171*, 194, 491, 501, 541, 543, **566**
Twitching, **566**
Tympanum, **566**
Typhoid fever, 105, 112, 115, 121, 324, 345, *347*, **566–567**
Typhus, 106, 114, 115, 279, 478, 550, 565, **567**
Tyrothricin, **567**

Ulcer, 121, 264, 277, 334, 349, 379, 388, 396, **568**
  peptic, 26, 126, 129–130, 224, 268–269, 275, 343, 354,
    568
  perforation of, 268
  types of, 568
Ulcerative colitis, 276–277, 388, 419, 568
Ulna, *20*, *58*, 338, **568**
Umbilical cord, *164*, *166*, 171, 173–174, 181, 323, 353, 517,
    568
  in emergency delivery, 303–304
Umbilical hernia, 277, 451
Unconscious, 532, **568**
Unconsciousness, **568**
Unconscious person:
  first aid for, 296, 307, 310, 311
  unknown problem, first aid for, 313
Undereating, 34, 338
Underweight, 27, 31, 38, 166, 216, 416, 481
Undulant fever. *See* Brucellosis.
United Cerebral Palsy Association, 272, 378
United States Pharmacopoeia (USP), 513, 570
Unsaturated fat, 383
Upper, 330
  See also Amphetamine.
Upper respiratory infection, 200–202, 283
Uremia, 93, **569**
Ureter, *40*, *62*, 63, 271, *271*, **569**, *569*
Urethra, *40*, 63, 101, 271–272, *271*, 354, 398, 399, 436, *559*,
    569, *569*, 570
Urethritis, 398, 532, **569**
Uric acid, 350, 439, 440, **569**
Urinalysis, **569**
  See also Urine test.
Urinary system, *569*
Urinary tract, *62*, 63, 271–272, 354, 437, **569–570**
  cystoscopy of, 399
  infection of, 209, 210, 435

Urinary tract stone, 371, 545
Urine, urination, *40*, 61, *62*, *62*, 94, 99, 104, 169, 170, 174, 209,
    230, 231, 264, 271, *271*, 354, 469, 488, 569, **570**
  albumin in, 325, 350
  difficulty in, 412, 533
  incontinence in, 461
Urine test, 139, 158, 159, 160, 271, 324, 405, 569
Urology, 134, 354, **570**
Urticaria. *See* Hives.
USP, 513, **570**
Uterotomy, **570**
Uterus (womb), 102, 103, 104, 152, 153, 155, *228*, *229*, 230,
    231, 232, 236, 358, 365, 379, **570**, *571*
  cancer of, 230, 261, 372, 570
  during labor, 170–171, *172–173*, 174, 303, 323, 381
  pregnancy and, 158, 159, *160–161*, *162*, *164*, 166, 169, 170,
    171, 173, 288

Vacation, 14, 117
  safety and, 121–124
Vaccination, 108–111, 114, 168, 210, 263, 279, 544, 563, **571**
  See also Immunization.
Vaccine, 335, 362, 369, 383, 462, 535, **571**
Vaccinia, **571**
Vacuum aspiration, 155
Vagina, 147, 148, 149, 150, 151–152, 153, 155, 157, 158, 181,
    228, 231, 278, 379, 387, 464, **571**, 577
Vaginal bleeding, 158, 168, 169, 170, 485
Vaginal diaphragm, 153, *154*, 231, 393, **405**, 512
Vaginal discharge. *See* Leukorrhea, Lochia.
Vaginal irritation, 64–65, 181, 231
Vaginismus, **571**
Vaginitis, 231, **571–572**
Vagotomy, 269
Vagus nerve, *46*, 269
Valium, 564, **572**
Valve, **572**, *572*
  in vein, *55*, 289, 360, 572, 573
  See also Heart valve.
Vaporizer, 123, 200, 201, 203, 367, 389, 396, 542, **572**
Varicella. *See* Chicken pox.
Varicose vein, 169, 225, 289–290, 334, **572–573**
Variola, **573**
Vas deferens, 155, 436, *559*, **573**, *573*
Vasectomy, 155, **573**
Vasoconstrictor, **573**
Vasodepressor, **573**
Vasodilator, 560, **573**
Vasomotor, **573**
Vasopressin, 98, 102, 517, **573**
Vastus muscle, *22*
Vector, 375, **573**
Vegetable and fruit group, 27–28
Vegetarian diet, 41
Vein, *50*, *54*, *84*, *141*, *166*, 169, 225, 260, 356, 360, 373, 374,
    573–574
  jugular, *54*, *55*, *467*
  See also Varicose vein.
Venereal disease, 114–116, 146, 149, 156, 278–279, 346, 391,
    439, 452, 480, 556, **574**
Venipuncture, **574**
Venom, 298, 312, 463, 544–545, 549, **574**
Venous, **574**
Venous blood, 573
Ventricle, 49, 50, 51, *51*, 374
Vermiform appendix, 64, 209, 277, 317, 337–338, *337*, 376,
    511
  See also Appendicitis.
Vertebra, *18–19*, 56, 134, *266*, 267, 291, 386, **574**
  See also Spinal column.
Vertebral disk, *18*, 19, 265–266, *266*, 375, **574**
  slipped, 266, 267, *267*, 291, 346, 538, 574
Vertigo, 230, **574**

Contributors

Robert Bahr
Rebecca Davenport
Arthur Freese
Nancy Gross
George Kemmerer
Zane Kotker
Carol Mankin
Joseph Morschauser III
Donald Pace
Lynne Rogers
Kim Waller